Textbook of
Physiotherapy

Textbook of Physiotherapy

Basanta Kumar Nanda BPT(Hons) MPT
Lecturer (Physiotherapy)
Swami Vivekanand National Institute of
Rehabilitation Training and Research
Cuttack, Odisha, India

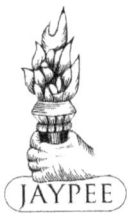

JAYPEE BROTHERS MEDICAL PUBLISHERS
The Health Sciences Publisher
New Delhi | London

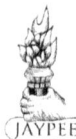 **Jaypee Brothers Medical Publishers (P) Ltd.**

Headquarters
Jaypee Brothers Medical Publishers (P) Ltd
EMCA House
23/23-B, Ansari Road, Daryaganj
New Delhi - 110 002, India
Landline: +91-11-23272143, +91-11-23272703
+91-11-23282021, +91-11-23245672
Email: jaypee@jaypeebrothers.com

Corporate Office
Jaypee Brothers Medical Publishers (P) Ltd
4838/24, Ansari Road, Daryaganj
New Delhi 110 002, India
Phone: +91-11-43574357
Fax: +91-11-43574314
Email: jaypee@jaypeebrothers.com

Overseas Office
J.P. Medical Ltd
83 Victoria Street, London
SW1H 0HW (UK)
Phone: +44 20 3170 8910
Fax: +44 (0)20 3008 6180
Email: info@jpmedpub.com

Website: www.jaypeebrothers.com
Website: www.jaypeedigital.com

© 2023, Jaypee Brothers Medical Publishers

The views and opinions expressed in this book are solely those of the original contributor(s)/author(s) and do not necessarily represent those of editor(s) and publisher of the book.

All rights reserved. No part of this publication may be reproduced, stored or transmitted in any form or by any means, electronic, mechanical, photocopying, recording or otherwise, without the prior permission in writing of the publishers.

All brand names and product names used in this book are trade names, service marks, trademarks or registered trademarks of their respective owners. The publisher is not associated with any product or vendor mentioned in this book.

Medical knowledge and practice change constantly. This book is designed to provide accurate, authoritative information about the subject matter in question. However, readers are advised to check the most current information available on procedures included and check information from the manufacturer of each product to be administered, to verify the recommended dose, formula, method and duration of administration, adverse effects and contraindications. It is the responsibility of the practitioner to take all appropriate safety precautions. Neither the publisher nor the author(s)/editor(s) assume any liability for any injury and/or damage to persons or property arising from or related to use of material in this book.

This book is sold on the understanding that the publisher is not engaged in providing professional medical services. If such advice or services are required, the services of a competent medical professional should be sought.

Every effort has been made where necessary to contact holders of copyright to obtain permission to reproduce copyright material. If any have been inadvertently overlooked, the publisher will be pleased to make the necessary arrangements at the first opportunity.

Inquiries for bulk sales may be solicited at: jaypee@jaypeebrothers.com

Textbook of Physiotherapy

First Edition: **2023**

ISBN: 978-93-5465-792-4

Preface

The *Textbook of Physiotherapy* is the fulfillment of a big dream of mine, which I thought to bring to lime light, after the book on electrotherapy, i.e., "Electrotherapy Simplified" successfully got its 3rd edition in 2020. The students across the country are my inspiration to motivate me to write more books, and ultimately, the success has reached the door step. The inspiration of Jaypee Brothers Medical Publishers (P) Ltd contributes significantly for bringing up this book.

I hope this book will fulfill the needs of students of Physiotherapy and Physiotherapists working in various disciplines.

Basanta Kumar Nanda

Acknowledgment

I, sincerely, acknowledge Dr Patitapaban Mohanty, Associate Professor Department of Physiotherapy and Director (Offg), Swami Vivekanand National Institute of Rehabilitation Training and Research, Olatpur, Bairoi, Cuttack, Odisha, for giving me continuous inspiration to work on this book and taking pain to go through the contents and give forewords. My sincere thank goes to my colleagues, students and patients of Swami Vivekanand National Institute of Rehabilitation Training and Research, who have continuously supported me to carry out this work.

I am very grateful to the whole team of M/s Jaypee Brothers Medical Publishers (P) Ltd, New Delhi, India, who helped and guided me, Shri Jitendar P Vij (Group Chairman), Mr Ankit Vij (Managing Director), Mr MS Mani (Group President), Dr Madhu Choudhary (Director-Educational Publishing), Ms Pooja Bhandari (Production Head), Ms Sunita Katla (Executive Assistant to Group Chairman and Publishing Manager), Ms Samina Khan (Executive Assistant to Director-Educational Publishing), Mr Rajesh Sharma (Production Coordinator), Ms Seema Dogra (Cover Visualizer), Mr Narsingh Kumar (Proofreader), Mr Kapil Dev Sharma (Typesetter), Mr Radhey Shyam Singh (Graphic Designer) and their team members, for all their support to work in this project and make it a success. Without their cooperation, I could not have completed this project.

I convey my sincere thanks to Mr Sabyasachi Hazra, Senior Business Manager (East) of M/s Jaypee Brothers Medical Publishers (P) Ltd, New Delhi, India, for his continous support and encouragement for continuing this work.

Contents

Section 1: Exercise Therapy and Massage

1. Exercise Therapy   3
- Warm-Up 3
- Cool Down 4
- Posture 5
- Balance 13
- Types and Ranges of Muscle Work 19
- Goniometry 21
- Classification of Exercises 34
- Relaxation 45
- Frenkel's Exercise 47
- Suspension Therapy 50

2. Hydrotherapy   56
- Principles of Hydrotherapy 56
- Objectives of Hydrotherapy 56
- Clinical Applications of Hydrotherapy 56
- Salient Features of Hydrotherapy Pool 57
- Contraindications and Precautions for Hydrotherapy 57

3. Proprioceptive Neuromuscular Facilitation   59
- Definition of Proprioceptive Neuromuscular Facilitation 59
- Basic Principles of Proprioceptive Neuromuscular Facilitation 59
- Basic Neurophysiologic Principles of Proprioceptive Neuromuscular Facilitation 59
- Philosophy of Proprioceptive Neuromuscular Facilitation 60
- Basic Procedures of Proprioceptive Neuromuscular Facilitation 60
- Techniques of Proprioceptive Neuromuscular Facilitation 63
- Clinical Application of Proprioceptive Neuromuscular Facilitation 67

4. Normal Human Locomotion, Walking Aids, and Gait Training   70
- Normal Human Locomotion 70
- Gait Analysis 72
- Walking Aids 74

5. Massage   79
- Classification of Massage 79
- Physiological Effects of Massage 83
- Therapeutic Uses of Massage 83
- Contraindications of Massage 84
- Massage Lubricants 84

Section 2: Physiotherapy for Musculoskeletal Conditions

6. Physiotherapy for Spinal Disorders   87
- The Lumbar Spine 87
- The Thoracic Spine 88
- The Cervical Spine 88
- Disorders of Spine 89
- Low Back Pain 105

7. Physiotherapy for Hip   137
- The Hip Joint 137
- Special Tests for Hip Joint 137
- Specific Disorders of Hip 139

8. Knee Joint   162
- Knee Joint 162
- Special Tests for Knee Joint 162

9. Physiotherapy for Ankle and Foot   192
- The Ankle Joint 192
- Special Tests for Ankle and Foot 193

10. Physiotherapy for Shoulder   209
- The Shoulder Joint 209
- Special Tests for Shoulder Joint 210
- The Common Shoulder Injuries and their Management 215

11. Physiotherapy for Disorders of Elbow   232
- The Elbow Joint 232
- The Superior and Inferior Radioulnar Joints 232
- Factors Contributing to Elbow Pain and Special Tests for Elbow Disorders 233

12. Physiotherapy for Disorders of Wrist and Hand   242
- Disorders of the Wrist and Hand 245
- Special Tests for Wrist and Hand 242

13. Physiotherapy in Scoliosis   256

14. Physiotherapy for Amputees   264
- Incidence of Amputation 264
- Causes/Indications of Amputation 264
- Phases of Amputee Rehabilitation 266
- Role of Physiotherapy in Amputee Rehabilitation 266
- Discharge Planning 270

15. Physiotherapy in Arthritis   271
- Arthritis 271
- Osteoarthritis 271
- Rheumatoid Arthritis 276
- Psoriatic Arthritis 280
- Syphilitic Arthritis 282
- Ankylosing Spondylitis 283

16. Physiotherapy in Fractures   288
- Fracture 288
- Fracture of Spine 288
- Fractures of Upper Limb 291

Lower Limb Fractures 298
Fractures around the Ankle and Foot 308
Fractures of Tarsals, Metatarsals, and Phalanges 309
Fracture of Talus/Navicular and Other Tarsal Bones 309

17. Physiotherapy for Burn 311
Causes of Burn 311
Types of Burn Injuries 311
Percentage of Burn 312
Clinical Features of Burn 312
Management of Burn 313
Rehabilitation of Burn Injury 314

Section 3: Physiotherapy for Neurological Conditions

18. Cerebral Palsy 319
19. Stroke/Cerebrovascular Accident 358
20. Physiotherapy for Spinal Cord Injury 388
21. Parkinson's Disease 412
Epidemiology and Etiology 412
Pathophysiology 412
Clinical Features 413
Stages of Parkinson's Disease 413
Diagnosis of Parkinson's Disease 414
Treatment 414

22. Traumatic Brain Injury 420
23. Physiotherapy in Multiple Sclerosis 427
Epidemiology 427
Etiology 427
Pathophysiology 427
Clinical Features 428
Diagnosis 428
Management 428
Physiotherapy Assessment 429
Prognosis 430

24. Physiotherapy for Muscular Dystrophies, Motor Neuron Disease and Spinal Muscular Atrophies 431
A. Muscular Dystrophy 431
B. Motor Neuron Disease 437
C. Spinal Muscular Atrophy 439

25. Physiotherapy for Peripheral Nerve Injuries 442
Brachial Plexus Injury 443
Obstetrics Brachial Plexus Injuries 448
Ulnar Nerve Injury 452
Median Nerve Injury 457
Radial Nerve Injury 461
Sciatic Nerve Injury 463

26. Physiotherapy in Guillain-Barré Syndrome: Acute Inflammatory Demyelinating Polyneuropathy and Chronic Inflammatory Demyelinating Polyneuropathy 467
Guillain–Barré Syndrome 467
Chronic Inflammatory Demyelinating Polyneuropathy 470

27. Physiotherapy in Ataxias (Ataxic Disorders) 471

Section 4: Physiotherapy in Obstetrics and Gynecology

28. Physiotherapy in Obstetrics 479
Pregnancy, its Complications, and Management 479

29. Physiotherapy in Gynecological Diseases 492
Physiotherapy after Radical Mastectomy 492
Physiotherapy after Hysterectomy 494
Physiotherapy in Pelvic Inflammatory Disease 496

Section 5: Physiotherapy for Pulmonary and Cardiac Conditions: Pulmonary Rehabilitation and Cardiac Rehabilitation

30. Pulmonary Rehabilitation 499
Introduction to Respiratory System 499
Mechanics of Ventilation/Breathing 499
Respiratory Physiology 500
Benefits of Breathing Exercise 515
Postural Drainage 516
Sarcoidosis 523
Idiopathic Pulmonary Fibrosis 524
Pulmonary Rehabilitation 524

31. Cardiac Rehabilitation 530
Indications of Cardiac Rehabilitation 531
Goal of Cardiac Rehabilitation 531
Benefits of Cardiac Rehabilitation 531
Assessment of Patient before Exercise Training for Cardiac Rehabilitation 531
Components of Cardiac Rehabilitation 533
Phases of Cardiac Rehabilitation 534

Section 6: Physiotherapy in Abdominal and Thoracic Surgeries

32. Physiotherapy in Abdominal Surgeries 539
Common Abdominal Surgeries 539
Physiotherapy in Abdominal Surgeries 540

33. Physiotherapy in Thoracic Surgeries 542
Thoracotomies and its Physiotherapy Management 543

Section 7: Ethics and Management and Special Techniques in Physiotherapy

34. Professional Ethics 551
Medicolegal Issues arising during Patient Treatments 551
Ethics in Physiotherapy 554
Code of Conduct for Physiotherapists 555

35. Management for Physiotherapists 557
Definition of Management 557
Functions of Management 557

Theories of Management 560
Management of Physiotherapy Department 560

36. Motor Control, Motor Learning and Special Techniques of Therapy to Improve Function in Neurological Diseases/Disorders   563

Motor Control 563
Motor Learning 567
Motor Relearning Program 570
Neurodevelopmental Treatment 585
Rood's Approach 592
Vojta Approach 593
Sensory Integration Therapy 595
Conductive Education Therapy 595

37. Manual Therapy   596

McKenzie Method 596
Maitland Approach 599
Cyriax Approach 601
Kaltenborn's Orthopedic Manual Therapy 604
Mennel's Approch 605
Muscle Energy Technique 606
Strain/Counter Strain (Positional Release Technique) 606
Myofascial Release 607
Mulligan's Approach 608

Index   *611*

SECTION 1

Exercise Therapy and Massage

Section Outline

Chapter 1: Exercise Therapy
Chapter 2: Hydrotherapy
Chapter 3: Proprioceptive Neuromuscular Facilitation
Chapter 4: Normal Human Locomotion, Walking Aids, and Gait Training
Chapter 5: Massage

Exercise Therapy

INTRODUCTION

Exercise therapy is the systematic, planned performance of bodily movements, postures, and activities, intended to provide to a patient/client to optimize the overall health status, fitness or sense of well-being by preventing/remediating impairments, improving/restoring physical function, preventing/reducing health-related risk factors, etc.

It is an essential tool used by therapists to treat patients/clients with neuromuscular, musculoskeletal, cardiopulmonary disorders with the objectives of:
- Improvement/maintenance of joint range of motion (ROM).
- Improvement/maintenance of muscle bulk, strength, and endurance.
- Decreasing pain of neuromusculoskeletal origin.
- Improvement of respiratory function/lung capacities.
- Improvement of cardiovascular function.
- Improvement of overall function.
- Prevention of impairment/activity limitation and participation limitation.

The exercise programs are designed by a qualified therapist to meet the unique need of the client. A patient/client who reports the therapist (Physiotherapist/Occupational therapist/Speech therapist) with a functional impairment causing activity and participation limitation is evaluated by the therapist using the internal classification of function (ICF) model (**Fig. 1.1**) and appropriate exercises are designed to remediate impairment, promote activity, restore participation in the society and community.

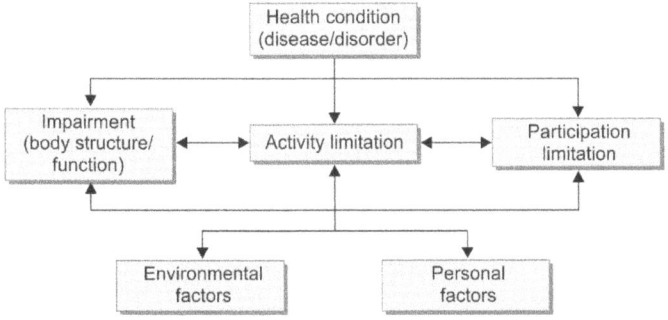

Fig. 1.1: The ICF model of patient management.

Impairment

Impairment is the consequence of pathology (i.e., injury/infection) involving body systems and organs, resulting in anatomical, physiological, and psychological alterations/losses, which if not reversed with interventions, may lead to activity and participation limitations. Physiotherapists provide care and services to patients with impairments of:
- Musculoskeletal system
- Neuromuscular system
- Cardiorespiratory system
- Integumentary system
- Cognitive/perceptual system

Activity Limitation

Activity limitation is the stage, where, due to the impairment, the individual fails to perform his normal activities for self-care and vocation. It is the difficulty the individual may have in executing activities in terms of quality and quantity.

Participation Limitation

Participation limitation is the stage where due to activity limitation, the person fails to participate in family and community activities/life situations.

The therapist designs the exercise techniques to deal local impairments such as a stiff knee after soft tissue injury or generalized movement disorders such as hemiplegia after brain stroke or movement dysfunction after myocardial infarction. In generalized movement disorders where significant impairment of posture and movement exists, a warm-up and cool down program is included in the therapeutic protocol for conditioning the body to bear the load imposed on the weaker systems of the body.

WARM-UP

The warm-up exercises enhance the numerous adjustment that take place before vigorous physical activity. It should be gradual and sufficient to increase muscle and core temperature without causing fatigue or reducing energy stores of body. A 10-minute period of total body movement, such as low intensity calisthenics (exercise consisting of a variety of movements, which exercise large muscle groups such as running, walking, and pushing, etc.), static stretching, slow walking (if possible) is performed. A heart rate increase by 20 beats per minute from the resting heart rate is desirable during the warm-up period.

COOL DOWN

Following vigorous aerobic training, a cool down period of 5–10 minutes is required to enhance the recovery with oxidation of metabolic waste and replacement of energy stores of the body. It prevents cardiovascular complications by promoting gradual return of blood to the heart and brain by allowing the muscles to maintain venous return, preventing pooling of blood in the extremities. A total body exercises such as low-intensity calisthenics (slow walking/running, dancing) are appropriate.

A clinician must understand that, to improve functional skills, which are impaired in clients with neuromuscular, musculoskeletal, cardiopulmonary as well as cognitive perceptual dysfunctions, various body systems need to work in co-ordination, resulting in achievement/restoration of functional skills, which can be understood from **Figure 1.2**.

Before discussing the various types of exercises and their clinical applications, a brief discussion on biomechanics of movement is discussed below:

Axis and plane: All body movements occur in different planes and around different axes **(Fig. 1.3)**.

* **Axis:** It is an imaginary line around which movement takes place. It is perpendicular to the plane, about which body/system rotates or spins. There are three types of axes:
  a. *Sagittal axis:* It lies parallel to sagittal suture of skull, i.e., in an anterior-posterior direction. Movement around this axis occurs in a frontal plane.

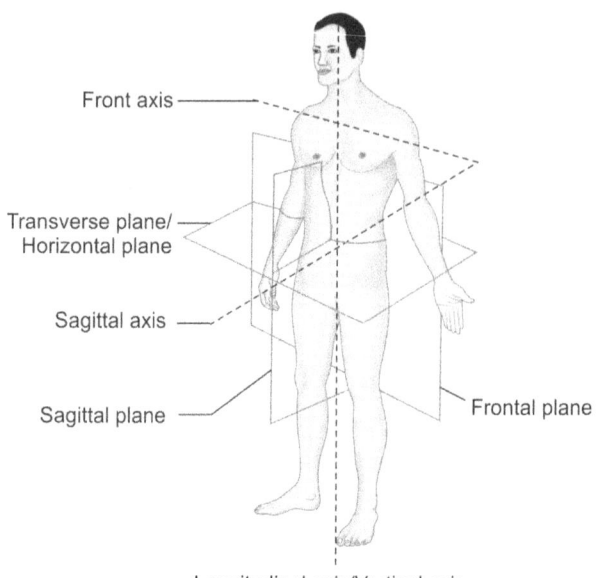

Fig. 1.3: The body axes and planes of movement.

  b. *Frontal axis:* It lies parallel to coronal suture of skull. It is aligned at right angles to sagittal axis. Movement around this axis occurs in a sagittal plane.
  c. *Longitudinal/Vertical axis:* It lies parallel to the line of gravity. Movement about this axis occurs in transverse/horizontal plane.
* **Plane:** It is the surface which lies at right angle to axis and in which the movement takes place. There are three types of planes.
  a. *Sagittal plane:* The sagittal plane lies vertically and divides the body into right and left parts. Movement in this plane occurs around frontal axis **(Fig. 1.4)**.
  b. *Frontal plane:* The frontal plane also lies vertically and divides the body into anterior and posterior parts. Movement in this plane occurs around sagittal axis **(Fig. 1.5)**.
  c. *Transverse plane/Horizontal plane:* The transverse plane lies horizontally and divides the body into superior and inferior parts. Movement in this plane occurs around longitudinal/vertical axis **(Fig. 1.6)**.

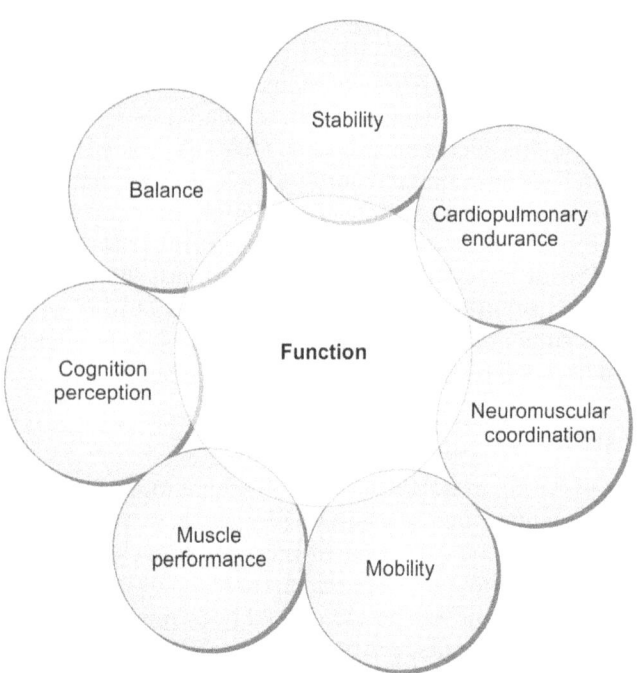

Fig. 1.2: Body systems involved in functional performance.

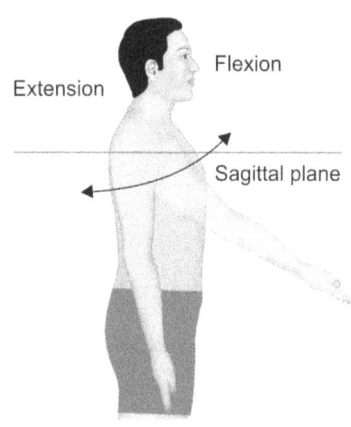

Fig. 1.4: Movement in sagittal plane.

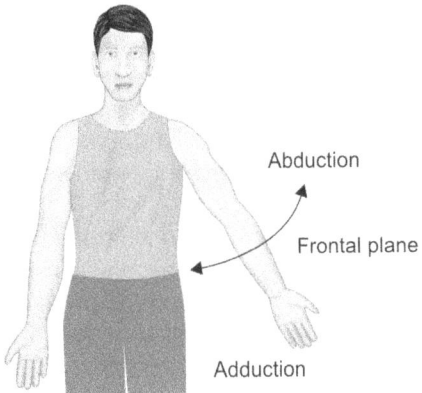

Fig. 1.5: Movement in frontal plane.

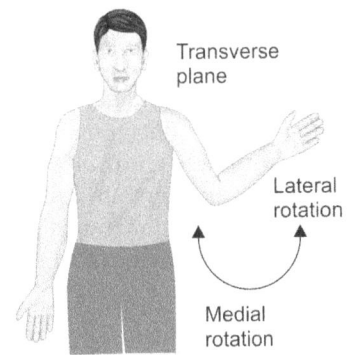

Fig. 1.6: Movement in transverse plane.

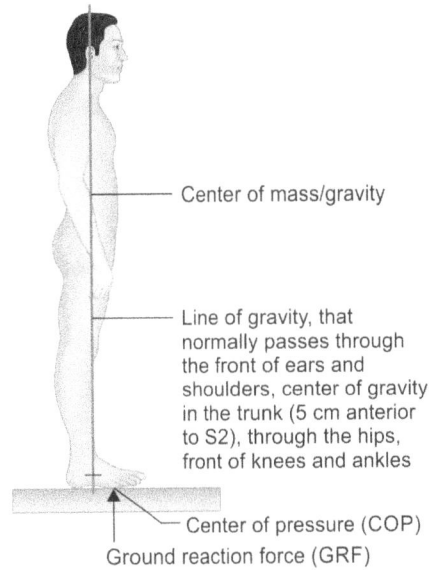

Fig. 1.7: Center of mass (COM), center of pressure, and ground reaction force.

Table 1.1: Movements in different planes and axes.		
Plane	Motion	Axis
Sagittal	Flexion/extension	Frontal
Frontal	• Abduction/adduction • Side flexion • Inversion/eversion	Sagittal
Transverse	• Internal rotation/external rotation • Horizontal adduction/abduction • Supination/pronation	Vertical/ Longitudinal

Examples of movements in different planes and axes are given in **Table 1.1**

POSTURE

Posture is the attitude assumed by the body either with support during muscular inactivity or by means of coordinated action of many muscles working to maintain stability.

It is the position from which movement can be initiated. It is often used to describe both biomechanical alignment of the body and the orientation of the body to the environment.

A good postural control mechanism is essential for maintenance of posture. As stated by Sherrington, posture follows movement like a shadow, i.e., every movement starts from a posture and ends in a posture.

Postural stability, also referred to as balance, is the ability to control the center of mass (COM), in relationship to the base of support (BOS).

- COM, is defined as a point that is at the center of the total body mass **(Fig. 1.7)**.
- The vertical projection of the COM is often defined as the center of gravity (COG).
- The BOS is defined as the area of the body that is in contact with the support surface.
- The center of pressure (COP) is the center of the distribution of the total force applied to the supporting surface. The COP moves continuously around the COM to keep the COM within the support base (Benda et al. 1994; Winter, 1990).

Postural Control

Postural control is the person's ability to maintain stability of the body and body segments in response to forces that disturb body's structural equilibrium. It involves controlling the body's position in space for the purposes of stability and orientation. It depends on the integrity of the central nervous system, visual, vestibular, and musculoskeletal system, that include information from receptors located in and around joints (i.e., joint capsule, tendons, and ligaments) and from cutaneous receptors located in the sole of foot.

Postural control emerges from an interaction of the individual with the task and the environment **(Fig. 1.8)**.

Postural control for stability and orientation requires a complex interaction of musculoskeletal and neural systems.

Musculoskeletal components include such things as joint ROM, spinal flexibility, muscle properties, and biomechanical relationships among linked body segments.

Neural components of postural control:
- **Sensory processes:** Organization and integration of visual, vestibular, somatosensory systems.
- **Central processing:** A higher-level integrative process, essential for mapping sensation to action, and ensuring anticipatory and adaptive aspects of postural control.

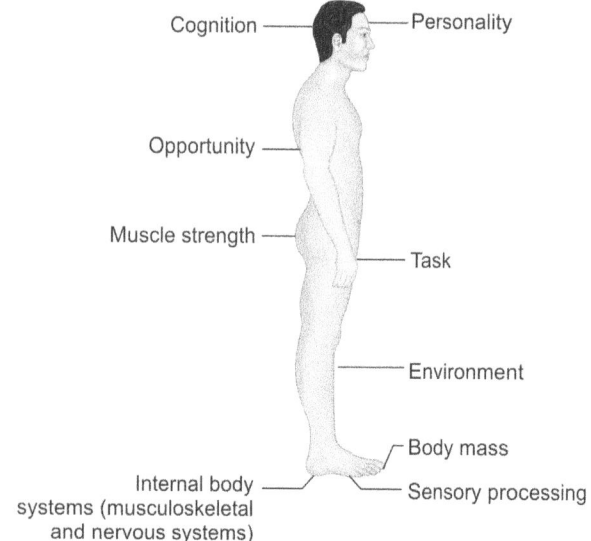

Fig. 1.8: The postural control mechanism.

- **Effector component:** Sometimes referred to as the neuromuscular component, which include organization of muscles throughout the body into neuromuscular synergies for postural alignment.

Postural control may develop by the postural reflex mechanism or may develop voluntarily as per the imposed demands of the task.

Individuals develop and maintain posture by mechanisms such as:

- **The postural reflex (Fig. 1.9):** A reflex is by definition, an efferent response to an afferent stimulus. The afferent stimuli from variety of sources of the body such as muscles, eyes, ears, and joint structures trigger the postural muscles to maintain postural tone for the development of the postures immediately during need. For example, when the legs slip on a slippery floor, and body tends to fall backward, the afferent information from the different receptors stated above trigger the postural reflex, which maintains erect position of the body by moving the upper body forward so that the line of gravity falls within the supporting base. The receptors in the following organs provide the necessary afferent input:
  - *Muscles:* Neuromuscular and neurotendinous spindles within the muscles record changing tension.
  - *The eyes:* Visual sensation records any alteration in the position of the body with regard to the surroundings.
  - *The ears:* Stimulation of the receptors of the vestibular nerve results from the movement of fluid contained in the semicircular canals of the internal ear.
  - *Joint structures:* In the weight-bearing position approximation of bones stimulates receptors in joint structures and elicits reflex reactions.
- **Adaptive postural control:** It requires modifying sensory and motor systems to changing tasks and environmental demands. The group of muscles most frequently the posterior chain antigravity muscles are recruited to maintain both static and dynamic posture as per the physical characteristic of the individual and nature of task to be performed by manipulating the environment.

Classification of Posture

Posture, which is the basic prerequisite for the movement are classified into:

- **Fundamental postures:** These are the basic positions of the body individuals adapt in their routine activities, e.g., standing, sitting, lying, kneeling, and hanging.
- **Derived postures:** These are the postures, where the positions of the arms, leg, or trunk may be altered in the fundamental postures to modify the positions of the body. These postures are derived from the fundamental positions such as: standing, kneeling, sitting, and lying. The derived postures are described as under:

Positions Derived from Standing

- Wing standing (Hands rest on the iliac crests, with the extended and adducted fingers placed anteriorly, and thumb placed posteriorly. The wrists are extended, forearms pronated, elbows flexed, and shoulders abducted) **(Fig. 1.10)**.
- Bend standing (The shoulders are laterally rotated and strongly adducted, the elbows are flexed, the forearms are supinated with wrist and fingers flexed to rest above the lateral border of the acromion process) **(Fig. 1.11)**.
- Reach standing (The shoulders are flexed with elbows in extension, so that the upper limbs remain parallel to each other perpendicular to the body) **(Fig. 1.12)**.
- Yard standing (The arms are straight and elevated sideways to horizontal position) **(Fig. 1.13)**.
- Stretch standing (The arms are fully elevated so that they are in line with the body, parallel to each other and with palms facing each other) **(Fig. 1.14)**.

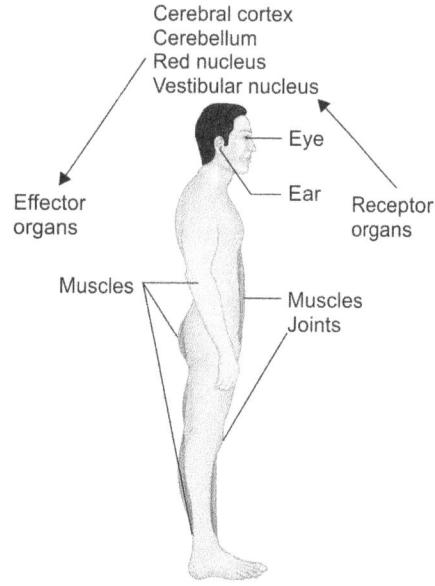

Fig. 1.9: The postural reflex.

- Walk standing (One leg is placed directly forward, so that the heels are two feet length apart and are on the same line. The body weight is equally distributed between them) **(Fig. 1.15)**.

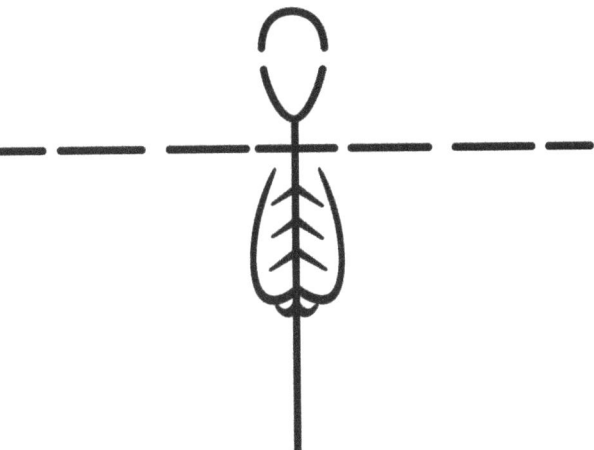

Fig. 1.13: Yard standing.

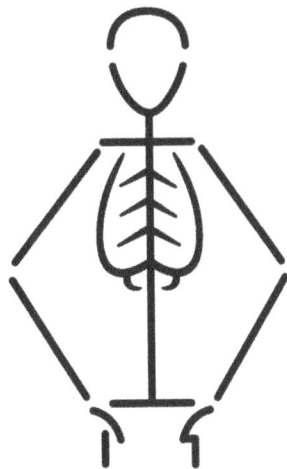

Fig. 1.10: Wing standing.

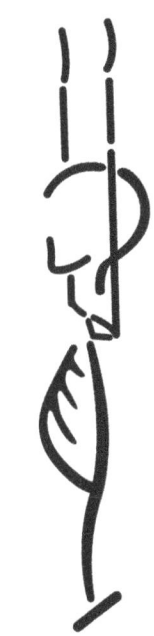

Fig. 1.14: Stretch standing.

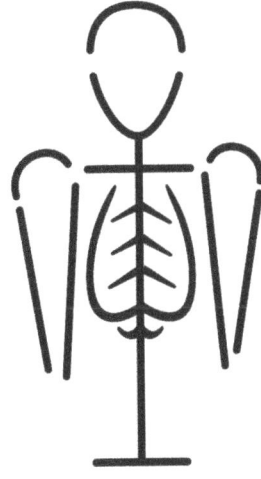

Fig. 1.11: Bend standing.

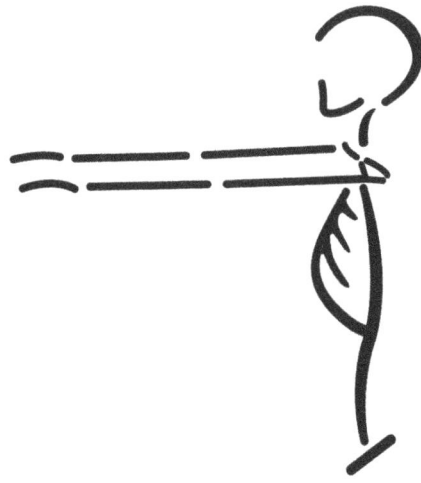

Fig. 1.12: Reach standing.

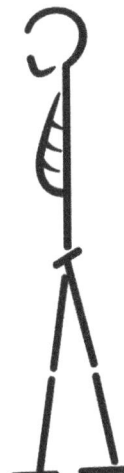

Fig. 1.15: Walk standing.

- Half standing (The whole weight of the body is supported on one leg, the other may be free or supported in a variety of positions) **(Fig. 1.16)**.
- Lax stoop standing (The hips are flexed and the trunk, head, and arms are relaxed, so that, they hang forward and downward. Balance is maintained by a slight plantar flexion of the ankle joints, causing a backward inclination of the leg) **(Fig. 1.17)**.
- Stoop standing (The hip joints are flexed, while the trunk, head, and arms remain in alignment and are inclined) **(Fig. 1.18)**.
- Fallout standing (One leg is placed directly forward to a distance of 3 feet length with the knee bent. The back leg remains straight and the body is inclined forward in line with it) **(Fig. 1.19)**.
- Lunge sideways standing (One leg is abducted at the hip with knee in extension and ankle plantar flexion, the other leg is abducted with knee in flexion and ankle in dorsiflexion. The trunk remains vertical) **(Fig. 1.20)**.

Positions Derived from Kneeling

- Half-kneeling (One leg is bent at the knee that supports most of the body weight, and the other leg is bent to a right angle at the hip, knee, and ankle so that the foot is supported on the ground in a forward direction) **(Fig. 1.21)**.

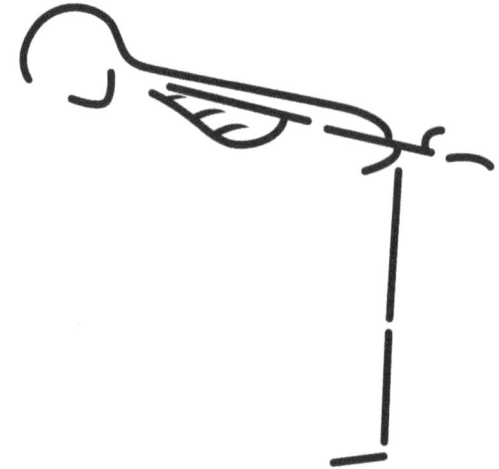

Fig. 1.18: Stoop standing.

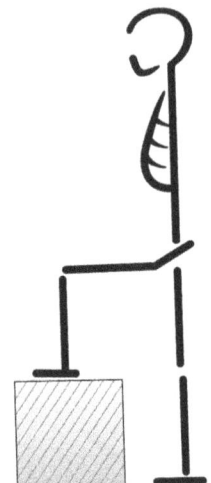

Fig. 1.16: Half standing.

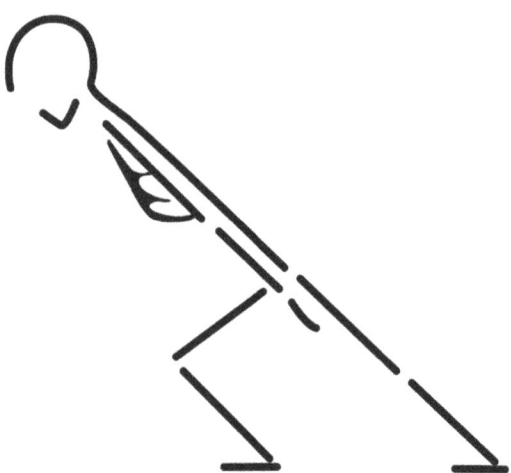

Fig. 1.19: Fall-out standing.

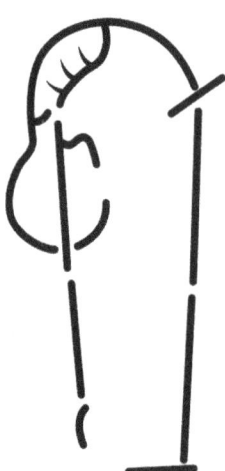

Fig. 1.17: Lax stoop standing.

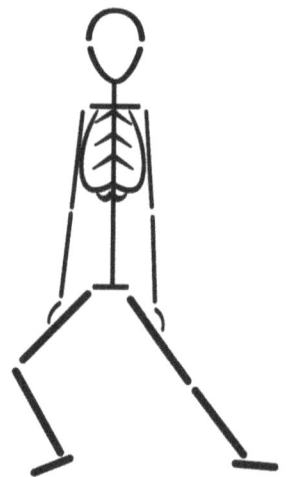

Fig. 1.20: Lunge sideways standing.

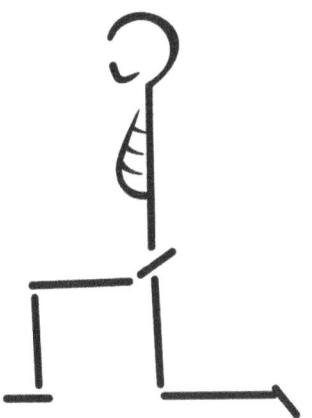

Fig. 1.21: Half kneeling.

- Kneel sitting (Both the hips and knees are flexed, so that the person sits over his heels) **(Fig. 1.22)**.
- Prone kneeling (The trunk is horizontal and the head is in line with the trunk. Body weight is supported both by the vertical arms with the elbow in extension and hands flat on the ground, as well as the thighs with hip and knees bent at right angles) **(Fig. 1.23)**.
- Inclined prone kneeling (From prone kneeling, the trunk is inclined forward, so that, head rests on ground over clenched hands) **(Fig. 1.24)**.

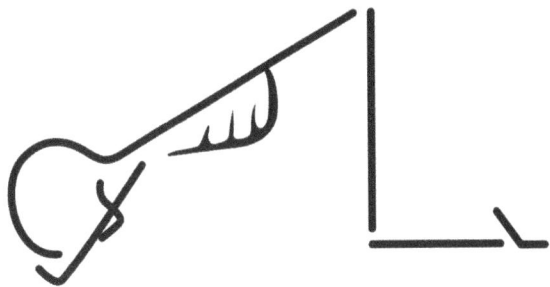

Fig. 1.24: Inclined prone kneeling.

Positions Derived from Sitting

- **Stride sitting:** This involves sitting with the hips abducted, so that the feet which usually rests on the floor, are usually 2-feet length apart **(Fig. 1.25)**.
- **Ride sitting:** This involves sitting on a table/gymnastic ball, so that, the apparatus is gripped strongly between the knees by the hip adductors making the posture very stable **(Fig. 1.26)**.
- **Side sitting:** This involves sitting on floor/bed, with one hip flexed, abducted with knee maximally flexed and ankle plantigrade and the other hip flexed, abducted

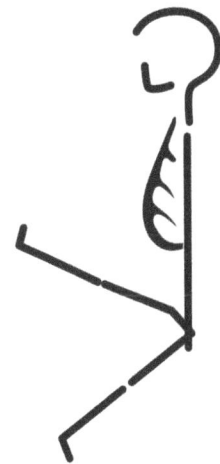

Fig. 1.25: Stride sitting.

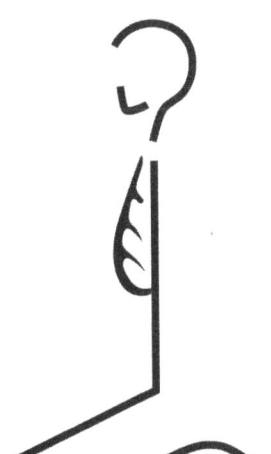

Fig. 1.22: Kneel sitting.

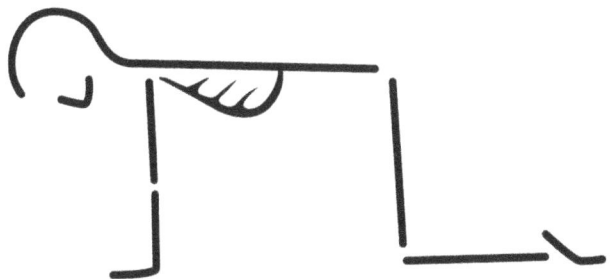

Fig. 1.23: Prone kneeling.

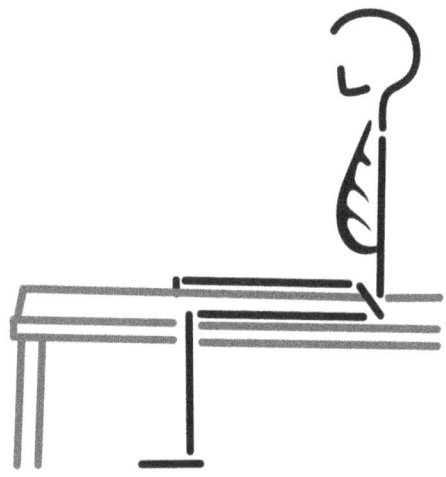

Fig. 1.26: Ride sitting.

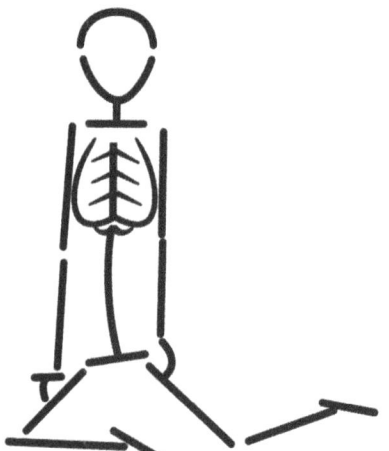

Fig. 1.27: Right side sitting.

and medially rotated with the knee partially flexed, and the ankle plantigrade. For right side sitting, the right leg remains as in cross-sitting and this hip supports the main weight of the trunk, while the left hip is abducted and medially rotated, so that the lower leg is bent and to the side **(Fig. 1.27)**.

- **Crooksitting:** This involves sitting on the floor with the hip and knees flexed, so that the feet are on the floor **(Fig. 1.28)**.

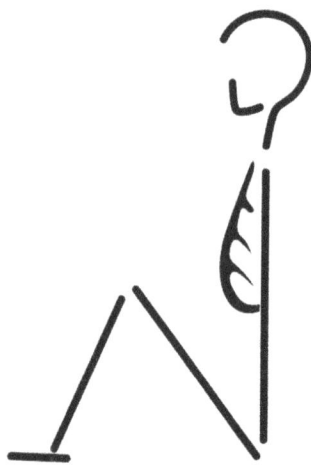

Fig. 1.28: Crook sitting.

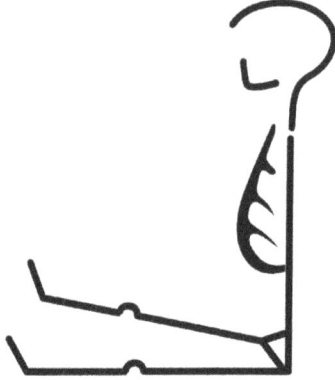

Fig. 1.29: Long sitting.

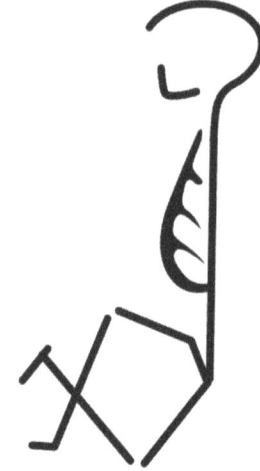

Fig. 1.30: Cross sitting.

- **Long sitting:** This involves sitting on the floor/bed with the hips flexed and the knees extended **(Fig. 1.29)**.
- **Cross-sitting:** This involves sitting on the floor/bed, with the hips flexed, abducted and laterally rotated, knees flexed, and ankles crossing each other **(Fig. 1.30)**.
- **High sitting:** This involves sitting on a plinth or high table, so that the feet remain unsupported **(Fig. 1.31)**.
- **Stoop sitting:** This involves sitting on a plinth/chair with the trunk inclined forward and the feet resting on the floor **(Fig. 1.32)**.
- **Fallout sitting:** This involves sitting on a stool/plinth with the trunk inclined, so that, the forward leg is supported across the stool, and the backward leg is extending straight with the knee extended and ankle plantar flexed **(Fig. 1.33)**.
- **Crouch sitting:** The hips and knees are fully flexed, and the straight trunk is inclined forward to allow the hands to rest on the floor **(Fig. 1.34)**.

Positions Derived from Lying

- **Crook lying:** In supine, the hips and knees are flexed, so that the feet rest on the bed/ground **(Fig. 1.35)**.

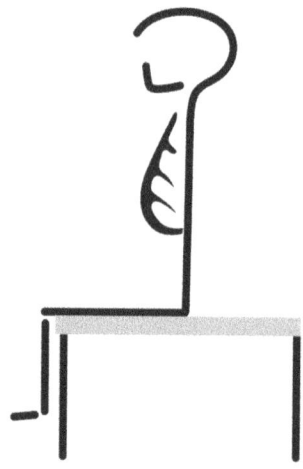

Fig. 1.31: High sitting.

Fig. 1.32: Stoop sitting.

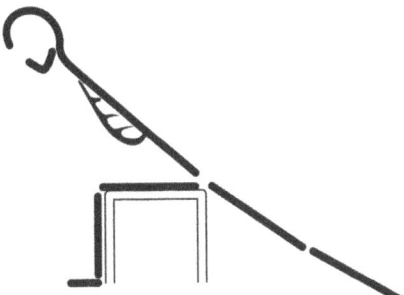

Fig. 1.33: Fallout sitting.

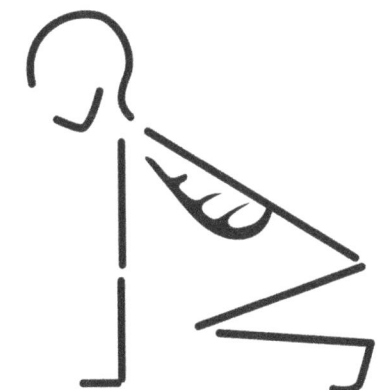

Fig. 1.34: Crouch sitting.

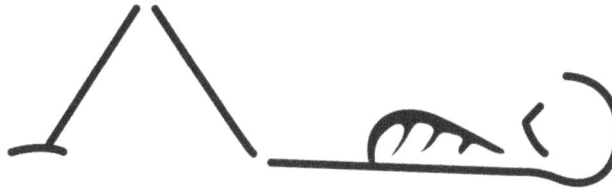

Fig. 1.35: Crook lying.

- **Half-lying:** In supine, the trunk is raised forward from the hips at an angle of 45 degrees, either by pillow positioning or elevating the head end of the bed. The lower limbs are supported on the bed horizontally **(Fig. 1.36)**.

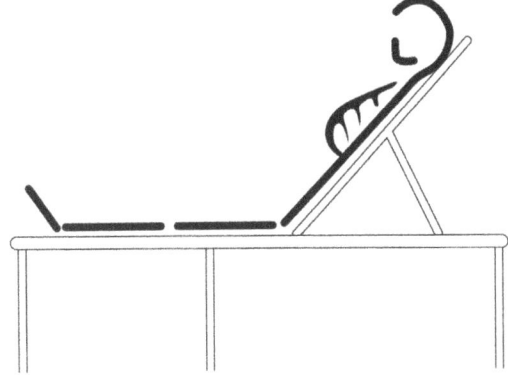

Fig. 1.36: Half-lying.

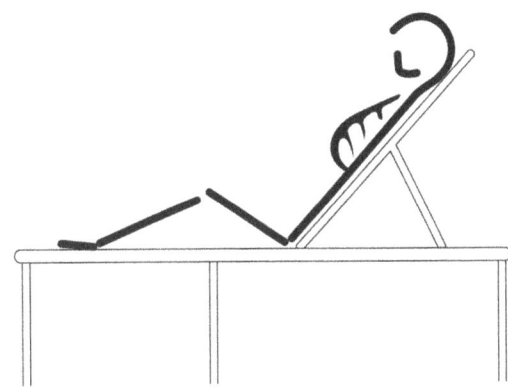

Fig. 1.37: Half-crook lying.

- **Half-crook lying:** In half-lying, the knees are flexed, so that the feet rest on the floor, to increase relaxation of the abdominals **(Fig. 1.37)**.
- **Prone lying:** Lying with face down and the body completely supported anteriorly on the plinth **(Fig. 1.38)**.
- **Leg-prone lying:** In prone lying, the lower limbs are supported on plinth and the trunk remains unsupported in space **(Fig. 1.39)**.

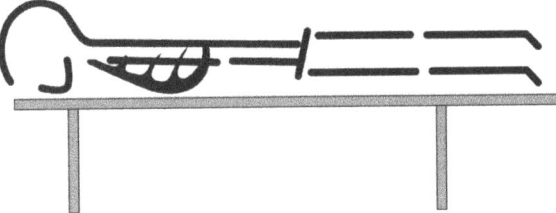

Fig. 1.38: Prone lying.

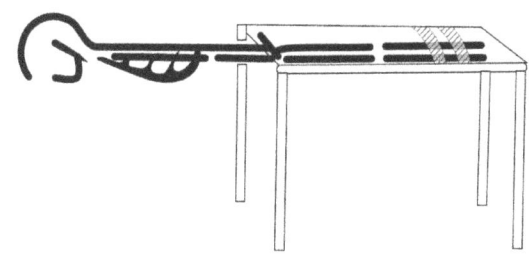

Fig. 1.39: Leg-prone lying.

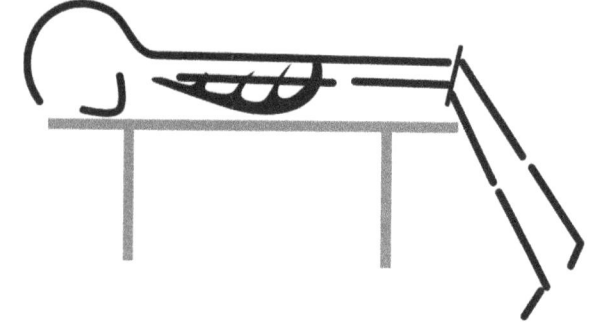

Fig. 1.40: Trunk-prone lying.

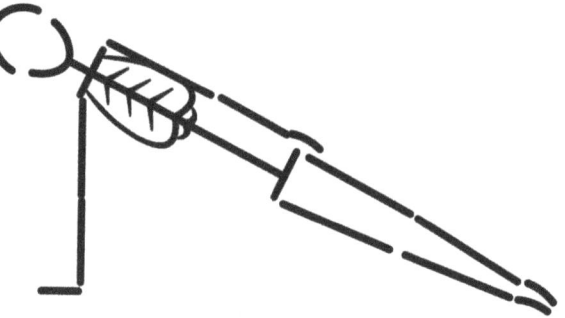

Fig. 1.43: Side falling.

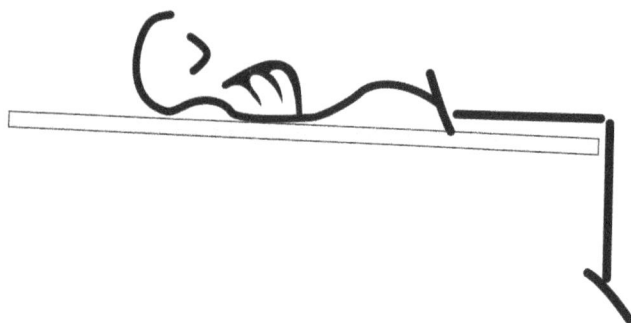

Fig. 1.41: Sit lying.

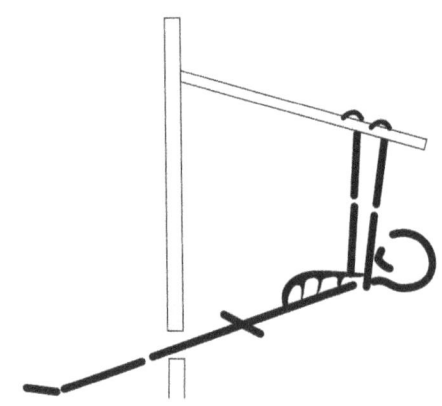

Fig. 1.44: Fall hanging.

- **Trunk-prone lying:** In prone lying, the trunk is supported on plinth, and the lower limbs remain hanging unsupported at the foot end of the bed **(Fig. 1.40)**.
- **Sit lying:** In supine lying, the lower limbs remain flexed at the knees and hang downward at the foot end of the bed **(Fig. 1.41)**.
- **Prone falling:** From crouch sitting, the legs are extended in line with the trunk, so that the body is supported on the vertical arms and toes **(Fig. 1.42)**.
- **Side falling:** In side lying, the upper body is raised by pushing through the lower side arms, so that the body is in an inclined position, with weight on the lower side hand and foot **(Fig. 1.43)**.

Positions Derived from Hanging

a. **Fall hanging:** The body is aligned in the oblique position by grasping a horizontal bar by the hands, and weight borne on the feet that rest on the floor **(Fig. 1.44)**.

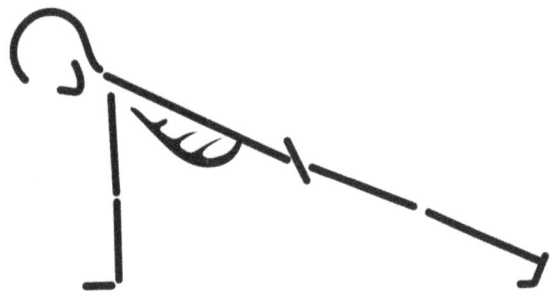

Fig. 1.42: Prone falling.

The fundamental and derived postures are further classified into:

- **Active postures:** These are the positions of the body, which are maintained by integrated action of many muscles. It could be static posture or dynamic posture:
  - *Static posture:* This is a constant pattern of posture, maintained by interaction of group of muscles that work more or less statically.
  - *Dynamic posture:* These are positions which are constantly modified and adjusted to meet the changing demands of body while performing movements for function.
- **Inactive posture:** These are attitudes assumed by the body while resting, where all the essential muscular activities required to maintain life are reduced to minimum.
- **Good posture/Efficient posture:** Posture is said to be good, when it fulfills the purpose for which it is used with maximum efficiency and minimum effort.

A good posture in lying, sitting, and standing, where normal alignment of the body is maintained with minimal effort is essential for efficient movement performance as well as prevention of musculoskeletal complications. Development of good posture depends upon:
  - Intact/efficient neuromusculoskeletal system.
  - Ergonomically designed working environment.
  - A stable psychological background.
  - Good hygienic conditions.
  - Opportunity of freedom for movement.

* **Poor posture/Inefficient posture:** Posture is said to be poor or inefficient, when it fails to serve the purpose for which it is designed, or if unnecessary amount of muscular effort is used to maintain it.

  A poor posture, which is always inefficient, leads to unnecessary muscle contraction and energy consumption, leading to early fatigue, deformities, pain, abnormal gait, etc., develops due to:
  – Psychological stress and mental attitude
  – Poor ergonomics in work place
  – Poor hygienic conditions
  – Prolonged fatigue
  – Pain
  – Muscle weakness
  – Occupational stress

Postural Re-education

As we know, posture precedes movement, hence a stable normal posture needs to be developed for production of efficient functional movements. A postural re-education program consists of:
* Measures to reduce pain, fatigue, occupational and psychological stress.
* Creation of ergonomically designed working environment.
* Relaxation programs that include breathing exercises, meditations, music therapy, relax passive exercises, and low intensity aerobic exercises.
* Strengthening of weak postural muscles.
* Postural awareness training through biofeedback devices such as postural mirror.

BALANCE

Balance is the ability to maintain the line of gravity of the body within the BOS with minimal postural sway. Balance requires keeping the "COM" over the "BOS" during static and dynamic situations.
* **Static balance/Static postural control:** It is the ability to maintain stability and orientation with the COM over the BOS with the body at rest.
* **Dynamic balance/Dynamic postural control:** It is the ability to maintain stability and orientation with the COM over the BOS, while the body/parts of the body are in motion.

In day-to-day activities, individuals require to maintain stable steady posture, called static balance, where the COM is constantly kept over the BOS. However, in certain activities such as reaching forward in sitting or standing, the COM, is made to move out of the BOS, still maintaining the body posture called dynamic balance.

Maintaining balance requires coordinated input from multiple sensory systems including the vestibular, somatosensory, and visual systems as described below.
* **Vestibular system:** This sense organ regulates equilibrium through directional information as it relates to head position.

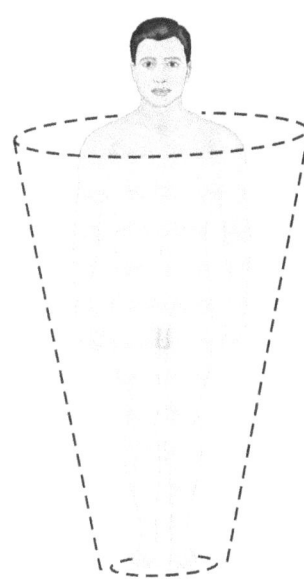

Fig. 1.45: The cone of stability/postural sway in quiet stance.

* **Somatosensory system:** The sensation of proprioception and kinesthesia of joints, information from skin and joints (pressure and vibratory senses), spatial position, and movements relative to the support surface, movements and positions of different body parts relative to each other, help in maintenance of postural tone-retaining balance.
* **Visual system:** The perception of verticality of head and body motion, spatial location relative to objects help in maintenance of balance.

During perturbation of balance, where the COM is displaced, the interaction of various sensory systems allows the modifications needed to maintain stability in a variety of environments.

During disturbance of balance:
* Adults rely on somatosensory inputs.
* Children rely more on visual input.

During quite stance, individuals have some displacement of COM within the limit of stability, where the balance is retained, even though the COM is displaced. Limit of stability is the maximum angle from vertical which can be tolerated. A cone of stability **(Fig. 1.45)**, which indicates the individual's ability to shift the COM of body from front to back and side to side without losing balance is exhibited by individuals during quite stance. This is manifested as postural sway.

A **"Postural Sway"** refers to small postural shifts from front to back and side to side, during quiet stance. However, while doing functional tasks, where there is shift in COM, normal individuals are able to maintain balance within the limit of stability. A "Limits of Stability" is defined as the distance a person can move, without losing balance or taking a step. When the balance is perturbed/lost individuals recruit different strategies described below to retain balance.
* **Ankle strategy:** The "ankle strategy" occurs with minimal perturbation of balance and involves shifting of COM at ankles **(Fig. 1.46)**. Control is distal-to-proximal. When perturbed from front to back, balance is retained by ankle

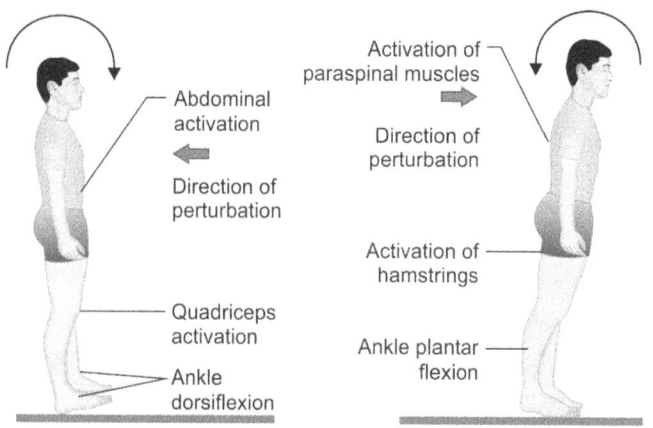

Fig. 1.46: The ankle strategy.

dorsiflexion followed by knee extension and activation of abdominals. When perturbed from back to front, balance is retained by ankle plantar flexion, followed by knee flexion and activation of paraspinal muscles.

- **Hip strategy:** The hip strategy (**Fig. 1.47**) involves shifting of COM by flexing or extending at the hips and is recruited when the ankle strategy fails (i.e., to larger perturbations). It has proximal to distal pattern of activation of muscles. With forward sway abdominals are activated first followed by the quadriceps. With backward sway, paraspinal muscles are activated first followed by the hamstrings.
- **Stepping strategy:** This strategy is recruited to larger perturbations, when ankle and hip strategies fail to retain balance. It realigns the BOS under the COM by rapid steps (**Fig. 1.48**) or hops in the direction of the displacing force, thereby increasing the base of support and retaining balance.

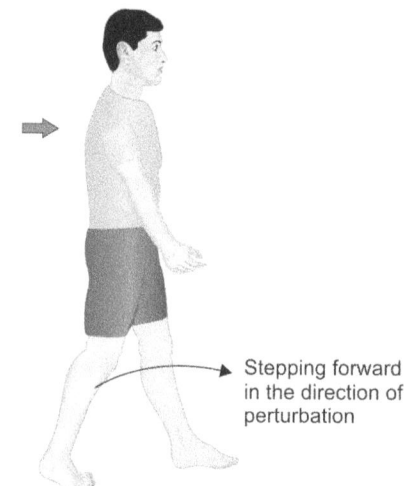

Fig. 1.48: The stepping strategy.

Assessment of Balance

Functional tests of balance focus on maintenance of both static and dynamic balance. Some of functional balance tests that are available are:

- **Romberg test:** This test is used to determine proprioceptive contribution to upright balance. The subject remains in quiet standing, feet together with the eyes open unaided for 20–30 seconds. If the patient demonstrates significant sway or instability with the eyes open, the test is over and said as positive suggesting vestibular or cerebellar pathology. If there is no difficulty in balancing, a Sharpened Romberg's test, where subjects are made to stand with eyes closed, arms crossed, and feet together. If the balance is compromised, this test is positive suggesting spinal pathology.
- **Functional reach test:** This test measures the maximal distance one can reach forward beyond arm's length, while maintaining feet planted in a standing position.
- **Berg balance scale:** This measures both static and dynamic balance abilities using functional tasks commonly used in everyday life.
- **Performance-oriented Mobility Assessment (POMA):** This test measures both static and dynamic balance using tasks testing balance and gait.
- **Timed up and go test:** This test measures dynamic balance and mobility.
- **Balance efficacy scale:** A self-reported measure that examines an individual's confidence while performing daily tasks with or without assistance.
- **Star excursion test:** A dynamic balance test that measures single stance maximal reach in multiple directions.
- **Balance Evaluation Systems Test (BESTest):** Tests for six unique balance control methods to create a specialized rehabilitation protocol by identifying specific balance deficits.
- **The functional balance grading scale:** In this grading system, both static and dynamic balance are graded using five grades such as:

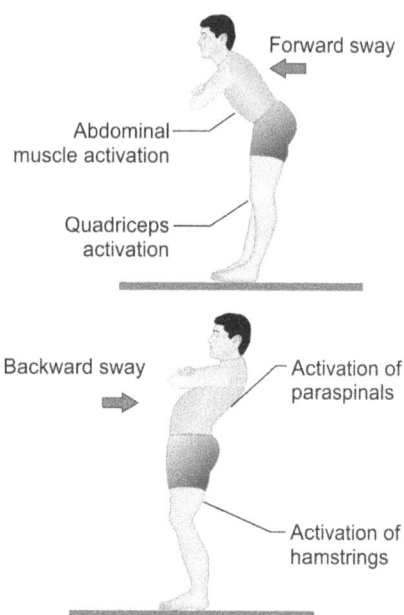

Fig. 1.47: The hip strategy.

- *Grade 4 (Normal):*
  - » Static: Patient is able to maintain steady balance without handhold support.
  - » Dynamic: Patient accepts maximal challenge and can shift weight easily within full range in all directions.
- *Grade 3 (Good):*
  - » Static: Patient is able to maintain balance without handhold support with minimal postural sway.
  - » Dynamic: Accepts moderate challenge. Able to maintain balance while picking up objects off the floor.
- *Grade 2 (Fair):*
  - » Static: Patient is able to maintain balance with handhold support, may require occasional minimal assistance.
  - » Dynamic: Patient accepts minimal challenge. Able to maintain balance while turning head/trunk.
- *Grade1 (Poor):*
  - » Static: Patient requires handhold support and moderate to maximum assistance to maintain position.
  - » Dynamic: Patient is unable to accept challenge or move without loss of balance.
- *Grade 0:* Patient is unable to maintain balance.

Balance Re-education/Balance Training

Before starting balance training, the therapist should make a comprehensive assessment for the prerequisites/missing components essential for maintenance of posture and balance. The motor/sensory (superficial and deep sensory modalities, visual, vestibular) system examinations and anthropometric measurements (ROM, limb length measurement) are to be done, before balance training/retraining is started.

Training activities are designed to improve:
- ❖ **Static postural control/Balance**: Postural alignment of the body in lying, sitting, and standing are described:
  - *Lying:* Supine/prone—head in midline, shoulders leveled, trunk symmetrically aligned over the leveled pelvis, hips and knees neutral and ankle plantigrade.
  - *Sitting (short sitting):* Head vertically aligned over the leveled shoulders, trunk vertically aligned over leveled pelvis, hips and knees flexed by 90 degrees, and ankles plantigrade.
  - *Standing:* Head vertically aligned over the leveled shoulders, trunk aligned over leveled pelvis, hips and knees in neutral, and ankles plantigrade.

Range of motion exercises, stretching exercises, strengthening of postural muscles, postural awareness training, use of training devices such as postural mirror, Biofeedback devices, and functional re-education (activities for ADL/IADL) help in the development of static postural control/balance.

- ❖ **Dynamic postural control/balance:** Dynamic postural control/balance in sitting and standing can be developed by using the Wobble board/Trampoline **(Figs. 1.49A and B)**, and dynamic balance in lying and sitting can be trained using a Swiss ball **(Fig. 1.49C)**. When the wobble board is perturbed with the patient on board, it is expected that, the normal response would be, there is abduction and extension response in the limbs with lateral bending of neck and trunk on elevated side, and protective extension of limbs on the lower side.

Trampoline is a very good modality to improve balance in children and adults. A trampoline with net boundary is used to improve sitting/standing balance in children. For adults, the patient is made to stand on trampoline and said to do mini hops, which is gradually progressed in intensity **(Fig. 1.50)**.

The fixed support strategies such as ankle strategy **(Fig. 1.51)** and hip strategies, as well change in support strategy (i.e., stepping strategy), etc., described earlier, are used to develop balance in standing. Single leg standing, walking, running, ball throwing/catching, etc., are used to develop balance in sitting and standing. All balance training programs should be repeatedly practiced through functional tasks for CNS adaptation.

Mechanical Principles Applied in Exercise Therapy

Lever

Lever is a rigid bar capable of moving around a fixed axis called fulcrum (F) **(Fig. 1.52A)**. Forces applied to levers produce movements such as rotation or translation. A work

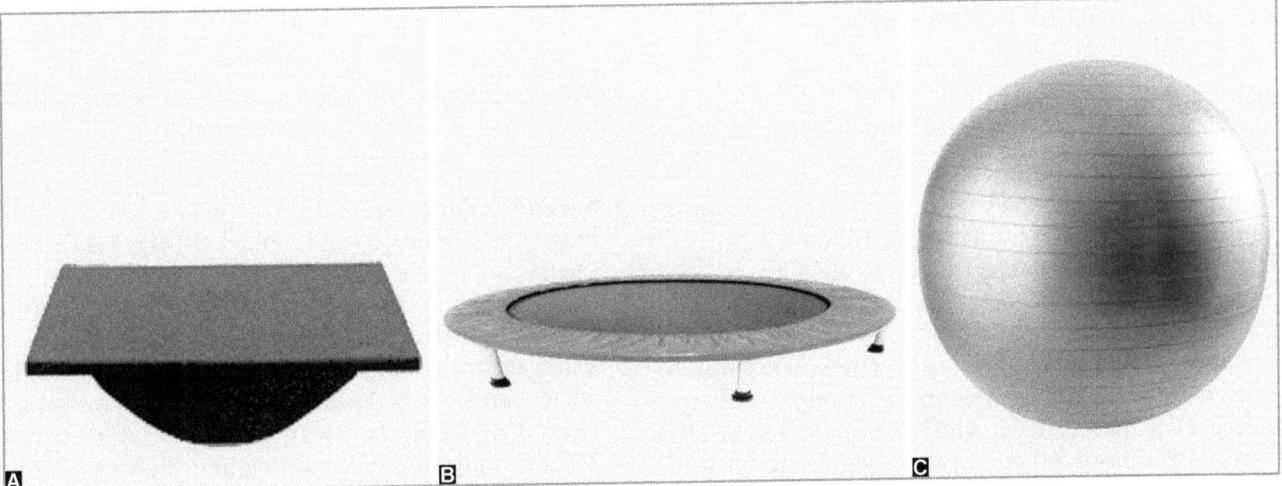

Figs. 1.49A to C: (A) Wobble board, (B) Trampoline, (C) Swiss ball.

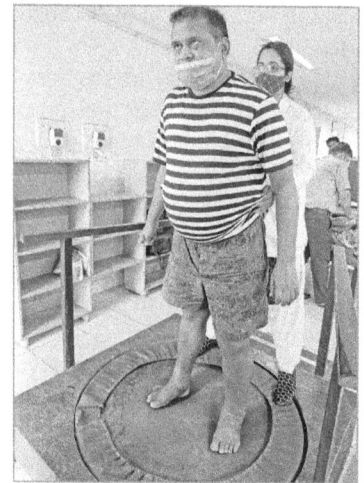

Fig. 1.50: Balance training on trampoline.

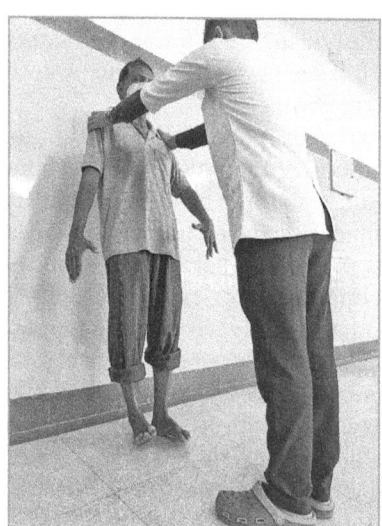

Fig. 1.51: Development of ankle strategy in a right hemiplegic patient.

is done when a force or effort (E), applied at one point on the lever, moves a load/weight (W) acting > on the other point. The distance from F (axis) to E (point at which force acts) is called effort arm, and the distance from fulcrum to the point of application of load (W), is the weight arm.

$$\text{Mechanical advantage (MA)} = \frac{\text{Effort arm (EA)}}{\text{Load arm/Weight arm (WA)}}$$

There are different classes (orders) of levers found mechanically as well as in human body. They are:

- **First-order lever**: In this type of lever, the fulcrum (F) is placed between the weight (W) and effort (E) **(Fig. 1.52B)**. It is the lever of balance.
  Examples of first order lever: (a) Mechanical example—Scissors **(Fig. 1.53A)**; (b) Anatomical example—Atlanto-occipital joint producing nodding movement **(Fig. 1.53B)**. In nodding of head, Atlanto-occipital joint is the fulcrum, weight is located anteriorly in face, and effort is supplied by the contraction of posterior neck muscles.

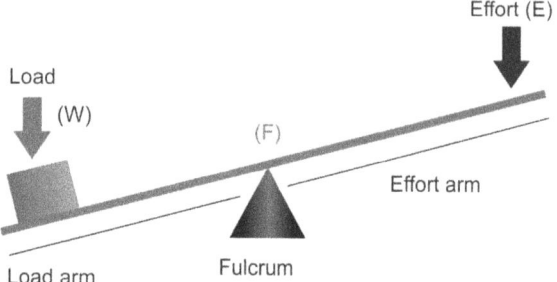

Fig. 1.52A: Lever.

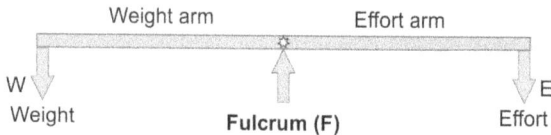

Fig. 1.52B: The first order lever.

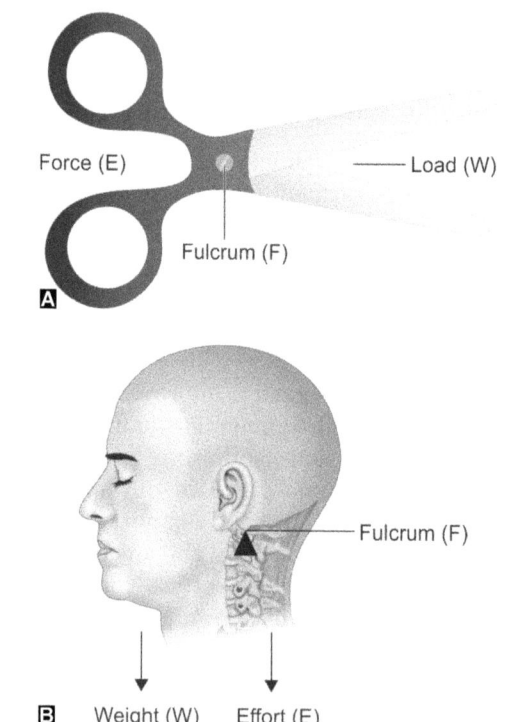

Figs. 1.53A and B: (A) First order lever (scissors), (B) First order lever (Atlanto-occipital joint).

- **Second-order lever:** In this type of lever, weight (W) lies between fulcrum (F) and effort (E) **(Fig. 1.54)**. This is the lever of power, as the weight is nearer to the fulcrum, thereby reducing the weight arm, and effort is away from the fulcrum, increasing the effort arm.
  Examples of second-order lever are: (a) Mechanical-wheel barrow **(Fig. 1.55A)** (b) Anatomical-Toe standing **(Fig. 1.55B)**. In toe standing, the fulcrum is the Metatarsophalangeal joint, weight is the weight of body transmitted through talus, effort is at the attachment of gastro soleus to calcaneus.

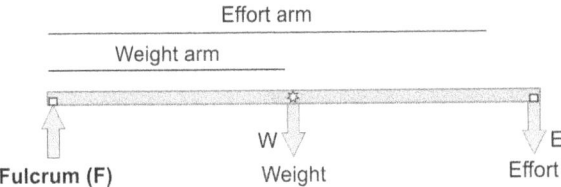

Fig. 1.54: The second-order lever.

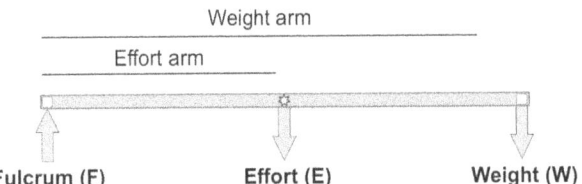

Fig. 1.56: Third-order lever.

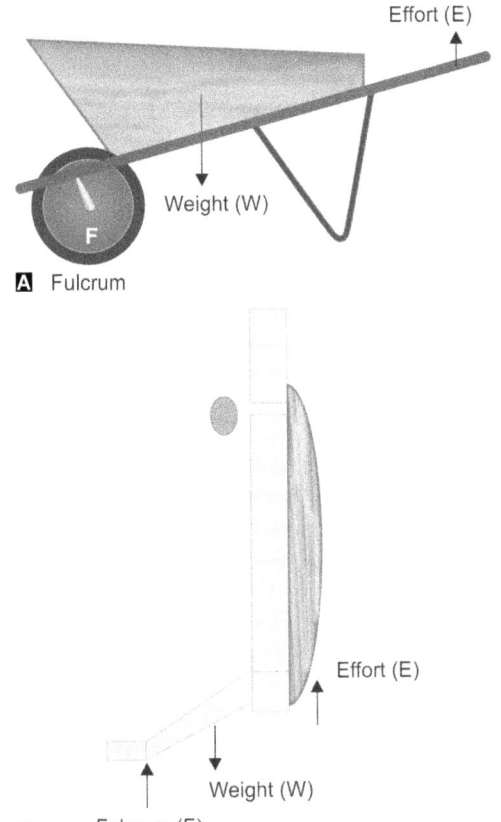

Figs. 1.55A and B: (A) Second-order lever (wheel barrow), (B) Second-order lever (toe standing).

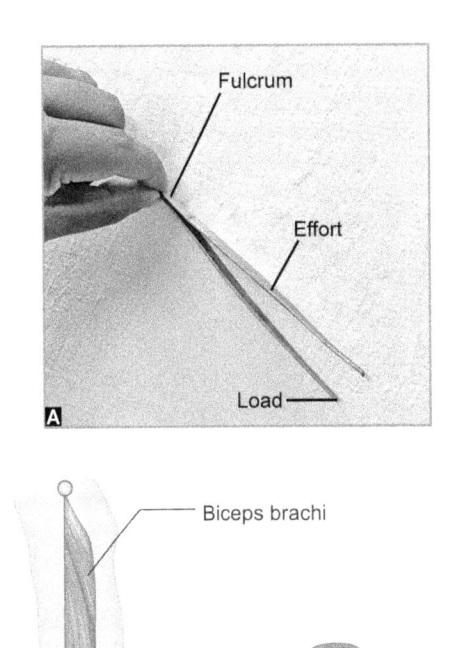

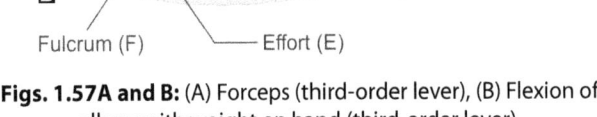

Figs. 1.57A and B: (A) Forceps (third-order lever), (B) Flexion of elbow with weight on hand (third-order lever).

- **Third-order lever:** In this type of lever, the effort (E), lies between fulcrum (F) and weight (W) **(Fig. 1.56)**. It is the lever of speed. Since, the length of the weight arm is always longer than the effort arm. This has poorer mechanical advantage and a force greater than the weight of the load need to be applied to move the system. As the weight is away from the fulcrum, a small movement produced by the force (effort), results in a large range of movement of the more distant weight. But the effort required to produce the movement is high, though the extra force required is compensated by a gain in speed.

Examples of third order lever are: (a) Mechanical-Forceps **(Fig. 1.57A)** (b) Anatomical: Flexion of elbow with weight on hand **(Fig. 1.57B)**. In flexion of elbow, with weight in hand, fulcrum is the elbow joint, effort is at the insertion of biceps brachii at radial tuberosity, weight is the load placed in the hand.

Significance of levers in physiotherapy: In human body all the three types of levers exist, making the person move and do functional activities. The principles of lever are used by the therapist, for designing, mobilization and strengthening exercises. For example, while strengthening weak deltoid (middle fiber), the patient is made to move the arm with the elbow in flexion, so that, the weight arm reduces **(Fig. 1.58A)** and mechanical advantage is increased causing a weak deltoid (middle fiber) to produce shoulder abduction. As strength of the muscle increases, the movement is done with elbow in extension, so that, increased weight arm gives load to contracting muscle, causing a gain in strength **(Fig. 1.58B)**.

Pulleys

A pulley is a grooved wheel that rotates about a fixed axis, by a rope, which passes around it. The pulley is supported on a frame or block. The pulleys are of two types:

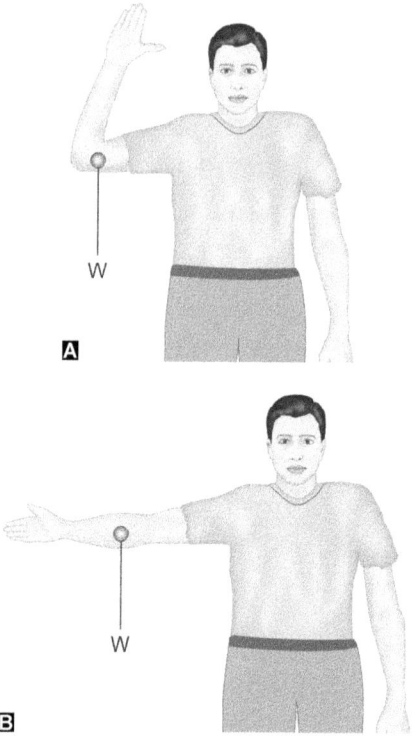

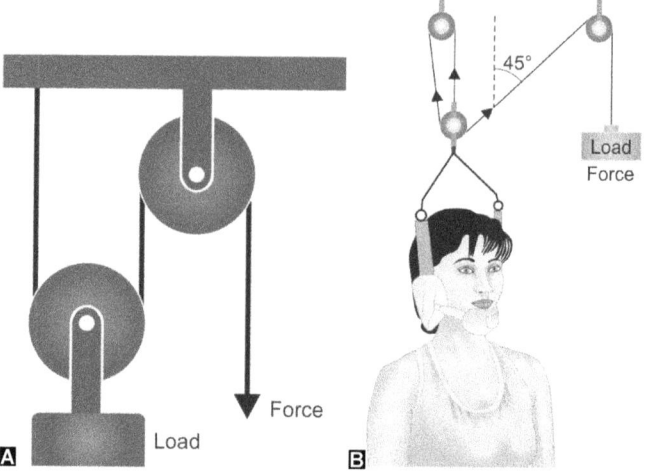

Figs. 1.60A and B: (A) The movable pulley, (B) Cervical traction using movable pulley.

is attached **(Fig. 1.60A)**. This pulley is commonly used for lifting the trunk for suspension exercises, application cervical traction using head halter **(Fig. 1.60B)**, etc.

Use of pulley in physiotherapy: Pulley systems are used in physiotherapy for mobilizing joints such as shoulder pulley, lifting body for suspension therapy, and for mechanical traction to joints, such as pelvic traction and cervical traction, etc.

Springs

Spiral springs are used either to resist or to assist the force of muscular contraction, or to produce passive movement of joint. It consists of a uniform coil of wire, which is extendible **(Fig. 1.61A)**. One end of the spring is attached to the body segment to move and the other end is attached to a rigid support. When the segment moves, the spring lengthens, there-by resisting movement, and when relaxed, the elastic recoil of the spring assists in moving the segment **(Fig. 1.61B)**.

Figs. 1.58A and B: (A) Abduction of shoulder in short weight arm, (B) Abduction of shoulder in long weight arm.

1. **Fixed pulley:** These are used to alter the direction of force. The pulley block is fixed and the rope, which passes round the wheel, is attached to the weight at one end and the effort is applied at the other **(Fig. 1.59A)**. In physiotherapy, a fixed pulley and rope system is used to mobilize stiff joints (e.g., Frozen shoulder) and strengthen weak muscles **(Fig. 1.59B)**.
2. **Movable pulleys:** These are used to gain mechanical advantage when lifting heavy weights. The upper pulley is fixed to an overhead support, to which one end of rope passes, which connects to the force/effort. The rope is then wound round the movable pulley, to which the weight

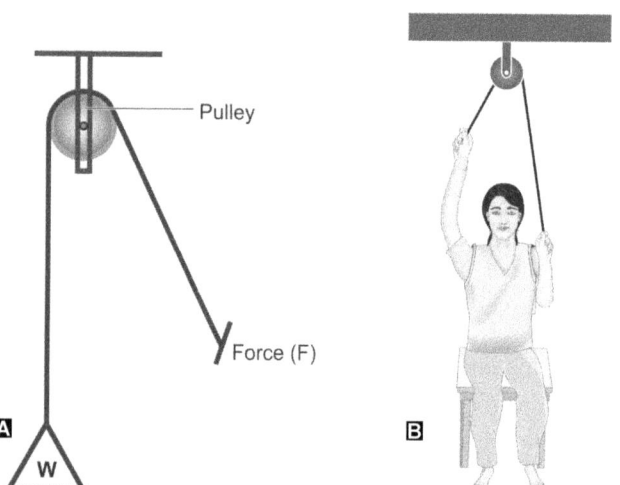

Figs. 1.59A and B: (A) Fixed pulley, (B) Fixed pulley for shoulder mobilization.

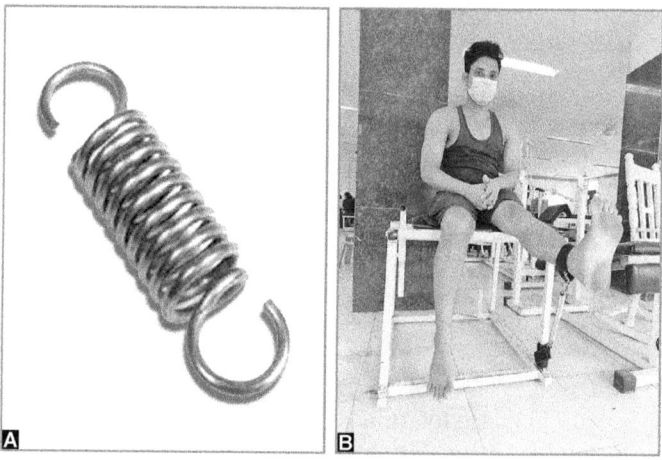

Figs. 1.61A and B: (A) Spring used in exercise therapy, (B) Resisted exercise using spring.

Chapter 1 : Exercise Therapy

Therabands are available in different elastic resistance capacities indicated by their colors **(Fig. 1.63B)**.

TYPES AND RANGES OF MUSCLE WORK

Types of Muscle Work

When muscles contract, force is produced and some work is done. Work is the product of force and the distance through which the force acts. The muscle works produced either help in holding a position (isometric/static muscle work), or lift a load (concentric muscle work) or lower a load (eccentric muscle work), which are briefly described below.

* **Isometric/Static muscle work (contraction):** This involves contraction of muscles isometrically (Shortening of muscles without producing joint movements) to balance opposing forces and maintain stability. Hence, no work is done. There occurs change in muscle tone without change in muscle length. For example, in isometric strengthening of the neck extensors, the clasped hands placed at the back of head are pushed by head, so that the neck extensors contract, without any movement of head **(Fig. 1.64)**.
* **Isotonic/Dynamic muscle work:** In this type of muscle work, there is change in length of the contracting muscles producing movement. The term isotonic (maintenance of an even muscle tone throughout the contraction period/movement) is not used now days, as muscle tone undergoes changes as muscle contracts to produce movement. Instead of isotonic, dynamic muscle work (contraction) is used now a days to explain the event. This type of muscle work is divided into two types:
  1. *Concentric muscle work:* The muscles contract with shortening of length to produce movement. The muscle attachments, i.e., origin and insertion are drawn closer. For example, while taking food to mouth, the elbow flexors contract concentrically to produce elbow flexion, enabling putting food in mouth **(Fig. 1.65)**.

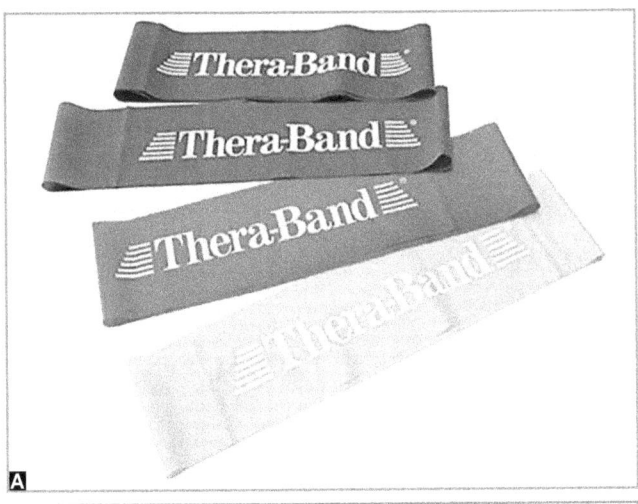
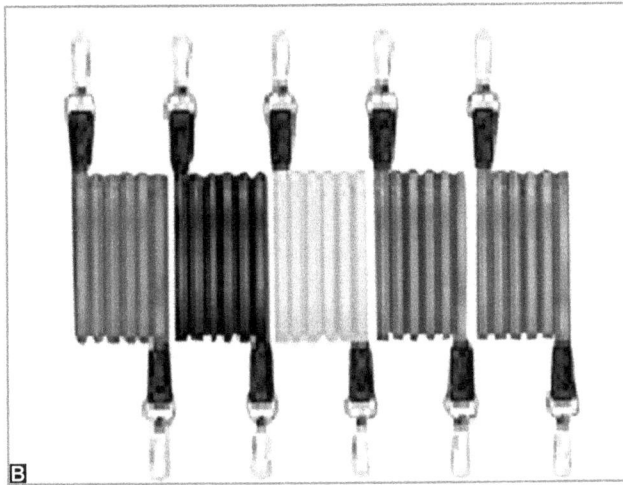

Figs. 1.62A and B: (A) Latex bands. (B) Latex tubes.

Theraband

Therabands or resistance bands are latex bands **(Fig.1.62A)** or tubes **(Fig. 1.62B)** that are used in physical therapy for light-strength training and joint mobility exercises. They are also commonly used by athletes, and people who are looking for a low-impact strength training workouts **(Fig. 1.63A)**.

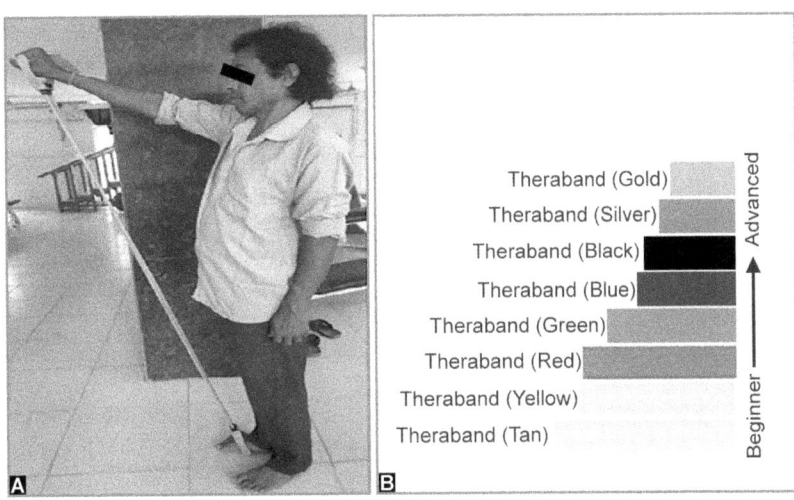

Figs. 1.63A and B: (A) Theraband exercise for shoulder. (B) Progressive use of therabands as per color.

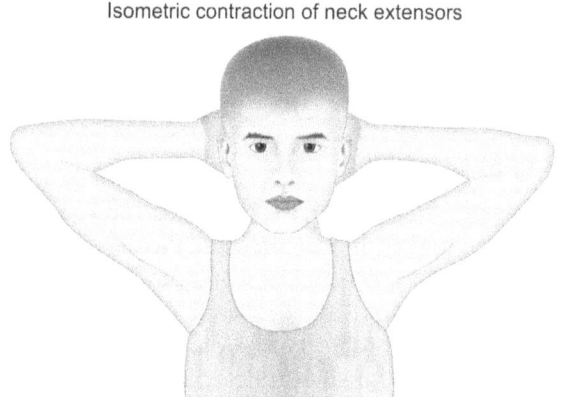

Fig. 1.64: Isometric muscle work (contraction) for neck extensors.

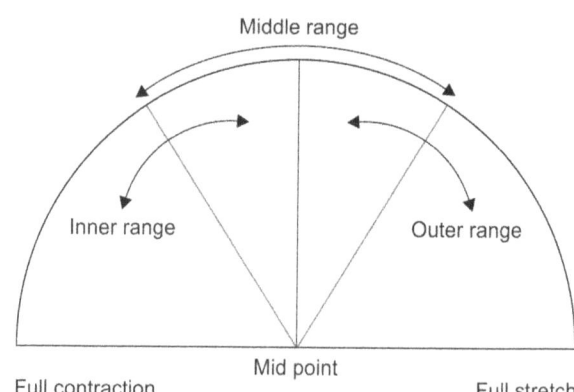

Fig. 1.67: Ranges of muscle work.

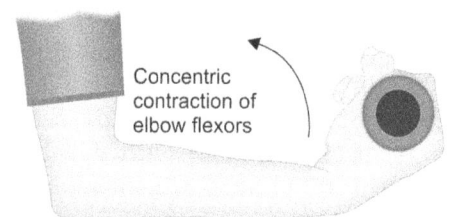

Fig. 1.65: Concentric work (contraction) of elbow flexors.

2. *Eccentric muscle work (contraction):* The muscles contract with lengthening to produce movements. The muscle attachments, i.e., origin and insertion are drawn apart, producing lengthening of the muscle as it contracts. For example, while lowering a load on the table, the elbow flexors work eccentrically **(Fig. 1.66)**.

Range of Muscle Work

As a muscle contracts, it undergoes shortening (concentric contractions) or lengthening (eccentric contractions). The amount of shortening or lengthening of muscle during contraction is about 50% of muscle's maximum length. The full range, in which the muscle works, refers to the muscle changing from a position of full stretch to contracting to a position of maximal shortening. The full range is divided into three parts as discussed below **(Fig. 1.67)**:

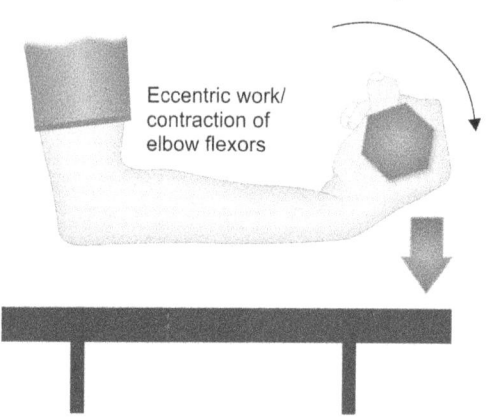

Fig. 1.66: Eccentric work (contraction) of elbow flexors.

a. **Outer range:** This is muscle contraction from a position where the muscle is in full stretch to a position half way through the full ROM, when muscle contracts concentrically or from halfway range to fully contracted position, when the muscle contract eccentrically. Use: Helpful for initiation of contraction (due to stretch reflex activity).
b. **Middle range:** This is the portion of the full range of muscle contraction between the midpoint of the outer range to the midpoint of the inner range. In this range, the muscle is neither fully shortened nor fully lengthened. This range is most functional and generally most efficient. Use: Helps for maintenance of muscle power and normal tone as most of the functional movements take place in this range.
c. **Inner range:** The muscle either shortens concentrically from half way of its range to a position where the muscle is fully shortened or is lengthened by eccentric contraction from fully contracted state to half way. Example: VMO strengthening in knee to stabilize the joint, where quadriceps is made to contract at the terminal part of knee extension, where VMO is recruited maximally.

Group Action of Muscles

Movement, which is the basic requirement of all living beings, is produced by integrated activity of many muscles. These muscles work in groups for the production of efficient functional movements. The muscle groups are categorized into:
a. **Agonist:** The agonist called prime mover is typically the muscle that is the largest, most superficial muscle crossing the joint in motion, that produces the maximum force to cause joint movement. An example of agonist muscle is the triceps brachii contracting during an elbow extension.
b. **Antagonists:** These are the muscles that oppose the action of the agonists, while movement is produced. These muscles relax progressively when the agonists contract. For example, during elbow flexion, the triceps brachii acts as the antagonist, that opposes elbow flexion.
c. **Synergists:** These are the muscles that assist the agonists (prime movers) to produce goal-directed movements.

These muscles act around a joint to help the action of an agonist muscle. These muscles can also act to counter or neutralize the force of an agonist and are also known as neutralizers/counteracting synergists when they do this. For example, during ankle dorsiflexion, Tibial is anterior muscle (prime mover), that produces ankle dorsiflexion and foot inversion is assisted by extensor. Digitorum longus that produces ankle dorsiflexion with foot eversion, to produce pure ankle dorsiflexion by neutralizing inversion and eversion. These two muscles are called neutralizing/counteracting synergists.

d. **Fixators:** These are the muscles that stabilize the bone of origin of the agonists to produce efficient movements. They serve as stabilizers of a part of the body during the movement of another part. They allows the agonist muscle to work effectively by stabilizing the origin of the agonist muscle. For example, during activities involving elbow flexion, the muscles of shoulder girdle contract strongly to stabilize the shoulder, so that, the elbow could flex efficiently to produce functional movements.

Simple Measurements Performed for Exercise Therapy

A. Goniometry

The term goniometry is derived from two Greek words, gonia meaning angle, and metron meaning measure. Goniometry refers to the measurement of angles created at human joints by the bones of the body. It is used to measure and document the amount of active and passive motion available in joints.

A universal goniometer is an instrument that measures an angle of the joint. It may be made of either plastic or metal. It has four parts, which are discussed in **Figure 1.68**.

1. **Body:** Either a full-circled protractor with scales from 0 to 360 degrees **(Fig. 1.69A)** or a half-circled protractor with scales from 0 to 180 degrees **(Fig. 1.69B)**.
2. **Fulcrum:** It is a rivet or screw-like device on the center of the body that allows the moving arm to move freely on the body of the goniometer. The fulcrum of the goniometer is placed over the axis of the joint to be measured.

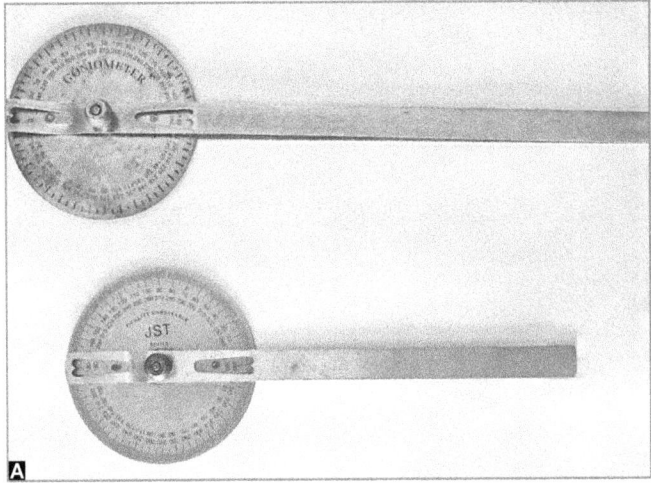
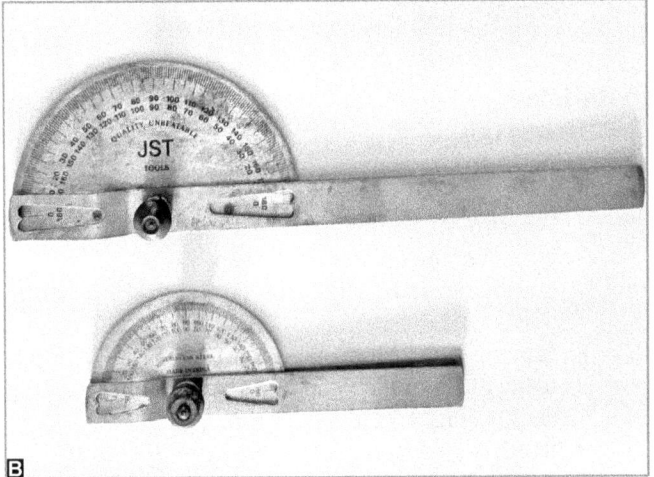

Figs. 1.69A and B: (A) Full circle bodied goniometer. (B) Half circle bodied goniometer.

3. **Stationary arm:** This arm is aligned over the inactive part (proximal segment) of the joint to be measured.
4. **Moving arm:** The moving arm is placed on the part (segment) of the limb that moves with the joint motion.

Technique of Goniometry

The patient/client is positioned in the test positions in such a way that the proximal segment of the joint is stabilized either by the weight of the part of the body or by therapist/assistant. The axis of the joint is located and the fulcrum of the goniometer is placed over the joint axis. The stationary arm of the goniometer is aligned along the proximal segment of the joint and the distal arm (called movable arm) is aligned over the distal segment of joint. The movable arm is made to move with the distal segment, as the joint moves either actively or passively. After the movement is completed the degree of angulation (Joint ROM) is recorded from the scales on the protractor/body of the goniometer.

Goniometry of joints of limbs and trunk are briefly described below:

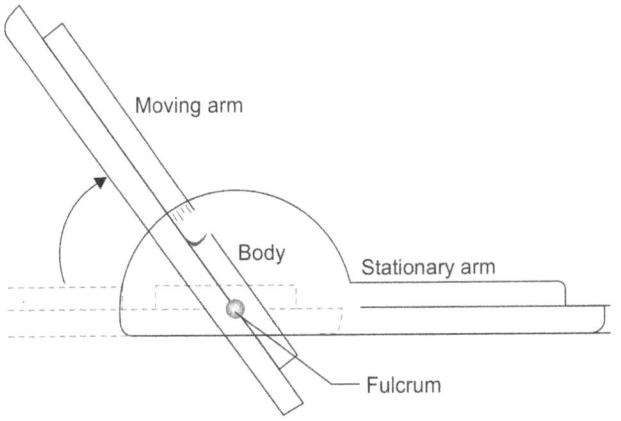

Fig. 1.68: The universal goniometer.

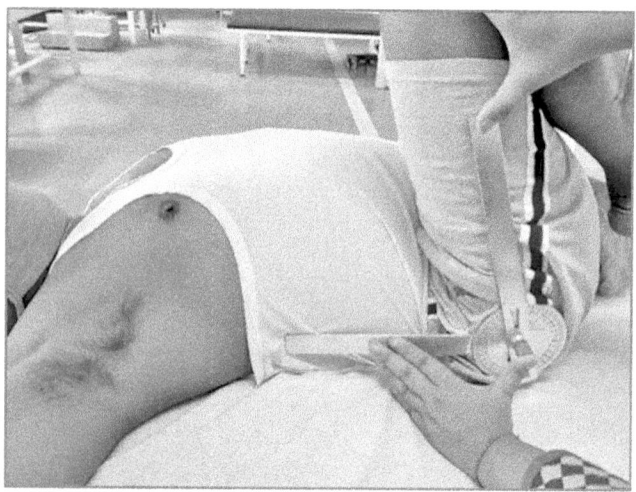

Fig. 1.70: Goniometry for hip flexion.

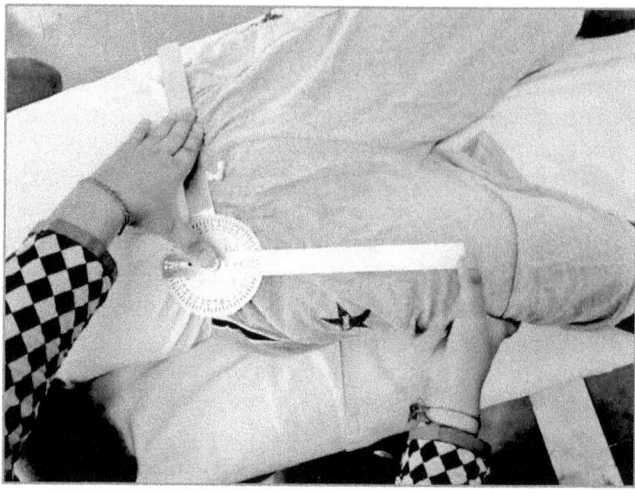

Fig. 1.72: Goniometry for hip abduction.

* **Hip joint:**
  - *Flexion* (**Fig. 1.70**):
    » ROM: 0–120 degrees (with knees flexed)
    » Position: Supine
    » Fulcrum of goniometer: Lateral aspect of the hip joint over the greater trochanter
    » Stationary arm: Along the lateral mid line of the pelvis.
    » Moving arm: Along the lateral mid line of femur using the lateral epicondyle as reference.
  - *Extension* (**Fig. 1.71**):
    » ROM: 0–30 degrees
    » Position: Prone
    » Fulcrum of goniometer: Lateral aspect of the hip joint over the greater trochanter.
    » Stationary arm: Along the lateral mid line of the pelvis.
    » Moving arm: Along the lateral mid line of femur using the lateral epicondyle as reference.
  - *Abduction* (**Fig. 1.72**):
    » ROM: 0–45 degrees
    » Position: Supine
    » Fulcrum of goniometer: Anterior superior iliac spine (ASIS).
    » Stationary arm: Along the opposite ASIS
    » Moving arm: Along the anterior mid line of femur with reference to mid line of patella.
  - *Adduction* (**Fig. 1.72**):
    » ROM: 0–30 degrees
    » Position of patient and placement of goniometer is same as described for hip abduction.
  - *Medial/lateral rotation* (**Fig. 1.73**):
    » ROM: 0–45 degrees
    » Position: Sitting on bed, with knees flexed to 90 degrees at the edge of bed.
    » Fulcrum of goniometer: Center of patella.
    » Stationary arm: Perpendicular to the floor/parallel to the supporting surface.
    » Moving arm: Along the anterior mid line of the leg with reference to crest of tibia and mid way between the two malleoli.

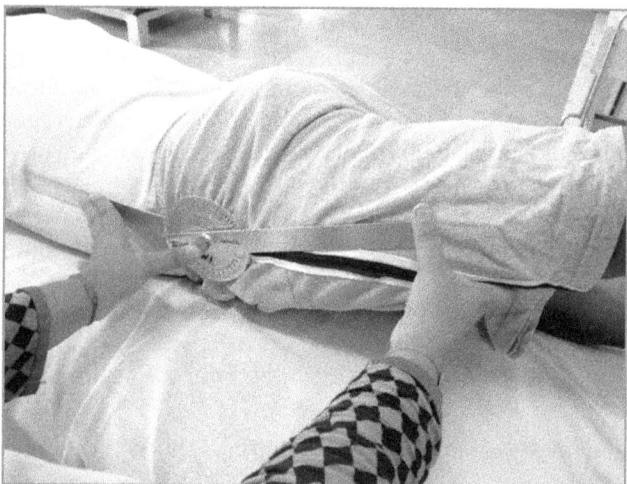

Fig. 1.71: Goniometry for hip extension.

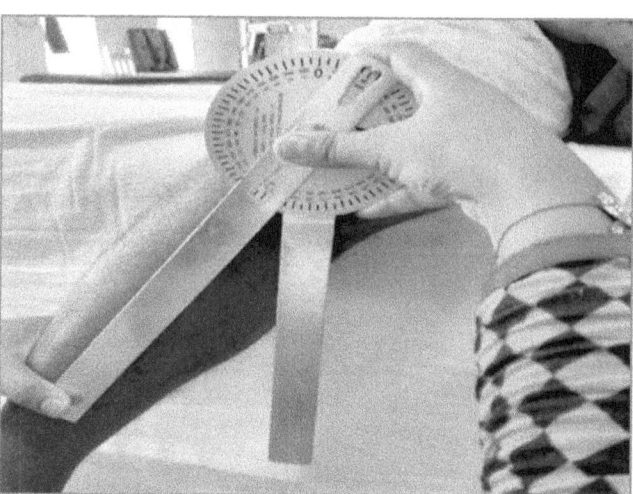

Fig. 1.73: Goniometry for hip medial rotation/lateral rotation.

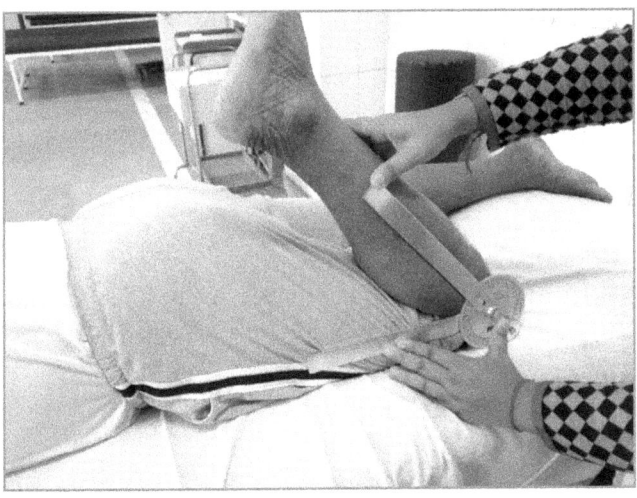

Fig. 1.74: Goniometry for knee flexion/extension.

- ❖ **Knee joint:**
  - *Knee flexion/extension* **(Fig. 1.74)**:
    » ROM: Flexion: 0-135 degrees, extension: 135-0 degrees.
    » Position: Prone lying
    » Fulcrum of goniometer: Over the lateral epicondyle of femur.
    » Stationary arm: Lateral mid line of femur using the greater trochanter as reference.
    » Moving arm: Along the lateral mid line of fibula with reference to the lateral malleolus.
- ❖ **Ankle and foot:**
  - *(A) Plantar flexion/(B) Dorsiflexion* **(Figs. 1.75A and B)**:
    » ROM: Dorsiflexion 0-20 degrees, plantar flexion: 0-50 degrees.
    » Position: Sitting/supine with knee flexed to 30 degrees.
    » Fulcrum of goniometer: Over the lateral aspect of the lateral malleolus.
    » Stationary arm: Along the lateral mid line of fibula using the head of fibula as reference.
    » Moving arm: Aligned parallel to the lateral aspect of 5th metatarsal.
  - *(A) Foot inversion/(B) Eversion* **(Figs. 1.76A and B).**
    » ROM: Inversion: 0-30 degrees, eversion: 0-20 degrees:
      ○ Position: Sitting on bed with flexed knee hanging at the edge and hind foot resting on the stool.
      ○ Fulcrum of goniometer: For inversion—the fulcrum of the goniometer is aligned over lateral aspect of head of 5th metatarsal, and for eversion, the fulcrum is aligned over the medial aspect of head of 1st metatarsal.
      ○ Stationary arm: For inversion, the stationary arm lies parallel to the anterior mid line of the lower leg along lateral aspect of head of 5th metatarsal. For eversion the stationary arm lies parallel to the anterior mid line of the lower leg along the medial aspect of head of 1st metatarsal.

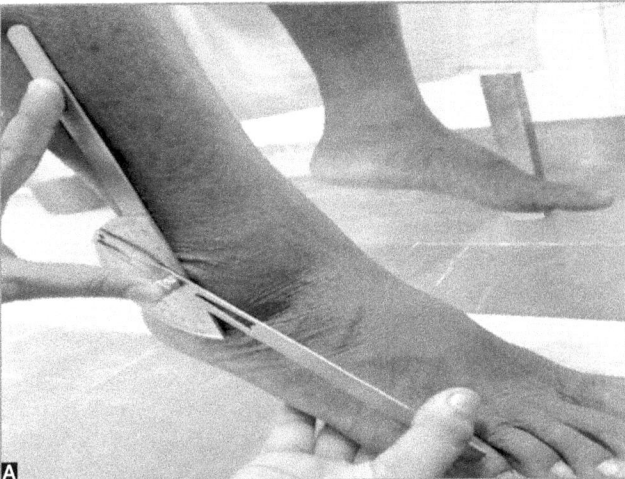

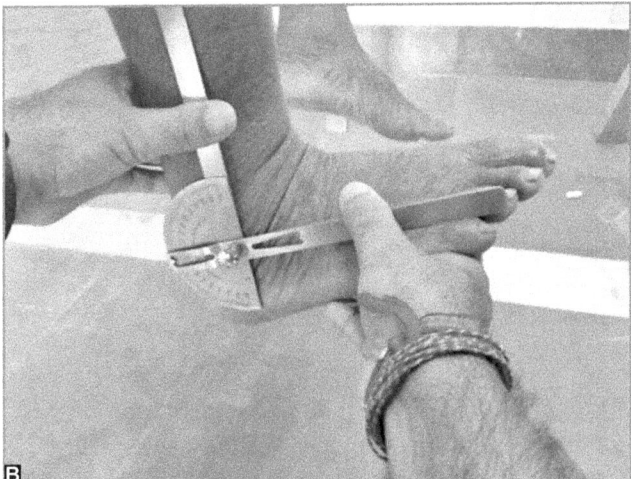

Figs. 1.75A and B: Goniometry for: (A) Ankle plantar flexion, (B) Ankle dorsiflexion.

  ○ Moving arm: For inversion and eversion—aligned along the plantar aspect 1st through the 5th metatarsal.
- ❖ **Goniometry for toes:** Goniometry for toes is performed by using small goniometers. Measurement of abduction ROM in metatarsophalangeal (MTP) joint of great toe is demonstrated in **Figure 1.77**, where fulcrum is placed over the MTP joint of great toe, fixed arm is aligned over the long-axis of the 1st metatarsal bone and movable arm is placed along the phalanges. However for complete goniometry of joints of toes, the reader is advised to refer some goniometry book.
- ❖ **Shoulder joint:**
  - *Flexion* **(Fig. 1.78A)**:
    » ROM: 0-180 degrees.
    » Position: Supine lying.
    » Fulcrum of goniometer: Close to the acromion process.
    » Stationary arm: Along the mid axillary line of thorax.
    » Moving arm: Along the lateral mid line of humerus with reference to the lateral epicondyle.
  - *Extension* **(Fig. 1.78B)**:
    » ROM: 0-60 degrees.
    » Position: Prone lying.

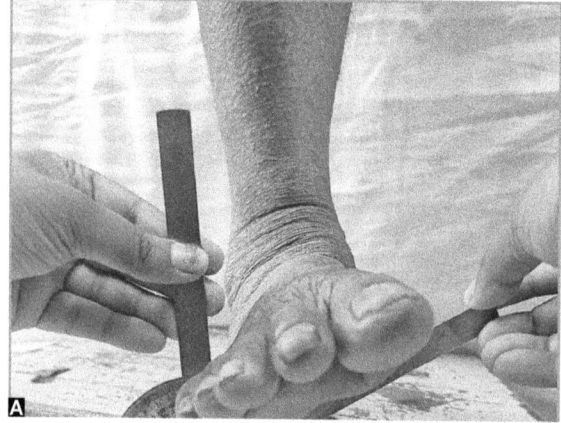

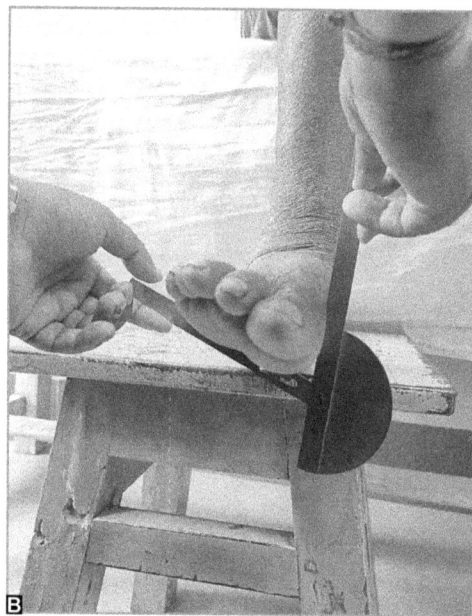

Figs. 1.76A and B: (A) Goniometry for inversion. (B) Goniometry for eversion.

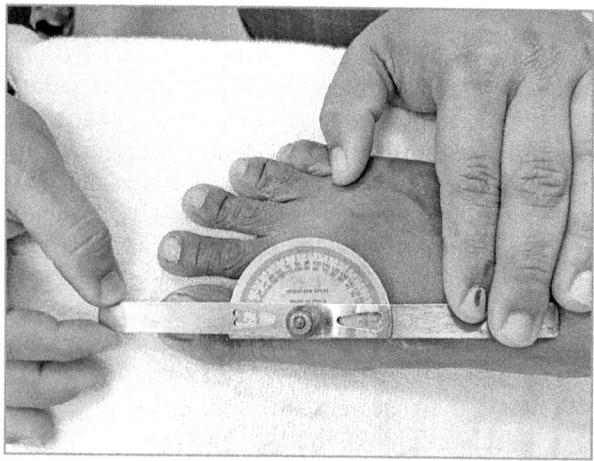

Fig. 1.77: Goniometry for abduction ROM of great toe.

- » Fulcrum of goniometer: Close to the acromion process.
- » Stationary arm: Along the mid axillary line of thorax.
- » Moving arm: Along the lateral mid line of humerus with reference to the lateral epicondyle.

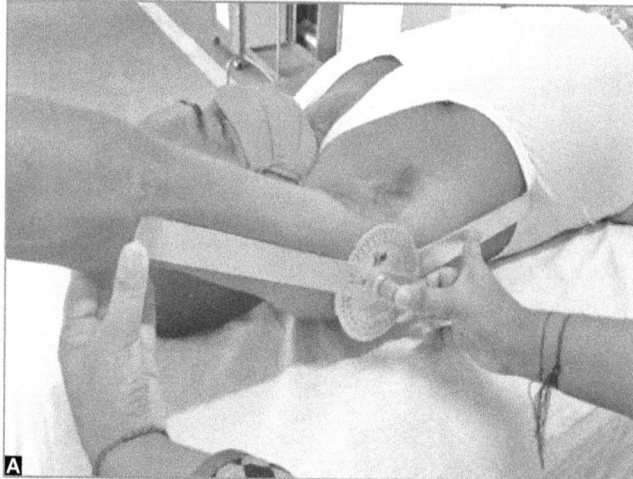

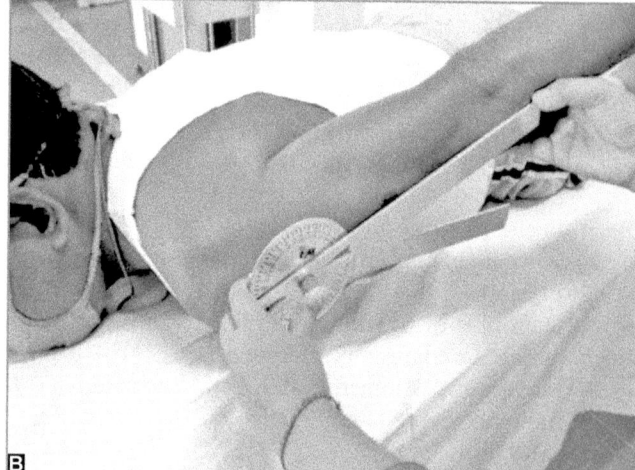

Figs. 1.78A and B: (A) Goniometry for shoulder flexion, (B) Goniometry for shoulder extension.

- *Abduction/Adduction* (**Fig. 1.79**):
  - » ROM: Abduction: 0–180 degrees, adduction: 180 degree–0
  - » Position: Supine lying.
  - » Fulcrum of goniometer: Close to the anterior aspect of acromion process.
  - » Stationary arm: Along the proximal arm, so that it is parallel to the mid line of the anterior aspect of sternum.
  - » Moving arm: Along the medial mid line of the humerus.
- *Medial rotation/Lateral rotation* (**Fig. 1.80**):
  - » ROM: Medial rotation: 0–70 degrees, lateral rotation: 0–90 degrees.
  - » Position: Supine lying, with shoulder in 90 degrees of abduction, forearm perpendicular to the supporting surface with palm facing toward the feet.
  - » Fulcrum of goniometer: Center of the fulcrum of the goniometer is placed over the olecranon process of ulna.
  - » Stationary arm: The stationary arm is aligned perpendicular to the floor.

Chapter 1 : Exercise Therapy

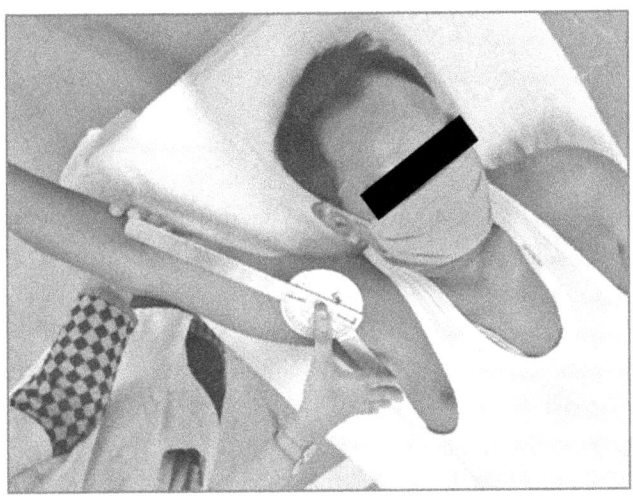

Fig. 1.79: Goniometry for shoulder abduction/adduction.

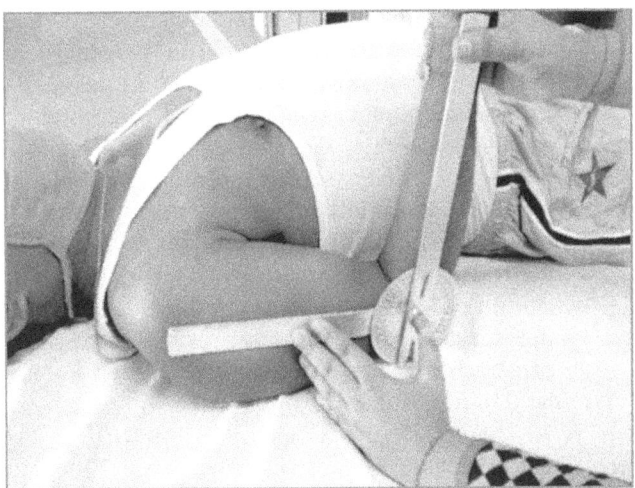

Fig. 1.81: Goniometry for elbow flexion/extension.

- *Forearm supination/Pronation* **(Figs. 1.82A and B, A: supination, B: pronation)**
  » ROM: Supination: 0–80 degrees, pronation: 0–80 degrees.

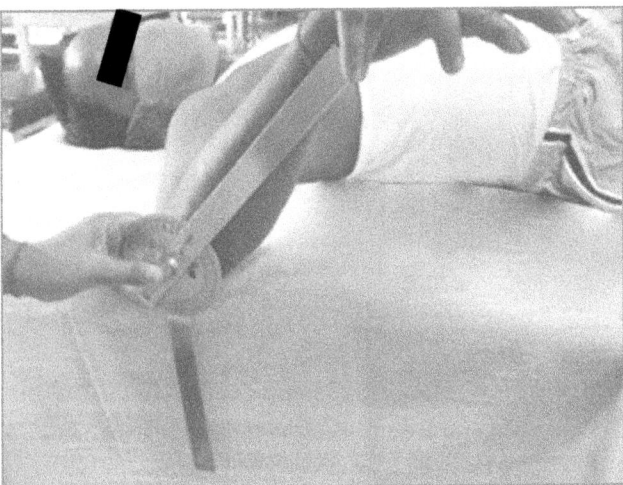

Fig. 1.80: Goniometry for shoulder medial rotation/lateral rotation.

» Moving arm: Aligned along the ulna, using the olecranon process and ulnar styloid process for reference.

❖ **Elbow and forearm:**
  - *Elbow flexion/Extension* **(Fig. 1.81):**
    » ROM: Flexion: 0–150 degrees, extension: 150–0 degrees.
    » Position: Supine lying, with arm by the side.
    » Fulcrum of goniometer: Center of fulcrum of the goniometer is aligned over the lateral epicondyle of humerus.
    » Stationary arm: Aligned along the lateral mid line of the humerus, using the center of acromion process as reference.
    » Moving arm: Aligned along the lateral mid line of the radius with reference to the radial head and radial styloid process.

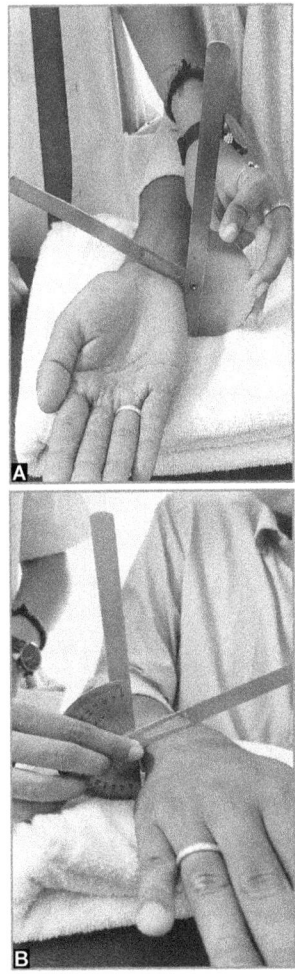

Figs. 1.82A and B: Goniometry for (A) Forearm supination, (B) Forearm pronation.

- Position: Sitting, arm by the side, elbow flexed to 90 degrees and forearm supported in mid prone position.
- Fulcrum of goniometer: For supination—aligned at medial to the ulnar styloid process. For pronation: Aligned at lateral to the ulnar styloid process.
- Stationary arm: For supination/pronation—aligned parallel to the anterior midline of the humerus.
- Moving arm: For supination; Place across the ventral aspect of forearm, just proximal to the styloid processes. For pronation: Place across the dorsal aspect of forearm, just proximal to the styloid processes of radius and ulna.

❖ **Wrist and hand:**
- *Wrist flexion/Extension* **(Figs. 1.83A and B):**
  - ROM: Flexion: 0–80 degrees, Extension: 0–70 degrees.
  - Position: Sitting, shoulder abducted, elbow flexed to 90 degrees and the pronated forearm resting on a pillow.
  - Fulcrum of goniometer: For flexion/extension: Place over the lateral aspect of the wrist on the triquetrum.
  - Stationary arm: For flexion/extension: Align over the lateral midline of ulna, using the olecranon and the ulnar styloid process as reference.

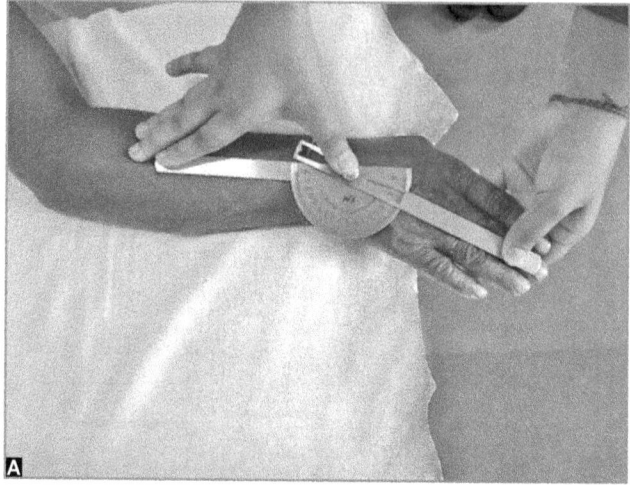

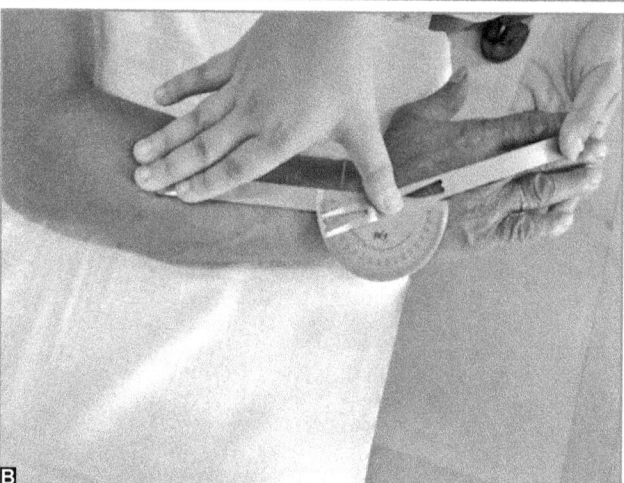

Figs. 1.84A and B: Goniometry for (A) Wrist ulnar deviation, (B) Wrist radial deviation.

  - Moving arm: Align along the lateral mid line of the fifth metacarpal.
- *Wrist radial/Ulnar deviation* **(Figs. 1.84A and B):**
  - ROM: Radial deviation: 0–20 degrees, ulnar deviation: 0–30 degrees.
  - Position: Sitting, shoulder abducted, and elbow flexed to 90 degrees and the pronated forearm resting on a pillow.
  - Fulcrum of goniometer: Center of fulcrum of the goniometer is aligned over the middle of the dorsal aspect of the wrist over the capitates.
  - Stationary arm: Aligned along the dorsal mid line of the forearm, using the lateral epicondyle of the humerus as reference.
  - Moving arm: Aligned along the dorsal mid line of the third metacarpal.

❖ **Thumb and fingers (Figs. 1.85A to D):** Measurements of ROM of small joints of the hand are made by using small goniometers made for the purpose. Examples of goniometry for the small joints, say PIP joint of finger, MCP and CMC joints of thumb are demonstrated below. However, for complete goniometry of hand, the reader is advised to refer some books on goniometry.

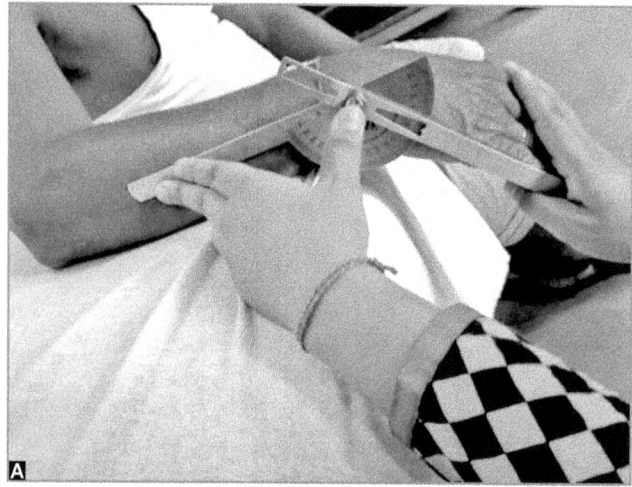

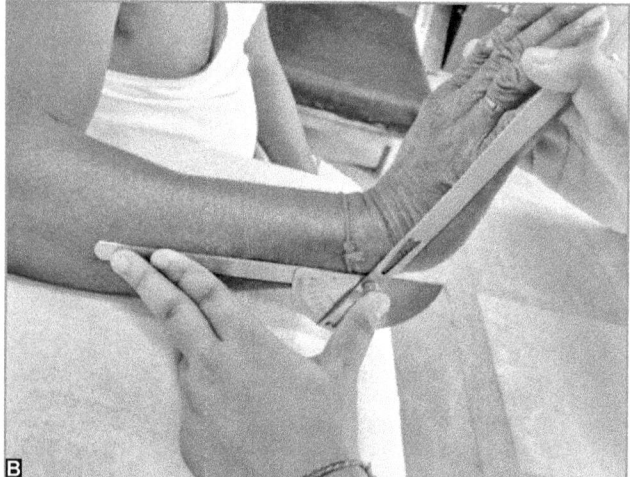

Figs. 1.83A and B: Goniometry for (A) Wrist flexion, (B) Wrist extension.

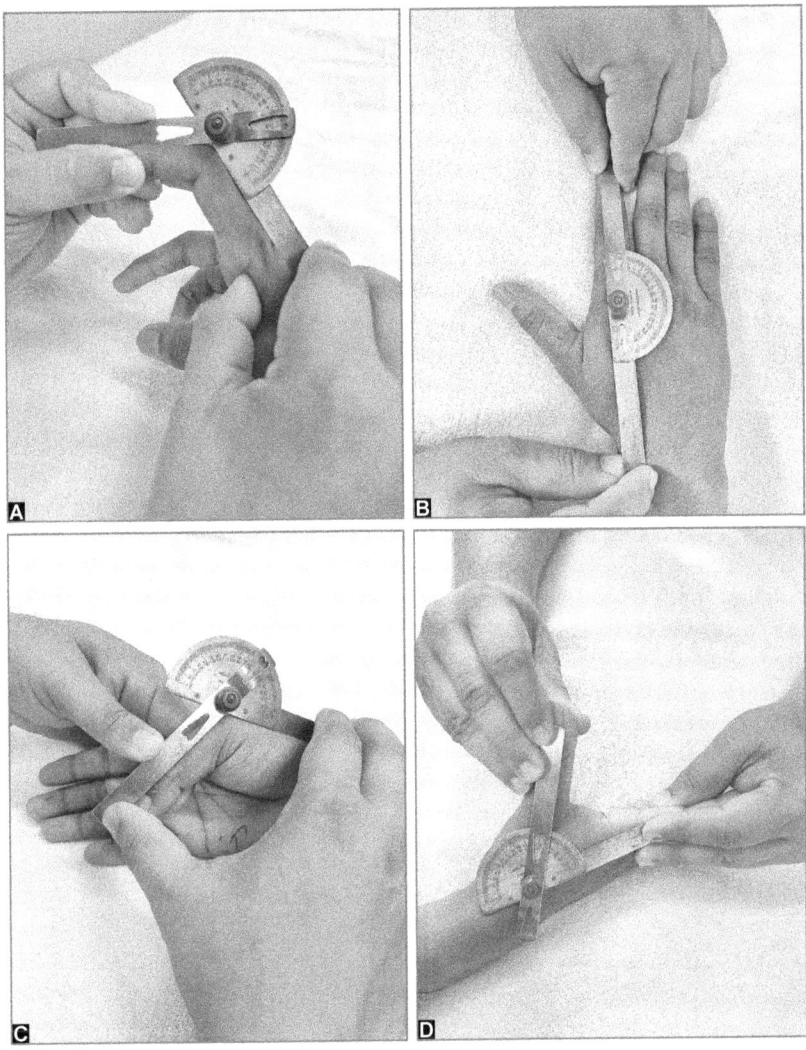

Figs. 1.85A to D: Goniometry for (A) PIP joint flexion of fingers, (B) Abduction/adduction in MCP joint of fingers, (C) MCP flexion of thumb, (D) Palmar abduction in CMC joint of thumb.

- **Cervical spine:**
  - *Flexion/Extension* (**Fig. 1.86**): ROM: Flexion: 0–45 degrees, Extension: 0–45 degrees.
    » Position: Sitting on a chair, thoracic and lumbar spine fully supported. A stick/tongue depressor may be held between the teeth.
    » Fulcrum of goniometer: Placed over the external auditory meatus.
    » Stationary arm: Aligned in such a way that, it is perpendicular to the ground.
    » Moving arm: Aligned parallel to the long axis of the stick/tongue depressor.
  - *Lateral flexion (Left/Right)* (**Figs. 1.87A and B**):
    » ROM: Lateral flexion to left and right: 0–45 degrees.
    » Position: Sitting on a chair, thoracic and lumbar spine fully supported and cervical spine is in vertical/neutral position.
    » Fulcrum of goniometer: Placed over the spinous process of C7.
    » Stationary arm: Aligned along the thoracic spine in such a way that, it is perpendicular to the ground.
    » Moving arm: Aligned in line with the dorsal midline of head, using the occipital protuberance as reference.
  - *Cervical rotation* (**Left/Right**) (**Fig. 1.88**):
    » ROM: Rotation to left and right: 0–60 degrees.
    » Position: Sitting on a chair, thoracic and lumbar spine fully supported. A stick/tongue depressor may be held between the teeth for reference.

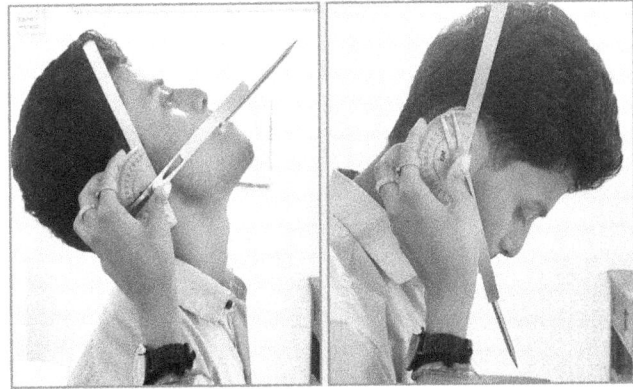

Fig. 1.86: Measurement of cervical extension/flexion.

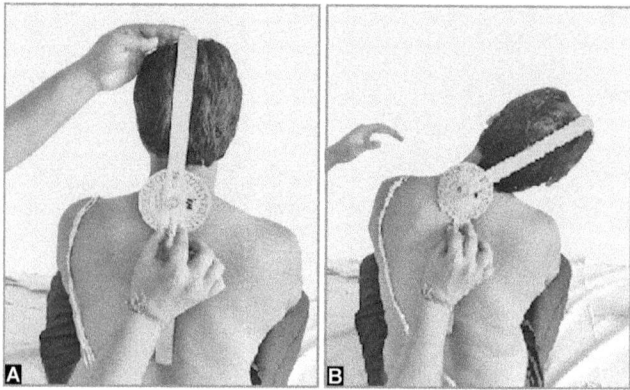

Figs. 1.87A and B: Goniometry for cervical lateral flexion: (A) Starting position, (B) Ending position.

» Fulcrum of goniometer: Placed over the center of the cranial aspect of the head.
» Stationary arm: Aligned parallel to the imaginary line between the two acromial processes.
» Moving arm: Aligned parallel to the longitudinal axis of the tongue depressor/stick. The range of motion of cervical spine can also be measured using measuring tapes as shown in the **Figures 1.88A to D**.

- **Thoracolumbar spine:** ROM: Flexion: 0–80 degrees. Extension: 20–30 degrees, lateral flexion (left and right): 0–35 degrees (each), Rotation (left and right): 0–45 degrees (each).
  - *Measurement of flexion/Extension:* ROM of flexion/extension is usually made through a measuring tape by using the following methods:
    » Patient standing, with the back exposed. The clinician marks the spinous processes of C7 and S1 and puts a measuring tape on the spine extending from C7 to S1 and measures the distance between these two points in upright posture. Then, the subject is asked to bend forward with the knees straight, and the distance between C7 and S1 is again measured. The difference in measured values between second and first procedures gives the ROM of thoracolumbar flexion. The same procedure is also followed to measure the extension ROM.
    » Measuring the distance between the middle finger and floor as the subject bends forward with knees straight documents flexion (**Fig. 1.88E**) and measuring the distance between the suprasternal notch and the floor/bed, as the subject extends the spine in prone helps to document extension range of motion (**Fig. 1.88F**).

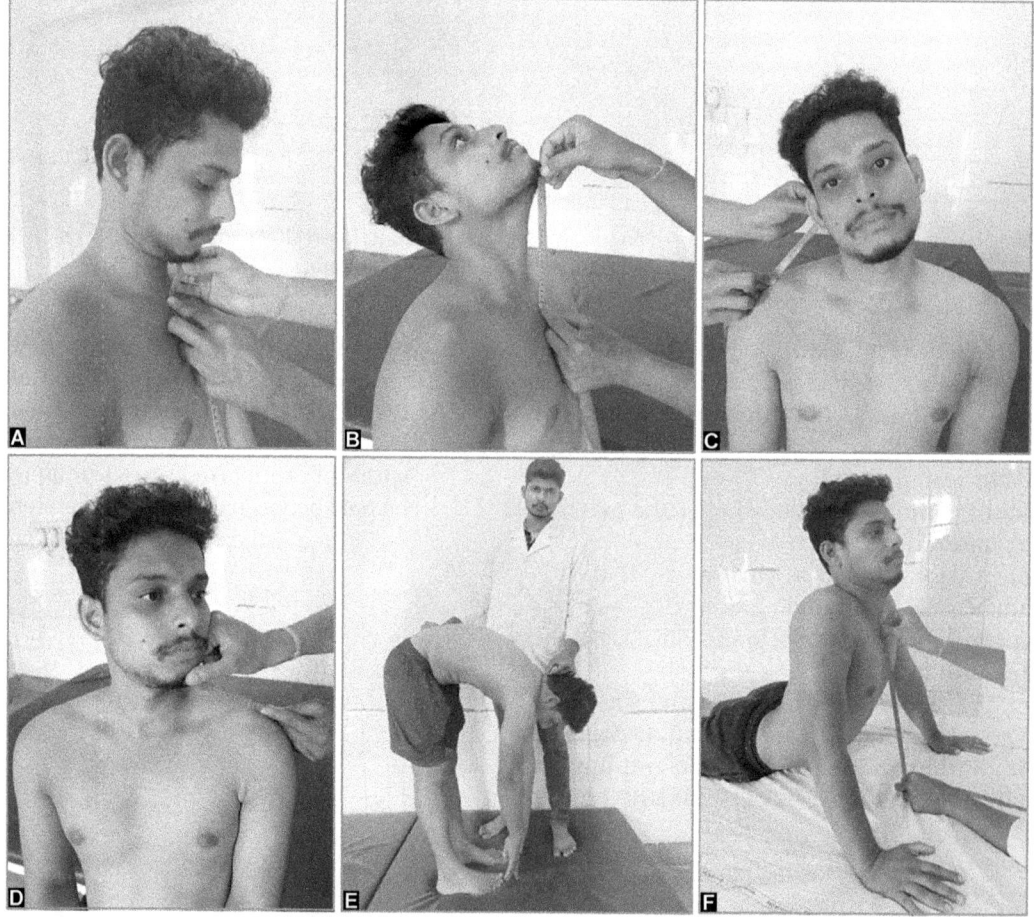

Figs. 1.88A to F: Goniometry for cervical rotation: (A) Tape measure for neck flexion; (B) Tape measure for neck extension; (C) Tape measure for neck side flexion; (D) Tape measure for neck rotation; (E) Tape measure for trunk flexion; (F) Tape measure for trunk extension.

» Modified Schober method: The patient standing with the back exposed, and feet 15 cm apart. Three marks as indicated below are made on the patients spine with some erasable marker:
  ○ One mark on the lumbosacral junction.
  ○ Second mark on the spinous processes 10 cm above L-S junction.
  ○ Third mark 5 cm below the first mark.
» Measuring tape is aligned on the spine, one end of the tape on second mark and the other on third mark and the subject is asked to bend forward (flexion)/backward (extension). The distance between the second and third points is noted. This distance minus 15 cm is the ROM (for flexion and extension, respectively) **(Fig. 1.89)**.
» The third method of measurement of ROM of D-L spine is measuring the distance between floor and tip of middle fingers as the subject bends forward (flexion)/backward (extension).
- *Measurement of lateral flexion:* The patient standing with back exposed. The fulcrum of the goniometer is aligned over the spinous process of S1, the stationary arm is aligned perpendicular to ground. The movable arm is aligned over the spine in line with C7. As the patient bends sideways the degree of lateral flexion is recorded from the body of the goniometer **(Fig. 1.90B)**. The measuring tape can also be used to measure lateral flexion, where the distance between the middle finger and floor is measured, as the patient bends sideways with the knees straight **(Fig. 1.90A)**.
- *Measurement of rotation:* The subject is sitting straight, so that the acromion processes are aligned directly over the iliac tubercles. The fulcrum of the goniometer is aligned over the center of the cranial aspects of head. The stationary arm is aligned parallel to the imaginary line between the two prominent tubercles on the iliac crests. The movable arm is aligned with an imaginary line between the two acromial processes. As the subject rotates, the body with cervicothoracic spine

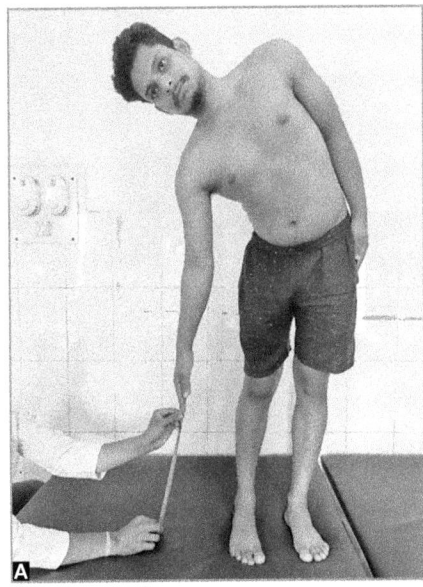

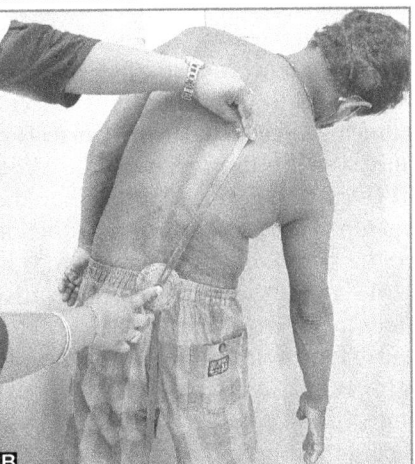

Figs. 1.90A and B: (A) Tape measure for trunk side flexion; (B) Measurement of lateral flexion of L-S spine.

as one unit, the angular displacement/measurement is taken from the body of the goniometer **(Fig. 1.91)**.

B. Limb length measurements (lower limbs): Leg length discrepancy can be divided into two etiological groups: True limb length discrepancy (LLD), defined as those which are associated with shortening of bony structures, and apparent LLD, defined as those which are the result of altered mechanics of the lower extremities.

A physiotherapist/clinician is very often asked to perform limb length measurements, mostly for the lower limbs (discussed further), though upper limb length measurement is also recommended, particularly, when limb lengthening procedures are warranted. The procedure for lower limbs involves:

- *Apparent limb length measurement:*
  Patient is in supine lying. Both the lower limbs are kept as straight and parallel as possible. Apparent limb length is measured from xiphisternum/umbilicus to the tip of medial malleolus **(Fig. 1.92)**. The length of both the lower limbs are to be measured, and difference

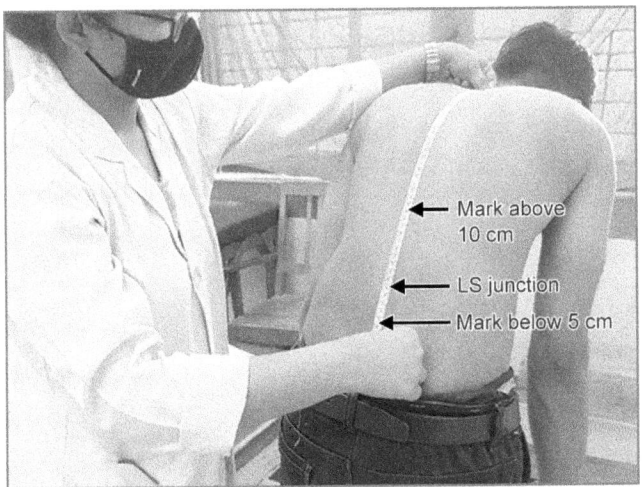

Fig. 1.89: The modified Schober test.

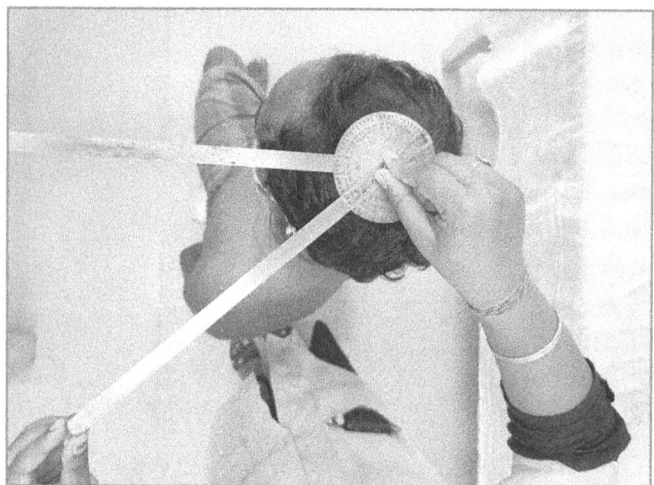

Fig. 1.91: Fixation of goniometer for D-L rotation.

to meet the 1st perpendicular). The vertical distance between the tip of the greater trochanter and the perpendicular line drawn from ASIS to bed, gives the supratrochanteric length.

» Infra-trochanteric length: Measurements are done from tip of greater trochanter to medial knee joint line (lateral knee joint line in case of grossly atrophied quadriceps), for the thigh component and

in reading between the two (if any) is the apparent shortening/lengthening.

- *Pelvis squaring:* Squaring of the pelvis is done by making both the ASIS at the same level. This is done by further adducting the affected hip in presence of an adduction deformity (where the pelvis on the affected side is raised) **(Figs. 1.93A and B)**, or further abducting the affected hip in the presence of an abduction deformity (where the pelvis on the affected side is lowered) till both ASIS are at the same level (i.e., distance from umbilicus to ASISs on both the sides are equal). If there is a fixed deformity in the hip, pelvis can not be squared.
- True LLD is measured from ASIS to tip of the medial malleolus (if the pelvis is squared) **(Fig. 1.94)**, If the pelvis could not be squared, or fixed deformities are present in hip and knee joints, segmental limb length measurements are done, which consists of:
  » Supra-trochanteric length from Bryant's triangle **(Fig. 1.95)**: The Bryant's triangle is a right-angled triangle formed by ASIS, tip of greater trochanter and junction of perpendiculars from the two points above (1st a perpendicular is drawn from ASIS to bed and another perpendicular from greater trochanter

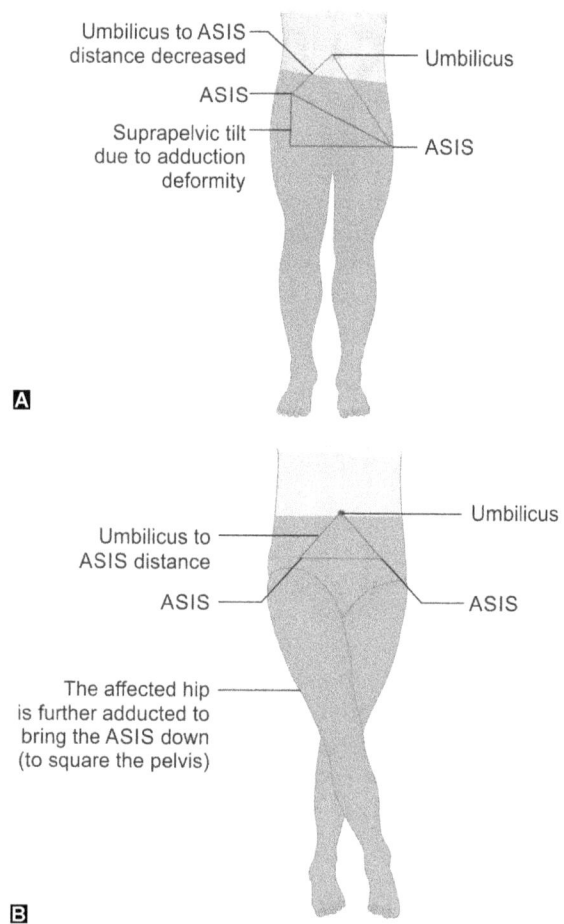

Fig. 1.93A and B: (A) Adduction deformity of hip, causing supra pelvic tilt, (B) Squaring of pelvis by further adducting the affected hip.

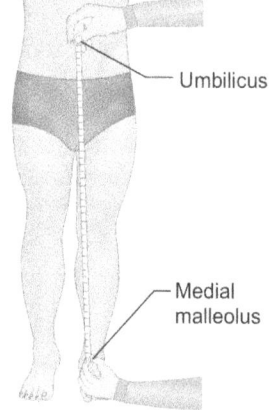

Fig. 1.92: Apparent limb length measurement.

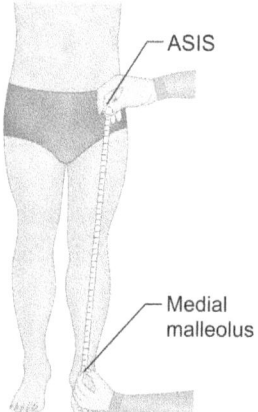

Fig. 1.94: Measurement of true limb length discrepancy.

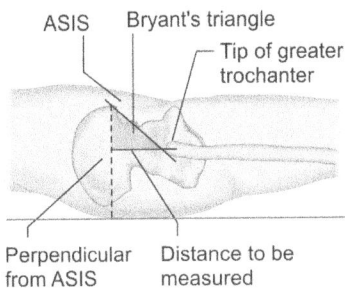

Fig. 1.95: Bryant's triangle.

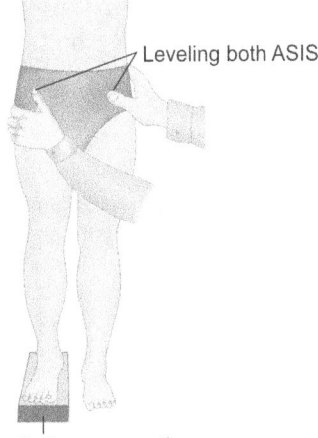

Fig. 1.96: Limb length measurement by wooden blocks/cork compensation.

Table 1.2: MRC grading scale.	
Grade	Criteria
0	No contraction
1	Flicker or trace of contraction
2	Full range of active movement with gravity eliminated
3	Full range of active movement against gravity
4	Full range of active movement against gravity with minimal resistance
5	Full range of active movement against gravity with maximum resistance

Note:
1. In case of stiff/deformed, joint, the available ROM is considered full range.
2. The maximum resistance is decided comparing with the sound side, or considering the patients age/general health and clinicians experience.
3. In case of power more than 1 and less than 2, a grade of 1+ or 2−, for power more than 2 and less than 3, a grade of 2+ or 3− is used.

Table 1.3: Myotomes of the body.		
Level (myotome)	Action to be tested	Muscle
C5	Shoulder abduction/ Shoulder flexion, elbow flexion	Deltoid middle fiber/ Deltoid anterior fiber, Biceps brachii
C6	Wrist extension	Extensor carpi radialis longus, extensor carpi radialis brevis
C7	Elbow extension	Triceps brachii
C8	Wrist ulnar deviation	Flexor carpi ulnaris
T1	Digit abduction/ adduction	Interossei, abductor digiti minimi
L2	Hip flexion	Iliopsoas
L3	Knee extension	Quadriceps
L4	Ankle dorsiflexion	Tibialis anterior
L5	Extension of great toe	Extensor hallucis longus
S1	Ankle plantar flexion	Gastrocnemius

from medial knee joint line to the tip of the medial malleolus for the leg component.

For patients who can stand, an alternative method to find the lower limb length is to put slices of wooden blocks under the short limb **(Fig. 1.96)**, till both the ASIS are leveled. The thickness of the wooden block used under the short limb, gives the amount of shortening present.

C Manual muscle testing: Wilhelmine Wright and Robert W. Lovett, Professor of Orthopedic Surgery at Harvard University Medical School, were the originators of the muscle testing system that incorporated the effect of gravity. Though different grading systems exist, the Medical Research Council (MRC) grading system is used by clinicians to grade muscle power. The MRC grading scale is given in **Table 1.2**.

D. Myotomes: A myotome is the group of muscles that a single spinal nerve innervates. The myotomes of the body are to be tested to determine the levels of injury in spinal cord disorders. The **Table 1.3** indicates the myotomes of upper and lower quarter of the body.

E. Grading of spasticity: Though different grading systems exist for grading of spasticity, presently, the modified modified Ashworth scale (MMAS) is used to grade spasticity. The grade 1 plus, which was used in the modified Ashworth scale (MAS) has been withdrawn in MMAS. It grades spasticity into:

Grades: 0: No increase in muscle tone, 1: Slight increase in muscle tone, manifested by a catch and release or by minimal resistance at the end of the ROM when the affected part(s) is moved in flexion or extension, 2: Marked increase in muscle tone, manifested by a catch in the middle range and resistance throughout remainder of the ROM, but affected part is easily moved. 3: Considerable increase in muscle tone, passive movement is difficult. 4: Affected part is rigid in flexion or extension.

F. Deep tendon reflex grading: By convention the deep tendon reflexes are graded as follows: 0 = No response; always abnormal. 1+ = A slight but definitely present response, may or may not be normal, 2+= Normal, typical reflex, 3+= Brisk reflex, possibly but not necessarily abnormal, 4+ = A tap elicits a very brisk repeating reflex (clonus); always abnormal. The **Figures 1.97A to E** demonstrates testing of ankle jerk **(Fig. 1.97A)**, knee jerk **(Figs. 1.97B and C)**, bicep jerk **(Fig. 1.97D)**, and triceps jerk **(Fig. 1.97E)**.

G. Examination of superficial reflexes (Table 1.4).

Table 1.4: Superficial reflexes.		
Superficial reflexes	Stimulus	Response
Plantar (S1, S2)	With blunt object (key or wooden end of applicator stick, or blunt end of the tendon hammer), stroke the lateral aspect of the sole, moving from the heel to the ball of the 5th metatarsal curving medially toward the ball of the 2nd metatarsal **(Figs. 1.98A and B)**. No part of leg/foot to be held during testing. Alternate reflex stimuli for plantar (for sensitive feet): • Chaddock: Stroke lateral ankle and lateral aspect of foot • Oppenheim: Stroke down tibial crest	Normal response is flexion (plantar flexion) of the great toe, and sometimes the other toes (negative Babinski sign). Abnormal response, termed a positive Babinski sign, is extension (dorsiflexion) of the great toe with fanning of the four other toes (indicates UMN lesions, if present in children above 2 years and adults). Equivocal response: A partial flexion, followed by extension of great toe, indicating minimal damage to corticospinal system
Abdominal reflex	Position patient in supine lying. Make brisk, light stroke over each quadrant of the abdomen above(T7-T9), and below (T11-T12) the umblicus/towards the midline **(Figs. 1.99A and B)**	Localized contraction under the stimulus, causing the umbilicus to move toward the stimulus is considered normal. Absence of response indicates UMN/LMN lesion and T7-T12 spinal cord injury. Tests integrity of T7-T9 segments (upper abdominals), when tested above umbilicus, and T11-T12 segments (lower abdominals), when tested below the umbilicus. Diminished reflex is found in obesity and pregnancy

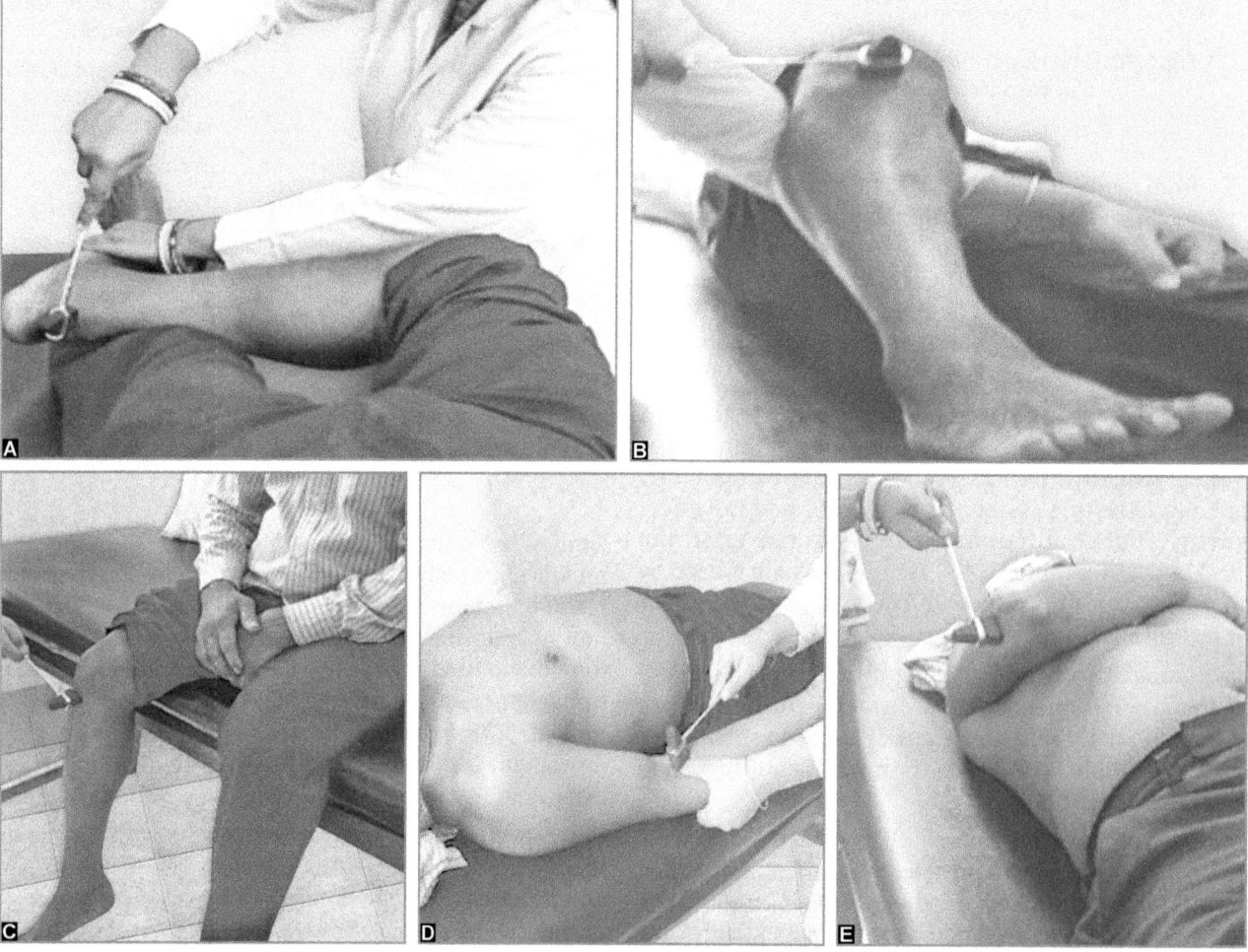

Figs. 1.97A to E: Deep tendon reflexes. (A) Ankle jerk, (B and C) knee jerk, (D) bicep jerk, and (E) triceps jerk.

H. Capsular pattern of movement limitations (Table 1.5).

Table 1.5: Capsular pattern of limitation.

Joint	Movements limited
Cervical spine	The capsular pattern of limitation from C2 to C7 is equal limitations of all motions except flexion, which is usually barely restricted
Thoracic spine	Greater limitation of extension, lateral flexion, rotation than of forward flexion
Lumbar spine	Marked and equal restrictions of lateral flexion, followed by restrictions of flexion and extension
Shoulder	Loss of external rotation, abduction and internal rotation
Elbow complex	Loss of flexion more than extension
Forearm	Loss of supination and pronation equally
Wrist	Loss of flexion and extension equally
Hand	
1st Carpometacarpal joint	Restriction of abduction and extension
2nd to 5th Carpometacarpal joint	Equal restriction of movements in all directions
Digits of hand	Flexion limitation is more than extension
Hip	Maximum loss of internal rotation, flexion and abduction. Minimal loss of extension
Tibiofemoral joint (knee)	Loss of flexion greater than extension
Ankle	Loss of plantar flexion greater than dorsiflexion
Subtalar joint/midtarsal joints	Restriction of inversion
1st MTP Joint	Extension loss is greater than flexion
2nd to 5th MTP Joints	Variable, flexion loss may be more
IP joint of digits	Variable, extension loss may be more

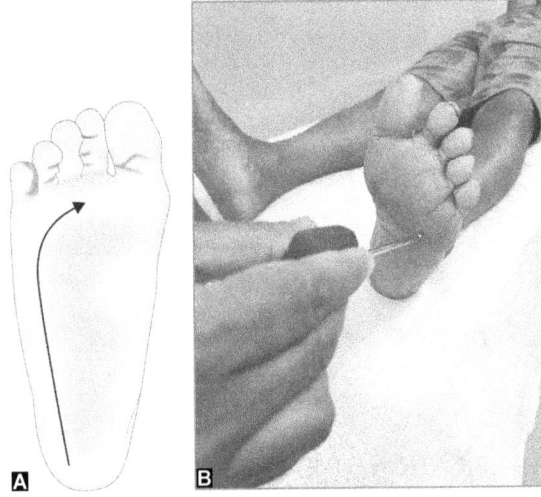

Figs. 1.98A and B: (A) Direction of stroking to elicit plantar response, (B) Testing for Babinski sign.

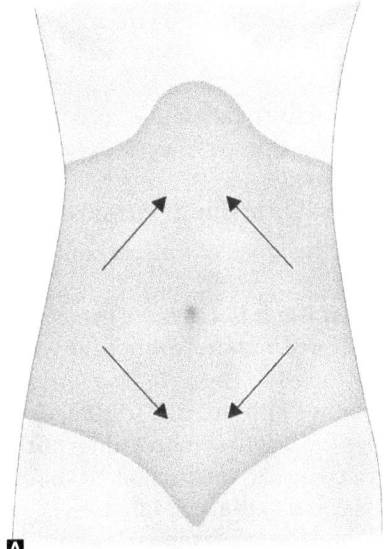

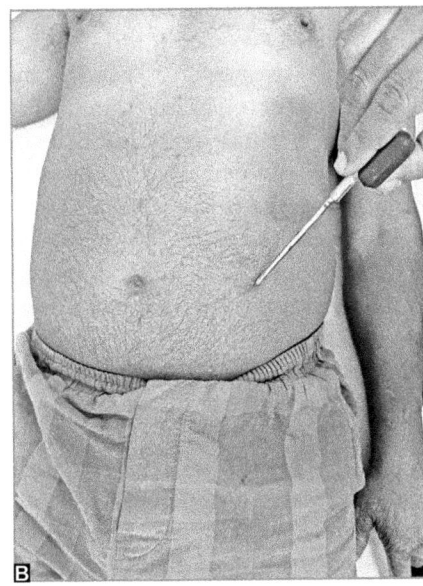

Figs. 1.99A and B: (A) Direction of stroking to (B) Elicit abdominal reflex.

I. End feels: End feel is a type of sensation or feeling, which the examiner experiences, when the joint is at the end of its available passive range of motion. **Tables 1.6 and 1.7** describe normal end feels and pathological end feels respectively.

Table 1.6: Normal end feel.

End feel	Structure involved
Soft	Approximation of soft tissue, e.g., Knee flexion, where calf muscles and hamstrings approximate
Firm	• Muscular stretch, e.g., Hip flexion with knee straight • Capsular stretch, e.g., Hyperextension of MCP joints of fingers • Ligamentous stretch, e.g., Forearm supination, where tension develops in the palmar radioulnar ligament of inferior radioulnar joint
Hard	Bone contacting bone, e.g., Elbow extension

Table 1.7: Pathological end feels.	
End feel	Examples
Soft: Feels boggy with fluid shift in a joint that has a firm or hard end feel	Synovitis/edema
Firm: Occurs in a joint that normally has a soft or hard end feel	Increased muscular tone, tightness of capsule
Hard: Grating or bony block present	Loose body in joint
Empty: Pain and muscle spasm restricts movement	Bursitis

J. **Results of resisted isometric tests (Table 1.8).**

Table 1.8: Resisted isometric tests.	
Results	Possible pathologies.
Strong and painless	There is no lesion or neurological deficit involving the tested muscle and tendon
Strong and painful	There is a minor lesion of the tested muscle or tendon
Weak and painless.	There is a disorder of the nervous system, neuromuscular junction, a complete rupture of the tested muscle or tendon, or disuse atrophy
Weak and painful	There is a serious, painful pathology such as a fracture or neoplasm. Other possibilities include an acute inflammatory process that inhibits muscle contraction, or a partial rupture of the tested muscle or tendon

K. **Four grading of ligament instability (Table 1.9).**

Table 1.9: Ligament instability.	
Grade	Amount of movement
I	0–5 mm
II	6–10 mm
III	11–15 mm
IV	>15 mm

L. **Grading of accessory joint movements and implications for treatment (Table 1.10).**

Table 1.10: Accessory joint movements and implications for treatment.		
Grade	Joint status	Treatment implications
0	Ankylosed	No indication for joint mobilization, surgery is the option
1	Considerable hypomobility	Joint mobilization to increase the extensibility of joint structures is indicated. Heat modalities before mobilization and ROM exercises after mobilization should be considered
2	Slight hypomobility	Joint mobilization to increase the extensibility of joint structures is indicated. Heat modalities before mobilization and ROM exercises after mobilization should be considered
3	Normal	No joint mobilization needed

Contd...

Contd...

Grade	Joint status	Treatment implications
4	Slight hypermobility	Joint mobilization is not needed. Taping, bracing, strengthening exercises, and education regarding posture should be considered
5	Considerable hypermobility	Joint mobilization is not needed. Taping, bracing, strengthening exercises, and education regarding posture should be considered
6	Unstable	Joint mobilization is not indicated; surgery/bracing should be considered as indicated

CLASSIFICATION OF EXERCISES

Exercises are classified into two types, such as:

I. Active Exercises

These are exercises/movements performed by the individual by his own muscular efforts. Active exercises are classified into several types:
a. Depending upon the types of muscle contraction,
b. Depending upon the assistance or resistance used to produce movements.

The active exercises are briefly discussed below:

Depending upon the types of muscle contraction exercises are classified into:

❖ **Isometric exercise:** It is a form of exercise, involving the static contraction of muscle, without any visible movement in the angle of the joint. The term "isometric", combines the prefix "iso" (same) with "metric" (distance), meaning that, in this exercise the length of muscle does not change. In this type of exercise/muscle contraction, the force produced by the muscle is equal to the load lifted.

There are several forms of isometric exercises, such as:
- *Muscle setting exercises:* Low-intensity isometric exercises, performed against little or no resistance. These exercises are primarily used to maintain the bulk and strength of the muscles, in the acute stage of disease or injury, where either joint movement is not allowed, or severe pain retards the movement of joints. Isometric quadriceps **(Fig. 1.100)** and gluteal sets are the common example of this type of exercise. Because muscle setting exercises are not performed, against any appreciable resistance, it does not increase the muscle strength, except in very weak muscles.
- *Stabilization exercise:* These exercises involve mid range isometric contraction against resistance in antigravity positions and in weight bearing postures, if the same is permissible. It is performed in different forms, such as rhythmic stabilization and alternating isometrics.
- *Multi angle isometrics:* It is a system of isometric exercise, where resistance is added manually or mechanically, at multiple joint positions within the available ROM. In situations, where dynamic resistance exercise is not

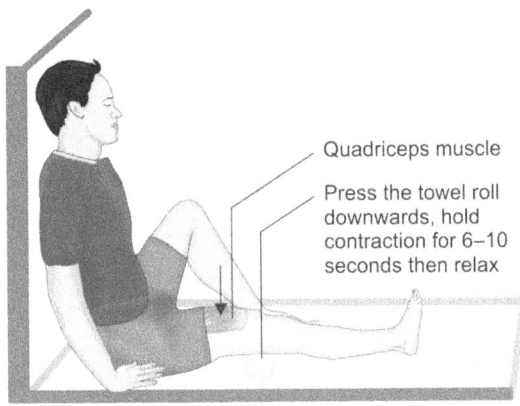

Fig. 1.100: Isometric quadriceps exercise.

- vagal tone and increased discharge of cardiac sympathetic nerves).
- Within a few seconds of the start of the exercise, both systolic and diastolic blood pressure rises.
- As the exercise produces a tourniquet effect on the underlying blood vessels, increasing a great demand on the heart, great caution need to be taken while treating cardiac patients, and the duration of isometric contraction should not exceed beyond 6 seconds.

❖ **Isotonic/Dynamic exercises:** These are the exercises in which shortening or lengthening contraction of muscles occur producing intramuscular tension resulting in joint movements.

These exercises are divided into:
- *Concentric exercises:* This exercise involves shortening contraction of the muscle producing joint movement, i.e., muscles undergo physical shortening causing the joint motion and overcoming an external load. In this contraction the force generated by the muscles are greater than the weight of the part or resistance applied.

  During a concentric contraction, a muscle is stimulated to contract according to the sliding filament mechanism. This occurs throughout the length of the muscle, generating force at the musculotendinous junction, causing the muscle to shorten, and changing the angle of the joint. For example in biceps curl in the upper limb, the biceps brachii muscles undergo shortening, causing elbow flexion **(Fig. 1.102)**.

- *Eccentric contraction/Exercise:* During an eccentric contraction/exercise, the muscles undergo lengthening contraction (sarcomere lengthens) producing movement in the joint **(Fig. 1.103)**. During this contraction, the force (load) opposing the contraction of the muscle is greater than the force produced by the muscle, causing physical lengthening of the muscle as it controls the load. Rather than, working to pull a joint in the direction of muscle contraction, the muscle acts as brake and slow the movement of joint and lengthens while generating force.

permissible [joint motion is permissible and strength gain is required throughout the ROM, this exercise is prescribed **(Fig. 1.101)**].

Factors to be considered for isometric training:
- ❖ **Intensity:** The intensity (exercise load/resistance), must be progressively increased to progressively over load the muscle for a gain in strength. It is sufficient to use an exercise load of 60-80% of a muscle's force developing capacity to gain strength.
- ❖ **Duration:** The muscle contraction should be sustained for 6-10 seconds, which should be repeated 6-10 times in one set and the number of sets in one session and the number of sessions in a day depends on the patients condition and the effect required.
- ❖ **Joint angle:** The angle of joint at which strength gain is desired, exercise should be performed at that angle. Therefore to achieve strength gain, muscle should be made to contract against exercise load at 4-6 points in the ROM.

Limitations of isometric exercise: The gain in strength in such exercise is angle specific without much carryover into dynamic activities. Resisted isometric exercise is not as effective for developing muscle endurance as dynamic resistance exercise.

Precaution of isometric exercise:
- The exercise prescription requires great caution, because it causes a rise in heart rate (due to decreased

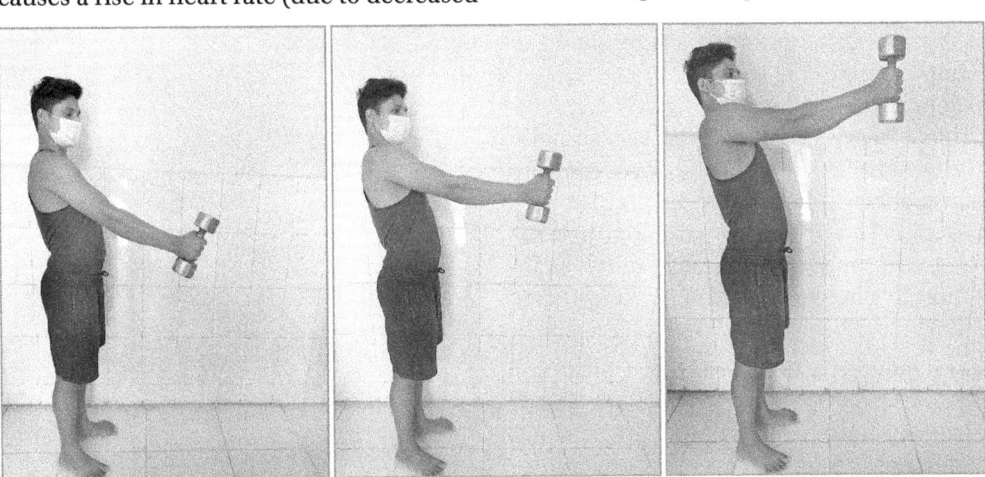

Fig. 1.101: Multiangle isometrics to shoulder flexors.

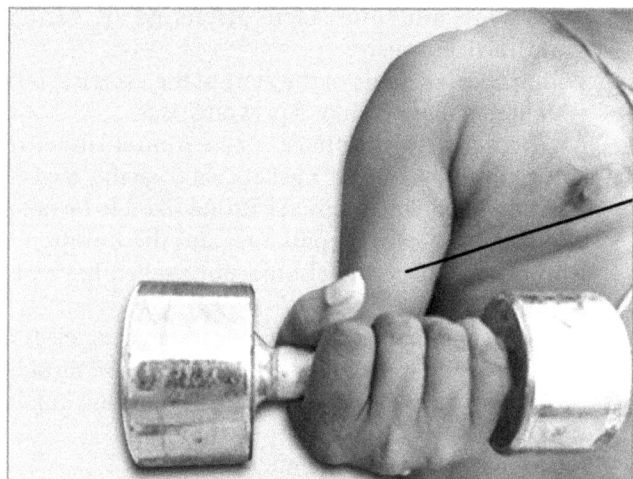

Fig. 1.102: Concentric exercise to biceps brachii.

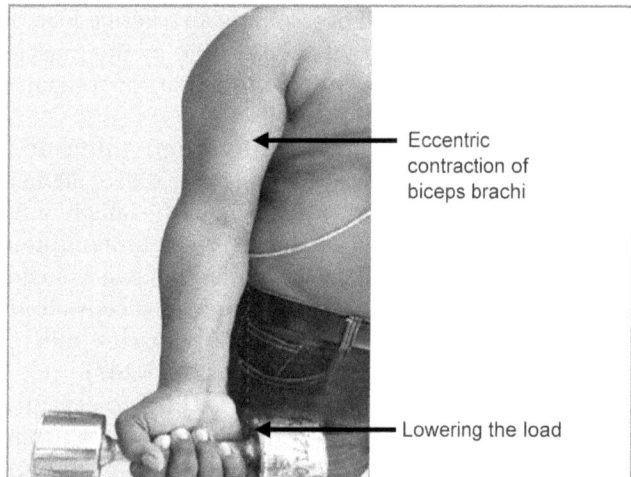

Fig. 1.103: Demonstrates eccentric contraction of biceps brachii.

The typical features of eccentric exercise include:
- It produces high-muscle force.
- It has lower metabolic demand as compared to concentric and isometric exercises, resulting in less fatigue, low cardiovascular demand.
- It involves less motor unit recruitment as compared to other types of contractions.
- It produces greater neural adaptations.

Exercise featuring a heavy eccentric load can actually support a greater weight (muscles are approximately 10% stronger during eccentric contraction than during concentric contraction). This type of muscle contraction/exercise results in greater muscular damage and results in delayed onset muscle soreness (DOMS), 1–2 days after training.

Difference between isometric and dynamic (isotonic) exercises (Table. 1.11):
- **Isokinetic exercise:** Isokinetic refers to " iso" means same and "kinetic" means motion. This exercise was first introduced by JJ Pemine in 1968.

Table 1.11: Difference between isometric and dynamic (isotonic) exercises.

Isometric exercise	Dynamic (isotonic exercise)
Tension in the muscle rises markedly	Tension in the muscle is either constant, or variable
Length of the muscle remains unchanged	The muscle either shortens/lengthens
Produces no external work	Produces external work
More energy expenditure	Less energy expenditure

It is a form of dynamic exercise in which the velocity of muscle shortening or lengthening and the angular limb velocity are predetermined and held constant by a rate limiting device known as an isokinetic dynamometer (**Fig. 1.104**). The term isokinetic refers to movement that occurs at an equal (constant) velocity. This type of exercise needs computer controlled equipment, which matches the resistance with the patient's effort. This type of exercise is used to increase muscular strength and endurance.

It is a type of strength training, where the speed of the limb movement remains constant, no matter how much muscle contraction one produces. The target exercise speed and ROM can be adjusted as per the need of the client.

In isokinetic resistance training, the speed of the limb movement, not the load is manipulated. The isokinetic dynamometers currently in use have the facility for testing and training of concentric, eccentric muscle work along with multi angle isometrics and passive ROM exercises.

These types of movements are usually applied in water sports, skating, climbing, running, etc.

Benefits of isokinetic exercise:
- Isokinetic exercises are often used for rehabilitation and recovery since it's a controlled form of exercise.
- Being able to control the resistance and speed it helps to prevent injury, increases muscle flexibility and controls muscle development.
- Isokinetic exercise is a form of strength training that can increase muscle tone, strength, and endurance. It can

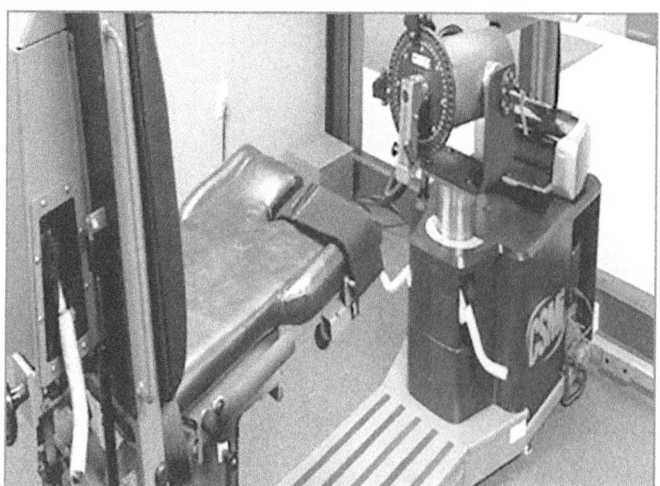

Fig. 1.104: Isokinetic dynamometer.

also help improve balance and coordination, and boost metabolism.
- ❖ Isokinetic exercise also has a beneficial impact on the core muscles that support the spine and stabilize the body.
- ❖ Isokinetic exercise allows muscles to gain strength consistently all through the range of movement.
- ❖ Isokinetic exercises were found to improve muscle strength, increase lean body mass, and reduce body fat, there by helps in reducing obesity.
- ❖ Isokinetic exercise has a positive effect on cognitive function and quality of life.

Open and closed kinematic chain exercises: The dynamic exercises are further typed into:
- ❖ **Open kinematic chain exercises:** In these types of exercises, distal end of the limbs are not fixed, and movement of any joint can occur isolately without movement of other joints in the chain. For example: Sitting, raising the arm upward is an open kinematic chain exercise **(Fig. 1.105)**.
- ❖ **Closed kinematic chain exercise:** In these types of exercises, the distal ends of the limbs are fixed, and movement of any joint brings about movement of other joints of the chain. For example: Squatting, where the distal lower limbs, i.e., feet are fixed on the ground **(Fig. 1.106)**.

Plyometric exercises: These are exercises involving eccentric and concentric contraction of muscles. Plyometrics, also known as jump training or plyos, are exercises in which muscles exert maximum force in short intervals of time, with the goal of increasing power (speed-strength). This training focuses on learning to move from a muscle extension (stretch/eccentric contraction) to a contraction (shortening/concentric contraction) in a rapid or "explosive" manner, such as in specialized repeated jumping **(Fig. 1.107)**.

These exercises are primarily used by athletes, especially martial artists, sprinters and high jumpers.

Depending upon the Assistance and Resistance used, Active Exercises are Classified into:

1. Active free exercise.
2. Active assisted exercise.
3. Active assisted/resisted exercise.
4. Active resisted exercise.

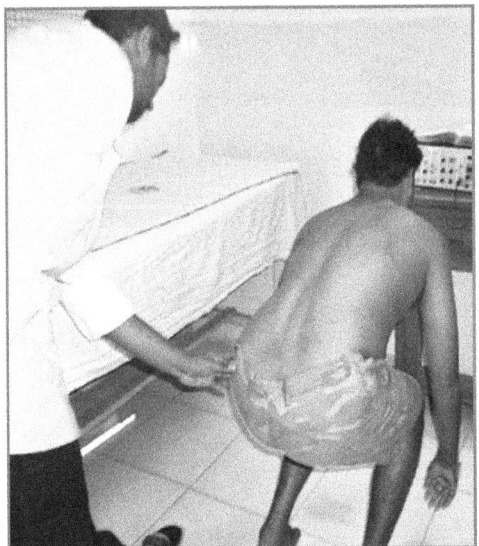
Fig. 1.106: Closed kinematic chain exercise.

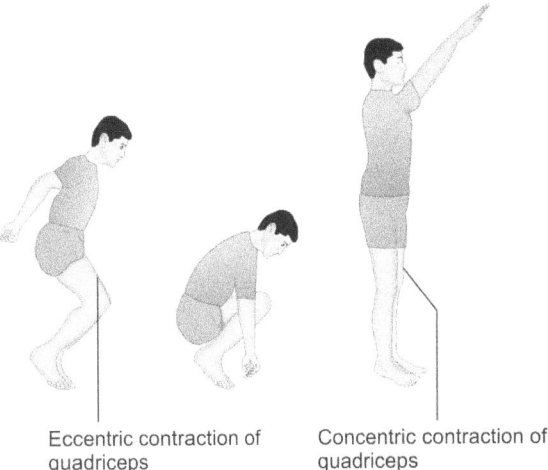
Eccentric contraction of quadriceps

Concentric contraction of quadriceps

Fig. 1.107: Plyometric exercises.

1. Active free exercise: Exercises performed by patients using own muscular effort, without the assistance or resistance except that of gravity **(Fig. 1.108)**. These are bodily movements that improve and maintain the physical fitness level of the individual. These exercises are indicated when the power of muscle is >2 as per MRC grading.

Advantage: It helps in maintaining ROM and muscle properties by the patient himself/herself without relying on others for this purpose.

Disadvantage: It frequently make insufficient demands on neuromuscular system to elicit the maximal response required for redevelopment of weak muscles.

The free exercises are classified, into the following types according to the extent of area involved such as:
- ❖ **Localized:** Localized exercises are designed to produce some local and specific effect, for example to mobilize

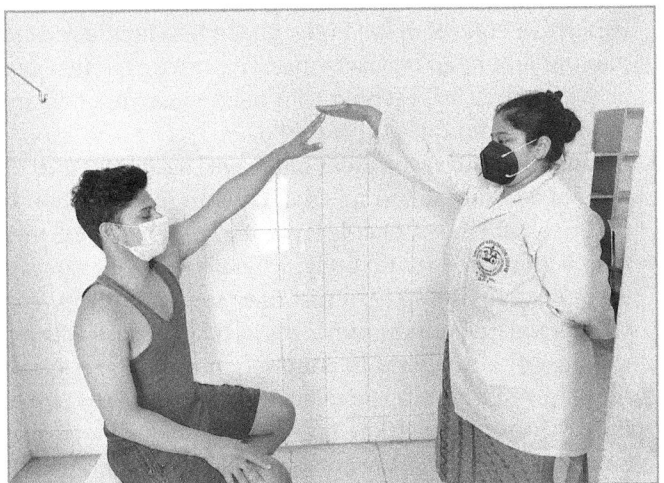
Fig. 1.105: Open kinematic chain exercise.

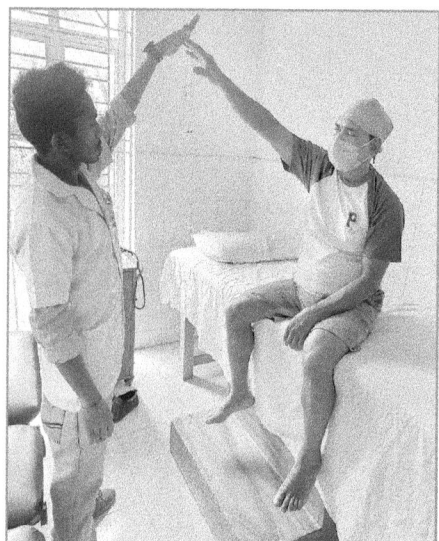

Fig. 1.108: Active free exercise for shoulder flexors.

a specific joint, say elbow joint following post fracture immobilization, or strengthening of a specific muscle say quadriceps in high sitting when the power of muscle is <3.
- **Generalized:** Generalized exercises are designed to produce movement in multiple joints of the body, such as walking, running, etc.

The character of free exercise may be:
- **Subjective:** These are the exercises, where the attention of the performer is focused on the form and pattern of exercise to ensure accuracy of performance. These exercises consist of more or less anatomical movements performed in full range. Example: hopping, jugging, and dancing.
- **Objective:** In this exercise, the patient's attention is concentrated on achievement of a particular goal such as arm stretching upward to hold a ball.

Techniques of free exercise:
- Explain the patient about the procedure and Dos and Don'ts.
- Select the starting position as per requirement of the goal.
- Give verbal command to move in the desired direction.
- Select the speed of the movement as per the effect required. Usually, the speed is kept low during learning period, slowly increasing as the strength and co-ordination increased.
- The duration of the exercise depends on the patient's capacity. Usually three repetitions of practice of each exercise, with short rest periods or change of activity in between, ensure sufficient practice without undue fatigue.

Effects and uses of active free exercise: The effect and consequent uses of any particular free exercise depend on the nature of the exercise, its extent and the intensity and duration of its performance which are discussed below.

- **Relaxation:** Rhythmical swinging movements, which are pendular in character assists the relaxation of hypertonic muscles in the region of the joint moved. The alternating and reciprocal contraction and relaxation of the opposing muscle groups, which is required to sustain the movement, helps to restore the normal state of relaxation, which follows contraction. This type of exercise is used in conjunction with other methods, which induce relaxation to reduce a state of wasteful tension in muscles, which limits the range of joint movement and reduces the efficiency of neuromuscular coordination. Exercises, which work particular muscle group strongly achieve reciprocal relaxation of the opposing groups, e.g., exercise of shoulder abductors and lateral rotators assists relaxation of the spastic shoulder adductors and medial rotators.
- **Joint mobility:** The normal ROM is maintained by exercises performed in full range. If and when the range of movement is limited, rhythmical swinging exercises incorporating overpressure at the limit of the free range may serve to increase it.
- **Muscle power and tone:** The power and endurance of the working muscles are maintained or increased in response to the exercise. A high degree of tension and consequent increase in power can be developed by free exercises when the muscles work for any time against the resistance offered by the body weight, or against the mechanical disadvantage of an adverse leverage provided by a long and heavy limb.
- **Neuromuscular coordination:** Coordination can be improved by repetition of an exercise. As the pattern of movement is established, it is simplified and becomes more efficient, and the conduction of the necessary impulses along the neuromuscular pathway is facilitated. Exercises or activities, which at one time required concentration and much effort, become with practice more or less automatic in character, and skill is developed, as e.g., in walking/running.
- **Confidence:** The achievement of coordinated and efficient movement assures the patient of his ability to maintain subjective control of his body, giving him confidence to attempt other and new activities. Objective exercises and activities such as reaching over head to catch a ball are usually used for this purpose.
- **Circulatory and respiratory changes:** During vigorous or prolonged exercise the speed and depth of respiration is increased, the heart beat is faster and more forceful, and heat is produced in the body, whereas in light exercises these changes are so light that they are not noticed. The venous and lymphatic return to the heart is increased during exercise due to alternate contraction and relaxation of muscles, resulting in an increase in cardiac output, which in turn increases arterial flow. Muscular contraction increases both the carbon dioxide content and the temperature of the blood, and both these factors stimulate the circulatory

and respiratory systems to further activity. The rise in temperature of the body is kept within normal limits by dilation of the skin capillaries and stimulation of the sweat glands, thus enabling heat to be lost from the surface.

2. Active assisted exercise: When the force exerted on one of the body levers by muscular action is insufficient for the production or control of movement, an external force is required to augment the muscle action **(Fig. 1.109)**. As the power of muscle increases, the assistance is decreased and progressed to active free exercise.

This is a good exercise in the early stage of nerve innervations, particularly, when the muscle has a grade of <2 as per MRC grading system. The assistive force to perform the movement can be given, manually by a therapist, or mechanically by using suspension devices (suspension therapy)/re-education board, etc., and electrically by applying faradic type stimulation. The exercise can also be performed by the patient himself by taking assistance from his sound limb (e.g., in high sitting, the patient can assist knee extension by taking assistance from his sound limb).

Technique of active assisted exercise:
- Explain the patient about the procedure and Dos and Don'ts.
- Support the part to be treated to minimize the effects of friction and gravity.
- Give a quick stretch to the muscle to be facilitated.
- Give verbal command to move in the direction of action of the muscle.
- Assist the patient to complete the movement by the combined action of his muscle and therapist's assistance.
- Design the assistance in such a way that, it should not be a substitute for patient's action, rather an augmentation for movement.
- Repetition should be done as needed, without inducing fatigue.

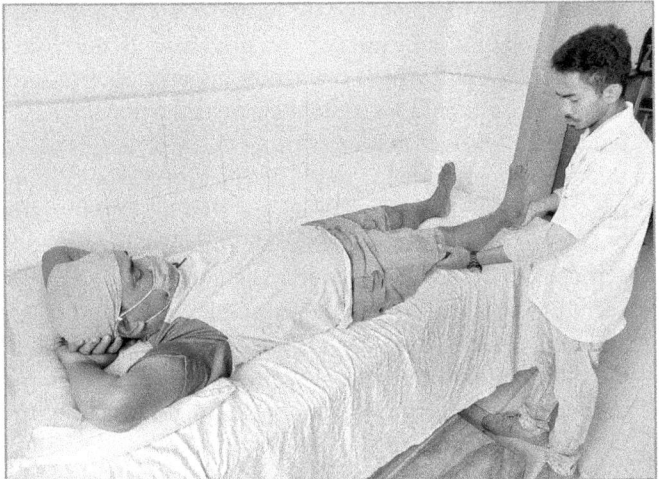

Fig. 1.109: Active assisted exercise to hip abductors.

Effects and uses of active assisted exercise:
- It increases the strength, power, and endurance of muscle.
- It increases the ROM of joints.
- It prevents adhesion formation of joints and breaks adhesions, if any.
- It reduces spasm of muscles.
- It maintains soft tissue flexibility and stretches tight structures.
- It reminds the pattern of movement to brain.
- It enhances venous and lymphatic return and increases arterial blood flow.

3. Active-assisted, resisted exercise: In this exercise, the muscle work is resisted through the initial part of the range and assisted through the remaining part of the range **(Fig. 1.110)**. For example, a patient with a power of quadriceps more than a grade of 3 with a quadriceps lag, is resisted through the initial part of range and assisted through the remaining part of the range, to make the muscle work through full range of knee extension. The techniques, effects, and uses of this exercise are as applicable to assisted and resisted exercises.

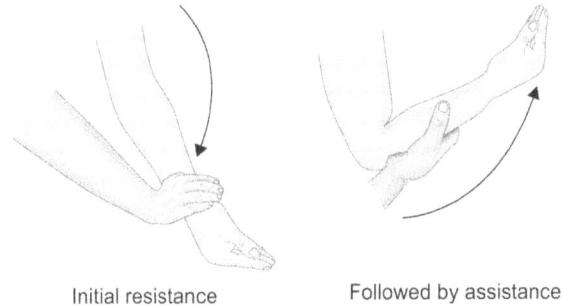

Initial resistance   Followed by assistance

Fig. 1.110: Active-assisted, resisted exercise.

4. Active resisted exercise: Resisted exercise is any form of active exercise in which dynamic or static muscle contraction is resisted by an outside force either applied manually by the therapist/caregiver or mechanically, to increase strength, power and endurance of the muscle. Dynamic resistance exercise involve movements (concentric/eccentric) with resistance.

Resistances/Resistive force: A resistive force other than that of gravity and friction may be provided by:
- Physiotherapist/Caregiver/Patient **(Fig. 1.111A)**.
- Weights (weight cuff/dumbbell/sand bag **(Fig. 1.111B)**.
- Elastic bands (theraband) **(Fig. 1.111C)**
- Springs **(Fig. 1.111D)**.
- Water (Buoyancy of water in hydrotherapy).

Resisted exercise is prescribed by a therapist to build strength, endurance, and power of a muscle in the terminal phase of rehabilitation of the patient.

Muscle strength: It is the ability of the muscle to produce tension and a resultant force, based on the demands placed upon the muscle. It is the greatest measurable force exerted by a muscle/muscle group to overcome resistance during a single maximum effort.

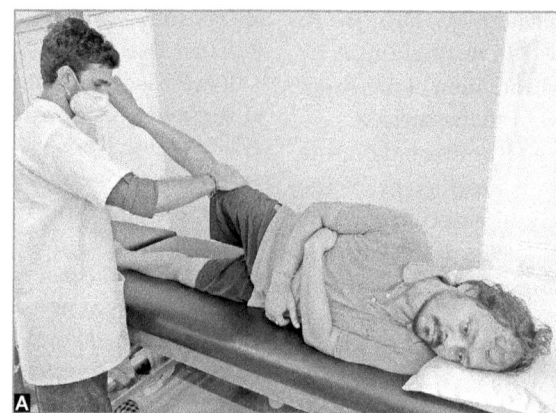
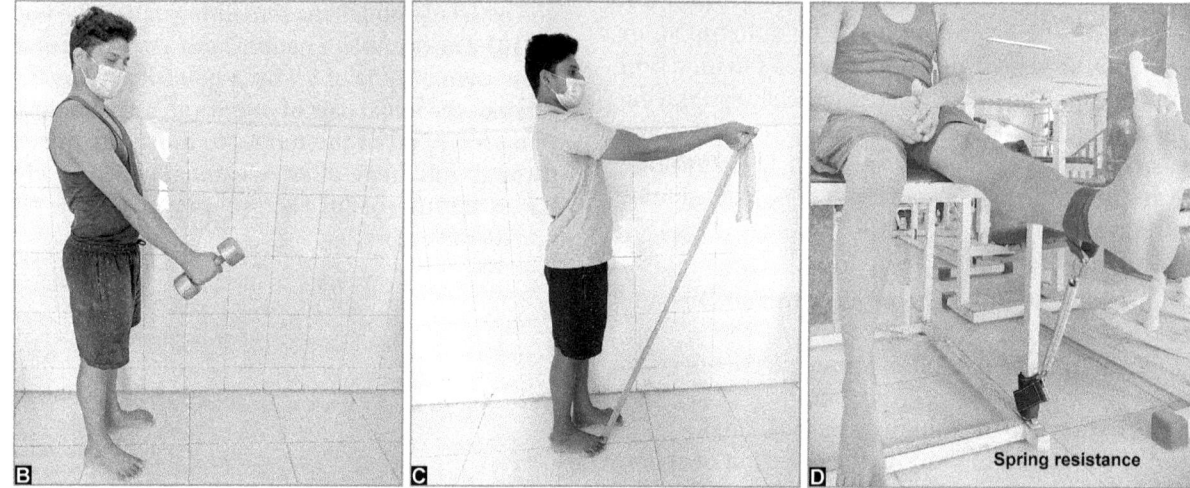

Figs. 1.111A to D: (A) Manual resisted exercise, (B) Resisted exercise using dumbbell, (C) Resisted exercise using theraband, (D) Resisted exercise using spring.

Strengthening exercises (called strength training/resistance training) is the systematic procedure of a muscle or muscle group, lifting, lowering, or controlling heavy loads (resistance), for relatively lower number of repetitions or over a short period of time. The increase in muscle strength in resistance training is usually brought about, as a result of both neural adaptations and hypertrophy of muscle fibers.

Muscle endurance: It is the ability of muscle to contract repeatedly, against a load (resistance), generate and sustain tension, and resist fatigue over an extended period of time. To develop muscular endurance a low load high repetitive exercise is prescribed.

Muscle power: It is the work (force × distance) produced by a muscle per unit time. In other words, it is the rate of performing work. Muscle strength is the necessary foundation for development of muscle power. The greater the intensity of exercise and shorter the time period taken to generate force, the greater is the muscle power.

Principles of strength training (resistance training):
- **Overload principle:** This is used for increasing muscle performance. This guiding principle of exercise prescription for resisted exercise to improve muscle performance (strength) states that, if muscle performance is to improve, a load that exceeds the metabolic capacity of the muscle (i.e., the load that is slightly higher than what the muscle can easily lift) must be applied to the muscle. Overload can be applied by increasing the intensity (load) or volume (frequency, repetitions, and time). In strength training intensity is increased, where as in endurance training, the volume of exercise is increased.
- **Specific adaptation to imposed demands (SAID) principle:** Adaptations produced by training are highly specific to the nature of the stimulus or over load applied. It suggests that, a framework of specificity is necessary foundation, upon which strengthening exercise program should be built up. This principle is an extension of Wolff's law (Body systems adapt over time to the stresses placed upon them), which help therapist to determine the exercise prescription. The adaptations are specific to strength, power, endurance, functional activity, joint angle, sequence of muscle activations, energy systems, and virtually all other variables present. As per the principle, if the functional activity requires strength, rather than endurance, then the intensity and duration of exercise should be designed to improve strength. The principle, also guides about the mode (type of contraction), velocity, and limb position (joint angle) to be selected for specific therapeutic benefit. For example, if quadriceps is weak in the terminal part of

knee extension, the resistance (as per over load principle) should be applied at that range in which the muscle is weak.

- **Transfer of training:** This principle, which is contrary to the SAID principle, speaks about carry over of training effects from one variation of exercise or task to another. For example, strength training in one speed of exercise has been shown to provide some improvement in strength at higher or lower speeds of exercise. Similarly, cross-training effect is found to occur, when strength is built up in one limb, where strength training is given to the contra lateral limb. Even though, small degree of transference of training occurs in strength training, it is advisable to design exercise programs that resemble the movement patterns required for the functional activities.
- **Reversibility principle:** The adaptations achieved through resistance exercise persist as long as the resistance exercise is performed regularly and go back gradually to the pre-exercise levels once the training is stopped. This means the effects of resistance training are reversible. The adaptive changes such as gain in strength and endurance, obtained in strength training is gradually lost, if the individual does not maintain the practice by performing regular activities or exercise programs. This detraining effect, which is reflected by a gradual reduction in muscle performance begins within a week or two of cessation of resisted exercise and continues until the training effects are lost. It is therefore recommended that to maintain strength and endurance after strength training, the individual should engage himself for routine functional activities or should perform regular resisted exercise.
- **Inter individual variability:** Every individual responds to resistance exercise in different way. Similar stimuli may bring about lot of changes in one person, but not in another.

Guidelines for prescription of resisted exercise:

- **Examination and evaluation:**
  - Determine the base line:
    » General physical examination.
    » Find the muscle strength: Manual muscle testing, dynamometry, repetition maximum (RM).
    » Find the ROM by Goniometry.
    » Asses the functional performance.
    » Periodic reassessment.
- **Preparation:**
  - Plan the regime according to the need and equipment available.
  - Give explanation and demonstration.
  - Ensure proper clothing, diet, and hydration.
- **Application:**
  - Warm up: Light repetitive dynamic exercise for the muscles to be exercised.
  - Placement of resistance distally.
  - Decide the direction of movement (concentric/eccentric).
  - Stabilize the proximal segment.
  - Cool down.
- **Techniques of resisted exercise:**
  - Explain the patient about the procedure and Dos and Don'ts.
  - Select the starting position as per requirement of the goal.
  - Give verbal command to move in the desired direction.
  - Stabilize the proximal or distal joint to prevent substitution.
  - Select the **mode** (manual/mechanical) types of muscle contraction (isometric, dynamic, and isokinetic), **position during exercise** (weight bearing/nonweight bearing), **intensity** (amount of resistance/load), **volume** (total number of repetitions and sets of a particular exercise during a particular exercise session), **frequency** (number of exercise sessions per day/week), **duration** (total number of weeks or months, during which resistance exercise program is carried out- 6–12 weeks of resistance training is ideal achieving muscle hypertrophy and increased vascularization of muscle), **rest interval** [dependent on intensity or volume of exercise, —e.g., between sets of moderate intensity and volume of exercise (8-12 RM levels), a 30-60 seconds rest period is selected, and for higher intensity exercises (at a 3-5 RM level) a longer rest period is selected before performing another set of same exercise], **speed of exercise** [(for concentric exercises, the speed is kept low to have higher force generation, and for eccentric exercises, it is found that initially, the force production in the muscle increases in proportion to the speed of muscle lengthening and subsequently it levels off), the training speeds should be geared to match the demands of desired functional activities], **periodization protocol** (systematic variation in exercise intensity and volume at regular intervals over a specific periods of time).
  - Follow a warm up protocol before starting moderate to high intensity exercise, and a cool down protocol at the end of the program
  - Integrate resistance training into functional activities to maintain carry over and prevent detraining effect.

Progressive Resistance Exercise

Progressive resistance exercise is a dynamic resistance training in which a constant external load is applied to the contracting muscle by some mechanical means, which is incrementally increased. This is performed to increase strength and endurance of muscle groups.

The repetition maximum (RM) is used as the basis of progression in the resistance. 1 RM is the maximum load the individual can lift once without fatigue. 10 RM is the maximum load the individual can lift 10 times without fatigue.

Techniques of Progressive resisted exercise: Various protocols/techniques, of progressive resisted exercise are used in strength training to build up strength and endurance. The techniques are:

- **DeLorme and Watkins technique:**
  - 10 lifts with ½ 10 RM.

- 10 lifts with ¾ 10 RM.
- 10 lifts with 10 RM.
  30 lifts 4 times weekly, progress 10 RM once weekly.
❖ **Zinovieff (Oxford technique):**
  - 10 lifts with 10RM.
  - 10 lifts with 10RM minus 1lb.
  - 10 lifts with 10RM minus 2lb.
  - 10 lifts with 10RM minus 3lb.
  - 10 lifts with 10RM minus 4lb.
  - 10 lifts with 10RM minus 5lb.
  - 10 lifts with 10RM minus 6lb.
  - 10 lifts with 10RM minus 7lb.
  - 10 lifts with 10RM minus 8lb.
  - 10 lifts with 10RM minus 9lb.
  - 100 lifts 5 times weekly, progress 10RM daily.
❖ **Mac Queen technique:**
  - 10 lifts with 10RM.
  - 10 lifts with 10RM.
  - 10 lifts with 10RM.
  - 10 lifts with 10RM.
    40 lifts 3 times weekly, progress 10 RM every 1-2 weeks.
❖ **DAPRE (Daily adjusted progressive resisted exercise) technique:** It is based on 6RM working weight. It is more systematic and takes into account the different rates at which individual progress during rehabilitation or conditioning program. The protocol includes the following **(Table 1.12)**.

Table 1.12: The DAPRE protocol.

Sets	Repetitions	Amount of resistance
1	10	50% of 6RM
2	6	75% of 6RM
3	Maximum possible	100% of 6RM
6	Maximum possible	100% of adjustable working weight

Effects and uses of resisted exercise (strength training):
❖ Enhances muscle performance: The exercise when practiced using the right protocol, helps in restoration, maintenance, and improvement of muscle strength, power, and endurance.
❖ Enhances blood flow to the working muscles.
❖ Enhances tissue temperature.
❖ Increases strength of connective tissues, like tendons, ligaments, and intramuscular connective tissues.
❖ Increases and maintains bone mineral density and prevents bone demineralization.
❖ Enhances joint stabilization, therefore decreases stress on joints during physical activity. This may reduce the risk of soft tissue injury or cumulative trauma disorder.
❖ Enhances the capacity of repair and healing of damaged soft tissues, due to positive effect on tissue remodeling.
❖ Promotes stable posture and improves balance.
❖ Enhances physical efficiencies for performance of self care, occupational, and recreational activities.
❖ Reduces obesity, by increasing lean body mass and decreasing body fat.
❖ Increases the feeling of physical well being by enhanced physical fitness.
❖ Reduces/reverses the impact of impairment, thereby promotes participation in society and improves quality of life.

II. Passive Movements/Passive Exercises

In clinical conditions, where active movements by the patient is not possible due to muscular inactivity/pain, or when active movement produced by the patient is insufficient to mobilize a stiff joint, the body segments need to be moved by an external system.

Passive movements are movements produced by an external force during muscular inactivity or when muscular activity is voluntarily reduced significantly to permit movements. The force/external agent used to produce movement could be:
❖ Manual force used by therapists/care giver, patient through use of the intact limb.
❖ Mechanical force, such as a continuous passive motion (CPM) exerciser **(Fig. 1.112)**.

Classification of Passive Movements

Passive movements are classified into:
I. Relaxed passive movements including accessory movements.
II. Passive manual mobilization techniques, that include:
   - Mobilization of joints.
   - Manipulation of joints.
   - Controlled sustained stretching of tight structures.
I. **Relaxed passive movements:**
   a. **Physiological movements:** These are bodily movements/exercises performed smoothly and accurately by the physiotherapist/clinician within the pain-free available range and in a direction same as the direction of active movements.
   Principles of relaxed passive exercise:
   » The patient is made fully relaxed during the procedure, and explained about the requirements and benefits.

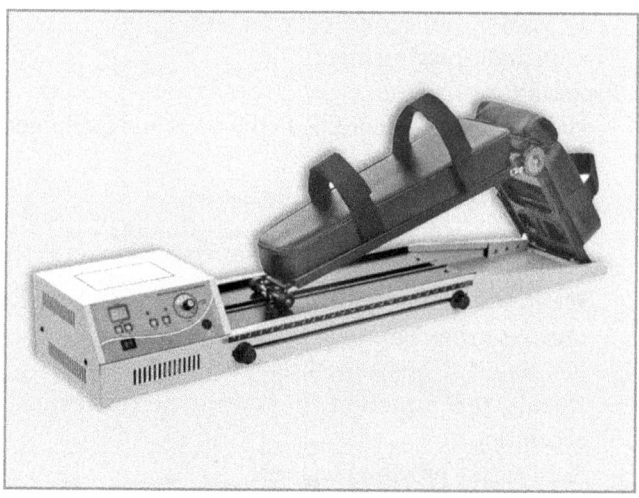

Fig. 1.112: The CPM machine for knee.

- » Fixation of the proximal segment should be done to localize the movement to the desired joint and to avoid compensatory movements.
- » The moving part is supported comfortably and fully, to develop confidence and promote relaxation.
- » Traction in the long axis of the joint is given to reduce intra-articular friction, there by promoting greater excursion of the joint.
- » Range of movement is as full as possible and no pain and spasm should be induced during the movement.
- » Speed of the movement performed should be uniform, slow and rhythmical to achieve relaxation.
- » Duration/number of repetitions of movement performed depend on the purpose for which the movement is performed.

Effects and uses of relaxed passive exercise:
- » Induces relaxation of the segment/whole body due to the soothing effects produced by continuous rhythmical movements, hence used before mobilization/stretching/strengthening exercises.
- » Maintains available ROM and extensibility of soft tissues and prevents adhesion formation, tightness (adaptive shortening), contracture and deformities in joints. One passive movement given to the joints at frequent intervals are sufficient for the purpose, however two movements to each joint performed twice daily is also adequate.
- » Helps to preserve the memory of movements by stimulating the kinesthetic receptors during the periods when active movements are not possible.
- » Assist in venous and lymphatic return and prevent formation of deep vein thrombosis (DVT), due to mechanical pressure created due to movement, as well as due to stretching of the thin-walled vessels that cross over the joints. This is used in conjunction with elevation of the body segment with edema, when active movement is not possible.

b. **Accessory movements**: These consist of gliding or rotational movements, which occurs in combination with physiological movements, but can not be performed in isolation actively. These movements are usually limited or absent in joint pathologies, and need to be restored by the therapists through mobilization techniques.

Principles of giving accessory movements:
- » Position the patient in a position as appropriate for restoration of movement.
- » Ensure that the patient is fully relaxed and the part is fully supported.
- » Fix the proximal segment.
- » Perform small amplitude gliding and rotational movements in a graded manner, comparing with such movements found on the sound side without traumatizing the joint.
- » Follow direction of movement as appropriate, i.e., when concave surface is made to glide over convex surface, the gliding is done in the direction of rolling of the distal segment of the joint **(Fig. 1.113)**, and when convex surface is moved over concave surface, gliding is given in the opposite direction of rolling of the distal segment of the joint **(Fig. 1.114)**.

Effects and uses of accessory movements:
- » Enhances joint play, hence beneficial for restoration of physiological movements of joints.
- » In stiffness of joints, accessory movements to joints are given before physiological movements.

II. Passive manual mobilization techniques: These are passive movements where controlled forces are applied either manually, or mechanically to stretch/mobilize soft tissues, enabling restoration of joint ROM in stiff joints affected by disease or trauma. These include:

- ❖ **Mobilizations of joints:** These are small repetitive rhythmical oscillatory movements (physiological/accessory) performed by the clinicians in various amplitudes under the patient's control to restore mobility. These are graded according to the part of the available range in which they are performed.
- ❖ **Manipulations of joints:** These are accurately localized, single, quick decisive movements of small amplitude and high velocity applied by the clinicians and are completed before the patient can stop it. These movements are done either by the Physiotherapists in a therapeutic environment

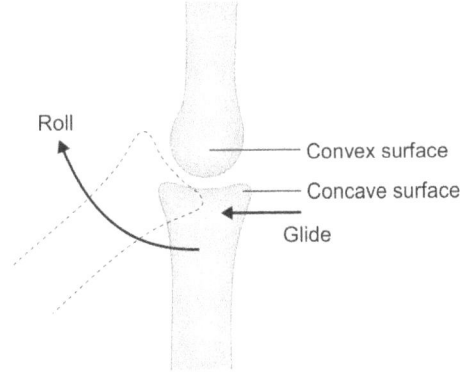

Fig. 1.113: Concave surface moving over convex surface.

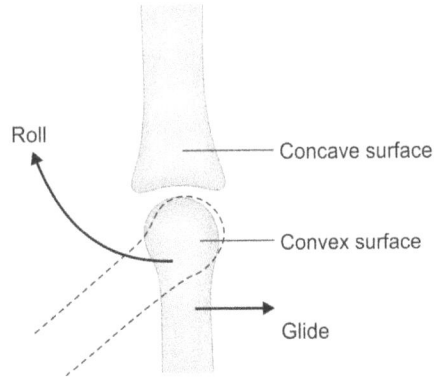

Fig. 1.114: Convex surface moving over concave surface.

or by the Orthopedic surgeon under general anesthesia. After the joint is manipulated by the Surgeon, the mobility is maintained and increased by the Physiotherapist either manually or by using CPM device.

- **Controlled sustained stretching of tightened structures/Passive stretching:** These are forceful passive movements, where sustained stretching force is applied to tight soft tissues either manually or mechanically by therapists using weight and pulley, weight cuffs, or devices like dynamometers, etc., to elongate tight structures to correct deformities, improve joint ROM, and to restore function. Before passive stretching is performed, the differentiation between tightness (a state of shortening of soft tissues, which can be elongated by passive force) and contracture (a state of shortening of soft tissues, which can not be elongated by passive force) should be made.

Principles of passive manual mobilization and stretching:

- Make an initial assessment of joint that includes ROM, joint play, end feel.
- Decide the position of the patient and the joint (loose pack position), technique (McKenzie, Maitland, Kaltenborn, Cyriax, etc.) and grades of mobilization/manipulation as appropriate.
- Stabilize the proximal segment to localize the force at the affected joint.
- For passive stretching, the patient should remain relaxed and the sustained stretching force should be applied for a minimum of 30 seconds. Repetition of stretches depends upon the tolerance of the patient and the effects required.
- The stretch/elongation should be maintained by suitable positional devices/orthoses to achieve permanent deformation/elongation (creep).
- Evaluate each joint mobilized/manipulated at the end of each session as well as at periodic intervals.
- Any gain in ROM and flexibility need to be maintained by regular exercises and functional integration.

Effects and uses of passive joint mobilization/manipulation and passive stretching:

- Mobilization of joints at low grades help in reduction of pain'
- Mobilization/manipulation break intra-articular/periarticular adhesions and correct positional faults in joints and restores mobility and function.
- Steady and sustained stretching helps in reduction of spasticity/spasm, elongates tight soft tissues, and corrects deformities.

Contraindications for passive stretching:

- Acute inflammation.
- Recent fracture.
- Hyper mobility.
- Severe osteoporosis.
- Loose body in joint.
- Hemophilic arthritis.
- Early tendon repair/transfer.

Types of stretching exercises: Stretching exercises are classified into the following types, depending upon the mode of their performance, such as passive or active, manual, or mechanical.

- **Passive stretching:**
  - *Static stretching:* This is the most commonly performed stretching exercise, where the tight soft tissues are lengthened past the point of tissue resistance and held in the lengthened position for an extended period of time preferably 30 seconds or more with a maintained stretch force. It is done manually by therapists or mechanically.
  - *Static progressive stretching:* In this type of stretching exercise, the tight soft tissues are held in the lengthened position, until a degree of relaxation is achieved. Then the shortened structured are further lengthened and held in the new lengthened position for some time.
  - *Cyclic stretching/Intermittent stretching:* In this type of stretching, a relatively short duration stretch force is applied repeatedly and gradually with intermittent release to cause elongation of tight tissues.
  - *Mechanical stretching:* In this type of stretching, devices like orthotics, weights (weight cuffs/sand bags), therabands, weight, and pulley circuits, traction devices, automated devices such as CPM, Dynamometers, etc., are used to apply a sustained stretch to elongate tight soft tissues.

- **Active stretching:**
  - *Self stretching:* This stretching exercise is carried out independently by a patient as advised by the therapists, to maintain/increase the flexibility of the tight tissues, as a home exercise program. For example, a straight leg raise is a self stretching done by the patient to maintain/increase flexibility of hamstrings.
  - *Ballistic stretching:* This is a rapid, forceful, high speed, high intensity intermittent stretch, performed by the patient as per instruction of the therapist to increase flexibility of soft tissues and increase joint ROM. The Codman's exercise used to mobilize shoulder joint, uses ballistic stretching (**Fig. 1.115**).
  - *Neuromuscular inhibition techniques/PNF stretching:* These procedures reflexively relax tension in shortened muscles prior to or during stretching.

These include:

- **Hold and relax:** The tight muscle is kept in a comfortably lengthened position and the patient is asked to isometrically contract the muscle against the resistance given by the therapist, and subsequently to relax the muscle voluntarily. As the patient relaxes, the therapist moves the extremity through the gained range. The procedure is repeated several times.
- **Hold relax with agonist contraction:** Follow the same procedure as done for hold and relax. After the patient contracts the tight muscle, have him/her contract the agonist (opposite of tight muscle) concentrically to achieve elongation of the tight muscle.

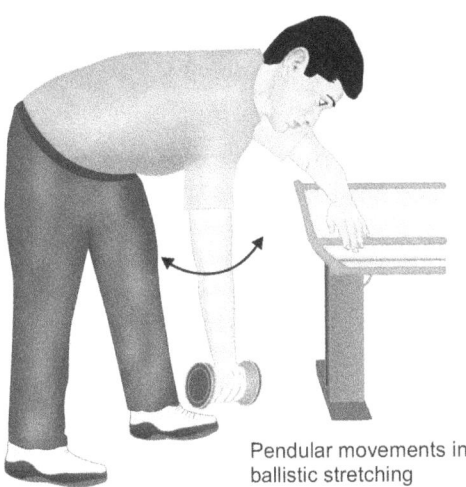

Fig. 1.115: Ballistic stretching.

- **Agonist contraction:** The tight muscle is passively lengthened to a comfortable position, and subsequently the patient is asked to contract the agonist muscle (opposite of tight muscle) concentrically. The therapist applies mild resistance to the contracting muscle. The tight muscle will relax and lengthen as a result of reciprocal inhibition.

Determinants of stretching exercises:
- **Intensity:** The lower the intensity, the longer the time the patient will tolerate stretching and soft tissues can be held in a lengthened position. The higher the intensity, the less frequently the stretching intervention can be applied.
- **Duration:** Stretch duration of 15, 30, 45, or 60 seconds or 2 minutes are effective, however, studies reveal that a long-duration stretch (say for 60 seconds) is no way more beneficial than a 30 seconds stretch. Most stretch durations are maintained at 30 seconds.
- **Frequency:** Frequency of stretching needs to occur a minimum of two times per week and depends upon the degree of tightness and functional integration of the affected segment.

RELAXATION

Relaxation is a state of body and mind, which is free from tension resulting in freedom for exercising smooth decision making and execution of function and leading to a pain-free and stress-free living.

Our muscles develop tension as they contract during strenuous activities, as well as in certain pathological states, such as upper motor neuron disorders. The normal tension developed in muscles subsides, as the individual takes rest, and relaxes the body. Mental stress developed in individuals, also lead to physical tension, causing alteration of muscle tone and posture.

Relaxation of body and mind is very essential for efficient functional performance with less and less consumption of energy. Recognition of a state of tension followed by voluntary relaxation of the muscles and mind, provide a mean of helping the patient to consume less energy, as in the state of relaxation, there is increased mobility of joints and a biomechanically efficient posture help in doing functional activities in an efficient way.

Degrees of Relaxation

Degree of relaxation implies the degrees to which existing muscular and mental tension is alleviated. Physiotherapists play a great role in alleviating tension and inducing voluntary relaxation. The procedures involved include:
- Creation of a regulatory environment conducive to both physical and mental rest.
- Recognition of a state of tension.
- Reassuring the patient and gaining confidence and co-operation.
- Designing Relaxation programs/strategies.

Techniques of Relaxation

I. **General relaxation:** Support, comfort and a regulatory and restful atmosphere are essential requirements for general relaxation of the body.
- **Support:** Proper support of the body contour and modifications of posture in lying and sitting are essential measures to induce relaxation. The weight of the body, when effectively counterbalanced, by the uniform upward pressure of a reciprocal surface, or by suspension, or by adapting a semi-flexed position of the lower limbs, eliminates mechanical tension in muscles and ligaments, helping in achieving relaxation. In lying or sitting, postural modifications need to be done as described here.
  - *Lying supine:* Select a bed that is firm and does not sag. Use a head pillow which is sufficiently soft to prevent the head from rolling to sides. Put a small pillow under the knees to relieve tension in the hamstrings and the iliofemoral ligaments and to allow the pelvis to roll backward, so that the lumbar spine is straightened and supported. The feet are held in the mid position by a sand bag or pillow used for the purpose. The upper limbs are supported on pillows with shoulders in slight abduction with elbows in slight flexion or hands may be placed relaxly on the body **(Fig. 1.116)**
  - *Half lying:* The plinth or bed should be firm and inclined vertically by an angle of 45 degrees. The pillow placements are same, as described for supine lying. The inclined posture is beneficial in facilitating breathing as there is less weight on the back, and abdominal pressure on the under surface of the diaphragm is reduced **(Fig. 1.117A)**. An arm chair with thighs supported on seat and feet supported on floor is also a good substitute for plinth **(Fig. 1.117B)**.
  - *Prone lying:* The head rests on a small pillow and turned to one side. A firm pillow is placed under the hips and lower abdomen to prevent the hollowing of the back. For adult females to avoid discomfort in anterior chest, the pillows may be extended up to the chest. The hips should be in medial rotation as much as possible, to keep the heels separated. The knees should be in slight

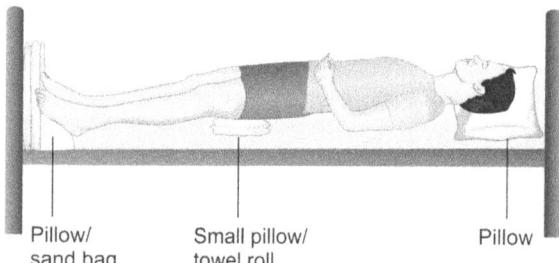

Fig. 1.116: Relaxed supine lying.

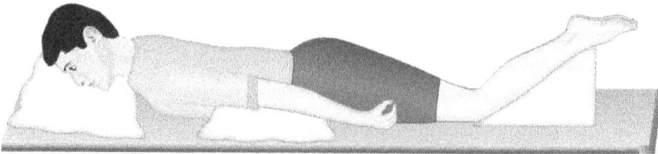

Fig. 1.118: Relaxed prone lying.

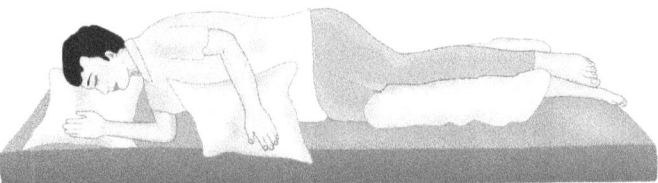

Fig. 1.119: Side-lying.

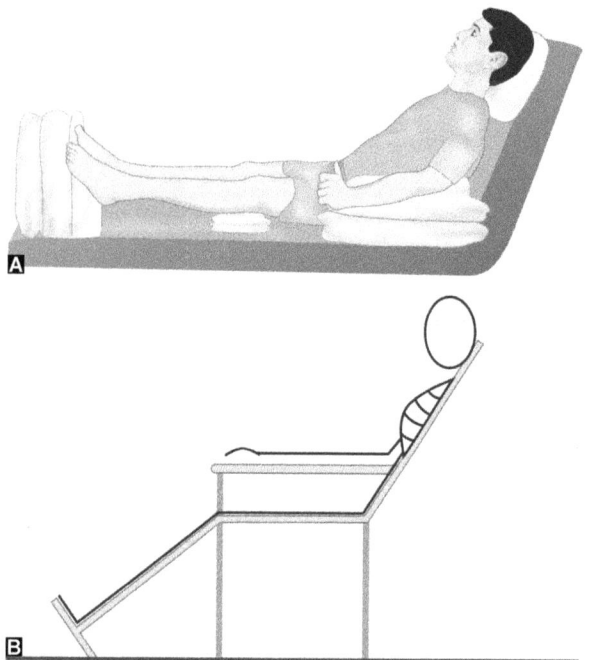

Figs. 1.117A and B: Relaxed half lying. (A) On bed. (B) On chair.

flexion, by placing pillows under the legs, so that the toes are free **(Fig. 1.118)**.
- *Side lying:* In this posture the degree of relaxation obtained, depends upon the stability of shoulder and pelvic girdles. The arm and legs on the upper side should be supported on pillows with the hips and knees flexed. The lower leg should be slightly extended at the hip with knee in slight flexion and the lower arm is flexed at the shoulder and so placed that, the body weight does not fall on it. This posture is used by majority of people **(Fig. 1.119)**.

❖ **Comfort:** Besides adequate support to body parts, comfort in terms of freedom to breath deeply, mild warmth, relaxation of abdominals, minimal physical activity are essential components for achieving relaxation. The dresses worn should not be too tight, and the room should have circulation of free air. A light well-balanced meal, timely voiding of bladder and bowel are conducive to achieve general relaxation.

❖ **Restful atmosphere:** As relaxation of body and mind are interdependent, effort is essentially required to establish a state of mental rest. As many patients such as Cerebral palsy, Head injury, Stroke and Cardiac patients, etc., are highly susceptible for disturbing influence of noise, the therapy/treatment room should be as quiet as possible. Bright lights and strong colors, such as red and bright yellow, are said to be stimulating, whereas a room with low well-diffused light with green and peach furnishings gives a soft and warm glow and provides an ideal setting for relaxation.

The behavior of the treating physician/physiotherapist plays a vital role in the creation of restful atmosphere. The voice of therapist should be low-pitched and clear.

Additional Methods of Relaxation

Even though, the conditions favoring relaxation are provided, to the patient, some times tension persists and additional methods for relaxation should be followed, as described under:

a. **Conscious breathing exercises:** During rest, very often the person's mind remains active generating so many unwanted thoughts resulting in anxiety and tension. Deep breathing exercises with a slight pause at the end of expiration may divert the attention of the person, making him concentrate on his own rhythm of breathing. During expiration, which is a phase of relaxation a feeling of "letting go" in the whole body should develop helping to eliminate anxiety and physical tension, there by inducing relaxation.

b. **Progressive relaxation:** Progressive muscle relaxation (PMR) is a deep relaxation technique that has been effectively used to control stress and anxiety, relieve insomnia, and reduce symptoms of certain types of chronic pain.

The technique of progressive muscle relaxation was described by Edmund Jacobson in the 1930s and is based upon his premise that mental calmness is a natural result of physical relaxation. This method is similar to the Yoga system and termed as "Savasana" or "Still Pose" **(Fig. 1.120)**.

It is based upon the simple practice of tensing, or tightening, one muscle group at a time followed by a

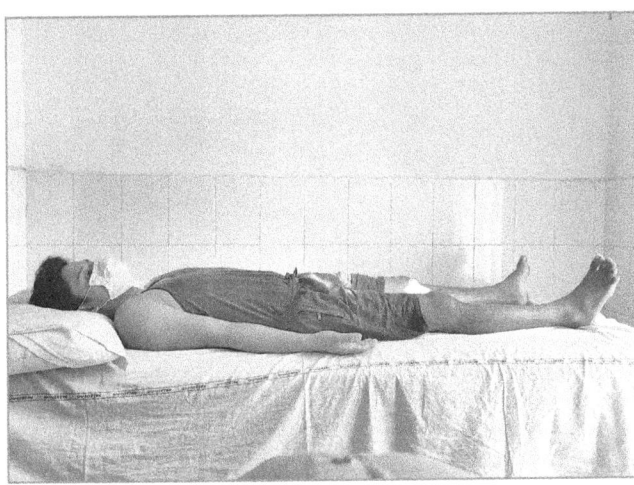

Fig. 120: The still pose.

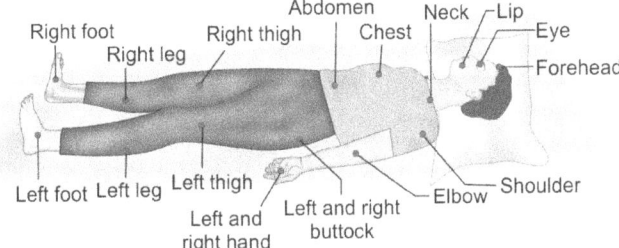

Fig. 121: Progressive relaxation.

relaxation phase with release of the tension **(Fig. 1.121)**. It can be learned by nearly anyone and requires only 10–20 minutes per day to practice.

c. **Contrast method**: In situations, where a patient is not able to feel the sensation of relaxation in tensed muscles, the contrast method, where the contrast between maximal muscle contraction and degree of relaxation which follows muscle contraction is demonstrated. The patient is told to contract any group or series of muscles, as strongly as possible and then to "let go" and "continue to let go".

d. **Physiological relaxation:** This method of relieving tension was devised by Laura Mitchell, in 1957, which is based on the physiological principle of reciprocal relaxation. The "Mitchell Method" of physiological relaxation—often known as the "simple method of relaxation"—is the name given to a technique of relaxing the whole, or parts of the body. Once learnt and practiced, it can be used easily and anywhere to relax and reduce the muscle tension produced by stress.

Principles of Mitchell Method of Relaxation:
- Tightening or contracting muscles results in movement.
- Movement causes repositioning of the joints and limbs.
- When we are awake, the brain will register a change in body position through muscle, joint, and skin sensation.
- The brain is only aware of the movement it causes. Movements are controlled by the nervous system; and if one group of muscles is "instructed" to tighten, the opposite group of muscles for that action receives an "instruction" to relax. One can learn to recognize and be aware of tense muscles and joints. Instructing or "ordering" the opposite muscle groups to tighten will automatically result in "relax" messages being received by the tense muscles and joints. This new "position of ease" can be learnt by registering the feeling in the muscles, joints, and skin. Finding the position of ease of all the joints will result in relaxation

Techniques of Mitchell methods of relaxation:
- Move away from the position of stress.
- Stop.
- Be aware of and feel the new position.

For example:

For relaxing the shoulders: The patient is asked to pull the shoulders toward the feet, so the neck becomes longer. Then, he/she should stop and feel that the shoulders are down and relaxed.

For relaxing the hips: The patient is asked to turn the hips outwards, then stop and feel that thighs and legs have rolled outwards.

In the same manner relaxation is achieved in the whole body.

e. **Relaxed passive movements**: Rhythmical passive movements of the limbs and head may assist in achieving relaxation. Mass movements of joints, e.g., flexion and extension of hip, knee and ankle, are preferable. The rhythm of small pendular movements is very effective in some cases.

II. Local relaxation. As we know, general relaxation takes time and sometimes is not required, Effort should be made to achieve local relaxation by the following methods.
- **Massage**: Massage such as, light stroking, gentle effleurage, and myofascial release help in inducing local relaxation.
- **Passive stretching:** Gentle stretching of the spastic, spasmodic muscles help in relaxing the segment of the body over which the muscle works.
- **Contract-relax and pendular movements:** These start in the free range and gradually increase in amplitude. It may restore confidence and achieve relaxation.
- **In case of tightness and deformity:** Relaxation techniques for the shortened muscles and strengthening techniques for their antagonists, followed by integration of their reciprocal action to establish the increase in the range of movement help to induce relaxation.

FRENKEL'S EXERCISE

Frenkel's exercises are a set of slow repetitious exercises developed by Professor Heinrich Sebastian Frenkel, Medical Superintendent of the Sanatorium Freihof, in Switzerland in 1889, to treat ataxias in patients of Tabes dorsalis and Cerebellar ataxia.

It is defined as a series of gradual progressive exercises designed to improve co-ordination. The exercises are systematic and graduated in nature, increasing in difficulty over the time. The patient watches his hand or arm movements (for e.g.) and corrects them as needed. The exercises are designed to establish the voluntary control of movements by the use of any part of the sensory mechanism which is intact, such as vision, hearing, touch, etc., to compensate for the loss of kinesthetic sensation. The visual sense is the most important supporting factor in the treatment. The ultimate aim is to establish control of movements, so that the patient is confidently able in his ability to carry out activities, which are essential for independence in everyday life. Daily treatment sessions for at least 6 weeks are effective.

The essential components of the program include:
- Concentration of attention.
- Precision.
- Repetition.

Indications of Frenkel's Exercise

- Cerebellar ataxia
- Sensory ataxia (tabes dorsalis)
- Stroke
- Cerebral palsy
- Multiple sclerosis
- Wilson's disease
- Parkinson's disease
- Other neurological disorders.

Technique of Frenkel's Exercise

- **Position and clothing:** The patient is positioned and suitably clothed, so that he/she can see the limbs throughout the exercise.
- **Explanation and demonstration:** A concise explanation and demonstration of the exercise is given before movement is attempted, to give the patient a clear mental picture of it.
- **Attention:** The patient must give his/her full attention to the performance of the exercise to make the movement smooth and accurate.
- **Speed of movement:** The speed of movement is dictated by the physiotherapist by means of rhythmic counting, movement of his/her hand, or the use of suitable music. The speed may be fast to start with, which is gradually reduced to make the movement more precise and accurate.
- **ROM:** The range of movement is indicated by marking the spot on which the foot or hand is to be placed (**Fig. 1.122**). Initially large ROM, which is easy to perform is emphasized, subsequently small range accurate movements are trained.
- **Repetition of exercise:** The exercise must be repeated many times until it is perfect and easy. It is then discarded and a more difficult one is substituted.
- **Rest periods:** As these exercises are very tiring at first, frequent rest periods must be allowed.

The exercises can be practiced in lying, sitting, and standing as required:
- **Frenkel exercises in lying:**
    - *Lying (Head raised):* Hip flexion and externsion—A weight cuff as shown may be applied, if there is severe incoordination, provided, if the patient has the ability to

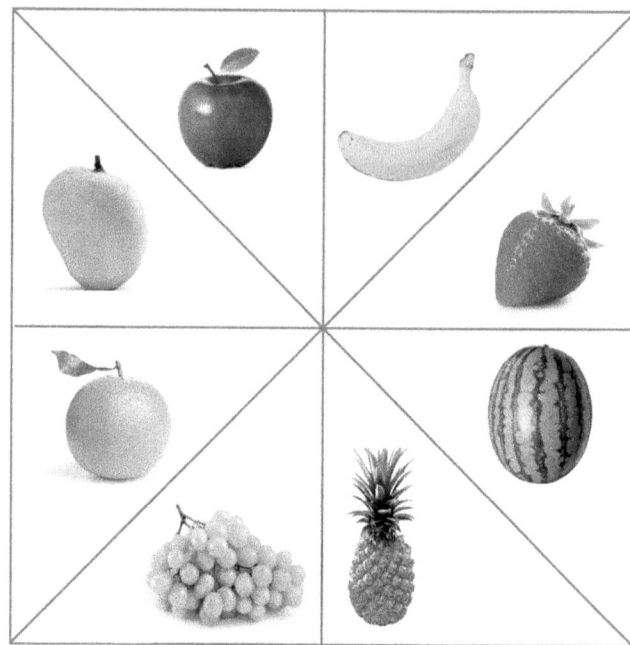

Fig. 1.122: Marks on the floor for Frenkel's exercise.

  lift the load (**Fig. 1.123**). In the same way, patient can be asked to do hip abduction and adduction.
    - *Lying (Head raised):* One hip and knee flexion and extension. The heel is supported throughout and slides on the plinth to a position indicated by the therapist (**Fig. 1.124**).
    - *Lying (Head raised):* One leg raised and placed over a specified mark on the plinth/therapist's hand/other foot/shin. The heel of the raised leg is moved up and down over the shin of the lower leg (**Fig. 1.125**).
    - *Lying (Head raised):* Bend one leg at the hip and knee, while straightening the other in a bicycling motion. Stopping and starting during the course of the movement may be introduced to increase the control required to perform the exercise/activity (**Fig. 1.126**).
- **Frenkel's exercises in sitting:**
    - Sitting, one leg stretched, to slide heel to a position indicated by a mark on the floor (**Fig. 1.127A**).
    - Sitting: lifting pegs from socket/bed as indicated by the therapist (**Fig. 1.127B**).
    - Standing from sitting and sit down as per instructions. The patient may be asked to hold a position, once the buttocks are off the bed, when instructed.
- **Frenkel's exercise in standing:**
    - Standing, taking the foot to marks on the floor, as instructed (**Fig. 1.128**).
    - Stride standing, walking side ways, placing feet on marks on the floor.
    - Standing, throwing and catching a cork ball.
    - Standing, performing peg board activities (**Fig. 1.129**)

Progression of Exercise

- **By altering speed, range, and complexity of movement:** As quick movements require less control than slow movements,

Chapter 1 : Exercise Therapy

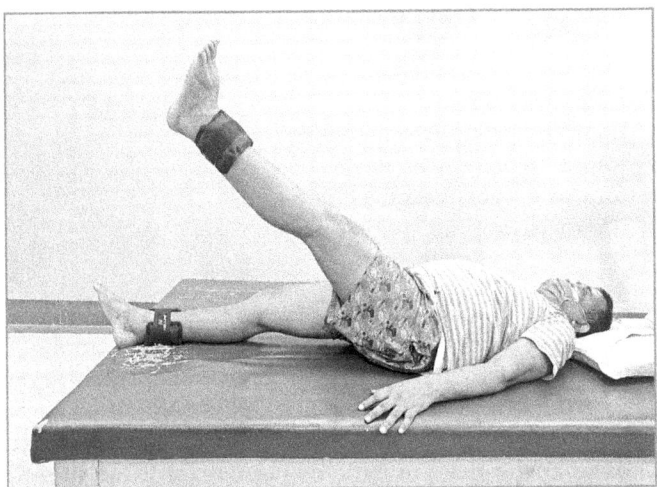

Fig. 1.123: Frenkel's exercise in lying.

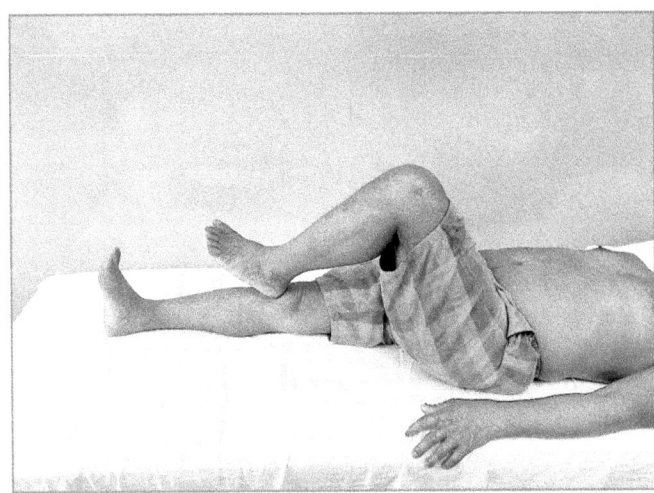

Fig. 1.125: Frenkel's exercise in lying.

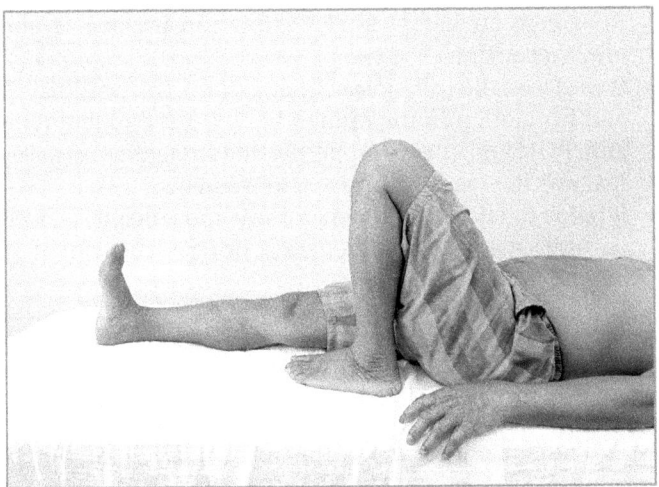

Fig. 1.124: Frenkel's exercise in lying.

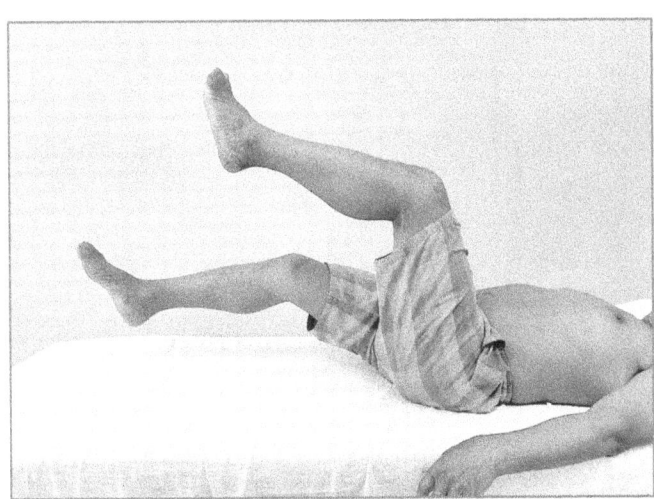

Fig. 1.126: Frenkel's exercise in lying.

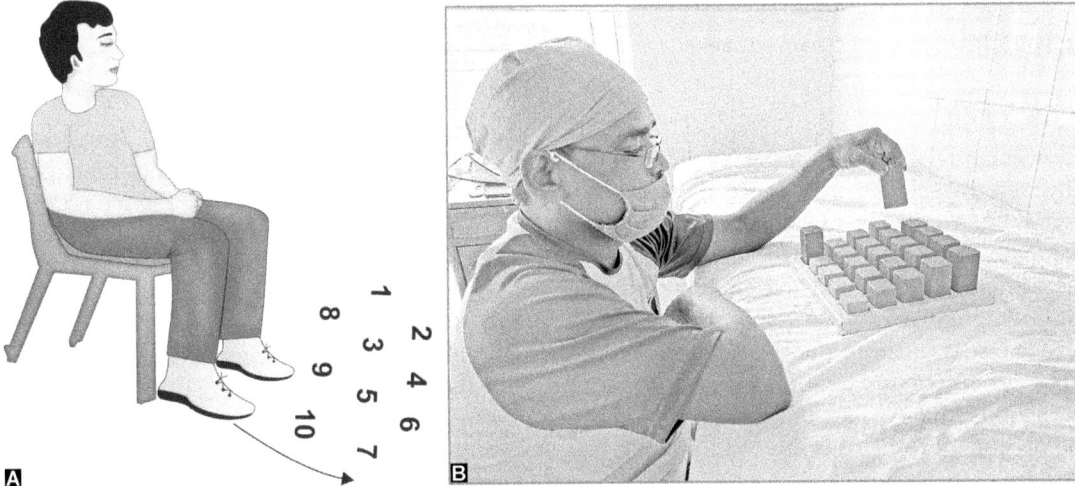

Figs. 1.127A and B: Frenkel's exercises. (A) Stretching the foot to numbers as indicated. (B) Lifting the peg from bed as per the instructions.

Section 1: Exercise Therapy and Massage

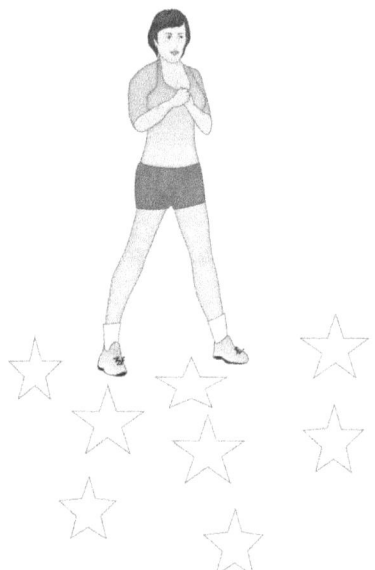

Fig. 1.128: Frenkel's exercise in standing.

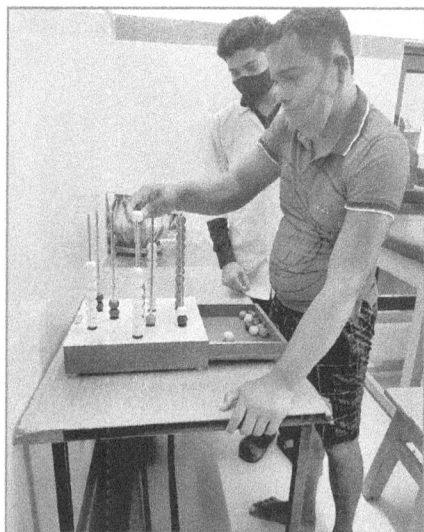

Fig. 1.129: Peg board activities in standing.

initially the movement should be fast, and gradually the speed should be decreased. Alteration of the speed of consecutive movements and interruptions, which involve stopping and starting to command, are introduced. Wide range movements involving large joints are performed first, gradually limiting the ROM and making use of small joints. The direction of movement is also frequently altered as a progression. Finally simple movements are built up into sequences to form specific actions which require the use and control of a number of joints and more than one limb, e.g., walking, ball throwing, etc.

- **According to the degree of disability**: Re-education exercises start in lying with the head propped up and with the limbs fully supported and progress is made to exercises in sitting, and then in standing.

Benefits of Frenkel's Exercise

- Improves co-ordination.
- Improves balance.
- Improves postural awareness.
- Improves body awareness.
- Improves selective movement.
- Improves proprioception (in a few cases)

SUSPENSION THERAPY

Suspension therapy is a special technique of therapeutic exercise in which a part or all of the body is suspended in the air in a special device called Guthrie-Smith Suspension frame by ropes and slings attached to a fixed point above the body. The therapy is given to patients to increase ROM, muscle power, and re-educate movement.

Principles of Suspension Therapy

- In suspension therapy friction is less, causing smooth and easy movement.
- It works on the principles of pendulum. The pendular to and fro motion in the human body is used to maintain joint ROM and muscle properties and strengthen muscles.
- It allows free/assisted/resisted movements.
- It helps to eliminate gravity for free movements, as well as, utilizes gravity to either assist or resist movement as per the need.

Advantages and Disadvantages of Suspension Therapy

- **Advantages:**
  - It reduces the burden of therapists.
  - Easy to lift and hold body parts for exercises.
  - Active movement can be performed easily with minimum friction.
- **Disadvantages:**
  - Quite complex procedure.
  - Requires many components/equipment.

The Suspension Unit and its Components

The suspension unit **(Fig. 1.130)**, invented by Late Mrs Guthrie smith, has the following components:

- **Suspension frame:** Shown in **Figure 1.130**.
- **Supporting ropes**: Connecting ropes provide the attachment of a sling to the frame and are adjustable in length. There are three types of supporting ropes: single rope, double rope, pulley rope.
  - *Single rope:* Has a ring fixed at one end by which it is hung up. The other end of the rope then passes through one end of the wooden cleat through the ring of a dog clip and through the other end of the cleat and then knotted. The cleat is for altering the length of the rope and should be held horizontally for movement and pulled oblique when supporting. The rope then "holds" on the cleat by frictional resistance. Length of rope required is 1.5 m **(Fig. 1.131)**.

Chapter 1 : Exercise Therapy

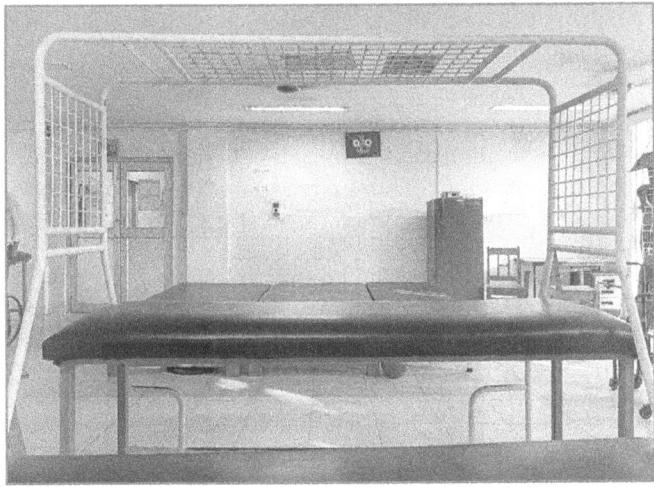

Fig. 1.130: The suspension frame.

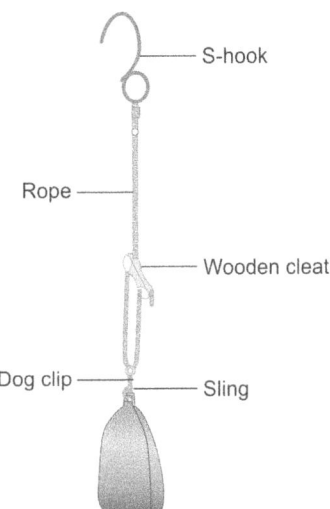

Fig. 1.131: The single rope system.

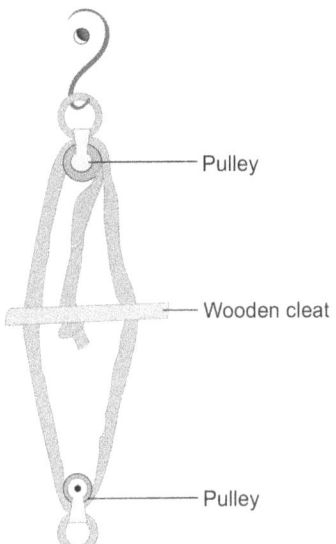

Fig. 1.132: The double rope system.

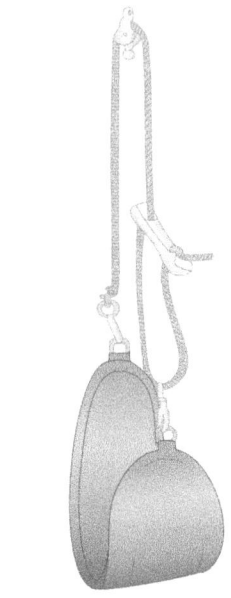

Fig. 1.133: The pulley rope system.

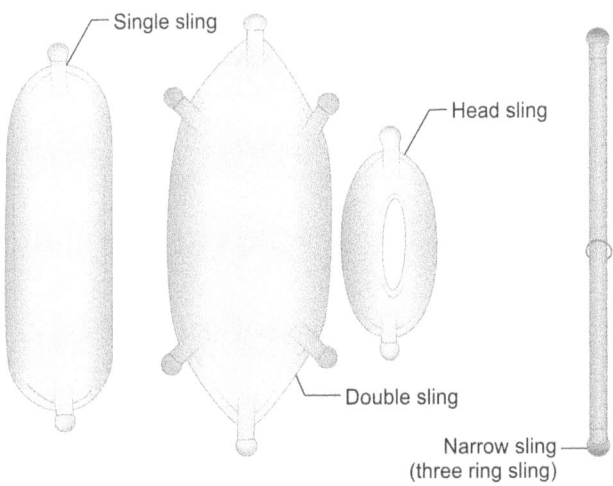

Fig. 1.134: Slings used for suspension therapy.

- *Double rope:* It consist of two pulleys at upper and lower attachments. This device gives a mechanical advantage of two as two pulleys are used. The rope is shortened by pushing the cleat down, allowing the lifter to move with gravity at the same time as it offers a mechanical advantage of two. Such a rope is used to suspend the heavy parts of the body, such as the pelvis, thorax, or heavy thighs when these are to be supported together **(Fig. 1.132)**.
- *The pulley rope:* This has a dog clip attached at one end of the rope, which then passes over the wheel of the pulley. The rope then passes through the cleat and a second dog clip. It is used for three-dimensional movements of a limb **(Fig. 1.133)**.
- ❖ **Slings:** There are four types of slings such as single sling, double sling, three ring sling, head sling **(Fig. 1.134)**.
- ❖ **Wooden cleat:** It is made of wood and is used for altering the length of the rope. It has two or three holes for the rope passage. The rope itself hold the cleat by friction resistance **(Fig. 1.135)**.

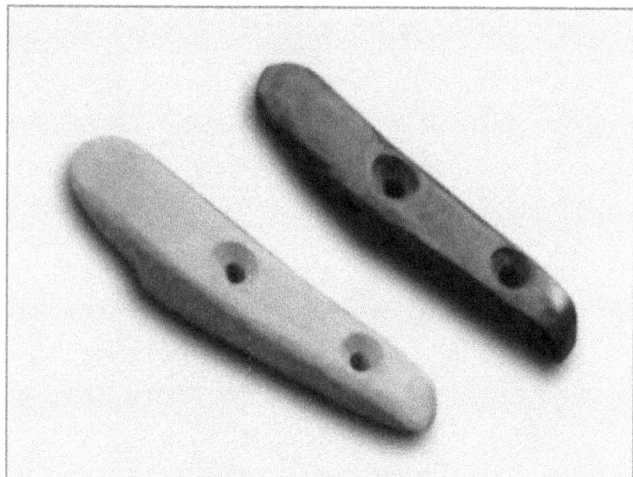

Fig. 1.135: Wooden cleat.

- **Dog clip and S-hook:** The dog clip attaches the rope to the slings supporting the body parts and the S-hook connects the rope to the wire mesh **(Fig. 1.136)**.

Types of Suspensions used in Therapy

Three types of suspensions used in therapy such as:
- **Vertical suspension**: COG of the body part or the body is taken as a point of suspension. In using vertical fixation the rope is fixed so that it hangs vertically above the COG of the part to be suspended. It is used for support as it tends to limit the movement of the part to a small-range penular movement on each side of the central resting point
- **Axial suspension**: It is the most common type of suspension used in therapy, where the joint axis is taken as the point of the suspension. The limb is supported by the slings above the axis of the joint. When the movement is initiated the limb is moved on both sides parallel to the floor. This suspension is used to maintain muscle properties, induce relaxation, and enhance blood flow and promote lymphatic drainage.
- **Pendular suspension:** In this type of suspension, the point of suspension is shifted away from the joint axis. When the axis is shifted opposite to the movement made by muscles, the muscles will be resisted, where as, if the axis is shifted in the direction of movement, the muscles will be assisted.

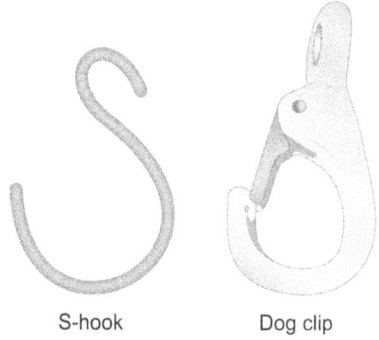

S-hook   Dog clip

Fig. 1.136: S-hook and dog clip.

This type of suspension is used to increase ROM, muscle strength, and endurance.

Indications for Suspension Therapy

- For re-education of weak muscles.
- For improvement of strength and endurance of muscles making the muscles contract against gravity, as in pendular suspension.
- For improvement and maintenance of joint ROM.
- For early neuromuscular co-ordination training.

Contraindications for Suspension Therapy

- Acute soft tissue injuries and fractures.
- Hyper mobile joints.
- Skin diseases.
- Open wound and sinuses.

Suspension Therapy for Trunk

I. **Upper trunk:**
   - **Side flexion**
     » Position of patient: Supine lying.
     » Fixation point: The ropes connecting the double sling supporting the thorax and head sling supporting the head should be connected to a point in the wire mesh just above the level of umbilicus. After the head and thorax are elevated the patient is asked to swing the body sideways **(Fig. 1.137A)**.
   - **Flexion and extension:** The subject is placed in side lying. The head sling supporting the head and large sling supporting the thorax are connected by ropes to a point on the wire mesh in line with the umbilicus. The head and trunk are elevated and the patient is asked to swing the body forward and backward.

II. **Lower trunk:**
   - **Flexion and extension (Fig. 1.137B):**
     » *Position of the patient:* Side lying.
     » *Fixation point:* The fixations of the ropes are done linearly in such a way that, the hooks should be in line at the level of the 3rd lumbar vertebra (level of the umbilicus). Two ropes, connecting the large sling/double sling under the pelvis are fastened to the outer ends of the line of hooks. The other two ropes connecting the single sling supporting the thighs are connected to the mesh through two hooks that are placed between two hooks connecting the pelvis. One single rope that is connected to the central-most hook in the line of hooks is connected with each three ring slings connecting each foot.

   If flexion is the desired movement, the thigh and foot ropes are moved to be fixed lateral to the front pelvic rope. If extension is the desired movement, then the thigh and the foot ropes are moved to outside the rear pelvic rope.
   - **Side/Lateral flexion (Fig. 1.138):** The patient in supine position lying with pillows placed under head and upper trunk. The arrangements of slings and ropes are done in same manner as described for flexion extension, i.e., the

Suspension Therapy for Upper Limb

- ❖ **Shoulder joint:**
  - *Abduction/Adduction* (**Fig. 1.139**):
    » **Position of the patient:** Supine.
    » **Fixation point:** Over the shoulder joint. Single sling is attached to the elbow and the narrow sling is applied to the wrist and hand.
  - *Flexion/Extension* (**Fig. 1.140**):
    » **Position of the patient:** Side lying
    » **Fixation point:** Over the shoulder joint. Single sling is attached to the elbow and the single sling supports the forearm, narrow sling is applied to the wrist and hand.
  - *Shoulder Rotation* (**Fig. 1.141**):
    » **Position of the patient:** Supine lying, elbow flexed to about 90 degrees.
    » *Fixation point:* Over the shoulder joint. Single sling is attached to the forearm and the narrow sling/single sling is applied to the wrist and hand.
- ❖ **Elbow joint: Flexion/Extension (Fig. 1.142):**
  - *Position of the patient:* Sitting on a chair with back support.

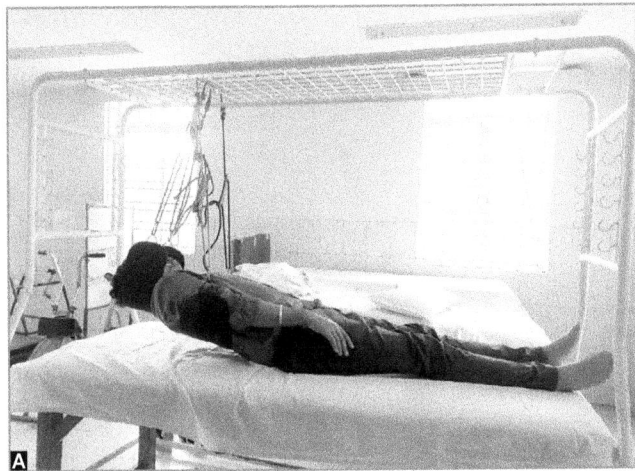
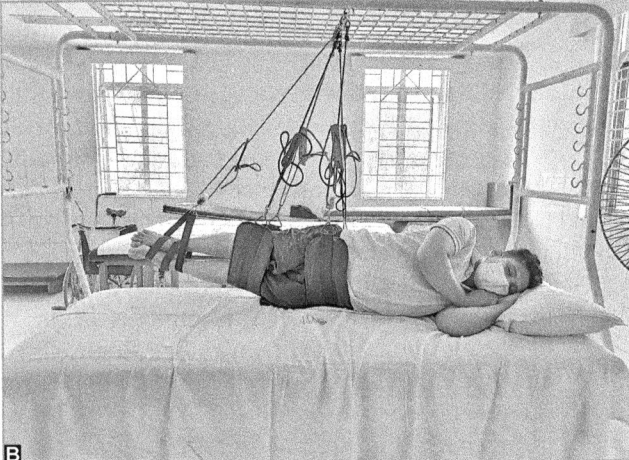

Figs. 1.137A and B: (A) Suspension therapy for upper trunk side flexion; (B) Suspension therapy for trunk flexion/extension.

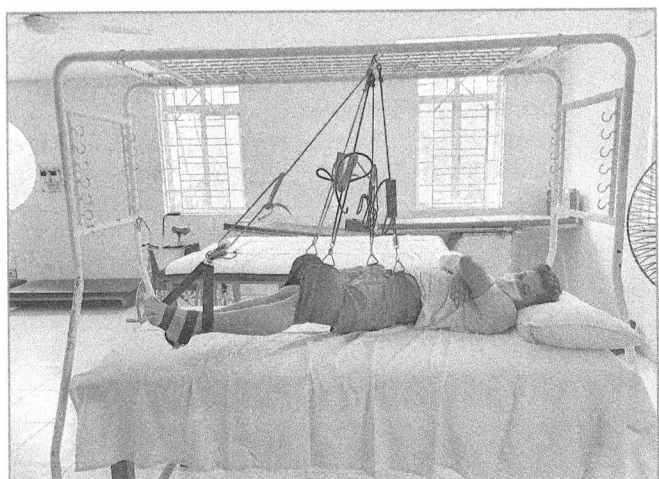

Fig. 1.138: Suspension therapy for trunk side flexion.

hooks are placed in one line over the L3 vertebra, with the two hooks for the pelvis being most outermost, followed by two hooks supporting the thighs and a central hook that supports the feet through the three ring slings. After arrangements of the slings, the ropes are shortened in an order, i.e., knee, followed by feet and pelvis to keep the lower body off the bed.

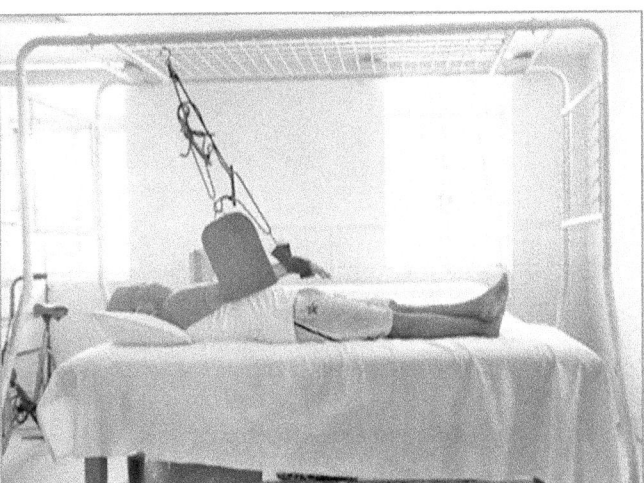

Fig. 1.139: Suspension therapy for shoulder abduction/adduction.

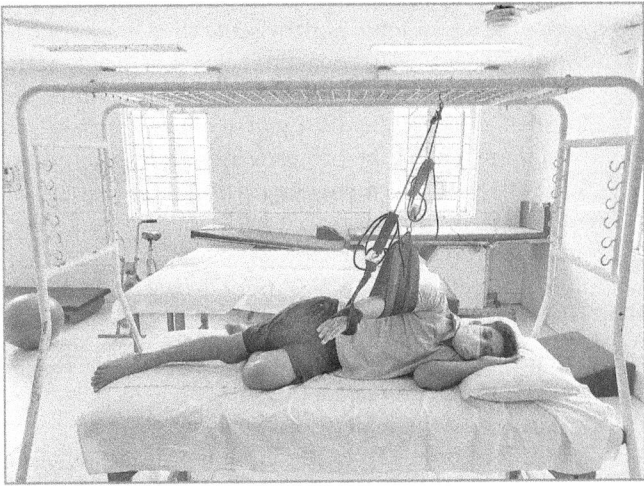

Fig. 1.140: Suspension therapy for shoulder flexion/extension.

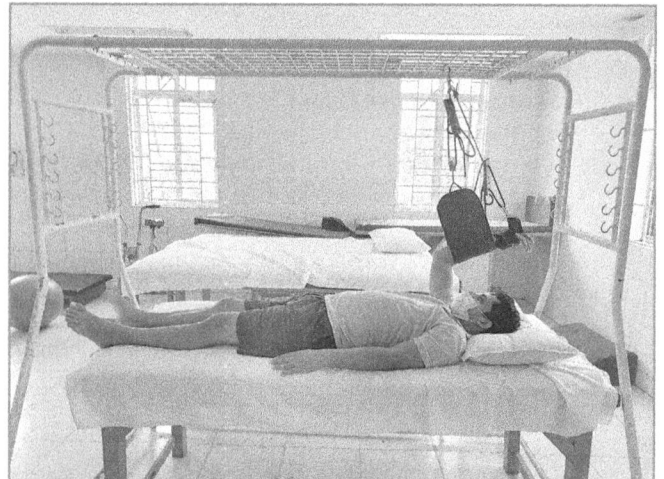

Fig. 1.141: Suspension therapy for shoulder rotation.

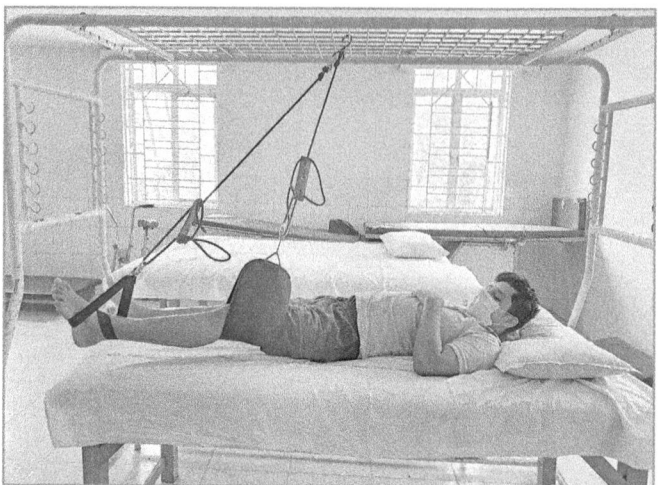

Fig. 1.143: Suspension therapy for hip abduction/adduction.

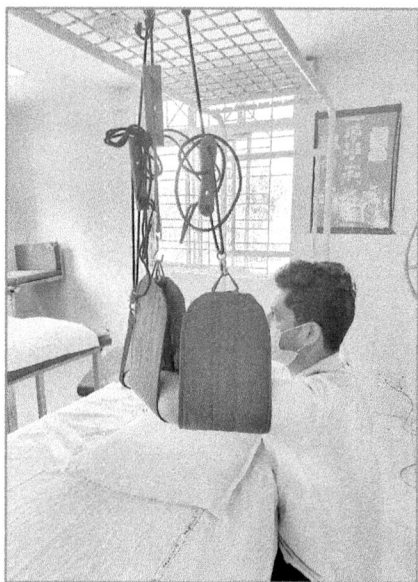

Fig. 1.142: Suspension therapy for elbow.

- *Fixation point:* The single sling supporting the forearm and the narrow sling supporting the hand are fixed through two separate ropes to a common point just above the elbow joint, and the other sling that supports the arm in vertical fixation, from center of gravity of the arm that lies at the junction of upper 1/3rd and lower 2/3rd of a line joining the tip of acromion process and lateral epicondyle of humerus are arranged, and the subject is asked to produce elbow flexion and extension.
- ❖ **Wrist joint:** Movement is usually performed on a polished/re-education board.

Suspension Therapy for Lower Limbs

- ❖ **Hip joint:**
  - *Abduction and adduction* (**Fig. 1.143**):
    » Position of the patient: Supine lying.
    » Fixation point: Over the hip joint (at the junction of medial 1/3rd and lateral 2/3rd of the line joining the ASIS and symphysis pubis, or 1/2 inch below the mid-inguinal point). The single sling is attached to the knee and one narrow sling is applied to the ankle and foot and they are attached to the rope hung from the fixation point.
  - *Flexion and extension* (**Fig. 1.144**):
    » Position of the patient: Side-lying.
    » Fixation point: Over the hip joint (i.e at the tip of greater trochanter of femur). The single sling is attached to the knee (lower thigh) and the narrow sling is applied to the ankle and foot. During flexion of hip both the hip and knee flexion should be allowed together to overcome passive insufficiency of hamstring muscle. When extension is performed the knee extension should be allowed to overcome the active insufficiency of hamstring muscle.
  - *Internal and external rotation* (**Fig. 1.145**)
    » Position of the patient: Supine lying with hip and knee flexed at 90 degrees.
    » Fixation point: Over the hip joint. A single sling is attached to the leg and the narrow sling is applied to the ankle and foot.

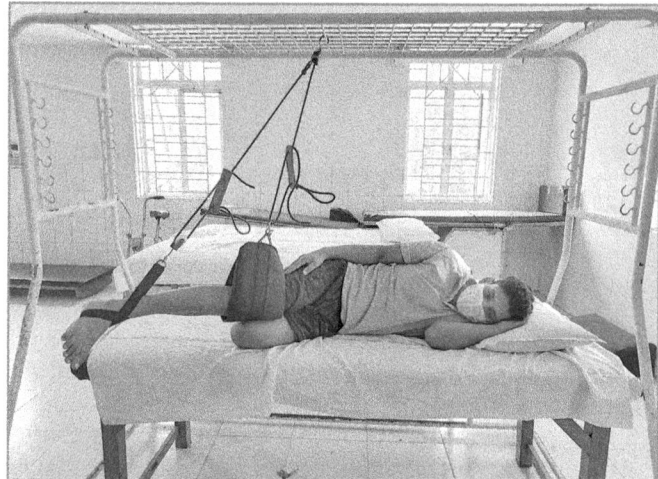

Fig. 1.144: Suspension therapy for hip flexion/extension.

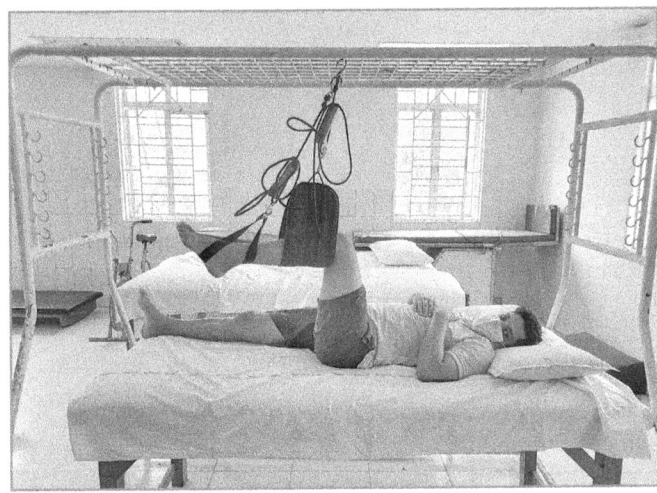 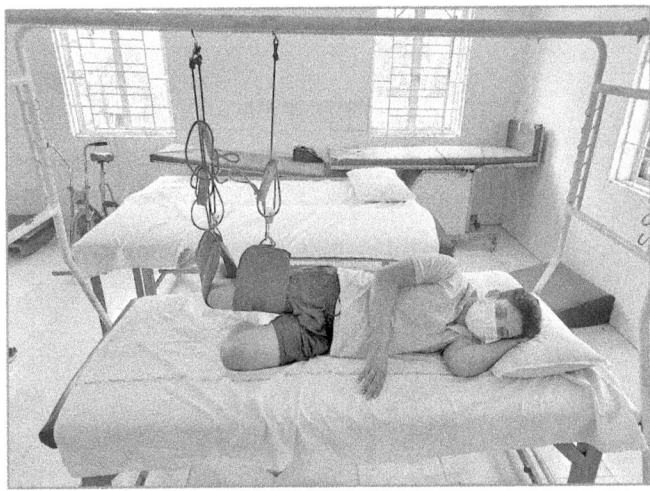

Fig. 1.145: Suspension therapy for hip rotation. **Fig. 1.146:** Suspension therapy for knee flexion/extension.

- ❖ **Knee joint: Flexion and extension (Fig. 1.146):**
  - *Position of the patient:* Side lying with hip slightly flexed and one or two pillows placed under the thigh.
  - *Fixation point:* Over the knee joint. Single sling is attached to the thigh and suspended from a point that is in line with the junction of proximal 1/3rd and distal 2/3rd of the thigh. A single single sling supporting the leg and the narrow sling supporting the ankle and foot are hung from wire mesh just above the axis of the knee joint.
- ❖ **Ankle joint:** It is rarely necessary to use suspension as in this case it is easier to perform the supported movements by using a polished board.

Hydrotherapy

INTRODUCTION

The term Hydrotherapy is coined from the Greek word—"Hydro" meaning "water" and "Therapeia" meaning "Healing". It is a method of using the physical aspect of water for medical and relaxing treatments. The buoyancy effect of water minimizes the effects of gravity on weight bearing joints, assists and resists muscle work, the hydrostatic pressure exerts a circumferential force that helps to reduce edema and stabilizes unstable joints, and the warmth of water enhances blood flow and induces muscle relaxation.

Hydrotherapy refers to the use of multi-depth immersion pools or tanks that facilitate the application of various established therapeutic interventions including stretching, joint mobilizations, strengthening, etc.

Water has an effect similar to a soothing massage on muscles by bringing more oxygen to the injured area. Movements that are extremely painful outside the water, can be conducted in water with minimum pain. Running, walking and floating in water have been found to be significantly effective.

PRINCIPLES OF HYDROTHERAPY

Hydrotherapy for treatment of diseases and disorders are based upon the properties of water and heat.

The properties of water that are used to assist or resist movement are as follows:

- **Buoyancy:** It is the upward force that works opposite to gravity when the body is placed in water. Buoyancy provides the patient with relative weightlessness and joint unloading allowing performance of active motion easily. It can be used to assist (when the body segment is made to move in a bottom to the top direction) or resist movement (when the body segment is made to move in the top to bottom direction).
- **Hydrostatic pressure:** It is the circumferential pressure exerted on the immersed objects inside water. This increased pressure reduces or limits effusion, assists venous return, centralizes peripheral blood flow.
- **Viscosity:** It is friction occurring between molecules of liquid resulting in resistance to flow. It creates resistance to all active movements.
- **Surface tension:** The surface of the fluid acts as a membrane under tension. Surface tension is measured as force per unit length. An extremity that moves through the surface will perform more work than if kept underwater.
- **Hydromechanics:** Hydromechanics is the physical properties and characteristics of the fluid in motion that affects movement. Its components include:
  - *Laminar flow:* These are the movements where all molecules move parallel to each other resulting in typically slow movements.
  - *Turbulent flow:* These are the movements where molecules do not move parallel to each other, resulting in typically faster movements.
- **Drag:** The cumulative effects of turbulence and fluid viscosity acting on an object in motion, which may be used to resist movements.
- **Warmth of water:** The properties of heat on body such as reduction of pain and spasm/spasticity, increase of metabolism, and nerve conduction velocity are used to achieve some desired therapeutic benefits in patients with diseases and disorders.

OBJECTIVES OF HYDROTHERAPY

Hydrotherapy has some prominent objectives, which are as follows:
- To relieve pain and swelling.
- To promote relaxation
- To increase range of motion
- To reduce muscle tone (spasticity)
- To strengthen muscles and enhance coordination stability and balance

CLINICAL APPLICATIONS OF HYDROTHERAPY

There are some conditions which require the treatment of hydrotherapy, they include:
- *Neck pain* and *back pain*
- *Head* and *spinal* injury sequel (except those having bladder and bowel incontinence)
- Cerebral palsy (children having no fear in water)
- Arthritic conditions (rheumatoid arthritis, ankylosing spondylitis, etc.)
- Sports injuries
- Amputees

- Orthopedic conditions
- Stroke sequel causing hemiparesis/quadriparesis
- Women during prenatal and postnatal stage.

SALIENT FEATURES OF HYDROTHERAPY POOL

The pool could be a stainless steel hydrotherapy pool, or a permanent concrete structure like a swimming pool **(Fig. 2.1)**. The swimming pool types has a floor with a slope which is shallow at one end and a deep at the other end. Hydrotherapy pools are often completely levelled with railings inside the pool to facilitate better physiotherapy.

The hydrotherapy pool room has a plant room, filtration system, and some kind of environmental control to provide air heating and dehumidification. The water temperature in the pool should be maintained at 28–30°C.

The water should be treated properly with disinfectants, filtration and heating. It should be tested in the laboratory to make sure and rule out that if there is no infection and risk of uprising infection.

Advantages of Hydrotherapy

There are certain collectible advantages of hydrotherapy which are as follows:
- It helps to handle the heaviest patients with great ease.
- It can treat cases that are traditionally difficult.
- It is applied to treat impairments like pain, swelling, decreased strength, and stiffness.
- It is used for treatment of disabilities to improve posture and mobility.
- It improves cardiovascular and respiratory functions.
- It positively influences overall as well as a local metabolism.
- It can easily be adapted to a patient's specific needs and can simply be applied in a progressive way from a nonweight bearing to a full weight bearing program.

Procedure of Treatment

The patient is advised to bring own costumes, swimming caps, etc. and should have a light tiffin before the hydrotherapy session. The contraindications for hydrotherapy such as fever, open wound, skin infections, epilepsy, etc. should be checked before each session. Patient should be asked to remove foot wear and take a shower before and after each hydrotherapy session. Patient should be advised to drink water before and after every hydrotherapy session. Individualized attention should be given to each patient in the pool. Use of floaters, and other exercise gadgets are made in the pool as required. The duration of each treatment session, is kept to about half an hour.

Therapeutic Effects and Uses of Hydrotherapy

- **Strengthening of muscle:** Water provides a remarkable environment to produce very fine exercise progression. Muscles are strengthened by resistance offered by upward force (buoyancy), turbulence force, etc. Even manual resistance can be applied along with these forces inside water.
  - *Uses:* Polyneuropathies.
- **Endurance training:** Exercises in water improves both cardiorespiratory and muscular endurance, hence considered as an important treatment modality for patients with poor endurance.
  - *Uses:* Ankylosing spondylitis.
- **To improve joint mobility:** Relief of pain and muscle spasm by the warmth of the water and by the support of buoyancy mobility of joints can be improved.
  - *Uses:* Polyarthritis like rheumatoid arthritis.
- **To improve co-ordination and balance:** The buoyancy of water relieves the patient from weight and makes the activities such as walking and step climbing easy. The hydrostatic pressure exerted on unstable joints produces a strong proprioceptive stimulation and helps in restoring stability of joints and balance of body.
  - *Uses:* Ataxic disorders like cerebellar ataxia.
- **For pain relief:** The enhanced joint movement due to augmentation of muscular activities, combined with the warmth of water improves circulation and enable removal of waste metabolites and improves nutrition. This phenomenon combined with the effect of reduction of muscle spasm helps in reduction of pain.
  - *Uses:* Low back pain.
- **For swelling reduction:** The hydrostatic pressure, combined with enhanced blood flow brought about by warmth of water and enhanced muscular contractions, help in reduction of swelling.
  - *Uses:* For stump edema.

CONTRAINDICATIONS AND PRECAUTIONS FOR HYDROTHERAPY

- **Contraindications:**
  - Infective wounds
  - Hyperpyrexia
  - Cardiac failure
  - Deep vein thrombosis

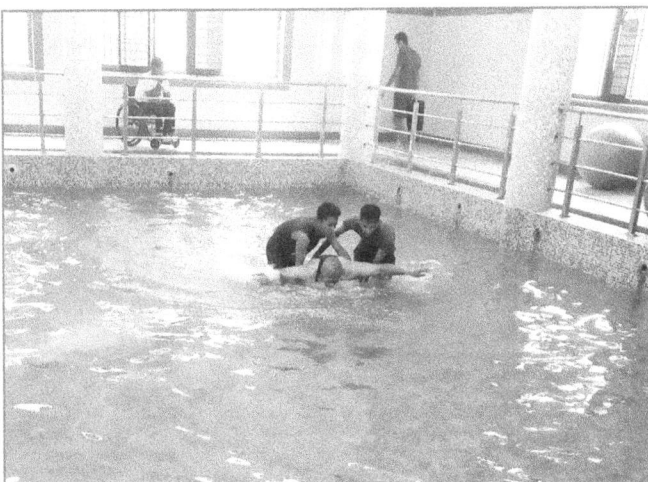

Fig. 2.1: The hydrotherapy pool.

- Gastrointestinal disorder
- Hypo- or hypertension
- Epilepsy
- Low vital lung capacity.

❖ **Precautions:**
- Mentally retarded
- Persons having fear for water
- Persons wearing contact lens
- Persons wearing hearing aids
- Persons with cardiorespiratory anomalies such as angina pectoris
- Small children.

Proprioceptive Neuromuscular Facilitation

INTRODUCTION

Proprioceptive neuromuscular facilitation (PNF) is a philosophy and a concept of treatment. It has been one of the most recognized treatment concepts in physiotherapy since the 1940s. Dr Herman Kabat and Margaret (Maggie) Knott started and continued to expand and develop the treatment techniques and procedures after their move to Vallejo, California in 1947. After Dorothy Voss joined the team in 1953, Maggie and Dorothy wrote the first PNF book that was published in 1956.

The technique can be understood from the following definitions:
- **Proprioceptive:** Having to do with any of the sensory receptors that give information concerning movement and position of the body.
- **Neuromuscular:** Involving the nerves and muscles.
- **Facilitation:** Making easier.

DEFINITION OF PROPRIOCEPTIVE NEUROMUSCULAR FACILITATION

Proprioceptive neuromuscular facilitation is a technique that involves stimulation of the proprioceptors for increasing the demand on the neuromuscular mechanism to obtain and facilitate its response for improving function.

The underlying philosophy of PNF signifies that all human beings, including those with disabilities, have untapped existing potential (Kabat1950), which could be unveiled by appropriate stimulation of the proprioceptors.

The primary goal of treatment using the technique is to assist the patients so that they can achieve their highest level of function, and to reach this highest level of function, the therapist integrates principles of *motor control* and *motor learning* and uses the International Classification of Functioning (ICF) model in the treatment.

BASIC PRINCIPLES OF PROPRIOCEPTIVE NEUROMUSCULAR FACILITATION (PNF)

- PNF as an integrated approach, is directed at the total human being, not just at a specific problem or body segment.
- It states that all human beings have potentials that are not fully developed.
- Based on the untapped existing potential of all patients, the therapist always focuses on mobilizing the patient's reserves.
- The treatment approach is always positive, reinforcing, and after using that the patient can actually perform, on a physical and psychological level.
- The technique recognizes that normal motor development proceeds in a cephalocaudal and proximodistal direction.
- It recognizes that early motor behavior is dominated by the reflex activity.
- The technique believes that, growth of motor behavior has some cyclic trends as evidenced by the shifts between *flexor* and extensor *dominances*.
- It identifies that goal-directed activity is made up of reversing movements.
- It states that normal movement and posture depend on "synergism" and a balanced interaction of antagonists.
- It states that developing motor behavior is expressed in an orderly sequence of total patterns of movement and posture.
- It states that normal motor development has an orderly sequence but lacks a step-by-step quality; overlapping occurs.
- It states that improvement of the motor ability depends on motor learning.
- Frequency of stimulation and repetition of activity are used for the promotion and retention of motor learning and for the development of strength and endurance.
- Goal-directed activities, coupled with facilitation techniques, are used to hasten learning of total patterns of walking and of self-care activities.

BASIC NEUROPHYSIOLOGIC PRINCIPLES OF PROPRIOCEPTIVE NEUROMUSCULAR FACILITATION

The work of Sir Charles Sherrington played a significant role in the development of the techniques of PNF. The neurophysiological principles abstracted from the work of Sherrington are:
- **After discharge:** The effect of stimulus continues after the stimulus stops. The feeling of increased power that comes after a static muscle contraction is a result of after discharge.

- **Temporal summation:** A succession of weak stimuli applied to the neuromuscular system combine to cause excitation of the said system.
- **Spatial summation:** Weak stimuli applied simultaneously to different areas of the body reinforce each other (summate) to cause excitation. This when combines with temporal summation produce increased activity of the neuromuscular system.
- **Irradiation:** This is the spreading and increased strength of a response that occur when either the number of stimuli or the strength of the stimuli is increased.
- **Successive induction:** An increased excitation of the agonist muscles follows the stimulation (contraction) of their antagonists. Techniques involving reversal of antagonists make use of this property.
- **Reciprocal innervations (reciprocal inhibition):** Contraction of the agonist muscles is accompanied by simultaneous inhibition of their antagonists. Relaxation techniques make use of this principle.

PHILOSOPHY OF PROPRIOCEPTIVE NEUROMUSCULAR FACILITATION

- Positive approach with a strong start, achievable tasks are set up for success in a pain less environment.
- A functional approach (ICF), which includes the treatment on body structure and activity level to promote participation.
- Mobilizes patient's potential by intensive training, active participation, motor learning and self-training.
- The technique considers the person as a whole, with his/her environmental, personal, physical and emotional factors.
- The technique makes use of principles of motor control and motor learning, uses repetition in different contexts, and respects stages of motor control and variability of practice.

BASIC PROCEDURES OF PROPRIOCEPTIVE NEUROMUSCULAR FACILITATION

- **Body position and mechanics:** The therapist's body should be in line with the desired motion or force (**Fig. 3.1**). The resistance comes from the therapist's body, while the arms and hands remain relaxed. By using bodyweight, the therapist can give prolonged resistance without any fatigue.
- **Manual contact:** Pressure of the physiotherapist's manual contact on the patient provides a means of applying maximal resistance to movement in patterns. Touch contributes to facilitation by stimulating the exteroceptors. Manual contacts must be:
  - *Purposeful:* Pressure must be firm so that the patient must be aware of it.
  - *Directional:* Pressure is applied only in the direction of the movement.
  - *Comfortable:* Manual contacts which produce painful stimuli must be avoided.
  - *Grip:* A lumbrical grip (**Figs. 3.2 A and B**) is used by the therapist.
- **Communication/command:** The therapist gives sensory cues by: touching, telling, and visual demonstration. The verbal command tells the patient what to do, and when to do the movements.

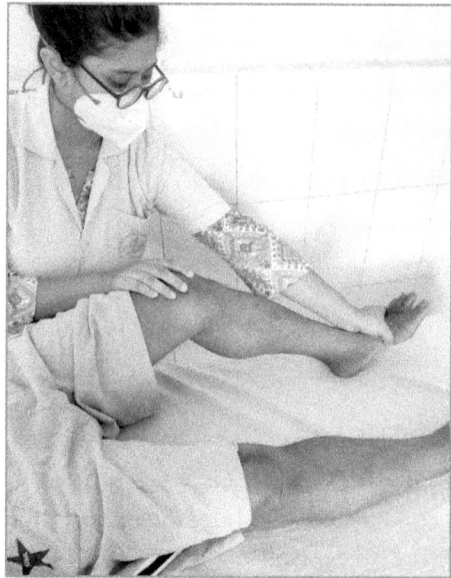

Fig. 3.1: Position of the therapist for applying proprioceptive neuromuscular facilitation (PNF).

- **Quick stretch:** It facilitates muscle contraction and associated synergistic muscles. It is used as a stimulus to initiate voluntary motion, enhance quicker response in weak muscles, and increase strength of muscles.
- **Traction and approximation:** Traction (separation of joint surfaces) is used to stimulate flexion movements, whereas approximation (compression of joint surfaces) is used to facilitate extension movements, therefore promoting stability and stimulating postural reflexes.
- **Maximal resistance:** It is the greatest amount of resistance that can be applied to an active contraction allowing full range of motion (ROM) to occur or to an isometric contraction without defeating or breaking the patient's hold. This facilitates muscle contraction, increases motor control, and learning, increases muscle strength and helps in the gain of awareness and direction of movements.
- **Normal timing:** Timing is sequencing of motion. It is the sequence of muscle contraction, which occurs in any motor activity, resulting in coordinated movement production. In normal developments, proximal control is evident before distal control, however, after coordinated purposeful movements have been acquired, timing and sequential contraction of muscles occur from distal to proximal. Hence normal timing is from distal to proximal.
- **Timing for emphasis:** Timing for emphasis involves changing the normal sequencing of motions to emphasize a particular muscle or desired activity. Kabat (1947) wrote that prevention of motion in a stronger synergist will redirect the energy of that contraction into a weaker muscle (**Fig. 3.3**). The best results come when the strong muscles score at least "good" in strength.
- **Irradiation and reinforcement:** Irradiation is spread of response from stronger muscles to weak muscles on stimulation. Reinforcement is to strengthen by fresh

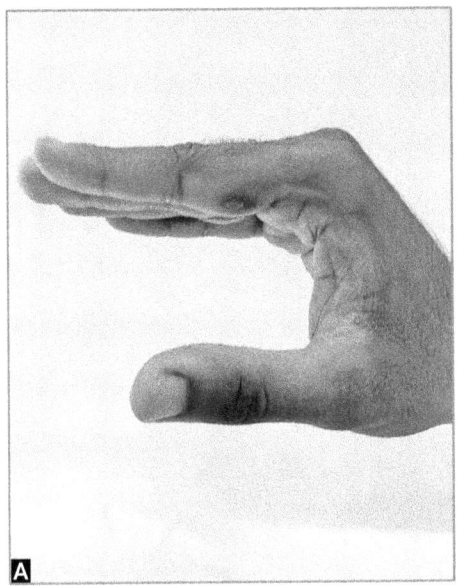 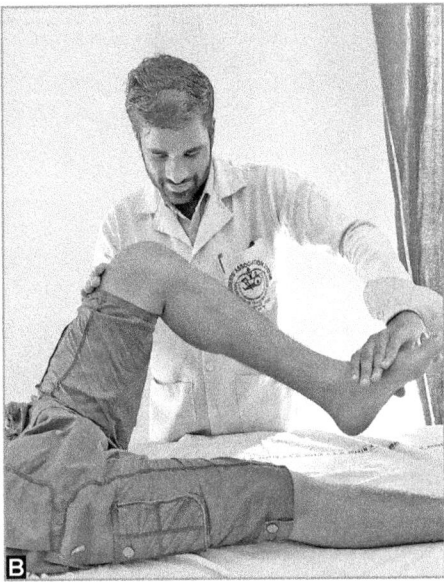

Figs. 3.2 A and B: (A) Lumbrical grip. (B) Manual contact using the lumbrical grip.

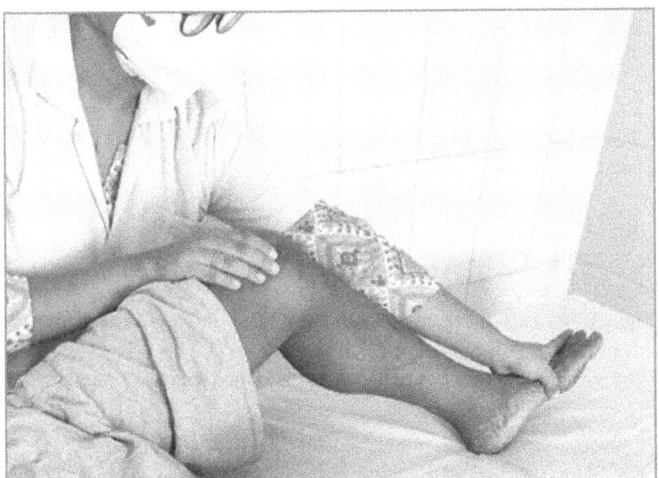

Fig. 3.3: Timing for emphasis–the strong motions of the hip and knee are blocked and the dorsiflexion-eversion of the ankle is promoted.

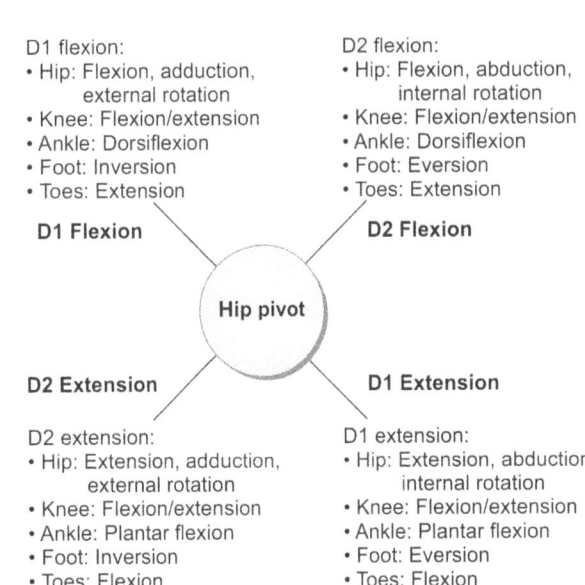

D1 flexion:
- Hip: Flexion, adduction, external rotation
- Knee: Flexion/extension
- Ankle: Dorsiflexion
- Foot: Inversion
- Toes: Extension

D2 flexion:
- Hip: Flexion, abduction, internal rotation
- Knee: Flexion/extension
- Ankle: Dorsiflexion
- Foot: Eversion
- Toes: Extension

D2 extension:
- Hip: Extension, adduction, external rotation
- Knee: Flexion/extension
- Ankle: Plantar flexion
- Foot: Inversion
- Toes: Flexion

D1 extension:
- Hip: Extension, abduction, internal rotation
- Knee: Flexion/extension
- Ankle: Plantar flexion
- Foot: Eversion
- Toes: Flexion

Fig. 3.4: PNF diagonal patterns for lower limbs.

addition. The therapist reinforces weak muscles by the amount of resistance given to stronger muscles.

The patterns of motion for proprioceptive neuromuscular facilitation are mass movement patterns, as mass movement is a characteristics of normal motor activity, which is used in accordance with Beevor's axioms, that the brain knows nothing of individual muscle action, but knows only of movements.

❖ **Patterns of facilitation:** Mass movement patterns are used as the basis for all the techniques of PNF as these movements are similar to the normal functional movements. The pattern of movement is spiral or diagonal (D1/D2) as shown in **Figures 3.4 and 3.5**, and they are observed in activities of everyday use such as taking the hand to the mouth, reaching for food, walking, etc.

The upper extremity, lower extremity, head/neck/upper trunk, and lower trunk patterns are described below:

A. Upper extremity patterns:
- *D1 flexion (D1 fl):* Shoulder flexion-adduction-external rotation, elbow flexion/ extension, forearm supination, wrist/fingers and thumb flexion. **(Fig. 3.6A)**.
- *D1 extension (D1 ex):* Shoulder extension-abduction-internal rotation, elbow flexion/ extension, forearm pronation, wrist/fingers and thumb extension. **(Fig. 3.6B)**.
- *D2 flexion (D2 fl):* Shoulder flexion-abduction-external rotation, elbow flexion/extension, forearm supination, wrist, fingers, and thumb extension. **(Fig. 3.7A)**
- *D2 extension (D2 ex):* Shoulder extension-adduction-internal rotation, elbow flexion/extension, forearm pronation, wrist, fingers and thumb flexion **(Fig. 3.7B)**.

D1 flexion:
- Shoulder: Flexion, adduction, external rotation
- Elbow: Flexion/extension
- Forearm: Supination
- Wrist/fingers/thumb: Flexion

D2 flexion:
- Shoulder: Flexion, abduction, external rotation
- Elbow: Flexion/extension
- Forearm: Supination.
- Wrist, fingers and thumb: Extension

D2 extension:
- Shoulder: Extension, adduction, internal rotation
- Elbow: Flexion/Extension
- Forearm: Pronation
- Wrist, fingers and thumb: Flexion

D1 extension:
- Shoulder: Extension, abduction, internal rotation
- Elbow: Flexion/extension
- Forearm: Pronation
- Wrist/fingers/thumb: Extension

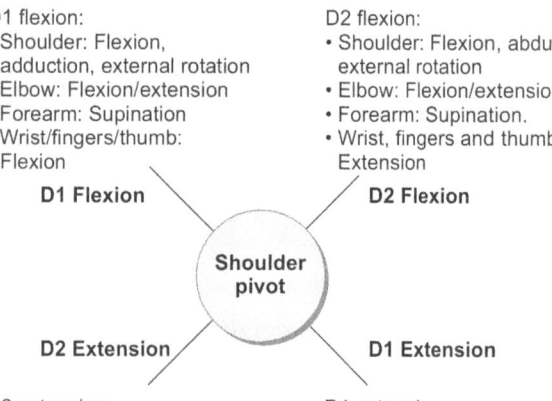

Fig. 3.5: PNF diagonal patterns for upper limbs.

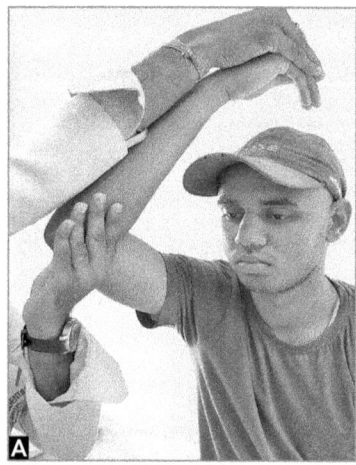

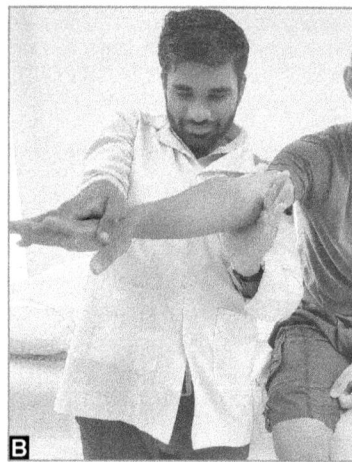

Figs. 3.6A and B: (A) D1 flexion with elbow flexion; (B) D1 extension with elbow extension.

Note: The pattern can be with elbow flexion or elbow extension, such as D1 flexion with elbow flexion/D1 flexion with elbow extension, D1 extension with elbow flexion/D1 extension with elbow extension-the patterns are selected and trained as per need of the client, i.e., -D1 flexion with elbow flexion is selected for training the task of taking food to mouth, combing hair, etc., and D1 extension with elbow flexion/ extension can be selected for the task of reaching for objects.

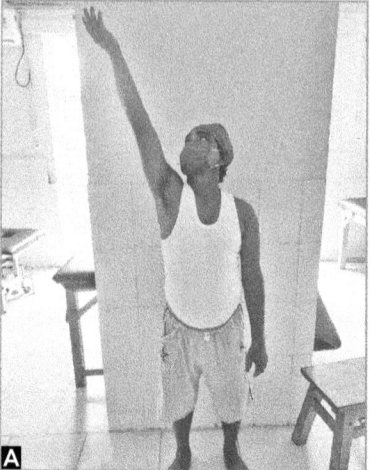

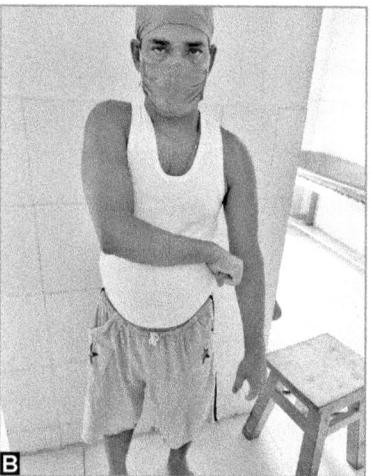

Figs. 3.7A and B: (A) D2 flexion with elbow extension; (B) D2 extension with elbow flexion.
Note: Like D1 pattern, D2 pattern can be performed with both elbow flexion and extension as per need.

B. Lower extremity patterns:
- *D1 flexion (D1 fl):* Hip flexion-adduction-external rotation, knee flexion/extension, ankle dorsiflexion, foot inversion, toes extension **(Fig. 3.8A)**.
- *D1 extension (D1 ex):* Hip extension-abduction-internal rotation, knee flexion/extension, ankle plantar flexion, foot eversion, toes flexion **(Fig. 3.8B)**.
- *D2 flexion (D2fl):* Hip flexion-abduction-internal rotation, knee flexion/extension, ankle dorsiflexion, foot eversion, toes extension **(Fig. 3.9A)**
- *D2 extension (D2 ex):* Hip extension-adduction-external rotation, knee flexion/extension, ankle plantar flexion, foot inversion, toes flexion **(Fig. 3.9B)**.

C. Head/neck/upper trunk patterns:
- Flexion with rotation to left (D fl.L) **(Figs. 3.10A and 3.11A)**.
- Extension with rotation to right (D ex. R) **(Figs. 3.10B and 3.11B)**.
- Flexion with rotation to right (D fl. R) **(Fig. 3.12A)**.
- Extension with rotation to left (D ex. L) **(Fig. 3.12B)**.
- Rotation to left (Ro. L).
- Rotation to right (Ro. R).

Chapter 3: Proprioceptive Neuromuscular Facilitation

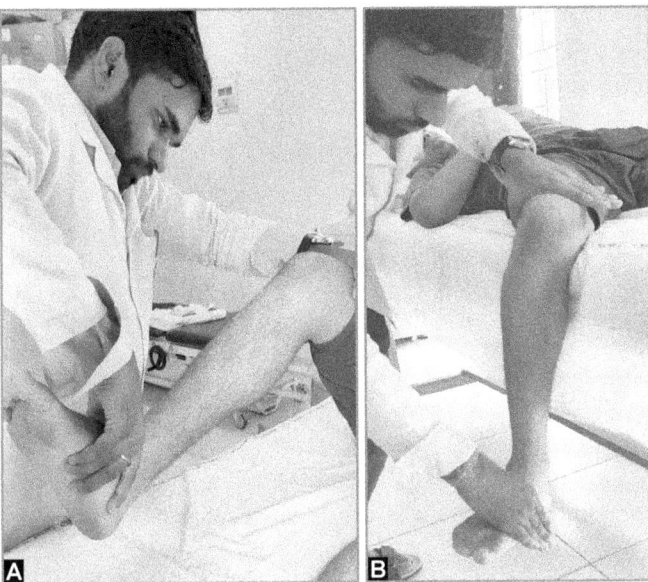

Figs. 3.8A and B: (A) D1 flexion with knee flexion; (B) D1 extension with knee flexion.

Note: The pattern can be with knee flexion or knee extension, such as D1 flexion with knee flexion/D1 flexion with knee extension, D1 extension with knee flexion/D1 extension with knee extension–the patterns are selected and trained as per need of the client, i.e., D1 flexion with knee flexion is selected for training the task clearing ground in the swing phase and D1 extension with knee extension can be selected for the task of heel striking on ground in stance phase.

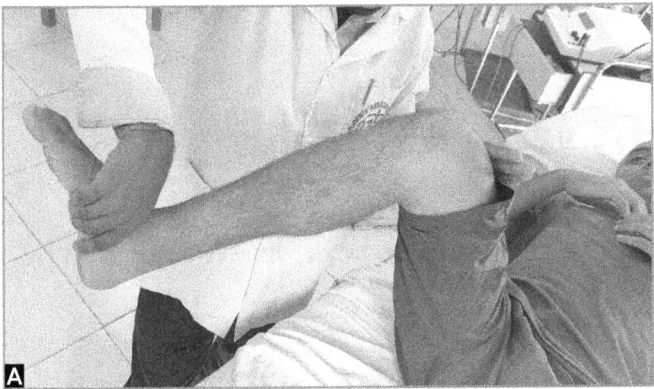

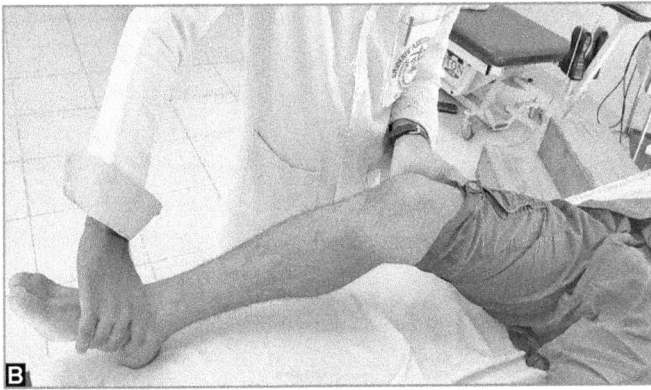

Figs. 3.9A and B: (A) D2 flexion with knee flexion; (B) D2 extension with knee extension.
Note: Like D1 pattern, D2 pattern can be performed with both knee flexion and extension as per need.

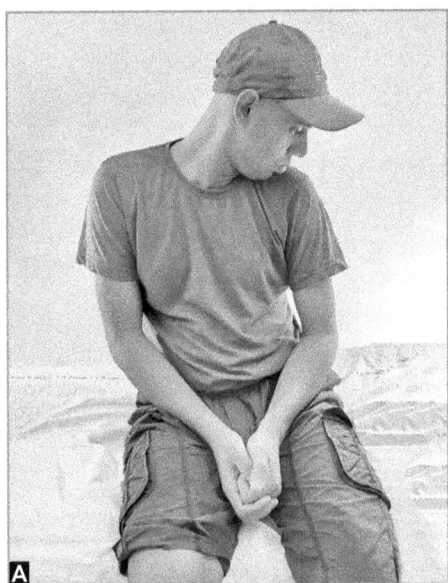

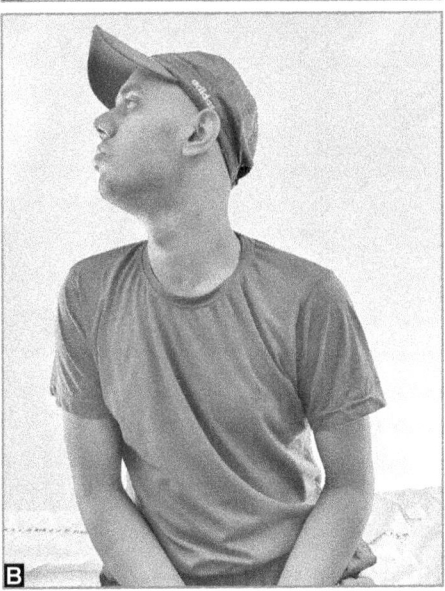

Figs. 3.10A and B: Neck pattern: (A) Flexion and rotation to left; (B) Extension and rotation to right.

D. Lower trunk patterns:
- Flexion with rotation to right (D fl. R) **(Fig. 3.13A)**.
- Extension with rotation to left (D ex. L) **(Fig. 3.13B)**.
- Flexion with rotation to left (D fl. L).
- Extension with rotation to right (D ex. R).
- Rotation to left (Ro. L) **(Fig. 3.14)**.
- Rotation to right (Ro. R).

TECHNIQUES OF PROPRIOCEPTIVE NEUROMUSCULAR FACILITATION (PNF)

- ❖ **Rhythmic initiation:**
  - **Characterization:** Rhythmic motion of the limb or body through the desired range, starting with passive motion and progressing to active resisted movement.
  - *Goals:*

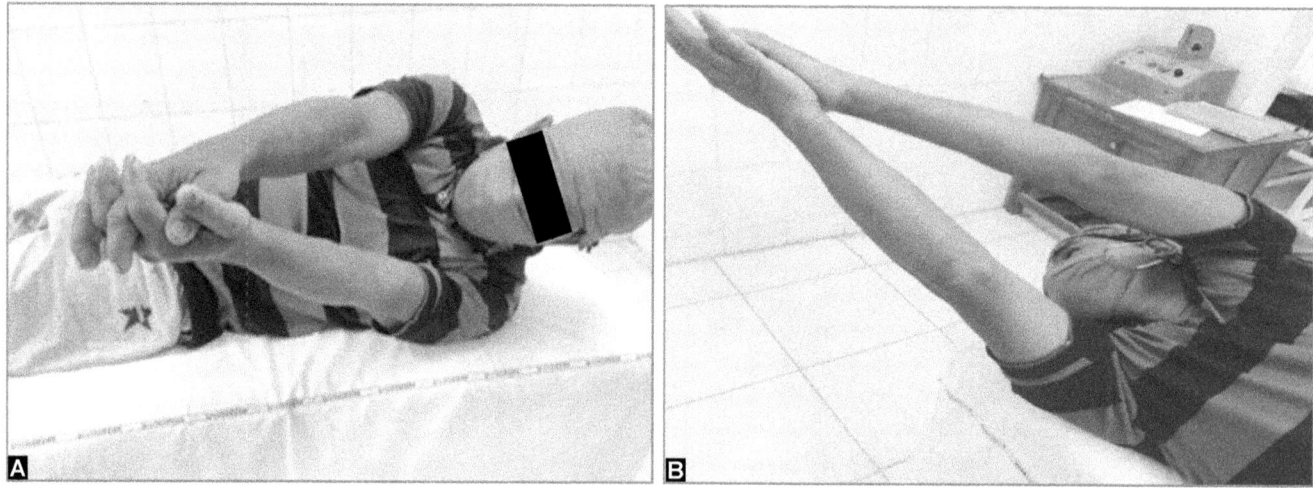

Figs. 3.11A and B: Head/neck/upper trunk pattern in lying: (A) Flexion and rotation to left; (B) Extension and rotation to right.

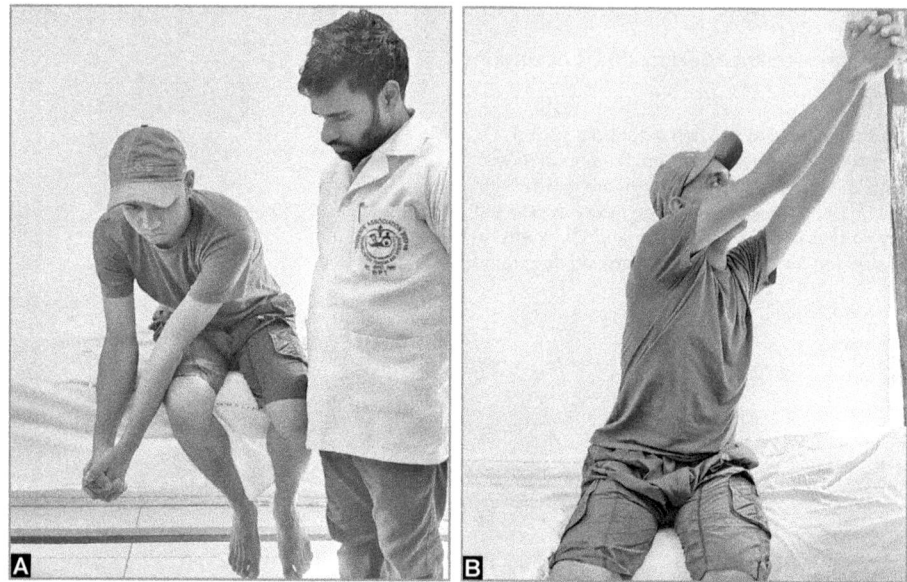

Figs. 3.12A and B: Head/neck/upper trunk pattern in sitting: (A) Flexion and rotation to right; (B) Extension and rotation to left.

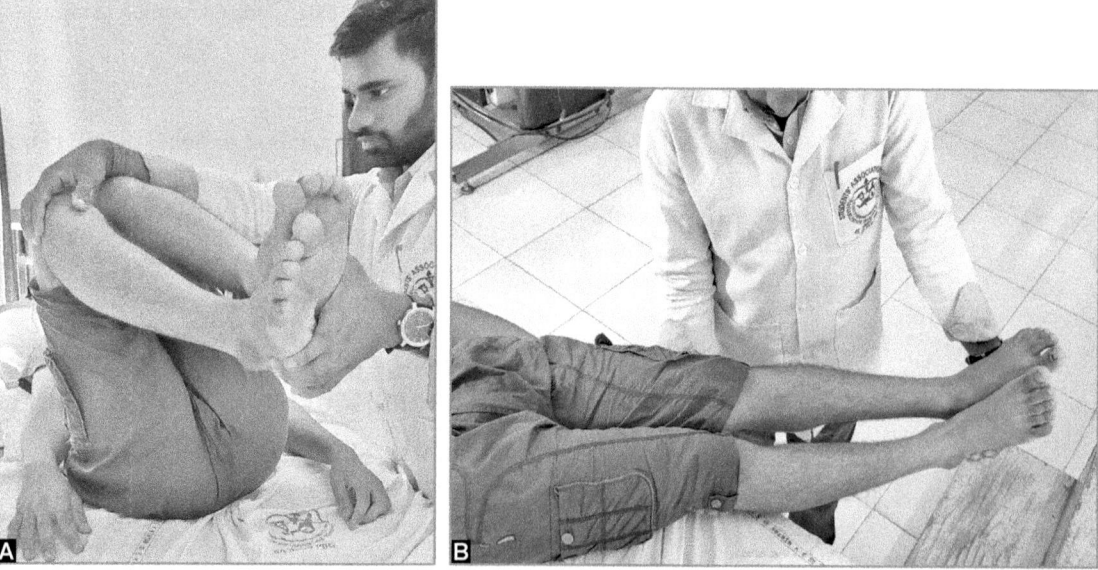

Figs. 3.13A and B: Lower trunk pattern: (A) Flexion and rotation to right; (B) Extension and rotation to left.

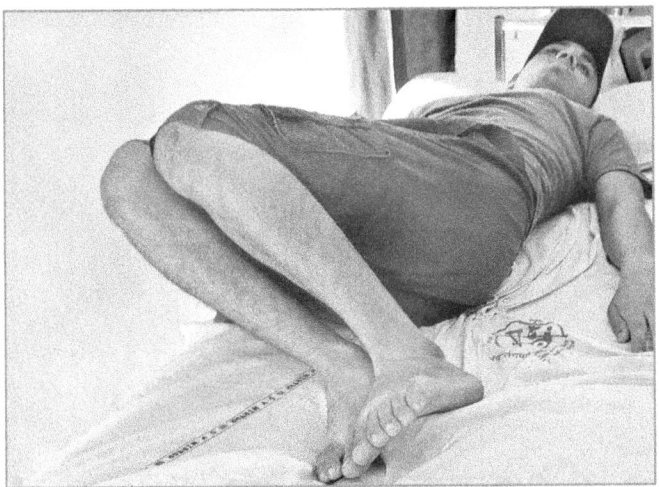

Fig. 3.14: Lower trunk rotation (Left-right).

- » To aid in initiation of motion
- » To improve coordination and sense of motion
- » To teach motion
- *Indications:*
  - » Difficulties in initiating motion.
  - » Conditions like Parkinson's disease, where movement is too slow (bradykinesia).
  - » Uncoordinated or dysrhythmic motion, i.e., ataxia and rigidity.
  - » To regulate or normalize muscle tone.
- *Procedure:* The therapist starts by moving the body segment passively, through the range of motion, using the speed of the verbal command to set the rhythm. The patient is asked to begin working actively in the desired direction. The return motion is done by the therapist. As movement is produced, the therapist resists the active movement, maintaining the rhythm with the verbal commands. At the end of the session, it is required that the patient should make the movement independently.

❖ **Combination of isotonics:**
- *Characterization:*
  - » Combined concentric, eccentric, and stabilizing contractions of one group of muscles (agonists) without relaxation.
  - » Treatment is started at a range, where the patient has most strength or best coordination.
- *Goals:*
  - » To achieve active control of movement and coordination.
  - » To promote functional training involving eccentric control of movement.
- *Indications:*
  - » Lack of coordination or the ability to move in the desired direction.
  - » Decreased eccentric control.
- *Procedure:* The therapist resists the patient's movements actively through the desired range of motion (concentric contraction). At the end of motion, the therapist tells the patient to stay in that position (stabilizing contraction). When stability is attained the therapist tells the patient to allow the part to be moved slowly back to the starting position (eccentric contraction). There is no relaxation between the different types of muscle activities and the therapist's hands remain on the same surface.

❖ **Reversal of antagonists:** These techniques are based on Sherrington's principle of successive induction (Sherrington 1961). They are of the following types:

Dynamic reversal/Slow reversal: Active motion changing from one direction (agonist) to the opposite (antagonist) without pause or relaxation.
- *Goal:*
  - » To increase active range of motion.
  - » To increase strength and endurance.
  - » To decrease muscle tone.
- *Indications:*
  - » Decreased active range of motion.
  - » Weakness of the agonistic muscles.
  - » Relaxation of hypertonic muscles.
- *Procedure:* The therapist resists the patient's movements in one direction, usually the stronger or better direction. As the end of the desired range of motion approaches, the therapist reverses the grip on the distal portion of the moving segment and gives a command to prepare for the change of direction. At the end of the desired movement, the therapist gives the action command to reverse direction, without relaxation and gives resistance to the new motion starting with the distal part. When the patient begins moving in the opposite direction the therapist reverses the proximal grip so all resistance opposes the new direction **(Figs. 3.15A to C)**.

❖ **Stabilizing reversals:** Alternating isotonic contractions opposed by enough resistance to prevent motion. The command is dynamic command ("push against my hands", or "do not let me push you") and the therapist allows only a very small movement.
- *Goal:*
  - » To increase stability and balance, increase muscle strength and coordination between *agonist* and *antagonist*.
  - » To increase muscle strength.
- *Procedure:* The therapist gives resistance to the patient, starting in the strongest direction while asking the patient to oppose the force. Very little motion is allowed. Approximation or traction should be used to increase stability. When the patient is fully resisting the force the therapist moves one hand and begins to give resistance in another direction. After the patient responds to the new resistance the therapist moves the other hand to resist the new direction.

❖ **Rhythmic stabilization:** Alternating isometric contractions against resistance to agonists and antagonists. No motion is desired and only stability is intended.
- *Goal:*
  - » Increase muscle strength and decrease pain. Increase stability and balance.
  - » To decrease muscle tone.

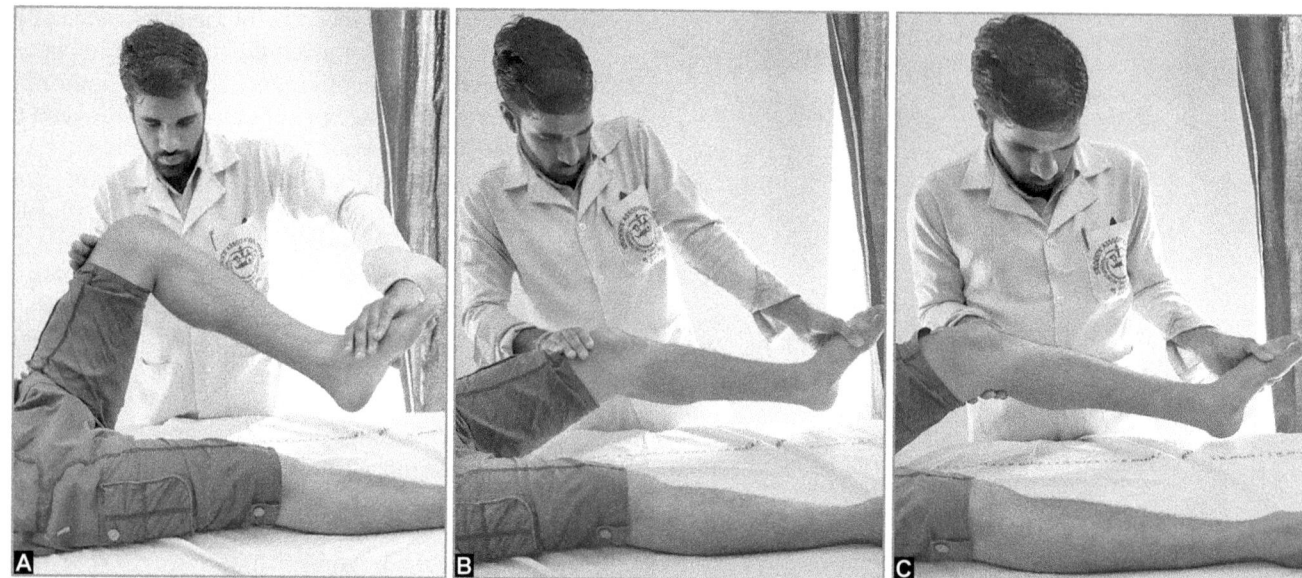

Figs. 3.15 A to C: Dynamic reversal/slow reversal of the leg diagonal: Hip flexion-adduction with knee flexion into hip extension-abduction with knee extension. (A) Resisting flexion adduction; (B) Distal grip changed and motion into extension-abduction started; (C) Resisting extension abduction.

- *Procedure:* The therapist resists an isometric contraction of the agonistic muscle group. The patient maintains the position of the part without trying to move. The resistance is increased slowly as the patient builds a matching force. When the patient is responding fully, the therapist moves one hand to begin resisting the antagonistic motion at the distal part. Neither the therapist nor the patient relaxes as the resistance changes. Traction or approximation to the joints is applied as required. The reversals are repeated as often as needed. While applying the procedure. The therapist uses commands such as "stay there", don't try to move **(Fig. 3.16)**.

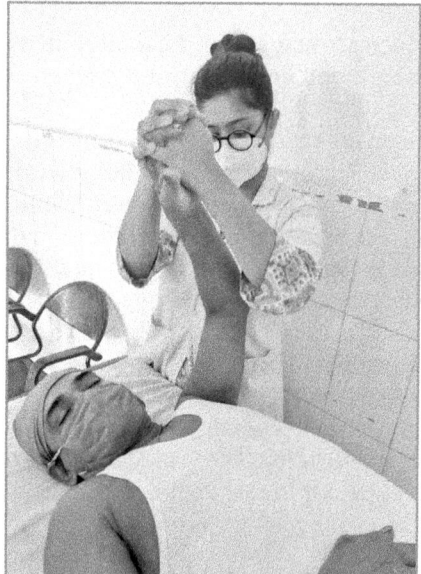

Fig. 3.16: Rhythmic stabilization of the shoulder in the diagonal of flexion-abduction/extension-adduction.

❖ **Repeated stretch (repeated contraction):**
  Repeated stretch from beginning of the range: The stretch reflex is elicited from muscles under the tension of elongation.
  – *Procedure:*
    » Lengthened muscle tension = stretch stimulus
    » Lengthened muscle tension + tap = stretch reflex
    The therapist gives a preparatory command while fully elongating the muscles in the pattern. Particular attention is given to the rotation. A quick "tap" is given to lengthen (stretch) the muscles further and evoke the stretch reflex. At the same time as the stretch reflex, a command is given to link the patient's voluntary effort to contract the stretched muscles with the reflex response. The resulting reflex and voluntary muscle contraction is resisted.
  – *Goal:*
    » To facilitate initiation of movement.
    » To increase active range of motion.
    » To increase muscle strength.
    » To guide motion in the desired direction.
    Repeated stretch through the range: The stretch reflex is elicited from muscles under the tension of contraction. The therapist resists a pattern of motion so that all the muscles are contracting and tense. The movement can start with an initial stretch reflex. A preparatory command is subsequently given to coordinate the stretch reflex, with a new and increased effort by the patient. At the same time, the therapist slightly stretches the muscles by momentarily giving too much resistance. A new and stronger muscle contraction is asked for and is resisted. The stretch reflex is repeated to redirect the motion as the patient moves through the range. The patient must be allowed

to move before the next stretch reflex is given and must not relax or reverse the direction of movement during the stretch.
  – *Goal:*
    » To increase active range of motion.
    » To increase muscle strength.
    » To prevent or reduce fatigue.
    » To guide motion in the desired direction.
* **Contract-relax/Hold-relax (direct treatment):** Resisted isotonic/ isometric contraction of the restricting muscles (antagonists) followed by relaxation and movement into the increased range.
  – *Goal:*
    » To increase range of motion.
  – *Procedure:* The therapist or the patient moves the joint or body segment to the end of the passive range of motion. The therapist asks the patient for a strong contraction (the contraction should be held at least for 5–8 seconds) of the restricting muscle or pattern. A maximal contraction in the most lengthened position of the muscle chain will provoke a structural change in the actin-myosin complex. After sufficient time, the therapist tells the patient to relax. The joint or body part is repositioned, either actively by the patient or passively by the therapist, to the new limit of the passive range. Active motion is performed by the patient at the new range and is resisted by the therapist. The technique is repeated until no more range is gained **(Fig. 3.17)**.
* **Contract–relax (indirect treatment):** The technique uses contraction of the agonistic muscles instead of the shortened muscles **(Fig. 3.18)**.
  – *Goal:*
    » To increase range of motion.
  – *Indication:* The indirect method is performed, when the contraction of the range limiting muscle is too painful or too weak to produce an effective contraction.

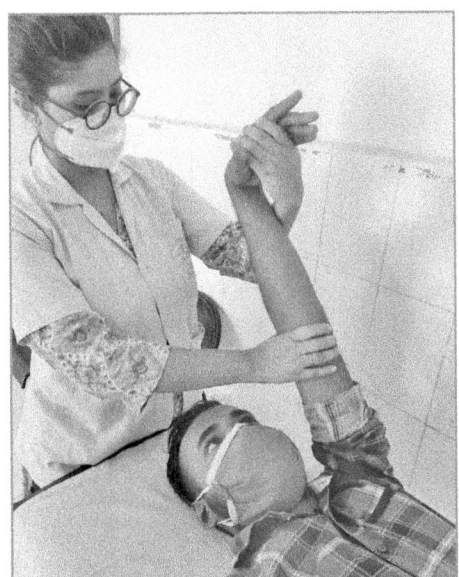

Fig. 3.17: Hold-relax or contract-Relax: Direct treatment for shortened shoulder extensor and adductor muscles.

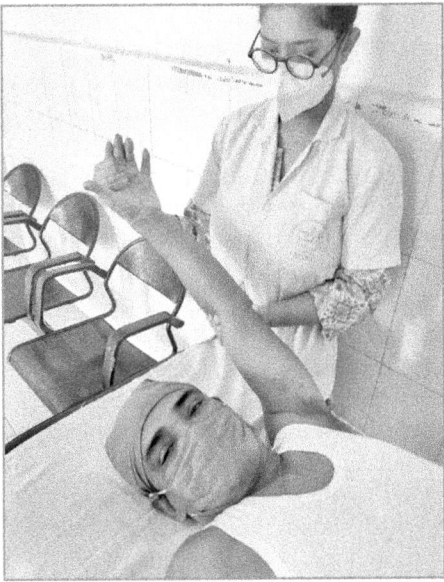

Fig. 3.18: Hold-relax or contract-relax: Indirect treatment for shortened shoulder extensor and adductor muscles.

* **Replication:** A technique to facilitate motor learning of functional activities. Teaching the patient the outcome of a movement or activity is important for functional work (for example sports) and self-care activities. The patient is placed in the "end" position of the activity where all the agonist muscles are shortened. The patient holds that position while the therapist resists all the components of movements. All the basic procedures are used to facilitate the patient's muscles. The patient is then asked to relax. The patient is then moved passively a short distance back in the opposite direction. Then he/she is asked to return to the end position. For each replication of the movement the patient is moved to the starting position (beginning of the movement), and movements are challenged through a greater range of motion. In the end, the patient should perform the activity or motion alone, without facilitation or manual contact by the therapist.
  – *Goal:*
    » Teach the patient the end position (outcome) of the movement.
    » Assess the patient's ability to sustain a contraction when the agonist muscles are shortened.

CLINICAL APPLICATION OF PROPRIOCEPTIVE NEUROMUSCULAR FACILITATION

1. **Stimulation of vital functions:** Proprioceptive neuromuscular facilitation may be specifically applied to facilitate motions of the parts necessary or responsible for vital functions such as:
   – *Respiration/Breathing:* Techniques of proprioceptive neuromuscular facilitation can be applied to stimulate breathing and to strengthen the muscles responsible for breathing.
   The patterns helpful for inspiration are:

a. Neck extension
b. Upper and lower trunk extension
c. Flexor patterns of upper limbs

The patterns responsible for expiration are:
a. Neck flexion
b. Upper and lower trunk flexion
c. Extensor patterns of the upper extremities

The neck and trunk patterns combined with bilateral asymmetrical upper extremity patterns (chopping and lifting) and bilateral symmetrical upper extremity patterns promote breathing.

Stimulation of muscles of respiration such as the diaphragm and intercostals can be facilitated using the technique. The accessory muscles that help in deep respiration can also be facilitated.

- *Swallowing:* PNF is used to promote movement of tongue, lips, and to stimulate the gag reflex (stimulation of the gag reflex is helpful, because it demands response of the pharyngeal muscles with the elevation of the soft palate, which is automatically followed by a swallowing response).

2. **To facilitate micturition and defecation:** The voluntary performance and control of micturition and defecation may be enhanced by performance of related patterns of facilitation against maximal resistance. The emptying of bowel and bladder can be promoted through flexor patterns of the lower limbs and lower trunk. However stopping of the bladder and bowel emptying can be achieved through extensor patterns of lower extremities and lower trunk. The muscles of perineal region could be facilitated through performance of bilaterally symmetrical extension-adduction-external rotation patterns of the lower limbs.

3. **To promote movement of eyeball:** The neck and upper trunk patterns promote the movement of the eye ball, for example, neck extension and rotation pattern enhances upward and lateral movement of the eye ball. PNF can also be used for the treatment of nystagmus, where decrements in the movement of the eye balls are emphasized for stabilization and visual tracking.

4. **To promote facial motion:** This helps in the promotion of facial motion with an ease.

5. **To reduce muscle tone:** As PNF patterns like D2 flexion with elbow extension in upper limb produces movements in an antispastic direction, hence reduces spasticity.

6. **To develop posture and balance:** Rhythmic stabilization technique help to promote postural stability, whereas the limb and trunk patterns help to restore balance.

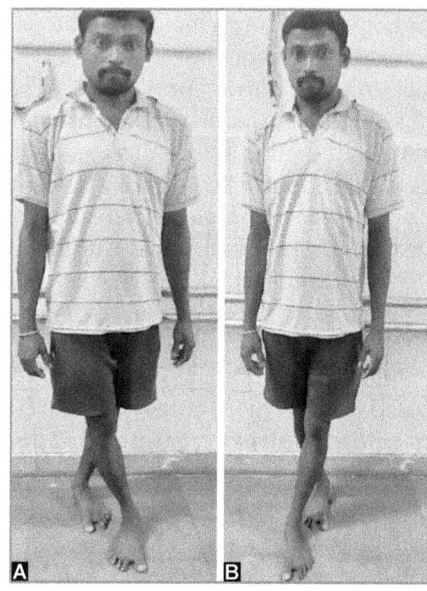

Figs. 3.20A and B: The braiding pattern.

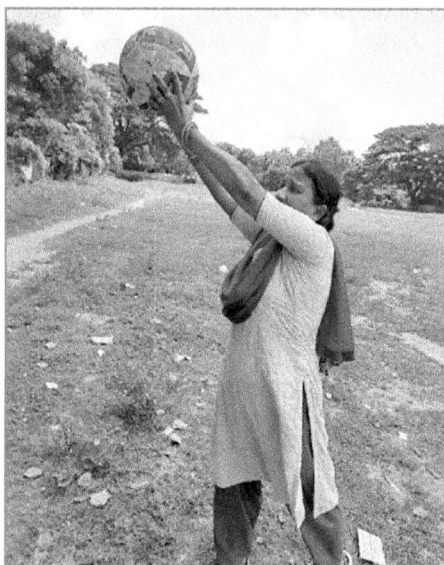

Fig. 3.19: The chopping pattern involving D2 flexion pattern in right upper limb and D1 flexion pattern in left upper limb.

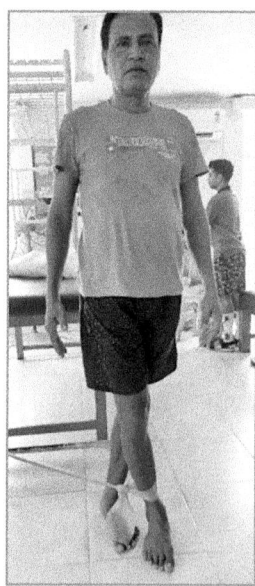

Fig. 3.21: Braiding with resistance.

7. **To promote mobility on bed:** In order to promote a smooth mobility on bed such as rolling, creeping, crawling as well as mobility out of bed like walking, where the flexor and extensor patterns of lower limbs are used in combination with neck and trunk patterns. The technique can be used to develop motor milestones in children with cerebral palsy and developmental delay.
8. **To improve functions:** For smooth functioning such as reaching for objects with the hand in an anterior direction, where D1 extension pattern of upper limb is used. For taking food to mouth, combing hair, etc., D1 flexion pattern with elbow flexion is used.

The chopping pattern which utilizes three dimensional movements referred to as spiral and diagonal patterns are used to improve activities like running, throwing, changing directions etc. It challenges the individual's ability to maintain spine and hip position in all three planes of movement, while transferring force between upper and lower body. The chop exercise, commonly used in functional training, utilizes both D1 and D2 PNF patterns for the upper extremity **(Fig. 3.19)**.

Braiding pattern/technique: This traditional PNF pattern involving cross over steppings of the lower extremities is used in functional training for the lower extremity **(Figs. 3.20A and B)**. This movement requires both D1 and D2 patterning from each hip when performing multiple steps. In order to increase difficulty in the PNF patterning, resistance bands can be used **(Fig. 3.21)**.

Normal Human Locomotion, Walking Aids, and Gait Training

NORMAL HUMAN LOCOMOTION

Normal human locomotion is the series of rhythmic alternating movements of the trunk and extremities, resulting in a forward progression of center of gravity. It is a cyclic motion of the body, called the *gait cycle*, which is measured from heel strike to heel strike of the same limb. The gait cycle consists of the following phases such as, stance phase and swing phase as shown in **Figure 4.1A**. There is also a period of double support, that occurs twice throughout one gait cycle. The relative contribution of different phases in the gait cycle are:
1. Stance phase: 60% of the gait cycle.
2. Swing phase: 40% of the gait cycle.
3. Double support: 20% of the gait cycle.

Biomechanics of normal gait: This has two components such as:
1. **Kinetics:** It is defined as the forces acting on the body, that are responsible for the movement. The factors are:
   - Forces acting on the foot by the supporting surface (Ground reaction force).
   - Forces acting in the joints.
   - Forces produced by the contracting muscles.
   - Moments produced by the muscles crossing the joints.
   - Mechanical power generated/absorbed by the muscles.
   - Energy pattern of the body while walking.
2. **Kinematics:** This is the term used to describe movements, without considering the internal or external forces that caused such movements. It includes:
   - Positions of body segment.
   - Velocity of body segments.
   - Acceleration of body segments.

The kinematics and kinetic factors of normal gait are discussed below:
❖ **Stance phase:** This is the period, when the limb is in contact with the ground. This phase constitutes 60% of the gait cycle having components such as:
  - *Heel strike/Initial contact:* Occurs when the foot contacts the ground.
    » Kinematics: *Hip:* 20 degrees flexed.
        Knee: Extended
        Ankle: Plantigrade
    » Kinetics:
       Hip: Single joint hip extensors and abductors contract vigorously to stabilize pelvis and trunk over femur.
       Knee: Low-amplitude contractions in hamstrings resist knee hyperextension.
       Ankle: Pretibial muscles, i.e., tibialis anterior, EDL, EHL contract eccentrically to decelerate foot lowering, and draw tibia forward following initial contact.
  - *Foot flat/Loading response:* Occurs after initial contact, until elevation of the opposite limb. The weight of the body gets transferred to the supporting limb in this phase.
    » Kinematics:
       Hip: 20 degrees flexed.
       Knee: 20 degrees flexed.
       Ankle: 5 degrees plantar flexed.
    » Kinetics:
       Hip: Same as initial contact.
       Knee: Quadriceps contract eccentrically to stabilize the knee and to counteract the flexion moment.

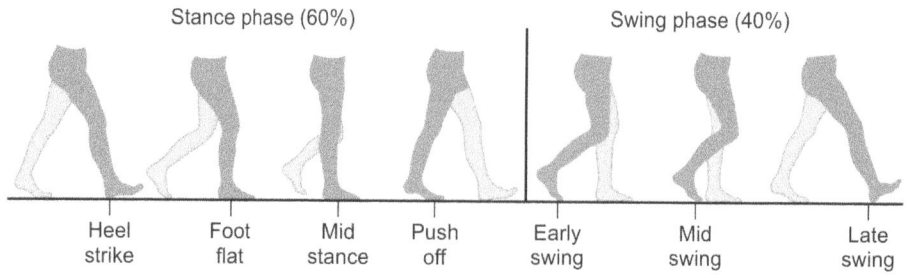

Fig. 4.1A: The gait cycle.

Ankle: Tibialis anterior contract eccentrically to control plantar flexion moment.
- **Mid stance:** This is the period of single limb support when whole body weight is borne on one limb.
  » Kinematics:
  Hip: Neutral extension.
  Knee: Appears fully extended.
  Ankle: 5 degrees dorsiflexed.
  » Kinetics:
  Hip: Residual hamstring activity assists for hip extension at the beginning, and low-level abductor activity stabilizes the pelvis.
  Knee: Quadriceps contract eccentrically to stabilize the knee in slight flexion (close to full extension).
  Ankle: Plantar flexors of ankle undergo eccentric contraction to allow controlled forward progression of tibia.
- **Push off: Heel off and toe off:**
  » *Heel off/Terminal stance:* Begins when the supporting heel rises from the ground.
  » Kinematics:
  Hip: 20 degrees extended.
  Knee: Appears extended.
  Ankle: 10 degrees dorsiflexed
  » Kinetics:
  Hip: Low amplitude tensor fascia lata activity.
  Knee: Quadriceps contract eccentrically to stabilize the knee in slight flexion (close to full extension).
  Ankle: Plantar flexors of ankle undergo eccentric contraction to allow controlled forward progression of the tibia.
- *Toe off/Preswing:* It starts from initial contact of opposite limb to just before the elevation of ipsilateral limb.
  » Kinematics:
  Hip: 10 degrees extended.
  Knee: 40 degrees flexed.
  Ankle: 15 degrees plantar flexed.
  » Kinetics:
  Hip: Rectus femoris assists with early thigh advancement.
  Knee: Rectus femoris modulates the rate of knee flexion.
  Ankle: Calf muscle activity cease in early pre swing. Stored elastic energy in tendo Achilles contributes to rapid plantar flexion as limb unloads.
- ❖ **Swing phase:** This is the period of time, when the foot is off the ground and limb advances forward. This phase constitutes 40% of the gait cycle, having components such as:
  - *Early swing (acceleration):* It starts from the elevation of a limb to point of maximal knee flexion.
    » Kinematics:
    Hip: 15 degrees flexed.
    Knee: 60 degrees flexed.
    Ankle: 5 degrees plantar flexed.
    » Kinetics:
    Hip: Iliacus, adductor longus, gracilis, sartorius advances the thigh producing hip flexion.
    Knee: Biceps femoris (short head), gracilis, and sartorius contribute to knee flexion.
    Ankle: Activity in pretibial muscles produces the required motion in the ankle.
  - *Mid swing:* It starts following knee flexion to the point where tibia is vertical.
    » Kinematics:
    Hip: 25 degrees flexed.
    Knee: 25 degrees flexed.
    Ankle: Neutral.
    » Kinetics:
    Hip: Increasing hamstring activity at end of the phase, restrains further thigh advancement.
    Knee: Activity in hamstrings modulates the rate of knee extension and thigh advancement.
    Ankle: Ankle dorsiflexors contract to ensure foot clearance, by maintaining the ankle in the neutral position.
  - *Terminal swing/Late swing:* It starts from the point where tibia is vertical to just prior to initial contact.
    » Kinematics:
    Hip: 20 degrees flexed.
    Knee: Appears fully extended.
    Ankle: Neutral.
    » Kinetics:
    Hip: Hamstrings continue to control thigh posture and decelerate the limb for heel strike.
    Knee: Hamstrings continue activity and vasti become active to prepare the limb for heel strike.
    Ankle: Activity in pretibial muscles, maintain ankle in neutral position.

Parameters of normal gait: The temporal (time taken for the event) and spatial (distance covered in space) parameters of gait are important parameters, that that help the clinician identify normal and pathological gaits, and to provide gait training.

The temporal parameters are:
- ❖ **Stance time:** Time taken for the stance phase.
- ❖ **Swing time:** Time taken for the swing phase.
- ❖ **Time for double support:** This is the time in one gait cycle, when both feet are supported on the ground.
- ❖ **Step time:** This is the time, that elapses from heel strike of one leg to the next heel strike of the opposite leg.
- ❖ **Stride time:** The time taken between two corresponding heel strikes in the same leg.
- ❖ **Cadence:** The number of steps taken in one minute. The normal value of cadence is: 80-130 steps per minute with an average value of 110 steps/min in adult female and 116 steps/min in adult males.

The spatial parameters are:
- ❖ **Step length:** The distance from heel strike of one limb to corresponding next heel strike of the other limb. The

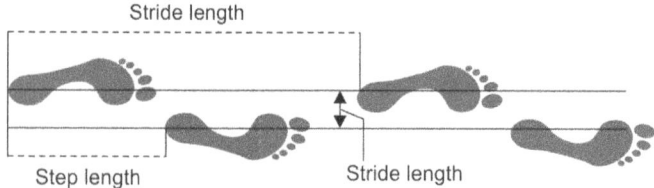

Fig. 4.1B: Spatial parameters of gait.

normal step length in adult female is about 65 cms and in adult male is about 75 cms.

- **Stride length:** This is the distance between two consecutive heel strikes of of the same leg. The average value of stride length for adult female is: 1.28 meter and for adult male is 1.46 meter,
- **Stride width/width of the walking base:** This is the transverse distance between centres of right and left heels during normal walking. The normal value being: 5-10 centimeters.
- **Degree of toe out:** This is the angle between the line of progression (line joining the centres of heels on the same side) and long axis of the foot. The normal value is about 10 degrees.

The spatial parameters of gait are shown in **Figure 4.1B**.

Characteristics of normal gait:

1. **Upward displacement of centre of gravity:** The centre of gravity of human body moves in a sinusoidal path in sagittal plane, with maximum upward displacement occurring during mid stance and maximum downward displacement occurring during double support. The amount of displacement is about 5 cm.
2. **Horizontal displacement of centre of gravity:** The centre of gravity which remains at the centre of the body during double support, gets displaces from side to side (i.e. from one limb to other at mid stance phases). The maximum displacement in the horizontal plane from right to left is about 5 cm.
3. **Pelvic dip/rotation of pelvis in coronal plane:** During normal walking, the pelvis dips by about 5 degrees on the swing phase side, which is counteracted by contraction of gluteus medius of the stance limbs with a reverse action, so that pelvis rotates about the same degrees over the femur of the stance limb, to assist effective ground clearance of the swing side limb.
4. **Knee flexion during stance phase:** Shortly after heel strike, flexion of the knee begins and continues, during the early part of the stance phase, until approximately 20 degrees of knee flexion is reached. This knee flexion, helps to smooth out the path of the center of gravity, by preventing its upward displacement.
5. **Width of the walking base:** The distance between the mid points of successive heel contacts of each limb, called width of the walking base normally has a value of 5-10 cm. Such narrow walking base helps to minimize the lateral displacement of center of gravity during normal walking.
6. **Cadence:** The number of steps taken in a minute, which normally ranges from 80-130 steps/min. If the cadence increases, walking turns into running.

Determinants of gait: The determinants of gait are supposed to represent the adjustments made by pelvis, hip, knee and ankle/foot, that helps to minimize the movements of body's center of gravity, resulting in an energy efficient gait. These determinants help for the followings:

- Minimizes the vertical and lateral displacement of body's center of gravity.
- Decreases energy expenditure.
- Makes the gait more efficient.

The six determinants of gait are:

1. **Rotation of pelvis in transverse plane:** The pelvis rotates in transverse plane upto an angle of 8 degrees total, i.e 4 degrees in a forward direction over the swing limb, and 4 degrees in a backward direction over the stance limb.
2. **Lateral pelvic tilt (drop of pelvis in the frontal plane):** The pelvis that tilts laterally by an angle of 5 degrees on the swing side, is controlled by contraction of gluteus medius on the supported side, there by helping in the prevention of too much upward displacement of body's center of gravity.
3. **Knee flexion during stance phase:** It occurs to prevent excessive upward displacement of the body's ceter of gravity, as the body is carried forward over the stance limb.
4. **Knee, ankle and foot interactions:** The combined movements of knee, ankle anf foot prevent the abrupt changes in the vertical displacement of the center of gravity from downward to upward direction.
5. **Physiological valgus of knee:** This reduces the width of the walking base, due to which minimal lateral displacement of the pelvis is required, to shift the COG, from one lower extremity to another over the base of support.
6. **Lateral displacement of the pelvis:** The pelvis that displaces laterally over the stance limbs can be kept to a minimum by a narrow walking base. By keeping the walking base narrow, little lateral movement of the pelvis is required to preserve balance.

GAIT ANALYSIS

When, a person is not able to walk normally, or has difficulty in walking, either due to neuromuscular/musculoskeletal diseases/disorders, then in this case the walking pattern (gait) of the person should be analyzed and some appropriate exercises, walking aids and orthotic devices should be provided to make walking (gait) energy efficient.

The methods of gait analysis are as follows:

Visual/observational gait analysis: This is the simplest form of gait analysis made by the unaided human eye. This, of course, neglects the remarkable abilities of the human brain to process the data received by the eye. Visual gait analysis is, in reality, the most complicated and versatile form of analysis available. Many clinicians include the observation of a subject's gait as part of their clinical examination. Visual gait analysis is entirely subjective and the quality of the analysis depends on the skill of the person performing it.

The limitations of this method are:

- It is transitory, giving no permanent record.
- The eye cannot observe high-speed events.

- ❖ It is only possible to observe movements, not forces.
- ❖ It depends entirely on the skill of the individual observer.
- ❖ It is subjective and it can be difficult to avoid assessor bias if the patient is undergoing treatment.
- ❖ Subjects may act differently when they know they are being watched (Hawthorne effect).
- ❖ A clinic or laboratory environment may be very different than the real world.

Gait analysis in gait laboratory that incorporates videography, force plates, etc., to gather kinematic and kinetic data.

- ❖ **Methods for kinematic analysis:**
  - *Videography:* This has provided one of the most useful enhancements to gait analysis in the clinical setting during recent years. Gait examination by video recording is not an objective method, since it does not provide quantitative data in the form of numbers. This helps to overcome two of the limitations of visual gait analysis such as—the lack of a permanent record and the difficulty of observing high-speed events. Two-dimensional (2D) and three-dimensional (3D) video-based motion analysis systems are available for gait analysis; however, their use is limited due to challenges with providing accurate data. It has the following advantages:
    » It can be used as a record for future reference.
    » The patient can be demonstrated about his/her gait pattern by showing the video of his walking.
  - *Electrogoniometry:* Electrogoniometers provide an affordable means of measuring joint motion during walking. Early electrogoniometer designs included two rigid links connected by a potentiometer that converted movement into an electrical signal that was proportional to the degree of movement. Recently, designs use a flexible shaft and two small end blocks that are affixed to the proximal and distal segments of the joint.
  - *Optical motion analysis systems:* These are computerized motion analysis systems, where markers are placed on body segments such as the hip, knee, and ankle that are tracked by automated systems **(Fig. 4.1C)**. Motion analysis systems primarily use either active [light emitting diodes (LED)] or passive markers (that requires an external source of illumination) for tracking motion.
  - *Electromagnetic motion analysis systems:* The challenges with optical tracking systems is that T-motion analysis cameras need to be able to "see" the markers to track their position and subsequently calculate kinematic data. This alternative motion analysis technology employs electromagnetic tracking capabilities to determine the 3D coordinates of location and angulation of each sensor.
- ❖ **Kinetic analysis of gait:**
  - *Force plate analysis:* This method focuses on analysis of the forces involved in gait, which include ground (floor) reaction forces (GRFs), joint torques, center of pressure (COP), center of mass (COM), mechanical energy, moments of force, power, work, joint reaction

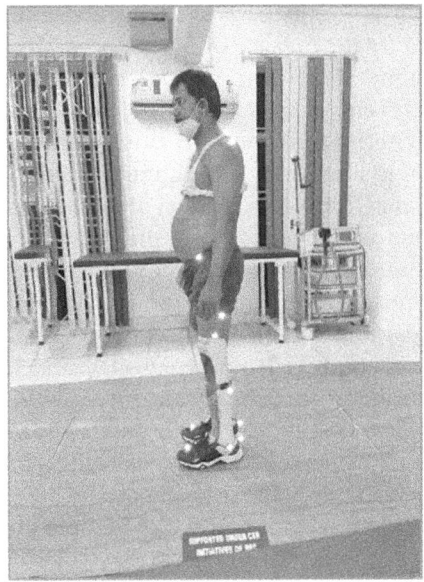

Fig. 4.1C: Shows automated motion analysis with markers attached to body in gait laboratory.

forces, and intrinsic foot pressure. The analysis usually starts with the forces being applied to the foot, which is determined by a force plates embedded in the floor. These plates contain load transducers that measure the COP, COM, and GRFs during gait.
  - *Plantar pressure measurement systems:* Pressure measurement systems may be used with force plates. Plantar pressure measurements are used most commonly in gait analysis to determine the pressure distribution under the foot such as—foot-to-ground contact, foot to- shoe contact, and shoe-to-ground contact.

Energy cost analysis (measurement of energy consumption) during gait: Energy expenditure is an important consideration in gait analyses, particularly in neurological conditions where muscular resources may be low. There are three general approaches in determining energy costs which are as follows:
- ❖ Physiological cost of energy expenditure.
- ❖ Mechanical energy analysis.
- ❖ Heart rate data.
- ❖ **Physiological cost of energy expenditure:** It is the measurement of oxygen uptake/maximum oxygen consumption volume of oxygen (VO_2 max), during walking, through open loop Spirometry, in which exhaled air is sampled and analyzed for its oxygen content. Physiological cost analysis methods are most useful in comparing the energy cost of walking with normal values, which helps for determining the effects of energy costs of interventions such as use of orthoses, prosthesis, and walking aids.
- ❖ **Mechanical energy cost analysis:** There are two methods of measurement of mechanical energy costs such as:
  - *Estimation of energy expenditure from the kinematic data:* The mass of the moving part and the COM are used to calculate the potential energy and translational and rotational kinetic energy levels of each body part

through basic equations of motion and anthropometric constants for masses of body parts. The difference between values obtained at each time increment indicates energy cost.
- *The kinetic approach:* In this energy changes in body parts between subsequent instants in time are calculated from—the product of forces on each end of the joint and the velocity of the point of application, and from the muscle power, which are the product of each muscle moment and the angular velocity of the body part.
- ❖ **Energy expenditure from heart rate data:** This focuses on the measurement of heart rate during ambulation. The physiological cost index, which determines the relative costs of walking per unit distance walked, calculated as the difference between walking heart rate and the resting heart rate divided by average speed, is a method of calculation of energy expenditure from heart rate.

The total heart beat index provides an alternative approach for determining the relative energy efficiency of walking. It is calculated by dividing the total (cumulative) number of heartbeats during exercise by the total distance traveled in a given time period

WALKING AIDS

Walking aids are the assistive devices provided to individuals with sensory and motor deficits to facilitate locomotion. These are useful to assist people who have difficulty in walking or people who cannot walk independently. These include crutches, sticks, rollators, and walking frames.

Crutches

These are devices, which are provided to patients to reduce weight bearing on one or both legs and to give support where strength, endurance, and balance are inadequate to support and move the body.

There are various types of crutches used in clinics, such as:

Axillary Crutches

These are either made of wood or aluminum, consisting of an axillary pad, a hand piece, and double uprights joined distally by a single leg and a rubber ferrule that covers the base of the device. The length of the crutch and position of the hand piece is adjustable as per the need of the individual (**Fig. 4.2**). The axillary pad should rest 5 cm beneath the apex of the axilla and the hand grip should be so aligned that, the elbow remains in approximately 15 degrees of flexion when weight is not fully taken. As weight is fully taken by the crutch, the elbow goes into extension, so that weight is transmitted down the arm to the hand piece (weight of body should not be transmitted to the crutch through the axillary pad to avoid complications like crutch palsy, where the radial nerve is compressed at the axilla, producing wrist drop). These crutches when used help to maintain standing balance with lateral stability.

Measurement of axillary crutch: It can be measured either with the patient in a lying position or standing, as follows.

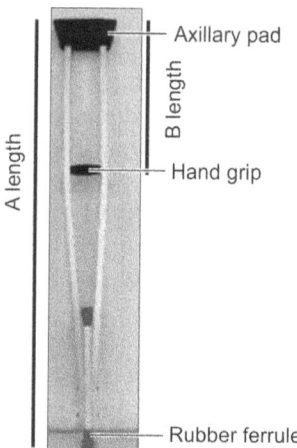

Fig. 4.2: Axillary crutch showing "A" and "B" lengths.

The measurements done in standing position comes out to be most accurate and is commonly performed.
- ❖ *Measurement in supine lying:*
  - Length of the crutch:
    » A length with shoes off: Measurement is taken with an inch tape from apex of axilla to the lower margin of medial malleolus.
    » A length with shoes on: Measurement is taken with an inch tape, from a point 5 cm vertically down from the apex of the axilla (from the anterior axillary fold) to a point 20 cm lateral to the heel of the shoes.
  - *Length from axillary pad to hand grip -B length:* With the elbow flexed to 15 degrees, measurement is taken from a point 5 cm below the apex of the axilla to the ulnar styloid process.
- ❖ *Measurement in standing:* Patient standing with support in front of a wall. Before standing, a general estimate of the length of the crutch can also be obtained by subtracting 16 inches from the patient's height.
  - *Length of the crutch (A length):* 2" below the apex of the axilla to a point 2" lateral and 6" anterior to the feet.
  - *Location of the hand grip from axillary pad (B length):* With the shoulder relaxed, the hand grip should be adjusted to provide 20-30 degrees of elbow flexion.

Preparation for Crutch Walking

- ❖ **Preparation of upper limbs:** Muscles of crutch walking such as scapula depressor, shoulder extensors and adductors and elbow extensors, wrist extensors must be assessed and strengthened before the patient starts walking. The hand grip must also be tested to see that the patient has sufficient power and mobility to grasp the hand piece. If the patient is found to have weaker grip, grip strength must be increased, before the patient is made to use the crutch.
- ❖ **Preparation of lower limbs:** The strength and mobility of both legs should be assessed and muscles, if weak should be strengthened. Main attention should be given to the hip abductors and extensor, the knee extensors, and the ankle plantar flexors.
- ❖ **Development of balance with crutches:** Patient's standing balance with the crutches must be assessed, and balance

training with crutches should be given before he/she is made to walk with the crutches.
- **Demonstration:** The physiotherapist should demonstrate appropriate crutch walking pattern/types of crutch gait to the patient, such as:
  - *Non-weight bearing crutch gait/3 point crutch gait:* This gait is generally used for unilateral lower limb amputees, acute fractures in one lower limb, joint replacement in one knee or hip and patients after surgery for fractures in lower limb, where weight bearing is not permitted. The patient is made to stand with a triangular base, i.e., crutches either in front or behind the weight bearing leg. The crutches serve as two points and the normal limb that bears load acts as the third point. While walking, the patient should take both the crutches with affected leg without the affected leg while touching the ground, followed by the normal/weight bearing leg **(Fig. 4.3)**.
  - *Partial weight bearing crutch gait:* This is a modification of the three point pattern. During forward progression of the involved lower extremity, weight is borne partially on both crutches and on the affected leg. In this, both the crutches and the affected leg are taken forward and put down together. Weight is then taken through the crutches and the affected leg, while the unaffected leg is brought through **(Fig. 4.4)**.
  - *4-point crutch gait:* This gait pattern is used when there is a lack of coordination, poor balance, and muscle weakness in both lower extremities. In this gait pattern, one crutch is advanced and then the opposite leg is advanced. For example, the left crutch is moved forward, then the right leg, followed by the right crutch, and then the left leg **(Fig. 4.5)**.
  - *2-point crutch gait:* This gait pattern is similar to the four point gait. However, it is less stable as only two points of floor contact are maintained and the use of such gait requires better balance. This pattern more closely simulates normal gait, i.e., lower extremity along with opposite upper extremity move together along with

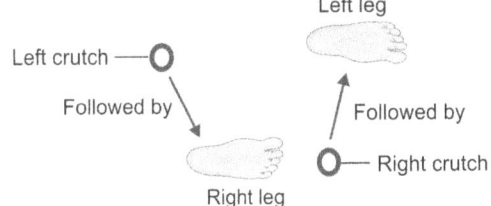

Fig. 4.5: 4-point crutch gait.

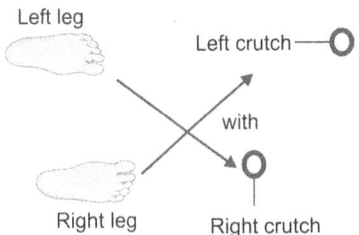

Fig. 4.6: 2-point crutch gait.

the crutch. That means left lower extremity and right upper extremity with the crutch moves as one point, and right lower extremity and left upper extremity with the crutch move as another point, making the two point gait pattern **(Fig. 4.6)**.
  - *Swing to gait:* This gait is commonly used for patients of spinal cord injury, who have bilateral lower extremity involvement. This gait involves forward movements of both crutches simultaneously, shifting weight to the hands and swinging the lower extremities to the crutches, not crossing the crutch line **(Fig. 4.7)**.
  - *Swing through gait:* In this gait which is also used for patients with spinal cord injury, the crutches are moved forward together, weight is shifted onto the hands and the lower extremities are swung beyond the crutches **(Fig. 4.8)**.

Elbow Crutch

It is also called as *Lofstrand* and *Canadian* crutch. It is usually made of aluminum. It consists of a single upright, forearm cuff, handgrip, and rubber ferrule **(Fig. 4.9)**. It can be adjusted both proximally to alter the position of the forearm cuff and distally to alter the height of the crutch. It is available with push button mechanism to alter the length. Forearm cuffs

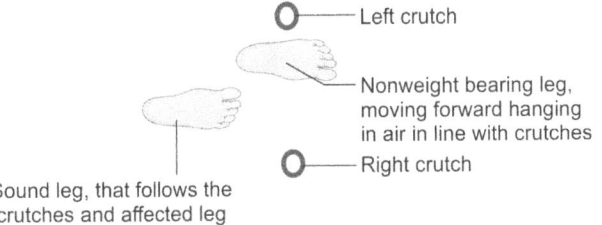

Fig. 4.3: Three point/non-weight bearing crutch gait.

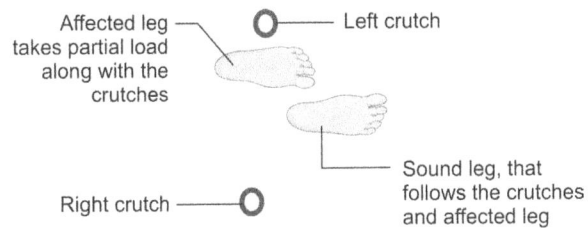

Fig. 4.4: Partial weight bearing crutch gait.

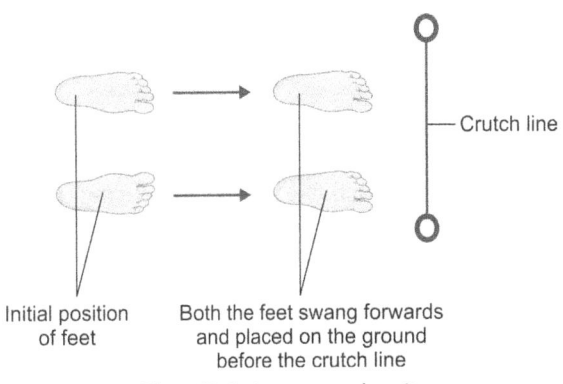

Fig. 4.7: Swing to crutch gait.

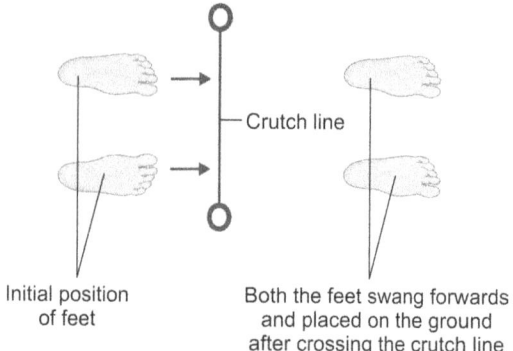

Fig. 4.8: Swing through crutch gait.

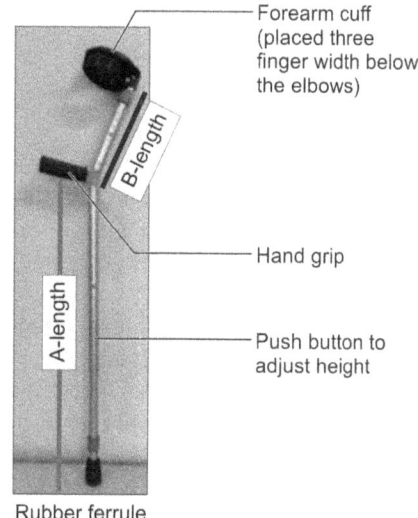

Fig. 4.9: The elbow crutch.

allow the use of hands without disengaging the crutch. The crutch is easily adjustable and allows functional stair climbing activity. It is more cosmetic than other crutches. This crutch has the disadvantage of providing less lateral support due to the absence of an axillary pad. These crutches are suitable for patients with good balance and strong arms.

Measurement of elbow crutch: As per the measurement of axillary crutch, standing is also a method of choice to measure the length of the elbow crutch for the patient. However, for those having difficulty in standing, supine measurement can also be performed.

- **In supine lying (with shoes on):** To get the length of the lower part of the crutch, i.e., from the handgrip to the lower end of the crutch (A-length), measurement is taken from the ulnar styloid process to a point of 20 cm lateral to the heel of the shoe, with the elbow flexed to 15 degrees. To get the length of the upper part of the crutch, i.e., forearm cuff to hand grip (B-length), measurement is taken from a point 1–1.5 inches below the elbow to the ulnar styloid process.
  In standing:
  Length of the lower part of the crutch from hand grip to the floor (A length): Patient standing tall with the back against the wall, shoulders back with the elbows flexed at 20-30 degrees. Measurement is taken in an inch tape from the floor up to the deep crease between the palm of the patient's hand and wrist and 1 inch is added to this length.
  or
  From a supported standing position, the distal end of the crutch should be positioned at a point 2 inches lateral and 6 inches anterior to the foot. With the shoulders relaxed, the height should then be adjusted to provide 20–30 degrees of elbow flexion.
- **Length of the upper part of the crutch (forearm cuff to hand grip-B length):** Measurement is taken from a point 1–1.5 inches below the elbow to the ulnar styloid process (the forearm cuff should be positioned over the proximal third of forearm, which is 1–1.5 inches below the elbow).

Gutter Crutch

This crutch is made of metal with padded forearm support and strap. It has an adjustable hand piece and rubber ferrule **(Fig. 4.10)**. It is used for patients who require support on the forearm due to deformities and pain in hands, such as Rheumatoid arthritis where, weight cannot be taken through the hands.

Measurements of Gutter Crunch:

- **Measurement of forearm support:** Measured from 3 inches below the elbow to the wrist.
- **Measurement of the vertical upright:** In supine lying, with shoes on—measurement is taken from the point of flexed elbow to 20 cm lateral to the heel of the shoe.

Walking Sticks/Tripod/Quadripod

Sticks may be made up of either wood or metal with curved or straight handpiece. Metal made sticks are adjustable while the wooden ones are nonadjustable. Tripod or quadripod sticks made of metal with three or four prolonged bases and gives more stable support than the simple walking stick **(Figs. 4.11A to C)**.

- **Measurement of the walking stick:** The stick or center of the broad based stick such as tripod/quadripod stick

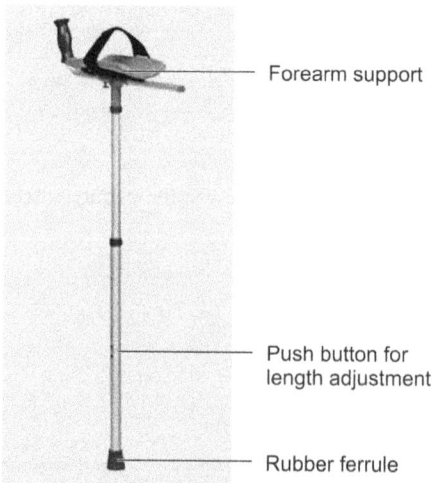

Fig. 4.10: The gutter crutch.

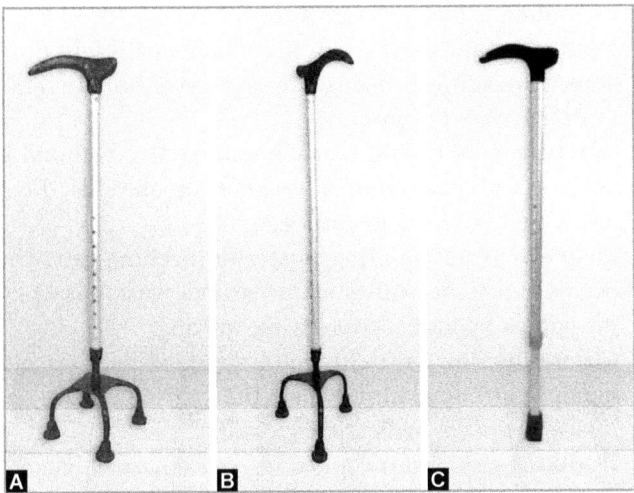

Figs. 4.11A to C: (A) Quadripod; (B) Tripod; (C) Walking stick.

is usually placed approximately 6 inches from the lateral border of the toes. The top of the stick/handgrip should remain at the level of greater trochanter and the elbow should be flexed to about 20-30 degrees.

* ❖ *Uses of sticks:* Sticks allow more weight to be taken through the legs than crutches, and used as a progression from crutch walking. The stick should be used on the strong side and move with the weak side, i.e., one stick may be used on the unaffected side, so that the stick and affected leg are placed forward together, taking some of the weight through the stick. Using the walking stick on the opposite side to the injury allows to shift weight more to the stronger side.
* ❖ **Gait training with walking stick:** While walking, the stick should be held in the hand opposite to the affected limb. For ambulation over ground on level surfaces, the stick and the involved extremity are simultaneously advanced. The stick should remain relatively close to the body and should not be placed ahead of the toes of the involved extremity to prevent lateral and anterior trunk bending.

Walking Frames

They are light weight frames with four supporting bases (**Figs. 4.12A and B**), which can be adjustable in height. Patient lifts the frame forward then leans on it and takes steps. Frames with wheels such as rollator frames which can be pushed are used for individuals with better trunk stability. The *reciprocal frame* where each side moves independently are useful for ataxic patients.

The walker/Rollator frame may be either anterior opening type or posterior opening type (most commonly used). The anterior opening type is usually attached with a seat over the posterior bar of the walker/Rollator (**Figs. 4.13 A and B**). The anterior opening type is selected for very weak patients with poor endurance, who fatigue very easily, as the seat attached with the posterior bar is used to make the patient rest on it when signs of fatigue are noticed.

* ❖ *Measurement of walker:* With the elbows flexed to 20-30 degrees, the handgrip or handle of the walker should come to approximately the level of greater trochanter of the femur.
  – *Gait training with conventional walker/walking frame:*

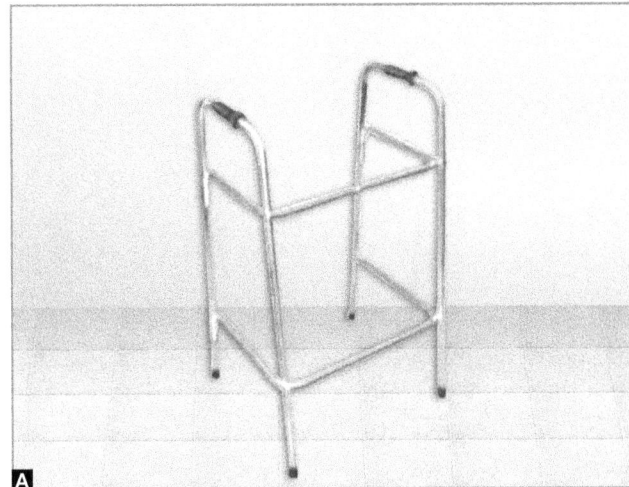

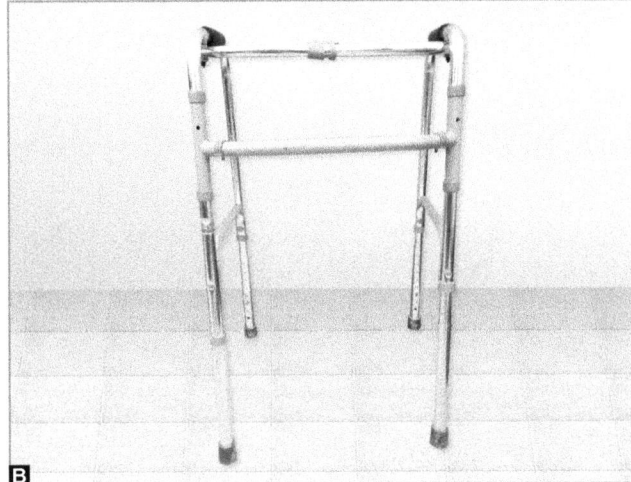

Figs. 4.12 A and B: (A) Simple walking frame; (B) Reciprocal walker.

The patient should remain as vertical a posture as possible. The walker should be picked up and placed down on all four legs simultaneously to achieve maximum stability. The patient should be cautioned not to step too close to the front crossbar, as it will reduce the base of support and may result in a fall. As needed, the patient may be taught non-weight bearing/partial weight bearing/full weight bearing gait patterns with the walker as follows:

» Full weight bearing gait training with walker: The walker is picked up and moved forward about an arm's length, followed by the forward movement of first leg. Subsequently, the second leg is moved forward and past the first. The cycle is repeated resulting in forward movement of the body.

» Partial weight bearing gait training with walker: The walker is picked up and moved forward about an arm's length. The involved partial weight bearing leg is moved forward, transferring part of the body weight onto this limb, and part of the body weight is transferred through the upper extremities to the walker. Subsequently, the normal leg is moved forward past the affected leg. The cycle should be repeated, resulting in partial weight bearing gait with the walker.

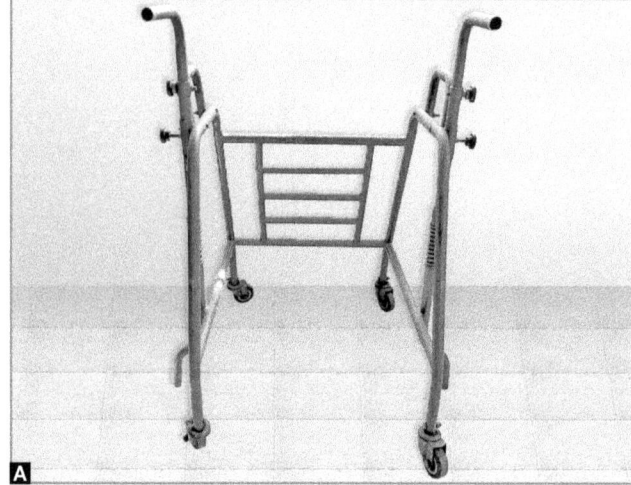

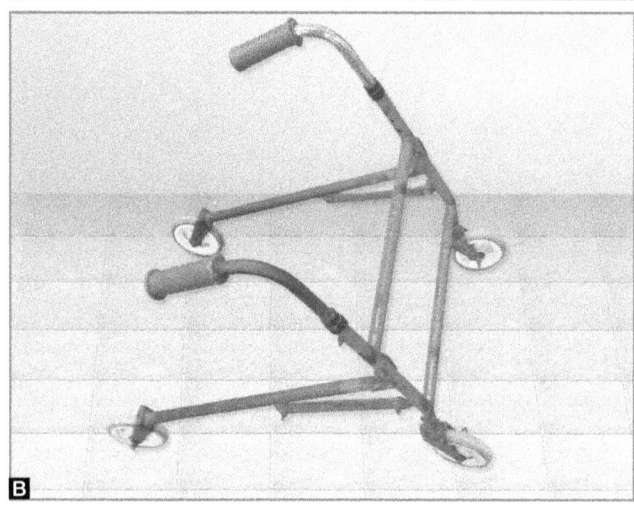

Figs. 4.13 A and B: (A) Anterior opening type walker rollator; (B) Posterior opening type walker rollator.

» **Non-weight bearing gait training with walker:** The walker is picked up and moved forward about an arm's length. Weight is then transferred through the upper extremities to the walker. The involved non-weight bearing leg is held anterior to the patient's body without making contact with the floor. Subsequently the uninvolved leg is moved forward and the cycle is repeated resulting in non-weight bearing gait with the walker.

Pathological gaits: The therapist/clinician should be able to identify pathological gaits, which will help him to evaluate the abnormal patterns and train normal walking as much as possible:

The common pathological gaits are:
- **High steppage gait:** Found in patients with foot drop, where the subject moves with excessive hip and knee flexion to clear the ground.
- **Lurching gait/lateral trunk bending:** This is found in subjects with hip abductor weakness on one side, this is also called as Trendelenburg gait.
- **Posterior trunk bending/posterior lurching gait:** This occurs in patients with gluteus maximus weakness where the patient bends backward while walking.
- **Circumduction gait:** This gait is found in patients with hemiplegia/hemiparesis, where the individual hikes and rotates the pelvis to clear the ground.
- **Waddling gait:** This occurs due to weakness of bilateral hip abductors where the subject lurches on both sides while walking.
- **Vaulting gait:** This gait is seen in individuals with shortening of one lower limb where the subject raises the heel on the shortened side to clear the ground on opposite side.
- **Antalgic gait:** This is found in individuals with painful joints where the individual tries to reduce the single stance period on the affected leg to avoid weight bearing on that side.
- **Scissoring gait:** This is found in individuals with spasticity of hip adductors and medial hamstrings commonly seen in spastic diplegic cerebral palsy. Both hips remain adducted while walking.
- **Hand to knee gait:** This is found in individuals with weak quadriceps where he/she leans forward and pushes the affected thigh posteriorly with own hand during single leg stance.
- **Anterior trunk bending gait:** This is seen in patients with weak quadriceps where the individual bends the trunk forward to bring the line of gravity more and more in front of the knee joint to create an extension torque during single leg stance.
- **Crouch gait:** Here the subject walks with hips and knees flexion and ankle dorsiflexion. This is commonly seen in spastic diplegic cerebral palsy.
- **Jump knee gait:** The individual walks with both hips and knees flexion and ankle plantar flexion as if he/she is going to jump. This is also seen in spastic cerebral palsy.

Massage

INTRODUCTION

Massage is the scientific manipulation of soft tissues of the body (muscle and connective tissues) to aid in healing, decrease tension, relieve stress, promote relaxation, reduce swelling, and enhance function.

It is one of the ancient methods used for healing of soft tissues. Massage therapy has been used in many cultures around the world for a long time. Presently, the therapy has received wide acceptance among clinicians for recognized therapeutic effects.

CLASSIFICATION OF MASSAGE

Massage is classified into various types on the basis of character of the technique, depth of the soft tissues manipulated, and part of the body massaged.

A. Classification on the basis of character of the technique:
1. *Stroking massage:* The uninterrupted linear movement of hand along the whole length of segment is called stroking.
    a. Superficial stroking: It is the rhythmical movement of hand or parts thereof over the skin with the least amount of pressure in order to obtain sensory stimulation. It can be applied from the proximal to the distal or vice versa **(Fig. 5.1)**.
    Uses: It is used to induce relaxation of the segment/body.
    b. Effleurage (deep stroking): Effleurage, a French word meaning "to skim" or "to touch lightly on," is a series of massage strokes used in Swedish massage to warm up the muscle before deep tissue work using petrissage. This is a soothing, stroking movement used at the beginning and the end of the facial and/or body massage. It is the movement of the palmar aspect of hand over the external surface of the body with constant moderate pressure, in the direction of the venous and lymphatic drainage **(Fig. 5.2)**.
    Uses: It aids relaxation, reduces stress, and increases lymphatic and venous drainage.
2. *Pressure manipulation/massage:*
    a. Kneading: In this group of techniques, the tissues are pressed down on to the underlying firm structure and intermittent pressure is applied in a circular direction, parallel to the long axis of bone. It can produce many physiological effects that include increased capillarization, increased vasodilation, and increased tissue elasticity.

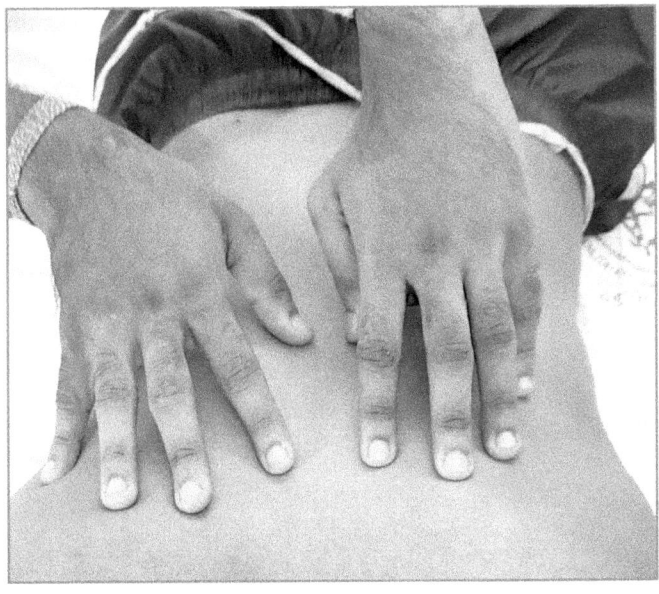

Fig. 5.1: Stroking massage.

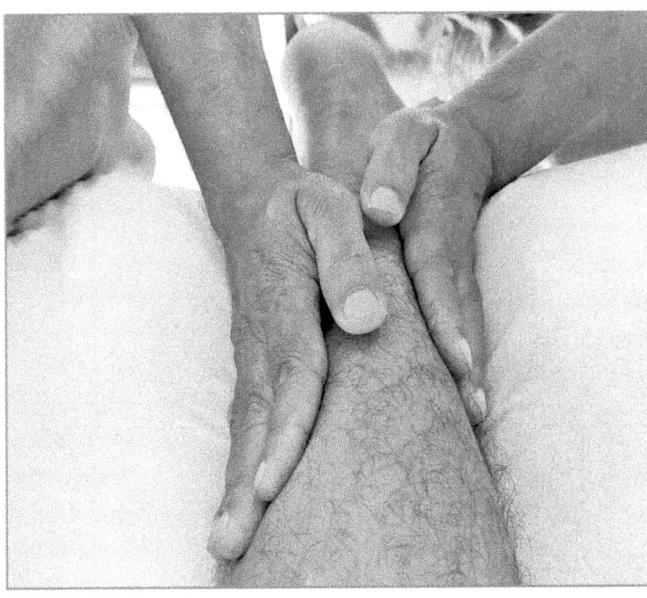

Fig. 5.2: Effleurage massage.

Uses: It is used to increase flexibility of tight soft tissues, to decrease muscle spasm and pain, and to reduce stress.

They are of the following types:
  i. Palmar kneading: Pressure is applied with the heel of palm **(Fig. 5.3).**
  ii. Elbow kneading: Pressure is applied with the olecranon process of elbow **(Fig. 5.4).**
  iii. Digital kneading: Pressure is applied with the fingers (finger kneading) or thumbs (thumb kneading) **(Fig. 5.5).**
  iv. Reinforced kneading: Both the hands, placed over one another, are used to apply pressure **(Fig. 5.6)**.
b. Petrissage: In this technique, the tissues are grasped and lifted away from the underlying structures and intermittent pressure is applied to the tissues in the direction that is perpendicular to the long axis of the bone.

Uses: It is used to improve blood circulation, loosen tight muscles, and enhance the flexibility/joint range of motion (ROM).

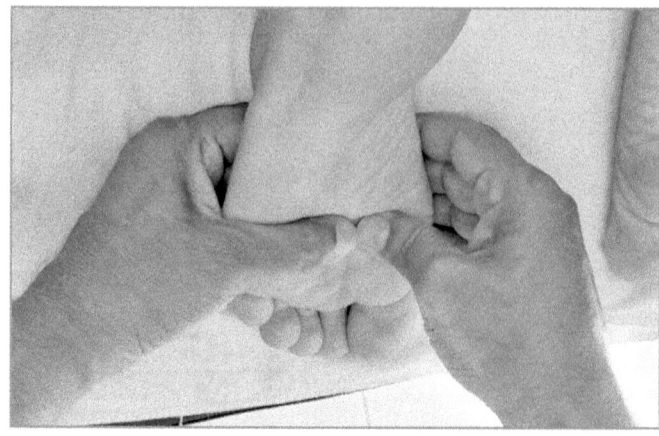

Fig. 5.5: Thumb kneading.

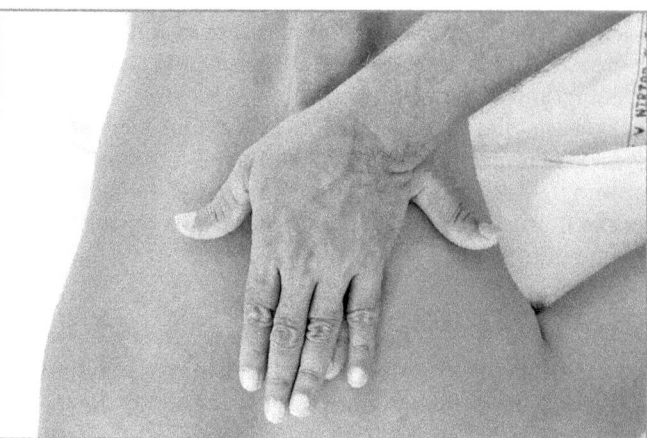

Fig. 5.6: Reinforced kneading.

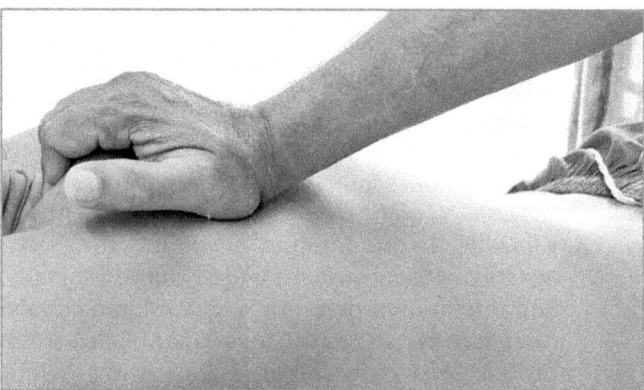

Fig. 5.3: Palmar kneading.

They are of the following types:
  i. Picking up: In this technique, the tissues are lifted away from underlying structures, squeezed, and then released using one or both the hands **(Fig. 5.7)**.
  ii. Wringing: In this the tissues are lifted away from the underlying structures, squeezed, twisted, and then released, using both the hands **(Fig. 5.8).**
  iii. Skin rolling: The skin and fascia are lifted up with both the hands and moved over the subcutaneous tissues by keeping a roll of lifted tissue continuously ahead of the moving thumb **(Fig. 5.9).**

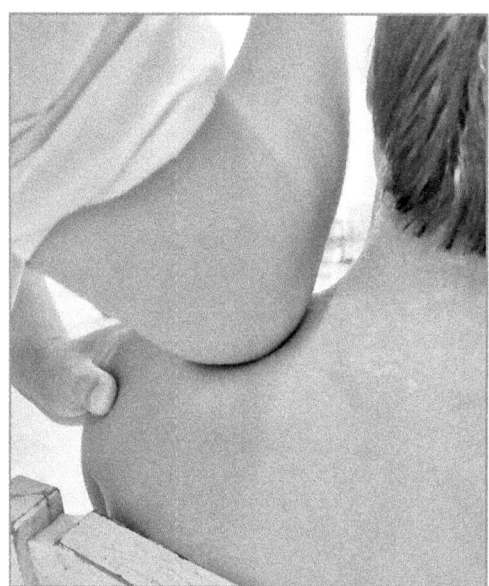

Fig. 5.4: Elbow kneading.

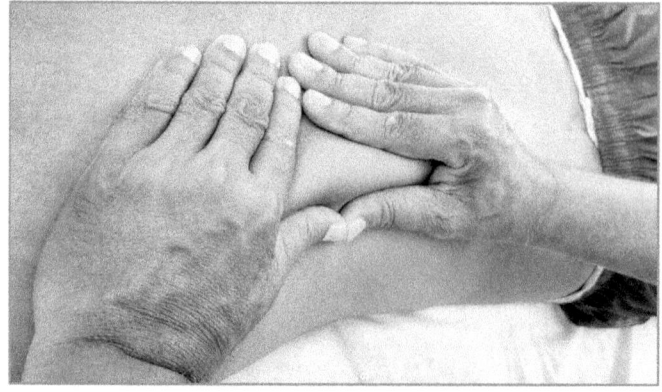

Fig. 5.7: Picking up massage.

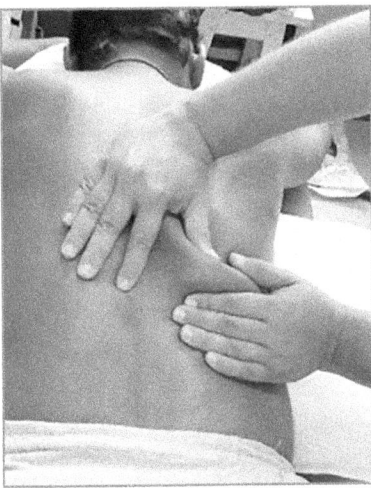

Fig. 5.8: Wringing massage.

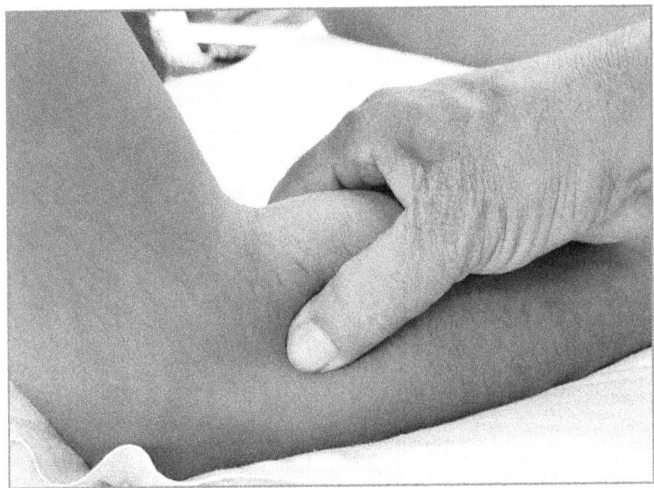

Fig. 5.10: DTFM, using thumb.

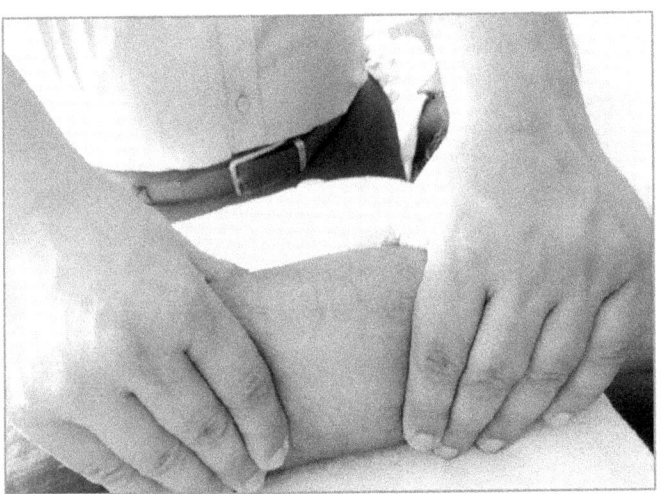

Fig. 5.9: Skin rolling massage.

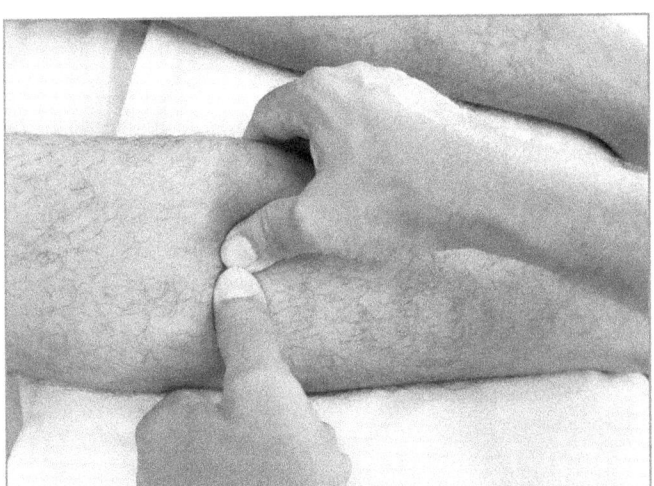

Fig. 5.11: Circular friction using thumb.

c. *Friction:* In this technique, the tissues are subjected to small range of to and fro movement performed with constant deep pressure of the finger or thumb.
Uses: Friction is a massage technique used to increase circulation and release areas that are tight, particularly around joints and where there are adhesions within the muscles or tendons. It also prevents formation of adherent scars.
It is of the following types:
   i. Deep transverse friction massage (DTFM): In this technique, to and fro movement is performed using the thumb or finger across the length of the structure **(Fig. 5.10)**.
   ii. Circular friction: In this, circular movements are given over the tissue using finger or thumb **(Fig. 5.11)**.
d. *Myofascial release:* It is a technique that combines traction with varying amount of stretch to the muscles and underlying fascia, to produce a moderate sustained force in these tissues. The goal of this technique is to produce viscoelastic lengthening and plastic deformation of the fascia **(Figs. 5.12A and B)**.
Uses: The technique is indicated to lengthen muscle and fascia, increase mobility between fascia layers, and break adhesions. It also decreases pain and increases flexibility (ROM).

3. *Percussion/Tapotement:* In this group of techniques, a succession of soft, gentle blows are applied over the body, which produce a characteristic sound. The striking hands are not in constant contact with the skin and strike the body part at regular intervals. This results in the application of an intermittent touch and pressure to the body during these manipulations.
Uses: It is used to loosen the muscle and fascia, increase ROM and flexibility, and decrease soreness/stiffness. It also helps loosening secretion from the airways.
It is of the following types:
   i. Clapping: The technique is applied with the cupped hand **(Fig. 5.13)**.
   ii. Hacking: The technique is applied using ulnar border of the 5th, 4th and 3rd digits **(Fig. 5.14)**.

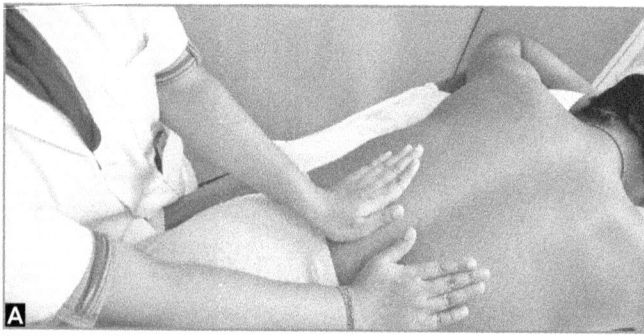
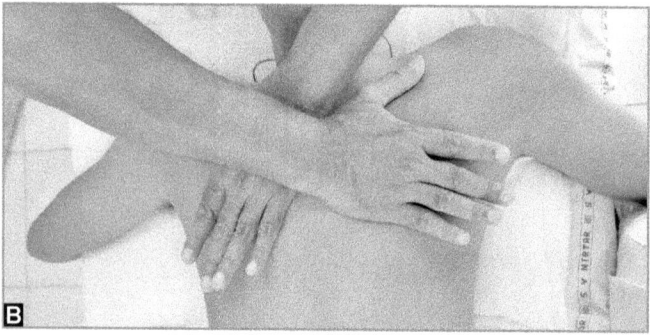

Figs. 5.12A and B: Myofascial release techniques.

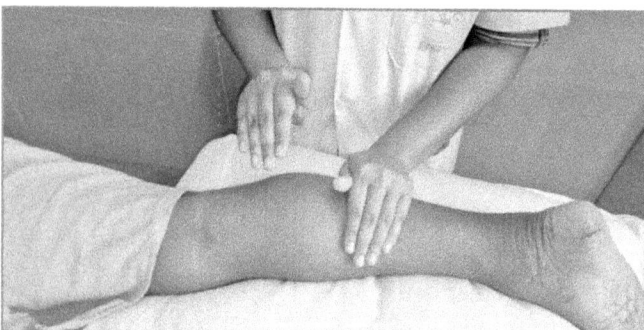

Fig. 5.13: Clapping massage.

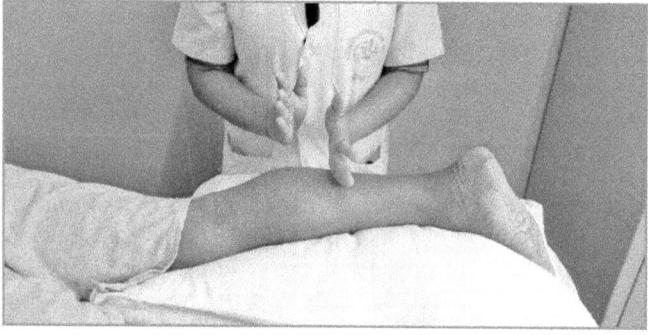

Fig. 5.14: Hacking massage.

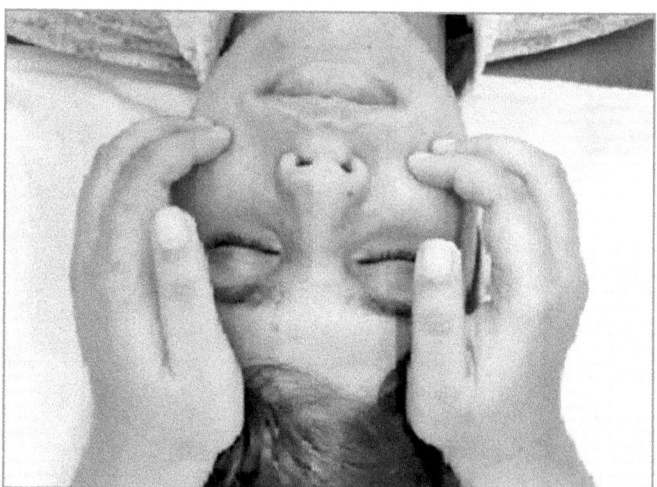

Fig. 5.15: Tapping massage.

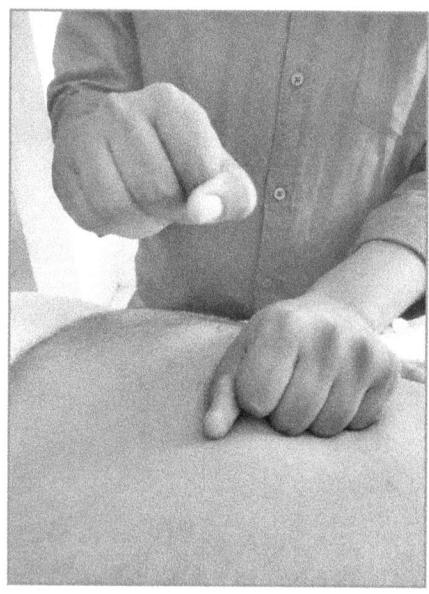

Fig. 5.16: Beating massage.

iii. *Tapping massage:* The technique is applied using the pulp of the fingers. It is ideally given for areas of the body, such as face, head and over painful neuromas at the end of the stump **(Fig. 5.15)**.

iv. *Beating:* The technique is applied using the anterior aspect of the clenched fist **(Fig. 5.16)**.

v. *Pounding:* The technique is applied using the medial aspect of the clenched fist **(Fig. 5.17)**.

4. *Vibratory massage:* In this group of techniques, the mechanical energy is transmitted to the body by the vibrations of the distal part of upper limb, i.e., hand and/or fingers, which are in constant contact with the subject's skin, using the body weight and generalized co-contraction of the upper limb muscles.

This technique is mainly directed toward the lung and other hollow cavities.

Uses: It is used to increase metabolism, increase ROM, improve vascularization, and release trigger points and loosen secretions in the lungs.

They are of the following types:

i. Vibrations: In this technique, the fine vibrations are produced, which tend to produce fine movement of hand in upward and downward direction.

ii. Shaking: In this technique, coarse vibrations are produced, which tend to produce fine movement of hand in sideway direction.

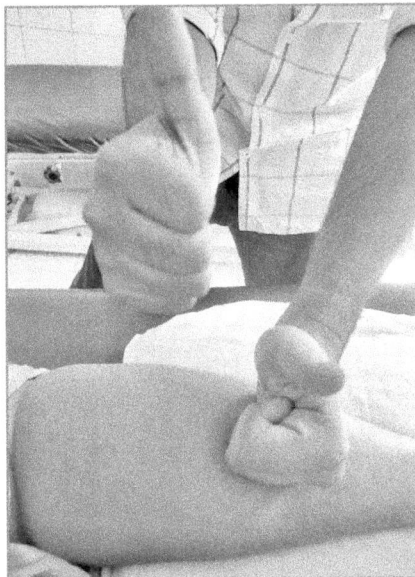

Fig. 5.17: Pounding massage.

B. Classification on the basis of depth of tissue:
 1. Gentle/light massage: The forces applied during the maneuver are light, so that the effect of massage is confined to the superficial tissue only, e.g., stroking, tapping.
 2. Deep massage: The forces applied during the massage are moderate to deep so that the effect of massage reaches to the deeper tissues like muscles, e.g., friction, kneading.
C. Classification on the basis of part of body massaged:
 1. Local massage: When massage is administered in a particular area of the body segment, it is termed local massage. For example, DTFM for lateral epicondylitis.
 2. General massage: Massage applied to the entire body/large body segment such as back or lower limb is usually termed general massage.

Swedish Massage

It is the use of five basic strokes put together in a sequence that will benefit the client. Pressure with a Swedish massage generally begins with light movements and increases gradually to medium to deeper pressure, and then returning to a lighter pressure to end body work in that specific area. The five basic strokes are effleurage, petrissage, friction, tapotement, and vibration.

PHYSIOLOGICAL EFFECTS OF MASSAGE

a. **Effect on circulatory system:** The mechanical effect of massage helps in pushing the venous blood and lymph toward the heart, resulting in prevention of pooling of blood and fluid in the distal body parts. The increased venous and lymphatic return also promotes increase of arterial blood flow, due to decrease of venous congestion, release of vasodilators, and activation of axon reflex.

b. **Effect on removal of waste metabolites:** As massage speeds up the lymphatic and venous flow, it promotes rapid disposal of the waste products of metabolism.
c. **Effect on nervous system:** Massage produces its effect on the sensory, motor as well as autonomic components of the nervous system such as:
 – *Sensory system:* Massage produces a strong sedative effect on the body when applied with slow rhythm. Deep stimulating massages, such as friction massage and kneading, etc., help in reducing pain due to the effects on the pain gate.
 – *Motor system:* Massage has the effects of inhibition and facilitation on the motor function. Massage techniques that inhibit the motor system causing a reduction of muscle tone include petrissage and gentle effleurage. Massage techniques that increase the muscle tone by stimulating the stretch reflex of the muscle spindle include—superficial stroking, tapping, hacking, etc.
 – *Autonomic nervous system:* Massage has definite reflex effect and it can influence the functioning of visceral organ by modulating the autonomic nervous system through peripheral sensory stimulation.
d. **Effect on soft tissues:** Massage has significant effect on certain properties of soft tissues such as elasticity, plasticity, and mobility. The adhesions present in the soft tissues are broken and mobility of soft tissues is promoted.
e. **Effect on the respiratory system:** Massage techniques such as percussion, shaking, and vibration assist in mobilization of secretions and drainage of the same toward the larger airways, when combined with postural drainage. This results in efficient gaseous exchange in the lungs.
f. **Effect on the skin:** Massage techniques such as stroking (effleurage), petrissage help in improvement of nutrition to the skin through increase of blood flow. As a result, the skin becomes soft, supple, and finer.

THERAPEUTIC USES OF MASSAGE

Massage is used as a therapeutic modality to treat various conditions such as:
1. **Edema control:** Effleurage technique combined with elastic bandaging, elevation, and active exercises is helpful for relief of both local and general edema. For example: Lymphedema after radical mastectomy.
2. **Scar mobilization:** Techniques such as deep transverse friction and kneading massages are helpful to mobilize tight scar that restrict joint ROM. For example: DTFM to postsurgical scar after quadricepsplasty.
3. **To increase circulation:** All types of massages and most particularly petrissage, deep stroking, light digital kneading, etc., can be applied to increase circulation to tissues to promote repair. For example: Light finger kneading to margins of ulcers to increase blood flow to the ulcer, accelerating healing of the ulcer.

4. **To reduce muscle spasm and pain:** Techniques such as myofascial release and petrissage manipulation are found to be effective in reducing muscle spasm and pain. For example: Spasm of paravertebral muscles in low back pain.
5. **To induce general and local relaxation:** Techniques such as light stroking is helpful to induce general relaxation of the body and techniques such as petrissage and myofascial release light percussion (tapping) are helpful to induce local relaxation of muscles. For example: Light stroking is applied in the state of tension of body to induce relaxation, whereas light percussion (tapping) is applied to the forehead to induce local relaxation, in case of tension headache.
6. **To mobilize secretions in lungs:** Certain percussion massage techniques such as clapping and hacking and the vibratory techniques such as vibration and shaking massages are applied to mobilize secretions in the lungs and drain them to the larger airways, when combined with postural drainage. For example: Chest shaking in chronic bronchitis to drain secretions from the lungs.

CONTRAINDICATIONS OF MASSAGE

A. General contraindications:
   i. High fever
   ii. Hypersensitive skin
   iii. Renal diseases
   iv. Cardiac diseases
   v. Deep X-ray therapy/Radiotherapy
   vi. Generalized osteoporosis
   vii. Severe spasticity
B. Local contraindications:
   i. Acute inflammation
   ii. Skin diseases
   iii. Recent fractures
   iv. Open wound (applicable to most of the techniques, except a few)
   v. Varicose veins
   vi. Atherosclerosis
   vii. Deep vein thrombosis

MASSAGE LUBRICANTS

Lubricants are used to decrease friction and control the amount of glide and drag that occurs between the therapist's moving hands and the patient's skin. The lubricants should be hypoallergenic and should be in the form of lotions, oils, creams, and powders.

SECTION 2

Physiotherapy for Musculoskeletal Conditions

Section Outline

- Chapter 6: Physiotherapy for Spinal Disorders
- Chapter 7: Physiotherapy for Hip
- Chapter 8: Knee Joint
- Chapter 9: Physiotherapy for Ankle and Foot
- Chapter 10: Physiotherapy for Shoulder
- Chapter 11: Physiotherapy for Disorders of Elbow
- Chapter 12: Physiotherapy for Disorders of Wrist and Hand
- Chapter 13: Physiotherapy in Scoliosis
- Chapter 14: Physiotherapy for Amputees
- Chapter 15: Physiotherapy in Arthritis
- Chapter 16: Physiotherapy in Fractures
- Chapter 17: Physiotherapy for Burn

6. Physiotherapy for Spinal Disorders

THE LUMBAR SPINE

Disorders of lumbar spine are variable and one of the most common spinal disorders affecting young to old individuals. There are five lumbar vertebrae, joining together by secondary cartilaginous joints formed by the vertebral bodies on the anterior side and zygapophyseal joints, which are plane type of synovial joints formed by the articular facets on the posterior side.

Among the five lumbar vertebrae, the 5th lumbar vertebra differs from the remaining four, having a wedge-shaped body, with anterior height greater than the posterior height. The intervertebral disc that lies between adjacent vertebrae, acts as shock absorber. The surfaces of the superior facets at the zygapophyseal joints are concave and face medially and posteriorly. The surfaces of the inferior facets are convex and face laterally and anteriorly. As the facets are aligned in the sagittal plane, it permits more flexion and extension with limited lateral flexion and rotation.

The stability of the lumbar spine is maintained by the strong ligaments like iliolumbar ligament that stabilizes the lumbosacral joints, the inter transverse ligament, that helps to limit lateral flexion, the anterior and posterior longitudinal ligaments (the PLL is not well-developed in the lumbar area, where as the ALL is quite strong), joint capsules of zygapophyseal joints, the intervertebral discs, and the paraspinal and abdominal muscles.

Osteokinematics of Lumbar Spine

Flexion, extension, lateral flexion (limited degrees), rotation (limited degrees) are the movements permitted by the intervertebral joints in the lumbar region. The zygapophyseal joints of L1 to L4 lie primarily in the sagittal plane, which favors flexion and extension and limits lateral flexion and rotation. The greatest amount of flexion takes place at the lumbosacral joints, where as lateral flexion and rotation is more in the upper lumbar region, with no or very less lateral flexion occurring in the lumbosacral region.

Capsular Pattern of Limitation

The capsular pattern of movement limitation of the lumbar spine is marked and equal limitation of extension and both side flexions.

Ranges of Motion of Thoracolumbar Spine

Ranges of motion (ROM) of thoracolumbar spine are given in **Table 6.1**.

Table 6.1: Ranges of motion of thoracolumbar spine.

Movement	Range of motion (in degrees)
Flexion	80
Extension	20–30
Lateral flexion (left)	35
Lateral flexion (right)	35
Rotation (right)	45
Rotation (left)	45

Lumbosacral angle

The 1st sacral segment, which is inclined slightly anteriorly and inferiorly, forms an angle with the horizontal, called the lumbosacral angle. This angle is determined by measuring the angle formed by a line drawn parallel to the superior aspects of sacrum and a horizontal line **(Fig. 6.1)**. The optimum physiological lumbosacral angle is about 30 degrees. The alteration of this angle has an impact on low back and may cause low back pain . It's value increases in individuals with increased lumbar lordosis and decreases in flat back as occurs in PIVD of lumbo sacral spine.

Lumbopelvic rhythm: Lumbopelvic rhythm refers to the relative pattern of lumbar and pelvic contributions to trunk

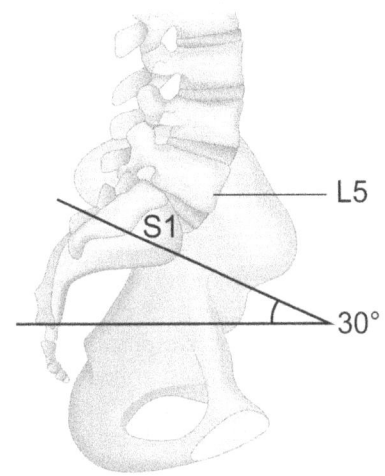

Fig. 6.1: The lumbosacral angle.

motion in the sagittal plane. It is a specific instance of co-ordinated simultaneous activity of lumbar flexion and anterior tilting of pelvis in the sagittal plane during flexion and posterior tilting of pelvis during lumbar spine extension to return to the erect posture.

The first part of the bending forward consists of lumbar flexion, followed next by anterior tilting of the pelvis at the hip joints. A return to erect posture is initiated by posterior tilting of the pelvis at the hips followed by extension of the lumbar spine. The integration of motion of the pelvis about the hip joints with motion of the vertebral column increases the range of motion (ROM) available to the total column, and also reduces the amount of flexibility required of the lumbar region.

THE THORACIC SPINE

The thoracic spine has 12 thoracic vertebrae, joined together and to the adjacent lumbar and cervical vertebrae through the intervertebral and zygapophyseal joints. There is an intervertebral disc between adjacent vertebral bodies. The superior facet surfaces of the zygapophyseal joints are slightly convex, where as the inferior facet surfaces are slightly concave. The superior facet surfaces face posteriorly, slightly laterally and cranially, whereas the inferior facet surfaces face anteriorly, slightly medially and caudally. The joint capsules are tighter than in the cervical region.

Osteokinematics

The zygapophyseal facets from T1 to T6 lie in the frontal plane, therefore limits flexion and extension in the upper thoracic segments. The facets in the lower thoracic region are oriented more in the sagittal plane; therefore permit some amount of flexion and extension.

A very few degrees of flexion, extension, and lateral flexion is permissible, whereas significant amount of rotation is present in thoracic spine.

Capsular pattern of limitation of thoracic spine: Equal limitation of both rotations.

THE CERVICAL SPINE

The cervical region is composed of seven cervical vertebrae, which are aligned in such a manner that a posterior concavity (cervical lordosis) exists. The joints in this region are:

- **Atlanto-occipital joint:** The atlas which forms the joint with the occiput of the skull has no vertebral body and spine. It has two lateral masses containing the articular facets. The lateral masses are connected by anterior and posterior arches. The anterior arch contains a facet for articulation with the dens of axis, which is secured by transverse ligament of atlas. The posterior arch has a groove for the vertebral artery and C1 spinal nerve. This joint is composed of right and left concave superior facets of atlas, articulating with right and left convex occipital condyles of skull. This joint is plane type of synovial joint, permitting flexion-extension (nodding) in the sagittal plane with very little lateral flexion and rotation.
- **Atlantoaxial joint:** The atlantoaxial joint is composed of three separate articulations such as, the median atlanto-axial joint and two lateral joints. The median atlanto-axial joint consists of an anterior facet on the dens (the odontoid process of C2), that articulates with a facet on the internal surface of the atlas (C1). The two lateral joints are composed of the right and left superior facets of axis (C2) that articulate with the right and left slightly convex inferior facets on the atlas (C1).

The median atlantoaxial joint is a pivot type of synovial joint, permitting rotation in the transverse plane around a vertical axis. The two lateral joints are plane type of synovial joints. The motions permitted at the three articulations of atlantoaxial joint are flexion-extension, lateral flexion, and rotation.
- **The intervertebral and zygapophyseal joints:** The intervertebral joints (secondary cartilaginous type) are made up of joints between the vertebral bodies and adjacent intervertebral discs. The zygapophyseal joints are formed by the right and left superior articular process (facets) of one vertebra and the right and left inferior articular processes of an adjacent superior vertebra. The facets in the cervical region are oriented 45 degrees to the transverse plane. These joints are plane type of synovial joints having their own capsules. The capsules in the cervical region are lax, permitting greater ROM.

Osteokinematics and Arthrokinematics

Flexion, extension, lateral flexion, and rotation are the movements permissible in cervical spines.

During flexion, the inferior facets of the superior vertebrae slide anteriorly and superiorly, on the superior facets of the inferior vertebrae. During extension, the inferior facets of the superior vertebrae slide posteriorly and inferiorly on the superior facets of the inferior vertebrae. During lateral flexion and rotation, one inferior facet of the superior vertebra slides inferiorly and posteriorly on the superior facet of the inferior vertebra on the side to which the spine is laterally flexed and rotated. The opposite inferior facet of the superior vertebra slides superiorly and anteriorly on the superior facet of the adjacent inferior vertebra. The ROM permissible are given in **Table 6.2**.

Table 6.2: Range of motion of cervical spine.	
Movements	**Range of motion (in degrees)**
Flexion	45
Extension	45
Lateral flexion (left)	45
Lateral flexion (right)	45
Rotation (left)	60
Rotation (right)	60

Cervical Nerves

The cervical nerves are the spinal nerves from the cervical vertebrae in the cervical segment of the spinal cord. Although there are seven cervical vertebrae (C1-C7), there are eight cervical nerves C1 – C8. All cervical nerves except C8 emerge above their corresponding vertebrae, while the C8 nerve emerges below the C7 vertebra.

Capsular Pattern of Limitation

A capsular pattern is the reproducible limitation of joint movements when the joint capsule is the limiting structure. The capsular pattern of limitation of movement of cervical spine include: Equal limitation of extension, both side flexions and both rotations.

The surface landmarks of the spine are given in the **Table 6.3**.

Table 6.3: Surface landmarks of spine.

Structure	Landmarks
Cervical vertebral bodies	Same level as transverse process
C1 transverse process	One finger's breadth inferior to mastoid process
C3-C4 vertebrae	Posterior to hyoid bone
C4-C5 vertebrae	Posterior to thyroid cartilage
C6 vertebra	Posterior to cricoid cartilage
C7 vertebra	Prominent posterior spinous process
T1 vertebra	Prominent protrusion inferior to cervical spine
T2 vertebra	Posterior from jugular notch of sternum
T3 vertebra	Level with the root of spine of scapula
T7 vertebra	Level with the inferior angle of scapula
L3 vertebra	Posterior to umbilicus
L4 vertebra	Level with the iliac crest.
L5 vertebra	Typically demarcated by bilateral dimples
S2 vertebra	Level with PSIS

DISORDERS OF SPINE

The common disorders of spine treated by physiotherapists are discussed below:

1. Cervical Spondylosis

Cervical spondylosis is a chronic degenerative condition of the cervical spine affecting the vertebral bodies and intervertebral discs characterized by thinning and hardening of the discs and formation of bone spurs (marginal osteophytes), that may have impact on the nerve roots in the intervertebral foramina or spinal cord in the spinal canal.

Spondylotic changes can produce stenosis of spinal canal that may affect the spinal cord producing myelopathy, or it may affect the lateral recess and foramina producing radiculopathy.

Epidemiology and Etiology

Cervical spondylosis is commonly found in individuals in the age group of 40–60 years, though secondary spondylosis may affect young individuals.

The disorder affects males and females equally; however, males are affected earlier as compared to females.

Primary cervical spondylosis is caused by aging process. However, secondary cervical spondylosis has the following etiologies:
- Trauma/fracture to cervical spine.
- Occupation: Those carrying load on head.
- Disc bulge.
- Spinal deformities.
- Metabolic bone disease (most commonly osteoporosis).
- Poor posture (head forward posture).

Pathophysiology

As an aging process, the intervertebral discs lose fluid and elasticity, resulting in cracks and fissures. The surrounding ligaments also lose their elastic properties and develop traction spurs. Due to collapse of the disc, the annulus bulges out, resulting in narrowing of the disc space and overriding of the facets. The hypermobility that develops in the affected spinal segment causes further damage to the disc. As the annulus bulges, facets hypertrophy and ligamentum flavum becomes thick, the cross-sectional area of the spinal canal is narrowed. Neck extension causes the ligamentum flavum to fold inward, reducing the anteroposterior diameter of the spinal canal.

As the disc degenerates, the uncinate process overrides and hypertrophies, compromising the venterolateral portion of the intervertebral foramina. This in combination of facet hypertrophy that causes decrease of dorsolateral aspect of the intervertebral foramina leads to radiculopathy, which is a common feature of cervical spondylosis.

Subsequently, marginal osteophytes that develop, stabilize the vertebral bodies adjacent to the degenerating discs and increase the weight-bearing areas in the spine.

Degeneration of joint surfaces and ligaments decrease motion, in the spinal segments preventing further damage. Thickening and ossification of the posterior longitudinal ligament (PLL) leads to narrowing of the spinal canal. A canal less than 13 mm diameter leads to the development of myelopathy.

Clinical Features

The course of cervical spondylosis may be slow and prolonged, and patient's may either remain asymptomatic or have mild-to-moderate cervical pain with or without pain radiating along one or both upper limbs (brachial neuralgia). The ROM of the cervical spine may be decreased, with more limitation of extension as compared to flexion. Decrease of cervical lordosis, a forward head posture, cervicothoracic scoliosis with convexity toward the painful side may be present. Headache (mostly due to involvement of upper cervical segments), brachial neuralgia, muscle weakness/myelopathy, sensory loss in a dermatomal distribution, sphincter dysfunction, etc., are the patient's presentation in this disorder.

Compression of the cervical roots in the intervertebral foramina, leads to ischemic changes that cause sensory dysfunction (radicular pain, numbness/paresthesia) and/or motor dysfunction (weakness). The C6 root is the most commonly affected, because of predominant degeneration at C5-C6 interspace. The next most common roots affected are C7 and C5. The pain some times even affects the patient's sleep. Vertebrobasilar insufficiency causing vertigo, gait disturbances may also be present.

Chronic spondylosis, sometimes leads to myelopathies. Cervical myelopathy has an insidious onset, which typically becomes apparent in persons in the age group of 50–60 years. Five categories of cervical spondylotic myelopathies exist, such as:

- **Transverse lesion syndrome:** Corticospinal, spinothalamic, and posterior columns are involved.
- **Motor syndrome:** This primarily involves the corticospinal tract, or anterior horn cells.
- **Central cord syndrome:** Motor and sensory impairment is greater in the upper extremities, than the lower extremities.
- **Brown-Sequard syndrome:** Unilateral cord lesion with ipsilateral corticospinal tract involvement and contralateral analgesia are present below the site of lesion.
- **Brachialgia and cord syndrome:** Predominant upper limb pain is present with involvement of some long tracts.

Findings at physical examination may include the followings.
- Decreased ROM of cervical spine more of neck extension.
- **Spurling sign/Positive spurling test:** On extension and lateral flexion of the neck towards the painful side with/ without vertical compression of head causes compromise of the neural foramina resulting in increase of symptoms **(Fig. 6.2)**.

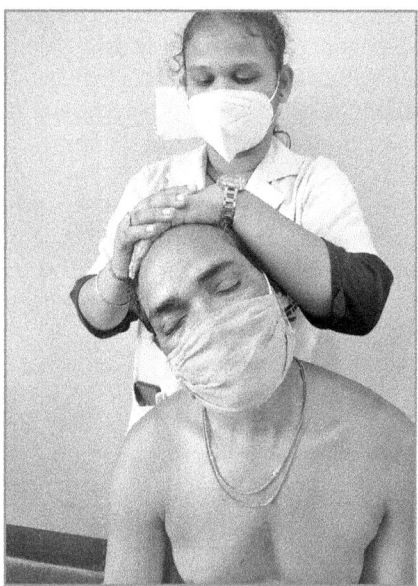

Fig. 6.2: The spurling test.

- **Positive neural tension tests for median/ulnar/radial nerves (Figs. 6.3A to D):** The upper limb tension tests (ULTTs) also known as brachial plexus tension tests or Elvey tests are designed to put stress on nerves (median/ulnar/radial) of upper limb. The shoulder, elbow, forearm, wrist, and fingers are kept in specific positions to put stress on particular nerve (nerve bias). Sensitizing addition like contralateral/ipsilateral neck side flexion is performed to put additional stress on the nerve. While performing the test, the order of joint positioning is shoulder followed by forearm, wrist, fingers, and lastly elbow. Each movement component is added until the pain is provoked or symptoms are reproduced. If no symptoms are produced, on positioning of the upper limb, side flexion of the cervical spine can be added as sensitizer.

If pain or sensations of tingling or numbness are experienced at any stage during movement into the test position or during addition of sensitization maneuvers, particularly reproduction of neck, shoulder, or arm symptoms, the test is positive. This confirms a degree of mechanical interference affecting neural structures, which could be at the intervertebral foramina level also.

Table 6.4 indicates the various upper limb neural tension tests and their procedure of performance.
- Root signs such as hypotonia, muscle atrophy and weakness, sensory loss, and diminished reflexes may be present in individuals with radiculopathy.
- Cord signs such as, hypertonia/spasticity, hyper-reflexia, extensor plantar response, hand clumsiness, clumsy/spastic gait, sensory loss, sphincter disturbances, etc., may be present in those with involvement of the spinal cord.
- Spasm of trapezius, levators, and rhomboids with myofascial bands are found in majority of patients.

Diagnosis

History, clinical findings, and radiological features [X-ray, CT scan/Magnetic resonance imaging (MRI)], and electro-diagnostic tests help for the diagnosis of this disorder.

X-ray and MRI features are:
- Reduction of intervertebral space.
- Facet hypertrophy and marginal osteophyte formation **(Fig. 6.4)**.
- Intervertebral foramina stenosis.
- MRI may also reveal cervical canal stenosis (if any).
- Electrodiagnostic tests such as NCV study, EMG study may be considered, if the client presents features of motor/sensory impairments.

Tests for vertebra basilar insufficiency (VBI)
- **In supine:**
  - *Vertebral artery compression test/Extension and rotation test:* It should be done to exclude compromise of vertebral arteries **(Fig. 6.5)**.
    » *Procedure:* The patient is placed in supine with head and neck at the edge of the bed. The clinician performs full passive extension and side flexion of

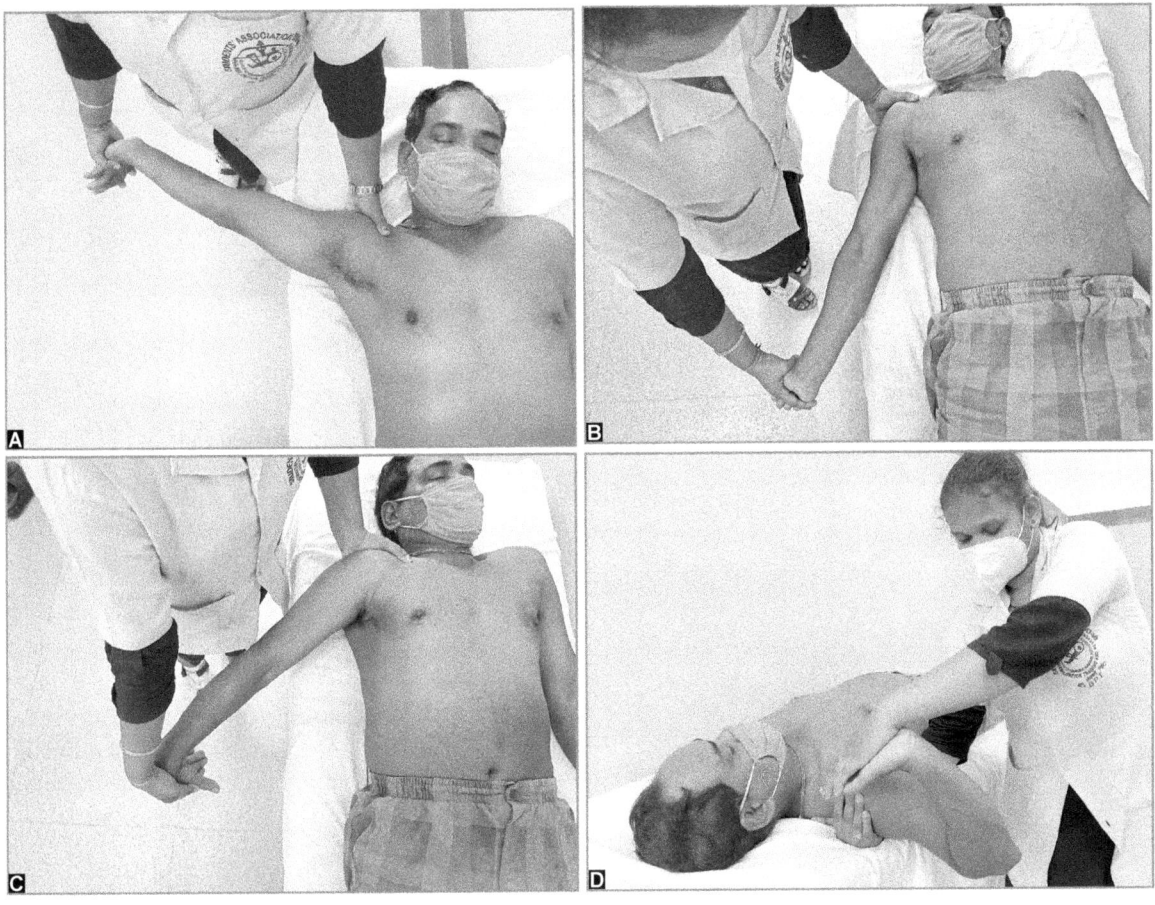

Figs. 6.3A to D: (A) ULTT-1, (B) ULTT-2a, (C) ULTT-2b, (D) ULTT-3.

Table 6.4: The various upper limb neural tension tests and their procedure of performance.

Component parts	ULTT-1 Median nerve/anterior interosseous nerve	ULTT-2a Median nerve, musculo-cutaneous nerve, axillary nerve	ULTT-2b Radial nerve	ULTT-3 Ulnar nerve
Scapula	Depression	Depression	Depression	Depression
Shoulder	Abduction to 110 degrees and laterally rotated	Abduction to 10 degrees and laterally rotated	Abduction to 10 degrees and internally rotated	Abduction to 90 degrees and lateral rotation
Elbow	Extended	Extended	Extended	Flexion
Forearm	Supinated	Supinated	Pronated	Supination
Wrist/fingers/thumb	Extended	Extended	Flexed.	Wrist extension and radial deviation, fingers and thumb extension
Cervical spine (Sensitizer)	Contralateral Side flexion	Contralateral Side flexion	Contralateral Side flexion	Contralateral Side flexion

head and neck to one side. Then the neck is rotated to the same side and held for 30 seconds. Presence of 5D's, i.e., dizziness, diplopia, drop attacks, dysphagia and dysarthria, nystagmus, nausea, etc., suggests compromise of the vertebral artery.

- *The Wallenberg/Underberg test:* The neck of the supine patient is taken to an end range position of rotation, extension or combination of both **(Fig. 6.6)**. At this point presence of vertebrobasilar artery symptoms such as dizziness, vertigo, light headedness, nausea, nystagmus, blurred vision, etc., suggests vertebrobasilar insufficiency.

❖ **In sitting:** Patient rotates head opposite to tested side maximally and holds position for 10 seconds. Patient returns to neutral for 10 seconds. Patient extends head for 10 seconds. Patient returns to neutral for 10 seconds.

Section 2: Physiotherapy for Musculoskeletal Conditions

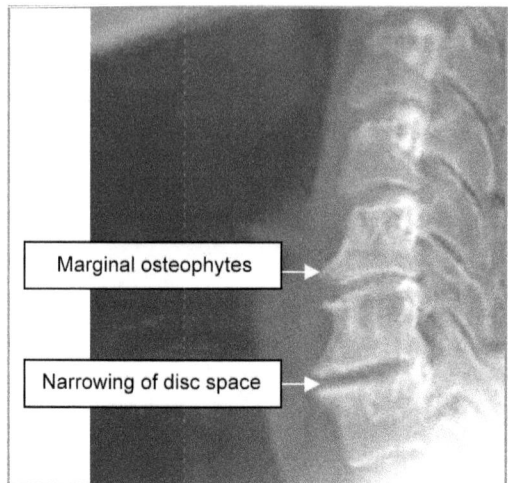

Fig. 6.4: X-ray of neck showing cervical spondylosis.

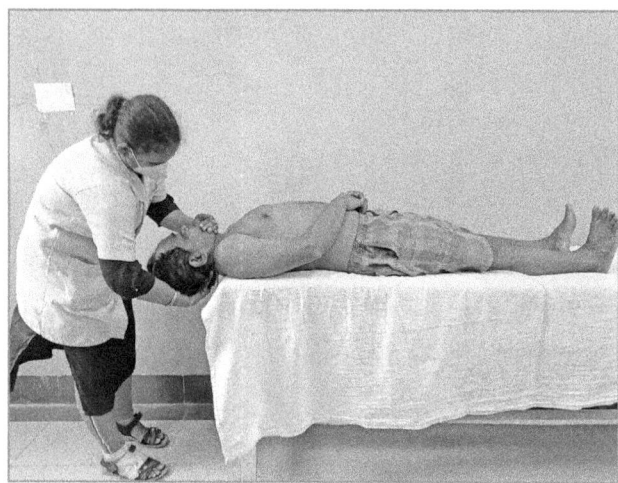

Fig. 6.5: Tests for VBI.

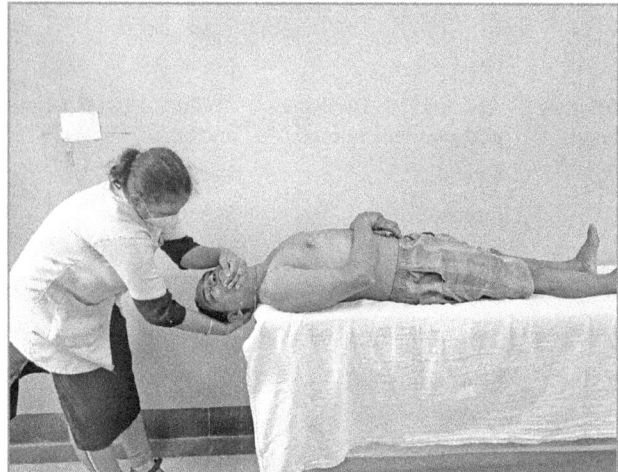

Fig. 6.6: The Wallenberg/Underberg test.

Patient extends and rotates head (again opposite to tested side) maximally for 10 seconds **(Fig. 6.7)**. Positive symptoms include (The 5 D's) dizziness, diplopia, dysarthria, dysphagia, drop attacks, nausea vomiting and sensory changes, nystagmus, etc.

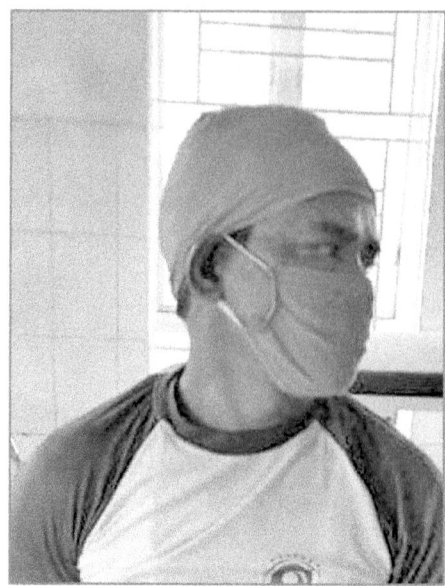

Fig. 6.7: Test for VBI in sitting extension/rotation test.

Management

* **Medical management:** Nonsteroidal anti-inflammatory drugs (NSAIDs), muscle relaxants, calcium supplements in those with osteoporosis, etc., may be considered by the physician.
* **Physiotherapy:**
  - *In acute case:*
    » Rest to cervical spine using either a soft/hard cervical collar, or a rigid support like Philadelphia collar **(Figs. 6.8A to D)** may be recommended during day time use. A cervical pillow or a thin pillow to be used during lying on bed (the patient should never be advised to lie in supine position without a pillow, as the head will fall backwards resulting in extended cervical posture), which may put stress on the degenerated facets and reduce the intervertebral foramina, enhancing local and radicular symptoms).

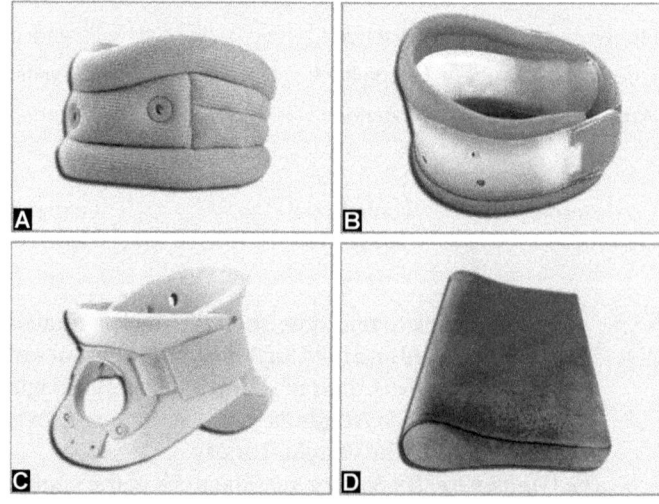

Figs. 6.8A to D: (A) Soft cervical collar, (B) Hard cervical collar, (C) Philadelphia collar, (D) Cervical pillow.

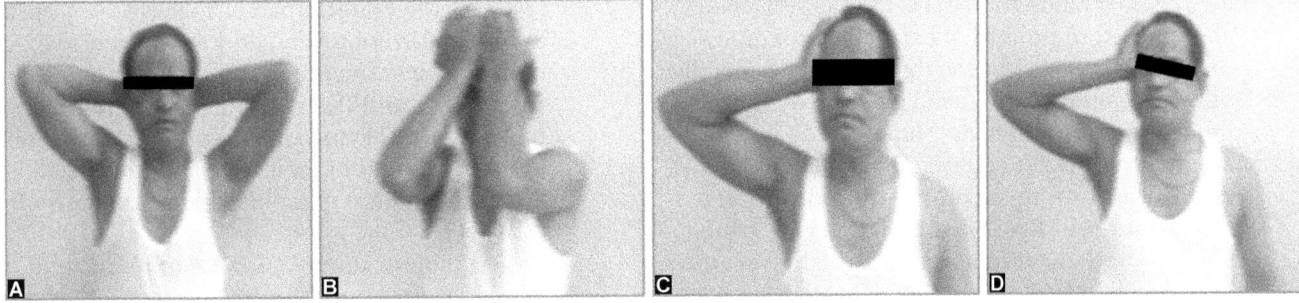

Figs. 6.9A to D: Isometric exercises to cervical spine: (A) Isometric extension, (B) Isometric flexion, (C) Isometric lateral flexion, (D) Isometric rotation.

- » Mechanical traction to cervical spine: Continuous traction to the cervical spine in supine lying and neck slightly flexed using a small pillow/pad of towel with a low load starting with 7% of body weight is helpful to provide relief from pain and spasm and immobilize the cervical spine. The duration of traction ranges from 5-20 minutes, several times in a day as per patients responses.
- » Passive modalities: Moist hot packs, IRR, PSWD/IFT/TENS are applied as indicated.
- » Exercises: Low intensity isometric cervical spine exercises help in strengthening the neck muscles, stabilizes posture, and reduces pain **(Figs. 6.9A to D)**.
- *In the late stage of the disease with/without brachial neuralgia:* Physiotherapy includes:
  - » Posture correction and joint protection techniques.
  - » Stretching/Myofascial release techniques to muscles of neck and upper back to relieve spasm and increase flexibility.
- Use of passive modalities such as Moist hot packs/IRR/SWD/MWD/therapeutic ultrasound/LASER therapy/IFT/TENS, etc., may be selected as appropriate.
  - » Traction: The efficacy of traction has not been conclusively proven in a randomized, controlled trial, but it is commonly used and thought to be beneficial in the treatment of cervical radiculopathy. The rationale for traction is based on elongation of the spine, resultant increase in intervertebral space, relaxation of spinal muscles, opening of the neural foramen, and relief of nerve root compression. Concerning duration of traction forces, Colachis and Strohm showed that nearly all vertebral separation occurs during the first 7 seconds of force application, but that up to 20-25 minutes is necessary to produce muscle relaxation. Intermittent traction produces twice the amount of separation as sustained traction and as a result it is currently the mode of choice. With regard to positioning, traction is typically performed with the patient sitting or supine **(Figs. 6.10A to C)**. The supine position has been shown to provide greater separation of intervertebral spaces from C4 to C7 than sitting, when the angle of pull and force were controlled. Flexion of 20-30 degrees is advocated to obtain the greatest benefit of posterior muscular elongation and enlargement of the intervertebral foramina It appears that at

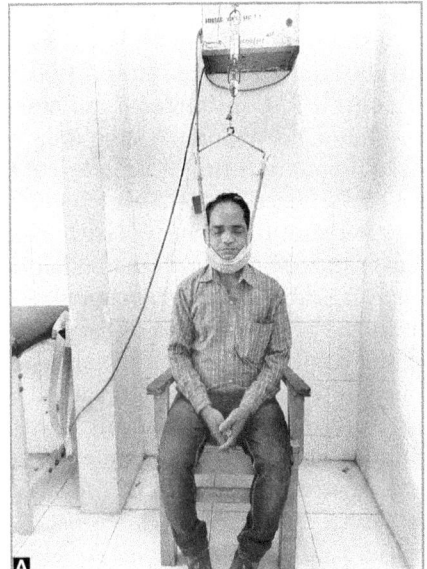
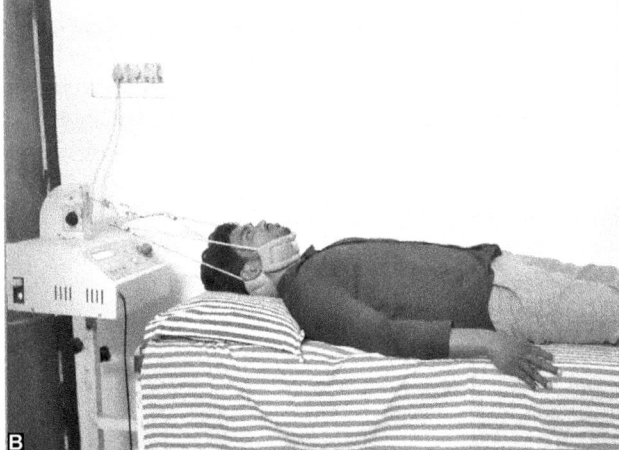
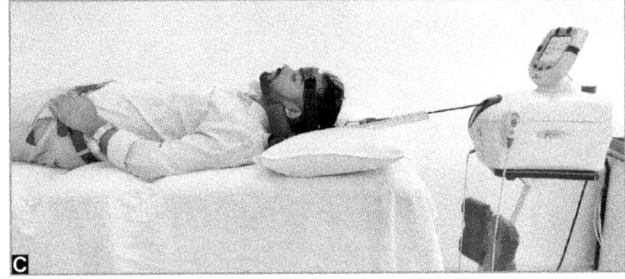

Figs. 6.10A to C: (A) Cervical traction in sitting using mandibular halter, (B) Cervical traction in lying using mandibular halter; (C) Cervical traction in supine using Saunder's halter.

least 25–30 pounds of force (11–13 kg approximately) are required to produce measurable separation of the cervical vertebrae. The traction force generally selected amounts to 1/6th to 1/8th of body weight to produce any significant decompression.

» Manual therapy: It could be high velocity thrust manipulations or nonthrust manipulations/mobilizations. Thrust manipulations are usually applied to thoracic spine, which usually becomes hypo-mobile. Mobilizations such as Maitlands grade 1 and 2 P/A can be applied during acute stage to reduce pain. In chronic stage, with movement limitations and radiculopathy, grade 3 and 4 unilateral P/A on contralateral side, lateral transverse glide on contralateral side in unilateral radiculopathies and central P/A in bilateral radiculopathies, if found relieving symptoms should be used. As far as manipulation (thrust techniques) of the cervical spine is concerned, moderate level evidence support the immediate effectiveness of such manipulations, however the safety of such manipulations remains unclear. It is advisable not to manipulate the cervical spine in the presence of osteophytes.

The McKenzie protocol for cervical spondylosis is applied to reduce dysfunction caused by adaptive shortening of certain structure associated with poor postural habits. The treatment is stretching of shortened structures **(Figs. 6.11A and B)** and postural correction.

» Mulligan's mobilization: Studies done by Pragassame et al., (International Archives of Integrated Medicine, Vol. 8, Issue 1, January, 2021), reveals Mulligan spinal mobilization with arm movement (SMWAM) technique with neurodynamics combined with conventional therapy has a positive effect in patients with cervical radiculopathy by reducing pain, increasing cervical ROM and reducing functional disability.

Natural apophyseal gliding movements (NAGs)/Sustained natural apophyseal gliding movements (SNAGs), which are the part of Mulligan's concept are also helpful in improving cervical ROM and reducing radicular pain including cervicogenic headaches **(Figs. 6.11C and D)**. NAGs mobilize joints mid way through range of movement, whilst SNAGs mobilize joints to the end of their range of movement. The SNAGs are a form of mobilization with movement (MWM)

» Neural mobilization: Graded mobilization of the nerves of the upper limb when combined with cervical traction has been found effective in reducing unilateral radicular pain as per a study done by Kattela et al., in 2017. Hence, it is recommended that neural mobilization should be carefully considered for non-remitting radicular pain in upper limbs in the absence of neurological deficits.

» Moderate intensity isometric strengthening to neck muscles and physiological neck movements are recommended as per the patient's tolerance. However, full range extension and rotation to the painful side should be avoided, if radicular pain persists.

» Advice on home exercise program, posture care, joint protection and energy conservation techniques form an integral part of management. The patient should be educated appropriately. The patient should be advised to use a large/extra large soft cervical collar during functional activities, if radicular pain continues. The collar should be removed periodically for performing exercises. A pocket TENS may be used to reduce intractable pain (if any), during night and while performing functional tasks.

❖ **Surgery:** Patients who do not respond to conservative treatment, and develop progressive neural involvement such as myelopathy (UMN features) or peripheral neuropathy may be recommended for surgery. The indications for surgery include:
  – Progressive neurological deficits.
  – Compression of cervical roots and/or spinal cord.
  – Intractable pain.

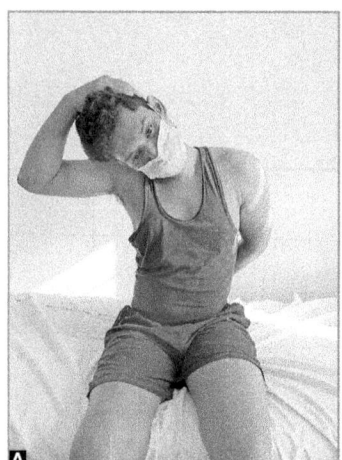 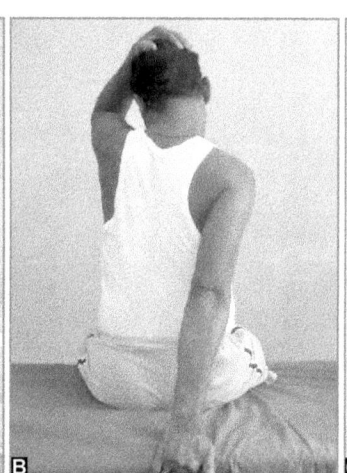 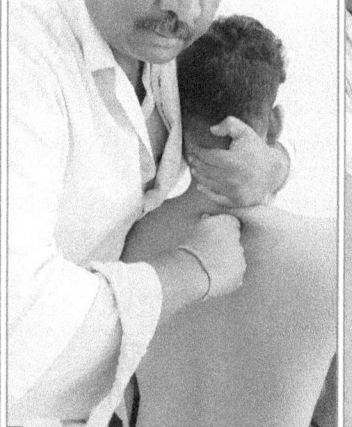 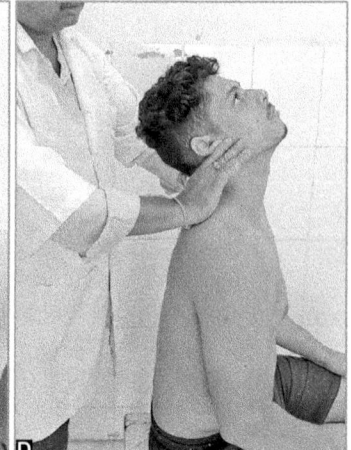

Figs. 6.11A to D: (A) Self-stretching of upper trapezius; (B) Self-stretching of levator scapulae to overcome dysfunction associated with cervical spondylosis; (C) C-NAG to cervical spine; (D) SNAG to cervical spine, with active neck extension.

The aims of surgery are to relieve nerve compression that causes pain and neural deficits such as upper and lower motor neuron features and to achieve spinal stabilization. The surgical approaches include:
- **Anterior approaches:** Discectomy with or without bone graft, cervical instrumentation.
- **Posterior approaches:** Decompressive laminectomy and foraminotomy, hemilaminectomy.

2. Cervical Prolapsed Intervertebral Disc (PIVD)

An intervertebral disc is a cartilaginous structure composed of three components (1) an inner nucleus pulposus, (2) outer annulus fibrosus, and (3) endplates **(Fig. 6.12)** that anchor the discs to adjacent vertebrae. It is an avascular structure. The discs are present throughout the cervical spine between the interbody joints, except between C1 and C2. The discs are connected to the vertebral bodies through 1 mm thick vertebral end plate, made of fibro and hyaline cartilage.

Disc herniations occur when part or all of the nucleus pulposus protrudes through the annulus fibrosus. This process can occur acutely or more chronically. Chronic herniations occur when the intervertebral disc becomes degenerated and desiccated as part of the natural aging process; this typically results in symptoms of insidious or gradual onset that tend to be less severe. In contrast, acute herniations generally are the result of trauma, resulting in the nucleus pulposus extruding through a defect in the annulus fibrosus. This injury will usually result in a sudden onset of more severe symptoms when compared to chronic herniations.

The central portion of the disc, called nucleus pulposus, is made of type-II collagen that contains water and proteoglycans. The annulus fibrosus is made of type-I collagen, and has a structure of 12 concentric layer of lamellae with alternate layers of collagen. It also contains water and proteoglycans.

The disc discharges the following functions:
- Acts as a shock absorber.
- It allows compressive, tensile, and rotational motion.

Epidemiology and Etiology of Cervical PIVD

The prevalence of cervical disc herniation increases with age for both men and women and is most common in people in their third to fifth decades of life. It occurs more frequently in females:
- Factors associated with injury are: Frequent lifting of heavy objects and carrying objects on the head, continuous

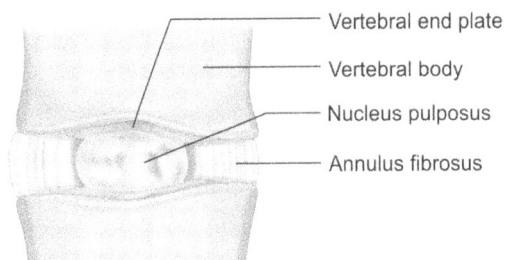

Fig. 6.12: The intervertebral disc.

forward head posture as occurs in Desk workers/IT professionals, as well as people using very thick pillows.
- Cigarette smoking.

Pathophysiology

The pathophysiology of herniated discs is thought to be a combination of mechanical compression of the nerve by the bulging nucleus pulposus and local increase in inflammatory cytokines. Compressive forces can result in varying degrees of microvascular damage, which can range from mild compression producing obstruction of venous flow that causes congestion and edema, to severe compression, which can result in arterial ischemia. Herniated disc material and nerve irritation may induce the production of inflammatory cytokines, which can include: interleukin (IL)-1 and IL-6, substance P, bradykinin, tumor necrosis factor-alpha, and prostaglandins. There may even be an additional role that stretching on the nerve root plays in the reproduction of symptoms. The trajectory of the cervical nerve as it exits the neural foramen makes it susceptible to stretch, in addition to compression from a herniation. This arrangement could, in part, explain why certain patients experience pain relief from the abduction of the arm, which presumably decreases the amount of stretch the nerve experiences.

Herniations are more likely to occur posterolaterally, where the annulus fibrosus is thinner and lacks the structural support from the PLL. Due to the proximity of the herniation to the traversing cervical nerve root, a herniation that compresses the cervical root as it exits can result in radiculopathy in the associated dermatome.

Types of Disc Bulge

The bulging of disc could be of four types **(Fig. 6.13)**:
1. **Protrusion:** It mostly causes neck pain.
2. **Prolapse:** It causes neck and arm pain.

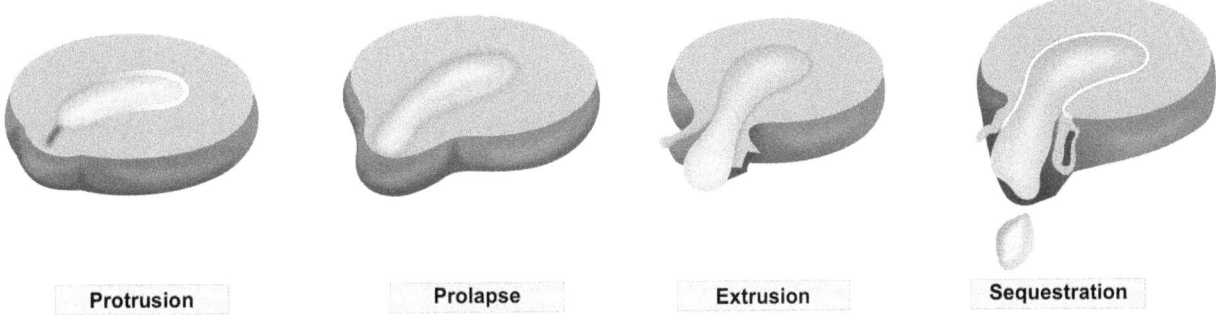

Fig. 6.13: Types of disc bulge.

3. **Extrusion:** It causes neck and arm pain.
4. **Sequestration:** It causes arm pain, but no neck pain.

The disc bulge in cervical spine could be:
- Central.
- Posterolateral.
- Foraminal.
- Extraforaminal.

Cervical disc prolapse is mostly posterolateral in nature, as the strong PLL prevents the central/posterior bulge from occurring **(Fig. 6.14)**.

Common sites of cervical disc prolapsed

The C5-C6 disc is more prone for prolapsed, as maximum movement in the cervical spine occurs at this site. However, in old people, prolapse of C6-C7 disc occurs. Depending upon the site of prolapse the nerve roots are affected, e.g., prolapse of C5-C6 disc will cause compression of C6 root, as the C6 root passes above C6, between C5 and C6. A herniated disc impinges upon the nerve root exiting above the disc and passing through the nearby foramen result in involvement of one specific neurological level **(Fig. 6.15)**.

Clinical Features of Cervical Disc Prolapse

The features depend on the type of disc bulge such as, posterior or posterolateral and whether the injury to the disc is a protrusion /prolapsed/ extrusion/ sequestration. In case of a posterior disc bulge, the patient may present with neck and bilateral arm pain with UMN features below the site of prolapse and LMN features in the muscles supplied by the root coming from the affected segment of the spinal cord. In the posterolateral disc bulge, the patient may show unilateral features (except when the prolapse has occurred bilaterally). The features of posterolateral disc bulge in the cervical spine are:

- Neck pain radiating to arm or chest in the dermatomal pattern.
- Pain is less at rest, but increases in upright posture.
- Increase of pain on forward and lateral bending of neck.
- In prolapse, extrusion and sequestration the pain in the neck or arm may increase on sneezing/coughing/laughing.
- Neurological deficiencies such as muscle weakness, sensory loss, and diminished reflexes may be present in the myotomal, dermatomal patterns as well as the nerve root affected. Depending upon the nerve roots affected, the following movements may be impaired **(Table 6.5)**.

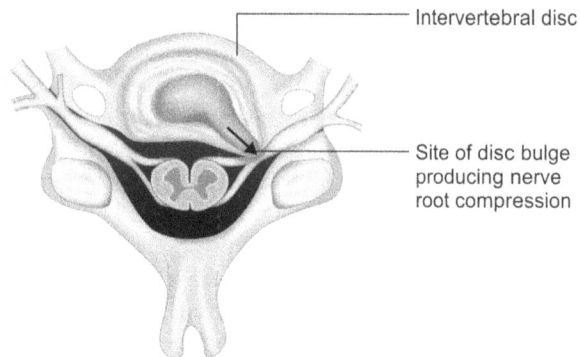

Fig. 6.14: Posterolateral disc bulge.

Table 6.5: Movements impaired depending upon the nerve roots affected.

Nerve root affected	Muscle weakness/movement impaired
C1/C2	Neck flexion/extension
C3	Neck lateral flexion
C4	Shoulder girdle elevation
C5	Shoulder abduction/elbow flexion
C6	Wrist extension
C7	Elbow extension/wrist flexion/finger extension
C8	Finger flexion
T1	Finger abduction

- In case of vertebral artery involvement patient may complain of dizziness, tinnitus, blurring of vision and retro-ocular pain.

In posterior/central disc bulge, the patient may present with UMN features, motor and sensory deficits and a clumsy gait.

Clinical Examination

The findings of examination reveal:
- Restriction of cervical ROM. Flexion more limited as compared to extension. However, in old people (> 40 years old) extension of cervical spine may be more limited than flexion.
- Cervicothoracic scoliosis, with convexity on the painful side.
- Muscle weakness/tingling numbness on the affected side upper limb.
- **Special tests such as:**
  - *Spurling test* **(Fig. 6.2)** may be positive, where the pain that arises in the neck, radiates in the direction of corresponding dermatomes ipsilaterally.
  - *Lhermitte's sign* **(Fig. 6.16):** This phenomenon is also called as Barber chair phenomenon. It is an

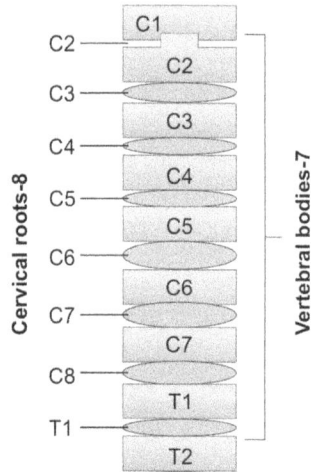

Fig. 6.15: Displays the different roots emerging from different cervical vertebral segments.

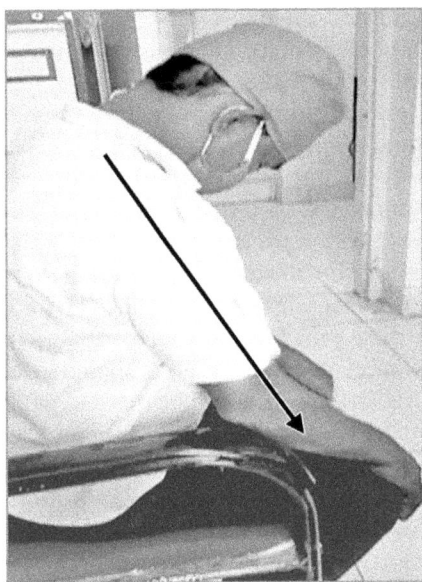

Fig. 6.16: The Lhermitte sign.

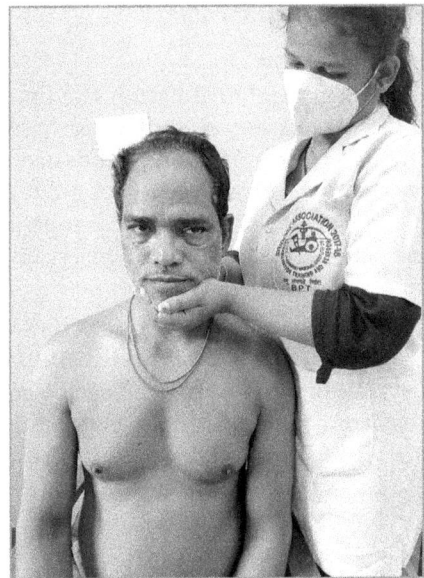

Fig. 6.18: Distraction test for cervical spine.

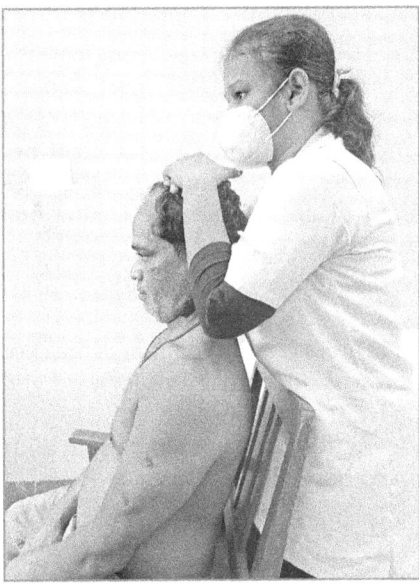

Fig. 6.17: Compression test.

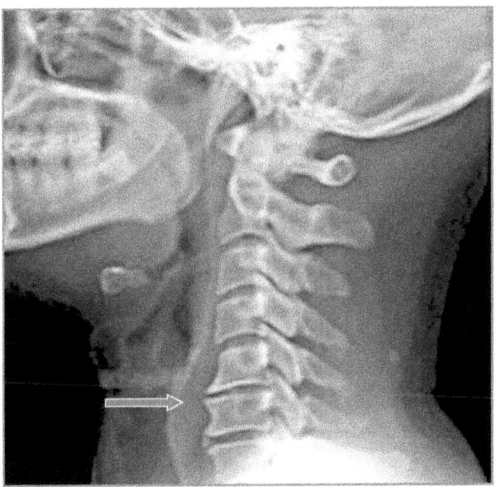

Fig. 6.19: X-ray of cervical spine showing C5-C6 disc bulge.

uncomfortable electrical sensation produced on neck flexion or extension, radiating from the spine to the limbs.
- *Compression test* **(Fig. 6.17)**: In lying/sitting, the patient's head is pressed downward. Any increase of pain suggests nerve root compression.
- *Distraction tes*t **(Fig. 6.18)**: This test evaluates the effect of traction on relief of pain. In sitting, the clinician pulls the head up by placing one hand under the chin and the other hand under the occiput. If the pain reduces in intensity, the patient is understood to get benefit with traction.

Confirmatory investigatory tests for cervical PIVD
- X-ray of cervical spine **(Fig. 6.19)**.
- MRI **(Fig. 6.20)**
- CT scan.
- Myelogram.

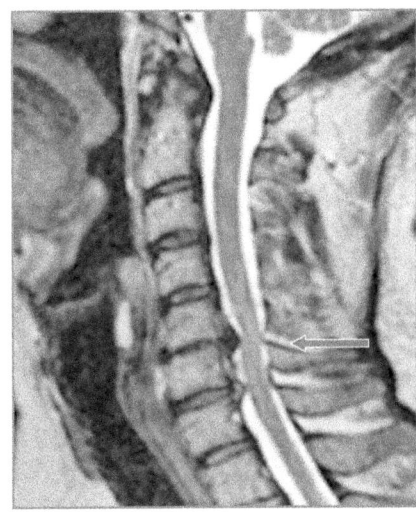

Fig. 6.20: MRI showing C5-C6 and C6-C7 disc bulge.

Management of Cervical Disc Bulge

Conservative management

Conservative/nonsurgical treatment is the first step to be followed to promote recovery in cervical disc herniation. The methods of treatment include: short periods of rest, NSAIDs, physiotherapy, and cervical orthosis. A great majority of people with cervical disc prolapse and arm pain recover in about 6 weeks and return to job. The conservative methods of management are described as under:

Medication: There is no evidence to demonstrate the efficacy of NSAIDs in the treatment of cervical radiculopathy. However, they are commonly used and can be beneficial for some patients. If oral medications and physiotherapy fails in reducing pain arising from a cervical disc bulge, therapeutic injections such as cervical epidural steroid injections, selective nerve root injections may be considered by the Physician/surgeon.

Rest and activity modification: A cervical herniated disc is very much painful when it first develops or during intermittent flare-ups, that occurs during activity. During the acute stage, when the pain in neck is severe and/or radiates down into the arm or hand, a short period of rest and/or activity modification is advised as follows:
- Refraining from strenuous activities, such as physical labor or playing sports
- Avoiding specific movements that worsen pain, like turning head to one side.
- Modifying sleep positions, by using the cervical pillow/using cervical roll **(Fig. 6.21)** and/or sleeping on the back instead of the side or prone.
- Relative rest to the cervical spine through use of cervical collar. A short course of continuous use of cervical collar may be beneficial during the acute stage. Subsequently, as the acute pain subsides, the patient should be advised to use the cervical collar during activity, if pain persists.

Physiotherapy: Commonly started after a short period of rest and immobilization. Modalities include cervical stabilization exercises (isometric neck exercises), graduated range of motion exercises focusing on flexion at last, heat, ultrasound, and electrical stimulation and traction.

Traction: Cervical traction has been used widely to help relieve neck pain from muscle spasm or nerve compression. Traction may be beneficial in reducing the radicular symptoms associated with disc herniations. Theoretically, traction would widen the neural foramen and relieve the stress placed on the affected nerve, which, in turn, would result in the improvement of symptoms. The traction should be given in supine lying as compared to sitting, as the muscles of neck remain relaxed in lying as compared to sitting. It can be applied in sustained/intermittent mode as per the patient's tolerance and benefits obtained. However, static traction with a low load (3-4 kg) should be applied initially in a position of neck that is comfortable **(Fig. 6.22)** for a short time (5-10 minutes). However, after the acute pain subsided, intermittent cervical traction with a load of 5-7 kg with neck in slight flexion (20-30 degrees, if comfortable) for 20-30 minutes is applied.

Use of passive modalities such as SWD/PSWD/MWD/IRR/Moist hot packs, IFT, TENS/ Therapeutic ultrasound, etc., should be selected as required.

McKenzie Approach: For most cervical disc disorders, studies support conservative treatment, such as the McKenzie approach and cervicothoracic stabilization programs combined with aerobic conditioning are helpful. The McKenzie protocol, and its use in the management of neck pain, is discussed below:

McKenzie method of assessment: The McKenzie mechanical assessment consists of:
- Evaluation of gross range of motion of the cervical spine.
- Cervical protrusion (maximum forward glide/anterior translation without rotation).
- Cervical retraction (maximal backward glide/posterior translation without rotation).

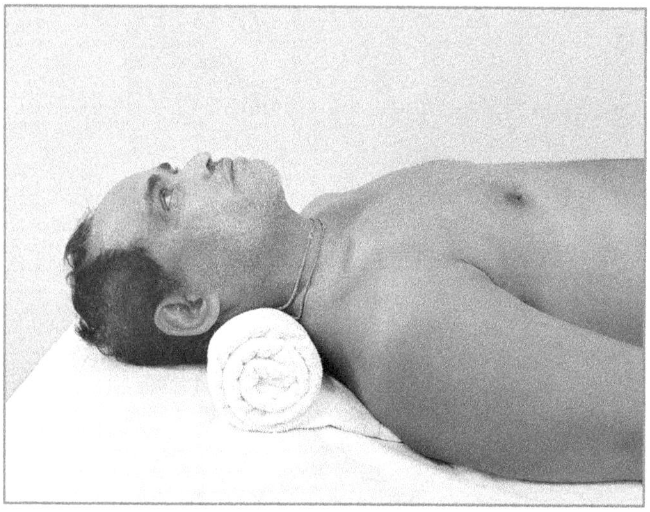

Fig. 6.21: Cervical roll.

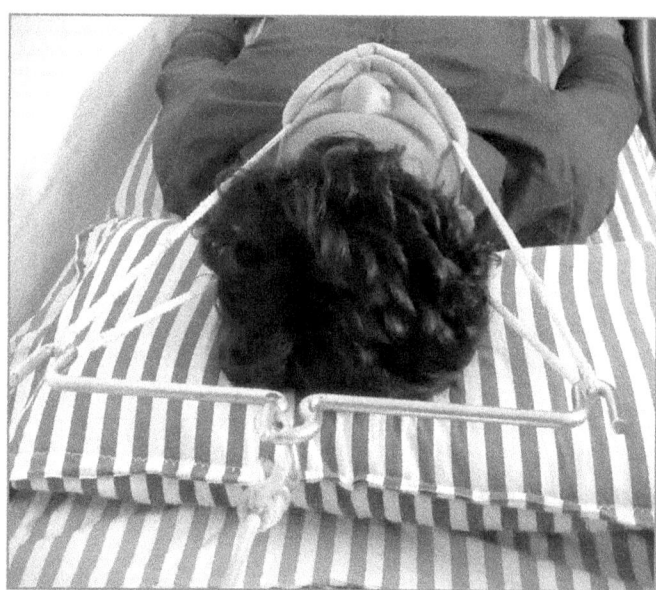

Fig. 6.22: Static cervical traction in acute PIVD.

The movements should be performed on a repeated basis (5-15 times) and the effects of symptoms (increased/decreased, peripheralized/centralized), should be noted.

If there is reduction/centralization of symptoms with test movements of end-range neck extension and retraction, the same movements should be considered for treatment, as cervical PIVD peripheralizes with neck flexion and protrusion and centralizes with neck extension and retraction. Neck retraction **(Fig. 6.23)** which has been advocated by McKenzie causes extension of the lower cervical segment and helps in alleviating stress on the posterior annulus, there by causing relief of pain.

McKenzie method of treatment: Flexion exercises of the cervical spine are to be avoided initially and the initial exercise consists of chin tuck/neck retraction exercises, progressing to chin tuck with neck extension exercises.

- In sitting/standing: The chin tuck is performed either in sitting or standing, where the patient is asked to look forward and tuck the chin toward the neck, hold for 10 seconds before coming to the neutral position.
- In supine, a small pillow is placed under the occiput to maintain slight flexion of neck. Patient is made to perform retraction of neck with overpressure applied by therapist at end range of retraction and the end position should be maintained for 1 second. 3-4 sets (10-15 repetitions in a set) of exercise are to be performed with advice to maintain proper posture (avoiding forward head posture) and to perform 10-15 repetitions of exercise in every waking hour.
- The exercises should be progressed by performing neck retraction with cervical extension in supine, neck retraction and extension in sitting with therapist applied overpressure, followed by neck retraction and extension combined with clinician applied traction at end range **(Fig. 6.24)**.

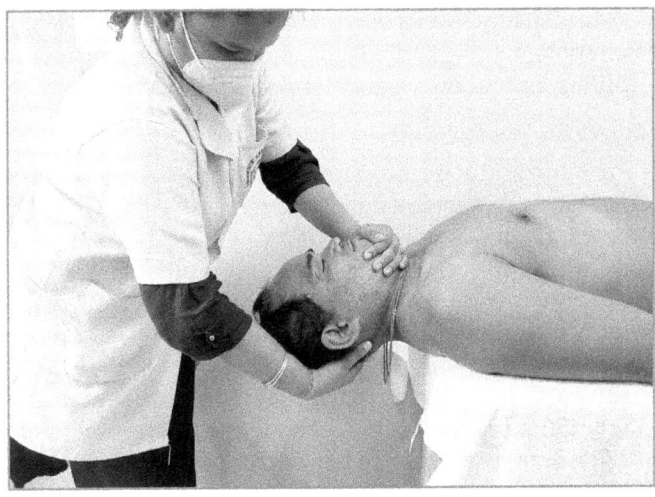

Fig. 6.24: Neck extension and retraction combined with manual traction.

- Cervicothoracic stabilization exercises **(Fig. 6.36A)**/isometric strengthening exercises **(Figs. 6.9A to D)** to increase strength of cervicothoracic muscles.
- Stretching exercises/massage/myofascial release techniques **(Fig. 6.25)** are performed to increase flexibility which in combination with strengthening exercises help to maintain normal biomechanics of the cervical spine.
- Aerobic exercises and functional re-education training are to be given as the pain subsides. The patient should be advised for neck care measures such as avoiding use of thick pillows and using cervical pillow/cervical roll/thin pillows, avoiding carrying of load on head, etc., and to perform home exercise program as per the advice of therapist/clinician.
- **Cervical manipulation:** There is limited evidence suggesting that cervical manipulation may provide short-term benefits for neck pain and cervicogenic headaches. Complications from manipulation are rare and can include worsening

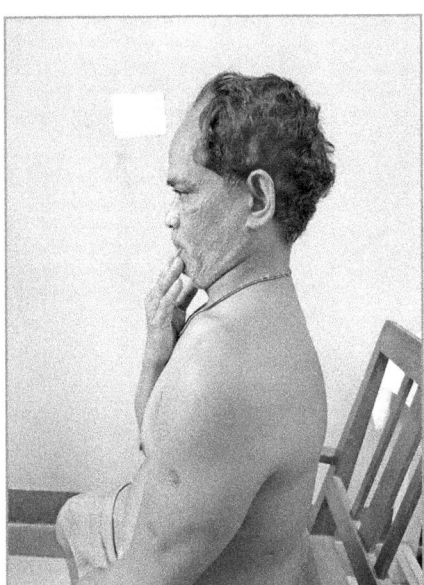

Fig. 6.23: Chin tuck (neck retraction exercise), that centralizes pain.

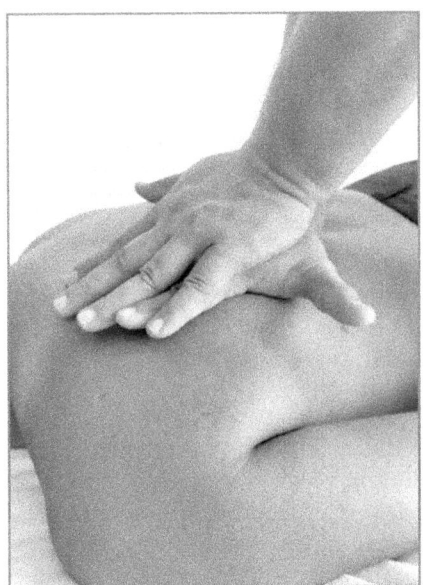

Fig. 6.25: Myofascial release for cervicothoracic muscles.

radiculopathy, myelopathy, spinal cord injury, and vertebral artery injury. A manipulation should only be considered during the chronic stage of the disease/ hard disc injuries.

Surgery for Cervical PIVD

If the symptoms do not subside and patient develops progressive neurological deficit, surgery is the next choice of intervention. It consists of:

- Anterior cervical decompression and spinal fusion: The purpose is to remove pressure on the spinal cord/nerve roots by removing the damaged disc and reconstructing the spinal column.
- Minimal invasive surgeries like microdiscectomy/ foraminotomy are performed to remove pressure on the exiting nerve root from a bulged disc. A microdiscectomy when performed does not require spinal fusion.
- Synthetic/artificial disc replacement is currently undertaken, which helps to maintain the normal biomechanics of the spinal column.
- Postoperative physiotherapy depends upon the method of surgery performed and aims at:
  - Improvement of breathing.
  - Improvement of range of motion and strength of cervical and affected muscles of trunk and limbs.
  - Reduction of pain (if any).
  - Improvement of endurance.
  - Improvement of function.
- Home care advice to a patient with cervical disc prolapse, managed conservatively/surgically: As recurrences of disc prolapse in the cervical region is frequently seen after conservative or surgical management without spinal fusion such as micro/ partial discectomy, the patient should be advised to follow ergonomic measures, such as use of proper chairs and work desks, avoid putting load on head and use cervical collar during activities requiring frequent forward bending and to perform regular exercises.

3. Postural Neck Pain (Forward Head Posture)

Postural neck pain is caused due to prolonged adaptation of poor posture such as a forward head posture. This puts stress on the soft tissues in the cervicothoracic region that stabilizes the neck and supports the head. The movement of the head forward results in stretch weakness, microtrauma, and subsequent myofascial band formation in the posterior neck muscles, resulting in neck pain. This pain can radiate down the back and also into the arm. This can also give pins and needles sensation as nerves are also irritated. The forward head posture is also called scholar's neck, where the chin protrudes and the neck is misaligned to the rest of the spine.

Etiology/Risk Factors

The factors that lead to the development of bad posture causing postural neck pain are:
- Frequent use of smart phone and computers.
- Inactivity/leading a sedentary living.
- Using inappropriate chairs, computer/ office tables and pillows.

Pathophysiology

Forward head posture that coexists with upper cross syndrome is the main factor for postural neck pain (**Fig. 6.26**).

There occurs hyperextension of the upper cervical vertebrae with forward alignment of the vertebrae. Thoracic kyphosis, causing rounded upper back and slouched forward shoulders is associated with the forward head posture. Subsequently, painful shortening of muscles of neck and upper back and compression of the upper cervical vertebrae develop. The muscles involved are the cervical flexor muscles (sternocleidomastoid, scalenus anterior, longus cervicis, and longus capitis), cervical extensor muscles (Semispinalis capitis, semispinalis cervicis, iliocostalis cervicis, longissimus cervicis, longissimus capitis, longissimus thoracis, iliocostalis thoracis, semispinalis thoracis, rectus capitis posterior major, and scalenus posterior), mid thoracic muscles (Rhomboid muscles, middle and lower trapezius, pectoralis major). The posterior cervical muscles such as semispinalis cervicis, levator scapulae undergo stretch weakness, where as semispinalis capitis, rectus capitis posterior major undergoes shortening (**Fig. 6.27**). The flexor muscles of the neck namely longus cervicis, scalenus anterior, sternocleidomastoid, undergoes shortening, and longus capitis undergoes lengthening. Pain in the neck and upper back is the common outcome of increased compressive forces as well as increased muscle tension produced in the neck.

Clinical Features of Postural Neck Pain

The patients exhibit the features such as:
- Neck pain.
- Occipital headache.
- Upper and mid back discomfort.
- Muscle tension in the neck, upper back and shoulders producing myofascial bands/myofascial trigger points.
- Shoulder stiffness.
- Temporomandibular joint pain.

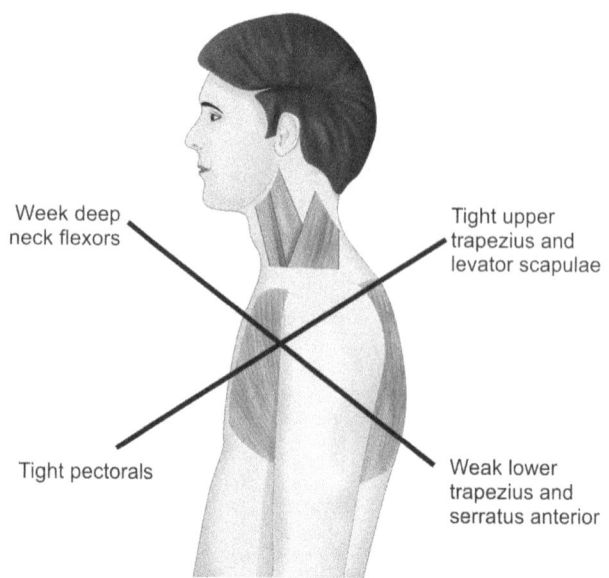

Fig. 6.26: The upper cross syndrome.

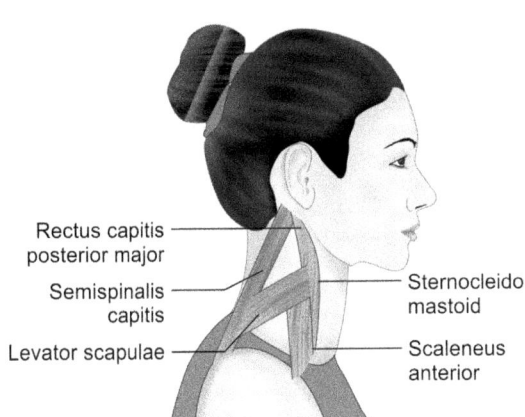

Fig. 6.27: Forward head posture and the muscles shortened/lengthened.

- Breathing difficulties due to weakness of the accessory muscles of respiration.
- Shortening of upper cervical extensors and lower cervical flexors.

Diagnosis of Forward Head Posture

The diagnosis of forward head posture is done by:
- Observation.
- Simple clinical test such as making the individual stand with the pelvis and back fully touching the wall. If the head (occiput) does not touch the wall, it indicates the presence of forward head posture (**Fig. 6.28**).
- X-ray examination.

Physiotherapy Management

The aim of physiotherapy for postural neck pain includes:
- To decrease pain.
- To improve posture.
- To provide ergonomic advice.
- To increase the flexibility of the tight muscles around the neck and upper trunk.
- To strengthen weak muscles around the neck and upper back.
- To restore normal function.

Physiotherapy treatment intervention
- Posture correction and ergonomic advice (**Fig. 6.29**).
- Passive modalities such as moist hot packs, IRR, therapeutic ultrasound (**Fig. 6.30**), High power LASER, are applied before stretching exercises.
- Soft tissue massage/myofascial release/soft tissue stretching (**Figs. 6.31A to C**).
- Positional stretching of rhomboids (**Figs. 6.32A and B**).
- Myofascial release (**Fig. 6.33**).
- Muscle energy technique (MET) to tight neck muscles (**Fig. 6.34**).
- Self stretching of neck extensors and pectoral muscles- corner stretch (**Figs. 6.35A and B**).
- Cervical spine stabilization exercises, strengthening of lower trapezius and serratus anterior muscles (**Figs. 6.36A to C**).
- Pain modulation by using IFT/TENS.

4. Upper Back Pain

Pain in the upper back is usually caused by soft tissue injuries such as sprains/ strains, muscle tension due to poor posture,

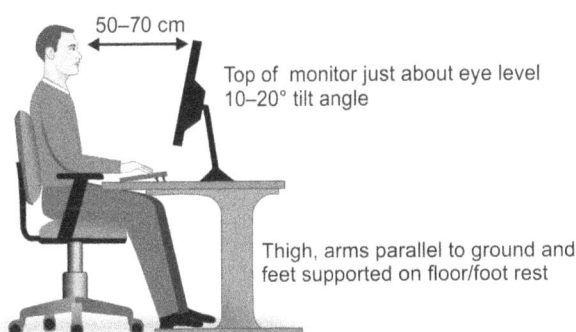

Fig. 6.29: Displays ergonomic arrangement of computer for office work in sitting.

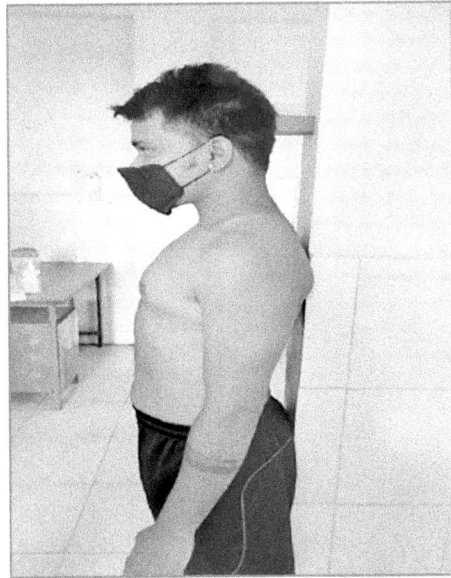

Fig. 6.28: Test for forward head posture.

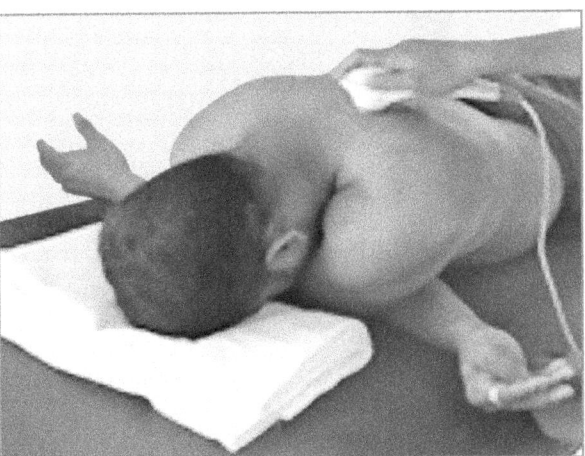

Fig. 6.30: Ultrasound therapy to rhomboids.

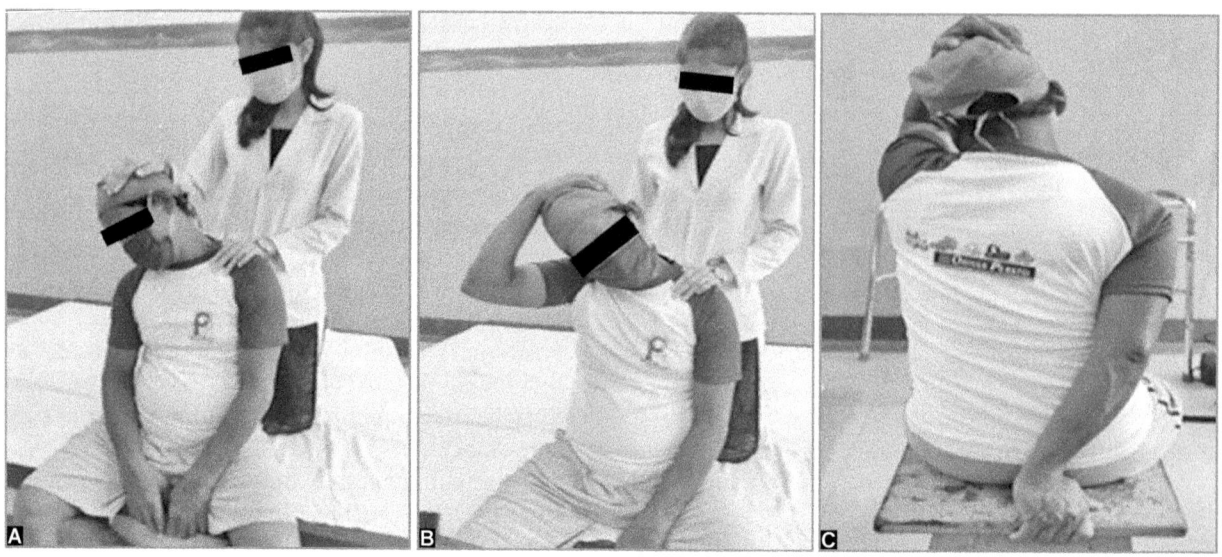

Figs. 6.31A to C: (A) Stretching of left upper trapezius muscle. (B) Self stretching of left scalene muscles (C) Self stretching of right levator scapulae.

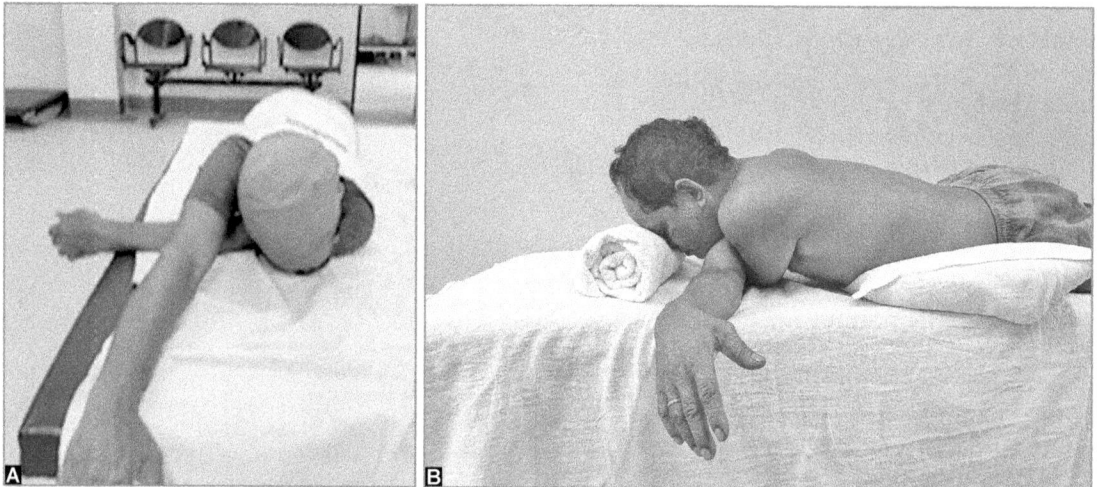

Figs. 6.32A and B: Positional stretching for rhomboids: (A) Unilateral (left), (B) Bilateral.

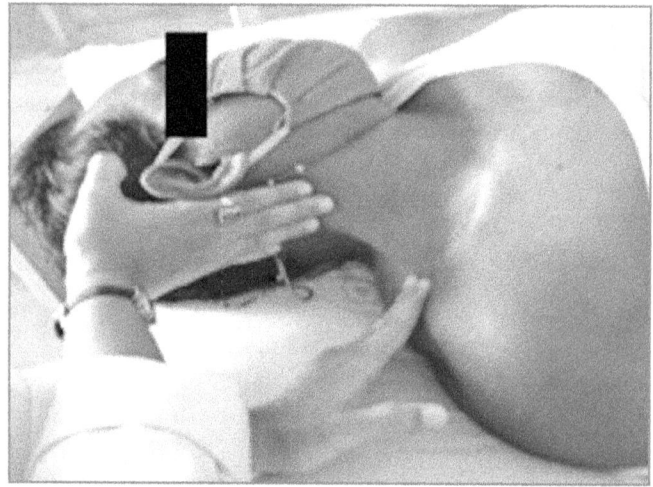

Fig. 6.33: Myofascial release to levator scapulae.

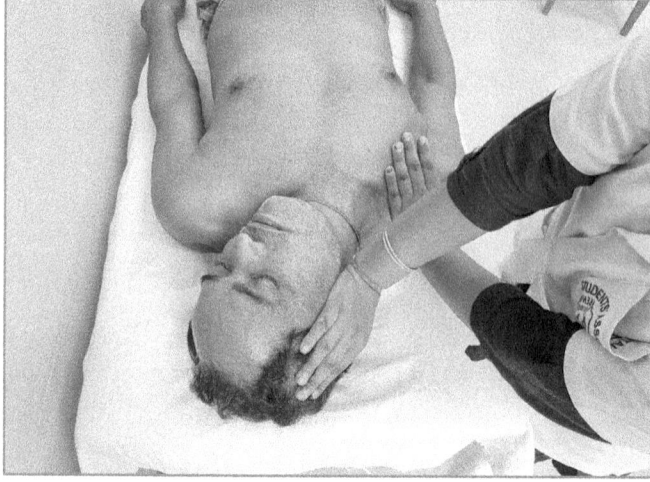

Fig. 6.34: MET to tight neck muscles.

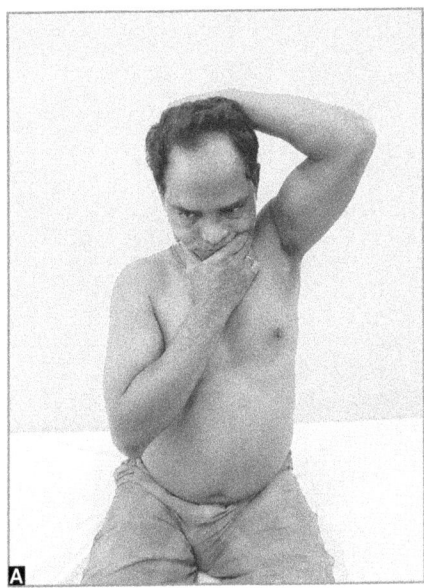

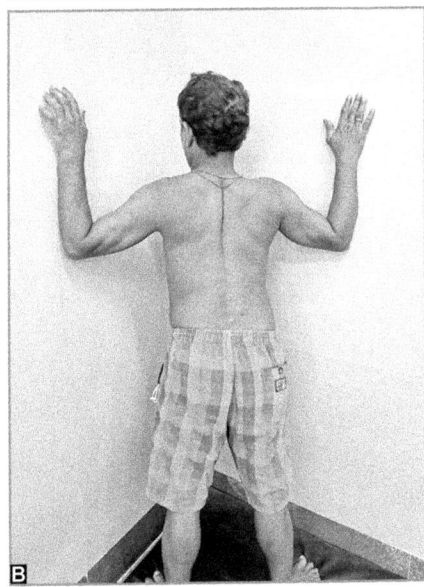

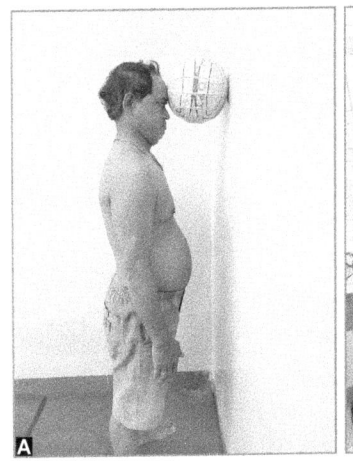 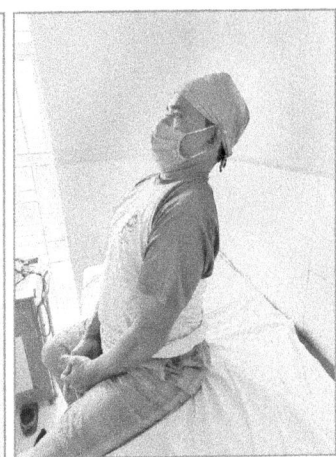

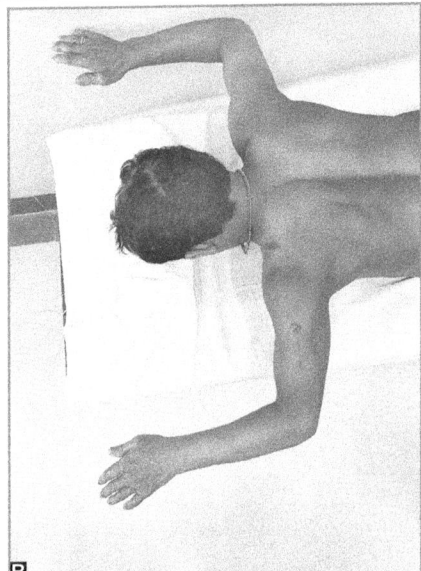

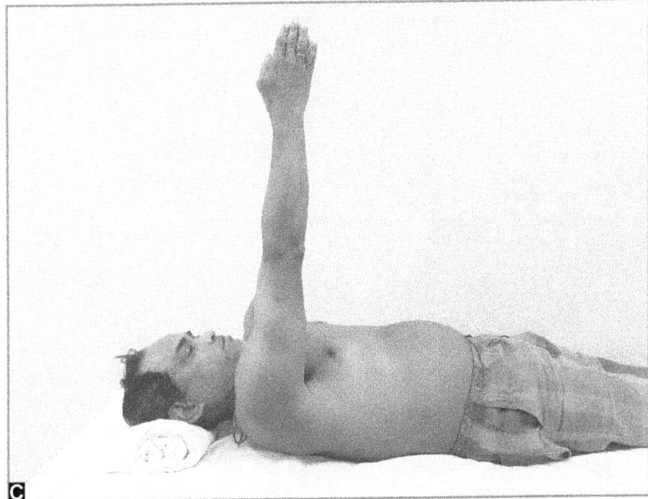

Figs. 6.35A and B: (A) Self stretching of neck extensors, (B) Self stretching of pectorals-corner stretch.

Figs. 6.36A to C: (A) Cervical stabilization exercises, (B) Strengthening of lower trapezius, (C) Strengthening of serratus anterior.

osteoarthritis, disc herniation, ergonomically unfavourable working environment etc. Besides the above in females long damp hairs falling on the posterior neck and upper back is also considered to cause spasm of muscles of neck and upper back and development of myofascial bands leading to upper back pain.

The pathophysiology and clinical features of upper back pain are similar to that of postural neck pain and the management is in the same lines that of postural neck pain. Modalities like ultrasound therapy **(Fig. 6.30)**, high power laser therapy **(Fig. 6.37)**, moist hot packs, SWD/MWD, IFT, etc., should be selected as needed.

A few points regarding management include:
- Deep breathing exercises, combined with upper limb elevation.
- Elbow kneading **(Fig. 6.38A)**/DTFM/Myofascial release **(Fig. 6.38B)**.
- Positional stretching for rhomboids **(Fig. 6.32)**.
- Functional stretching of muscles of upper back **(Figs. 6.39A to C and 6.35B)**.
- Shoulder shrugs **(Fig. 6.39D)**.

Section 2: Physiotherapy for Musculoskeletal Conditions

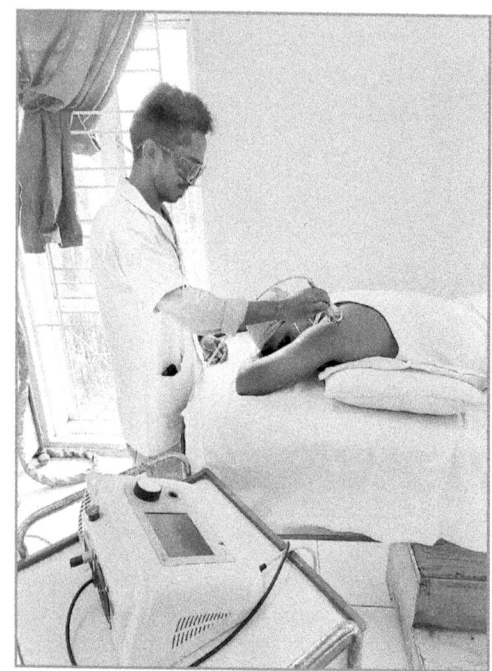

Fig. 6.37: High power laser therapy to parascapular muscles.

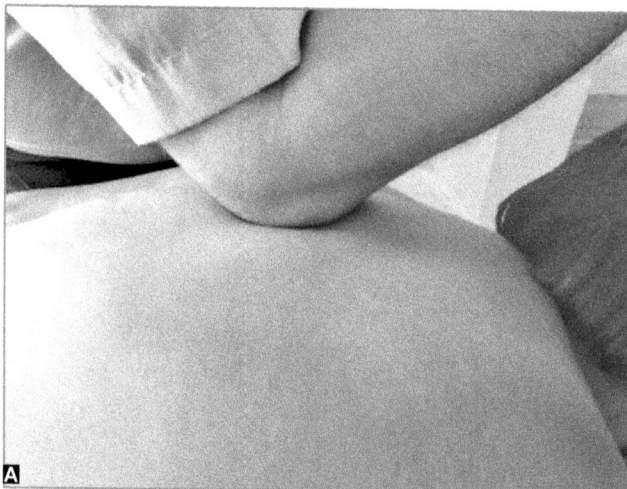

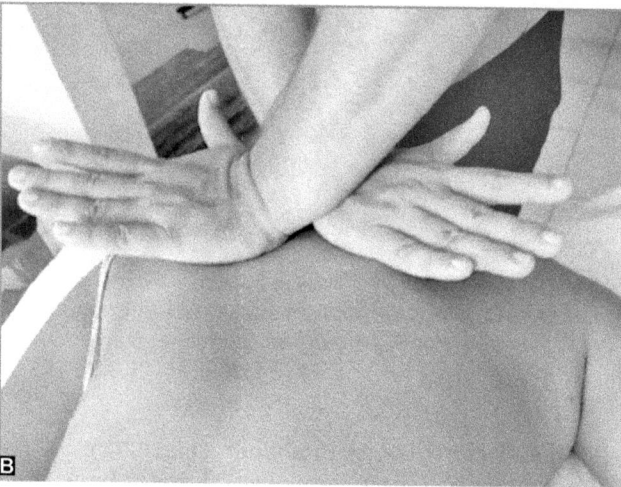

Figs. 6.38A and B: (A) Elbow kneading to muscles of upper back, (B) Myofascial release to rhomboids.

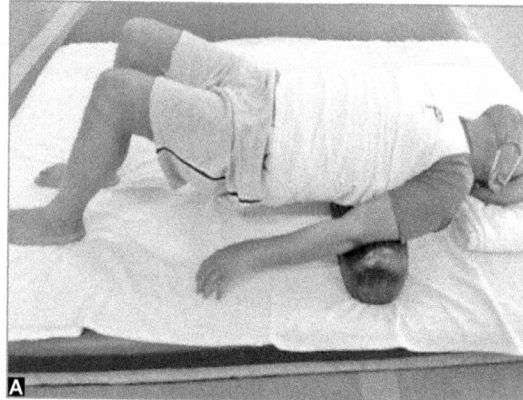

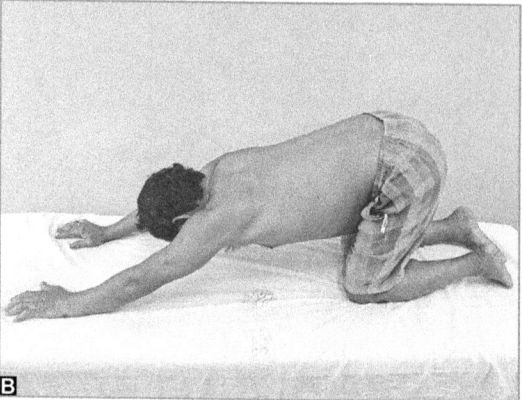

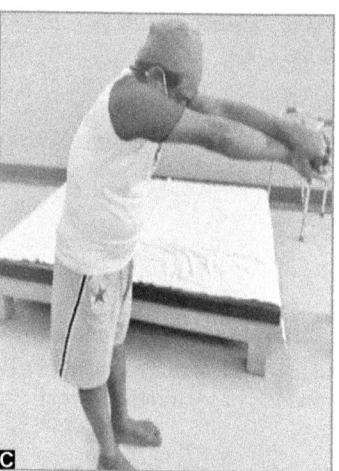

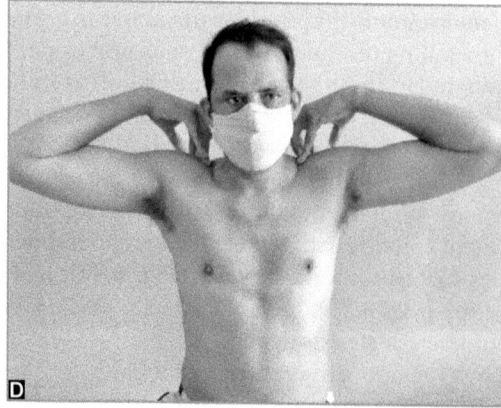

Figs. 6.39A to D: Functional stretching of upper back: (A) Crook lying with bolster under upper back, (B) Stretching in quadruped, (C) Active stretching in standing; (D) Shoulder shrugging exercise.

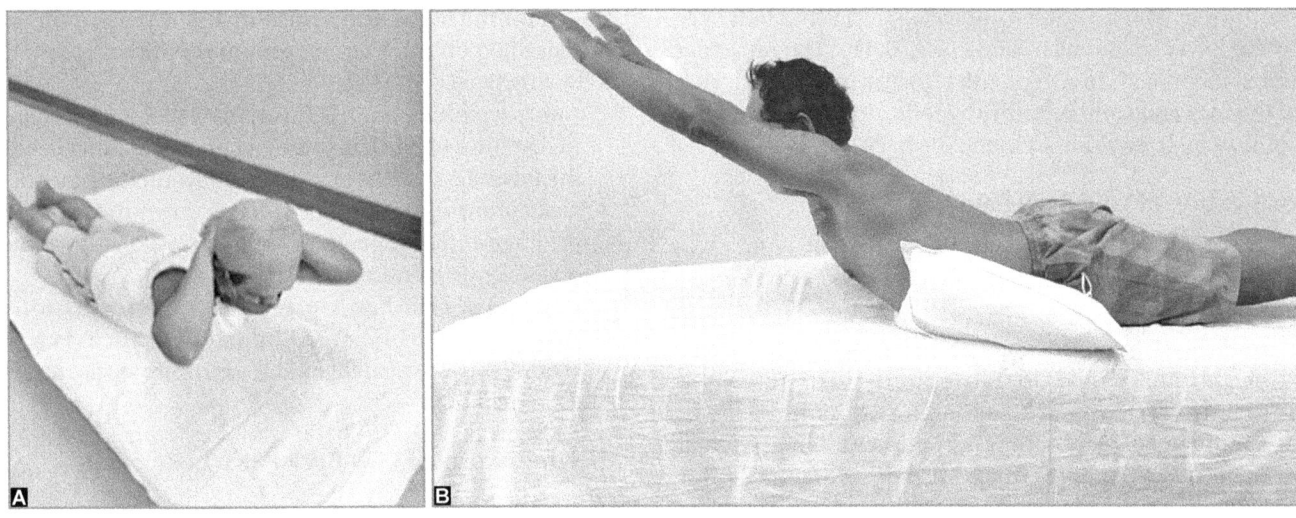

Figs. 6.40A and B: Upper back strengthening exercises.

- Upper back strengthening exercises **(Figs. 6.40A and B)**
- Mobilization exercises such as Mulligan's techniques (NAGs/SNAGs), Maitland's accessory central P/A mobilization etc may be applied.

LOW BACK PAIN

Low back pain is the common disorder affecting, the muscles, bones, nerves, and joints of the low back. The pain varies from dull constant aches to sudden sharp feeling. Very often, the pain also radiates from the back down the lower limbs.

It is the most common cause of job related disability. Almost every body in their lives suffers from some sort of back pain affecting their function. Sometimes, the low back pain becomes so intense that, the person fails to perform his duties including self care resulting significant impairment of quality of life.

Low back pain once developed, should be given attention to identify the underlying pathology, as the pain is one symptom and there is an underlying pathology that is producing the pain. If the low back pain is ignored, sometimes it aggravates to such an extent that, it produces neurological deficits in the form of motor weakness, sensory loss, bladder bowel incontinence, sexual dysfunction, etc. Very often patients with low back pain necessitate, surgical intervention to remove a fragment of the intervertebral disc (in case of disc bulge/PIVD), or to stabilize a displaced vertebra as found in lumbar spondylolisthesis. Some times low back pain is the manifestation of severe illness like Ankylosing spondylitis or malignancy (life-threatening condition). It is always emphasized that, the clinician should not end his/her duty by simply prescribing/recommending some analgesics or muscle relaxants or the physiotherapist should not end his duty by advising some exercises. Rather the patient with low back pain should be thoroughly evaluated to establish the underlying cause and accordingly medical and therapeutic managements be provided.

Epidemiology of Low Back Pain

Approximately 9-12% of people have low back pain at any given point in time, and 40% of people have the pain at some point in their lives. Difficulty most often begins between 20 and 40 years of age. Men and women are equally affected. Low back pain is a common presentation in individuals between 40 and 80 years, though currently adolescents and very young adults are also found to suffer from this disorder.

Etiology of Low Back Pain

Though the majority of low back pain is due to bad posture and cumulative trauma (PIVD), this is not always the case. Other causes of low back pain include:
- Poor posture.
- Aging.
- Poor working environment.
- Spinal stenosis: When the spinal canal narrows, it puts pressure on the spinal cord and nerves and also causes pain at the low back,
- Spinal deformities such as scoliosis, kyphosis, hyperlordosis.
- Fibromyalgia: Long-term pain and tenderness in the joints, muscles, and tendons.
- Spondylitis: Inflammation of the joints between the spinal bones.
- Spondylosis: A degenerative disorder that sometimes leads to loss of normal spinal structure and function.
- Cancer of the spinal column, e.g., multiple myeloma.
- A herniated disc/PIVD.
- Spondylolysis/spondylolisthesis.
- Compression fractures.
- Arthritis.
- Inflammatory spinal diseases, e.g., ankylosing spondylitis.
- Kidney infections
- Infections of the spine such as tuberculosis.
- Bladder problems
- Endometriosis
- Ovarian cysts
- Uterine fibroids.
- Lower cross syndrome: This is also known as Unterkreuz syndrome/pelvic crossed syndrome/distal crossed

syndrome, which is due to muscle strength imbalances in the lower segments of body **(Fig. 6.41)**. The muscular imbalance results in anterior tilt of pelvis, increased flexion of the hips and compensatory hyperlordosis in the lumbar spine, which may cause pain in the back.

Classification of Low Back Pain

A. Based upon the pathology, low back pain is classified into the followings:
   - *Musculoskeletal/Mechanical back pain:* It include muscle strain, muscle spasm, degenerated disc/vertebrae (spondylosis), spondylitis, herniated disc (PIVD), spinal canal stenosis, spondylolysis, spondylolisthesis, compression fracture, etc. A great majority of patients with back pain come under this category, though in some of the sufferers no underlying pathology are identified, it is believed that some stress/strain to the ligaments and muscles of the spine is responsible for causation of back pain.
   - *Nonmechanical back pain:* It is of the following types:
     » Inflammatory back pain: HLA-B27 associated arthritis including ankylosing spondylitis, reactive arthritis, psoriatic arthritis, and inflammatory bowel disease, etc., cause nonmechanical back pain.
     » Back pain due to malignancy: Multiple myeloma, bone metastasis from lung, breast, prostate, thyroid, etc., are also causes of back pain.
     » Back pain due to infection: Tuberculosis, osteomyelitis; abscess also cause low back pain.
     » Referred pain from internal organs: Kidney and bladder problems, endometriosis, ovarian cysts, uterine fibroids, etc., also refer pain to low back.

B. Based upon the duration of development and persistence of symptoms, low back pain is classified into the following types:
   - Acute low back pain: Pain lasting for a period lesser than 6 weeks.
   - Subacute low back pain: Pain lasting for a period between 6 and 12 weeks.
   - Chronic low back pain: Pain persisting beyond 12 weeks. It should be noted that a chronic low back pain may also cause acute relapse.

C. **Based on the signs and symptoms:** Low back pain may be classified on the basis of signs and symptoms into the following types:
   - *Nonspecific back pain:* Diffuse pain that does not change in response to particular movements and is localized to the lower back without radiating beyond the buttock.
   - *Radicular pain:* Pain that radiates down the leg below the knee and changes the severity in response to certain positions or maneuvers.
   - *Back pain that needs urgent/specialized attention:* Pain that is accompanied by red flags such as fever, trauma, history of malignancy, and more severe muscle weakness.

Pathophysiology of Low Back Pain

The structures surrounding and supporting the vertebrae and pelvis can be sources of low back pain. The lumbar region made of five vertebrae, and the fibro cartilaginous disc between the adjacent vertebrae. The stability of the spine depends on the ligaments of spine, muscles of the back and abdomen, the intervertebral disc, and the facets on the superior and inferior aspects of the vertebral bodies. The multifidus muscles that run up and down along the back of the spine, is important in keeping the spine straight and stable. Due to dysfunction or derangement of the spine, the back pain that develops, causes the person to use the back muscles inappropriately (may be due to a sciatic scoliosis or a decreased lumbar lordosis). The problem with the multifidus muscle continues even after the pain subsided. Due to dysfunction of the multifidus muscle, the patient may have a relapse of the back pain, even after the primary pathology is corrected.

The intervertebral discs have a gelatinous nucleus pulposus, surrounded by the fibro cartilaginous annulus fibrosus. The intervertebral disc has no blood supply. It derives its nutrition from the circulating blood in the adjoining structures through osmosis. The intervertebral disc is innervated through the sinuvertebral nerves. The nerve fibres are mainly restricted to the outer lamellae in the endplate. As the nucleus pulposus is not having its own nerve and blood supply, and over time, as the person ages, the disc loses its flexibility and ability to absorb physical forces. When the disc fails to absorb physical stresses, the physical forces increase stress on the other parts of the spine causing the ligaments of the spine thicken and bony spurs developing on the vertebrae. As a result of thickening of the ligaments (most commonly PLL and ligamentum flavum), and bony spur formation the spinal cord and/or nerve roots may be compressed causing back pain with or without radiation of pain to the lower limbs.

When a disc degenerates due to injury/disease, the structure of the disc is altered, pushing directly on the nerve root. There is also reduction of the intervertebral space, causing increased loading on the facets, resulting in facet hypertrophy, and further compromising intervertebral foramina producing both back pain as well as radicular symptoms.

A displaced vertebra, as occurs in spondylolisthesis, a defect in the pars interarticularis, as seen in spondylolysis, sacralization/lumbarization, etc., affects the normal

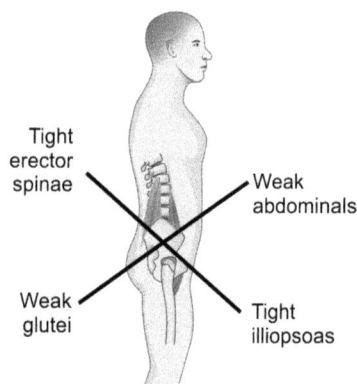

Fig. 6.41: The lower crossed syndrome.

biomechanics of spine, causing inflammation at or in the nearby segments of the spinal column causing pain.

Inflammatory and infective disorders of spine such as spondylitis, Caries spine, etc., also produce pain which is produced both by chemical factors as well as altered biomechanics.

Clinical Features of Low Back Pain

The clinical features of low back pain depend on the causes and pathologies involved producing the symptoms. The different disorders of the spine and their manifestations are described separately. However, the features common to all are discussed here.

The individuals between the ages of 20–40 years usually experience acute back pain, which in due course of time, as the individual ages becomes chronic with or without acute relapses. The common presentations of acute mechanical low back pain are pain in the back with spasm of the paravertebral muscles, while the sufferer produces movement of the spine involving beding and twisting movements. The common presentation of non mechanical/ inflammatory back pain are: pain during rest, with a diurnal variation, i.e, pain while taking rest at night hours with some morning stiffness, which reduce significantly after doing some activities, such as walking. If the individual complains of severe night pain, it indicates serious pathologies like malignancy, infection etc.

In case of PIVD with involvement of annulus fibrosus only, the pain is initially experienced in the low back, later on it may/ may not radiate to the lower limbs, where as if the disc injury involve bulging of the nucleus pulposus, the sufferer may get radiating pain in the lower limbs as initial symptoms, with or without lowback pain subsequently. In patients with a nuclear bulge, the pain the low back/ leg increases on sneezing and coughing. The symptoms may range from tenderness at a particular point to diffuse pain in the back with or without radiation to lower limbs. It may or may not worsen with certain movements, such as raising a leg, or positions, such as sitting or standing.

Postural deviations, such as sciatic scoliosis/listing and decreased lumbar lordosis (**Fig. 6.42**), may develop as an attempt by the body to relieve the foramina off pressure. In some patients neurological deficits in the lower limbs in the form of foot drop, sensory impairment in dermatomal distribution, loss/diminution of deep tendon reflexes, bladder/bowel and sexual dysfunction may develop. Chronic low back pain is associated with sleep problems, anxiety, depression, and a decreased quality of life.

Diagnosis

Diagnosis of low back pain is made from the history of onset of pain such as sudden in onset (PIVD), or gradual in onset (Spondylolisthesis/spondylosis/postural), aggravating factors (sitting-PIVD, standing-Spondylosis/Spondylolisthesis), relieving factors (Exercise- Inflammatory pain, rest-PIVD, sitting-spondylosis/spondylolisthesis), clinical features,

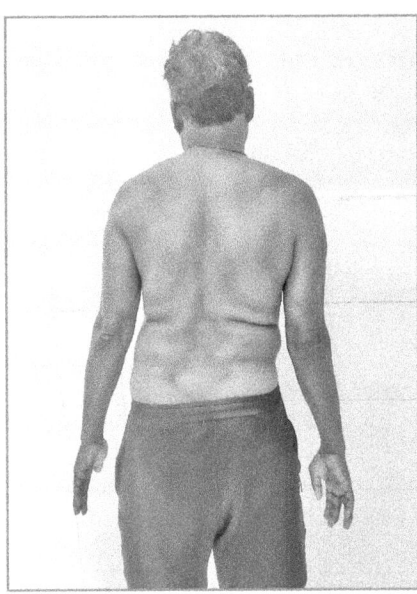

Fig. 6.42: Right-sided sciatic scoliosis with convexity to right with compensatory left sided T-L scoliosis in a patient of lumbar PIVD with right sciatica.

clinical examination, and radioimaging such as X-ray, CT scan, MRI (**Figs. 6.43A to F**). Imaging is indicated when there are red flags, ongoing neurological symptoms such as spinal canal stenosis, causing neurogenic claudication, that do not resolve with therapy.

Assessment of Low Back Pain

Once a patient is referred to the physiotherapist, for the management of low back pain, the therapist performs detail assessment of the patient to establish the cause of pain and the present physical and neurological status, which guides him/her for planning the management. Subjective pain behavior, movement testing, neurological examination (Sensory/Motor/Deep tendon reflexes) are performed by the therapist/clinician which are briefly discussed below:

* **Subjective examination:** It includes complain of patient, demographic data, and history. The history taken includes:
    - *History of present illness:*
        » Mode of onset: Whether sudden or gradual: It should be noted that, most of the PIVDs are sudden in onset, where the individual while doing some activities in forward bent posture, such as lifting some heavy load, experiences a catch in the low back with back pain with or without pain radiating along the lower limb (s) after some times, suggesting tear of the annulus fibrosus. Less often, some patients may get pain in the leg at first followed by pain in the back, suggesting bulging of the nucleus pulposus.
        » Duration of the symptoms: Whether the pain is recent in origin (acute) or persisting for long time (chronic).
        » Aggravating/relieving factors: Whether rest gives relief and activity aggravates the symptoms (found in PIVD) or the reverse (found in inflammatory back pain like that seen in ankylosing spondylitis).

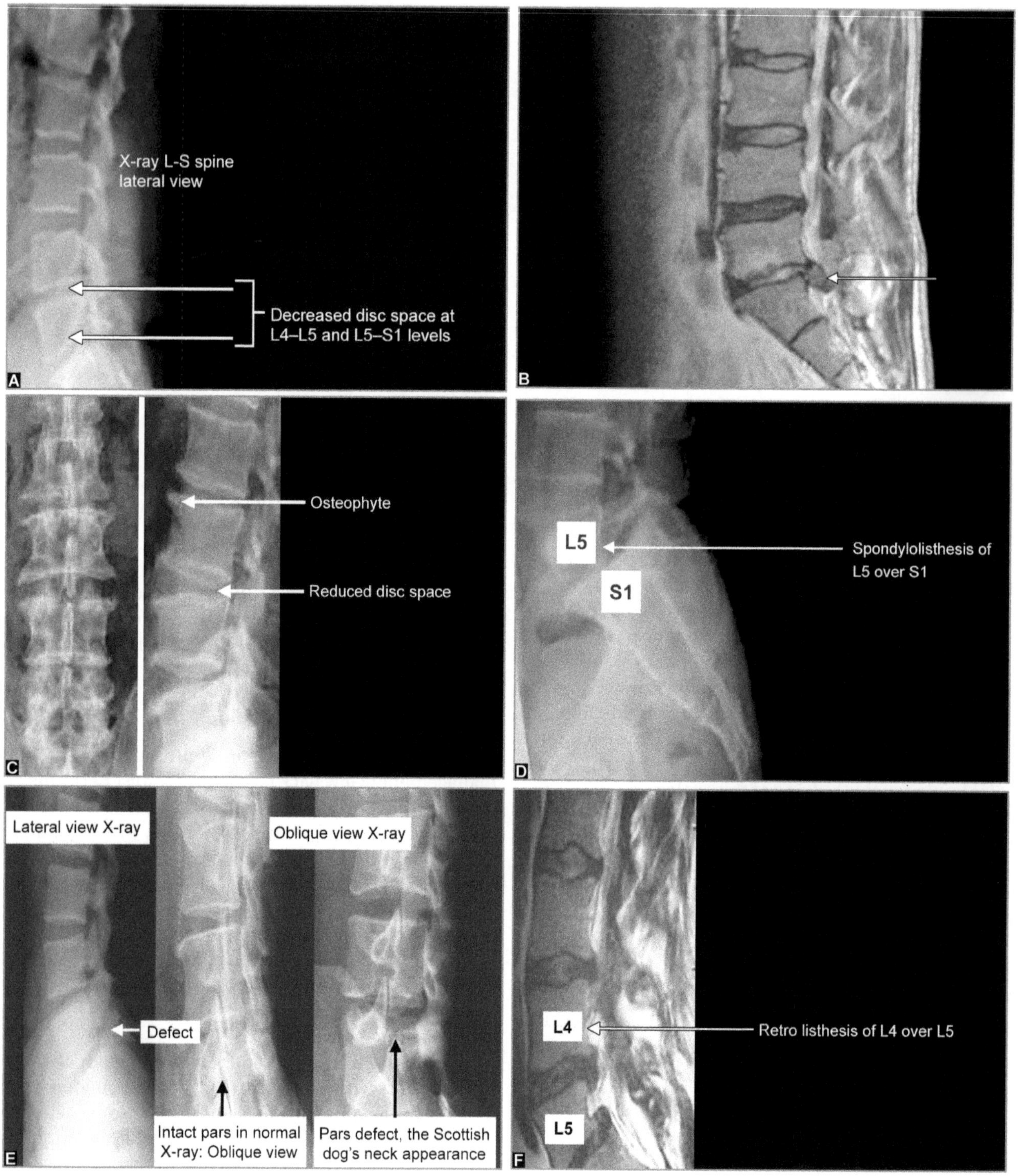

108 Section 2: Physiotherapy for Musculoskeletal Conditions

Figs. 6.43A to F: (A) Shows X-ray lateral view showing reduction of joint space due to PIVD, (B) MRI showing disc bulge at L5-S1, (C) X-ray showing lumbar spondylosis, (D) X-ray showing spondylolisthesis of L5 over S1, (E) X-ray showing spondylolysis, (F) MRI showing retrolisthesis of L4 over L5.

Note should be made, whether the pain increases in sitting (PIVD), or standing (lumbar spondylosis/ Spondylolisthesis), and whether pain increases on sneezing and coughing (nuclear bulging).

» Assessment of intensity of pain: The Visual Analogue Scale (VAS) **(Fig. 6.44)** that grades pain from 0 (zero)

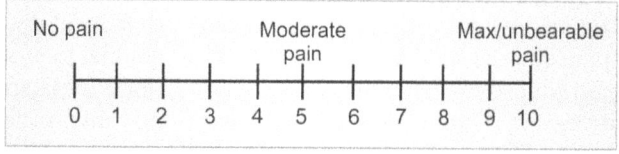

Fig. 6.44: The VAS scale.

no pain to 10 (maximum pain) helps to grade the intensity of pain felt by the patient.
- *Past history:* History of trauma/previous episode of back pain.
- *Personal history:* Marital status, smoking history, etc.
- *Occupational history:* Nature of job, the individual performs helps in establishing the cause of pain and to provide ergonomic advice.
- *Treatment history:* Whether, previous back pain (if any) was managed conservatively/surgically.

❖ **Objective examination:** It includes:
- A listing is an undefined spastic reflex mechanism that the body designs to splint the injured disc and to diminish painful stimulation on the nerve roots, that result from pressure from the injured disc. There occurs tilting of the affected spinal segments without any rotation. The direction of concavity describes the side of listing.
- A sciatic scoliosis is a protective mechanism, body produces to keep the intervertebral foramina free of pressure from a herniated disc or an osteophyte. There occurs tilting of vertebral segments away from the affected side with some degree of rotation of the spine towards the painful side. The direction of convexity describes the side of sciatic scoliosis.
- *Observation:* Observation of posture for listing/sciatic scoliosis/flattening of lumbar lordosis, paravertebral muscle spasm (if any).
- *Range of motion of lumbosacral spine:* It includes both active and passive physiological movements with or without terminal overpressure **(Figs. 6.45A and B)** and accessory movements (joint play) in the lumbar and thoracic segments. Any reproduction/remission of pain locally/peripherally with movement should be noted. While testing physiological movements extension should be tested first and flexion should be tested last (as testing of flexion first may aggravate the pain in the presence of disc bulge, which may affect further movement testing). When the original pain is not reproduced on single movement testing, combined movements such as extension with rotation toward the painful side to test for foramen compromise should be performed.

McKenzie method of movement testing where, repeated movements in the direction of extension in case of flexion derangement like PIVD centralizing the symptoms **(Fig. 6.46A)**, repeated flexion in case of conditions like spondylolisthesis, spondylosis with foramina stenosis and lumbar canal stenosis **(Fig. 6.46B)**, that reduces peripheral symptoms, should be performed as test movements for considering the same as therapeutic exercises. End-range stressing to elicit pain in dysfunction, and production of movements in opposite direction to painful postures that produces pain relief helps in establishing dysfunction and postural syndromes and planning exercises accordingly. While testing joint play/accessory movements, the grade of joint

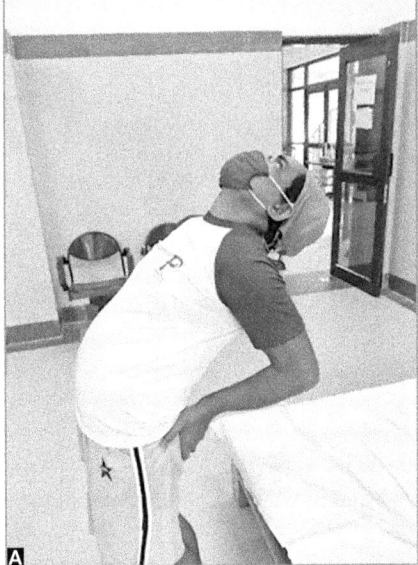
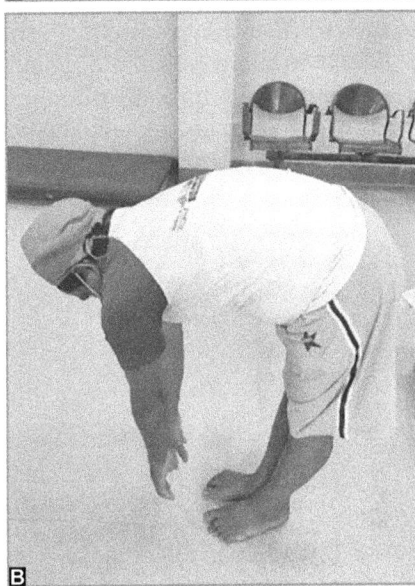

Figs. 6.45A and B: (A) Testing of extension, (B) testing of flexion.

play that reduces the symptoms should be found and documented for treatment application.
- *Performance of special tests:*
  » **Straight leg raise test** (sciatic nerve tension tests): Patient supine and relaxed, with no pillow under the head. If a patient can not lie in supine, it can be done in side lying. Therapist/Clinician explains him about the procedure and tells him/her to report when back or leg pain appears, as he/she (Clinician) will be raising his/her (Patient's) leg passively off the bed **(Fig. 6.47A)**. The angle of leg raise, when pain appears at back/leg is noted through observational method and documented. If there is confusion to interpret, pain from the hamstrings stretch can be ruled out by making sensitive additions like hip adduction and medial rotation, or performing Lasegue test/Fajersztajn test. If there is no increase of pain on hip adduction and medial rotation and/

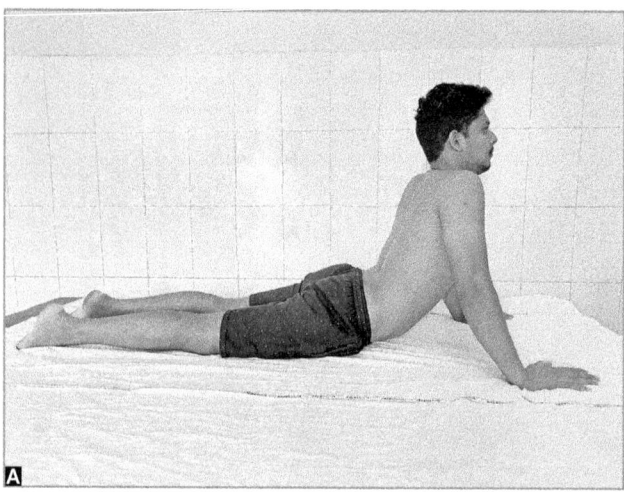
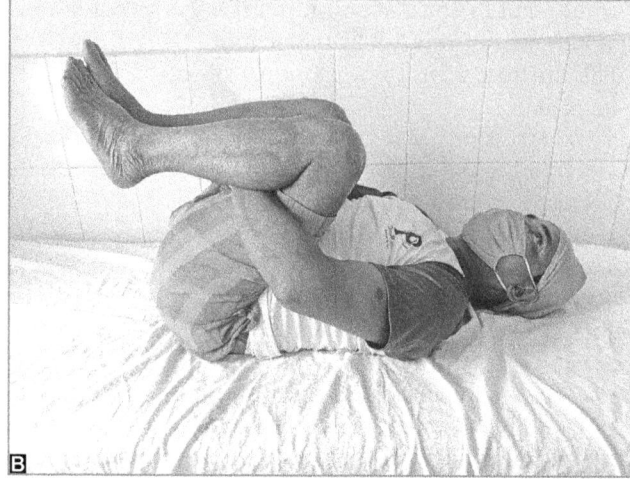

Figs. 6.46A and B: McKenzie method of testing for centralization/peripheralization: (A) Repeated extension, (B) Repeated flexion.

or Lasegue test/Fajersztajn test, it is the pain coming from stretch of hamstrings muscles. The normal value of SLR is 80–90 degrees. Radiating pain/paresthesia suggests lumbar disc prolapse/lumbar root canal stenosis with root impingement. The normal stress on the sciatic nerve as the leg is raised is shown in **Figure 6.47B**.

Interpretations

- Pain up to 35 degrees is suggestive of severe intervertebral disc prolapsed.
- Pain between 35 and 70 degrees is suggestive of disc prolapse/intervertebral foramina stenosis.
- Pain beyond 70 degrees is equivocal, i.e., may be due to tightness of hamstrings or may be due to neural tension.
  - *Fajersztajn test-Bragards sign:* This test is highly indicative of PIVD of lumbar spine. First straight leg raise test (SLRT) is done to the point, where the symptoms are produced. Then the limb is slightly lowered and the ankle is dorsiflexed **(Fig. 6.48)**. If this reproduces the pain, then the test is considered positive and Bragards sign is present.
  - *Lasegue test:* Lasegue test or Lazarevic's sign is a test done during physical examination to determine, whether a patient with low back pain, has the underlying nerve root sensitivity, often to L5 root.
    With the patient supine, the examiner lifts the patient's leg with the knee straight. Once some pain is elicited, the

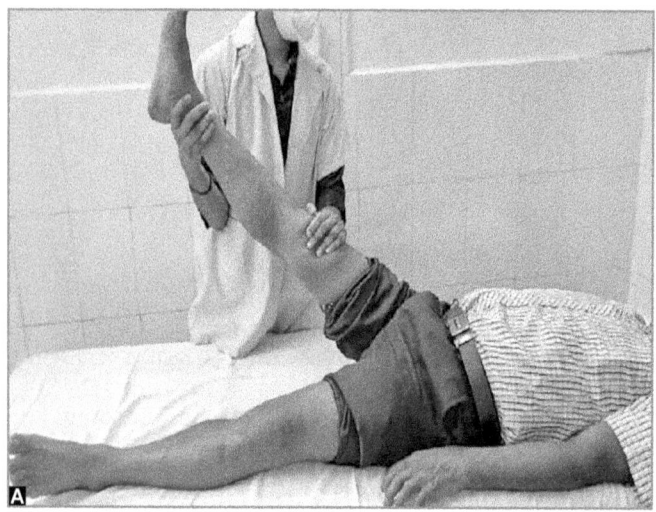
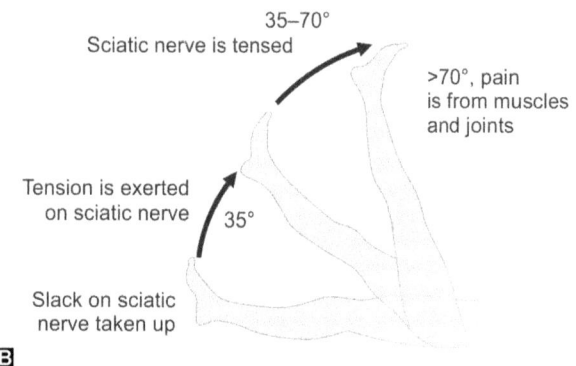

Figs. 6.47A and B: (A) Testing of SLR, (B) Displays normal tension in the sciatic nerve as leg is raised.

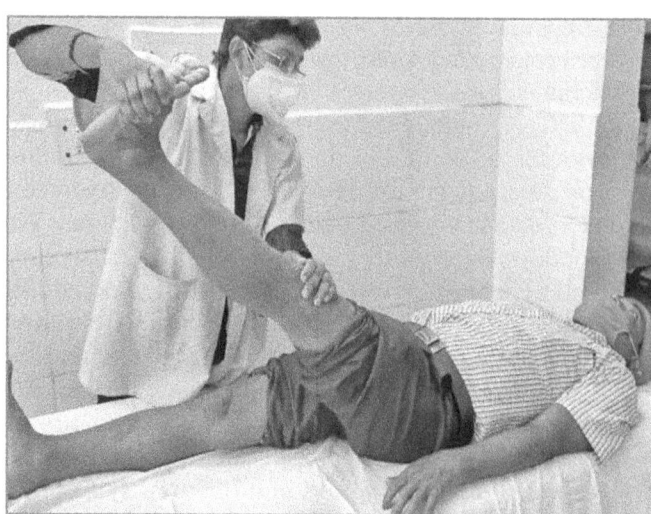

Fig. 6.48: The Bragards sign.

Chapter 6: Physiotherapy for Spinal Disorders | 111

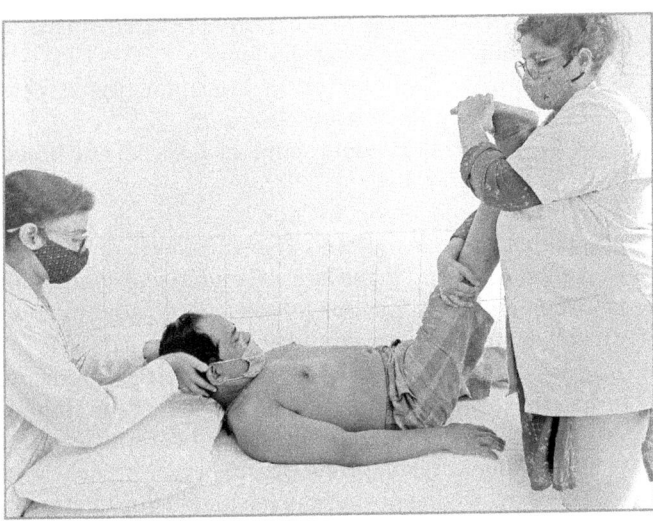

Fig. 6.49: Lasegue test.

leg is slightly lowered and then the ankle is dorsiflexed and cervical spine flexed **(Fig. 6.49)**.

If the patient experiences sciatic pain, more specifically, pain radiating down the leg, when the straight leg is at angle of between 30 and 70 degrees, then the test is positive and a herniated disc is the possible cause.

- *Prone knee bend test (femoral nerve tension test)/ Reverse SLR test:* The patient in prone lying. The examiner flexes the knee as far as possible, and holds the position for 45-60 seconds. If no pain is experienced, gradually additions like hip extension and ankle plantar flexion are added. If pain in the front of thigh increases with ankle plantar flexion, when knee is flexed and hip extended, it indicates positive femoral nerve tension **(Fig. 6.50)**.
- *Crossed SLR test/Well leg-raise sign:* This test is also known as well leg raising test or cross over sign. This test, when positive suggests medial disc bulge, i.e., bulging medial to the root.

The patient is in supine lying. The examiner performs a SLR test on the unaffected side up to 75 degrees, or till pain is felt on the affected leg. The angle of SLR on the unaffected side, at which pain is felt on the affected side is documented.

- *Bow string test:* After a positive SLR test, the knee is flexed. If the knee flexion reduces the pain in the leg, it could be due to nerve root compression. It can be further confirmed by pressing over the lateral popliteal nerve behind the lateral tibial condyle, to tighten it like a bow string. If no change in pain status with this maneuver, the pain could be of hip origin. However, with bow stringing, if the pain increases, it could be due to neural tension from disc bulge
- *The Slump test:* It is used to evaluate for lumbar nerve root impingement or irritation. It begins with the patient seated on the table with both hips and knees positioned at 90 degrees. The examiner stands to the side of the patient **(Fig. 6.51)**. The patient is instructed to slump forward while maintaining the head and neck in neutral position. The clinician extends patient's one knee with one hand while using the other hand to apply overpressure to the patient's thoracic spine; thus exacerbating the curvature of the spine. Once in this position, the patient is instructed to lower the chin to the chest, producing cervical flexion. A positive Slump test result is demonstrated with the reproduction of radicular symptoms.
- *Neurological examination:* It includes sensory examination, motor examination, reflex examination (knee jerks, ankle jerks, and plantar response Babinski sign). A decrease of muscle power (Hip flexor-L2, knee extensor-L3, ankle dorsiflexor-L4, great toe extensor-L5, and ankle plantar flexor-S1), a decrease of knee jerk-L3, ankle jerk-S1 and sensory impairments in dermatomal distribution in the lower limbs suggests neurological impairments. Involvement of bladder and bowel, sexual

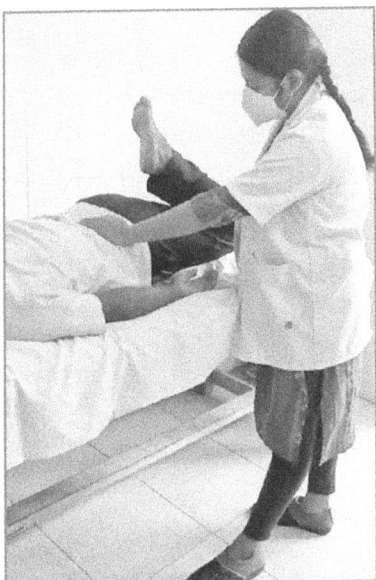

Fig. 6.50: Prone knee bend test (femoral nerve tension test).

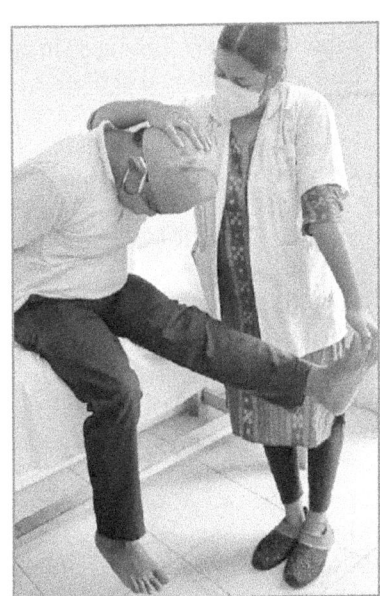

Fig. 6.51: The slump test.

function (if any) indicates involvement of sacral roots (S2, S3, S4).
- *Assessment of function and gait:* As many individuals with low back pain have impairment of function and walk with antalgic gait, evaluation of function and gait should be done.
- ❖ **Evaluation of the patient**: After completing clinical examination, and correlating with radiological/laboratory examinations (say HLAB27 to rule out early ankylosing spondylitis as a cause of back pain), the clinician makes a diagnosis of the condition that causes low back pain and plans management accordingly. Certain tips to make clinical diagnosis are:
  - Pain in low back sudden in onset, while lifting weight, with or without leg pain subsequently, which is more in sitting and supine lying as compared to standing and prone lying suggests PIVD (Annular tear).
  - Pain in leg (radiating pain) occurring first followed by pain in low back, increasing on sneezing and coughing, which may be sudden or gradual in onset, and more in sitting and supine lying and reduces in standing and lying prone, suggests PIVD (nucleus pulposus bulging).
  - Pain in low back with a gradual onset, with or without radiation to lower limbs, occurring after the age of 40 years, aggravated in standing, but reducing in sitting with a history of morning stiffness, suggests lumbar spondylosis.
  - Pain in the low back with increased lumbar lordosis, with or without radiation to lower limbs in multiparous females, suggests spondylolisthesis, necessitating X-ray examination before any therapy.
  - Pain in the low back, with negative SLR test and neurogenic claudication, making difficult to walk, suggests lumbar canal stenosis.
  - Pain in the back, that increases on rest (night), suggests inflammatory pathology (malignancy, tuberculosis, ankylosing spondylitis) necessitating necessary investigations before therapeutic intervention.
  - Pain in the low back, that is produced in holding certain posture during occupational activities, say computer works, but reduces when posture is normalized/corrected suggests postural back pain.
- ❖ **Making a problem list:** After, evaluation of the patient, a problem list that includes pain, limitation of movement and function etc., should be made by the treating therapist/clinician.
- ❖ **Planning the management.**

Management of low back pain: Management of low back pain depends on its pathology, which are briefly discussed below:
1. **Management of lumbar PIVD**: The management of PIVD of lumbar spine is mostly made conservatively. If conservative management fails and patient develops intolerable pain and progressive neurological deficit, surgery may be considered. The management depends on the stage of the disorder, when the patients report such as acute stage, subacute stage, and chronic stage.

- *Acute lumbar PIVD management:* The aim of management in this stage include:
  » To prevent further injury to disc and neural tissues.
  » To reduce pain and muscle spasm.
  » To educate the patient about the disorder and how it can be controlled.

Methods of management include:
- ❖ NSAIDs and muscle relaxants prescribed by the Physician.
- ❖ **Rest**: Controlled rest in the form of bed rest and continuous traction with a low load for 2 weeks. While advising rest, the following measures should be observed.
  - *Positioning:* As prone lying is a position of extension, this position may be adopted while lying on bed. If the patient can tolerate the prone position, a pillow under the thorax in prone may be the best position, if tolerated, as this position helps the nucleus pulposus move anteriorly reducing the herniation **(Fig. 6.52)**. However, if the patient can tolerate supine lying, supine position with a pillow under the knee to relax the abdominal muscles and reduce tension on the sciatic nerve may be considered.
  - Avoiding postures that aggravate the symptoms: Postures such as prolonged periods of sitting.
  - Local support to the spine such as lumbosacral belt **(Fig. 6.53)**: A lumbosacral belt may be advised for providing support to the spine, when the patient is out of bed and to maintain the lumbar lordosis that accelerates healing of the torn annulus fibrosus.

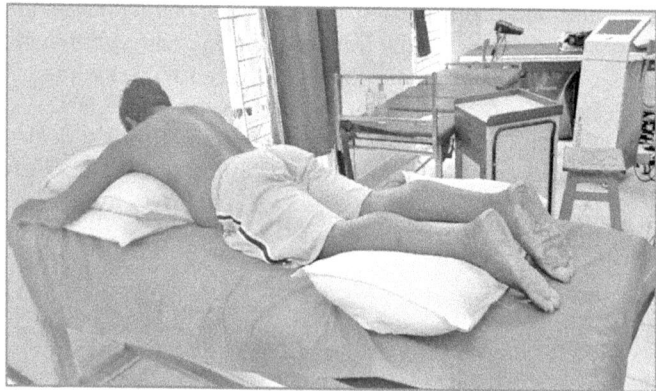

Fig. 6.52: Prone positioning in acute PIVD.

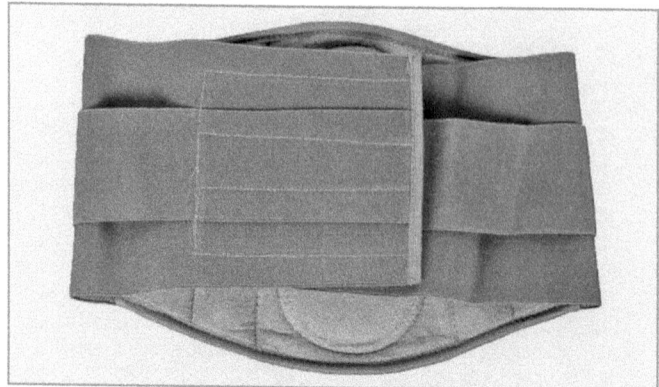

Fig. 6.53: The lumbosacral belt.

- Controlled walking: If the symptoms are less severe, after a short period of bed rest, patient may be advised to walk intermittently as tolerated with the use of a lumbosacral belt. Walking with the belt makes the sufferer remain extended and also helps in reduction of the disc by stimulating fluid mechanics.
❖ **Physiotherapy:** Besides measures to provide rest, the following therapeutic modalities are also helpful in the acute stage when applied judiciously.
    - *Traction:* Traction in the sustained mode at a load of 25% body weight may be applied for 10 minutes to help in relieving nerve root pressure **(Fig. 6.54B)**. The duration of traction in the acute phase should be shorter as it may increase the symptoms due to fluid imbibition. It may help in reducing nuclear protrusion by reducing pressure on the disc, and tension in the PLL as well as inhibits muscle spasm. There is evidence that, the bulging/protrusion of the disc can be reduced, and spinal nerve root compression symptoms relieved, when spinal traction is applied. Traction can indeed separate lumbar vertebrae; lead to a decreased pressure at the disc space with a resulting suction force; and that the disc material can be drawn from the epidural space into the disc space. If traction using a motorized machine can not be given, due to any cause, traction at home **(Fig. 6.54C)**, can also be arranged by the physiotherapist. Traction is usually contraindicated, if the disc bulge is medial to the root. Before traction is applied mechanically, the patients response to traction in various positions of body (i.e., supine/prone) should be tested manually **(Fig. 6.54A)**. If there is increase of symptoms with traction, it should not be applied or the load should be reduced.
    - *Heat therapy:* To reduce muscle spasm, that produces pain as a result of pain spasm vicious cycle, superficial heat therapy (moist hydrocollator packs) may be helpful.
    - *PSWD* is also helpful in the acute stage for promoting repair and reducing inflammation.
    - *Iontophoresis:* Iontophoresis with anti-inflammatory drugs may help in reducing muscle spasm and local inflammation.
    - TENS/IFT, etc., may be applied to modulate the pain **(Fig. 6.55)**.
    - *Exercises:* The McKenzie program can be started from the acute stage to reduce nuclear protrusion and related signs and symptoms, provided that, the test movements and posture demonstrate a reduction of symptoms. Extension exercises are beneficial in reducing signs and symptoms. In the acute stage, the objective of exercises and postural adaptation is to cause a reduction of disc bulge. The exercises performed include:
❖ **Autoassisted lumbar extension:** This is suitable for patients with a posterior/posterolateral disc bulge. The patient is in prone lying. A pillow may be placed

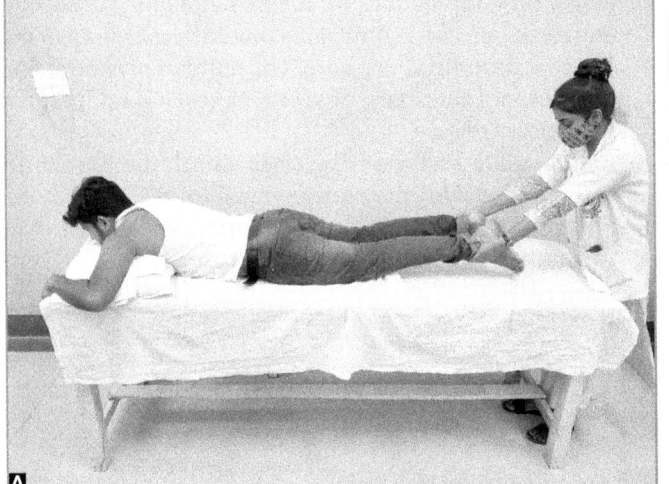
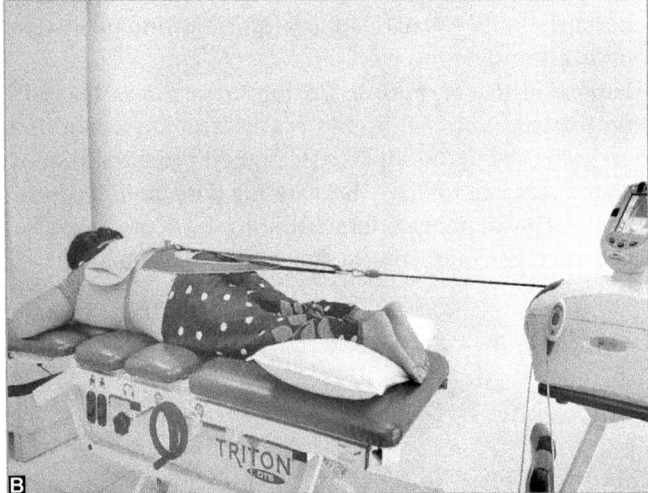
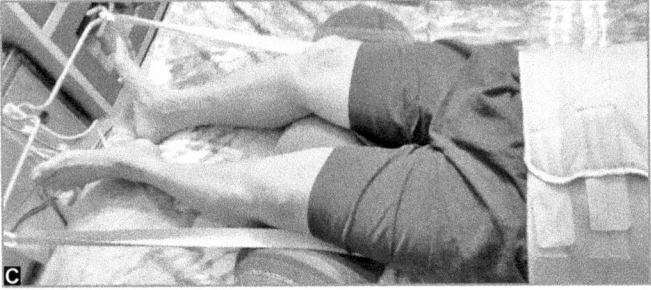

Figs. 6.54A to C: (A) Testing for benefits of traction manually (B) Motorized lumbar traction in prone, (C) Lumbar traction at home.

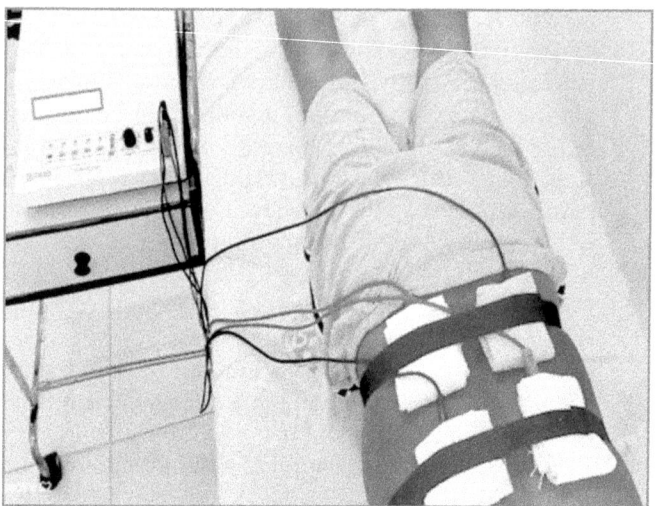

Fig. 6.55: Application of IFT to low back.

under the abdomen for support, if he/she has extreme pain and this pillow support gives relief. As tolerance to position improves, the pillow can be removed and the patient is asked to prop himself/herself up on the elbows, i.e., to attain prone on elbow, allowing the pelvis to sag down **(Fig. 6.56A)**. The position may be held for 5–10 minutes to allow reduction of water content and size of the disc bulge. This is progressed by allowing the patient to prop on the hands and maintain full spinal extension for 5–10 minutes with pillow support under thorax, if required **(Fig. 6.56B)**. If sustained extensions of the spine are not tolerated by the patient, he/she should be advised to perform prone push-ups intermittently.

❖ **Lateral shift correction**: Listing/correction of sciatic scoliosis should be done before extension exercise program, using the McKenzie method provided that, if the patient can tolerate the standing position (However, traction/positioning performed during this acute stage also helps in correcting listing to some extent). If the patient can not tolerate standing, and hip flexion and adduction are not painful, Cyriax method of correction in supine lying/crook lying can be performed.

– *Correction by therapist:*
  » The McKenzie method **(Fig. 6.57)**: The therapist stands on the side of the patient toward which the thorax is shifted and places his/her shoulder against the patient's elbow, which is placed against the rib cage. The therapist wraps his arms around the patient's pelvis and pulls pelvis toward him, while pushing patient's thorax away.
  » Cyriax method: Those, who can not stand cyriax listing correction is followed in crook lying position. The clinician stands on the convex side. The convex side limb is placed over the concave side and is pushed away and the concave side limb is pulled toward **(Fig. 6.58)**.

– *Self correction:* Patient is asked to place his hands on the side of the shifted rib cage on the lateral side, and places the other hand over the crest of the opposite ilium. He/she then gradually push these regions toward mid line and hold **(Fig. 6.59A)**.

Self correction can also be done by the patient, standing with the shoulder on the shifted side of thorax resting against the wall. He/she is asked to glide the hips on the convex side of the deviation laterally toward the wall **(Fig. 6.59B)**.

❖ Isometric gluteal contractions/isometric spinal extension exercise in supine can be started with the patient supine with a pillow under the knees. He/she should be asked to gently raise the buttock off the bed, hold for 3–6 seconds and relax. Forceful contractions should be avoided as it may increase intradiscal pressure. The number of contractions in a set and numbers of sets and sessions depend on patient's tolerance.

❖ Active ankle and foot exercises should be performed without provoking the patient's symptoms.

❖ Stretching of piriformis, if required should be done through myofascial release technique in side lying

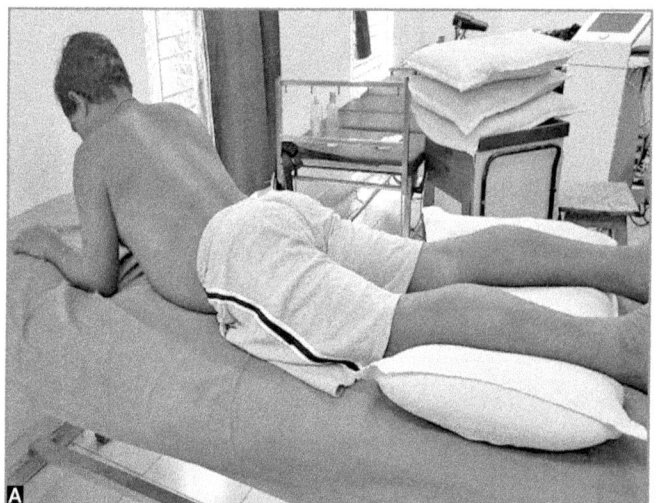
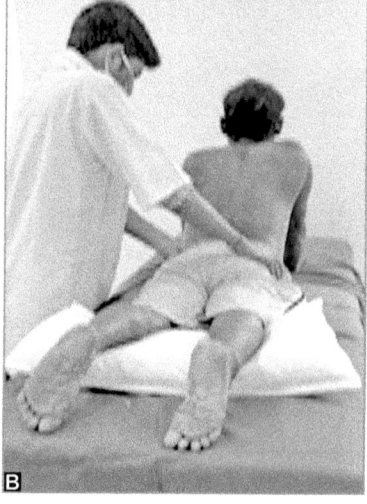

Figs. 6.56A and B: (A) Prone on elbow, (B) Prop on hands prone extension.

Chapter 6: Physiotherapy for Spinal Disorders

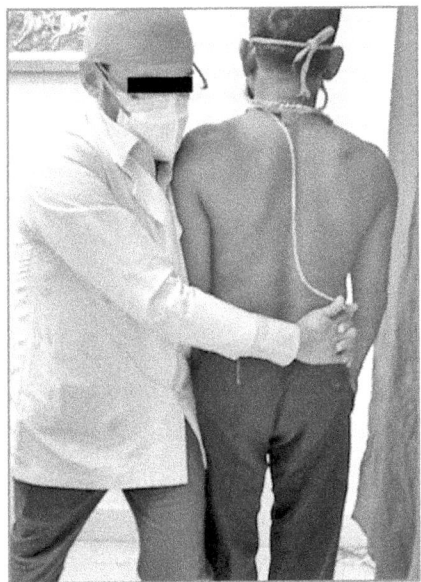

Fig. 6.57: Listing correction by therapist.

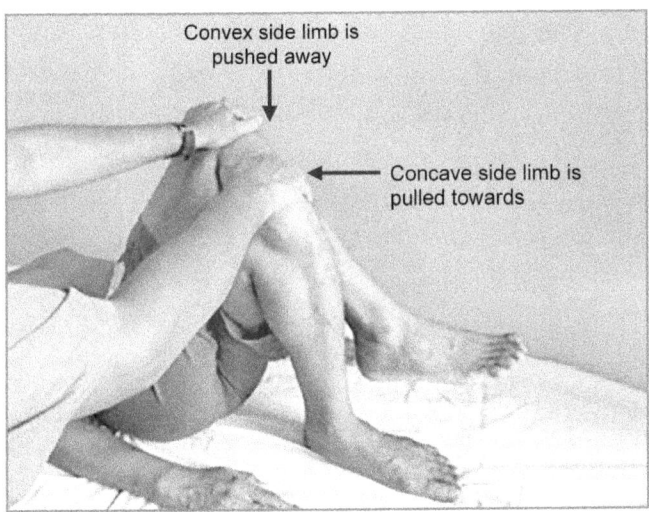

Fig. 6.58: The Cyriax listing correction.

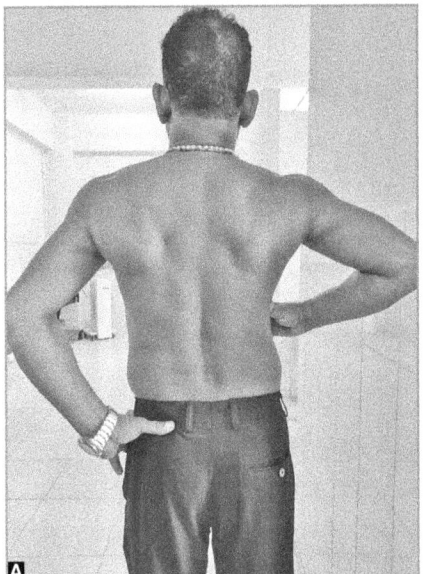

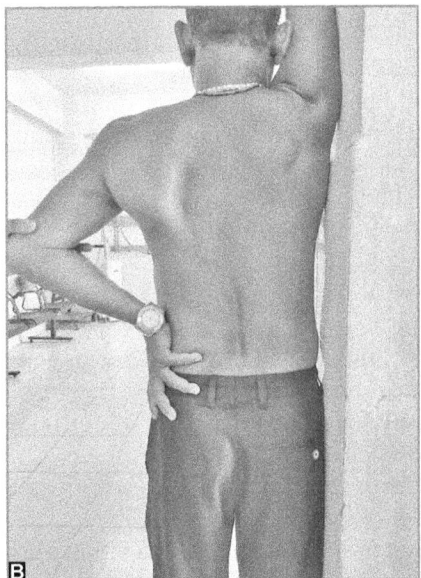

Figs. 6.59A and B: Listing correction by self.

(**Fig. 6.60**), as conventional stretching with hip flexion/adduction/medial rotation may produce neural tension in sciatic nerve and aggravate the symptoms.
* If there is any stiffness of upper trunk, it should be mobilized as discussed under upper back pain.
* **Hydrotherapy:** Breast stroke swimming using floaters may helpful to promote extension with assistance from buoyancy (**Fig. 6.61**). The warmth of water also helps in reducing muscle spasm.
* **Patient education:** Nachemson's work on intradiscal pressures should be taken into account when educating the patient concerning unsafe positions and activities for them while convalescing. He found that sitting causes more intradiscal pressure than standing. Forward bending also increases intradiscal pressure and causes posterior movement of the nucleus pulposus. The patient should avoid these positions and activities during early treatment of the herniated disc. Return to normal

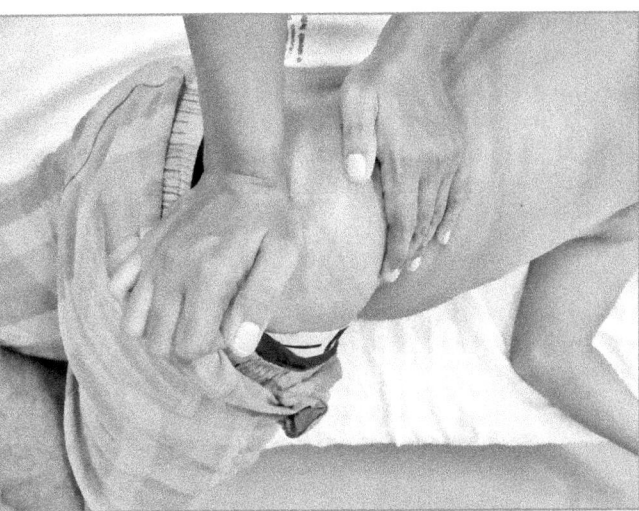

Fig. 6.60: Myofascial release to piriformis.

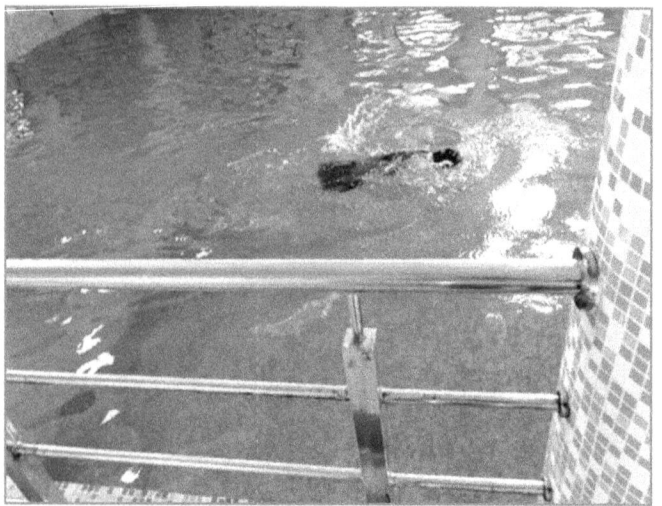

Fig. 6.61: Hydrotherapy—Breast stroke swimming in PIVD.

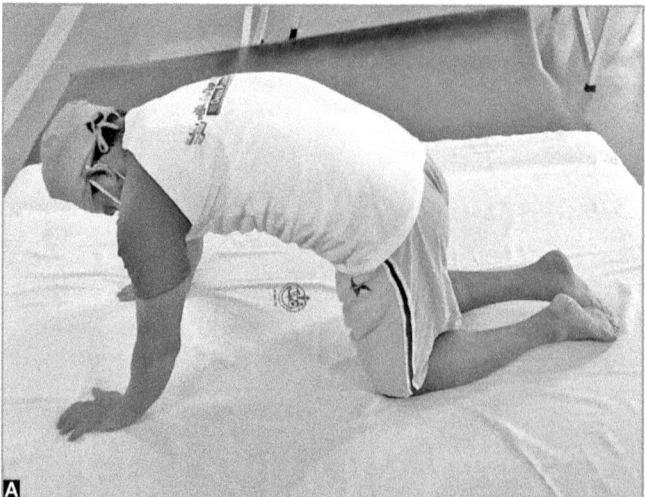

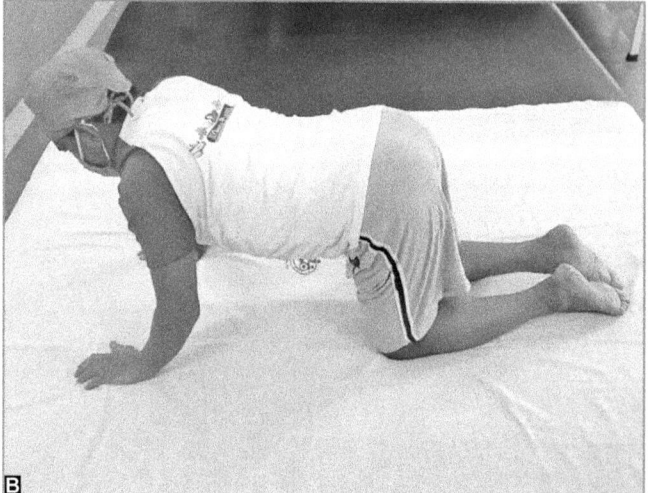

Figs. 6.62A and B: Cat-camel exercises.

activities should be gradual and only after the injured disc has healed and stabilized.

The patient should be educated for the do's and don'ts such as:
- Avoiding forward bending and weight lifting.
- Avoid squatting.
- Avoid cycling.
- Avoid lying on sponge mattresses.
- Avoid prolong sitting.
- Avoid exposure to cough irritants.
- Avoid jerks to spine.
- Use pillow under knee in supine and as tolerated place pillow under chest in prone and lie down.
- Use L-S belt while performing activities, to prevent unintended movements.
- Do exercises and follow precautions as advised by physiotherapist/clinician.
- **Management of lumbar PIVD in subacute stage:** With proper medical and therapeutic management and ergonomic advice, the acute pain usually subsides by 4–6 days in most of the cases. The exercises and modalities used in the acute stage are continued in this stage with few additions.

Prone push ups, pelvic rocking in supine, sitting, prone lying, and quadruped (cat-camel exercise, **Figs. 6.62A and B**), with emphasis on anterior pelvic tilt are performed. Isometric strengthening of back extensors are continued without holding breath (avoiding Valsalva maneuver). Aerobic exercises such as walking, swimming, static bicycling, etc., are progressed in this stage.

- **Management of chronic PIVD:** The intensity of pain is significantly reduced in this stage, i.e., the symptoms from disc is less due to stabilization of the disc. However, there is significant stiffness in spine with weakness of spinal muscles. The aims of physiotherapy in this stage are:
  - To reduce pain.
  - Restore functional range of motion of lumbosacral spine.
  - Increase spinal muscle strength, endurance and function.
  - Retrain kinesthetic awareness.
  - Educate the patient about correct posture and measures to be taken for prevention of recurrence.

The interventions given include:
- **Gentle active range of motion exercises in pain free range:** By about 3 weeks after onset of PIVD, when the disc symptoms are reduced, gentile active side flexion and extension of lumbar spine (**Fig. 6.63B**), and flexion in supine (**Fig. 6.63A**) are started within the pain-free range (flexion in supine, i.e., pulling the knee to chest should be performed with caution without provoking leg pain-peripheral symptoms). After flexion exercises, extension exercises such as prone push ups, standing spinal extension exercises should be performed actively to correct any derangement that develop due to flexion. However, it is recommended that, flexion exercise such as supine, pulling the knees to chest should be started, if the patient has developed severe flexion dysfunction and doing such exercise does not produce any increase of symptoms. Careful decision to start flexion exercise should be taken after a thorough patient evaluation.
- **Core muscle strengthening exercises:** The aim of the core strengthening exercises is to support the back by strengthening the muscles of the spine. The exercises are:

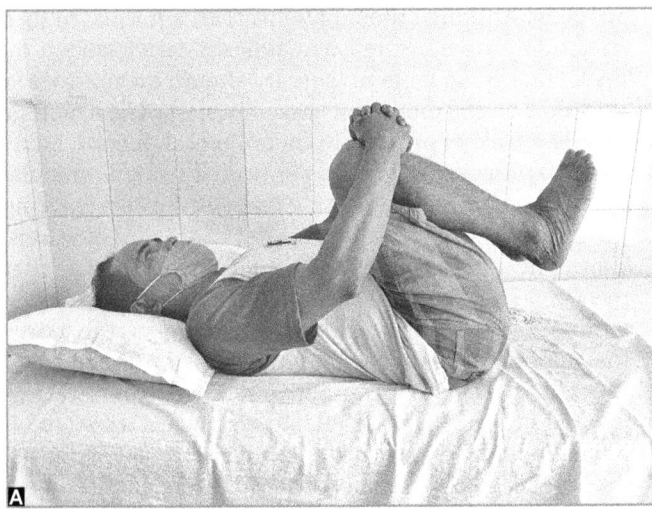

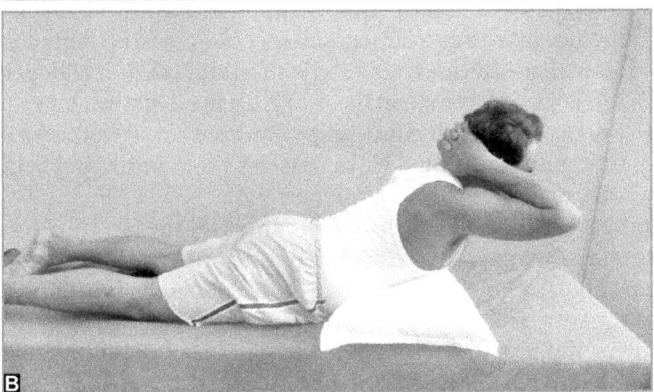

Figs. 6.63A and B: (A) Lumbar flexion in supine, (B) Lumbar extension exercise.

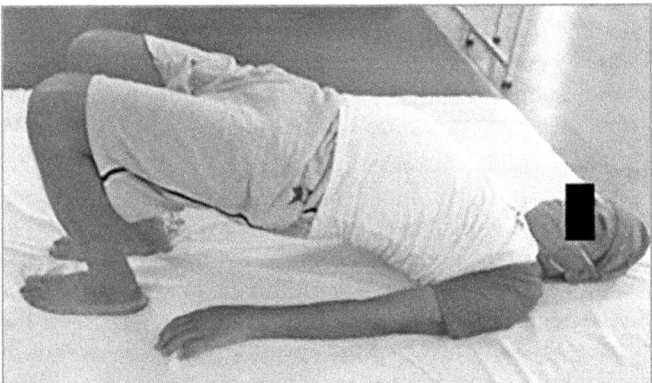

Fig. 6.64: Pelvic bridging exercise.

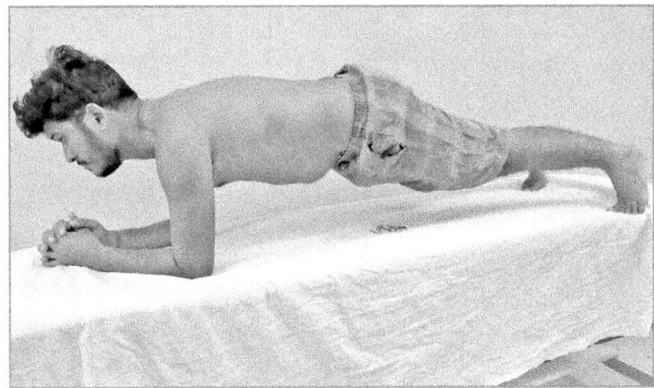

Fig. 6.65: The plank exercise.

- *The Bridging exercise:* This exercise strengthens several core muscles, such as muscles of buttock/back/abdominals. The procedure involves lying in crook lying, feet flat on the floor. Patient is advised to tighten the abdominals and raise the buttocks off the floor, keeping the abdominals tight and hold the position for a count of five. The buttocks should then be lowered to bed slowly and the exercises should be repeated for 5-15 times in a session **(Fig. 6.64)**.
- *The plank:* The patient is made to lie prone on elbows and tries to balance on elbow and toes. He/she is asked to keep the back and legs straight like a plank. He should tighten the abdominals and hold the position for 10 seconds, and the same should be repeated for 5-10 times **(Fig. 6.65)**.
- **The side plank:** This exercise strengthens the oblique muscles of trunk. Patient in side lying position with elbow and forearm on bed. He/she should be advised to tighten the abdominals and push the body up laterally until the shoulder is on the elbows and the pelvis is raised laterally. Only the forearm and the side of the down side foot are on the floor **(Fig. 6.66)**. The position should be held for 10 seconds and performed five times in each side.
- **Wall squats:** The patient is asked to stand with the back against the wall and heels about 18 inches away from the wall and the feet shoulder width apart. Patient is asked to tighten the abdominals and slide the back slowly down the wall into a crouch with knees bent to 90 degrees. The position is held for five counts and reverted again to the vertical position and repeated for 5-10 times.
- **Back extensor strengthening exercises:** Patient lies in prone with the arms over head and the palms and forehead on the floor. He/she is asked to lift the head and trunk upward along with lifting of arm and opposite leg off the floor at a time stretching them away from each other **(Fig. 6.67)**. The position is held for 5 seconds and then head, trunk, arm, and leg are lowered to bed and the same are repeated on the other side. Total of 5-10 repetitions are performed in one session. The same type of exercises can also be performed in quadruped position.

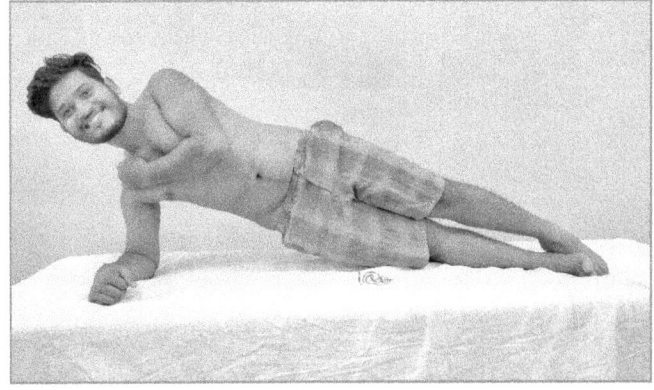

Fig. 6.66: The side plank exercise.

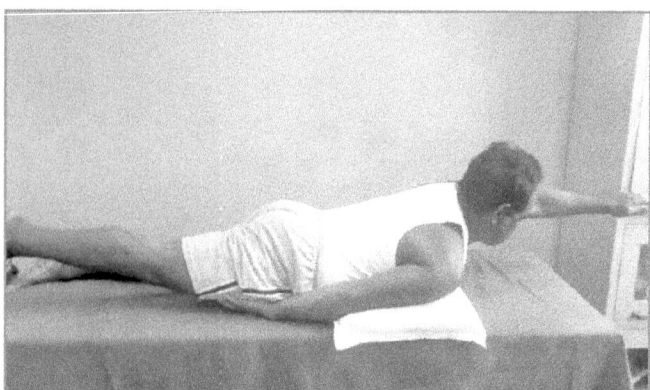

Fig. 6.67: Spinal extensor strengthening exercise.

- **Upper abdominal muscle strengthening exercises:** Patient supine. A rolled up towel is placed under the lumbar spine. The hands are placed under the head with the elbows pointing outward. The patient is asked to tighten the abdominals and raise the head and shoulders off the floor by 3–6 inches with exhalation and lower the elbows to the bed with inspiration. Total 10–15 repetitions of exercise are performed.
- **Isometric strengthening of lower abdominals:** Raising both legs together off the bed through an angle of 45 degrees in supine lying, holding for 3–5 seconds, followed by lowering. The exercises are performed 10 times in a session.
- Hip extension exercises, hydrotherapy, and static cycle exercises, etc., are advised to perform.
- Modalities like SWD **(Fig. 6.68)**/MWD/IFT/TENS/Lumbar traction, etc., may be applied as per requirement after clinical reasoning. Combined therapy using SWD/MWD with static lumbar traction in supine with a pillow placed under the knees is sometimes found beneficial and may be considered, if the patient shows symptomatic relief. The suction effect produced due to decreased pressure in the intervertebral spaced, as a result of separation of vertebral bodies due to traction, combined with increased pressure in the disc as a result of fluid absorption from increased blood flow caused by the effect of SWD/MWD, helps in movement of the nucleus pulposus into the intervertebral space, correcting the derangement.

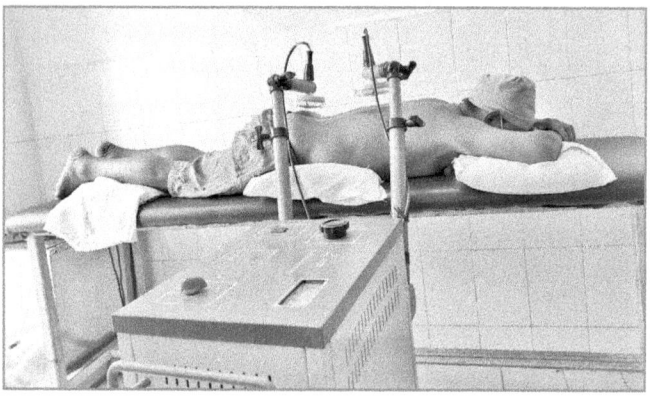

Fig. 6.68: SWD to lumbar spine.

- **Surgery:** Although most patients with a herniated disc respond well to nonsurgical treatments, some patients do need surgery. In general, surgery should be considered only after several months of nonsurgical treatment or if the patient develops progressive neurological deficits. Many surgical procedures can be performed using minimally invasive techniques (meaning less cutting and entering the body). These techniques result in smaller incisions, shorter hospital stays, less pain after surgery, and a faster recovery. The most typical surgery for a herniated disc is laminectomy with discectomy. This is a surgical procedure that removes all or part of the damaged intervertebral disc. Recently, surgeons are performing discectomies using various less invasive techniques (sometimes known as micro, mini-open, minimally invasive, or percutaneous discectomies). In these techniques, surgeons perform the entire surgery through a very small incision, or through a tube which allows them to insert a tiny camera and special surgical instruments. Sometimes the disc is replaced with an artificial disc, although this is more common in the neck than in the low back.
- **Postoperative physiotherapy:** Focuses on strengthening the muscles of spine (core muscles), and imparting back care measures to prevent recurrence.

2. **Management of lumbar spondylosis:** Lumbar spondylosis, also known as spinal osteoarthritis, is a medical condition in which chronic pain is experienced by the patient in the lower back, with or without pain radiating along the lower limbs and motor/sensory weakness in a few cases leading to disability.

Epidemiology/Etiology

The disorder commonly affects individuals above the age of 40 years (primary spondylosis), though young individuals who have/had a primary pathology such as a PIVD or spine fracture may also be affected from this disorder (secondary lumbar spondylosis). Males are affected more than females with a male to female ratio of 2:1.

The causes of this disorder include:

- **Aging:** This is the most common cause of this disorder. As the individual ages, with passage of time, can lead to changes in the bones of the spine. Being over the age of 40 years increases one's risk for lumbar spondylosis.
- **Abnormal spinal movements:** Frequent overuse of the back as seen during sports or other physically strenuous activity can put increased amounts of stress on the lumbar vertebrae, leading to injury and start of degeneration.
- **Genetics:** Those genetically predisposed to weak bones and ligaments may be at increased risk for injury to the lumbar spine.
- **Sedentary lifestyle:** Sedentary living, abnormal posture, smoking (decreases the amount of water in the discs), etc., also lead to this disorder.
- **Prolonged sitting posture:** Puts more load on the discs and lumbar vertebrae, leading to degeneration.
- **Obesity:** Increase of body weight, puts excess load on the joints leading to wear and tear and subsequent degeneration.
- **Old trauma:** Any previous injury that alters the biomechanics of the spine also leads to abnormal loading of the vertebrae and degeneration.

Pathophysiology of lumbar spondylosis

The degenerative effects of ageing can cause the fibers of the discs to weaken and there occurs reduction of water content from the discs, making the discs hard, stiff, and decreased in size, causing wear and tear. Constant wear and tear and injury to the joints of the vertebrae causes inflammation in the joints. Degeneration of the discs leads to the formation of mineral deposits within the discs. There is also an increased risk of disc herniation.

The end plates that attach the disc to the vertebrae and supplies nutrition to the disc, degenerate causing stiffness and reduction of sizes of these end plates. Movement of the spine stimulates the pain fibers in the facet joints as well as in the annulus fibrosus. There is also thickening and hardening of the facets.

Degenerative changes can cause ligaments to lose their strength. In degenerative spondylosis, one of the main ligaments (known as the ligamentum flavum) can thicken or buckle, making it weaken.

Abnormal bone growths (known as bone spurs or osteophytes) can form in the vertebrae. In more severe cases, these bone spurs can compress nerves coming out of the spinal cord causing pain in the legs and neurological deficits.

Clinical features

All patients with lumbar spondylosis do not complain of symptoms of pain in the back, even though they have degenerative changes in the radiographs of spine. Those who have symptoms, present with back pain, ranging from mild to severe as well as morning stiffness lasting for more than 30 minutes.

Additions symptoms of lumbar spondylosis include:
- Localized pain.
- Limitation of spinal movements, extension more painful and limited than flexion.
- Pain after prolonged sitting and standing.
- The pain is usually more in standing as compared to sitting.
- Worsening pain after repeated movements
- Muscle spasms
- Regional tenderness
- Tingling, numbness in the limbs
- Weakness of affected limb due to possible nerve compression.
- Bladder bowel dysfunction.

Diagnostic tests: It includes

- Physical examination that reveals a decreased lumbar lordosis and painful movement limitation more in the direction of extension than flexion. A positive SLR is a common association **(Fig. 6.47A)**.
- X-ray of lumbosacral spine: Usually show bone spurs on the vertebral bodies of the spine, thickening of the facet joints, and narrowing of the intervertebral disc spaces **(Fig. 6.43C)**.
- CT scan: Provides greater image detail and can diagnose narrowing of the spinal canal, if present.
- MRI: Sometimes required in patients with progressive neurological deficits.
- SPECT: Single-photon emission computed tomography bone scintigraphy can be used to further evaluate patients with suspected spondylolysis.

Management of lumbar spondylosis

- **Acute stage:**
    - *Medical management:* Managed in the same lines as acute PIVD, with relative rest, anti-inflammatory, and muscle-relaxant drugs. A lumbosacral belt is also recommended for use. The use of the lumbosacral belt should gradually be decreased as acute symptoms subside.
    - *Physiotherapy:* Consists of the followings:
        » Positioning the spine in flexion (supine lying, pillow placed under the knees), if patient has radicular pain.
        » Traction: Sustained traction in the position of ease, usually given in the semi-Fowler position.
        » Posture re-education.
        » Modalities such as hot pack, IRR, ultrasound, PSWD, IFT, etc., can be applied to reduce pain and spasm.
        » Relaxation techniques like breathing exercises, myofascial release to paraspinal muscles **(Fig. 6.69)** can be applied.
        » Manual therapy: Maitlands grade-I, II PA glides can be applied to inhibit muscle spasm and provide synovial movement within the joint for healing.
        » Gentle active ROM exercises such as trunk rotation in crook lying (knee roll) **(Fig. 6.70)**, Isometric spinal

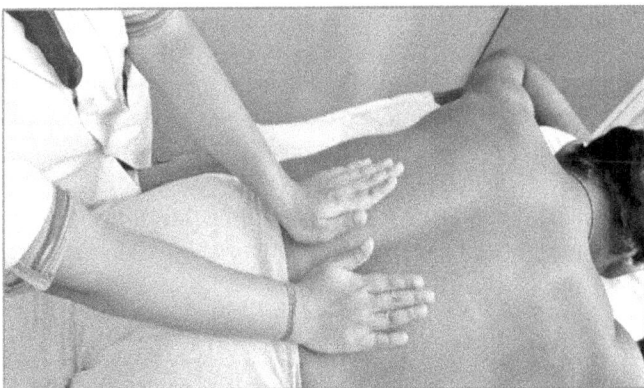

Fig. 6.69: Myofascial release to paravertebral muscles.

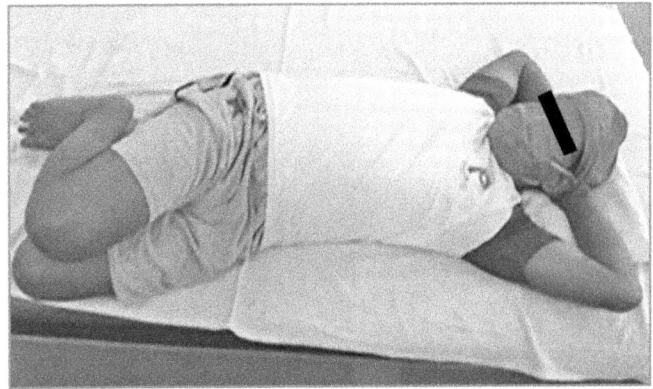

Fig. 6.70: Knee roll in supine.

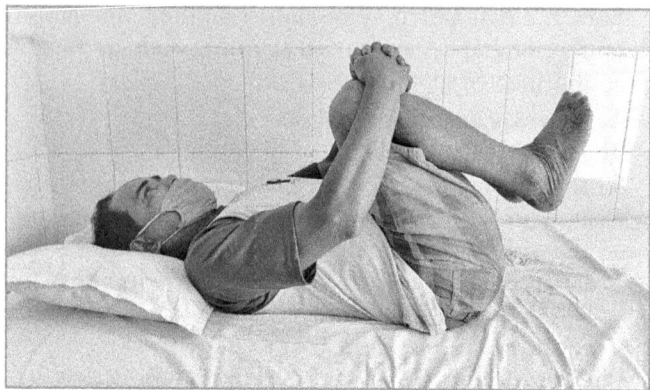

Fig. 6.71A: McKenzie flexion exercise.

exercises, spinal flexion exercises/McKenzie flexion exercise **(Fig. 6.71A)**, can be started within the limits of pain.

* **Subacute/Chronic stage:** After acute pain subsided, physiotherapy is started with the following goals:
  – Relief of pain.
  – Restoration of lumbosacral ROM and reduce dysfunction.
  – Strengthening of spinal muscles.
  – Education of posture.
  – Prevention of acute relapse.

Procedures of physiotherapy

* Mobilization exercises such as, Maitland's lateral P-A glide in grade-III/IV on the contralateral side/lateral transverse glide toward the painful side is helpful in opening the compromised IV foramina, to cause the nerve roots free of pressure, in unilateral radicular symptoms. Maitland's central PA mobilization may be applied in case of bilateral radicular symptoms, if relief occurs.
  – McKenzie mobilization in the direction of dysfunction [McKenzie flexion exercise **(Fig. 6.71A)**], Mulligan's mobilizations with movements are helpful in restoring the ROM of the lumbosacral segments **(Figs. 6.71B and C)**.

  – Stretching the paraspinal muscles through myofascial release technique.
  – Strengthening the core muscles to increase spinal stability.
  – Stretching the piriformis, hamstrings, if the muscles are tight **(Figs. 6.72A and B)**
  – Traction: Intermittent lumbar traction in semi-fowler position **(Fig. 6.73)**, positional traction at home **(Fig. 6.74A)** for radicular/sciatic pain are applied. In the **Figure 6.74A**, below, for positional traction, the patient has been made to lie on the right side over pillow, for radiating pain in left lower limb. If the pain radiates to both lower limbs and, the patient does not have soft disc lesion, positional in trunk prone lying **(Fig. 6.74B)**

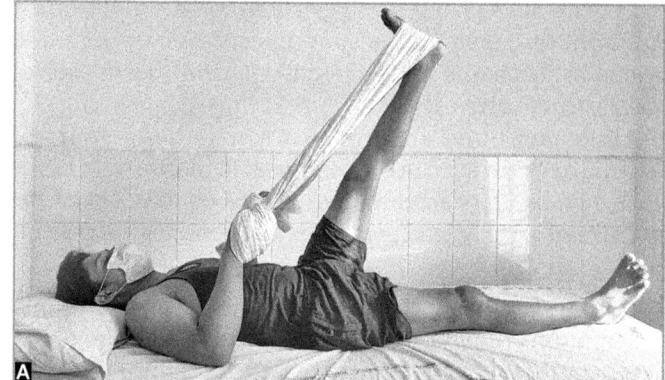

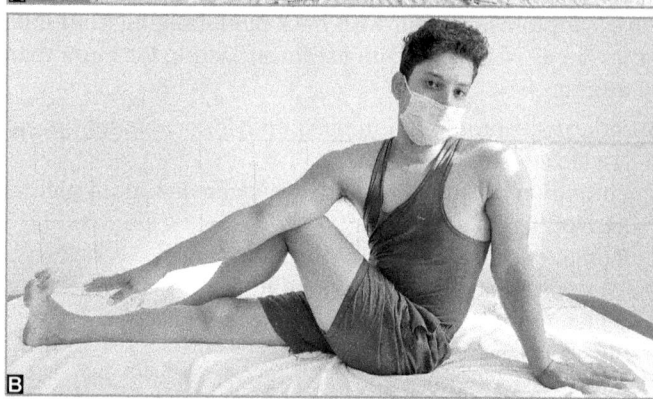

Figs. 6.72A and B: (A) Self stretching of hamstrings, (B) Self stretching of piriformis.

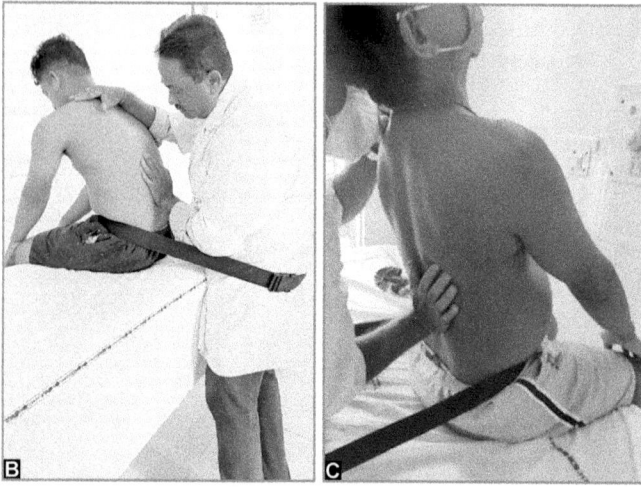

Figs. 6.71B and C: (B) Mulligan mobilization to increase lumbosacral flexion; (C) Mulligan mobilization to increase lumbosacral extension.

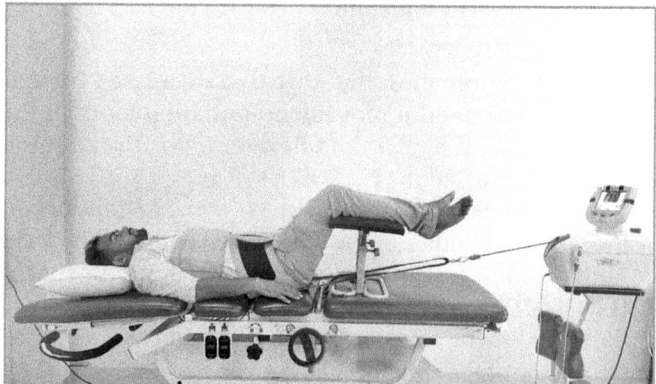

Fig. 6.73: Intermittent lumbar traction in semi-fowler position.

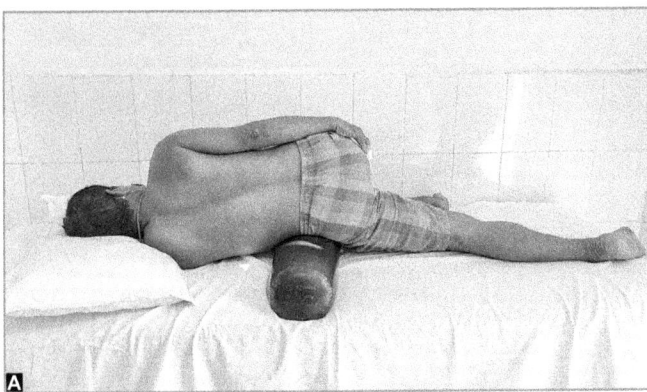

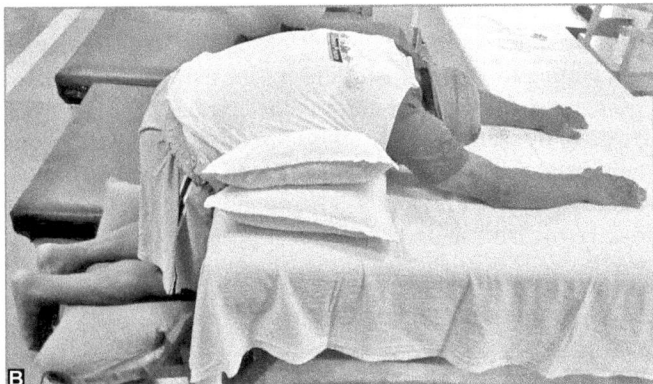

Figs. 6.74A and B: (A) Positional traction in side lying, (B) Positional traction in trunk prone lying.

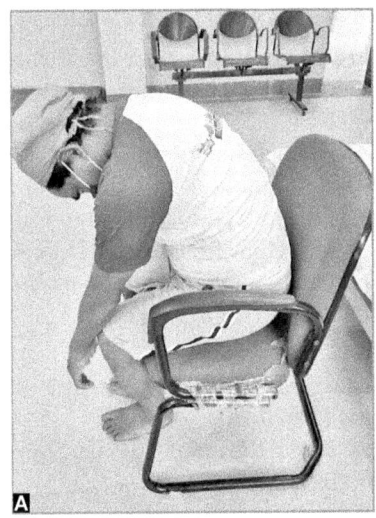

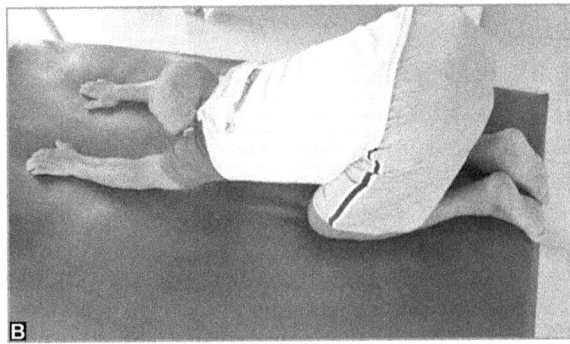

Figs. 6.75A and B: (A) Sitting flexion exercise, (B) Prone kneeling to kneel sitting.

may be advised, if tolerated and found beneficial. Sitting flexion exercise **(Fig. 6.75A)**, if tolerated, prone kneeling to kneel sitting **(Fig. 6.75B)** can be advised to get relief from radicular pain.
- Passive modalities such as ultrasound, IFT/TENS, hot packs should be applied as indicated.
- Advice on posture correction and ergonomic measures to be followed, so that spinal degeneration could be prevented. Joint protection and energy conservation techniques are emphasized.
- Life style modification such as regular exercises and fat free diets to reduce weight, and changing the pattern of activities like avoiding constant standing and performing activities that require repeated bending and twisting should be avoided.
- A spinal support such as a lumbosacral belt may be used, if found beneficial.
- **Surgery:** If the patient has progressive neurological deficits such as bladder/bowel dysfunction, motor and sensory loss in the lower limbs due either to neural canal stenosis or spinal canal stenosis, or the pain is not relieved after prolong conservative management, surgery is the option. The surgeries commonly performed in lumbar spondylosis are:

Spinal decompression surgeries:
- **Facetectomy:** It involves surgical removal of the facet joint to cause pressure relieved from the nerve roots.
- **Foraminotomy:** It involves widening the intervertebral foramen, so that, the nerve roots can pass easily through it.
- **Laminectomy:** All or part of the lamina is removed to relieve pressure from the spinal cord as occurs in lumbar canal stenosis.
- **Laminotomy:** This is a spinal canal widening procedure, performed for patients with a lumbar canal stenosis.
- **Spinal stabilization surgery:** After the spinal decompression procedure, if the surgeon feels for any instability in the spine, spinal fusion procedure is carried to achieve a stable spine.

The Physiotherapist involved with the management of the patient post operatively need to clearly understand the procedure undertaken, before providing therapy to increase mobility and function.

3. Lumbar Spondylolisthesis

The word Spondylolisthesis is derived from two parts, such as "spondylo", which means spine, and "listhesis", which means slippage. The disorder is very common in lower lumbar spine, though, it is also found in lower cervical and thoracic spine (rare).

Spondylolisthesis is herein defined as a disorder of spine, where one vertebra with vertebrae above it, is displaced anteriorly over the vertebra below it **(Fig. 6.43D)**. When the upper vertebra is displaced posteriorly, it is called retrolisthesis **(6.43F)**.

Epidemiology and Etiology of Spondylolisthesis

Males are more likely to develop the disorder than the females due to more involvement in physical activities. In females, increased lumbar lordosis during pregnancy and weak abdominal muscles after child birth is the important factor for the development of this disorder. Degenerative spondylolisthesis is more commonly found in females than males. Isthmic Spondylolisthesis, which is commonly seen in adolescents and young adults is found more in males.

The causes of the disorder include:
- A birth defect.
- Trauma causing fracture of pars interarticularis.
- Spondylolysis **(Fig. 6.76)**.
- Degenerative spinal disorders due to aging/overuse.
- Tumors of vertebrae.
- Multiparity (repeated child birth).
- Spinal surgeries.

Types of Spondylolisthesis

Wiltse classification is one of the most commonly used classification systems based on the etiology of spondylolisthesis. It has five major types such as:
- **Degenerative:** Degenerative spondylolisthesis occurs from degenerative changes in the spine without any defect in the pars interarticularis. It is usually related to combined facet joint and disc degeneration leading to instability and forward movement of one vertebral body relative to the adjacent vertebral body.
- **Isthmic:** Isthmic spondylolisthesis results from defects in the pars interarticularis. The possible etiology includes microtrauma in adolescence related to sports such as wrestling, football, and gymnastics, where repeated lumbar extension occurs.
- **Traumatic:** Traumatic spondylolisthesis occurs after fractures of the pars interarticularis or the facet joint structures due to trauma.
- **Dysplastic:** Dysplastic spondylolisthesis is congenital and secondary to variation in the orientation of the facet joints to an abnormal alignment. In dysplastic spondylolisthesis, the facet joints are more sagittally oriented than the typical coronal orientation.
- **Pathologic:** Pathologic spondylolisthesis can be from bone or connective tissue disorders or a focal process, including infection, neoplasm, or iatrogenic origin.

Table 6.6: Grading of spondylolisthesis.

Grade of spondylolisthesis	Criteria
1	25% forward slipping of vertebra
2	50% forward slipping of vertebra
3	75% forward slipping of vertebra
4	100% forward slipping of vertebra
5	Vertebral body completely fallen off (spondyloptosis)

Grading of spondylolisthesis: Spondylolisthesis can be graded into five grades **(Table 6.6)** based on severity. Grade-1 being less severe and grade-5 being most severe. Grading is done by measuring percentage of slippage of vertebral body over the underlying vertebra.

Clinical Features of Lumbar Spondylolisthesis

Many people with a spondylolisthesis may have no symptoms and only become aware of the problem when it is revealed on an X-ray for a different problem. However, there are several symptoms that often accompany spondylolisthesis, which are discussed below:
- Localized and intermittent low back pain.
- Increased lumbar lordosis is a common association.
- Pain is increased by movement of L-S spine and extension is more difficult and painful than flexion. However, if there is an associated PIVD, flexion also may be more painful.
- Inspection of the low back reveals increased lumbar lordosis and a sill like capital letter "L" (the sill sign). Palpation of the spine reveals local tenderness and a step sign may be present **(Fig. 6.77)**.
- Phalen Dickson sign (increased slippage of lumbar vertebra may make the sacrum more vertical resulting in limitation

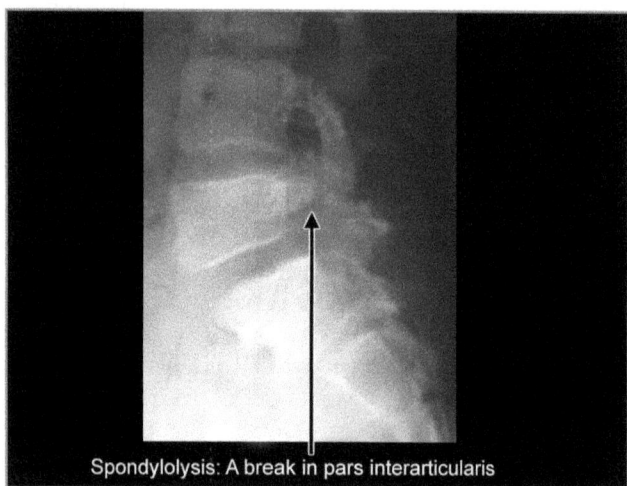

Fig. 6.76: Showing a break in pars interarticularis.

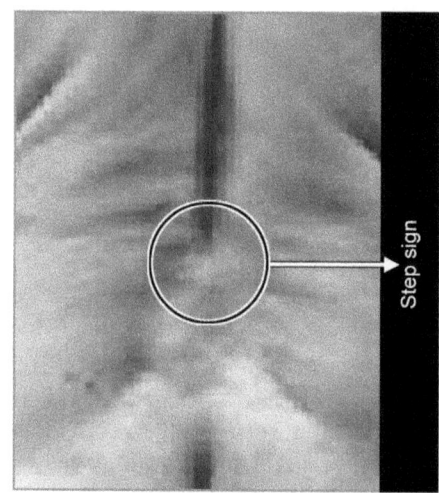

Fig. 6.77: The step sign/Sill sign.

of hip extension and the patient walking with hip and knee in flexion) may be present in high-grade spondylolisthesis.
- ❖ The patient may also exhibit radicular symptoms in the lower limb (sciatica), with neurological deficits (lower/upper motor neuron features) depending upon the site (UMN features above L1 and LMN features below L1).
- ❖ Spasm of lumbar paravertebral muscles, hamstrings, and tightness of psoas major muscle is usually associated.
- ❖ Sometimes the patient may also have bladder/bowel dysfunction and gait abnormalities.

Diagnostic Tests

- ❖ **X-ray of lumbosacral spine:** A lateral view is commonly recommended. An oblique view is recommended to rule out spondylolysis **(Fig. 6.43E)**.
- ❖ MRI/CT scan may be requested, when the patient develops progressive neurological features (cauda equina syndrome) **(Fig. 6.78)**.

Diagnosis: Diagnosis is mostly done from complain, clinical, and radiological examinations.

Management of Spondylolisthesis

A. Conservative management: Patients with grade-I and II, Spondylolisthesis are managed conservatively by the following methods:
  - Relative rest:
  - *Medical management:* NSAIDs, Epidural steroid injections are sometimes applied by the physician/surgeon to reduce low back/radicular pain.

Physiotherapy: Physiotherapy in the form of, moist heat/SWD/MWD/IRR to reduce local inflammation and muscle spasm Exercises to stabilize the spine and correct the displacement, sustained traction in semi fowler position/positional traction to reduce the displacement, IFT/TENS to modulate back pain and radicular pain, back care, etc., are advised by the therapist. A spinal brace may be advised to decrease segmental spinal instability and pain **(Fig. 6.79)**.

Traction: Sustained lumbar traction in semi-fowler's position **(Fig. 6.80A)** may be tried in patients with grade-I and II

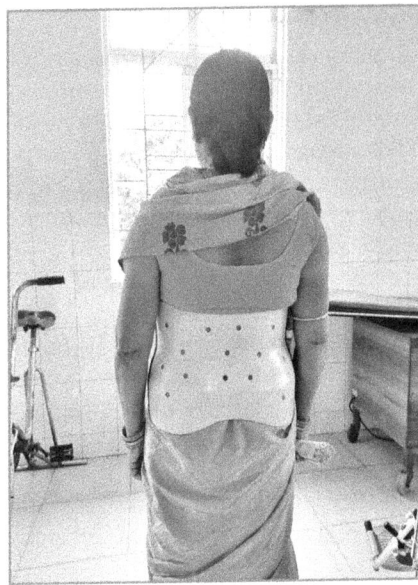

Fig. 6.79: Patient with lumbar spondylolisthesis using L-S brace.

spondylolisthesis, if symptomatic relief takes place. Further, if the patient is benefited by traction, positional traction in trunk prone lying position **(Fig. 6.80B)**, may also be advised to do at home. A moist hot pack may be applied to the low back during positional traction.

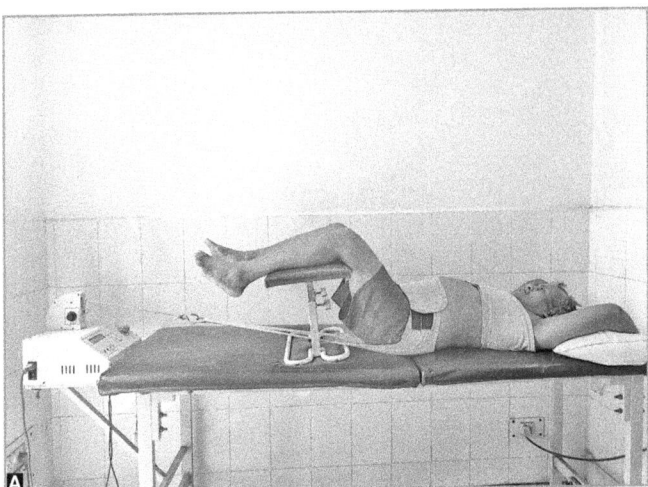

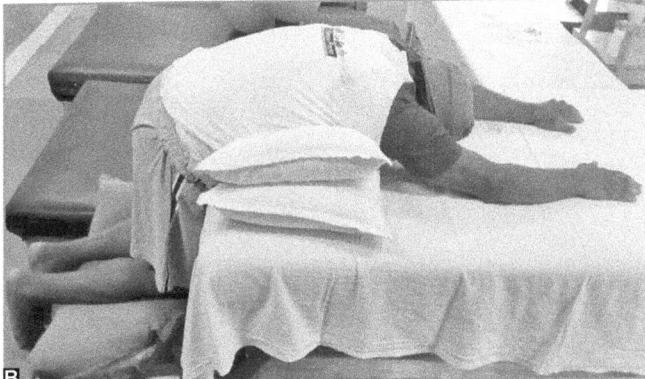

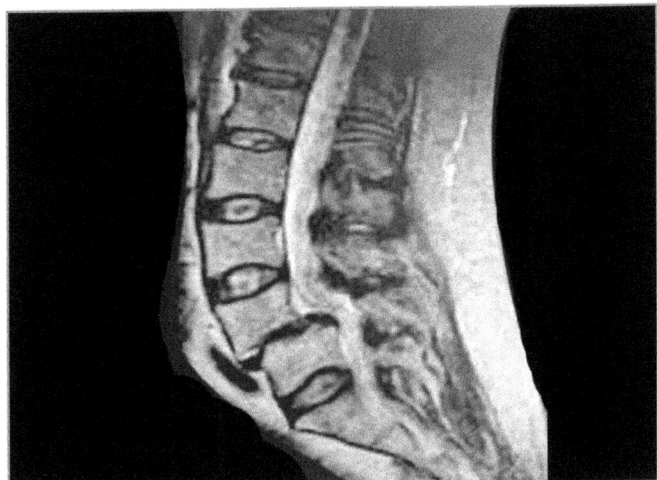

Fig. 6.78: MRI showing spondylolisthesis of L4-L5 with cauda equina involvement.

Figs. 6.80A and B: (A) Lumbar traction in semi-fowler position, (B) Positional traction to decompress the spine.

Section 2: Physiotherapy for Musculoskeletal Conditions

Exercises for spondylolisthesis

Stretching of spinal extensors, hamstrings, hip flexors, and strengthening of spinal flexors, extensors, and the core muscles are required to increase stability of the spine and reduce pain. The strengthening exercises should be performed both in isometric and isotonic mode. Aerobic exercises including hydrotherapy are also beneficial to make the patient return to sports and function.

- Isometric exercises for strengthening of spinal extensors and flexors **(Figs. 6.81A to C)**.
- Pelvic tilt exercise: Patient is made to lie on the back with the knees bent and the feet flat against the floor. He/she is asked to pull the belly button toward the spine using the abdominal muscles and focus on pressing the low back flat against the floor **(Fig. 6.82)**. This position should be held for 10-15 seconds, followed by relaxation. Total 10 repetitions of this exercise in sets of three are performed in one session.
- **Dead bug:** This is a more advanced version of the pelvic tilt **(Fig. 6.83)**. The patient begin this exercise in the same fashion as described for pelvic tilt such as lying on the back with the knees bent, feet flat against the floor and arms at the sides. He/she is asked to draw the belly button toward the spine and tighten the abdomen. Keeping the legs bent, one of the legs are lifted off the floor and held for 5 seconds before lowering it to the ground followed by lifting the other leg for 5 seconds. Next, one arm is lifted over the head; held for 5 seconds then lowered, followed by lifting of the other arm. Once this becomes easy, the patient should be asked to lift one leg and the opposite arm at the same time. This sequence should be repeated for 5-10 repetitions in sets of three.
- **Partial curl:** The patient lies on back with knees bent and feet on floor. He/she is asked to tuck the chin to the chest and curl the upper body forward to lift the shoulders off the floor with the hands straight out in front of the body. This position is held for three seconds before relaxing the abdominals and uncurling the upper back down to the floor **(Fig. 6.84)**. Breathing out can help to lift the shoulders off the floor. This exercise is repeated 10 times for 3 sets. To make this more difficult, one can clasp the hands behind the head with the elbows pointed out to the sides (like a crunch) while performing this exercise.
- **Erector spinae stretch:** Patient lying on the back with both knees bent. He/she rests the ankle of one leg against the knee of the other and grabs onto the thigh of the bottom leg and pull it toward the chest until feeling of a stretch in the

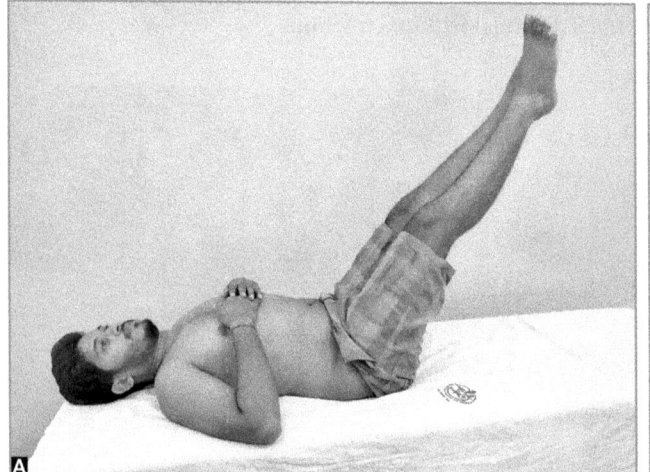
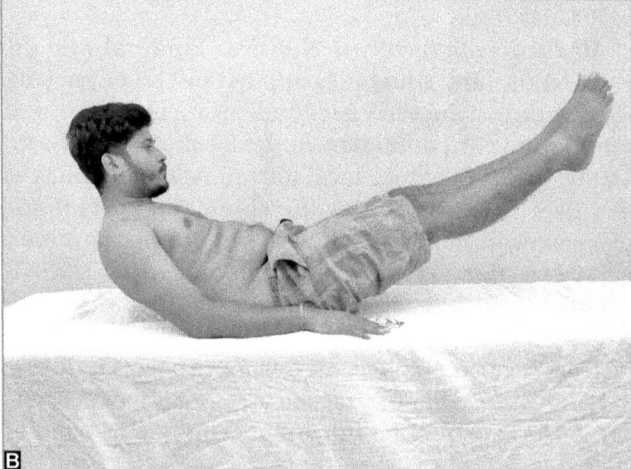
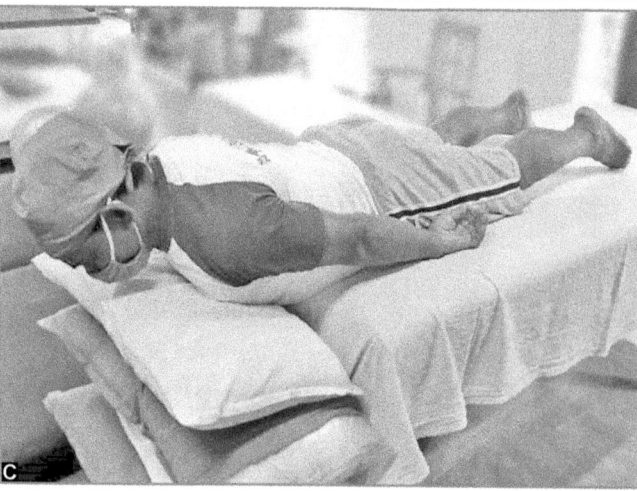

Figs. 6.81A to C: (A) Isometric exercise to lower abdominals, (B) Isometric exercise to both lower and upper abdominals, (C) Isometric spinal extension exercise (extending the neck and lifting the shoulder girdle just off the bed).

Chapter 6: Physiotherapy for Spinal Disorders

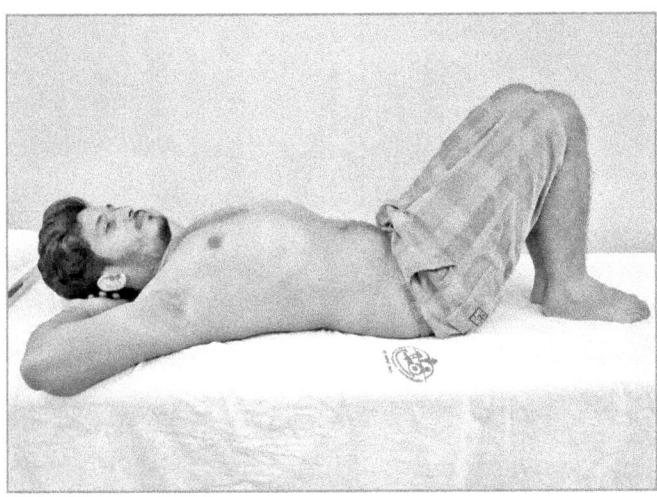

Fig. 6.82: Posterior pelvic tilt exercise.

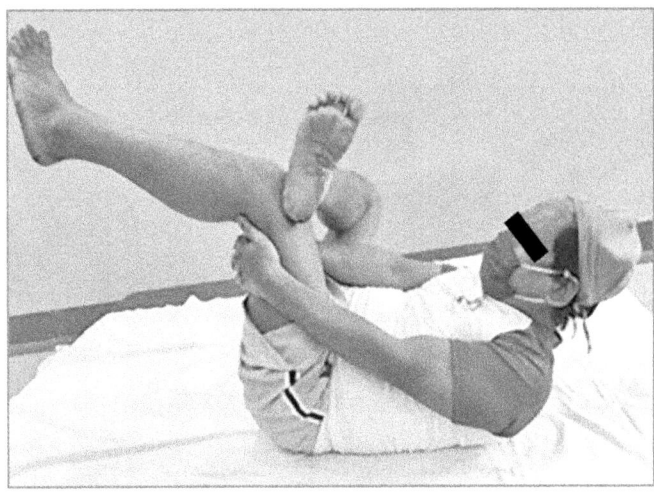

Fig. 6.85: Erector spinae stretch.

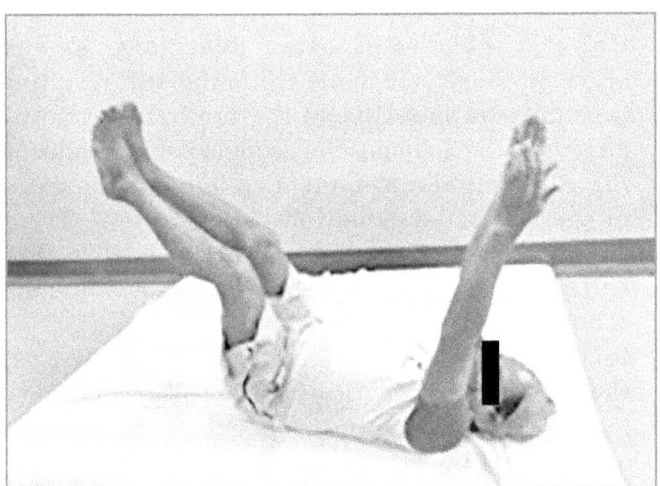

Fig. 6.83: The dead bug exercise.

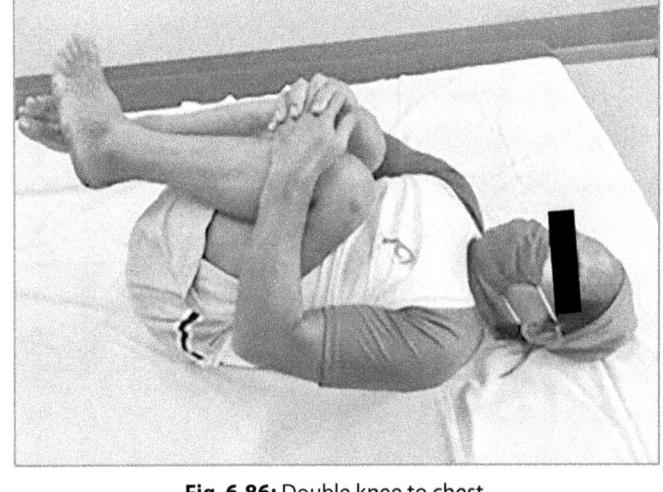

Fig. 6.86: Double knee to chest.

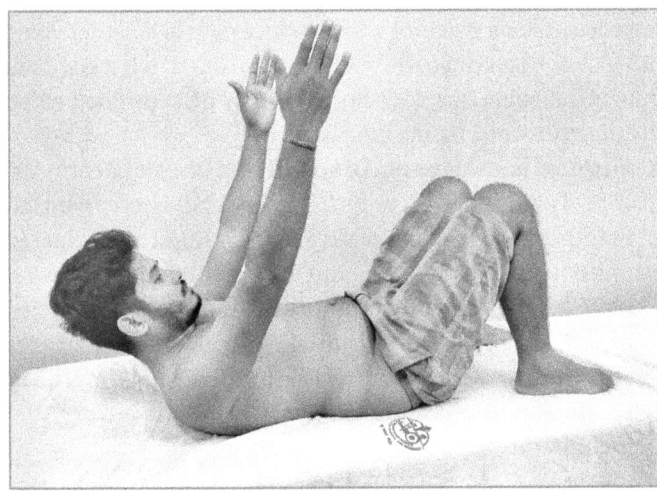

Fig. 6.84: The partial curl.

buttocks and possibly the back **(Fig. 6.85)**. This position is held for 15–30 seconds followed by switching over to the opposite side. These stretches for spondylolisthesis should be repeated three times for each leg.

- ❖ **Double-knee to chest:** The patient supine with the knees bent and feet flat against the floor. He/she is asked to tighten the abdomen to push the low back against the floor and then lift both legs off the ground and pull them to the chest **(Fig. 6.86)**. This position is held for 5 seconds then legs are lowered back down to the ground. 10–20 repetitions of the exercises are performed in a session.
- ❖ **Quadruped arm/leg raises:** The patient is in quadruped, i.e., on hands and knees. He/she is asked to tighten the abdominals and while doing so, and raise one arm and the opposite leg **(Fig. 6.87)**. This position is held for 5 seconds and then arm and leg are lowered, followed by raising of the opposite arm and leg. Ten repetitions on each side are performed.
- ❖ Core muscle strengthening/core stability exercises: Strengthening of the deep abdominals. **(Fig. 6.88A)**, side plank exercise **(Fig. 6.88B)**.
- ❖ Stretching of glutei and hip flexors **(Fig. 6.89)**.
- ❖ Theraband exercise: This exercise **(Fig. 6.90A)** should be advised for patients who do not have associated disc bulge, as it increases intra abdominal pressure enhancing the bulge (if any).

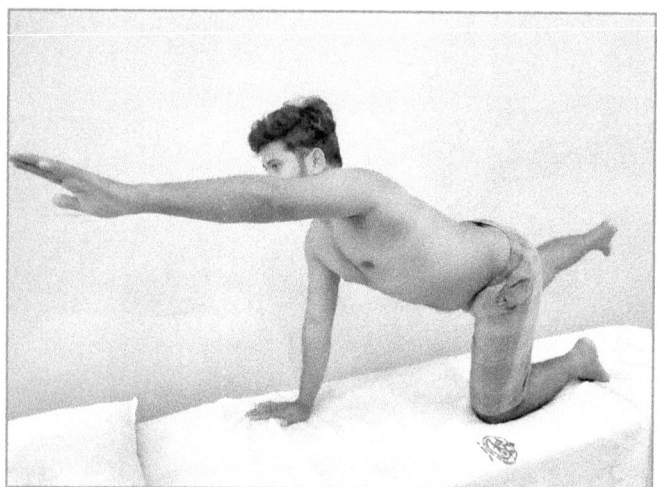

Fig. 6.87: Quadruped arm and leg raises.

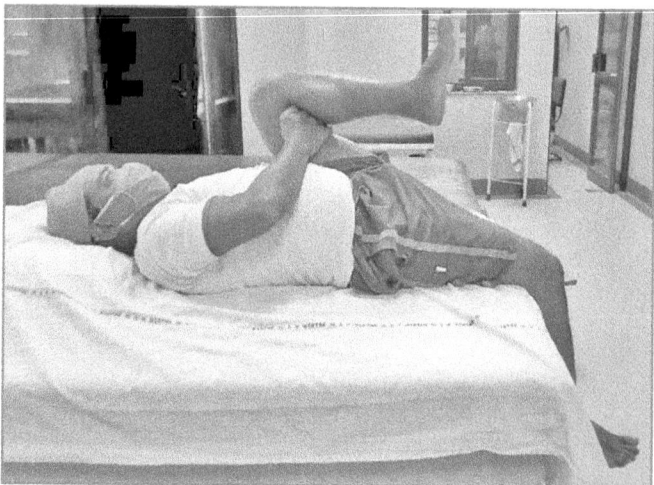

Fig. 6.89: Self stretching of left gluteus maximus and right hip flexors.

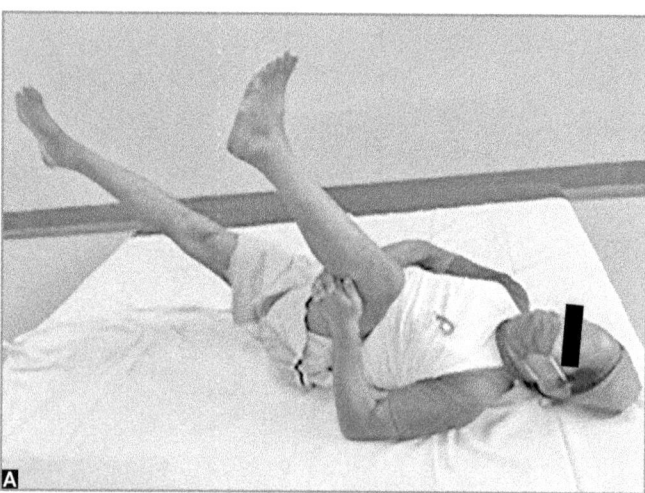

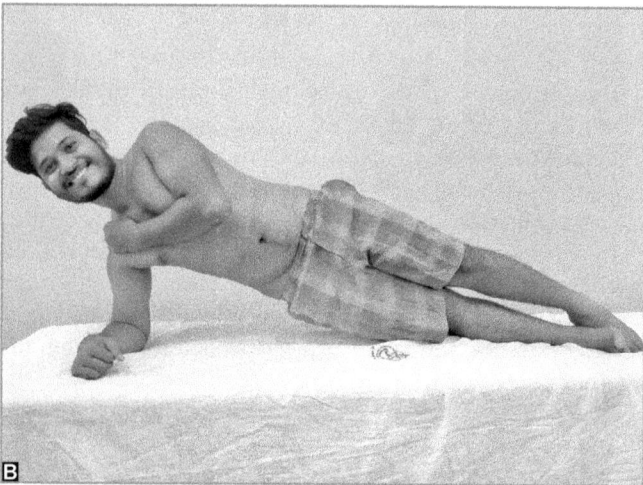

Figs. 6.88A and B: (A) Strengthening of deep abdominal muscles, (B) Side plank exercise.

- Williams flexion exercises, also called Williams lumbar flexion exercises are a set or system of related physical exercises **(Fig. 6.90B)** intended to enhance lumbar flexion, avoid lumbar extension, and strengthen the abdominal and gluteal musculature in an effort to manage low back pain nonsurgically.
- Upper back mobilization exercises, as the cervicothoracic segments are found stiff resulting in increased mobility of the lumbar segments. Stretching the tight muscles of upper back, mobilizing the cervicothoracic spine also helps in stopping progression of the spondylolisthesis.
- Stretching of hip flexors **(Fig. 6.91A)**/hamstrings **(Fig. 6.91B)** should be performed both in therapy clinics and at home.
- Pain modulating modalities such as IFT/TENS **(Fig. 6.92)** should be applied to the low back for pain modulation.

Spinal brace: A rigid custom made spinal brace, made of polypropylene **(Fig. 6.79)**/or readymade braces available in market **(Fig. 6.93)** may provided to the patient during functional activities to stabilize the spine. According to Prateepavanich et al., a lumbosacral corset can be used to improve walking distance and to reduce pain in daily activities but it does not reduce the shift of the vertebra. It is a good aid during the painful periods but should be discontinued when the patients' complaints are reduced.

A. **Surgical management of spondylolisthesis:** Nearly 10–15% of patients with grade-I, II Spondylolisthesis, who fail to improve with conservative management and selected patients with grade: III, and IV, Spondylolisthesis who have severe spinal instability and neurological deficits, are candidates for spinal stabilization procedures **(Fig. 6.94)**. Core strengthening exercises without producing lumbosacral spinal movements are advised postoperatively.

4. Spinal Canal Stenosis

Spinal stenosis is one of the most common causes of nontraumatic spinal cord injuries in people older than 50 years. The spinal canal that contains the spinal cord **(Fig. 6.95)** is severely compromised causing progressive neurological deficits.

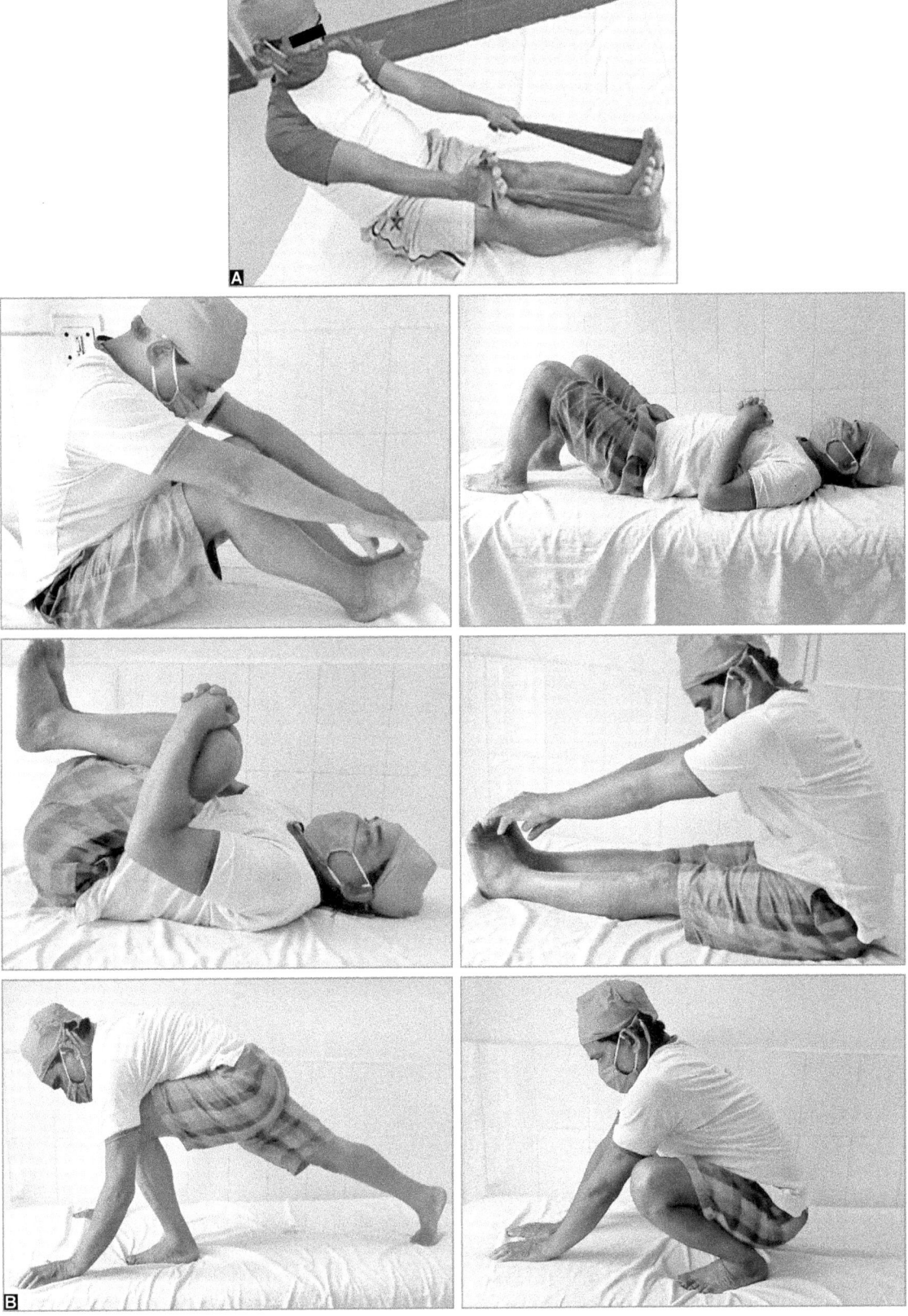

Figs. 6.90A and B: (A) Theraband exercise for abdominal strengthening (B) A set of William's lumbar flexion exercises for lumbar spondylolisthesis.

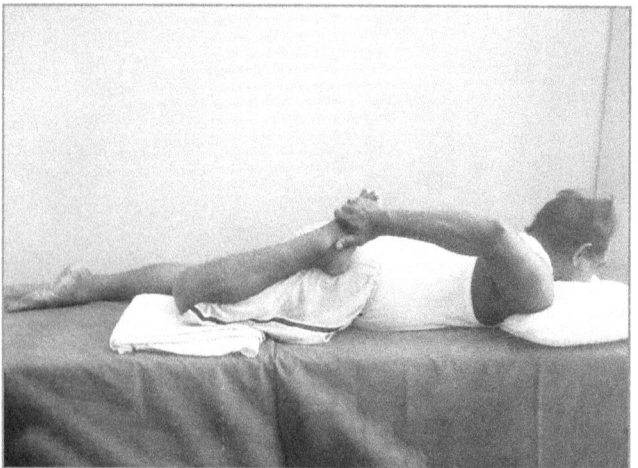
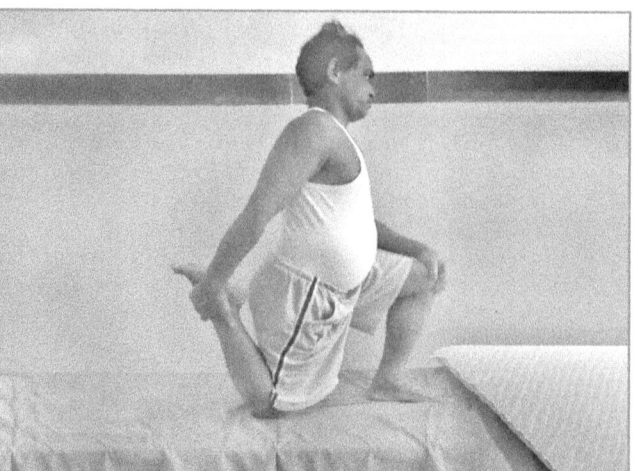
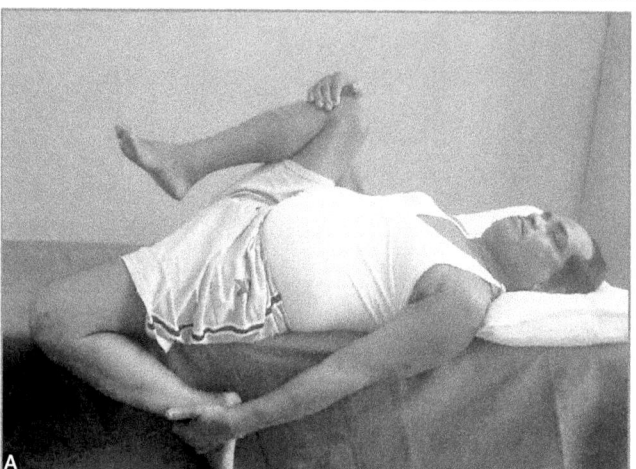
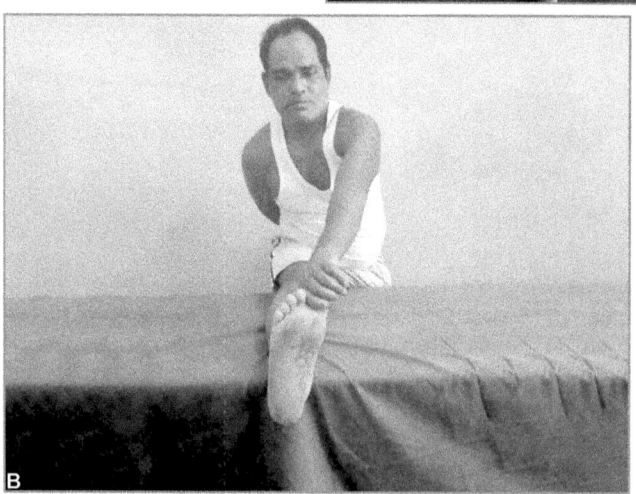
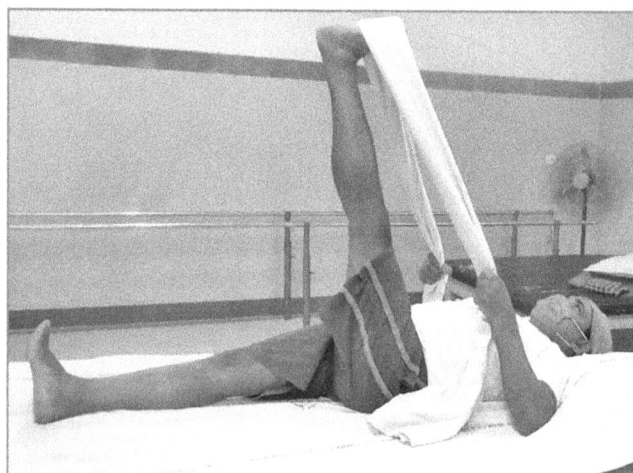

Figs. 6.91A and B: (A) Stretching of hip flexors in various postures. (B) Self stretching of hamstrings.

Etiology of Lumbar Canal Stenosis

Lumbar canal stenosis is caused by the following factors:
- Degenerative spondylosis: A posteriorly formed osteophyte, and ligamentum flavum hypertrophy may compromise the lumen of the spinal canal.
- Spondylolisthesis: The displacement of vertebrae that occurs lead to narrowing of the spinal canal.
- Central disc bulge: A central/posterior disc bulge pushes the PLL into the spinal canal causing narrowing of the lumen of the spinal canal.
- Space occupying lesions, diffuse idiopathic skeletal hyperostosis, inflammatory spinal diseases such as ankylosing spondylitis, and burst compression fractures in vertebral body with posterior displacement of the fracture fragment can also lead to this disorder.

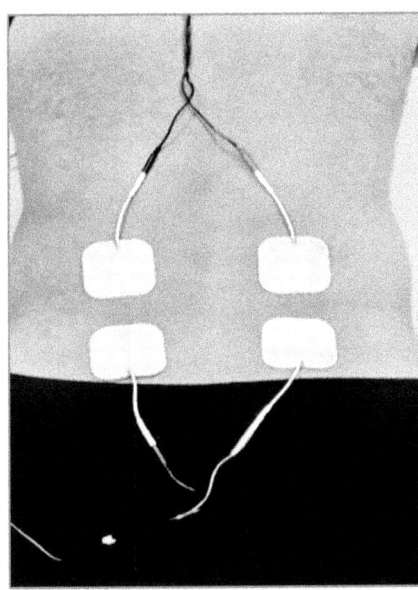

Fig. 6.92: Placement of TENS electrodes to low back.

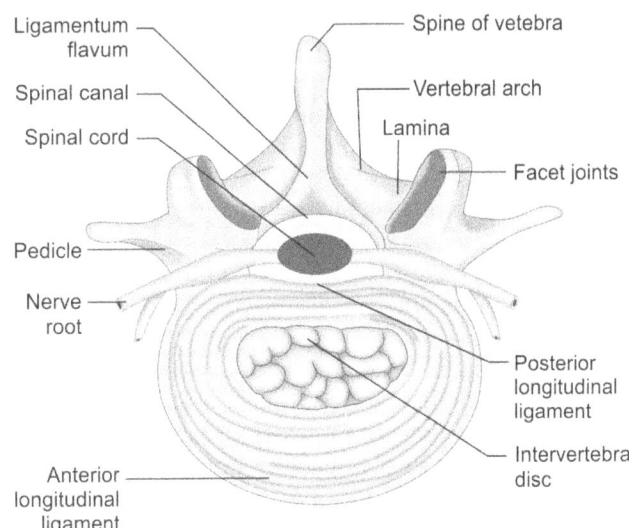

Fig. 6.95: The spinal canal containing the spinal cord.

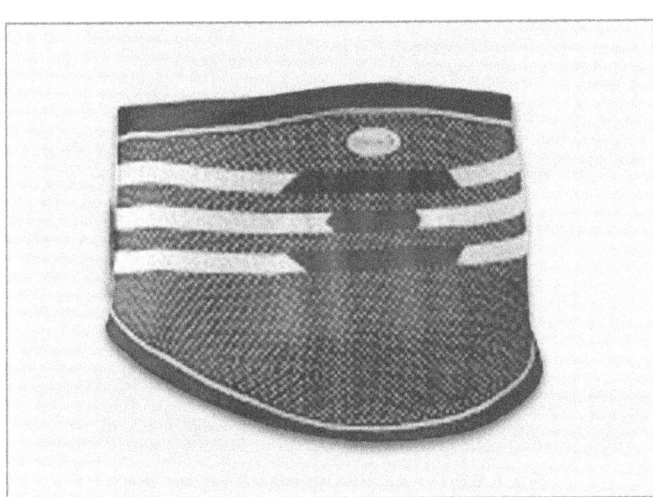

Fig. 6.93: Readymade lumbosacral brace.

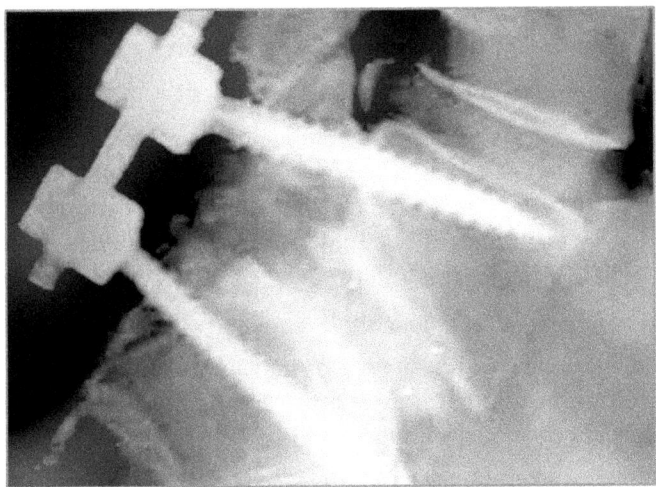

Fig. 6.94: X-ray of L-S spine showing spinal stabilization for spondylolisthesis through application of pedicular screw.

❖ Metabolic bone disorders that cause bone growth such as Paget's disease.

Clinical Features

❖ Gradual onset of tingling numbness in the lower limbs, which may or may not be associated with low back pain.
❖ Decreased lumbar lordosis and spasm of the paravertebral muscles may be present.
❖ Pain is exacerbated by prolonged ambulation, standing, and with lumbar extension, and is relieved by forward flexion and rest.
❖ Neurogenic claudication (also referred to as pseudo-claudication) is an important feature of lumbar canal stenosis. Pain in the legs may become so severe that walking, even short distances, is unbearable. Frequently, patients sit or lean forward to temporarily ease pain. Symptoms are typically bilateral, but usually asymmetric.
❖ Patients also report walking upstairs is easier, as the spine is flexed, than walking down the stairs.
❖ Extension of the spine increases the symptoms and flexion causes a relief (except when the stenosis is due to a central disc bulge, where extension of lumbar spine may decrease pain and flexion causes an increase of pain).
❖ Straight leg raise test is usually negative.
❖ Symptoms progressively worsen when standing and walking and are relieved on sitting.
❖ Side-lying is more comfortable than prone and supine lying as the lumbar spine is flexed.
❖ Patients often present with nocturnal cramps in the lower limbs.
❖ Bowel or bladder dysfunction, saddle anesthesia, bilateral lower extremity weakness are the presentations when there is progressive stenosis affecting the conus medullaris/cauda equine.

Diagnosis

Diagnosis of lumbar canal stenosis is done from:
a. Clinical features (signs and symptoms).
b. Physical examination: The findings may include:
   - Extension of spine more painful and may produce leg pain in most of the patients, however, if the stenosis is due to a central disc bulge, extension gives relief and flexion increases the symptoms.
   - The straight leg-raise test and other neural tension signs are usually negative unless there is accompanying disc herniation.
   - Patients with stenosis often have lumbar, paraspinal, or gluteal tenderness, which is usually related to underlying degenerative changes, muscle spasms, and poor posture.
   - Bicycle stress test is usually positive: During this test the patient first pedals on a cycle ergometer in upright position with preservation of neutral lumbar lordosis. The distance the patient has pedaled in a certain amount of time is recorded. The patient has to pedal a second time in a slumped position. The distance the patient has pedaled in the second time is recorded again. If the patient can pedal more distance in slumped position than in upright position, lumbar spinal stenosis is indicated.
   - Two-stage Treadmill test is positive: The patient is made to walk on a flat tread mill (0 degree inclination) with the spine extended (straight). The distance covered and time taken are recorded. Then the patient is made to walk on the same treadmill with the walking surface inclined and trunk in flexion. The time taken to cover the previous distance is recorded. If the time taken to cover the distance, when the treadmill is inclined (spine is flexed) is less, the patient is likely suffering from lumbar canal stenosis.
   - Positive extension loading test: The lumbar extension-loading test is used to evaluate symptoms due to lumbar canal stenosis. The lumbar extension-loading test involves maintaining the lumbar region in moderate extension, while standing for as long as possible **(Fig. 6.96)**. Increase of symptoms in the lower limb indicates a positive test.
   - Passive lumbar extension test: The subject is laid in the prone position. The clinician passively lifts both thighs to a height of about 30 cm from the bed while maintaining the knees extended and gently pulling the legs **(Fig. 6.97)**. Increase of symptoms suggests a positive test, revealing severe spinal instability such as degenerative spinal canal stenosis.
c. **Radiological tests:**
   - *X-rays:* An X-ray of the spine can reveal bony changes, such as bone spurs that may be narrowing the space within the spinal canal.
   - *Magnetic resonance imaging (MRI):* The test can detect damage to discs and ligaments, as well as the presence of tumors (if any).
   - *CT or CT myelogram:* In the absence of MRI, a CT scan may be performed. In a CT myelogram, the CT scan is conducted after a contrast dye is injected. The dye outlines the spinal cord and nerves, and it can reveal herniated discs, bone spurs and tumors.

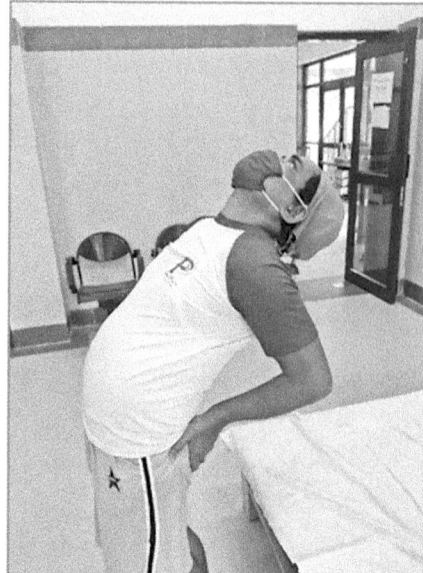

Fig. 6.96: Extension loading test.

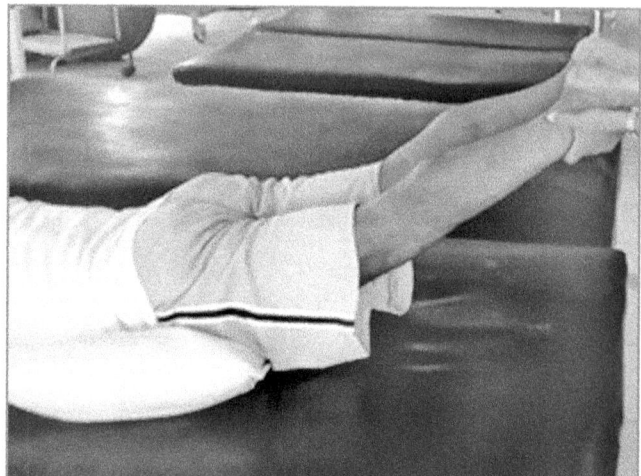

Fig. 6.97: The passive lumbar extension test.

Differential Diagnosis

Lumbar canal stenosis with neurogenic claudication should be differentiated from vasculogenic claudication and lumbar spondylosis with radiculopathy to establish the diagnosis and plan the management. The **Table 6.7** describes the differences found in different conditions.

Management of Lumbar Canal Stenosis

Conservative management: Conservative treatment options include oral anti-inflammatory medications, epidural steroid injections, and physiotherapy.

Physiotherapy: Physiotherapy is associated with reduced likelihood of patients requiring surgery within 1 year. Low quality evidence is available regarding benefits with

Table 6.7: Differential diagnosis between spinal canal stenosis, peripheral vascular diseases, and lumbar spondylosis.

Nature of pain	Neurogenic claudication (lumbar canal stenosis)	Vasculogenic claudication (thromboangiitis obliterans)	Lumbar spondylosis
Type	Vague, cramping, aching, sharp, burning in the lower extremities	Tightness, cramping, dull aching in the lower limbs (more in calf)	Dull aching in the back with or without shooting pain in the legs
Exacerbations	Standing with trunk extended, walking, rare with bi-cycling (if the trunk is extended, while cycling, pain may increase)	With walking and bi-cycling	Prolonged standing, bending and twisting
Relief	With flexing, sitting and squatting	With rest	With reduced activity and rest
Back pain	Common	Uncommon	Common
Limitation of spinal movements	Common	Uncommon	Common
Straight leg raise test	Negative	Negative	May be positive
Femoral nerve tension test	Negative	Negative	May be positive
Pulses in lower limbs	Normal/symmetrically diminished	Diminished/absent, often reduced asymmetrically	Normal
Bi-cycle test	Positive, if performed with the spine in extension	Positive when performed in any position	Usually negative

modalities such as ultrasound, TENS/IFT/hot packs, manual therapy, traction/lumbosacral belts, etc., for patients with lumbar canal stenosis. However, hot packs/TENS/IFT is recommended to reduce paraspinal muscle spasm and modulate pain, and a lumbosacral belt may be recommended for patients with lumbar canal stenosis due to a central disc bulge for use during functional activities.

Exercise: Flexion based exercises are usually recommended for patients with lumbar canal stenosis. However extension exercises are beneficial for patients with lumbar PIVD, causing lumbar canal stenosis from a central disc bulge. However, the clinician should do a detailed movement testing of the L-S spine and decide the type of exercises to be performed after a thorough clinical reasoning.

The exercises recommended include:

- **Knee to chest:** In supine lying, the patient is asked to pull both the knees toward the chest holding the legs at the upper legs (or at the lower thighs, if holding the legs produce knee pain), hold for 2 seconds and lower the legs to bed one after the other. The exercise is repeated 10 times in one session and number of sessions depends on the benefits obtained **(Fig. 6.98)**.
- **Sitting flexion exercise:** The patient is made to sit on a chair with knees bent and feet resting on the floor. He is asked to lower both the hands and bend forward, hold the bent position for 2 seconds and then come to upright position. The exercise is repeated 10 times **(Fig. 6.99)**, and is recommended, if the cause of stenosis is not a central disc bulge.
- **Standing lumbar flexion exercise:** Standing lumbar flexion is a great exercise to treat spinal canal stenosis, except when it is from a central disc bulge. The patient is

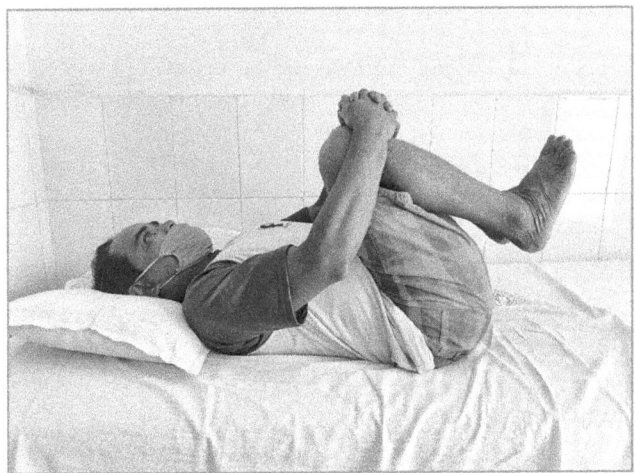

Fig. 6.98: Knee to chest lumbar flexion exercise.

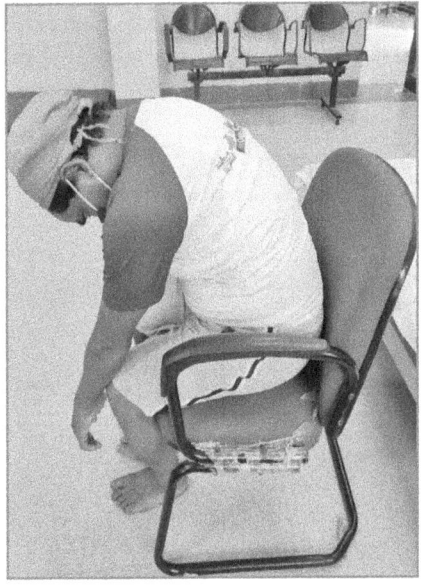

Fig. 6.99: Sitting flexion exercise.

made to stand with the feet apart and asked to bend slowly to reach the floor with the hands **(Fig. 6.100)**. When, fully bent the position is maintained for 2 to 3 seconds and after maintaining the position, he/she is asked to slowly return to the upright standing. The exercise should be repeated 10 times.

- **Lumbar flexion in kneel sitting:** The patient is in kneel sitting. He/she is asked to bend the trunk forward toward the bed so that the head touched the bed and arms move forward **(Fig. 6.101)**. The position is held for 2 to 3 seconds and are repeated for 10 times. The exercise is recommended, if the cause of stenosis is not a central disc bulge,
- **Standing lumbar extension:** This exercise should be performed by patients with a central disc bulge, and if extension exercise causes a relief from symptoms. The patient is in standing with the hands resting on buttocks. He/she is asked to bend the trunk backward, hold for 2 to 3 seconds and again come back to erect position **(Fig. 6.102)**. The exercise is repeated for 10 times in a session.

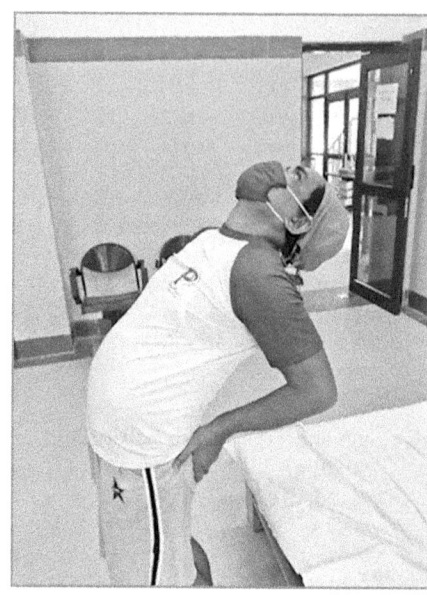

Fig. 6.102: Standing extension exercise.

- **Core strengthening exercises:** The patient is asked to lie on the back with hips and knees bent to 90-90, arms stretched forward **(Fig. 6.103)**. He/she is asked to slowly roll the pelvis backwards (produce posterior pelvic tilt), as if flattening the lumbar spine and hold the position for 3 seconds and then return to the starting position. Ten repetitions of this exercise are performed.
- **Stretching of piriformis (Figs. 6.104A and B)**, hamstrings, etc., should be done to increase flexibility and reduce pain.

Surgery: If the patient develops progressive neurological deficits surgery is the only option. Common surgical procedures involved are:

- **Laminectomy:** This procedure removes the back part (lamina) of the affected vertebra. A laminectomy is sometimes called decompression surgery because it eases the pressure on the nerves by creating more space around them.

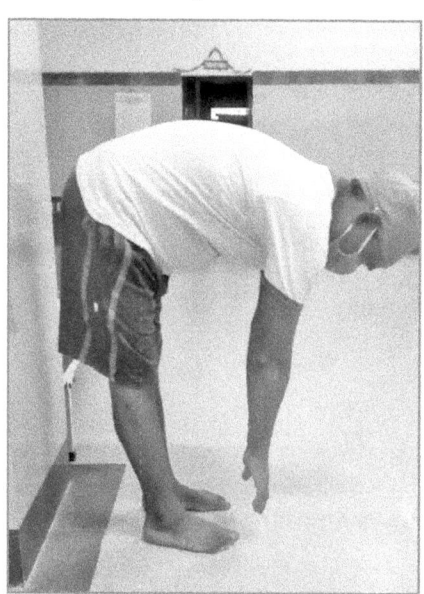

Fig. 6.100: Standing lumbar flexion exercise.

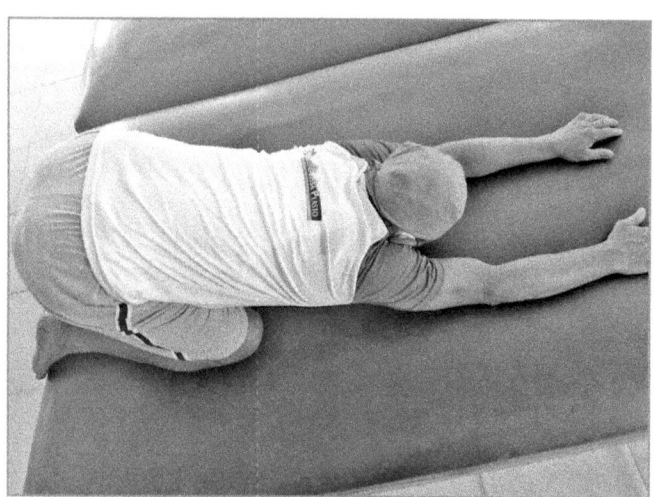

Fig. 6.101: Lumbar flexion in kneel sitting.

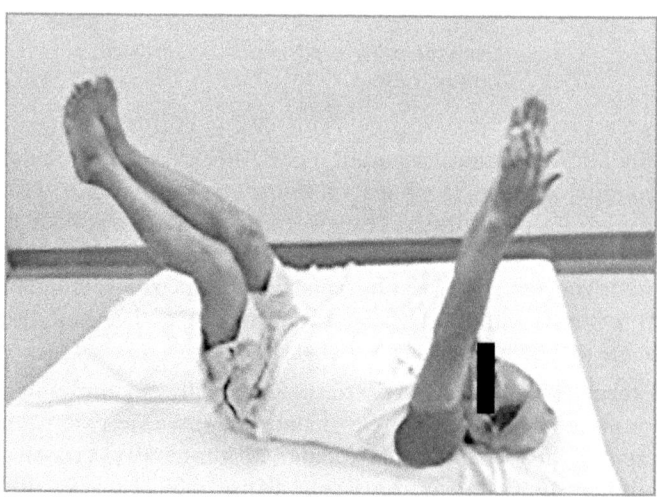

Fig. 6.103: Core strengthening exercise.

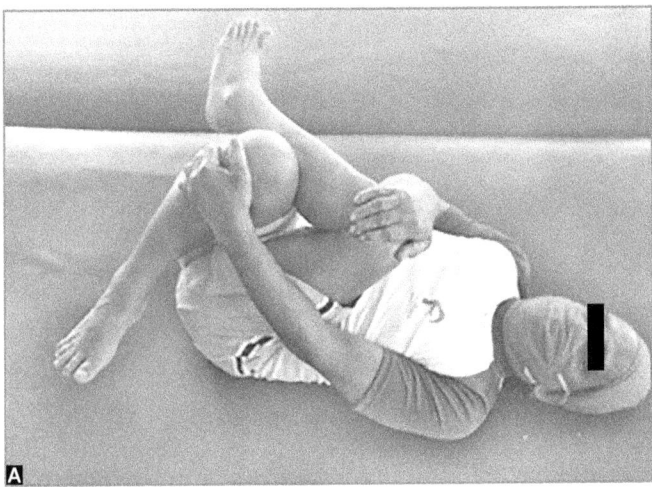

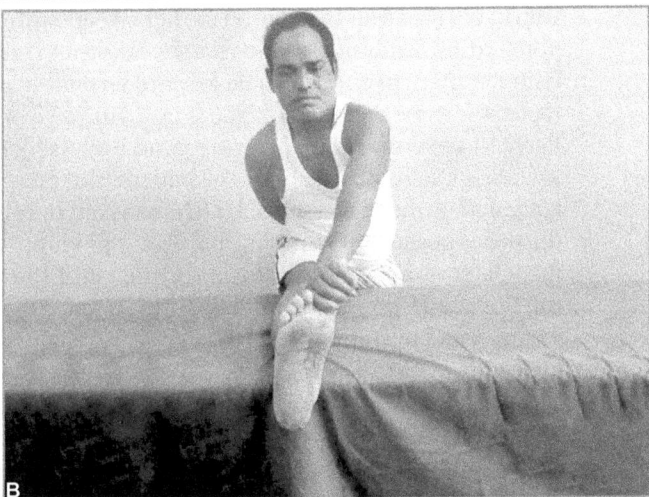

Figs. 6.104A and B: (A) Piriformis stretching exercise, (B) Hamstrings stretching exercise.

- **Laminotomy:** This procedure removes only a portion of the lamina, typically carving a hole just big enough to relieve the pressure in a particular spot..
- **Minimally invasive surgery:** This approach to surgery removes bone or lamina in a way that reduces the damage to nearby healthy tissue. This usually does not need fusion of spine.

Postoperative physiotherapy: Chest care, pain reduction, core strengthening, and management of residual deficits in the lower limbs are the areas need intervention postoperatively. Endurance activities such as walking, static cycle exercises are performed to make the individual gradually return to function.

5. Sacralization/Lumbarization

Sacralization is a common irregularity of the spine, where the fifth lumbar vertebra (L5) is fused to the first sacrum bone at the bottom of the spine. The fusion may be full or partial and located to either one side or both sides in the base of the spinal column.

Lumbarization of 1st sacral bone(S1), which is less common, results in assimilation of S1 to lumbar spine partially (unilateral) or completely (bilateral). It is a condition, where the 1st segment of the sacrum, fails to fuse with the 2nd sacral bone, so that it appears to be a part of the lumbar bone. It presents as if there are 6 lumbar vertebrae, instead of 5.

Etiology

Both Sacralization and Lumbarization are congenital anomalies that develop during the embryonic stage of development. They are considered as genetic disorders, developing at about 8 weeks of intrauterine life, when vertebra begins to ossify.

Pathophysiology

The sacralization or lumbarization of S1 cause stress concentration on L4-L5, which can accentuate development of back pain including disc bulge in upper lumbar segments and degenerative Spondylolisthesis. Due to fusion of L5 to S1, the intervertebral disc at L5-S1 is thinned and the discs at L1-L4, cannot cope with the assigned load resulting in increased compressive load and back pain. Compressions of the nerve roots that exit through L5-S1 inter vertebral foramina causes pain in the leg and neurological deficits. Increased strain on the ligaments produce inflammation of the ligaments leading to pain in the entire spine.

Clinical Features

Patients with sacralization/lumbarization usually complain of low back pain. The association between sacralization and low back pain was first described in 1917 by Italian physician Mario Bertolotti and was called as Bertolotti syndrome.

The features of sacralization/lumbarization are:
- Back pain (localized to opposite side of fusion in unilateral type and both sides of low back in bilateral type).
- Upper back pain due to hypermobility in the upper segments.
- Paravertebral muscle spasm.
- Lumbosacral scoliosis.
- Pain in the buttock, sometimes radiating down the leg.
- Limitation of lumbar spinal movements such as not able to bend forward and touch the floor with the tip of the middle finger. Extension, lateral flexion may also be limited and painful.

Types of Sacralization

Sacralization has several forms, classified according to whether the fusion seen on an X-ray is partial or total, and whether the fusion is on only one side (unilateral) or both (bilateral). The commonly used Castellvi classification is:
- Type 1: A fusion of at least 19 mm in width on one (1a) or both sides (1b)
- Type 2: Incomplete fusion with a pseudo joint created on one side (2a) or both sides (2b)
- Type 3: Complete fusion of the L5 to the sacrum on one side (3a) or the other (3b)
- Type 4: Combination of type 2 and type 3.

Types of lumbarization: Lumbarization could be of the following 2 types:
1. **Partial lumbarization:** Where a part of the 1st sacral bone is separated from rest of the sacral vertebrae and remains attached to L5.

2. **Complete lumbarization:** Where the 1st sacrum is completely separated from rest of the sacral vertebrae and is attached to 5th lumbar vertebrae, giving appearance of 6 lumbar vertebrae.

Diagnosis
- Clinical presentations.
- X-ray of L-S spine **(Figs. 6.105A and B)**
- MRI.

Management

The treatment for sacralization/lumbarization is usually conservative. The conservative treatment given for pain associated with sacralization/lumbarization is the same as for other lower back pain. It includes:
- **Medical management:** It includes:
  - NSAIDs.
  - Muscle relaxants.
  - Steroid injections, if inflammation is very acute.
- **Physiotherapy:** It includes:
  - *Modalities such as:*
    » Pulsed US/IRR/High power LASER/Moist hot packs may be selected and applied after a thorough clinical reasoning. However, the use of deep heating modalities like SWD/MWD should be avoided in early stage, when sacralization/lumbarization starts to develop.
    » IFT/TENS to modulate pain **(Fig. 6.55)**.
  - *Exercises:* Exercises to increase the mobility and stability of the lumbosacral spine and hips are to be performed to reduce symptoms and increase function. The exercises recommended include:
    » Knee to chest exercise: The patient in supine lying with back flat on floor. He/she is asked to bend one knee toward the opposite shoulder and hold it for 5 seconds, keeping the abdominals tight and pressing the back into the floor. Then he/she is asked to return to the starting position and repeat with the opposite leg **(Fig. 6.106)**.

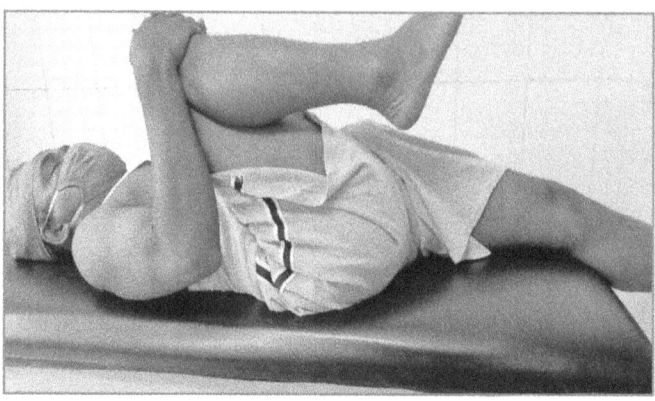

Fig. 6.106: Knee to chest exercise.

» Knee roll (Lower trunk rotation): Patient in supine lying with knees flexed and feet flat on the floor. Keeping the upper trunk firmly on the floor, he/she is asked to roll both the knees to one side, hold for 5-10 seconds and repeat the same on the other side **(Fig. 6.70)**.
» Pelvic tilt exercise: This is a very good exercise for sacralization/lumbarization. The patient is in crook lying with arms at the sides. He/she is asked to roll the pelvis posteriorly resulting in a strong abdominal muscle contraction, hold for 3 seconds and then roll the pelvis anteriorly holding for the same time. Anterior and posterior tilts of the pelvis are repeated alternatively **(Fig. 6.107)**
» Cat and camel exercise: This is a core strengthening exercise, found very much beneficial for sacralization/lumbarization **(Fig. 6.62)**
» Hamstrings stretching exercise: This exercise increases flexibility of the patient and stabilizes the lumbar spine **(Fig. 6.91B)**.
» Alexander technique: The Alexander technique is an educational program that teaches movement patterns and postures, with an aim to improve coordination and balance, reduce tension, relieve pain, alleviate fatigue. A typical Alexander technique **(Fig. 6.108)** program teaches topics such as:

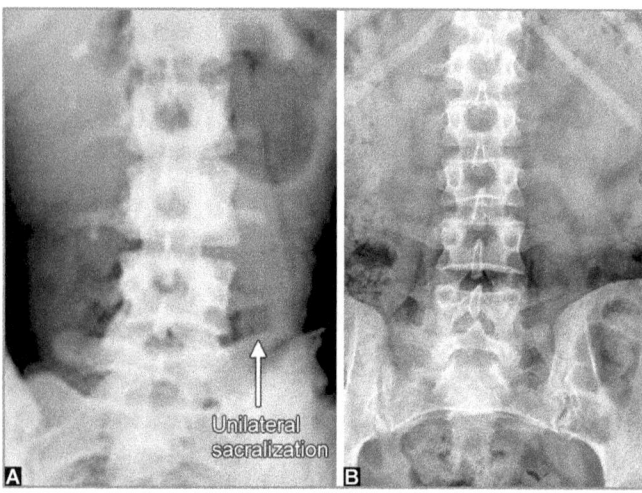

Figs. 6.105A and B: X-ray showing: (A) Unilateral sacralization; (B) Completely lumbarization.

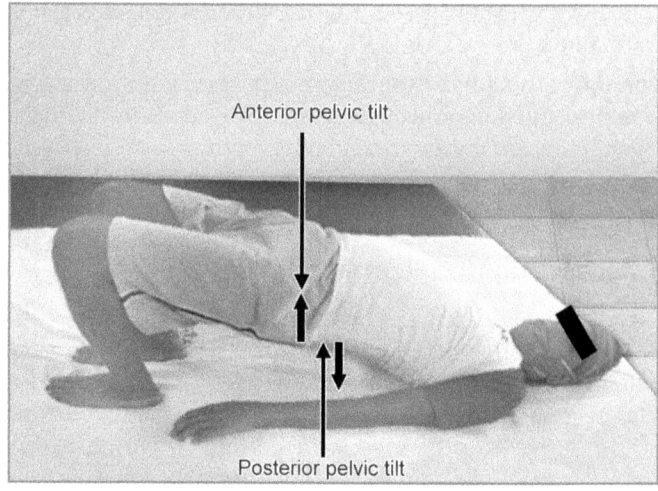

Fig. 6.107: The pelvic tilt exercise.

Chapter 6: Physiotherapy for Spinal Disorders

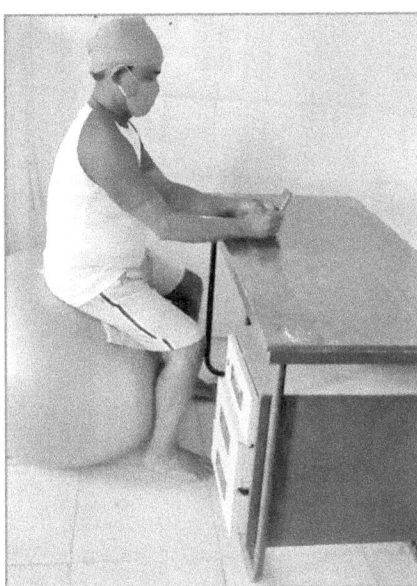

Fig. 6.108: The Alexander technique.

- How to comfortably sit up straight
- How to reduce overuse of superficial musculature in upright postures.
- How to increase proprioceptive awareness
- How to become more attuned to the body's warning signs of tension and compression.

Surgery

Surgery is not usually required for patients with sacralization/lumbarization. Physiotherapy is found to have a significant yield in such patients both in improving mobility and pain as well as improving the quality of life. However, very severe cases may be managed by surgical intervention.

6. Coccygodynia/Coccydynia

Coccygodynia, also called as coccydynia, coccalgia, coccygeal neuralgia, or tailbone pain, is the term used to describe pain that occur in the region of the coccyx. The pain is mostly triggered, when the individual sits on a hard surface for long period. The pain very often resolves within a few weeks/months. However, in some people chronic pain persists for long time making sitting difficult and significantly affecting the quality of life.

Postacchini and Massobrio (1983) classified the variations in morphology of the coccyx associated with the disorder into four different configurations:

- **Type I:** The coccyx is slightly curved forward, with its apex positioned downward.
- **Type II:** The forward curvature of the coccyx is more exaggerated, with the apex positioned in a straight forward direction.
- **Type III:** Sharp angulation of the coccyx forward.
- **Type IV:** Subluxation of the coccyx at the sacrococcygeal or intercoccygeal joint.

Clinical Features of the Disorder

- Pain (pulling/cutting type) around the coccyx.
- Palpable tenderness over coccyx.
- Pain is more during sitting and transition from sitting to standing.

Diagnosis: Made from complain, clinical features and dynamic X-ray examinations **(Fig. 109)**/MRI studies. In dynamic X-ray examination, X-ray of coccyx is first taken in sitting, and then in standing. The angulation/change in position of the coccyx (if any) from sitting to standing indicates coccydynia.

Management

Conservative management that includes the followings is considered gold standard for the management of Coccydynia. This method of management is found to be successful in most of the sufferers. However, those found to have consistent pain are managed by surgery (coccygectomy), where part of the coccyx is removed surgically.

- **Conservative management:** It consists of:
  - NSAIDs. Corticosteroid injections may be tried in patients having intolerable pain.
  - *Physiotherapy:*
    » Ergonomic advice: Using coccydynia cushions over chair **(Fig. 6.110A)**.
    » Sitz bath **(Fig. 6.110B)**.
    » Physical modalities such as extracorporeal shock wave therapy (ESWT), SWD, pulsed ultrasound, IFT are also applied as per indications, and available evidences.
    » Manual therapy: Massage, stretching, mobilization, manipulation techniques are performed, which may involve external or internal contact with the coccyx. External contact technique involves manipulation

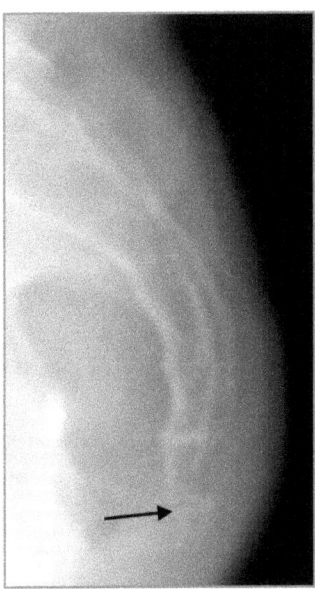

Fig. 109: X-ray of patient with coccydynia, showing displacement of tip of coccyx.

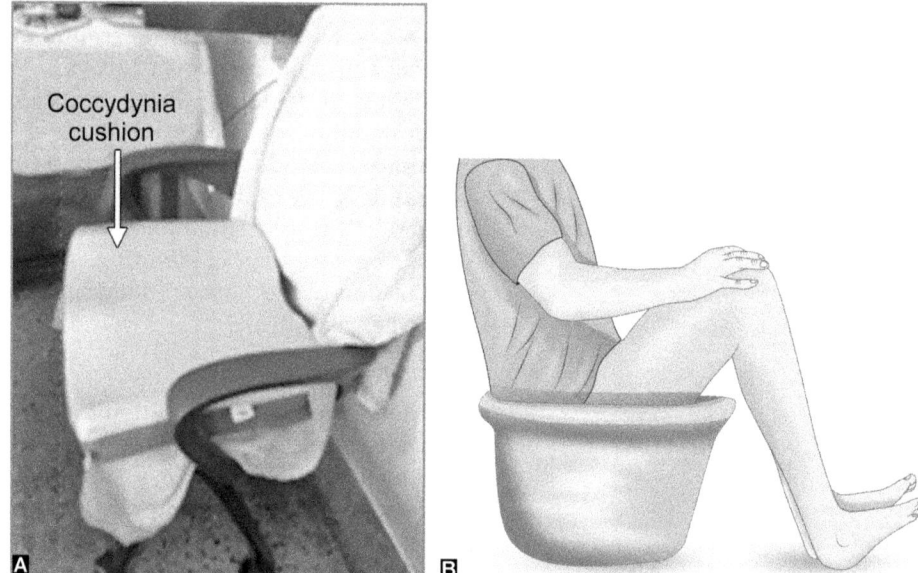

Figs. 6.110A and B: (A) Coccydynia cushion on chair, (B) Sitz bath.

of the coccyx or sacroiliac joint, stretching of the piriformis and iliopsoas muscles, thoracic mobilization (to improve thoracic extension, helping to reduce load on coccyx) are performed. Internal contact techniques involve massage to levator ani and coccygeus muscles, mobilization exercises when the coccyx is hyperextended or rotated.

❖ **Surgery:** Coccygectomy (partial removal of the coccyx) is done in few subjects not benefited by conservative management. After surgery postoperative physiotherapy to mobilize tight scar and reduce pain are applied.

CHAPTER 7: Physiotherapy for Hip

THE HIP JOINT

Osteokinematics

The hip joint, also called coxa, is a synovial joint of ball and socket type, with three degrees of freedom. Flexion-extension is produced in the sagittal plane and around the mediolateral axis. Abduction–adduction is produced in frontal plane and around the anteroposterior axis. Medial-lateral rotation is produced in the transverse plane and around the vertical/longitudinal axis.

Arthrokinematics

In an open kinematic chain (nonweight-bearing position), the convex femoral head, slides on the concave acetabulum, in a direction opposite to the movement of shaft of femur. In flexion, the femoral head slides posteriorly and inferiorly on the acetabulum. In extension, the femoral head slides anteriorly and superiorly. In abduction, the femoral head slides inferiorly, and in adduction, the femoral head slides superiorly. In medial rotation, the femoral head slides posteriorly on the acetabulum and during lateral rotation, the femoral head slides anteriorly.

Capsular Pattern

Marked limitation of medial rotation, abduction and flexion, and slight limitation of extension. No limitation occurs in adduction and lateral rotation.

Range of Motion

The ranges of motion of hip joint are given in the **Table 7.1**.

Table 7.1: Ranges of motion of hip joint.

Movement	Range of motion
Flexion	0–120°
Extension	0–30°
Abduction	0–45°
Adduction	0–30°
Medial rotation	0–45°
Lateral rotation	0–45°

SPECIAL TESTS FOR HIP JOINT

Trendelenburg Test

Trendelenburg's sign is named after Friedrich Trendelenburg who was a German surgeon. This sign is positive in individuals whose abductor muscles of the hip, i.e., gluteus medius and gluteus minimus, have become weak or paralyzed.

During test patient is advised to stand on one leg (affected leg). Trendelenburg sign is considered positive, if upon standing on the affected leg, the patient's pelvis drops on the opposite side (**Fig. 7.1**). A positive Trendelenburg sign indicates muscular dysfunction, i.e., weakness of the gluteus minimus or medius.

Telescopic Test

Telescopic sign is found to be present in dislocated hip. The patient is made to lie supine or flat on their back on an examination table. The examiner stands on opposite side of the leg, which is tested. The tested side hip and knee are bent at 90°. Gentle pressure is applied in a downward motion toward the table and then lifted back up (**Fig. 7.2**). The test is positive, if the patient does not exhibit any movement or if there is excessive movement due to hip dislocation. During test patient complains of increased pain. The test is negative

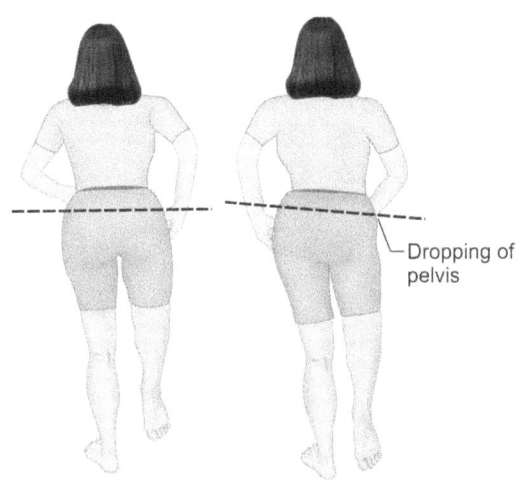

Normal hip   Positive Trendelenberg test due to weak hip abductor on left side

Fig. 7.1: Positive Trendelenburg test.

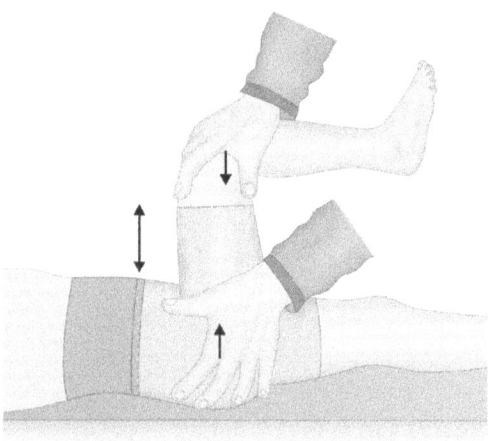

Fig. 7.2: The telescopic test.

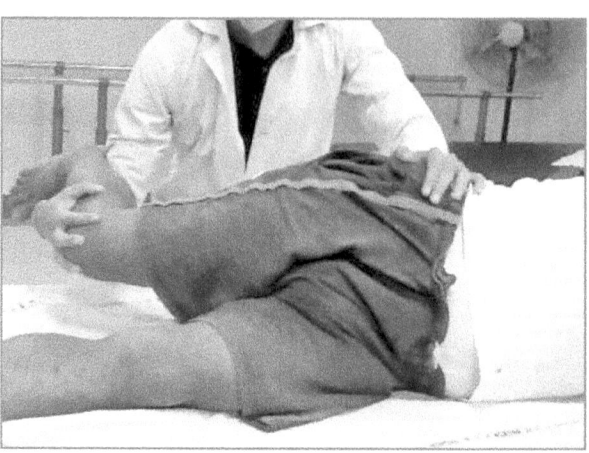

Fig. 7.4: The Ober test.

if there is only a little bit of movement and patient does not complain of increase of pain.

Ortolani Test

The maneuver was described by Marino Ortolani to diagnose congenital dysplasia of the hip joint. The Barlow Maneuver dislocates the hip joint and Ortolani maneuver reposition the hip joint by adjusting head of femur in the acetabulum. Barlow Maneuver is done first then Ortolani maneuver is performed.

The procedure is known as relocating a dislocated hip joint. The position of both knee and hip joint is maintained at 90° during entire period of test. The examiner palpates the greater trochanter with index finger and abducts the leg at hip joint using thumb. The maneuver places the head of femur into hip joint socket with a click sound. The test confirms the diagnosis of congenital hip joint dysplasia **(Fig. 7.3)**.

Barlow Maneuver

Examiner supports both legs with hand with flexion of both knee joints. Then hip joints are also flexed at 90°. Examiner while continuing his hands on knee joint adduct the leg at hip joint while leg is pushed posteriorly toward the examining bed to dislocate one or both hips. Examiner may feel or hear click while hip joint is dislocated indicating positive test.

Ober's Test

Ober's test is performed to find tightness of Iliotibial (IT) tract. The patient is made to lie on the examination table in side lying over the sound side. The normal leg is flexed at hip and knee and placed forward.

Examiner stands on the back of the patient and holds the affected pelvis with the left hand, while the right hand abducts and extends the tested hip supporting at the knee. The examiner then releases the hand that was supporting the knee. If the clinician fails to adduct the hip, then it is a positive test and indicates IT band tightness **(Fig. 7.4)**.

Thomas Test

Thomas test was described by Orthopedic surgeon Dr Hugh Thomas from Great Britain. The test helps to diagnose hip flexor tightness/contracture. The patient is asked to lie supine on examination bed with both legs hanging over the side of the examination bed. Both the legs are maintained in flex position at knee joint. Examiner stands on side of patient that has pain/tightness. Examiner then assists patient to flex both hips with knees flexed and pulls the knees toward the chest. While the examiner/patient holds the other hip flexed, the tested hip is extended, actively by the patient/passively by the examiner **(Fig. 7.5)**. After noting any deformity/tightness on

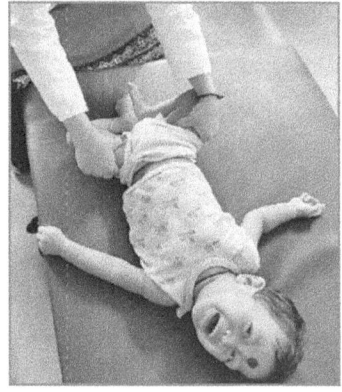

Fig. 7.3: The Ortolani maneuver.

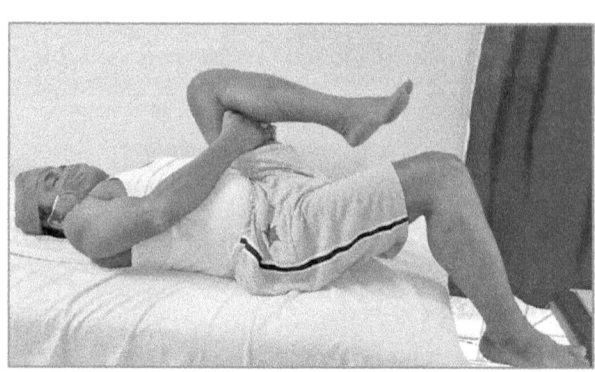

Fig. 7.5: The Thomas test.

the affected hip, the other hip is tested to find any tightness/deformity.

Patrick's Test

The test is performed to evaluate hip and sacroiliac joint diseases. The patient is made to lie supine on examination bed. Both the legs are tested alternately. Examiner stands on side that is being tested. The affected side lower limb is flexed at knee and hip joint simultaneously. Then the lower limb is abducted and laterally rotated. The knee is pressed towards the bed while foot is rested on thigh of opposite leg **(Fig. 7.6)**. Patient suffering with hip or sacroiliac joint disease will complain of moderate to severe pain.

Ely's Test

Patient is advised to lie on examination bed in prone position. Examiner stands on side of the examination bed. The patient is asked to flex the tested side knee actively, or the examiner passively flexes the tested side knee, if active flexion is not possible. If on knee flexion, the buttock on the test side is elevated **(Fig. 7.7)**, the test is positive indicating tightness of rectus femoris.

SPECIFIC DISORDERS OF HIP

a. Piriformis Syndrome

Piriformis syndrome is a painful musculoskeletal condition, characterized by buttock or hip pain sometimes causing radiation of pain along the back of thigh and leg along the course of the sciatic nerve.

The piriformis muscle (PM) originates from the pelvic surface of the sacral segments S2-S4 and passes through the greater sciatic notch to insert onto the greater trochanter of the femur.

The muscle is functionally involved with external rotation, abduction, and partial extension of the hip. The

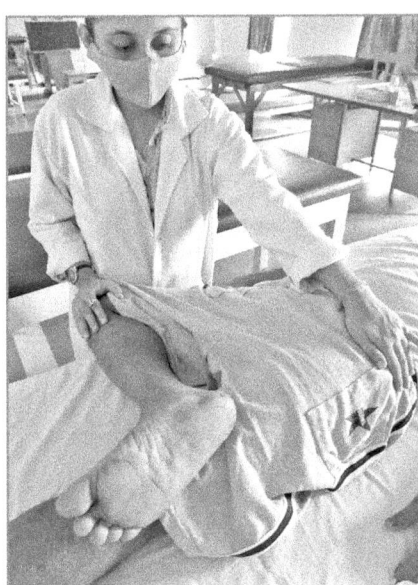

Fig. 7.6: The Patrick test.

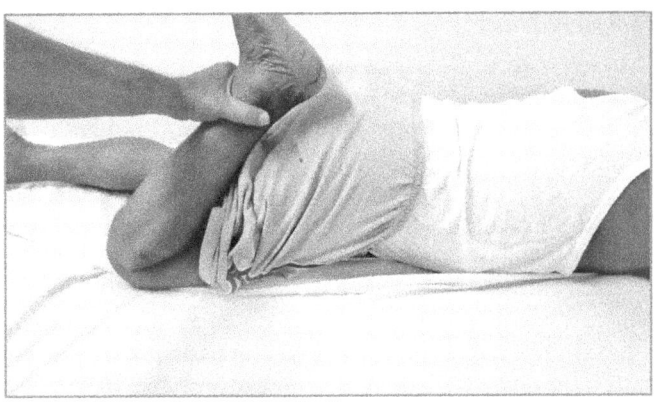

Fig. 7.7: The Ely's test.

sciatic nerve generally exits the pelvis below the belly of the muscle **(Fig. 7.8)**.

Though, the sciatic nerve usually exit the greater sciatic foramen, along the inferior surface of the piriformis, some times the nerve also exits the greater sciatic foramen along the superior surface of the PM, may also divide proximally, and a division of the nerve passes through the belly of the muscle.

Epidemiology/Etiology

The condition is found more in females than males, with a female to male ratio of 6:1. According to Boyajian O' Neill et al., there are two types of piriformis syndrome such as primary and secondary:

1. **Primary piriformis syndrome**: This accounts to less than 15% of individuals suffering from this syndrome. Anatomical factors such as a split PM, split sciatic nerve resulting in an anomalous sciatic nerve path (one branch passing above the muscle, one branch passing through the muscle belly), is responsible for this disorder in some individuals.
2. **Secondary piriformis syndrome**: It occurs as a result of macrotrauma to the buttock, due to over use, such as long distance walking, leading to inflammation of soft tissues, muscle spasm or both resulting in compression of sciatic nerve. Spasm of the PM that result from direct trauma, postsurgical injury, or lumbar and sacroiliac pathologies are also an important cause of the disorder in some individuals. Altered biomechanics of lumbosacral spine/lower limbs also contributes significantly to the causation of the disorder.

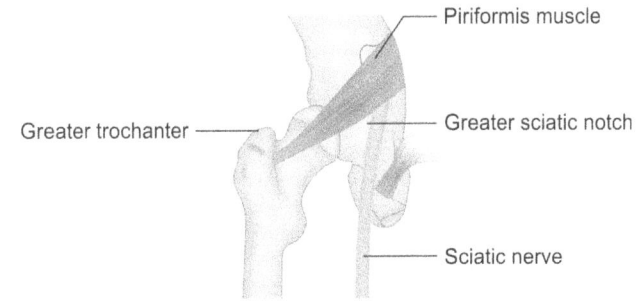

Fig. 7.8: The piriformis muscle and sciatic nerve.

Clinical Features

Patients with piriformis syndrome have many symptoms that typically consist of pain in the buttock, tenderness over the sciatic notch, and persistent and radiating low back pain, numbness, paresthesia, difficulty with walking (limping on the affected side) and other functional activities such as pain with sitting, squatting, standing, with bowel movements and dyspareunia in women.

The syndrome is not characterized by neurological deficits typical of a radicular syndrome, such as declined deep tendon reflexes and myotomal weakness. The patient may present with a limp when walking. The lower limb may remain in an externally rotated position while supine, called a positive piriformis sign. It can be the result of a contracted/spasmodic PM.

Investigations/Examinations

Piriformis syndrome appears as a controversial diagnosis for low back and sciatic pain. Radiographic studies have limited application in its diagnosis, only helping to exclude pathologies involving lumbosacral spine and hip joints.

Electromyography (EMG) examination of muscles supplied by sciatic nerve, combined with FAIR (flexion, adduction, internal rotation) test **(Fig. 7.9)** is helpful in establishing diagnosis of piriformis syndrome. Besides FAIR test, other clinical tests performed to establish diagnosis are:

- **Pace sign:** It consists of pain and weakness on performing resisted abduction and external rotation of hip in sitting position.
- **Straight leg raise test:** The patient reports buttock and leg pain during passive straight leg raise performed by the examiner.
- **Freiberg sign:** Involves pain on passive forced internal rotation of the extended hip in the supine position. The pain is thought to be a result of passive stretching of the PM and pressure placed on the sciatic nerve at the sacrospinous ligament.
- **Beatty's Maneuver:** This is an active test where in the patient lying on the sound side is asked to abduct the flexed hip on the painful side. Deep buttock pain on the affected buttock is suggestive of piriformis syndrome, where as pain in the leg and back is suggestive of lumbar disc disease.
- **The Hughes test:** Isometric external rotation of the affected lower extremity from maximal internal rotation is painful suggesting positive test.
- **The hip abduction test:** The patient lies on the sound side with the sound lower limb in flexed attitude for better body support. The patient is asked to abduct the affected hip. The examiner standing in front of the patient, if observes the affected lower limb rotates externally, it indicates tightness of PM.
- **Trendelenburg test:** This test may also be positive in patients with piriformis syndrome, when tested with the patient standing on the affected side.
- **Palpation:** Tenderness over greater sciatic notch and spasm of the PM is detected through palpation.

Differential Diagnosis

The condition need to be differentiated from other disorders affecting hip, such as Gluteus medius syndrome, IT band friction syndrome, and lumbosacral disorders causing low back and radiating pain.

Management of Piriformis Syndrome

- **Medical management:** NSAIDs, muscle relaxants.
- **Physiotherapy:** Physiotherapy is one noninvasive method of management of piriformis syndrome, which when combined with lifestyle/activity modification helps significantly in improving function. According to Tonley et al., the most commonly reported physical therapy interventions include: ultrasound therapy, soft tissue mobilization, piriformis stretching **(Fig. 7.10)**, hot packs or cold spray. The electrotherapy applied for treatment include:
  - *Ultrasound therapy:* For ultrasound therapy, the patient must lie on the sound side, with the affected hip in FAIR position. Ultrasound treatment at a dose of 2.0–2.5 W/cm^2, for 10–14 minutes, is applied along the length of the PM.
  - Extracorporeal shock wave therapy.

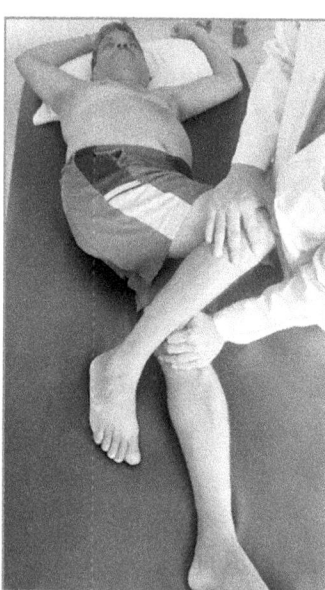

Fig. 7.9: The FAIR (flexion-adduction–internal rotation) test.

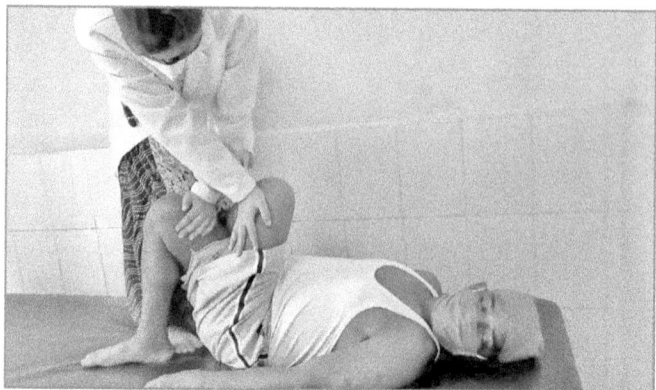

Fig. 7.10: Stretching of left piriformis.

- SWD (Monoplanar method).
- IFT/TENS applied over the buttock/affected lower limb helps to reduce pain.

Before stretching exercises are performed, either moist hot packs or cold packs/cold sprays are applied for 10 minutes to reduce pain, so that the patient co-operates for effective stretching. Besides self stretching **(Fig. 7.11A)**, positional stretching **(Fig. 7.11B)**, myofascial release muscle energy technique (MET), stretching by therapist/ caregiver, kneading/ DTFM, etc. are also applied.

Besides the therapeutic interventions described above, the therapist also gives several tips to avoid an aggravation of the symptoms. This includes:
- Avoid sitting for a long period; stand and walk every 20 minutes/or as possible.
- Make frequent stops when driving to stand and stretch.
- Prevent trauma to the gluteal region and avoid further offending activities.
- Periodic stretching should be done to prevent recurrences.

Surgical Interventions

Surgical interventions should be considered only when nonsurgical treatment has failed and the symptoms are becoming intractable and disabling. Surgical release with tenotomy of the piriformis tendon to relieve the nerve from the pressure of the tense muscle results in immediate pain relief.

The postoperative management consists of partial weight-bearing using crutches for 2 weeks and unrestricted range of motion exercises.

b. Iliotibial Band Syndrome

Iliotibial band syndrome is a common nontraumatic overuse injury that usually presents with pain and/or tenderness on lateral aspect of the thigh, along the band **(Fig. 7.12)** superior to the knee joint line and inferior to the lateral femoral epicondyle.

Etiology

It includes:
- Friction between the posterior edge of the IT band and underlying lateral femoral epicondyle occurring during flexion/extension of knee.
- Weakness of the hip abductors is also associated with IT band syndrome as this causes increased hip internal rotation and knee adduction. This is commonly found in athletes.
- Other etiologies for IT band syndrome include compression of the fat and connective tissue that is deep to the IT band, as well as chronic inflammation of the IT band bursa, excessive foot pronation, internal tibial torsion, medial compartment arthritis of knee, causing genu varum.

Clinical Features

The condition is found more in males than females. The main symptom is a sharp burning pain and mild swelling on the outer aspect of the knee, at the level of the lateral femoral epicondyle. The patient complains of pain in activities that require repetitive knee flexion and extension. The pain at the outer aspect of the knee is felt most commonly when the heel strikes the floor, and can also radiate to outer thigh or calf. The pain tends to be worse when running or descending stairs. There may be an audible snapping sensation in the knee,

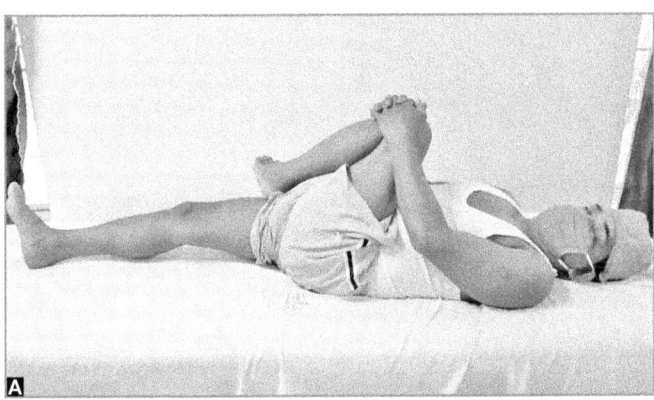
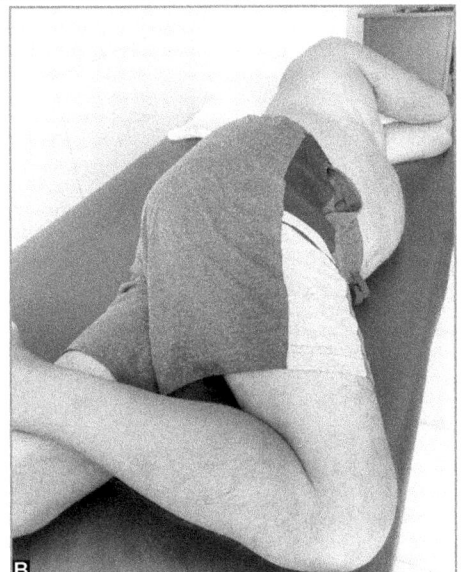

Figs. 7.11A and B: (A) Self stretching of piriformis, (B) Positional stretching of piriformis.

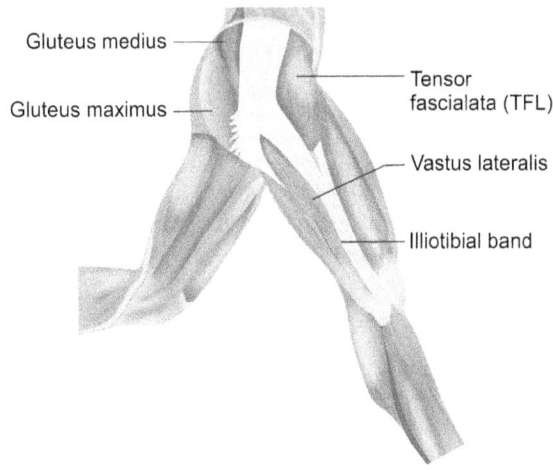

Fig. 7.12: The iliotibial band.

during bending activities, due to slipping of the band over the bony tubercle.

Diagnosis

The patient's complain, pain history, combined with clinical tests help the clinician to make a diagnosis of the disorder.

The following tests when performed give positive result:

- **Strength testing for hip abductors**: The hip abductor strength is usually decreased in this disorder.
- **Treadmill test:** If running on treadmill produces pain over the lateral side of the knee, the test is considered positive.
- **Noble compression test:** This test starts in supine posture with a knee flexion of 90°. As the patient extends the knee the assessor applies pressure to the lateral femoral epicondyle. If this induces pain over the lateral femoral epicondyle near 30–40° of flexion, the test is considered positive. A goniometer is used to ensure the correct angle of the knee joint.
- **Ober's test:** The patient is lying on his side with the injured extremity facing upward. The knee is flexed at 90° and the hip in abduction and extension, the thigh is maintained in line with the trunk. The patient's hip is adducted either actively by the patient or passively by the examiner. If there is pain and movement limitation, the test is positive. A positive Ober test **(Fig. 7.4)** indicates a short/tense IT band or tensor fasciae latae, which is frequently related to the friction syndrome.

Management

- **Medical management:** It includes NSAIDs and muscle relaxants.
- **Physiotherapy management:** The treatment of IT band friction syndrome is usually nonoperative and physiotherapy is usually considered as the best line of treatment.
- **Acute management:** In the acute stage, protection, rest, ice, is the early intervention applied. The patient should be advised to modify the activity and take rest usually for a period of 3 weeks. After the acute pain/swelling subsided, the following interventions can be applied after a thorough clinical reasoning.
  - Moist hot pack.
  - Ultrasound therapy.
  - Iontophoresis or phonophoresis with anti inflammatory medications. Iontophoresis with dexamethasone may be useful as an anti-inflammatory modality. Phonophoresis using 10% hydrocortisone applied to the subcutaneous tissue on the IT band is helpful.
  - Radial shock wave therapy (RSWT) is the treatment of choice in some nonremitting cases. RSWT is believed to stimulate healing of soft tissue and inhibit nociceptors. It increases the diffusion of cytokines across vessel walls into the painful area and stimulates the tendon healing response.

As the inflammation and pain get controlled, the physiotherapist designs a set of stretching and strengthening exercise to improve the condition and facilitate early return to activity/sports. The exercises recommended include:

Gentle static stretching exercises to IT band **(Fig. 7.13A)** to be done, in few repetitions, three times a day. Stretching of the band can also be done with a firm roll **(Fig. 7.13B)**.

- Myofascial release **(Fig. 7.14)** can be considered in the early stage, when static stretching is painful.
- Strengthening of hip abductors and extensors (i.e., Gluteus medius and Gluteus maximus), using therabands **(Fig. 7.15)**/weight cuff.

As the patient improves, multidimensional movement patterns, such as, running, jumping, balancing, agility drills, etc., may be started and the individual should be made for a gradual return to sports/ functional activities.

Surgical Management

In cases, where medical management and physiotherapy fails, surgery is the treatment for consideration. During surgery, a small piece of the posterior part of the IT band that covers the lateral femoral epicondyle is resected. Z-lengthening of the

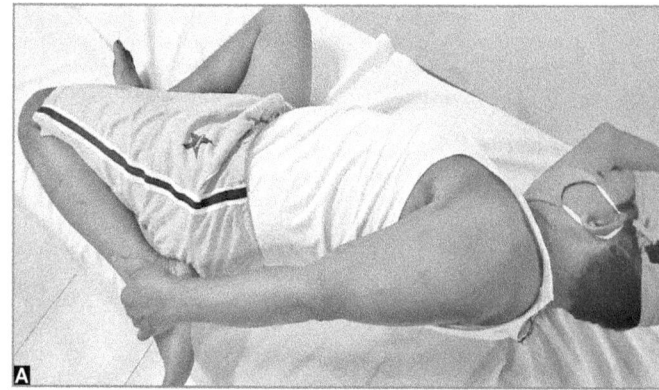

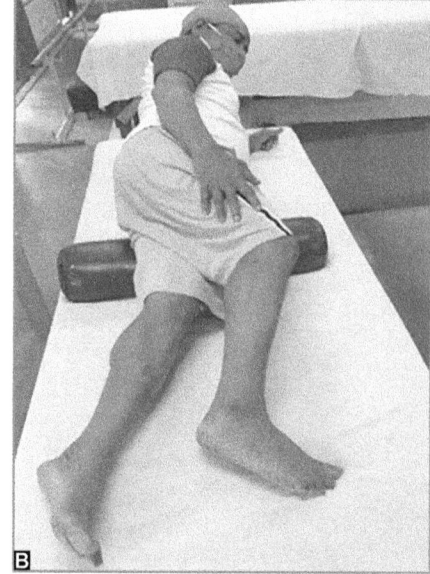

Figs. 7.13A and B: Stretching of IT band: (A) Auto stretch, (B) Using firm roll.

Chapter 7: Physiotherapy for Hip

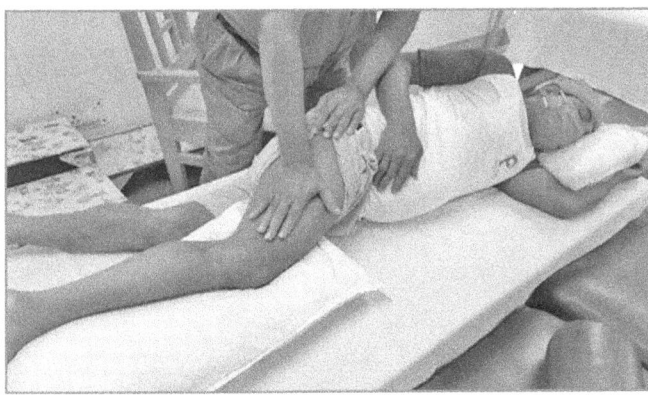

Fig. 7.14: Myofascial release to IT band.

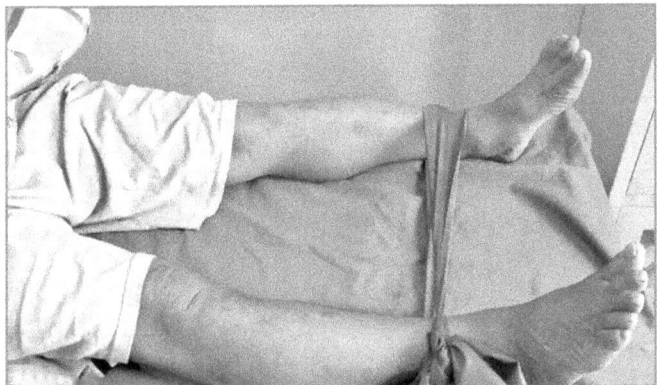

Fig. 7.15: Strengthening hip abductors using theraband.

IT band at the level of the lateral epicondyle has also been proposed.

Appropriate postoperative physiotherapy is given after surgery to restore mobility and function.

c. Transient Synovitis of Hip

Transient synovitis of the hip, also called toxic synovitis, is an inflammation and swelling of the tissues around the hip joint. Usually, only one hip is affected. This condition is called "transient" because it lasts only for a short time. Transient synovitis of the hip is the most common cause of sudden hip pain in children.

Epidemiology and Etiology

Transient synovitis of the hip usually occurs in children between 3 and 10 years of age. Sometimes, it occurs in children younger than 3 years of age. It is more common in boys than in girls.

The exact cause of transient synovitis of the hip is unknown. It might be caused by a virus or it might be from an allergic reaction to an infection somewhere else in the body.

Clinical Features

The main symptom of this disease is pain in the hip joint, resulting in difficulty in walking, causing a limp on the affected side. A very few children complain pain in the inner thigh and knee joint. The affected child prefers to lie supine with the affected hip in flexion, abduction and lateral rotation, and foot moving away from the body. Internal rotation and adduction of hip is generally limited and painful. The symptoms typically last for 1–3 weeks.

Investigations

Blood tests, may reveal normal WBC count, however, the ESR may be slightly elevated. X-ray and ultrasound imaging are the investigations performed in this condition. MRI may help to differentiate this condition from septic arthritis.

Management

Rest at home is the most important way to help the child's hip get better. The child may need to take a nonsteroidal anti-inflammatory medicine to reduce the swelling and inflammation around the hip joint.

Skin traction may be applied to provide rest and prevent complications. Moist heat packs may be applied to reduce pain. Graduated active exercises are applied to maintain/promote mobility/muscle power.

PSWD/Pulsed Microwave Diathermy may be applied to reduce inflammation and promote healing. IFT/TENS as appropriate may be indicated to modulate pain.

d. Meralgia Paresthetica

Meralgia paresthetica is a condition characterized by tingling numbness and burning pain in the outer aspect of thigh, as a result of compression of lateral cutaneous nerve of thigh under the inguinal ligament.

Etiology

Meralgia paresthetica occurs when the lateral femoral cutaneous nerve, which supplies sensation to the surface of the outer thigh, becomes compressed, or pinched. The lateral femoral cutaneous nerve is purely a sensory nerve and does not affect motor power in the lower limb.

In most people, this nerve passes through the groin to the upper thigh without trouble. But in meralgia paresthetica, the lateral femoral cutaneous nerve becomes trapped—often under the inguinal ligament, which runs along the groin from the abdomen to the upper thigh.

Common causes of this compression include:
- Tight clothing, such as belts, corsets and tight pants.
- Obesity.
- Wearing a heavy tool belt.
- Pregnancy.
- Scar tissue near the inguinal ligament due to injury or postsurgery.

Clinical Features

Pressure on the lateral femoral cutaneous nerve, which supplies sensation to the upper thigh, leads to the following symptoms. The symptoms commonly occur on one side of the body and may increase after standing/walking. It includes:
- Tingling and numbness in the outer (lateral) part of the thigh.

Section 2: Physiotherapy for Musculoskeletal Conditions

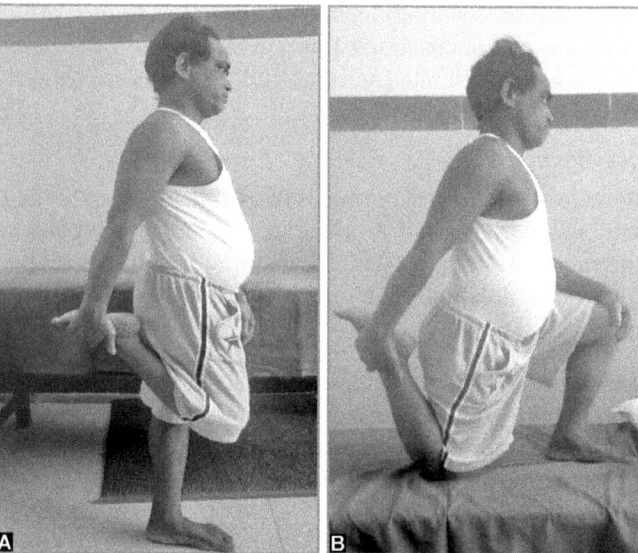
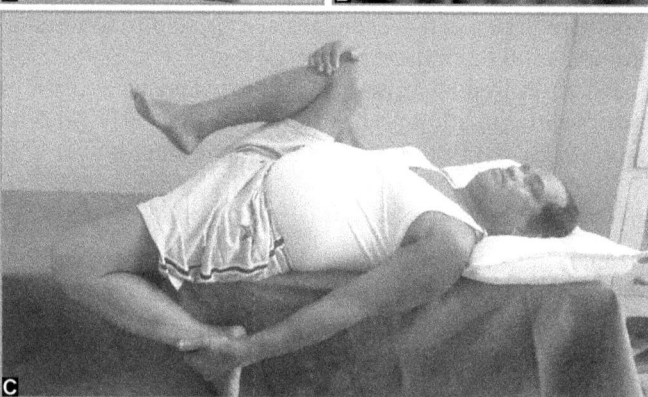

Figs. 7.16A to C: (A) Stretching of right hip flexors in standing, (B) Stretching of right hip flexors in half kneeling, (C) Stretching of left hip flexors in supine lying.

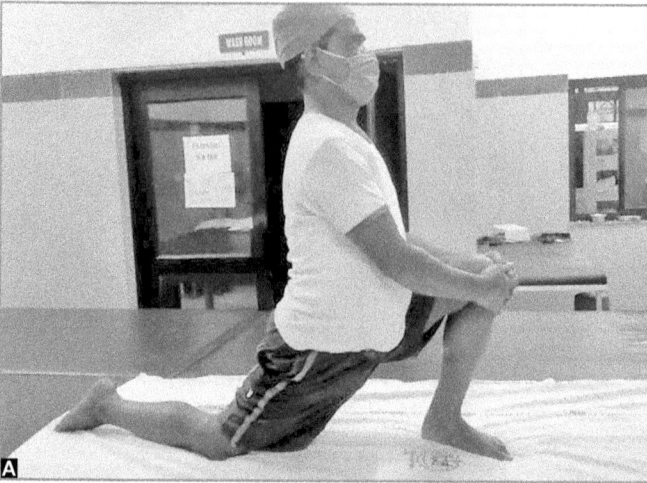
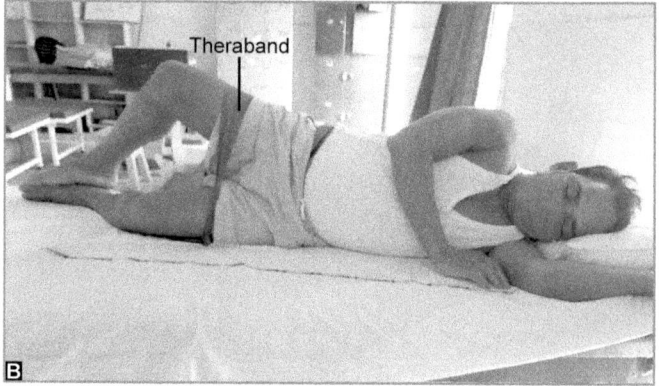

Figs. 7.17A and B: (A) Lunge exercise (B) Resisted clam shell exercise.

* Burning pain on the surface of the outer part of the thigh.

Diagnosis
The diagnosis of meralgia paresthetica is done basing on medical history and a physical examination. Testing the sensation over the affected thigh to find numbness, in the absence of any motor weakness helps in establishing the diagnosis.

Treatment
For most people, the symptoms of meralgia paresthetica subside within a few months. The treatment is usually conservative, focusing on relief of nerve compression and reduction of pain. The treatment includes:
* Loosening of compressive agents such as tight garments.
* Reduction of weight.
* **Medical management:** NSAIDs.
* Stretching of structures in the inguinal region through hip flexor stretches **(Figs. 7.16A to C)**, lunges **(Fig. 7.17A)**, and clam shell exercises **(Fig. 7.17B)** The other exercises include:
  - Brisk walking.
  - Low impact aerobics.
  - Hydrotherapy.
  - Static cycle exercises.
  - TENS.

Surgery
Rarely, in long-standing cases not responding to conservative management, decompression of the nerve under the inguinal ligament is considered.

e. Snapping Hip Syndrome
Snapping hip syndrome, called as dancer's hip, is a medical condition characterized by snapping/popping sensation felt when the hip is flexed and extended, accompanied by pain in the hip, which decreases with rest.

Etiology
The causes of snapping hip syndrome are not fully understood. The onset is often insidious with reports of a "nonpainful" sensation or audible snapping, clicking, or popping with certain activities. Athletes such as ballet dancers, gymnasts, horse riders, track and field athletes, and soccer players, appear to have an increased risk of snapping hip syndrome due to repetitive and physically demanding movements. In excessive weight lifting or running, the cause is usually attributed to extreme thickening of the tendons in the hip region. Snapping hip syndrome most often occurs in people who are 15–40 years old.

Clinical Features

In some cases, an audible or popping noise is heard during flexion and extension of the hip, as the tendon at the hip flexor crease moves in flexion to extension. After prolong activities, pain or discomfort in the hip may be felt. The pain often decreases with rest/diminished activities. Symptoms often last from months to years without treatment and may be very painful. Depending upon the structures affected, snapping hip syndrome can be typed into following categories:

Extra-articular

The more common extra-articular type of snapping hip syndrome is lateral type, that result in sliding back and forth of the thickened tendons of IT band, TFL, and gluteus medius across the greater trochanter. The underlying bursa may also be inflamed, causing painful external snapping hip syndrome. Less commonly the iliopsoas tendon, catches on the anterior inferior iliac spine, lesser trochanter, or the iliopectineal ridge during hip extension, as the tendon moves from an anterolateral to posteromedial position.

Intra-articular

As the iliopsoas crosses directly over the anterior superior labrum of the hip, an intra-articular hip derangement (i.e., labral tears, hip impingement, and loose bodies) can lead to an effusion that subsequently produces internal snapping hip symptoms.

Diagnosis

- Ultrasound during hip motion may visualize tendon subluxation and any accompanying bursitis when evaluating for iliopsoas involvement in medial extra-articular causes.
- MRI can sometimes identify intra-articular causes of snapping hip syndrome.

Management

Medical management

Patients may require intermittent NSAIDS, as they perform exercises and activities. If persistent pain due to bursitis persists, corticosteroid injections may be applied.

Physiotherapy

Rest and ice is applied during 48-72 hours after the onset of the pain. Rest involves avoiding activities and exercises such as running, squatting, etc. As the acute symptoms subside, stretching of the tight muscles, such as piriformis **(Fig. 7.18A)**, hip flexors **(Fig. 7.18B)**, hip abductors may reduce the symptoms. Massage or myofascial release to the tight soft tissues may help in improving the disorder. Light aerobic activities, such as jugging, followed by stretching and strengthening of hamstrings, iliopsoas, IT band is performed to reduce recurrences.

Ultrasound therapy/shock wave therapy may be beneficial for extra-articular types of the disorder. Intense pain if persists should be modulated by TENS/IFT.

Surgery

If medicine and/or physical therapy are ineffective, surgery may be recommended. Iliopsoas and IT band lengthening can be done arthroscopically. Postoperatively extensive physiotherapy is started to regain full strength and mobility.

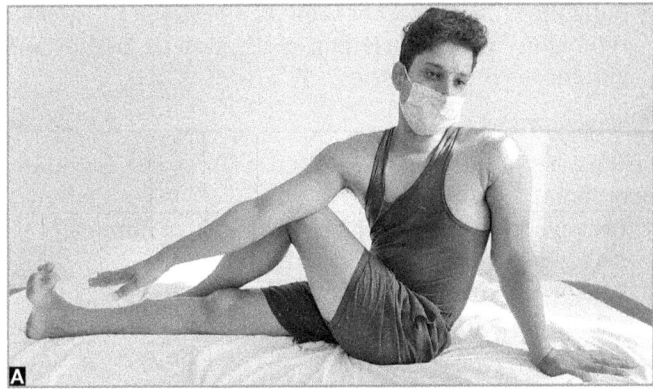
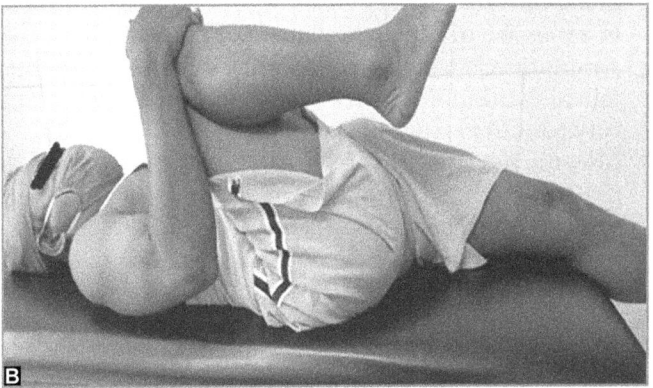

Figs. 7.18A and B: Self stretching of: (A) Piriformis in sitting, (B) Hip flexors in supine lying.

f. Trochanteric Bursitis

Trochanteric bursitis is inflammation of the bursa (fluid filled sac) at the outer aspect of the hip, i.e., over the greater trochanter. This is one of the common causes of hip pain.

Etiology/Epidemiology

Inflammation of the bursa is a slow process, which progresses over time. This bursitis most often occurs because of friction, overuse, direct trauma or too much pressure. Bursitis is more common in women and in middle-aged or elderly people. The disorder results from the following events:

- Direct injury to the hip.
- Repetitive activities such as outdoor sports, causing overuse injuries.
- Faulty posture such as scoliosis.
- Other diseases, such as Rheumatoid arthritis, gout, psoriatic arthritis, thyroid disease and rarely infection.
- Surgeries around hip, such as replacement arthroplasties.
- Osteophytes in hip, calcific deposits over tendons that are attached to greater trochanter.

Pathophysiology

In trochanteric bursitis, two bursae are commonly involved:

- Subgluteus Medius bursa located above the greater trochanter and underneath the insertion of the gluteus medius.

- Subgluteus Maximus bursa located between the greater trochanter and the insertion of the gluteus medius and gluteus maximus muscles.

Clinical Features

Trochanteric bursitis typically produces the following symptoms:
- Pain over the outer side of the hip, thigh, or buttock.
- Pain when lying on the affected side.
- Pain on walking upstairs.
- Pain while getting up from chair of lower height.

There are two types of bursitis:
- **Acute bursitis:** Acute bursitis occurs because of trauma or a massive overload. Just after a few days of the event, symptoms like pain, swelling, and a warm feeling, when touching the affected area can be noticed. It will also be very painful to move the joint.
- **Chronic bursitis:** This is caused by overuse, too much pressure on the structures or extreme movements. Wrong muscle strain can also be a cause of chronic bursitis. The main symptom—which is always present—is pain.

Diagnosis

Diagnosis of lateral hip pain (Trochanteric bursitis) is made thorough history, inspection, palpation, range of motion, stability and strength of hip joint. Hip abductor weakness is a common finding and testing the abductors can provoke lateral hip pain during the examination. Palpation around the greater trochanter that produces pain is considered as one important diagnostic test for this condition.

Diagnostic tests performed include:

Ober's test: The reproduction of pain or the reduced range of motion observed during the test is significant to diagnose trochanteric bursitis.

MRI: If there is still any doubt about the diagnosis it is advisable to make an MRI, which will give more specific information **(Fig. 7.19)**.

Differential Diagnosis

Trochanteric bursitis need to be differentiated from other conditions that cause lateral hip pain such as, IT band syndrome, snapping hip syndrome, Gluteus medius syndrome, Meralgia paresthetica, and Referred pain from lumbosacral spine.

Management of Trochanteric Bursitis

There are various approaches in the treatment of trochanteric bursitis, depending on whether or not the bursa has an infection, and whether it is necessary to treat the lesion with or without surgery. In most cases trochanteric bursitis is treated without surgery.

Medical management

Focuses on control of infection (for bursitis caused by infection), and inflammation.

Physiotherapy

Focuses on reduction of pain, improvement of ROM of hip and strengthening the muscles, particularly hip abductor and extensors. For bursitis caused by overuse, activity modification, and energy conservation techniques are advised to the patient.

In the acute stage, cryotherapy, pulsed ultrasound, low intensity laser therapy (LILT), iontophoresis, etc., may be used as per evidence. Subsequently, after acute pain subsided, moist heat, continuous ultrasound, and high power laser therapy may be considered along with stretching and strengthening exercises to help the patient for gradual return to function.

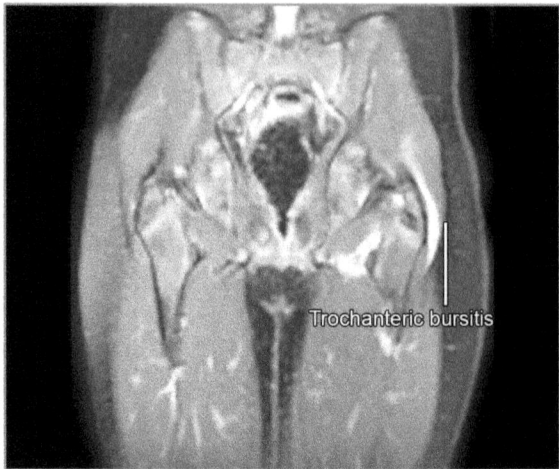

Fig. 7.19: MRI of hip showing trochanteric bursitis.

g. Ischial Bursitis

Ischial bursitis, also called as Weaver's bottom is a rare and infrequently recognized bursitis of the buttock region, occurring mostly due to chronic and continuous irritation of the ischial bursa, developing in individuals who remain seated for prolong periods in a day, as well as sports men who get injury to the hamstring muscle while running or bicycling.

The ischial bursa is a deep located bursa over the bony prominence of ischium and lies between the gluteus maximus and ischial tuberosity.

Etiology
- Injury to bursa due to prolonged sitting/ direct trauma/ sports activities like running.
- Arthritic conditions (e.g., Rheumatoid arthritis).
- Infection.
- Crystal deposits (e.g., Monosodium urate crystal deposit in gout).

Clinical Features
- Pain and swelling in the region of ischial tuberosity.
- Radiating pain to lower limb.
- Pain on prolong sitting.
- Tenderness over ischial tuberosity.
- Atrophy and weakness of glutei.

Diagnostic Tests:
- **Clinical examination:**
  - Palpation reveals a soft tissue mass, not mobile and tender in the gluteal region.

- Straight leg raise test may be painful.
- Resisted extension of the affected hip is painful.
- **Radiographic examination**:
  - X-rays may show any injury to ischial tuberosity/calcification of bursa.
  - *MRI:* T1-weighted images show an injury with intermediate intensity. T2-weighted images show a higher intensity of this lesion, suggesting a space filled with fluid.

Management

Medical: NSAIDs. Steroid injections are advised for patients who do not respond to NSAIDs and physiotherapy.

Physiotherapy:
- **Acute case:**
  - *Protection/Rest and ice:* Protection and rest by minimizing the duration of sitting and intensity and duration of activities such as running in sports. Ice pack application should be for about 20–30 minutes, as the bursa is located deep and prolong icing can only cool the bursa. Vapocoolant sprays can also be applied instead of ice pack. Pulsed ultrasound therapy may also be applied in the acute stage using 1 MHz output to promote healing of the bursa.
  - *Chronic stage:*
    » Electrotherapy: Continuous ultrasound therapy with 1 MHz output, high power laser therapy, hot packs can be applied as per availability and evidence.
    » Friction massage: It is recommended to use friction massage to stretch the adhesions in chronic bursal problems It breaks down scar tissue, increases extensibility and mobility of the structure, promotes normal orientation of collagen fibers, increases blood flow, reduces stress levels, and allows healing to take place.
    » Therapeutic exercises: Static stretching of hamstrings, gluteus maximus **(Figs. 7.20A and B)** may be performed several times a day to improve flexibility of hamstring/gluteus maximus muscle and to reduce pressure on the bursa. Strengthening exercises starting from low-intensity isometric sets to progressively resisted glutei and hamstring strengthening exercises should be performed to prevent recurrence and promote return to sports/function.

h. Avascular Necrosis of Head of Femur

Avascular necrosis (AVN) of head of femur, also known as osteonecrosis, is characterized by variable areas of dead trabecular bone and bone marrow, extending to and including the subchondral plate in the head of the femur.

Etiology

This condition is categorized under the multifactorial disease that means multiple causes/pathologies lead to this condition. The common causes include:

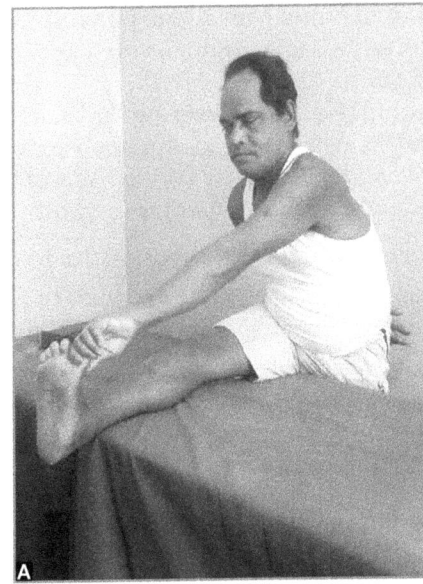
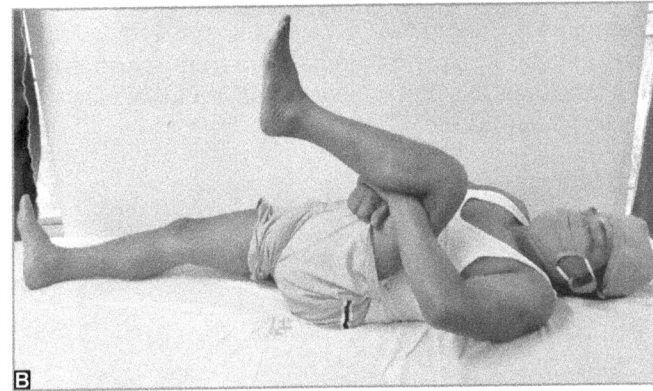

Figs. 7.20A and B: (A) Self-stretching of hamstrings, (B) Self-stretching of gluteus maximus.

- Trauma (leading to fracture neck of femur).
- Genetic disorder (sickle cell disease).
- Prolonged intake of steroids.
- Chronic alcoholism/chronic smoking.
- HIV infection.
- Pregnancy (rare).

Pathophysiology

Pathophysiology of AVN is not fully understood. Most of the time, it is the anterolateral region of the femoral head that is affected but no area is necessarily spared. This disease is often seen in patients in the third, fourth, and fifth decades. The older the patients, the less the chance of revascularization.

Clinical Feature

The patients usually complain of pain in the groin, often radiating to buttock or knees. The ROM of hip becomes limited and painful resulting in difficulty in walking and squatting.

Diagnostic Tests

- **X-ray:** In the X-ray, the earliest sign of this mechanical failure is the crescent sign **(Fig. 7.21A)**, which represents the separation of the subchondral plate from the

underlying necrotic cancellous bone. In progressive lesions, there is radiographic evidence of collapse of femoral head.
* MRI of the hip **(Fig. 7.21B)** help the clinicians to establish the diagnosis. When standard anteroposterior and frog-leg lateral radiographs show obvious AVN of the femoral head, it is not necessary to perform an MRI.

Management of Avascular Necrosis of Head of Femur

The management of AVN of the femoral head ranges from conservative (nonoperative) to invasive (operative).

Conservative management

It includes physiotherapy, restricted weight-bearing (nonweight-bearing crutch gait/walking stick on opposite side) pain control medication. Decisions regarding surgery depend on patient's age, amount of damage to femoral head, and comorbidities associated.

Physiotherapy for Avascular Necrosis of Head of Femur

As soon as the condition is diagnosed, protected weight-bearing in the form of nonweight-bearing crutch gait, partial weight bearing gait with crutches, walker, and walking stick, etc., are practiced.

Electrotherapy in the form of PSWD may be tried. Nonweight-bearing active mobilization of hip in the pain-free range is taught to maintain ROM.

Exercises recommended include:
* Isometric gluteal exercises.
* Isometric quadriceps exercise.
* Active free exercises/assisted exercise.
* Suspension therapy.
* Exercise on rowing machine.

Surgical Management

There are several possible surgical methods to treat AVN of the hip such as core decompression, osteotomy, bone-grafting, and arthroplasty. The joint preservation interventions are core decompression, osteotomy, bone grafts, while reconstructive interventions are arthroplasty. After surgery weight-bearing and postoperative physiotherapy is followed as per protocol.

i. Hip Dislocations

Dislocation of hip joint is the disruption of the joint between the femur and pelvis.

Etiology/Epidemiology

Hip dislocations are uncommon, as compared to dislocations of shoulder. Males are usually more affected than females, which may be due to the fact that, males are more and more involvement in driving and doing work at heights as compared to females. Traumatic dislocations occur most commonly in the age group of 16–40 years.

Dislocation of hip is usually caused by trauma from motor vehicle accidents and fall from height.

Clinical Features

Symptoms of a hip dislocation include pain and instability of the hip resulting in inability to move the joint. A dislocated hip may lead to complications like AVN of head of femur, lesion to sciatic nerve, and arthritis of hip joint.

Types of Hip Dislocations

Dislocations of hip are categorized as either posterior or anterior, or central, based on the location of the head of the femur, which are briefly discussed below:

Posterior dislocation of hip

This is the most common dislocation in hip. The affected lower limb, remains in a position of flexion, adduction, and medial rotation. Sciatic nerve palsy may be present in such dislocations.

Anterior dislocation

This dislocation, which is less common, the limb is held by the person, externally rotated, with mild flexion and abduction. Femoral nerve palsy may develop in such dislocations.

Central fracture dislocation

A central dislocation, which is not very common in hip, is always a fracture dislocation. A strong lateral force against an adducted femur, fractures the acetabulum, and places the femoral head medial to the fractured acetabulum.

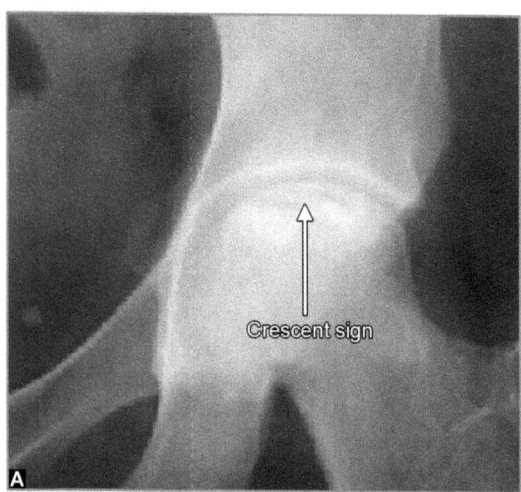
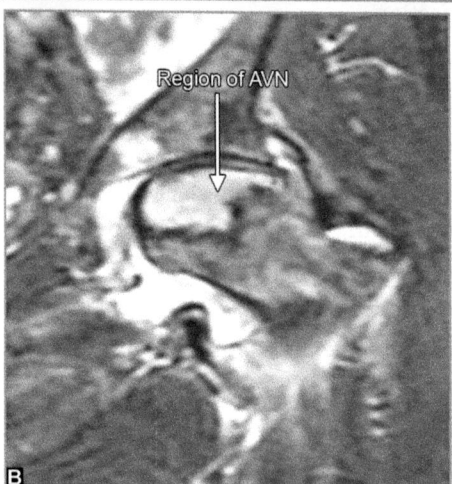

Figs. 7.21A and B: (A) X-ray of hip showing AVN of head of femur with crescent sign. (B) MRI showing AVN.

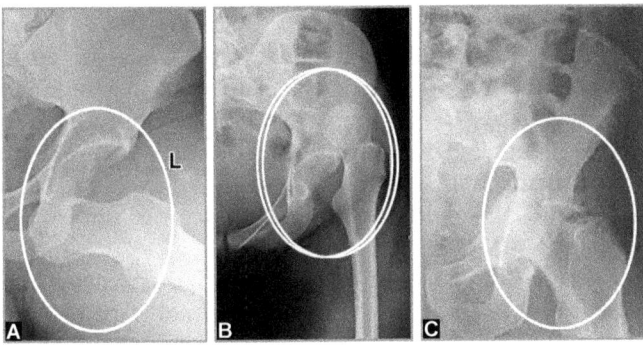

Figs. 7.22A to C: X ray hip showing: (A) Anterior dislocation, (B). Posterior dislocation, and (C) Central dislocation.

Diagnosis

History of trauma and attitude of the lower limb, combined with X-ray **(Figs. 7.22A to C)**/CT scan help in establishing a hip dislocation.

Anteroposterior and lateral radiographs of both hips help to confirm both posterior and anterior dislocation of hip. In posterior dislocation, the femoral head looks smaller as compared to the sound side, and in anterior dislocation, the femoral head looks larger as compared to the sound side.

A central fracture dislocation can best be identified from a CT scan.

Management of Hip Dislocation

Reduction

The dislocation should be reduced as quickly as possible by the orthopedic surgeon to reduce the risk of osteonecrosis and possible nerve damages. Closed reduction of the hip is the choice of treatment for uncomplicated dislocations. However, for complicated dislocations, where reduction is not achieved by closed manipulation, open reduction is the choice.

Physiotherapy

Rehabilitation of hip dislocation may take 2–3 months, depending on the type of dislocation and nature of reduction (closed/open). After the dislocations are reduced, rehabilitation therapy starts with protection, rest, and ice. As the pain allows, graduated weight-bearing starting from nonweight-bearing crutch gait, progressing to partial weight bearing with crutches/stick on opposite side is started followed by full weight bearing as the joint becomes stable and pain reduces.

Exercises

Gentile passive exercises of the hip are started after 5–7 days of reduction to maintain/increase flexibility of soft tissues and mobility of hip joint. Subsequently, the Physiotherapist designs a set of active exercises for the patient to improve stability of hip joint and return to function. The exercises are first performed as free exercises, and subsequently progressed to resisted exercise. The exercises performed include:

- **Bridging of pelvis (Fig. 7.23):** In crook lying, feet in line with the hips, the patient is advised to lift both hips slowly upward, hold for 3–5 seconds and lower. The exercises meant to strengthen glutei, are repeated 10 times in one session and the number of sessions in a day depends on the patient's tolerance to exercise.

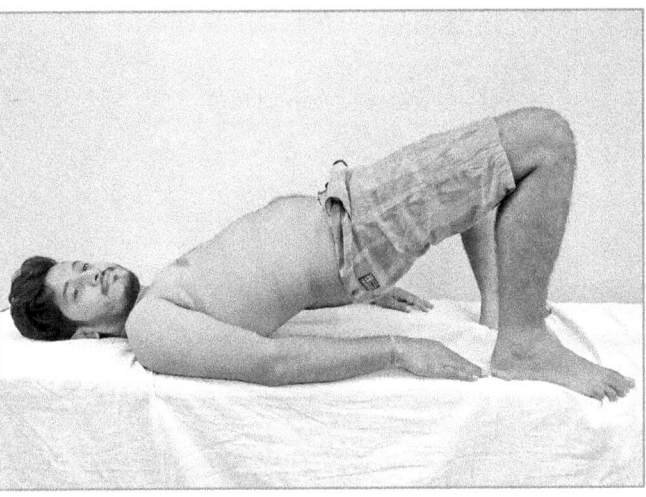

Fig. 7.23: Pelvic bridging exercise.

- Supine hip abduction with knee straight initially with no resistance, progressing to resisted abduction by using theraband to strengthen the hip abductors **(Fig. 7.15)**.
- Side lying hip abduction, initially performed freely, followed by resisted hip abduction using theraband **(Fig. 7.24)**, as a progression from supine hip abduction to strengthen the hip abductors.
- Standing hip abduction **(Fig. 7.25A)**, as a progression from side lying hip abduction to strengthen the hip abductors.
- **Standing knee raise (Fig. 7.25B):** Standing, holding on to a support, the patient is advised to flex and raise one knee and slowly lower it down.
- **Standing hip flexion and extension:** Holding on a stable support, the patient swings one leg forward away from body, holds the position for 3–5 seconds, and then swings the body backward behind the body, holds for 3–5 seconds, and then lower to ground. The exercises are repeated 10 times in a session and number of sessions depends on the patient's tolerance to the exercise.
- Supine hip flexion by adding weight to the ankle **(Fig. 7.26)**.

Electrotherapy

During the early stage, PSWD can be applied to promote resolution of inflammation and repair. Subsequently, SWD/

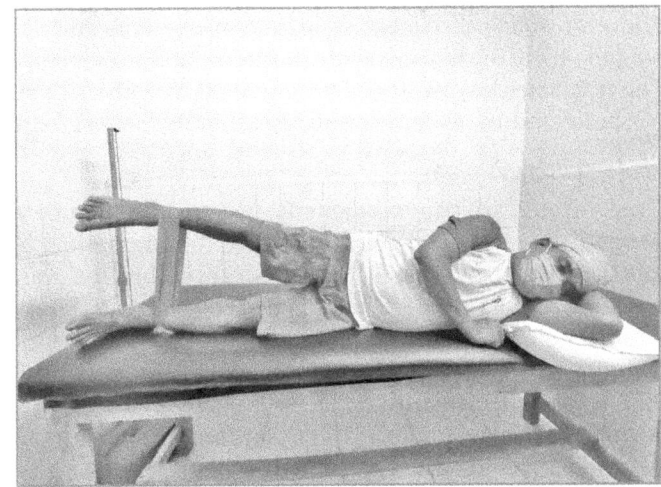

Fig. 7.24: Hip abductor strengthening in side lying.

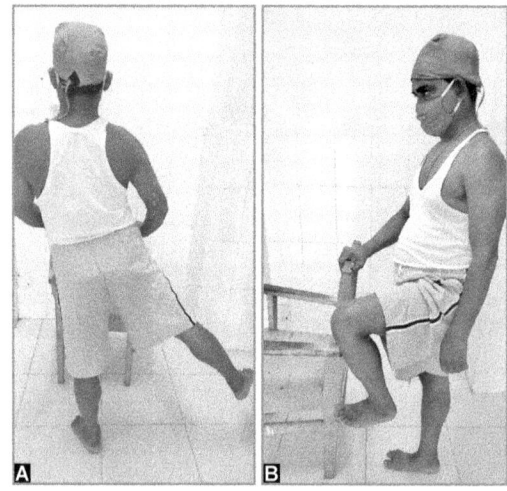

Figs. 7.25A and B: (A) Standing hip abduction, (B) Standing knee raise.

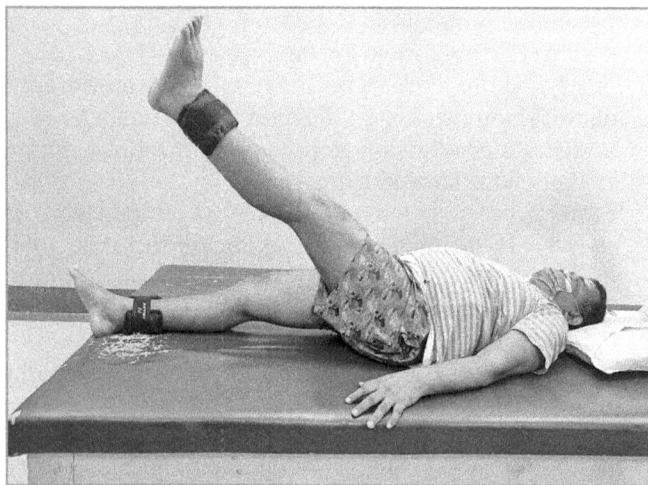

Fig. 7.26: Resisted hip flexion with weight cuff.

MWD may be applied to enhance flexibility of soft tissues and reduce pain. Pain (if any) affecting function can be managed by IFT/TENS.

j. Adductor Strain/Groin Strain

Adductor strain called groin strain is an injury to the muscle/tendon unit of the hip adductors, mostly the adductor longus. The groin muscles consist of three large groups of muscles that can be injured: the abdominals, iliopsoas, and adductor group.

Epidemiology/Etiology

Groin strains are common among athletes who compete in sports that involve repetitive twisting, turning, sprinting, and kicking. Strain injuries to the groin are among the most common groin injuries in adult male soccer players. Groin strains are also known from other sports such as hockey, running, tennis, etc.

The exact incidence of groin muscle strains in most sports is unknown because athletes often play through minor groin pain and the injury goes unreported.

Clinical Features

The main sign of the adductor muscle injury is intense pain in the groin. The patient presents with pain in the inner thigh and tenderness along the muscle belly/tendon of insertion. The pain is exacerbated by adduction. There is no loss of strength or range of movement of the hip. There is a documented and well-established grading system of adductor muscle injury such as:

- **Grade 1:** No loss of function or strength. Muscle tears can show normal appearances or a small area of focal disruption with hematoma and perifascial fluid relatively common on imaging with ultrasound and MRI. There is intense pain in the groin area like the stabbing sensation, when the athlete continues activities.
- **Grade 2:** It is the partial tear with disruption of few muscle fibers, resulting in weakness of the muscle. There is also intense pain in the groin area like stabbing sensation. Locally, a hemorrhage and swelling can be seen a few days after the injury.
- **Grade 3:** Complete muscle tear and complete functional loss. The strain is most often found in the distal musculotendinous junction located toward the insertion on the femur.

In chronic cases, the symptoms of groin injury are often complex. There is a tendency for the pain to radiate out distally along the medial aspect of the thigh or proximally toward the rectus abdominis. The most common symptoms are pain during exercise, stiffness after exercise and in the morning, as well as pain at rest.

Diagnosis

Diagnosis is made from history and clinical examination. On examination, there is tenderness on palpation and focal swelling at the site of pain in the adductor muscles. On resisted adduction (RIC of hip adductors) of hip there is pain and weakness.

Confirmatory investigations like ultrasonography and MRI help to establish the lesion and differentiate it from other conditions.

Management

The treatment of musculotendinous groin injuries is generally conservative, and depends on the stage of injury:

- **Acute stage:** Management consists of rest and application of ice/vapocoolant spray and NSAIDs (prescribed by physician). Protected weight bearing with crutches is recommended in this stage. Modalities such as pulsed ultrasound, low intensity LASER, and TENS are effective in this stage. As the acute pain subsides, therapy consists of:
  – Resisted isometric exercises to muscles of hip, within the limits of pain.
  – Active assisted/ free exercises to hip in the pain free range.
  – Strength training and endurance training are gradually progressed as acute pain subsided.

- Sports specific training and gradual return to sports and activities are promoted.
- **Chronic stage:** In chronic groin strain, where pain persists, Holmich et al., demonstrated an 8–17 weeks active strengthening program, consisting of progressive resistive adduction and abduction exercises **(Figs. 7.27A and B)**, balance training, abdominal strengthening exercises are effective. Passive treatments like TENS, LASER, etc., should be combined with active treatment for early return to sports/function.

k. Gluteus Medius/Dead Butt Syndrome

Gluteus medius is a condition, where in weakness of gluteus medius muscle pulls, pinches, or compresses nerves resulting in numbness on the buttocks, accompanied by loss of strength and stiffness in the hips and legs, resulting in both hip and lower back pain as the weakened gluteus medius is unable to adequately support the hips and pelvis. This can ultimately affect balance and overall stability.

Etiology

The main cause of this syndrome is inactivity that results from prolonged activities in sitting. The lack of activities that result from continuous sitting, causes shut down of the gluteal muscles, resulting in over activity of other muscles in the hip and pelvis to compensate for the work done by the glutei.

As mentioned by Vladimir Janda, gluteus medius is one of the phasic muscles that tends to be inhibited in our body by many causes:

- Standing with body weight shifted mainly on one lower limb with the pelvis swayed sideways and hip joint adducted.
- Sleeping in side lying with no pillow in between two lower extremities will lead to the top leg flexed and adducted over the other leg.
- Sitting with crossed legs for a long period of time.

Pathophysiology

When Gluteus Medius is inhibited body tries to compensate by other muscles to maintain frontal plane stability and preventing pelvis from dropping, so the activity of ipsilateral tensor fascia latae and contralateral quadratus lumborum increase causing these muscles to become tight and overactive.

Clinical Features

The onset is insidious. The patient complains of pain and numbness in buttock, sometimes radiating downward. The weakness of gluteus medius also results in limping (Trendelenburg gait).

Management

It focuses on strengthening of gluteus medius, and increasing the flexibility of other muscles of hip and pelvis, that have become tight due to weak hip abductors. Pressman and colleagues described a progressive program for strengthening gluteus medius muscle, which is discussed below:

- **Nonweight-bearing and basic weight bearing exercises:** Side lying hip abduction, standing hip abduction **(Fig. 7.28)**, and basic single leg balance exercises.
- Weight-bearing exercises such as translating the center of gravity horizontally via stepping and/or hopping exercises.
- Sport-specific movement patterns.

Any pain that is coexisting is reduced by selecting appropriate modalities such as moist heat, IFT, TENS, etc.

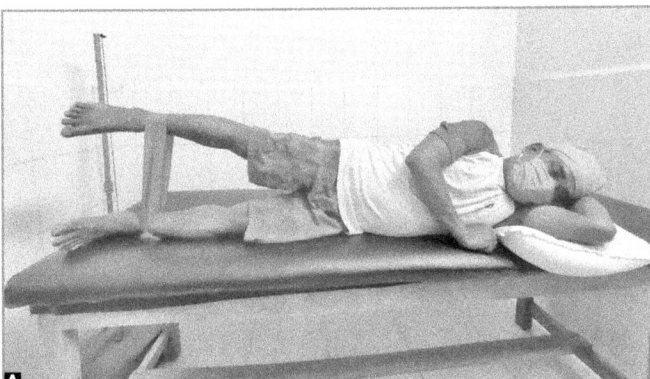
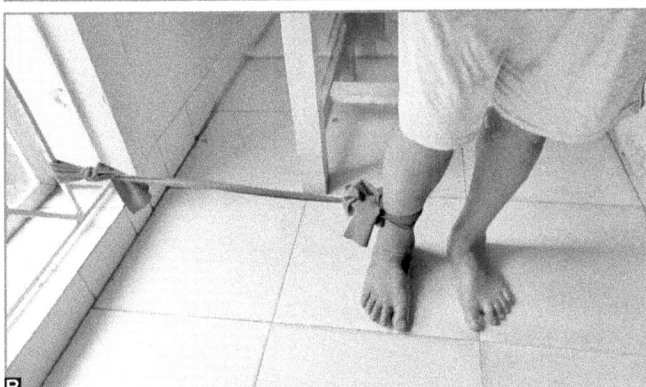

Figs. 7.27A and B: (A) Hip abductor strengthening, (B) Hip adductor strengthening using theraband.

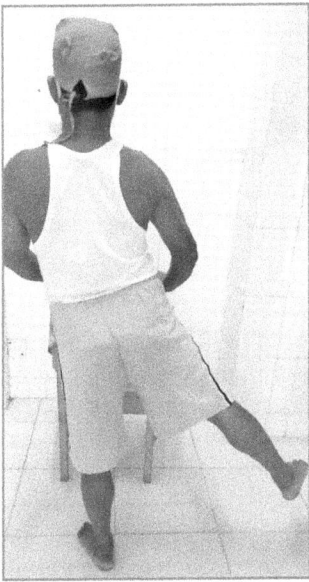

Fig. 7.28: Standing hip abduction exercise.

I. Congenital Dislocation of Hip (CDH)/Developmental Dysplasia of Hip

Developmental dysplasia of hip (DDH) also known as a congenital dislocation of hip (CDH) is a general term used to describe certain abnormalities of the femur, or the acetabulum, or both, nearly always diagnosed within the first 2 years of life, that results in inadequate containment of the femoral head within the acetabulum, resulting in an increased risk for joint dislocation, dislocatability, or inadequate joint development.

Early detection and timely treatment is essential for prevention of permanent disability.

Epidemiology/Etiology/Risk Factors

Congenital hip dislocation is one of the most severe orthopedic pathologies in children with an incidence rate of 3-4 cases per 1,000 normal deliveries. The condition affects females more than males. The left hip is usually affected more than the right hip, and bilateral dislocations also exist.

The etiology/risk factors include:
- **Genetic:** Hereditary predisposition, generalized joint laxity and shallow acetabulum.
- **Hormonal:** Maternal relaxin, high estrogen and progesterone produce this disorder more in females.
- **Intrauterine malposition:** Breech position.
- First born child (primigravida).

Pathophysiology

The affected hip is either dislocated at birth (classic DDH) or dislocates after birth (due to generalized joint laxity). The epiphysis is small and the femoral head is displaced upward and laterally. The acetabulum is shallow and there may be excessive femoral anteversion. The acetabular labrum may be folded and the joint capsule may be stretched. Adaptive shortening of the muscles of hip may be present.

Clinical Features

The disorder may be present at birth, or found soon after child started to walk. Routine screening of the new born reveals signs of the disorder. In early child hood, asymmetric groin fold, click on movements of hip and movement limitations are the features. In old children, gait disturbances, high buttock fold/asymmetric thigh fold, shortening of affected limb, external rotation of the limb, limitation of hip abduction, and increase of lumbar lordosis are the features.

Diagnosis

a. **Clinical tests:**
   - *Barlow test:* The Barlow maneuver identifies the unstable hip that is in a reduced position that the clinician passively dislocates.
   - *Ortolani's test* (**Fig. 7.3**): This test is performed following Barlow's test to relocate the hips and helps to determine, if the hips are actually dislocated.
   - *Klisic's test:* The clinician, places the middle finger over the child's greater trochanter and index finger on the ASIS. In normal hip, imaginary line between the two fingers point to umbilicus, where as in dislocated hip, where the greater trochanter is elevated, the line passes between umbilicus and the pubis (**Figs. 7.29A and B**).
   - *Galeazzi test* (**Fig. 7.30**).
   - *Trendelenburg gait.*

b. **Imaging studies:**
X-ray shows broken Shenton's line (**Fig. 7.31**), ultrasonography, MRI, CT scan.

Management

The treatment should be performed early, as restoration of anatomical structure and functions of the hip joint in children is only possible, if early diagnosis and timely treatment is provided at infancy.

The aim of management is to reduce the dislocation, so that the head of femur is stable inside the acetabulum. Age-specific management of children are discussed briefly below:

- **Infants (0-6 months):** Closed reduction is the treatment of choice. Application of splints such as the Von Rosen splint (**Fig. 7.32A**)/Pavlik harness (**Fig. 7.32B**), Craig nappy splint are used to maintain reduction in the position of flexion/abduction. The Pavlik harness is most preferred, as it allows small amount of movements within the splint, facilitating spontaneous reduction.
- **6 months to 2 years:** Closed reduction followed by application of hip spica for 3 months. If the child has adductor contracture, adductor tenotomy followed by application of skin traction/application of plaster of Paris (POP) hip spica for 3-6 months, is helpful. If conservative methods fail open reduction is the choice.

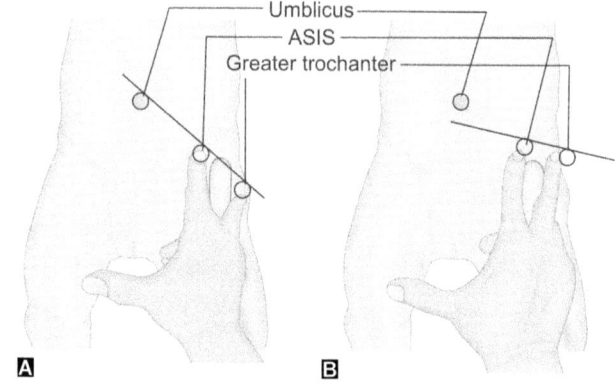

Figs. 7.29A and B: Klisic's test: (A) Normal, (B) Dislocated hip.

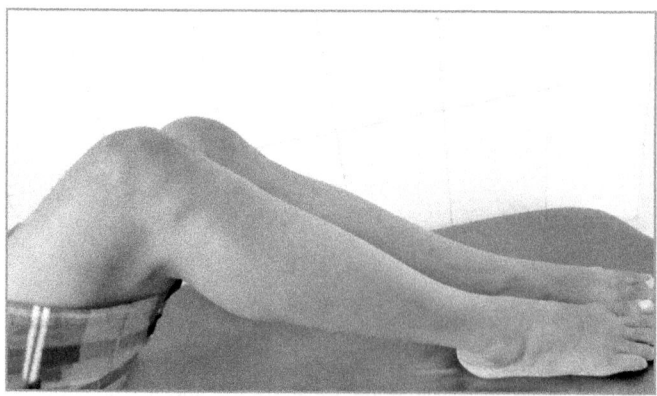

Fig. 7.30: Positive Galeazzi sign.

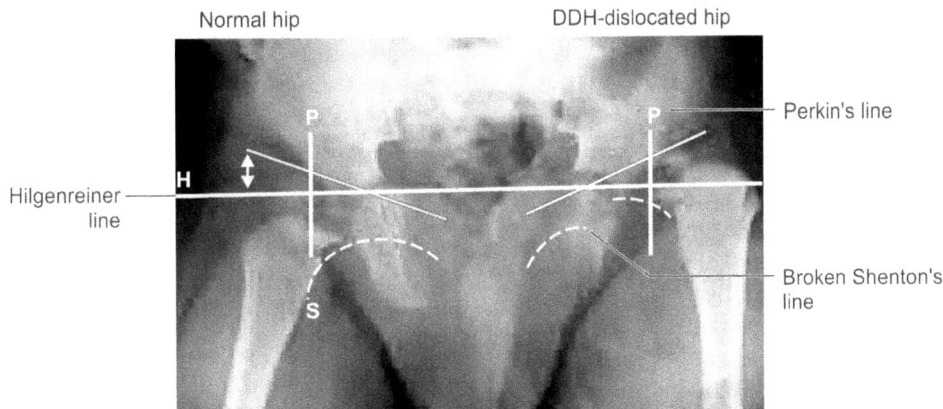

Fig. 7.31: X-ray showing normal and dislocated hips.

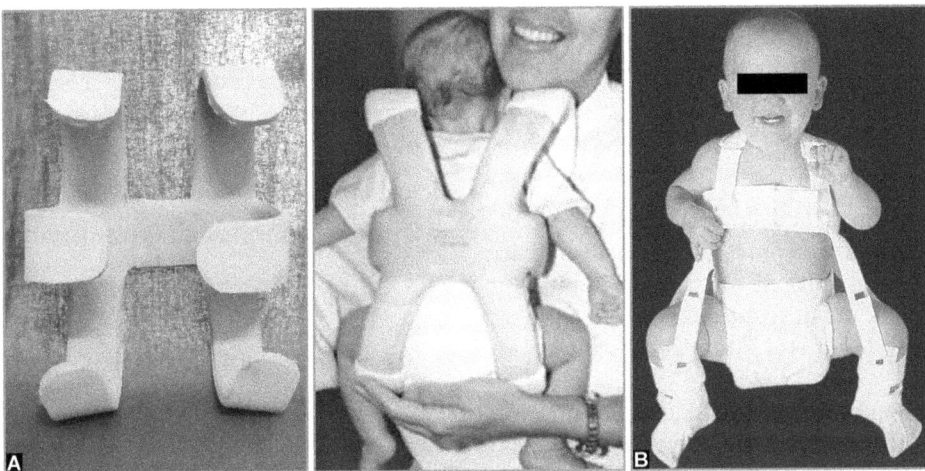

Figs. 7.32A and B: (A) Von Rosen splint, (B) The Pavlik harness.

❖ **2–8 years:** It requires open reduction with/without pelvic osteotomy (Salter's osteotomy). The Chiari pelvic osteotomy is more suitable for older children. POP immobilization is continued till osteotomy is united. After removal of the POP, graduated mobilization exercises and controlled weight bearing with walker/crutches are started.

❖ **Above 8 years:** These children do not respond to any form of treatment. They are prone to develop secondary osteoarthritis of hips, necessitating total hip replacement surgery in a later age.

Physiotherapy for Congenital Dislocation/Developmental Dysplasia of Hip

❖ For infants below the age of 6 months, the emphasis is on positioning the hips in flexion, abduction and internal rotation using Pavlik harness. Isometric gluteal and quadriceps exercises are taught to the parents.

❖ For children who undergo surgery, preoperative therapy focusing on strengthening of muscles over the hip, information about the role of mobilization and strengthening exercises after surgery, information regarding the use of walking aids, such as walker/crutches to have graduated weight-bearing ambulation after the cast removal following surgery are given for an effective postoperative rehabilitation.

❖ Graduated mobilization of the hip after cast removal, emphasizing on gradual regaining of hip adduction range.

❖ Strengthening of muscles of hip, hydrotherapy, TENS to reduce pain are considered.

❖ Assisted ambulation with walker/crutches, progressing to full weight bearing as muscle strength improves.

❖ Hippotherapy (making the child sit on horse back) is shown to motivate the child to engage in therapy, maintain the child's willingness to participate and provide a playful environment while facilitating pain-free movement.

m. Hip Arthroplasty

Hip arthroplasty is the surgical reconstruction of the hip joint, which has lost its mobility and function due either to pathologies involving the hip such as fusion (as occurs in ankylosing spondylitis), AVN, unbearable pain, etc.

Arthroplasties in hip are of the following types:

Fibrous Arthroplasty (Girdle Stone Arthroplasty)

In this mobility in the joint is restored by creating a joint through interposing soft tissues. The surgeon resects superior margin of the acetabulum, along with resection of the femoral head and neck up to the base of the trochanter and interposes some soft tissues in the gap. This sort of arthroplasty has lesser stability, as compared to replacement arthroplasty.

Postoperatively, the person is given skeletal traction for 5–6 weeks, with mobilization of hip and knee while on traction after 4 weeks of immobilization in traction. Nonweight-bearing crutch gait is started after 6 weeks, while full weight bearing ambulation is started after 3–4 months. Strengthening the muscles of hip is required to improve stability.

Replacement Arthroplasty

Replacement arthroplasty is commonly performed in the hip joint as it is more stable, as compared to girdle stone arthroplasty. Replacement arthroplasty and its types and therapeutic management are briefly discussed below:

Hip Replacement Arthroplasty

This arthroplasty could be of the following types:
- **Partial hip replacement arthroplasty/Hemiarthroplasty**: It is mostly done for displaced fractures involving the neck of femur, where only the femoral part is replaced **(Fig. 7.33A)**. Austin Moor and Thomson prosthesis are commonly used.
  Postoperatively, patient is nursed in bed in supine position, with hip maintained in abduction using abduction pillow to prevent dislocation of prosthesis. Flexion and adduction of hip for 4–6 weeks is avoided. Partial weight-bearing crutch gait is started after 3 weeks and full weight bearing is allowed after 4–6 weeks.
  The pre- and postoperative physiotherapy is followed in the same lines of total hip replacement arthroplasty described below.
- **Total hip replacement arthroplasty:** In this type of procedure, the head of the femur is replaced with a prosthetic head on a shaft, and the joint surface of the acetabulum is lined with a bowl-shaped synthetic joint surface **(Fig. 7.33B)**.

Total hip arthroplasty (THA) can be broadly divided into those hips fixed with cement and those fixed without cement. Cemented THA use polymethylmethacrylate (PMMA) to function as a grout producing an interlocking fit between cancellous bone and prosthesis. Uncemented hips rely on biological fixation of bone to a surface coating on the prosthesis. Biologic fixation uses either porous coated metallic surface to stimulate bone in growth or grit-blasted surface to allow bone on growth. The prosthesis can also be coated in hydroxyapatite, which is an osteoconductive agent.

There is a tendency to use noncemented femoral stems in younger patients, due to higher reported rates of loosening of cemented stems in long-term follow up. Cemented fixation is usually followed for older patients. A cemented or a hybrid prosthesis (consisting of a cemented femoral component and an uncemented acetabular component) is used in men older than 70 years and in women older than 60 years, and in younger patients in whom adequate initial fixation could not be obtained without cement.

Indications of Total Hip Arthroplasty:
- End stage symptomatic hip osteoarthritis.
- AVN
- Ankylosis of hip (commonly seen in Ankylosing spondylitis).
- Rheumatoid arthritis.
- Failure of internal fixation in hip.
- Congenital dislocation of hip.

Types of Surgical Approaches

There are two major surgical approach methods for performing a total hip replacement:
- The posterior approach (more common).
- The anterior approach (sometimes called the "mini-anterior approach" or "muscle-sparing hip replacement").

Physiotherapy for Total Hip Replacement Arthroplasty

Physiotherapy in total hip replacement arthroplasty is broadly divided into:
- **Preoperative assessment:** It consists of:
  - Subjective examination: It includes demographic data, history, examination of pain using scales such as VAS.

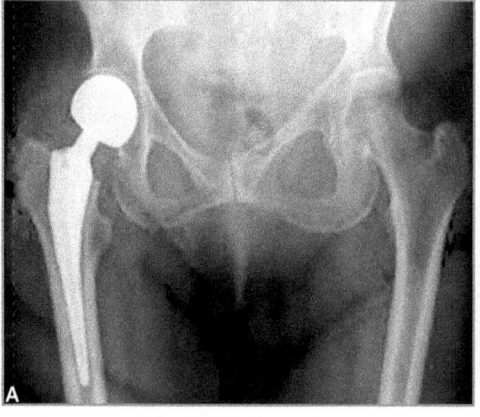
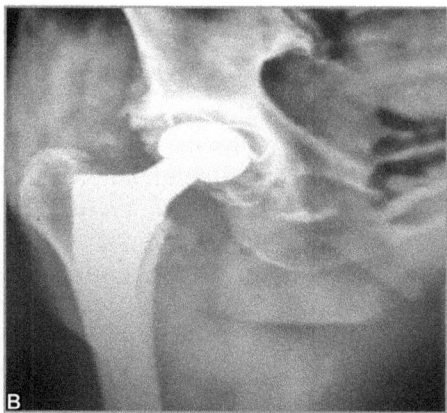

Figs. 7.33A and B: X-ray showing (A) Hemiarthroplasty of hip, (B) Total hip replacement.

- *Objective examination:* It includes:
    » ROM of hip joint.
    » Muscle power.
    » Limb length discrepancy (if any).
    » Functional examination.
    » Gait examination.
- ❖ **Preoperative physiotherapy:** It consists of the followings:
    - Patient education regarding precautions to be taken and the need for postoperative exercises. The procedure involves:
        » Teaching hip precautions as per the surgical approaches to be followed, such as:
            ○ For posterolateral approach: Advice given for avoiding the followings postoperatively:
                ◊ Flexion of hip beyond 90°.
                ◊ Extreme internal rotation of hip.
                ◊ Adduction of hip past body's midline.
            ○ For anterolateral approach: Advice given to avoid the followings postoperatively:
                ◊ Extension of hip.
                ◊ Extreme external rotation of hip.
                ◊ Adduction of the hips past the body's mid line.
            ○ For direct anterior approach: Advice given to avoid the followings postoperatively:
                ◊ Pelvic bridging.
                ◊ Extension.
                ◊ Extreme external rotation.
                ◊ Adduction of hip beyond mid line.
            ○ Preoperative exercises: It includes:
                ◊ Deep breathing exercise.
                ◊ Isometric gluteal and quadriceps exercise.
                ◊ Active hip abduction exercise.
                ◊ Active ankle/foot exercise.
                ◊ Bed mobility training.
                ◊ Stair climbing with/without support.
                ◊ Gait training with walker/crutches/stick.
- ❖ **Postoperative physiotherapy:** Postoperative physiotherapy should start on the day of surgery, which helps to decrease the length of hospital stay, reduces pain and improves function. The aims of postoperative rehabilitation are:
    - To reduce pain and swelling.
    - To improve mobility and ambulation.
    - To improve muscle strength.
    - To improve flexibility.
    - To improve lungs function.
    - To improve function.

The postoperative protocols (adapted to meet the needs of the patient) used for rehabilitation and weight bearing (started early in cemented than uncemented fixations) is surgeon specific, and the therapist should discuss with the surgeon for progressing therapy (weight bearing).

For some enhanced recovery after surgery protocols, patients are mobilized out of bed within the first 6 hours, postsurgery, where as other settings start mobilizing patients out of bed on day 1 or 2 postsurgery. Early weight bearing and physical activity have benefits for the quality of bone tissue, as it improves the fixation of the prosthesis and decreases the incidence of early loosening. The patient can be made to stand up with support, as early as on the third postoperative day, with consent of the surgeon.

Initially, nonweight-bearing gait with walker/axillary crutches are started, gradually progressing to toe touch weight-bearing with walker/crutches.

- ❖ **Partial weight bearing on walker/crutches:** The patient is asked to move the walker followed by the operated leg touching the ground, followed by the normal leg.
- ❖ **Full weight bearing:** Full weight bearing is allowed after 8 weeks after achieving consent of the surgeon, provided there are no complications. Patient should be independent functionally by end of 12 weeks. However, sitting on floor should be avoided, and if pain persists a walking stick may be given on the contralateral side till pain reduced.

A common postoperative protocol after THA is discussed below:

A. **Week 1:**
  - *Day 1:*
      » Reminding the patient about the precautions to be followed as taught during preoperative period.
      » Positioning on bed with an abduction pillow, between the thighs and a knee roll to maintain knee in slight flexion.
      » Application of cryopack avoiding the incision wound to reduce pain and swelling. Ice/cryopack should be applied for 10 minutes every hour as needed.
      » Deep breathing exercises.
      » Ankle and foot exercises.
      » Active free exercises to upper limb.
      » Isometric quadriceps and gluteal exercises **(Figs. 7.34A and B)**. Each exercise is repeated 10–15 times in a session for 2–3 times a day.
      » Active free exercises to the unaffected lower limb.
  - *Day 2:* Bed exercises as described above are continued, progressing repetitions and decreasing assistance given to patient. Besides the above, other exercises/activities include:
      » Getting in and out of bed **(Figs. 7.35A to C)** with affected limb supported through theraband/rope.
      » Sitting up by gradually raising the back rest.
      » Turning on the bed towards the sound side, under supervision is emphasized, with pillow between the thighs to prevent hip adduction.
      » Transfer training from bed to chair/wheelchair, and wheel chair to parallel bar/walker is emphasized.
      » Brief periods of partial weight bearing/toe down weight bearing on parallel bar/walker/axillary crutches is performed, if no pain is felt.
  - *Day 3–7:*
      » The exercises as described above, progressing in increasing repetitions and decreasing assistance given to patients are performed.

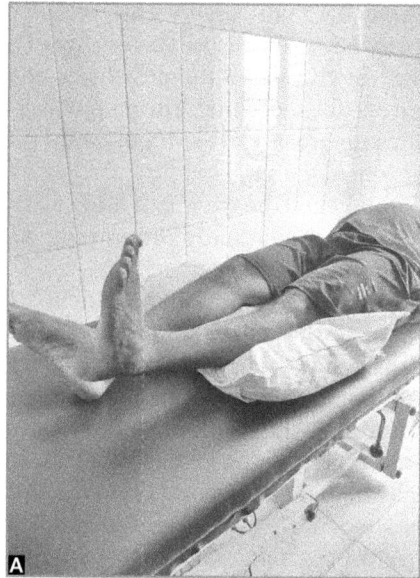

- » Resisted isometric quadriceps, strong isometric glutei are emphasized.
- » Brief periods of prone lying are emphasized.
- » Relaxed passive movement/active assisted exercise to hip flexors are initiated, as tolerated, with caution for not moving the hip beyond 90° of hip flexion. CPM/Suspension therapy **(Fig. 7.36)**/foot skater may be employed to exercise the affected hip.
- Assisted hip abduction with a pillow between the thighs **(Fig. 7.37A)**, to prevent hip adduction and dislocation of the prosthesis. Suspension therapy **(Fig. 7.37B)** is a very good method of assisting hip abduction. Hip abduction exercises, should be repeated ten to 15 times, in a session and performed 2–3 times in a day.
- Standing on sound leg and performing hip abduction **(Fig. 7.38)**, hip/knee flexion, hamstring curls on the affected side.
- Progression of partial weight bearing ambulation with mobility assistive device.
- Reminding about hip precautions and planning for discharge after 3 days, if patient is fit for discharge, with advice to continue home exercise program or attend physiotherapy on outpatient basis. However, the patient's home environment need to be modified as discussed below, for facilitation of recovery and function.

Home modifications needed for the patient:
- ❖ Staircase and toilet having hand railings.
- ❖ Facility for a raised toilet seat.
- ❖ Chair with stability.
- ❖ Availability of a dressing stick and sock aid, etc., to manage self care activities without excessive bending of the hips.

B. **Week 2:**
- Relaxed passive exercise/active assisted exercise are progressed to achieve hip flexion to 90°.

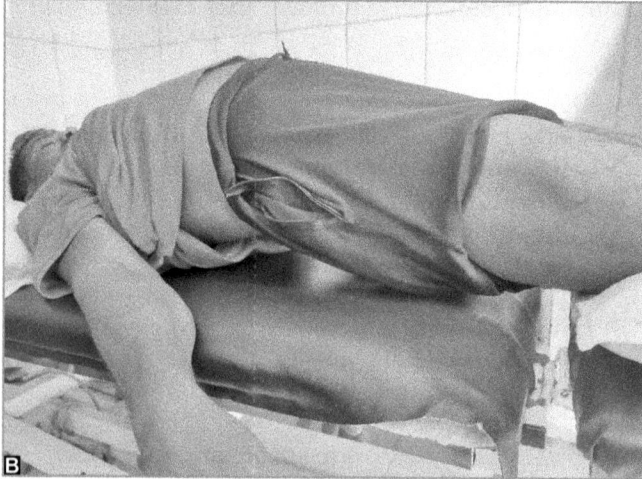

Figs. 7.34A and B: (A) Isometric quadriceps exercise, (B) Isometric gluteal exercise.

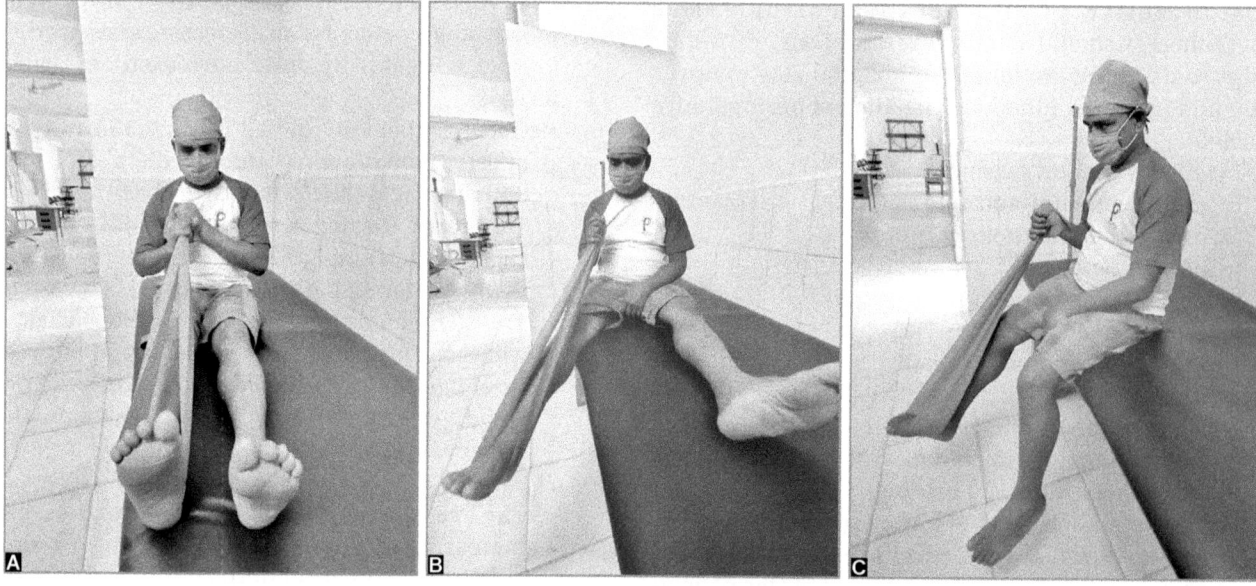

Figs. 7.35A to C: Getting in and out of bed with auto assistance using theraband/rope.

Chapter 7: Physiotherapy for Hip

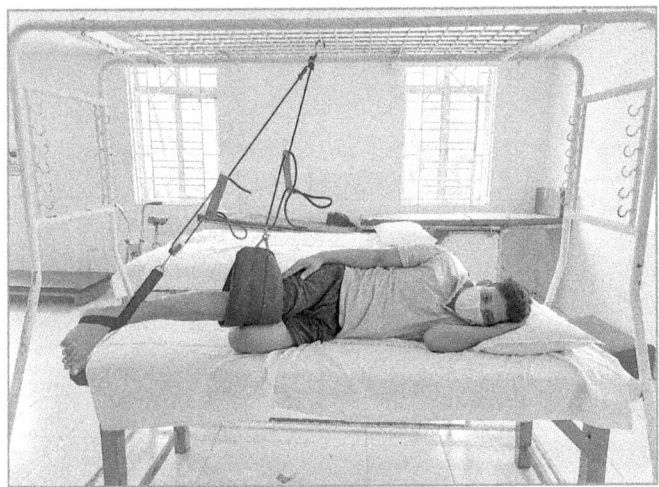

Fig. 7.36: Suspension therapy for hip flexion.

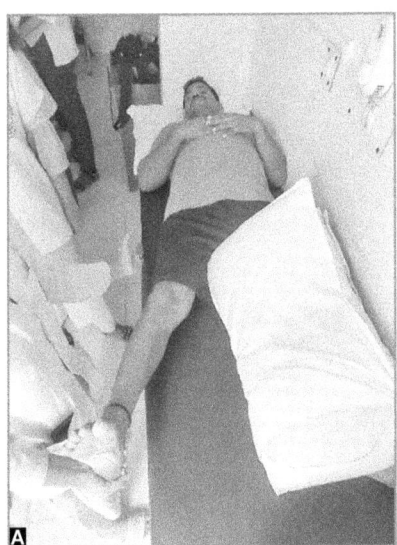

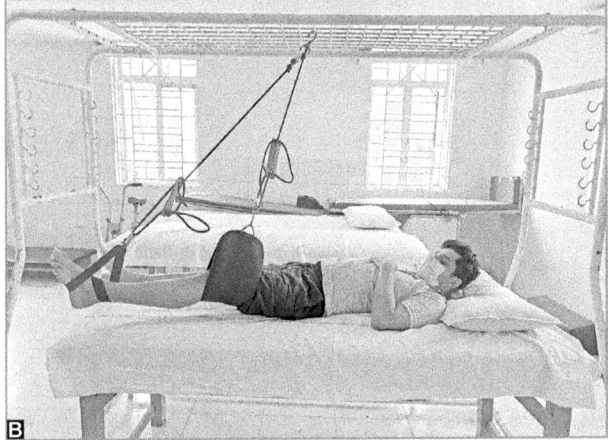

Figs. 7.37A and B: (A) Assisted hip abduction exercise, (B) Suspension therapy for hip abduction.

- Strengthening of TFL to enhance stability of the hip, by reinforcing gluteus maximus through the IT band is emphasized.
- Independent turning on bed over the sound side with a pillow between the thighs is promoted.

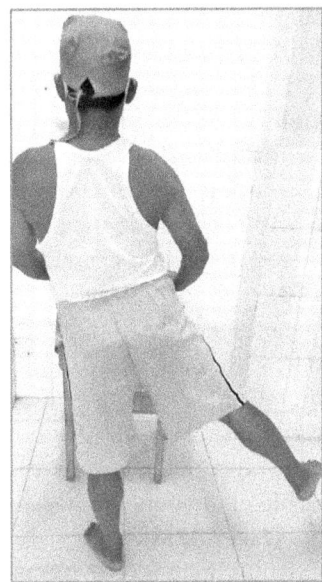

Fig. 7.38: Hip abduction in standing.

- Independent transfer from bed to wheel chair/chair and chair to parallel bar/walker is emphasized.
C. **Week 3-6:** All the exercises the patient was performing before are gradually progressed, in addition to the followings:
   - Partial weight-bearing ambulation is continued.
   - Static cycle exercises, stair climbing are added by about 4 weeks. For stair climbing, the patient is given an axillary crutch on the affected side and made to climb stair up with sound leg first, followed by the affected leg. While descending the stair, the affected leg is lowered first, followed by the sound leg.
D. **Week 6-8:** The following exercises and activities are advised after 6-8 weeks. The Surgeon and therapist decides, whether weight-bearing restrictions are to be fully withdrawn, or patient should be allowed to use a walking stick on the contralateral side. The exercises advised are:
   - Auto mobilization exercises, such as supine heel drag (**Fig. 7.39**).

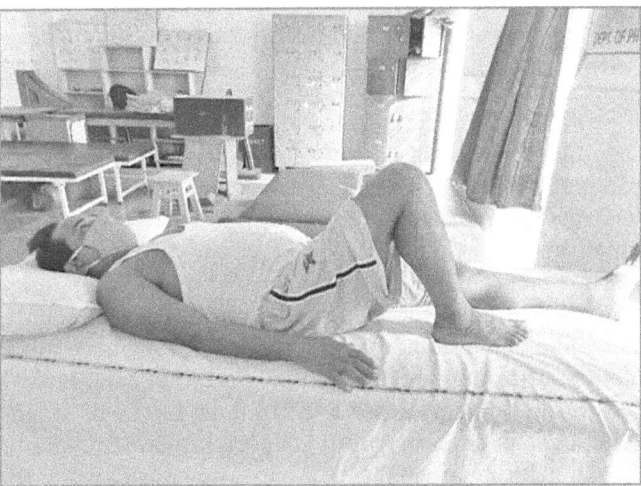

Fig. 7.39: Supine heel drag exercise.

- Strengthening and endurance exercises such as:
  » Pelvic bridging exercises, bilateral, followed by unilateral.
  » Clam shell exercise: Lying over the sound side, affected foot over the sound foot. The patient is asked to open the affected knee as much as possible, without rotating the thigh outwards. This is progressed to resisted exercise with therabands **(Fig. 7.17B)**.
  » Sitting on bed/chair. Performing hip flexion without followed by with resistance.
- Resisted hip abduction (with pillow between the thighs), knee extension and ankle plantar flexion **(Figs. 7.40A to C)**, with gentle hip rotation in supine is started.
  » Standing hip abduction with resistance applied by theraband **(Fig. 7.41)**.
  » Partial squatting holding on to support, with both feet on floor **(Fig. 7.42)** followed by affected foot on floor and sound foot off the floor.
  » Marching on floor in supported standing.
  » Crab walking: Standing feet shoulder distance apart, with hip and knees slightly flexed and a crepe bandage/ theraband applied to thighs. Maintaining the squat position, the patient is asked to take side steps on each foot and bring feet back, without adducting thighs **(Fig. 7.43)**.
  » Supine- hip flexor stretch **(Fig. 7.44)** sitting-hamstring stretch, standing-hip adductor stretch, standing-trunk lateral flexor stretch, etc., are practiced.
  » Balance/co-ordination and proprioceptive training is given.
  » Gradually returned to function and driving and is able to walk independently or with a walking stick, if required by about 12 weeks.

n. Legg-Calve-Perthes Disease

Legg–Calve-Perthes disease is an idiopathic juvenile AVN of the head of the femur found in children. This disease was first described by Legg-Calve and Perthes, hence the name Legg-Calve Perthes disease.

Etiology/Epidemiology

Legg-Calve Perthes disease affects children between the age group of 7–14 years. The incidence is between 4 and 32 per 100,000 children. Males are affected more than females with a male to female ratio of 5:1.

The exact cause of the disease is not known (idiopathic). However, some of the factors thought as causes include: congenital, environmental, traumatic, and socioeconomic factors. Thrombosis, fibrinolysis, and abnormal growth patterns of bone, repeated microtrauma, low birth weight, genetic factor such as type-II collagen mutation, maternal smoking during pregnancy, etc., are also considered as the causes of this disease.

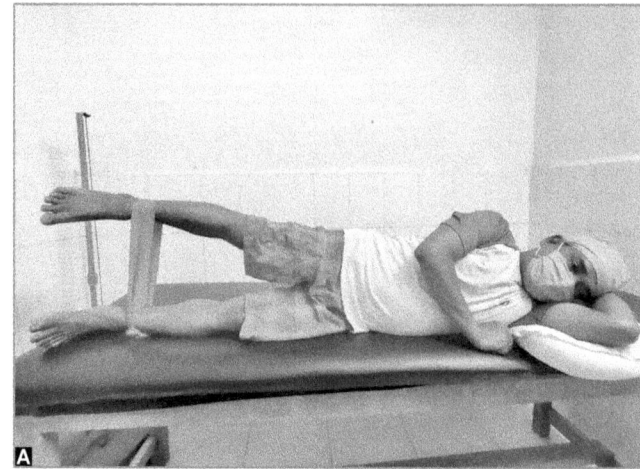

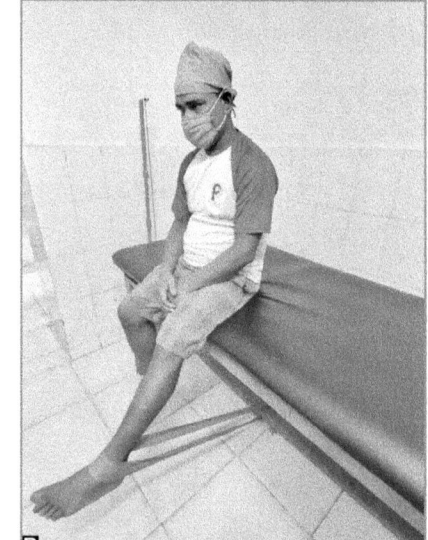

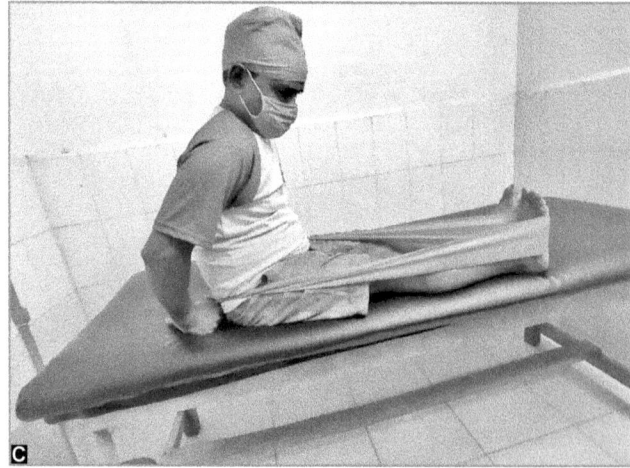

Figs. 7.40A to C: (A) Resisted hip abduction exercise, (B) Resisted knee extension exercise, (C) Resisted ankle plantar flexion exercise.

Pathogenesis

Disruption of blood flow through the medial and lateral circumflex arteries that supply the capital femoral epiphysis and head of femur, result in ischemic necrosis of the femoral head, which results in cessation of endochondral ossification and decreased mechanical strength of the head

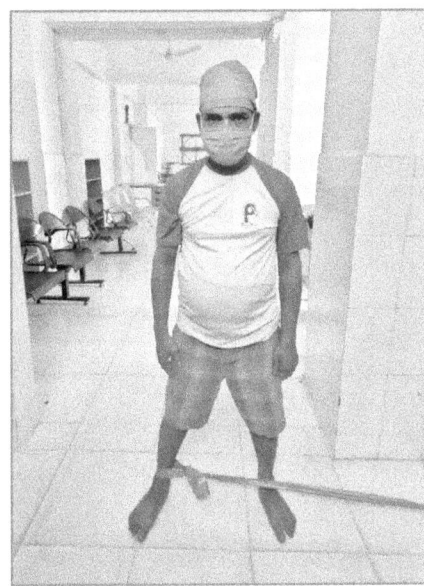

Fig. 7.41: Resisted hip abduction in standing.

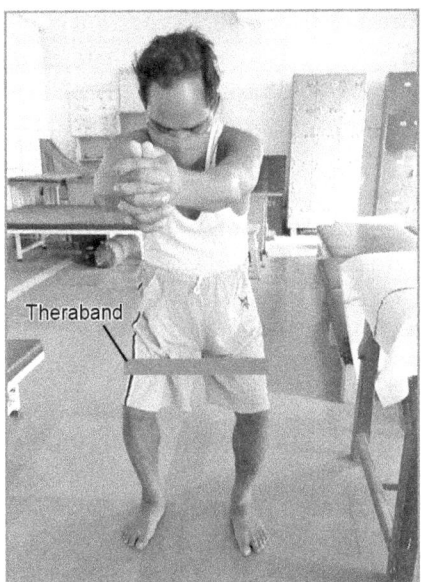

Fig. 7.43: The crab walking.

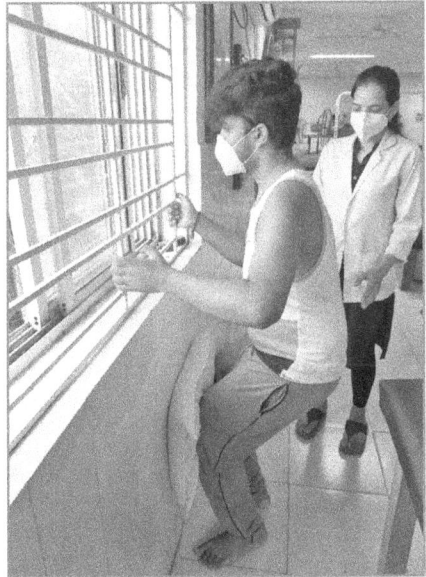

Fig. 7.42: Partial squatting, holding on to support.

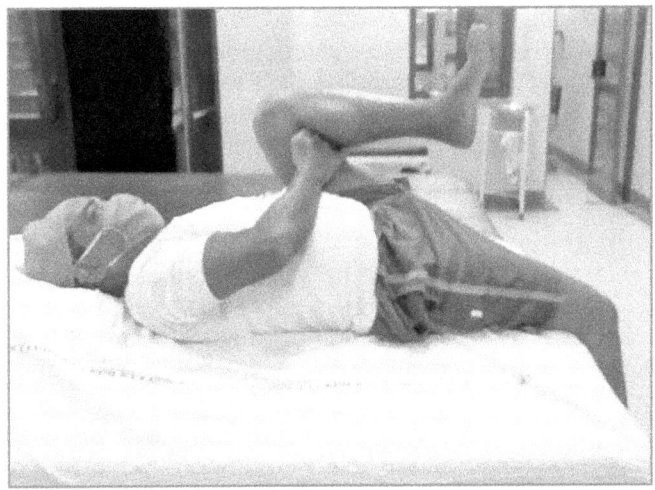

Fig. 7.44: Supine hip flexor stretching exercise by self.

of femur. The femoral head becomes soft and necrotic. The femoral head when stressed due to weight-bearing, gets deformed. Even though, the head of femur revascularizes and hardens after some days, it never regains the normal shape, if deformed.

The hip assumes flexion, abduction, and lateral rotation, due to distension of joint capsule following synovitis.

Clinical Feature

As already stated before, the disease is more common in boys as compared to girls, within the age group of 7–14 years, with an average age of onset of 6 years. The features typical to the disease are:

- The hip assumes flexion abduction and lateral rotation, leading to flexion deformity of hip (if not treated).
- **Pain:** During the acute stage of the disease, the child suffers from significant pain, which is more while walking and during night hours.
- **Limp:** The child shows marked limping during late hours in the day, after a period of prolonged walking.
- The child shows a decrease of ROM of hip, particularly abduction and internal rotation during early phase of the disease.

Diagnosis

The child who developed normal walking, but started to limp after 2 years of age attracts attention of parents/clinician toward Perthe's disease. The disease is confirmed by X-ray examination, which progresses through four stages. Catterall Classification, which differentiated the hips into four groups/stages based on radiographic appearance of the femoral epiphysis, is discussed below:

- **Stage I/Grade I-Initial phase**: Avascular necrosis leads to formation of cyst on the anterolateral aspect of the femoral capital epiphysis **(Fig. 7.45)**. The condition is benign requiring only symptomatic treatment.
- **Stage II/Grade II-Fragmentation/resorption stage**: Involvement of about half of portion of femoral capital epiphysis **(Fig. 7.46)**. The condition is benign requiring only symptomatic treatment.
- **Stage III/Grade III**: Most of the femoral capital epiphysis (nearly 3/4 of head of femur) is involved **(Fig. 7.47)**. There is extensive head involvement resulting in less favorable outcome.
- **Stage IV/Grade IV**: Extensive femoral head involvement with less favorable outcome, i.e., complete involvement of femoral capital epiphysis **(Fig. 7.48)**.

Management

The management of the disease can be made conservatively or surgically (if conservative management fails or the patient reports in the late stage (stage III/IV). The management schedule includes:
- NSAIDS to reduce pain and inflammation.
- Skin traction to immobilize the joint in the early stage when the joint is irritable and painful. Weight bearing on the affected limb should not be allowed. If the disease progresses to grade III/IV, the following procedures may be followed.

In grade III/IV, when the head is not deformed, containment of the femoral head in acetabulum is achieved by keeping the hip in abduction by POP cast/weight relieving orthosis (trilateral hip abduction orthosis) **(Fig. 7.49)**, or varus osteotomy of the proximal femur/ osteotomy of pelvis.

When head of femur is deformed, containment of the head in acetabulum is not possible, resulting in development of

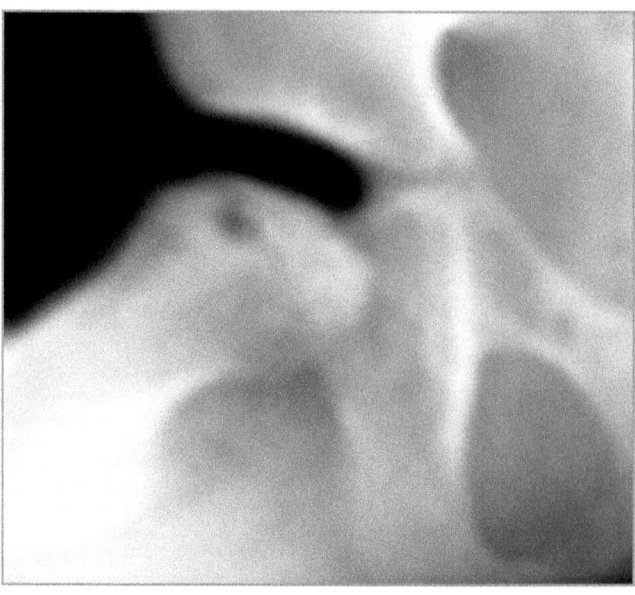

Fig. 7.46: X-ray of stage II.

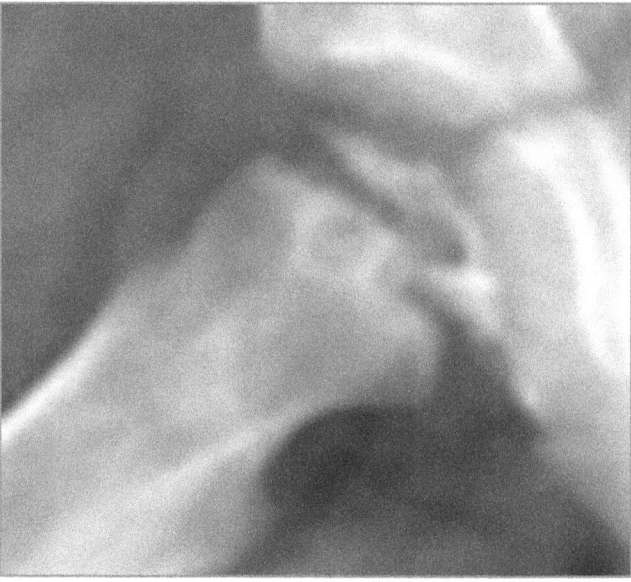

Fig. 7.47: X-ray of stage III.

hip osteoarthritis. It should be managed accordingly with hip replacement arthroplasty in a later age.

Physiotherapy

Physiotherapy is part of management of the child, whether the child is managed with simple bed rest, skin traction/ skeletal traction, or orthosis. The physiotherapy strategies include:
- Isometric exercises to the hip abductors, extensors and quadriceps hamstrings on the affected side should be performed during periods of immobilization with traction, combined with active ankle and foot exercises.
- Relaxed passive exercises/active-assisted exercises to the affected hip should be given as pain allows improving nutrition and maintain joint ROM. Full range of movement of hip extension, abduction and internal rotation is emphasized.

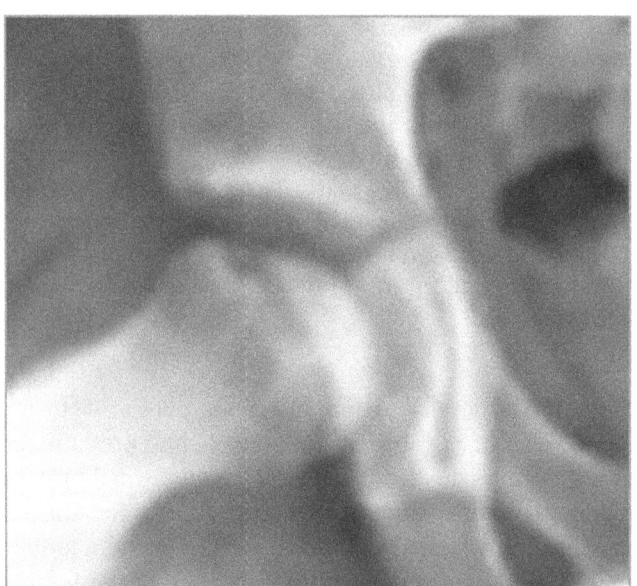

Fig. 7.45: X-ray of stage I.

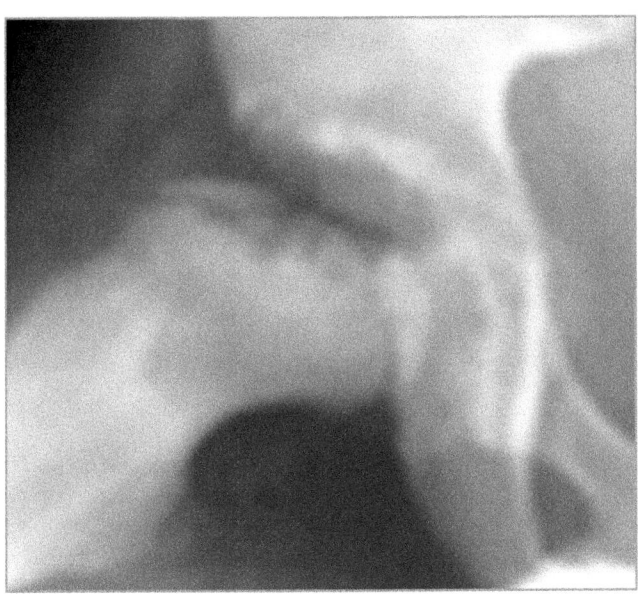

Fig. 7.48: X-ray of stage IV.

- Gentle stretching of muscles of the involved hip to prevent T/C/D. Frequent sessions of assisted prone lying helps in prevention of hip flexion deformity.
- Strengthening the muscles of the involved hip for the flexion, extension, abduction, and adduction. Exercises are started with isometric exercises progressing gradually to dynamic exercises (concentric and eccentric exercises).
- Ambulation training should be given initially in nonweight-bearing manner using trilateral hip abduction orthosis **(Fig. 7.49)**, progressing to partial weight bearing with walker/crutches as applicable.
- Hydrotherapy.
- Pain modulation with IFT/TENS.

For children over 6 years at diagnosis with more than 50% of femoral head necrosis, proximal femoral varus osteotomy gives a significantly better outcome than orthosis and physiotherapy. After surgery, the hip is immobilized in a hip spica for 6 weeks followed by physiotherapy.

Postoperative physiotherapy to mobilize the hip and knee, strengthening the muscles of hip are emphasized. Nonweight-bearing gait progressing to partial weight-bearing ambulation with walker/crutches are emphasized. Pain (if any) is managed by IFT/TENS.

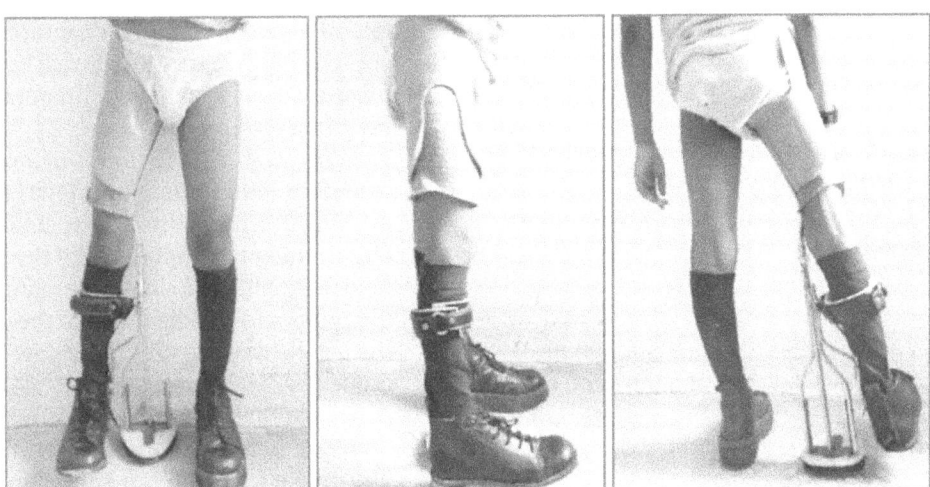

Fig. 7.49: The trilateral hip abduction orthosis.

Knee Joint

KNEE JOINT

The knee joint is composed of two distinct articulations, such as tibiofemoral joint and patellofemoral joint enclosed within a single joint capsule.

Osteokinematics of Knee Joint

The tibiofemoral joint is a synovial double condyloid/modified hinged joint having 2 degrees of freedom. Flexion-extension occurs around a medial-lateral axis in the sagittal plane. Rotation occurs in the transverse plane around the vertical/longitudinal axis.

Ranges of motion of knee joint are given in **Table 8.1**.

Arthrokinematics of Knee Joint

In nonweight-bearing position:
- During flexion, the tibial condyles slide posteriorly on the femoral condyles.
- During extension from full flexion, the tibial condyles slide anteriorly over the femoral condyles.
- The patella slides superiorly during extension, and inferiorly during flexion.

Capsular Pattern

The capsular pattern of knee is greater limitation of flexion, lesser limitation of extension, and no limitation of rotation.

Special Tests for Knee Joint

- **Tests for effusion in knee:** The knee joint undergoes effusion (**Fig. 8.1**) in trauma, infection, and arthritis, affecting movement and function. The tests for effusion are:
  - *Bulge test:* The examiner gently presses the medial aspect of the patella, and then moves the hand in an ascending motion. Then he/she presses firmly on the lateral aspect of patella. Commonly no fluid will be appreciated. A medial aspect that bulges out after lateral pressure is consistent with moderate amount of fluid, revealing positive bulge sign.
  - *Patellar tap:* This is done for large effusions. The examiner slides one hand down the patient's thigh, pushing down over the suprapatellar pouch (**Fig. 8.2**). On reaching the upper pole of the patella, the hand is held there with maintained pressure. The examiner uses the index and middle finger of the other hand, to push the patella down gently. If the patella bounces, the test is positive.
- **Tests for patellar instability:**
  - *Measurement of Q-angle:* It is the angle between a line drawn from anterior superior iliac spine (ASIS) to

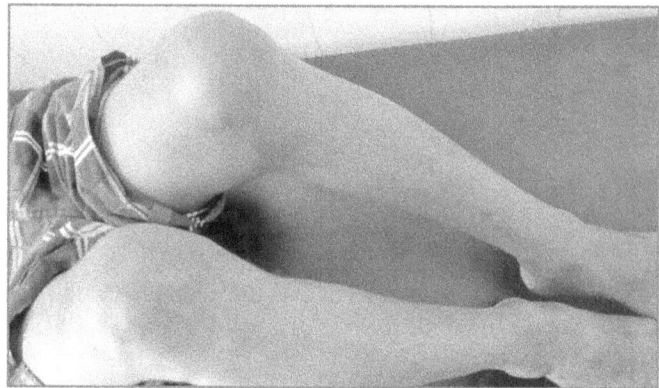

Fig. 8.1: Knee effusion.

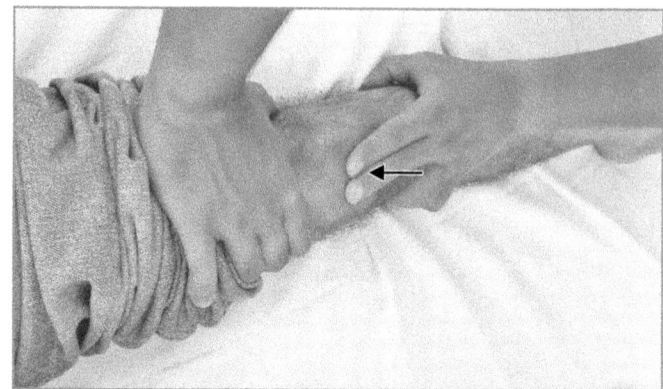

Fig. 8.2: The patellar tap test.

Table 8.1: Ranges of motion.

Movement	Range of motion
Flexion	0–130 to 140 degrees
Hyperextension	5–10 degrees
Rotation at 90 degrees of knee flexion	Lateral rotation –45 degrees Medial rotation –15 degrees

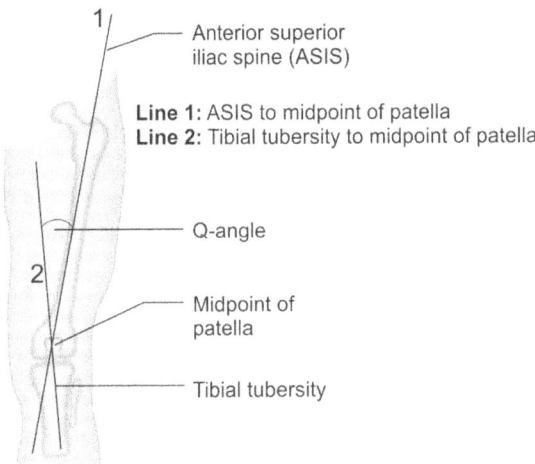

Fig. 8.3: Measurement of Q-angle.

center of patella to a line drawn from center of patella to tibial tuberosity **(Fig. 8.3)**. For males this angle is 8–10 degrees, and in females the value is 15 ± 5 degrees.

- *Apprehension test for patella:* The patient in supine lying, the knee is flexed by 20–30 degrees and supported on examiner's lap/pillow. The examiner laterally subluxates the patella manually **(Fig. 8.4)**. Pain and resistance to the lateral motion of patella is a positive apprehension test.

❖ **Tests for meniscus injury:**
  - *Joint line tenderness:* Tenderness over medial joint line of knee suggests injury to medial meniscus, and tenderness over lateral joint line **(Fig. 8.5)** of knee suggests injury to lateral meniscus.
  - *McMurray test:*
    » For medial meniscus: The examiner quickly flexes the knee, palpates the posteromedial margin of the knee joint, rotates the knee externally, and quickly extends the knee **(Fig. 8.6)**. A palpable click and/or pain is suggestive of injury to medial meniscus.
    » For lateral meniscus: The examiner quickly flexes the knee, palpates the posterolateral margin of the knee joint, rotates the knee internally, and quickly extends

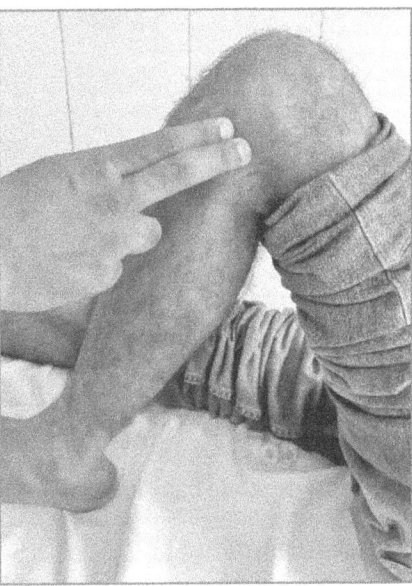

Fig. 8.5: Eliciting joint line tenderness.

the knee. A palpable click and/or pain is suggestive of injury to lateral meniscus.
  » Apley's grinding test: This test named after Alan Graham Apley, British Orthopedic surgeon. It is used for individuals with a problem in the meniscus of knee. The test is performed with patient in prone lying, knee flexed to 90 degrees. The leg is rotated medially (for lateral meniscus) and laterally (for medial meniscus) by the examiner **(Fig. 8.7)**. First a distraction force is applied, and then a compressive force is applied to the knee, from tibia. If rotation and distraction is more painful, the fault lies with the ligaments of the knee. However, if rotation combined with compression produces pain in the knee the fault lies with the meniscus.

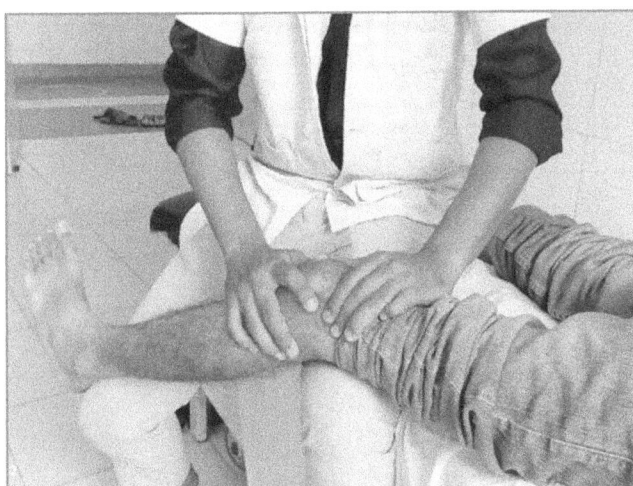

Fig. 8.4: Apprehension test for patella.

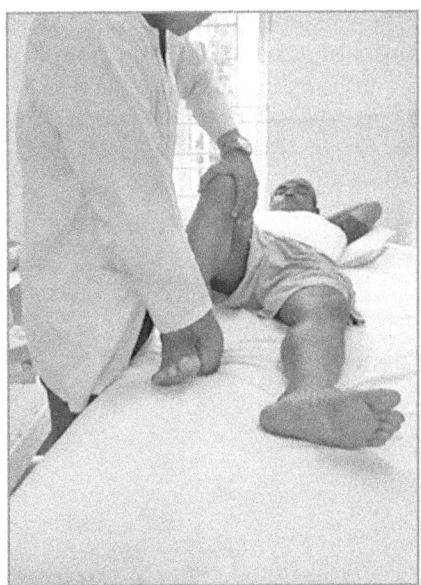

Fig. 8.6: McMurray test for medial meniscus.

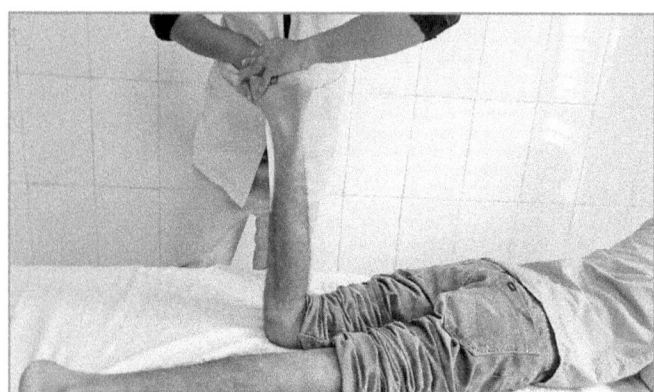

Fig. 8.7: Apley's grinding test.

- **Tests for anterior cruciate ligament (ACL) injury:**
    - *Anterior drawer test:* The patient in supine on a plinth, with the affected hip flexed to 45 degrees with the knee flexed to 90 degrees and the foot is flat on the bed. The examiner attempts to translate the tibia anteriorly, by holding the upper leg just below the tibial plateau. The test is considered positive, if there is excessive anterior translation of tibia relative to the contra lateral side **(Fig. 8.8)**.
    - *Lachman test:* The patient supine, knee in 15 degree flexion. The examiner places one hand behind the tibia with the thumb on tibial tuberosity, and the other hand grasps the thigh **(Fig. 8.9)**. The tibia is pulled forward to assess the amount of anterior motion of tibia over the femur. An intact ACL prevents forward translation of tibia, where as, in ACL deficient knee, there is increased forward translation of tibia.
    - *Pivot shift test:* The patient lies supine with the legs relaxed. The affected hip is passively flexed to 30 degrees, and abducted to relax the iliotibial (IT) band. The examiner grasps the heel of the involved leg with one hand, and the proximal tibia at the level of the superior tibiofibular joint, below the knee with the other hand. The examiner then applies a valgus stress and an axial load, while internally rotating the tibia as the knee moves into flexion from fully extended position **(Fig. 8.10)**. A positive test is indicated by subluxation of tibia while the femur rotates externally, followed by reduction of tibia at 30–40 degrees of flexion. A positive test is an indication of tear of ACL.

- **Tests for posterior cruciate ligament injury:**
    - *Sag sign/Godfrey test:* Patient supine, knee flexed to 90 degrees, heel supported by the examiner. If tibia sags visibly posteriorly, as compared to the other side, the test is positive, suggesting laxity of PCL **(Fig. 8.11)**.

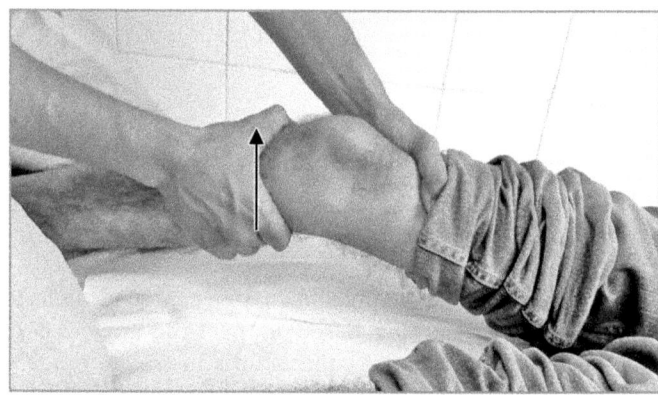

Fig. 8.9: The Lachman test.

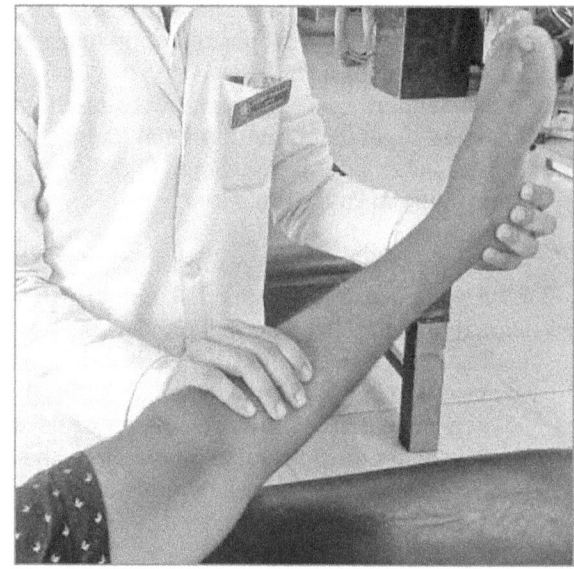

Fig. 8.10: The pivot shift test.

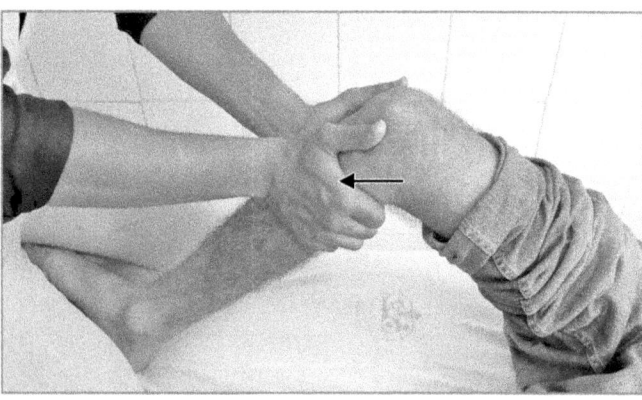

Fig. 8.8: Anterior drawer test.

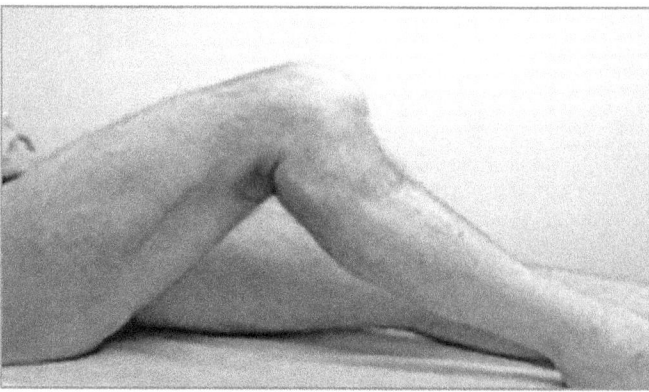

Fig. 8.11: Sag sign.

Chapter 8: Knee Joint

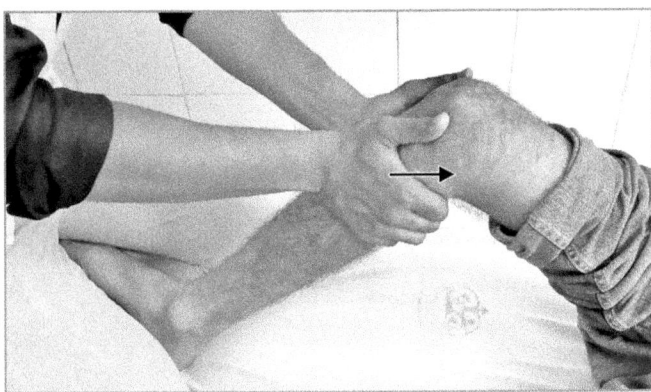

Fig. 8.12: The posterior drawer test.

- *Posterior drawer test:* The patient is supine. The affected knee flexed to 90 degrees and foot flat on bed. The examiner stabilizes the tested extremity by sitting over the foot lying flat on bed. The examiner, while holding the proximal leg at the tibial plateau or joint line, attempts to translate the tibia posteriorly **(Fig. 8.12)**. The test is positive, if there is lack of end feel or excessive posterior translation of tibia.
- *Quadriceps Active test/Muller test:* This test is used to find posterior cruciate ligament (PCL) disruptions and posterior knee laxity.
  The test is performed with the patient supine, knee flexed to 90 degrees, and foot flat on the bed **(Fig. 8.13)**. The patient is asked to raise his/ her foot off the table. A positive test reveals posterior sag of proximal tibia initially, and anterior translation of the proximal tibia prior to the foot leaving the table with attempted elevation of foot. This anterior translation could be quantified and compared to the opposite knee.

❖ **Tests for medial and lateral collateral ligament injury:**
- *Valgus stress test [for medial collateral ligament (MCL) injury]:* The patient in supine, knee flexed to about 30 degrees. The examiner, stabilizes the lower thigh by placing hand over the lateral aspect of thigh, and applies a valgus force to knee by holding the lower leg/ankle of the affected limb with the other hand **(Fig. 8.14A)**. In case of MCL tear, the joint will open up in the medial side.
- *Swain test:* The Swain test is performed with the knee flexed to 90° and the tibia externally rotated. When the tibia is externally rotated in flexion, the collateral ligaments are tightened while the cruciate are relatively lax. If there is tearing of MCL, the external rotation range will increase **(Fig. 8.14B)**.
- *Varus stress test (for lateral collateral ligament injury):* The patient in supine. Affected knee is flexed to 20-30 degrees. The examiner stabilizes the thigh by holding the medial aspect of thigh with one hand. A varus force is applied to the knee by holding the lower leg/ankle with the other hand **(Fig. 8.15)**. If the knee adducts excessively/excessive opening of lateral aspect of the knee, the test is considered positive.

❖ **Test for anterior rotator instability of knee:**
- *Slocum's test:* The Slocum's test, which is a modification of Anterior Drawer test, is used to find anteromedial and anterolateral rotator instability of the knee.
  The patient is in supine with the knee flexed to 90 degrees and foot stabilized to the examination table by the examiner. The examiner applies 30 degrees of internal rotation to the tibia by rotating the foot. The tibia is pulled anteriorly along with the medial rotation

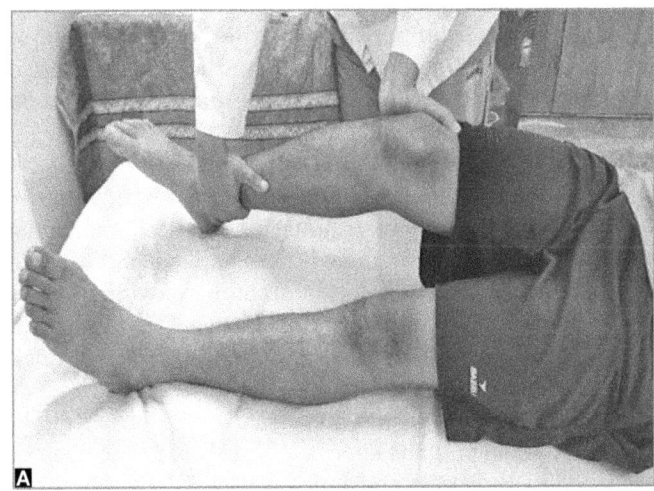

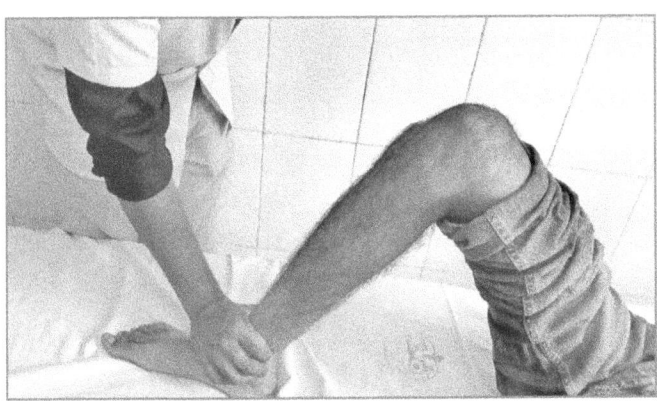

Fig. 8.13: Quadriceps active test-Muller's test.

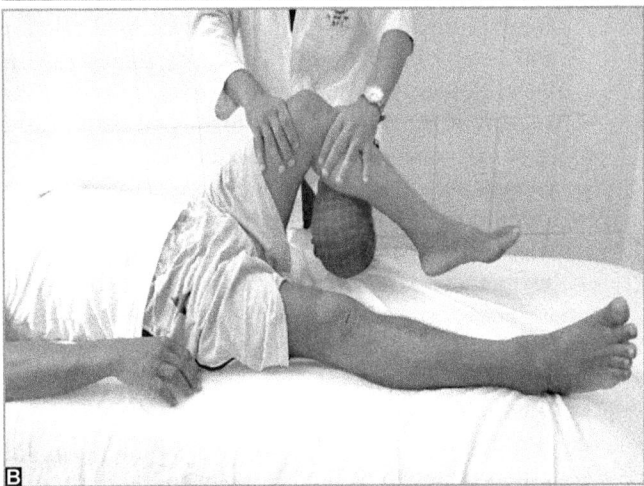

Figs. 8.14A and B: (A) The Valgus stress test. (B) The Swain test.

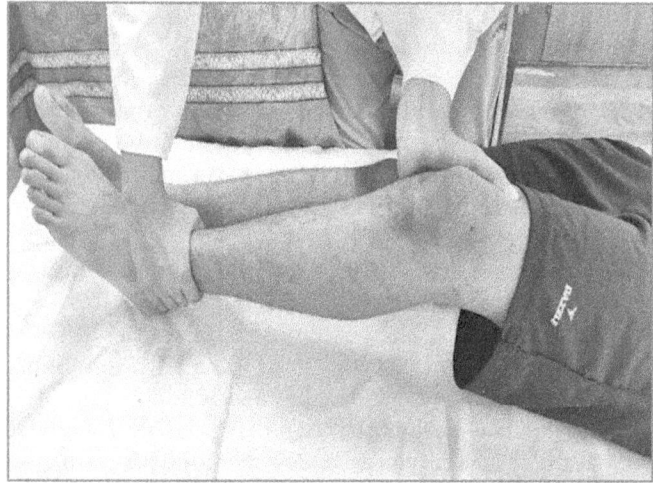

Fig. 8.15: Varus stress test for knee.

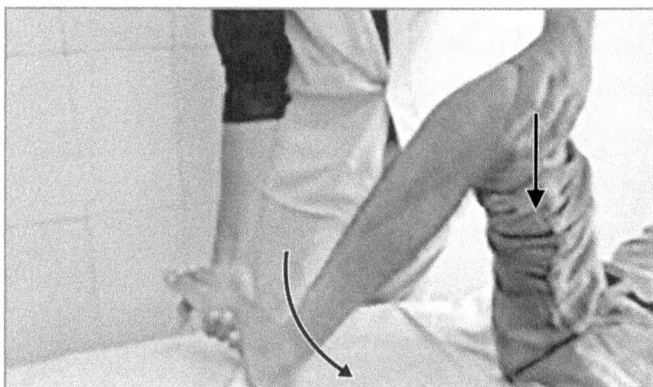

Fig. 8.16: The Hughston's Plica test.

to asses for anterolateral instability. The test is positive, if there is increased amount of tibial anterior translation with tibial internal rotation, indicating ACL deficiency.

- ❖ **Test for posterolateral knee instability:**
  - *Dial test:* This test is performed to diagnose posterolateral knee instability, as well as to differentiate between isolated posterolateral corner (PLC), and combination of PLC with PCL injury.

    The test can be performed either in prone lying or supine lying. The goal of the test is to inspect the external rotation at the knee joint, while the knees are in 30 degrees and 90 degrees flexion.
    » Test in prone lying: The clinician flexes the patient's knee to 30 degrees and place both hands on the feet of the patient, cupping his/her heel. A maximal external rotation force is then applied, and the foot thigh angle is measured and compared with the other side. The knee is now flexed to 90 degrees and again external rotation force is applied, and the foot thigh angle is measured.
    » Test in supine lying: The test can be performed either holding both the knees together flexed at 30 degrees and 90 degrees and applying external rotation to the knees and measuring the angle of external rotation and comparing the range of external rotation of the tested knee with the normal knee, or flexing the knee by 30 degrees over the side of bed, rotating the knee externally, followed by external rotation of the knee flexed by 90 degrees in the same position. The amount of external rotation found in the affected knees is compared with the sound knee.

    If the tibia rotates less at 90 degrees, than at 30 degrees, an isolated posterolateral column injury is more likely. If the knee rotates more at 90 degrees, injury is expected in both posterolateral column and PCL.

- ❖ **Tests for Plica syndrome:**
  - *Hughston's Plica test:* The patient in supine lying. The examiner flexes the knee with medial rotation of tibia and pushes the patella medially with the heel of the hand. He/she then palpates the region of the knee medial to the patella **(Fig. 8.16)**.

    A positive test is feeling/ hearing of snapping or popping sound, while flexing and extending the knee.
  - *Plica Stutter test:* The patient sits at the edge of the examination table with both knees flexed to 90 degrees. The examiner places one finger over the patella for palpation during movement. The patient is then instructed to slowly extend and flex the knee **(Fig. 8.17)**. The test is positive, if the patella stutters/ jumps somewhere between 60 and 45 degrees of flexion.

    The test is effective only if there is no joint swelling.

The disorders affecting knee include:

i. Chondromalacia Patella

Chondromalacia patella is also called as the disorder of anterior knee pain due to physical and biomechanical changes occurring over the under surface of patella, as a result of degenerative changes to the articular cartilage of the posterior surface of the patella.

There develops softening, swelling, fraying, and erosion of the hyaline cartilage underlying the patella and sclerosis of the underlying bone. This is one of the most commonly encountered disorders of knee pain among young people.

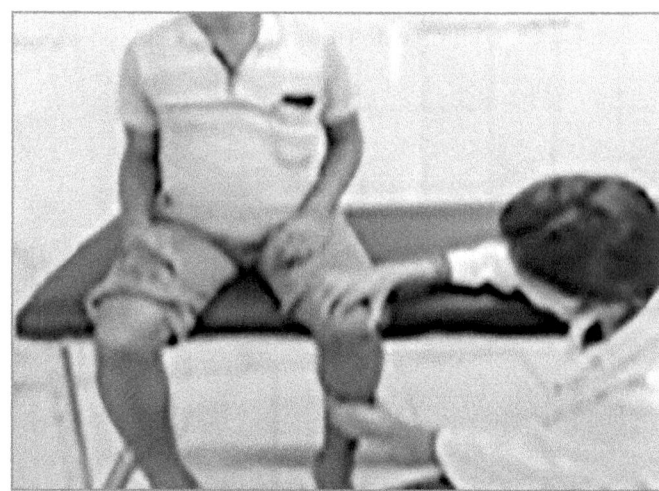

Fig. 8.17: The Plica Stutter test.

Epidemiology/etiology

Chondromalacia is common in adolescent females, though, idiopathic chondromalacia is usually seen in young children and degenerative type of the disorder is most common in the middle-aged and older population.

The etiology of chondromalacia patella is poorly understood. However, the following factors can be considered as the cause of this disorder:
- Trauma to chondrocytes in the articular cartilage under the patella.
- Instability or maltracking of the patella, which softens the articular cartilage.
- Mal alignment of the femur to the patella and tibia resulting in over load injury: Main reasons for patellar malalignment are:
  - Abnormal Q-angle: Q-angle greater than 14 degrees in males and 17 degrees in females, results in increase lateral pull on the patella.
  - Tightness of rectus femoris (affecting patellar movement during knee flexion), Tensor fascia lata (produces tightness of IT band), Hamstrings (causing increased knee flexion), Gastrocnemius (causing compensatory pronation of subtalar joint).
  - Excessive foot pronation, results in internal rotation of leg and mal alignment of patella.
  - Patella alta: The abnormal higher placement of the patella also results in damage to the articular cartilage under the patella.
  - Quadriceps [vastus medialis oblique (VMO)] weakness: The VMO, that stabilizes patella centrally during knee extension, when weaker leads to lateral displacement of patella, as muscular imbalance develops between vastus lateralis and VMO.

Pathology

Chondromalacia patella is a softening of the articular cartilage on the posterior surface of the patella, which may eventually lead to fibrillation, fissuring, and erosion of articular cartilage. In the early stages, chondromalacia shows areas of high sensitivity on fluid sequences. This can be associated with the increased thickness of the cartilage and may also cause edema. In the latter stages, there will be a more irregular surface with focal thinning that can expand to and expose the subchondral bone. The pathological process proceeds through the following four stages:
- **Stage 1:** Softening and swelling of the articular cartilage due to broken vertical collagenous fibers.
- **Stage 2:** Blister formation in the articular cartilage due to the separation of the superficial from the deep cartilaginous layers.
- **Stage 3:** Fissures ulceration, fragmentation, and fibrillation of cartilage extending to the subchondral bone but affecting less than 50% of the patellar articular surface.
- **Stage 4:** Crater formation and eburnation of the exposed subchondral bone more than 50% of the patellar articular surface exposed, with sclerosis and erosions of the subchondral bone. Osteophyte formation also occurs at this stage.

As the articular cartilage does not have free nerve endings, the pain in this condition does not arise from the cartilage. The pain usually arises from the inflammatory reactions under the patella and subchondral bone damage.

Clinical Features

Patients affected by chondromalacia patella are usually young females between the age of 15 and 35 years. Though they remain active, very often symptoms of aching pain behind the patella, recurrent effusion of the knee, knee instability, and crepitus, affect their function significantly. The main symptom of chondromalacia patella is anterior knee pain, which is exacerbated by common daily activities that load the patellofemoral joint, such as squatting, running, cycling, stair climbing, kneeling, etc. The pain in the knee is also felt in activities such as sitting to standing. The pain often causes disability affecting short-term participation in daily and physical activities. Other features such as tenderness under the medial and lateral border of patella, crepitation on knee movements, minor swelling in knee, a weak VMO, and an increased Q-angle. A significant number of individuals are asymptomatic, but complain of crepitus in knee on movements.

Pain and crepitus will be felt, if the patella is compressed against the femur, either vertically or horizontally, with the knee in full extension. Tenderness of one or other margin of patella may be elicited and more frequently the tenderness is felt medially. Resisting a static quadriceps contraction will generally produce a sharp pain under the patella.

Differential diagnosis

Chondromalacia patella should be differentiated from other conditions causing knee pain such as osteoarthritis, rheumatoid arthritis, patellofemoral pain syndrome, subluxation of patella, etc.

Diagnostic procedures

Though the diagnosis of chondromalacia patella is difficult; clinical tests, X-ray **(Fig. 8.18)**, arthrography, and MRI are useful in establishing the diagnosis.

Special tests

- **Patellar grinding test or Clarke's sign:** Patient is positioned in supine or long sitting with the involved knee extended. The examiner places the web space of his hand just superior to the patella while applying

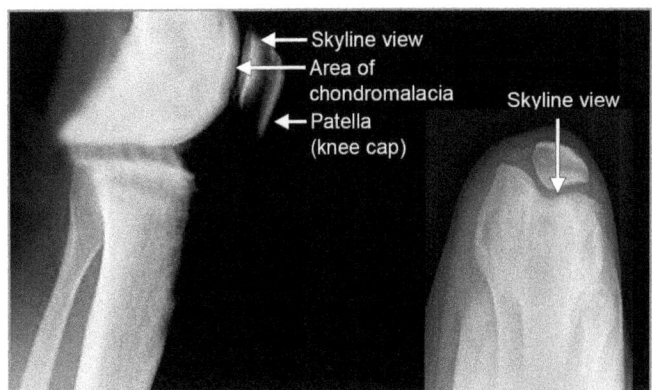

Fig. 8.18: X-ray showing chondromalacia patella (skyline view).

pressure or directly applies pressure over the patella. The patient is instructed to gently and gradually contract the quadriceps muscle. A positive sign on this test is pain in the patellofemoral joint. This test detects the presence of patellofemoral joint disorder.

* **Extension-resistance test:** This test is used to perform a maximal provocation on the muscle-tendon mechanism of the extensor muscles and is positive when the affected knee demonstrates less power when trying to maintain the pressure against resistance.
* **McConnell's test:** The patient is made to sit with legs hanging over the end of the table. The clinician sits in front of the client and instructs patient to externally rotate the femur of the affected leg while performing active resisted isometric contractions of the quadriceps muscles at 0, 30, 60, 90, and 120 degrees of flexion and notes the range at which pain is felt.

Then, the clinician passively brings the patient's knee to full extension, resting the heel on a small pillow, so that, the quadriceps muscle is relaxed. He/she then glides the affected patella medially and holds the patella in that position. The patient is again instructed to produce isometric contraction to quadriceps at the knee ranges that were painful before. If pain decreases significantly, after holding patella medially, it indicates patellofemoral lateral tracking problems.

Like the previous maneuver, the clinician now glides patella laterally and make the patient produce isometric contraction of quadriceps at the knee ranges that were painful before. If pain decreases significantly, after holding patella laterally, it indicates patellofemoral medial tracking problems.

Management:

* **Conservative management:** PRICE (Protection, rest, ice application, compression, and elevation) is the choice of treatment in the acute stage. NSAIDs prescribed by the physician/surgeon helps in reducing inflammation and pain. A patellar-alignment brace **(Fig. 8.19)** helps to maintain patellar alignment. McConnell taping/Kinesio taping is helpful in some cases.

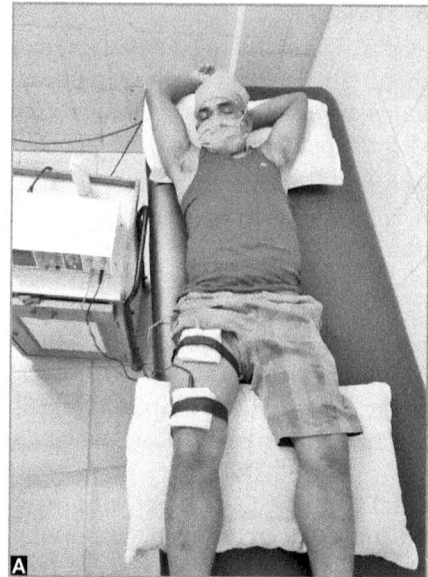
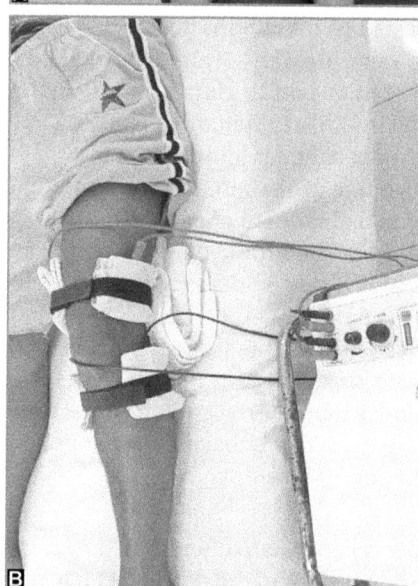

Figs. 8.20A and B: (A) Strong faradic stimulation to quadriceps, (B) IFT to knee joint.

Physiotherapy: It consists of exercises and application of modalities.

Modalities: Cryotherapy/low intensity laser therapy/pulsed ultrasound/Interferential therapy (IFT), etc., can be considered in the acute stage to reduce pain and inflammation. In chronic states, SWD/MWD/Strong-surged faradic stimulation **(Fig. 8.20A)**/IFT **(Fig. 8.20B)**, etc., are selected to improve blood flow, reduce pain and strengthen quadriceps muscle.

Exercises

* Restoration of adequate strength of quadriceps is essential for achieving good recovery. Isometric quadriceps sets/resisted-SLR exercises **(Figs. 8.21A and B)** are performed initially, followed by dynamic exercises to quadriceps in the inner range. Stretching of vastus lateralis and strengthening of vastus medialis is the

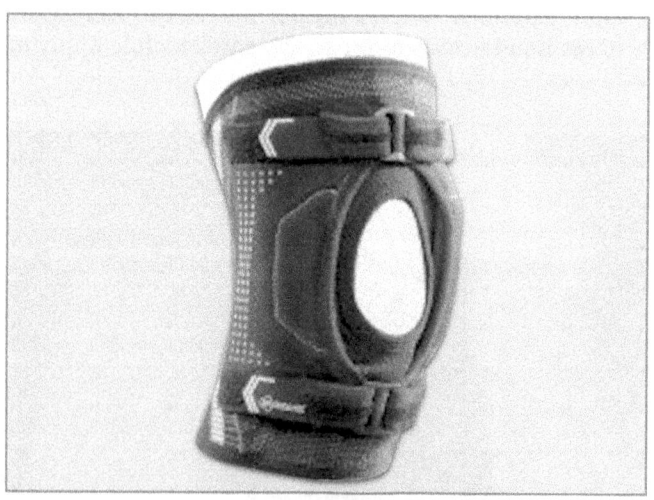

Fig. 8.19: Patellar alignment brace.

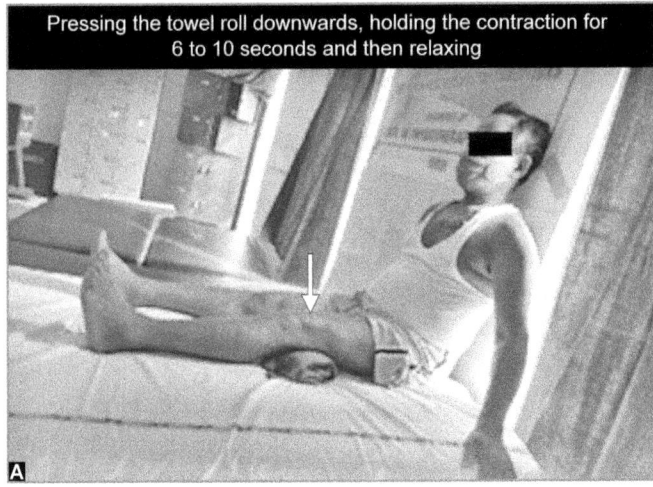

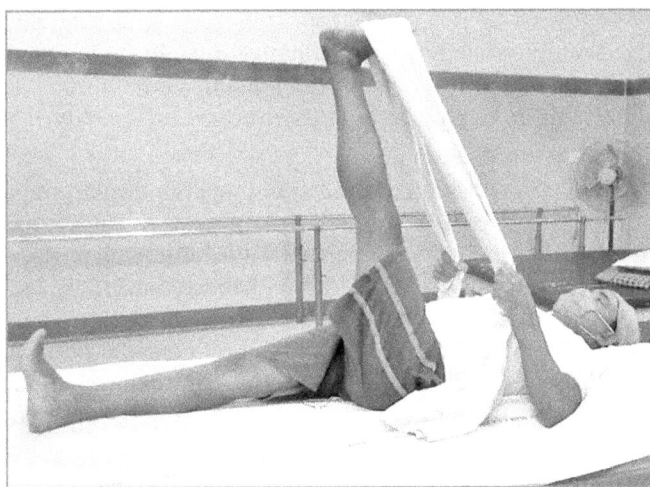

Fig. 8.22: Hamstring stretching by the patient.

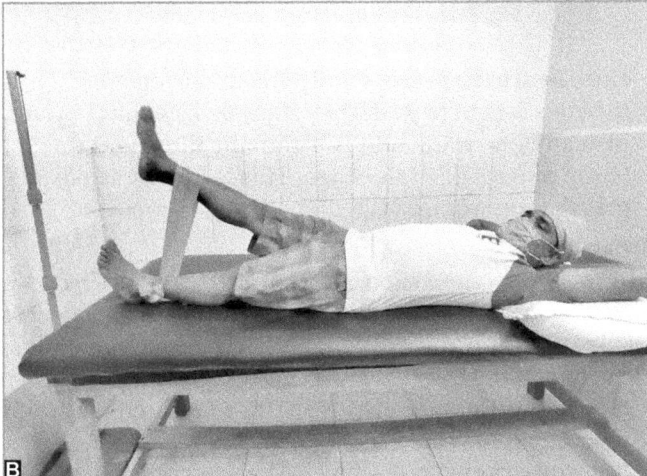

Figs. 8.21A and B: (A) Isometric quadriceps strengthening exercise, (B) Resisted SLR exercise.

recommendations. Closed kinematic chain exercises for improving the strength of quadriceps is found to be effective in improving patella femoral alignment and joint performance.
- Hamstrings stretching exercises are advised **(Fig. 8.22)**

Orthotic management
Besides the patellar alignment brace, discussed above, those who have associated foot deformity (pronated foot), need to be given foot orthosis either in the form of medial heel and sole raised with medial arch support or UCBL orthosis.

Surgical management:
- Chondrectomy, also known as shaving the damaged cartilage. The success of this treatment depends on the severity of cartilage damage.
- Drilling.
- Full patellectomy.
- Replacement of the damaged cartilage.
- Autologous chondrocyte transplantation.

ii. Patella Alta
Patella alta or high-riding patella refers to a disorder in knee, where the patella is located at an abnormally higher position in relation to the femur. This condition has been associated clinically with patellofemoral dysfunction and is a factor for development of patellofemoral pain.

When, the patella is placed at a lower position, it is called patella baja, which is also a cause of knee pain.

Etiology
This condition can occur due to trauma (sports injuries), though in majority of patients, it is found to have congenital/developmental cause rather than traumatic cause. The causes are listed as under:
- Defective fetal developments.
- Sports injury.
- Loose ligaments.
- Studded foot wear, as this type of foot wear when used, puts the foot firmly in contact with the ground, resulting in the displacement of patella.
- Body type (tall and thin people)
- Tendon rupture (rupture of ligamentum patellae).
- Quadriceps tendinitis.
- **Long patellar tendon:** People with a patellar tendon length more than 52 mm, usually suffer from patella alta **(Fig. 8.23)**.
- **Cerebral palsy:** It is a commonly associated problem in children with cerebral palsy, particularly those walking with flexed knees (Crouch gait).

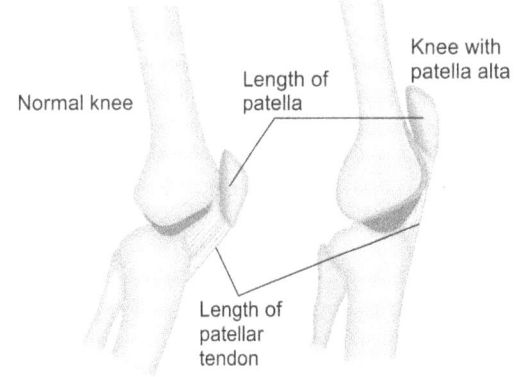

Fig. 8.23: Length of ligamentum patellae and patella alta.

Pathophysiology

The pathophysiology of the condition is not fully understood. However, one of the factors producing this condition is an abnormally long-patellar tendon.

Clinical features

Patella alta is a positional fault causing superior displacement of the patella within the trochlear groove of the femur. Anterior knee pain progressing slowly, increased with physical activity is the characteristic feature. Leung et al. (1996) and Kannus (1992) reported that subjects with anterior knee pain demonstrated a significantly more superior patellar position in the affected knee relative to healthy, control knees. Knee pain that improves during physical activity and returns after activity is suggestive of ligamentum patellae tendinitis, rather than pain due to patella alta.

Typical symptoms of patella alta are:
- Instability: Patients complain of instability of knee while walking and running.
- Recurrent dislocation of patella.
- Anterior knee pain: Especially when walking up and down slopes, squatting, stair climbing, prolonged sitting.

Diagnostic procedure

Diagnosis is made through physical and radiological examination. A lateral radiograph of knee (**Figs. 8.24A and B**) and/or sagittal MRI of knee may be helpful in diagnosing the disorder. The knee is flexed at an angle of 30 degrees and the radiograph is taken to find Patella alta.

Physical examination:

- **Full knee extension and patellar movement:** Normally when the knee is fully extended and relaxed, the patella can be moved slightly from side to side. However if, it moves further than normal, a patella alta is suspected.
- **Slight knee flexion and patellar movement:** When the knee is flexed to 30 degrees, the **"camel back"** sign (**Fig. 8.25**) is produced by the displaced patella. When looked from the side, two hump-like structures, one formed by the displaced patella and the other by the infra patellar pad of fat/or enlarged infrapatellar bursa are seen looking like the back of the camel.

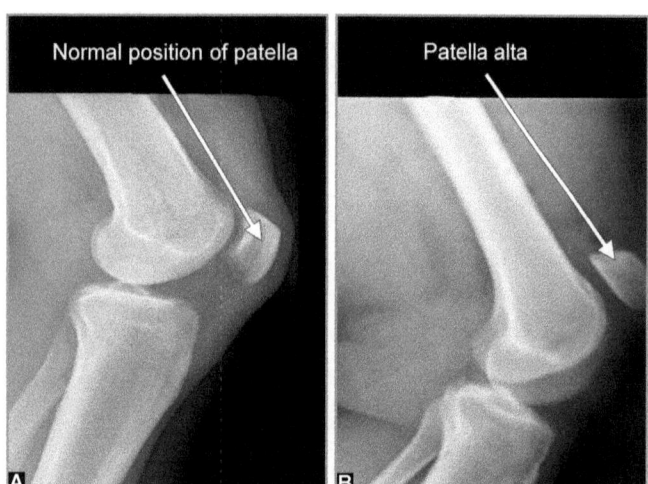

Figs. 8.24A and B: (A) Normal knee, (B) Knee with patella alta.

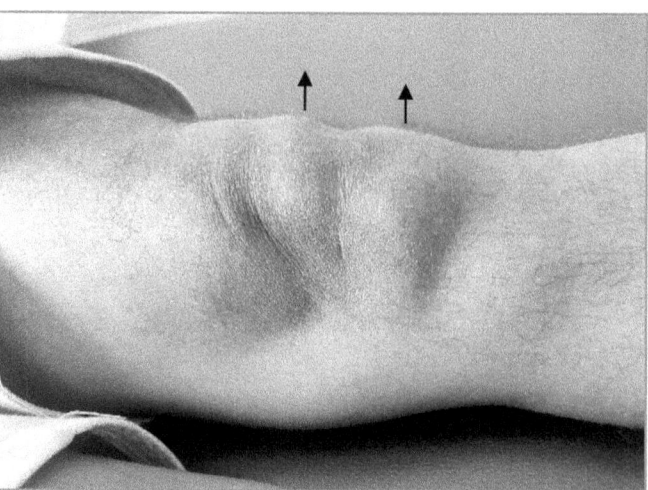

Fig. 8.25: The camel back sign on knee.

- **Knee bent to 90 degrees and patellar movements:** When the knee is bent to 90 degrees, the patella points upward, instead of forward, and is externally tilted and rotated to the outer side of the knee. This is known as positive **grasshopper sign**.

Management

RICE (rest, ice, compression, and elevation), and knee muscles strengthening exercises is the best way for the management of Patella alta. If nonsurgical methods fail to treat the condition, surgery may be advised.

- **Medical management:** NSAIDs to reduce pain and inflammation.
- **Physiotherapy:** Ice therapy in the acute stage to reduce pain and swelling. As acute pain subsides, physiotherapy should consists of:
  - Superoinferior glides to patella.
  - Stretching of quadriceps (**Fig. 8.26A**).
  - Strengthening of quadriceps, initially eccentric, progressing to isometric exercise.
  - Strengthening exercises for knee flexors (**Fig. 8.26B**).
  - Maintenance of patellar alignment using taping/patellar alignment brace (**Fig. 8.26C**).

Surgical management

If nonsurgical methods fail to treat the condition, it may be necessary to use surgical procedures, such as:
- Arthroscopy.
- **Patellectomy:** Some times considered for permanent relief from knee pain with this disorder.
- **Lateral release:** This procedure helps loosen the tight structures over the lateral aspect of patella and restores normal alignment.
- **VMO advance:** VMO advancement adjusts the position of the patella with in the groove and improves knee stability.
- **Tibial tuberosity osteotomy:** Tibial tuberosity osteotomy can be performed in patients with patella alta. With this surgery the surgeon moves the attachment of the patellar ligament downward to the tibia. The patella is also attached to this ligament, so the patella moves downward.

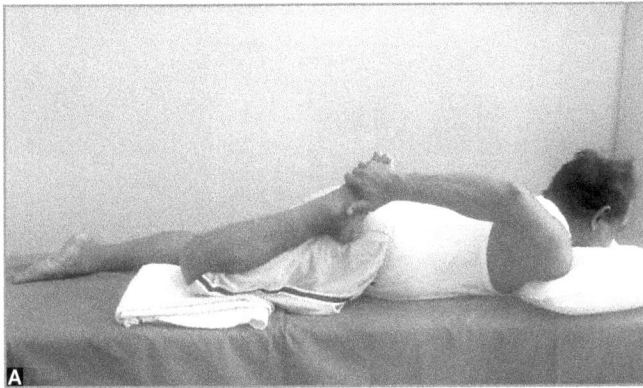
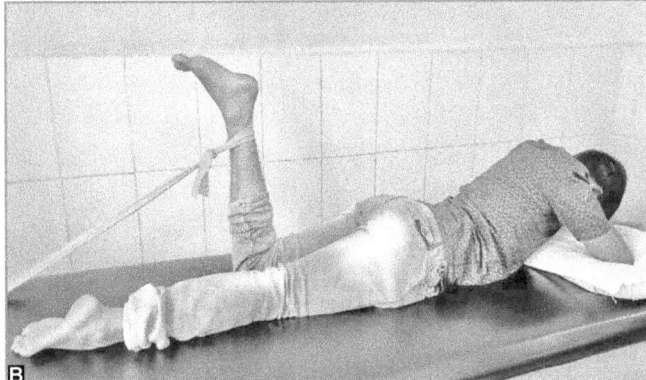
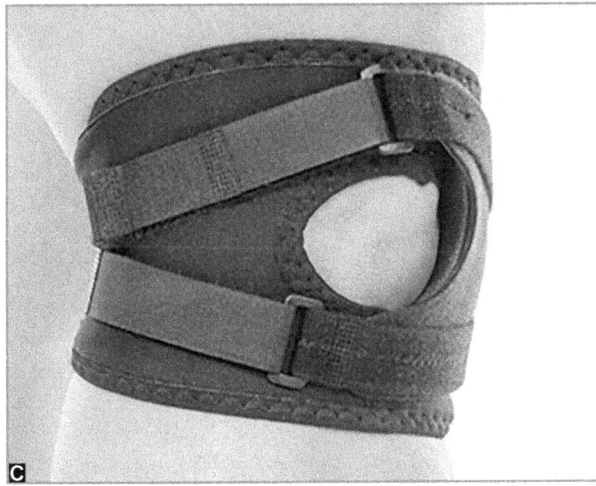

Figs. 8.26A to C: (A) Stretching of quadriceps, (B) Strengthening of hamstrings, (C) Patellar alignment brace.

iii. Dislocation of Patella

A patellar dislocation is the lateral shift of the patella leaving the trochlear groove of the femoral condyles. A dislocation of patella could be recurrent (where the patient gets dislocated again and again), or habitual (where every time, the knee flexes, the patella dislocates).

Epidemiology/etiology

The condition is more prevalent in females and athletes. Primary patellar dislocations are traumatic in nature. The other factors that lead to dislocation are:
* Ligament laxity.
* Reduced osseous constraints from the lateral condyle of femur.
* Patella alta.
* Increased Q angle.
* Genu recurvatum.
* Patellar hypermobility.
* Imbalance between stronger lateral structures (vastus lateralis and lateral retinaculum) and weaker medial structures (medial patellofemoral ligament and vastus medialis).
* Rotational deformities of femur and tibia.
* Pes planus deformity.

Clinical feature

The patient presents with the followings after a patellar dislocation:
* In acute primary traumatic dislocation of patella, hemarthrosis of knee with increased swelling in the medial aspect is the presentation, which could be due to rupture of the medial restraints of patella.
* Pain and instability
* Spontaneous reduction of dislocation by knee extension might be the presentation in some sufferers.
* After traumatic dislocation locking of knee may be a presentation.

Diagnosis

Diagnosis is done by considering history (history of trauma/past dislocation), X-ray examination **(Figs. 8.27A and B)**. CT scan/MRI may be performed to establish associated injuries such as osteochondral fractures, rupture of soft tissues in the medial aspects of knee.

Management

* **Conservative:** A conservative management is the choice of management for acute primary dislocations of patella. It consists of:
  – Spontaneous reduction by repeated knee extension and application of cryotherapy. If spontaneous reduction is not possible, reduction by the Surgeon under local anesthesia is the consideration. This is followed by immobilization of knee in a cylindrical plaster of Paris cast/knee immobilizer **(Figs. 8.28A and B)** for 6 weeks.

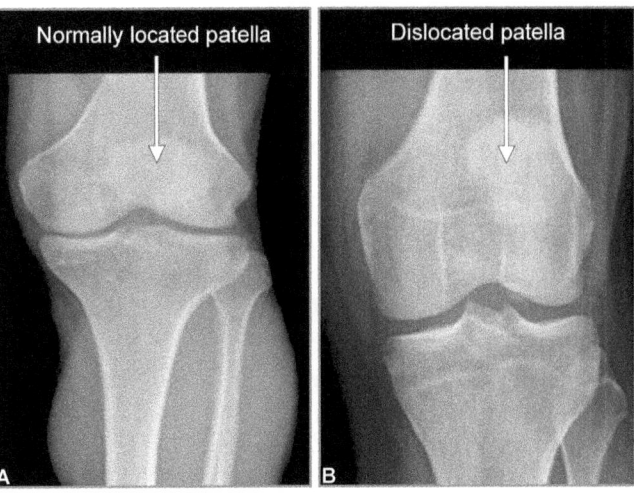

Figs. 8.27A and B: X-ray of knee showing: (A) Normally located patella, (B) Dislocated patella.

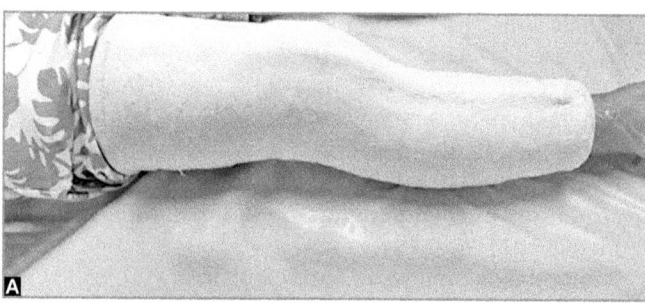

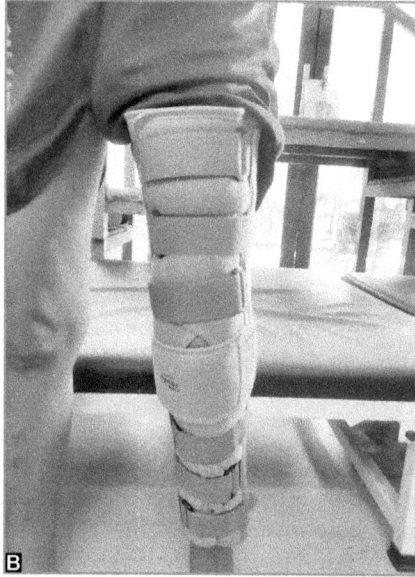

Figs. 8.28A and B: (A) Cylindrical POP cast, (B) The knee immobilizer.

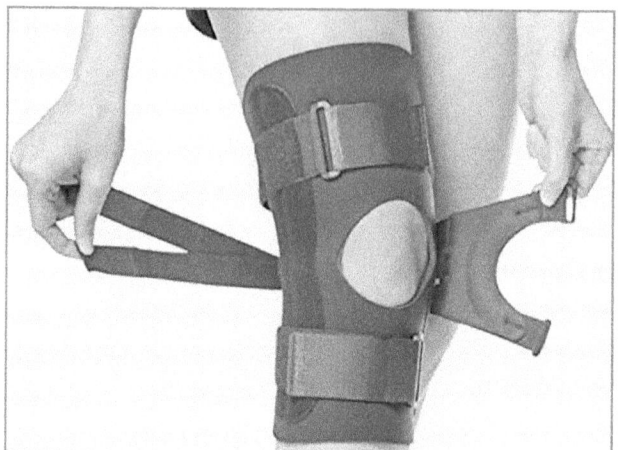

Fig. 8.29: Patellar stabilization brace.

- NSAIDs may be prescribed by the Surgeon to reduce pain and inflammation.
- A nonweight-bearing crutch gait using walking frame/axillary crutches can be started after the pain reduced.
- After 6 weeks, the immobilizer is removed and the patient undergoes a course of physiotherapy, partial weight-bearing ambulation progressing to full weight-bearing ambulation.

Physiotherapy

The aims of physiotherapy are:
- Reduction of pain.
- Increase of range of motion of knee (flexion of knee is gradually achieved and performed using the patellar stabilization brace to prevent further dislocation).
- Strengthening of the quadriceps (mostly VMO).
- Maintain the alignment of patella in the trochlear groove by using: Elastic crepe bandage/Patellar stabilization brace (knee cap with hole for patella) **(Fig. 8.29)**/Taping.

Methods of physiotherapy
- Modalities such as Paraffin Wax Bath (PWB), Surged faradic stimulation of VMO, IFT **(Figs. 8.30A to C)** ultrasound therapy, cryotherapy (cryokinematics to achieve active knee movement as the ice significantly reduces pain during movement), high power laser therapy, etc., may be selected by the therapist after a thorough clinical reasoning.

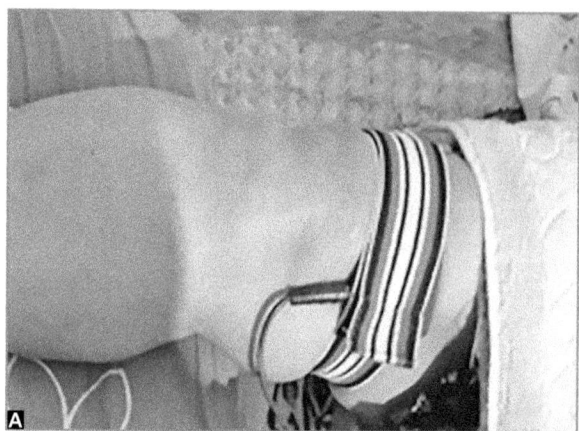

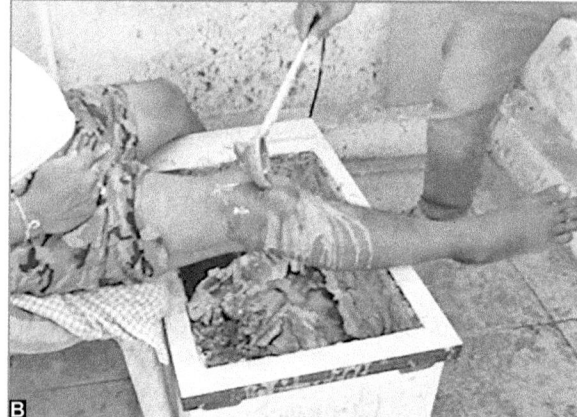

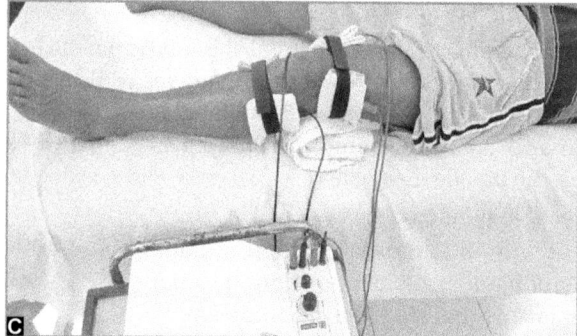

Figs. 8.30A to C: (A) Faradic stimulation to VMO, (B) PWB to knee, (C) IFT to knee.

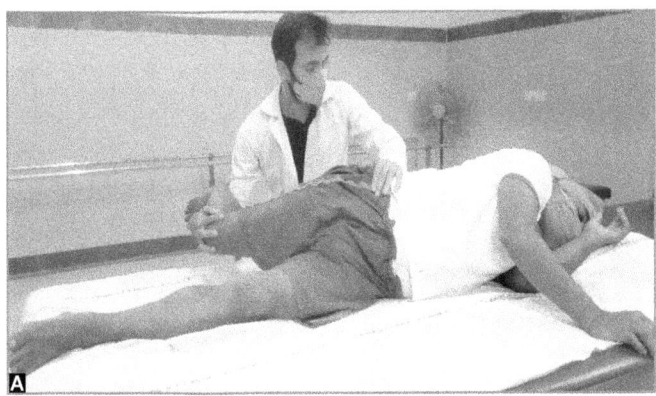
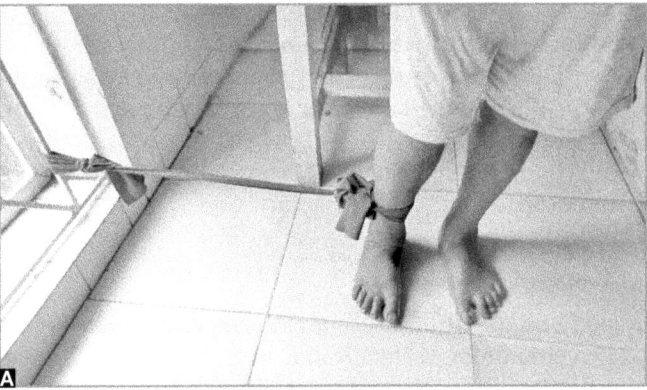

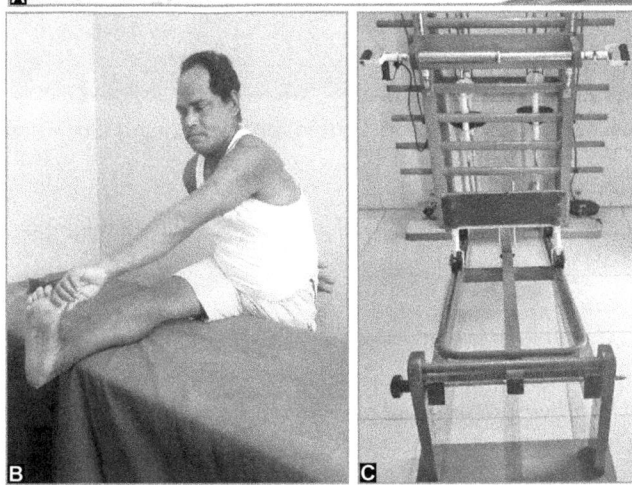

Figs. 8.31A to C: (A) Stretching of IT band by therapist, (B) Self stretching of hamstrings; (C) Rowing machine as a part of Mennel's apparatus.

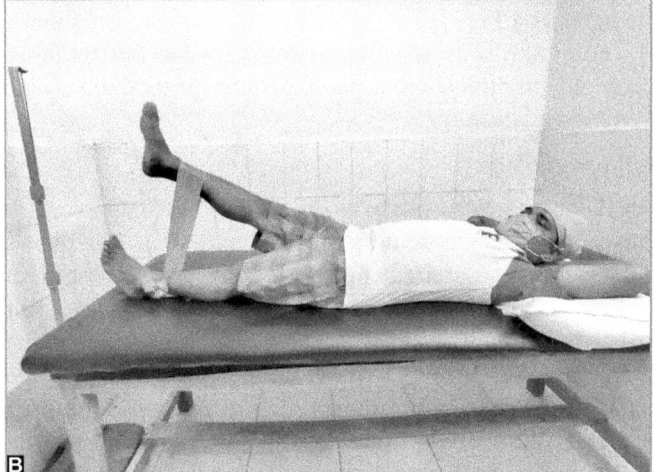

Figs. 8.32A and B: (A) Concentric resisted adductor strengthening using theraband, (B) Resisted SLR with theraband.

- **Exercises:**
  - Stretching exercises to improve flexibility of IT band, Hamstrings **(Figs. 8.31A and B)**.
  - Range of motion exercises progressing from nonweight-bearing mobilization exercisers such as heel drag to buttock, prone knee flexion, to partial weight-bearing closed kinematic mobility exercises such as static cycle exercise, exercise in rowing machine, mini squats holding on to support are performed as tolerated.
  - *Strengthening exercises:* Isometric VMO sets, isomteric hip adductor strengthening, progressing to resisted concentric strengthening exercises **(Fig. 8.32A)**, resisted SLR **(Fig. 8.32B)**, closed kinematic chain exercises such as squatting (graduated), are performed.
  - *Proprioceptive training:* Ball kicking, Hopping, Zig-zag walking (Agility drills), etc., are performed.
  - *Prophylactic measures:* As the patella once dislocated, may have recurrences, it is essential that, the patient must perform regular stretching exercises to hamstrings, IT band and strengthening exercises to Quadriceps (VMO), Hip adductors. He/she also need to be taught to use a dynamic patellar stabilization brace for few days, if engaged in sports or heavy work in standing. The patient should be advised to avoid full squatting, cross sitting till complete knee stability is achieved.

If conservative methods fail and recurrent dislocation results, surgery followed by protected weight bearing and a course of physiotherapy in the same line that done for conservative management are followed.

The surgeries performed are:
- **Lateral release:** Release of tight lateral retinaculum to allow more medial movement of patella. This is performed in mild patellar instability.
- Medial patellofemoral ligament reconstruction. This is sometimes combined with lateral release and is performed in severe patellar instability.
- **Distal realignment/anteromedialization:** The bony attachment of the tendon of quadriceps over the tibial tuberosity is moved more medially to allow normal alignment of patella. This is sometimes combined with lateral release and medial patellofemoral ligament reconstruction and is performed in severe patellar instability. A trochleoplasty, if required may also be considered.

iv. Osgood-Schlatter Disease

Osgood Schlatter disease is a traction apophysitis at the level of the tibial tuberosity due to repetitive strain on the secondary ossification center of the tibial tuberosity. The repetitive strain is from the strong pull of the quadriceps muscle produced during sporting activities. This is inflammation of the patellar ligament at the tibial tuberosity (apophysitis of tibial tuberosity), characterized by a painful bump just below the knee, that is worse with activity and better with rest.

This condition has been named after Robert Bailey Osgood, an American Orthopedic surgeon, and Carl B Schlatter a Swiss Surgeon.

Epidemiology/Etiology

Osgood Schlatter disease is one of the most common causes of knee pain in the skeletally immature, adolescent athlete. Onset coincides with adolescent growth spurts between the ages 10–15 years for males and 8–13 years for females. The condition is more common in males and occurs more frequently in athletes that participate in sports that involve running and jumping.

Pathophysiology

The tibial tubercle develops as a secondary ossification center that provides attachment for the patellar tendon. The physis is the weakest point in the muscle-tendon-bone-attachment (as opposed to the tendon in an adult) and therefore, at risk of injury from repetitive stress. With repeated contraction of the quadriceps muscle mass, especially with repeated forced knee extension as seen in sports requiring running and jumping (basketball, football, gymnastics), softening and partial avulsion of the apophyseal ossification center may occur with a resulting osteochondritis.

Clinical Features

The patient typically an adolescent male, complains of intense pain in one or both knees, which is more with activities such as running, jumping, squatting and especially while ascending and descending stairs as well as on kneeling, and relieved on rest. Episodes of pain typically last from few weeks to few months. The pain is localized to anteroinferior aspect of the knee.

The pain can be reproduced by extending knee against resistance and stretching the Quadriceps or striking the front of knee. In the acute state, the pain is severe and continuous, though initially it is mild and intermittent.

Types of Osgood Schlatter Disease

The condition may result in avulsion fracture, with the tibial tuberosity separating from the tibia (but remains attached to the tendon of quadriceps). The fracture on the tibial tuberosity can be complete or incomplete, depending upon which of the following types are described:

- **Type I:** A small fragment is displaced proximally, and does not require surgery.
- **Type II:** The articular surface of the tibia remains intact, and the fracture occurs at the junction where the secondary center of ossification and the proximal tibial epiphysis come together. It may or may not require surgery.
- **Type III:** Complete fracture through articular surface. This type usually requires surgery.

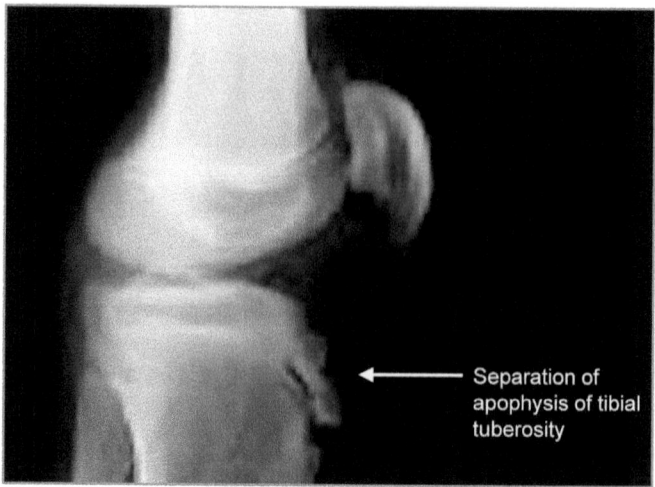

Fig. 8.33: X-ray showing pathology in apophysis of tibial tuberosity.

Diagnosis

Diagnosis is made from clinical presentation, ultrasonography, and X-ray (**Fig. 8.33**).

Treatment

Treatment is generally conservative consisting of NSAIDs, rest, ice, and physiotherapy to reduce pain and inflammation and improve function and prevent recurrence. Physiotherapy is generally recommended after initial symptoms subsided. Surgery is performed for those, who still have symptoms after the growth is completed.

Physiotherapy

Low intensity, isometric and dynamic quadriceps strengthening gradually progressing in intensity (**Fig. 8.34**), stretching of quadriceps and hamstrings, cryotherapy, knee ROM exercises, IFT/TENS are the treatment applied to prevent deconditioning of quadriceps and to reduce symptoms. Extracorporeal shockwave therapy, though is applied sometimes, has no strong evidence supporting its use.

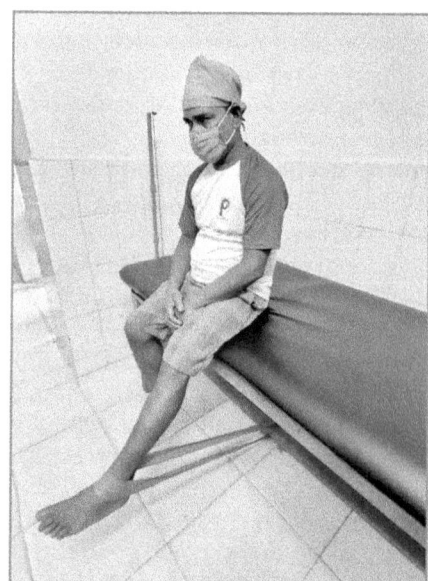

Fig. 8.34: Resisted knee extension exercise using theraband.

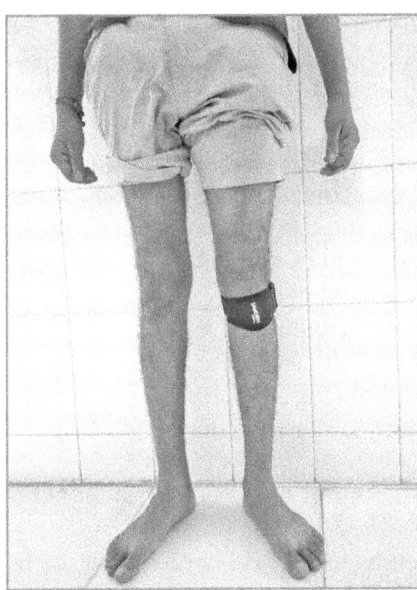

Fig. 8.35: The protective knee pad.

A knee support in the form of protective knee pad (**Fig. 8.35**), or knee cap, or crepe bandaging may provide some relief, while walking and doing activities. Activity modification, with observation of joint protection and energy conservation techniques are greatly helpful.

Surgery

The surgical options include excision of the ossicles together with reduction osteotomy or debridement of the tibial tuberosity, drilling of the tubercle, autogenous bone peg insertion through the tubercle, or sequestrectomy (i.e., excision of the ununited ossicles and free cartilaginous pieces).

v. Anterior Cruciate Ligament Injury Rehabilitation

Anterior cruciate ligament injury is a tear or sprain of the ACL. Anterior cruciate ligament is one of the major ligaments of the knee and contributes significantly for knee stability (**Fig. 8.36**).

Etiology

The ACL injury most commonly occurs in sports that involve sudden stops or change in direction, jumping, and landing, such as soccer, basket ball, foot ball, and down hill skiing. Besides injuries encountered during sports, road traffic accidents, fall from heights, direct blow to the knee, pivoting around the knee with foot planted firmly on the ground, etc., also lead to such injuries.

Risk Factors for ACL Injuries

The factors that increase the risk to sustain an ACL injury include:
- Females are three times more prone to sustain an injury than males due to anatomical configuration, muscle strength and hormonal influences, resulting in ligament laxity.
- Participating in sports that involve sudden twisting, turning, etc.
- Poor fitness.
- Improper foot wear.
- Using poorly maintained sports equipment.
- Playing on artificial turf surfaces.

Clinical Features

The signs and symptoms of ACL injury are:
- A loud "pop" or a popping sensation in the knee at the time of injury.
- Severe pain and instability or "giving way" in the knee with difficulty in bearing weight.
- Rapid swelling/Hemarthrosis.
- Loss of range of motion.

Diagnosis

Diagnosis of ACL injury is made from:
- History of injury.
- Clinical features.
- Tests made by clinicians for integrity of ACL such as: Anterior drawer test, Lachman test, Pivot shift test (**Figs. 8.8 to 8.10**), etc.

Besides the clinical examination, imaging studies described below are performed:
- **X-rays:** X-rays may be needed to rule out a bone fracture. However, X-rays don't show soft tissues, such as ligaments and tendons.
- **Magnetic resonance imaging (MRI):** The MRI can show an ACL injury (**Fig. 8.37**) and signs of damage to other tissues in the knee, including the cartilage.
- **Ultrasound:** Diagnostic ultrasound may be used to check for injuries in the ligaments, tendons and muscles of the knee.

Grading of ACL Injury

Three grades of ACL injuries have been described as under:
- **Grade-I sprain:**
    - The fibers of the ligament are stretched, without any tear.
    - There is a little tenderness and swelling.
    - The knee does not feel unstable or give way during activity.
    - No increased laxity and there is a firm end feel.

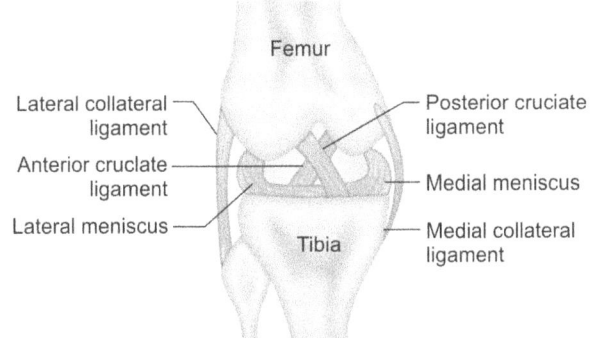

Fig. 8.36: The knee ligaments.

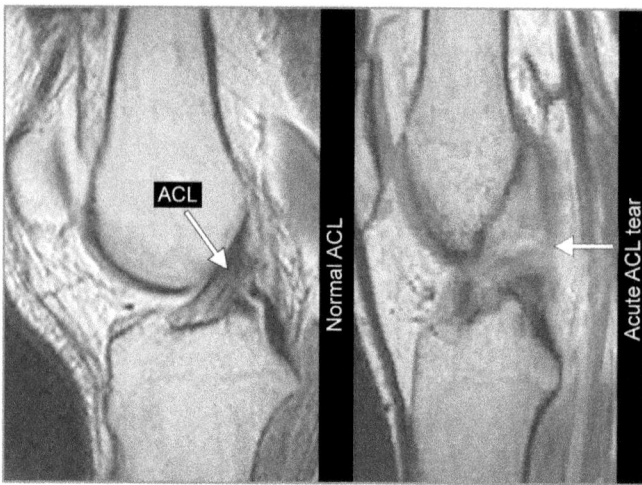

Fig. 8.37: MRI showing normal and injured ACL.

- ❖ **Grade-II sprain:**
  - The fibers of the ligament are partially torn or incomplete tear with hemorrhage.
  - There is a little tenderness and moderate swelling with some loss of function.
  - The joint may feel unstable or give way during activity.
  - Increased anterior translation, but there is still a firm end point.
  - Painful and pain increase with Lachman's and anterior drawer tests.
- ❖ **Grade-III sprain:**
  - The fibers of the ligament are completely torn (ruptured).
  - There is tenderness, but limited pain, especially when compared to the seriousness of the injury.
  - There may be a little swelling or a lot of swelling.
  - The ligament cannot control knee movements. The knee feels unstable or gives way at certain times.
  - There is also rotational instability as indicated by a positive pivot shift test.
  - Hemarthrosis occurs within 1–2 hours.

Treatment

PRICE, i.e., Protection, Rest, Ice, Compression, Elevation, is the immediate treatment that is given to the patient as under:
- ❖ **Protection:** Immediately, following injury a knee immobilizer should be applied and no weight bearing should be allowed on the affected limb. A nonweight-bearing crutch gait is advised.
- ❖ **Rest:** General rest is necessary for healing, hence the person should be advised to remain absent from sports/out door activities, till the acute symptoms subside.
- ❖ **Ice:** As long as swelling persists, the patient should be advised to apply ice packs/cold packs for 20 minutes at 2 hourly intervals.
- ❖ **Compression:** An elastic bandage or compression wrap should be applied around the affected knee.
- ❖ **Elevation:** The patient should be advised to keep the limb supported on pillow with the foot slightly raised.

NSAIDs are prescribed by the physician/surgeon to reduce pain and inflammation.

Rehabilitation

Anterior cruciate ligament rehabilitation has undergone considerable changes over the past decade. Intensive research into the biomechanics of the injured and the operated knee have led to a movement away from the techniques of the early 1980s characterized by postoperative casting, delayed weight bearing and limitation of ROM, to the current early rehabilitation program with immediate training of ROM and early weight bearing exercises.

Goal of ACL rehabilitation

The goal of rehabilitation is to reduce pain and swelling, restore knee's full range of motion, and strengthen muscles, and early return to sports/ activities, which are listed below:
- ❖ Reduction of pain and swelling.
- ❖ Restoration of full range of motion of knee to prevent arthrofibrosis.
- ❖ Strengthening muscles of knee, mostly the hamstrings.
- ❖ Gaining good functional stability.
- ❖ Reaching the best possible functional level and promote early return to sports/activities.
- ❖ Decreasing the risk for reinjury.

Physiotherapy for ACL injury

After ACL injury, regardless of whether surgery will take place or not, physiotherapy management focuses on regaining range of movement, muscle strength, joint proprioception, and stability. The physiotherapist applies PRICE discussed above and designs a set of exercises, selects appropriate electrotherapeutic modalities to improve stability, reduce pain, and early return to function.

A knee brace/knee immobilizer (**Fig. 8.38**) is applied and nonweight-bearing crutch ambulation is started gradually progressing to partial and full weight bearing ambulation as pain and stability improves.

Modalities such as PSWD to knee are applied to reduce inflammation and promote repair. Surged Faradic Stimulation

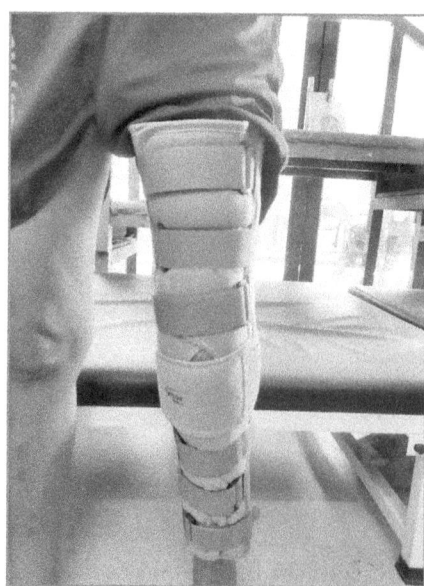

Fig. 8.38: The knee immobilizer.

to Quadriceps is applied to strengthen quadriceps eliminating quadriceps inhibition. IFT, 1-10 Hz rhythmic is also helpful in reducing pain and swelling.

Exercises:

Exercises are designed to increase range of movement, strengthen quadriceps and hamstrings, and improve proprioception. The exercises recommended are:
- Static quadriceps exercise/Straight leg raises exercise, without or with resistance **(Figs. 8.21 and 8.39)**.
- Active ankle/foot exercise.
- Active free knee flexion and extension in sitting.
- Patellar mobilization exercise.
- Active knee flexion in prone without and with resistance **(Figs. 8.40A and B)**.
- Gluteus medius work in side lying, without and with resistance **(Fig. 8.41)**.
- Gluteus maximus work in prone lying, without and with resistance **(Fig. 8.42)**.
- Weight transfer in standing holding on to support and with the knee brace on.
- Closed kinetic chain (CKC) exercises, such as mini wall squats **(Fig. 8.43A)**/lateral stepping/side lunges/leg press **(Fig. 8.43B)** and Open kinetic chain (OKC) exercises, such as, standing hamstring curls, prone lying, knee flexion, etc., play an important role in regaining muscle strength in and knee stability. Closed kinetic chain exercises are more popular than open kinetic chain exercises in ACL rehabilitation, as the CKC exercises place less strain on the injured ACL than OKC exercises.
- Stationary bicycle exercise **(Fig. 8.44)**, hydrotherapy, low-impact exercise on machines, such as an elliptical cross-trainer, leg curl machine, and treadmill, etc., are used to improve strength and endurance.

As the patient improves, before discharge, sports specific/function specific exercises should be performed under the supervision of the therapist, and he/she should be advised to use a hinged knee brace **(Fig. 8.45)** during activities/sports for a period of 6 months and continue home exercise program.

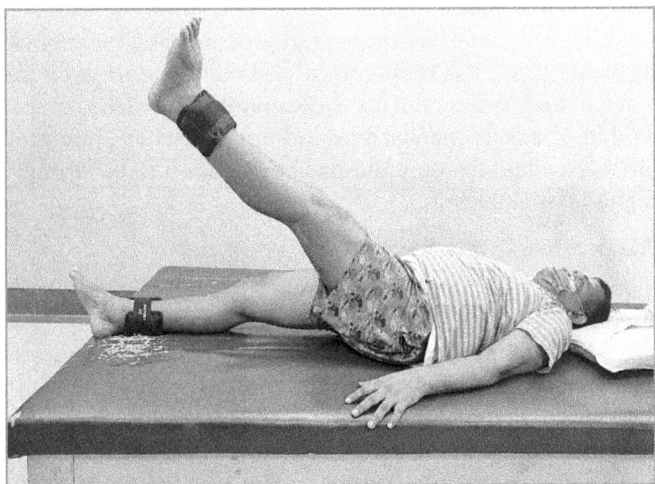

Fig. 8.39: Resisted SLR exercise using weight cuff.

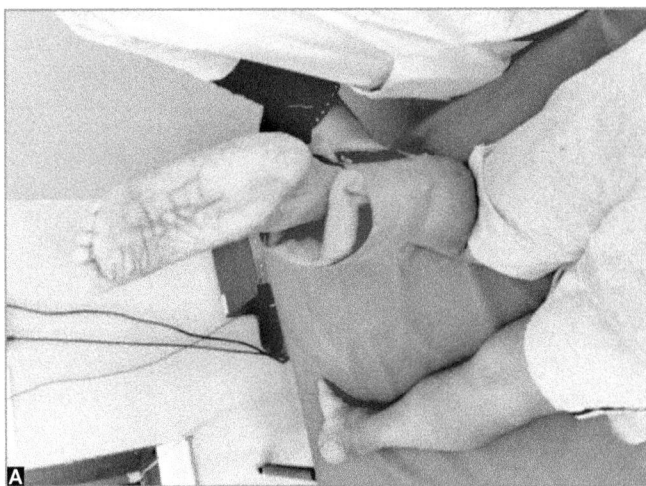

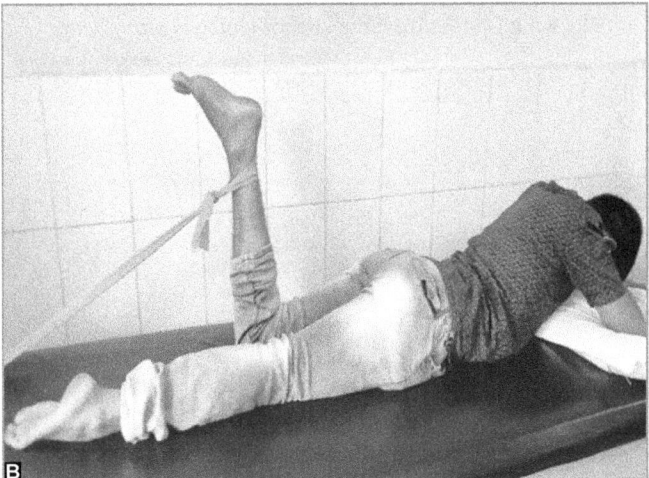

Figs. 8.40A and B: Resisted knee flexor strengthening using: (A) Weight cuff, (B) Theraband.

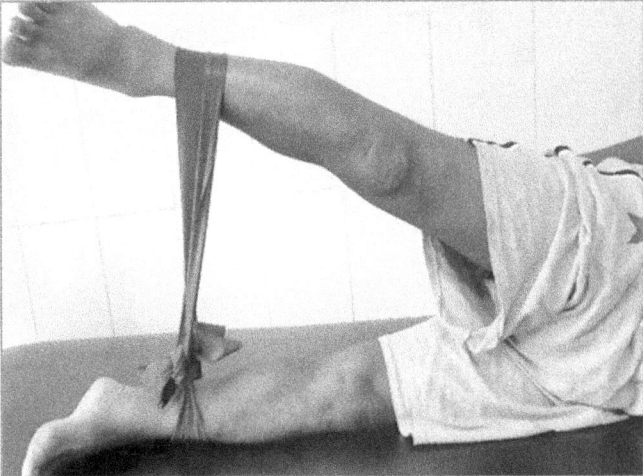

Fig. 8.41: Gluteus medius strengthening using theraband in side lying.

Surgical Management for ACL Injury

Grade-II and Grade-III, injuries to ACL, with significant knee instability are managed by surgical intervention. An arthroscopic procedure for repair of ACL is currently followed by surgeons. It must be understood by all who deal with such patients that, surgery should only be performed, after

Section 2: Physiotherapy for Musculoskeletal Conditions

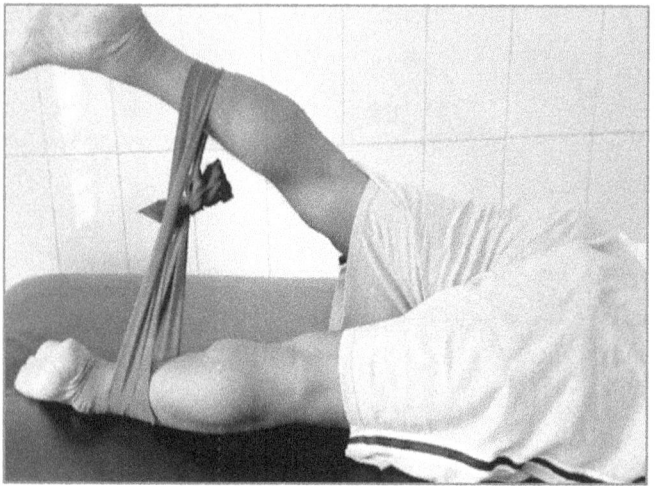

Fig. 8.42: Gluteus maximus strengthening in prone lying.

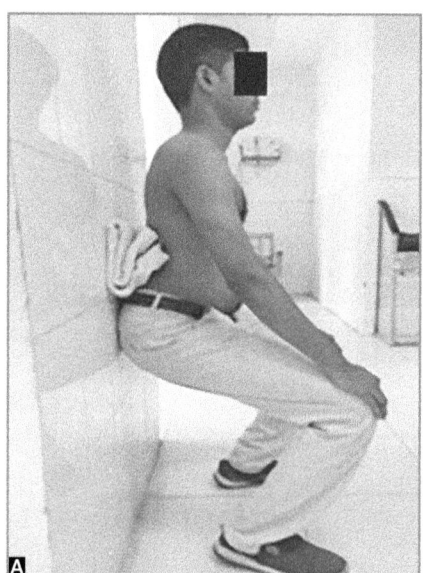

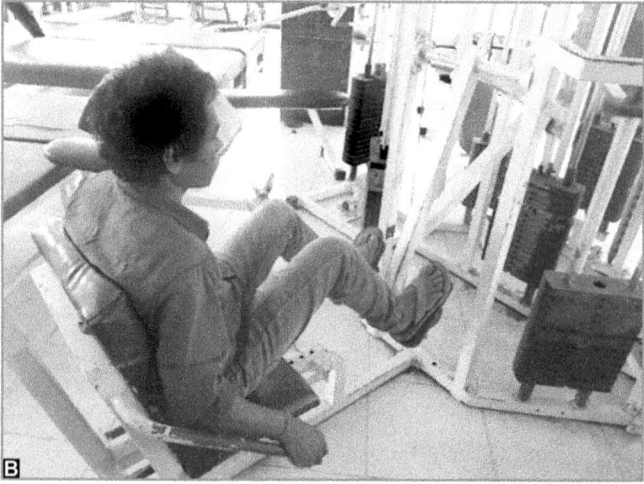

Figs. 8.43A and B: (A) Mini wall squats, (B) Leg press exercise.

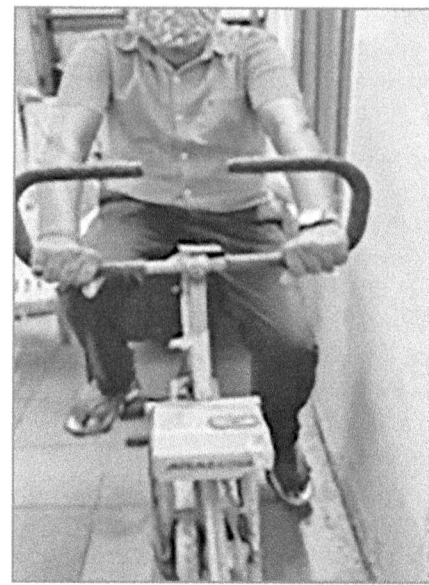

Fig. 8.44: Stationary bicycle exercise.

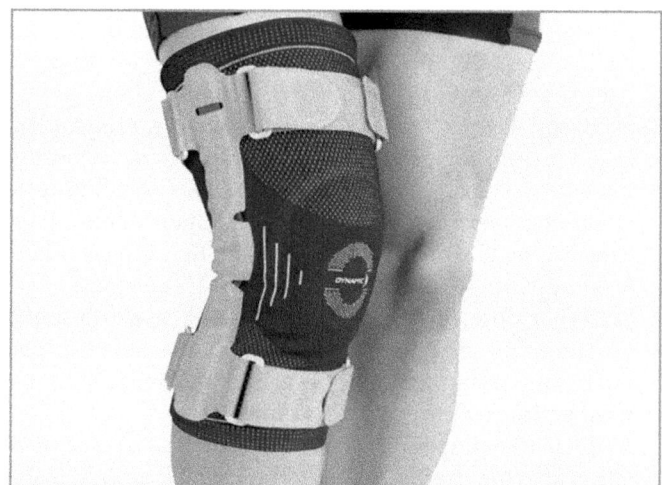

Fig. 8.45: The hinged knee brace.

result in significant arthrofibrosis postoperatively making it difficult to achieve full knee movements postoperatively.

Surgeries performed

A number of materials and techniques are used for surgical reconstruction. The most common surgery performed is the patellar tendon autograft using the middle third of the patellar tendon. The bone-patellar tendon-bone graft when performed offers excellent fixation and has been shown to be stronger than the original ACL.

Preoperative Physiotherapy

Before proceeding with surgery, the acutely injured knee should be in a quiescent state with little or no swelling, have a full range of motion, and the patient should have a normal or near normal gait pattern. The physiotherapist needs to prepare the patient for surgery.

PRICE and electrotherapy can be applied during several weeks ahead of the surgery in the similar manner for conservative management of Grade-I injury in order to

reduction of joint effusion and restoration of full knee range of motion, as surgeries performed without remitting knee effusion and without achieving full range of motion of knee,

reduce swelling and pain, to achieve full range of motion and to increase strength of muscles of hip and knee. This helps the patient to regain better movement and strength after the surgery.

The preoperative exercise program should consist of the followings:
* Isometric quadriceps exercise.
* Supine/sitting heel drag to improve knee flexion (**Fig. 8.46**).
* SLR exercise.
* Resisted knee flexion in prone (**Fig. 8.40**)
* Static cycle exercise (**Fig. 8.44**).
* Hydrotherapy.

Postoperative Physiotherapy

Three factors are important during postoperative period such as:
1. Gain of early terminal knee extension equal to the contralateral side.
2. Early weight bearing.
3. Closed and open kinetic chain strengthening exercises.

Achievement of early knee extension is the foundation for the entire rehabilitation process of postoperative ACL rehabilitation. Exercises to achieve knee ROM and muscle strength in quadriceps and hamstrings, as well as advising on a functional knee brace for use during the first few postoperative days are the main components of postoperative management. Though, the use of a functional knee brace is controversial as revealed from a study done by Harilainen et al., who compared the effects of functional bracing after ACL reconstruction against no bracing postoperatively. No significant difference in functional outcome, degree of stability, or isokinetic muscle torque was detected at 1 and 2 years postoperatively between the two groups. In a similar study, Risberg et al., found no significant differences in knee-joint laxity, range of motion, muscle strength, functional knee tests, or pain in patient's using brace and those not using brace. However, in the opinion of this Author, it is advisable to use a functional knee brace till knee stability is achieved and pain reduced following surgery, particularly when performing sports activities/function.

The postoperative ACL rehabilitation protocol
* **Week-1-2**: The patient is applied with a knee immobilizer, and made to walk using a walker/pair of axillary crutches, initially in nonweight-bearing crutch gait. Regular icing at 2 hourly interval and limb elevation are followed to reduce swelling. Relaxed passive exercises followed by active assisted exercises within the pain-free range are practiced several times a day to achieve full knee extension and 70 degrees of knee flexion by the end of first week. Isometric quadriceps exercise, active knee flexion in the form of heel drag, active ankle and foot exercise are performed. While performing knee extension, care should be exercised to prevent knee hyperextension from occurring.
* **Week-3-4**: The exercises performed during the first 1-2 weeks are continued in this period with emphasis on more knee flexion and partial weight-bearing crutch gait using walker/axillary crutches.
* **Week-5-10**: During this period, the use of the brace is progressively reduced. Exercises to improve knee flexion and strength of quadriceps and hamstrings are continued. Closed chain exercises from less responsible positions, such as static bicycle, leg press, stepping at lower exercise intensities are started initially, progressing to more difficult positions such as squatting against the wall (**Fig. 8.43A**). If strength of the muscles are good, proprioceptive training in form of balancing over balance board are started. Full weight bearing is started by this time; however, a functional knee brace may be used.
* **Week-10**: Isokinetic exercises, forward, backward, and side way walking are started.
* **After 3 months**: Functional exercises in the form of running and jumping are started. Agility drills such as figure-of-8 walking/running are practiced as tolerated. Hopping on trampoline, single-leg standing, etc., are practiced.
* **Months 4-5**: During this time, the emphasis is maximization of strength and endurance of the knee muscles. Plyometric exercises, sports/activity specific exercises, exercises involving acceleration/deceleration such walking up and down inclination, progressive agility drills, etc., are performed to help return to function and prevent further injury.

vi. Posterior Cruciate Ligament Injury Rehabilitation

The PCL is one of the two cruciate ligaments that act as the major stabilizing ligament of the knee (**Fig. 8.36**). It prevents the tibia from excessive posterior displacement in relation to the femur. It also functions to prevent knee hyper-extension and limits internal rotation, adduction and abduction at the knee joint. This ligament suffers less injury as compared to ACL, as it is stronger and two times thicker than ACL.

Epidemiology/Etiology

The mean age of people suffering from acute PCL injuries range between 20 and 30 years. The most common mechanism

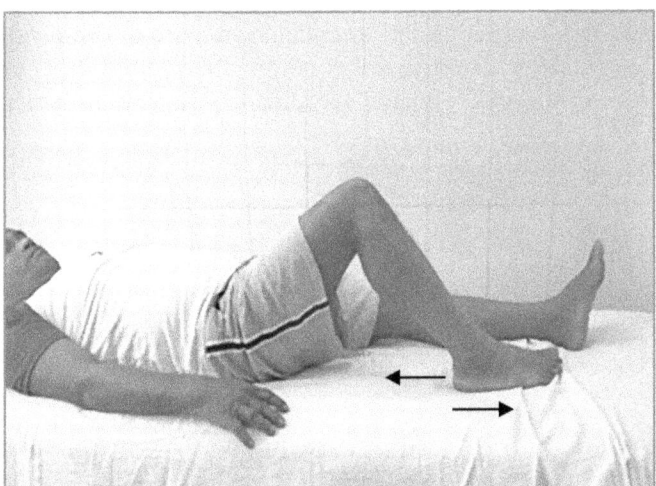

Fig. 8.46: Supine heel drag.

of injury is a direct blow to the anterior aspect of proximal tibia on a flexed knee with ankle in plantar flexion, as it occurs in dashboard injuries during motor vehicle accidents. Hyperextension and rotational or valgus/varus stress mechanism may also be responsible for PCL injuries.

The injuries occur mostly during sports such as playing foot ball, as well as activities involving jumping from height. Activities requiring faster change of direction, missing a step while stepping down also result in PCL injuries.

Clinical Feature

- ❖ **Acute PCL injury:**
  - Isolated PCL injury: Symptoms are usually minimal, sometimes patient's fail to notice that an injury has been caused. Minimal pain, swelling, instability may be present.
  - PCL injury in association with other ligament injuries: Symptoms depend upon the severity of injury. Most commonly patients present with pain, swelling, knee instability, movement limitation in knee. Bruising over the knee might be present.
- ❖ **Chronic PCL injury:** Patients sometimes fail to recall a mechanism of injury. They complain of pain and instability with weight bearing over the leg in a semiflexed knee, such as squatting or stair climbing. Walking long distance produces aching pain, whereas walking over uneven surface produces knee instability. Retro patellar pain and pain in the medial compartment of knee may also be present. The knee may be swollen and may become stiff.

Grades of PCL Injury

Depending on the severity of injury, PCL injury can be graded into:

- ❖ **Grade-I:** Limited damage to ligament mostly due to over stretch. Function and stability of knee is maintained.
- ❖ **Grade-II:** The ligament is partially torn with feeling of instability.
- ❖ **Grade-III:** Complete tear of the ligament with accompanying sprain of the ACL and/or collateral ligaments.

Diagnosis

History of injury, clinical presentation (difficulty in weight bearing and reduced ROM), special tests, and radiographic findings help in establishing the diagnosis.

Special tests performed include posterior drawer test, posterior Lachman test, posterior sag sign, and quadriceps active test **(Figs. 8.11 to 8.13)**.

Radiographic Examination

- ❖ **X-ray:** X-ray is done in standing as well as weight bearing on the leg with knee in 45 degrees of flexion. Lateral view detects the sagging of tibia.
- ❖ **MRI:** It is considered gold standard for the diagnosis of PCL tear **(Fig. 8.47)**.

Management

Nonoperative treatment is usually followed for acute isolated grade-I or II sprains of PCL. However, acute grade-III injury can also be managed conservatively, but grade-III injury of the PCL when combined with other soft tissue injuries in the knee, surgical reconstruction of the ligaments need to be done, often within 2 weeks from the injury.

When managed conservatively individuals with grade-I and II PCL injury are expected to return to play/works within 2-4 weeks, whereas those with grade-III, injury are expected to return to play/work by 3-4 months.

- ❖ The conservative management consists of:
  - Immobilization of knee in a knee immobilizer locked in extension for 2-3 weeks, for grade-I and II, and 2-4 weeks for grade-III injuries.
  - Nonweight-bearing/Partial-weight bearing (if tolerated) gait for 2 weeks using walker/axillary crutches, gradually progressing to full weight bearing for grade-I and II injuries, and nonweight bearing/partial weight-bearing gait using walker/crutches for 2-4 weeks, gradually progressing to full weight bearing as the pain allows for grade-III injuries are advised.

During the period of immobilization NSAIDs, physiotherapy, and the knee immobilizer **(Fig. 8.38)** constitute the components of conservative management.

- ❖ **Physiotherapy:**
  - *In acute stage(during immobilization)/Subacute stage*
- ❖ Physiotherapy for grade-I and II injuries consists of the followings:
  - *Cryotherapy:* To reduce inflammation.
  - *PSWD/PMWD:* To reduce inflammation and promote healing.
  - *IFT:* To reduce pain and swelling.
  - *Surged faradic current to quadriceps:* To overcome quadriceps inhibition.
  - Isometric quadriceps **(Fig. 8.21A)**/hamstrings exercise **(Fig. 8.48)**, isometric glutei exercises are performed for several sessions in a day.
  - Active ankle and foot exercises are advised.
  - Nonweight-bearing/partial weight bearing ambulation with walker/crutches are advised.

After 2 weeks the knee immobilizer is removed as per the advice of the treating Orthopedic Surgeon and full weight-bearing mobilization and ambulation are started. Along with the acute care managements described above, proprioceptive training on balance boards, coordination exercises involving

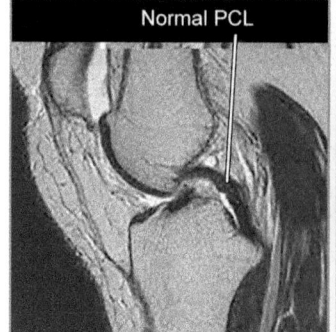 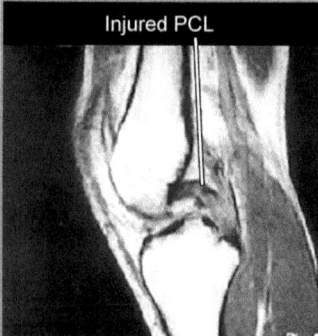

Fig. 8.47: MRI of knee showing normal and injured PCL.

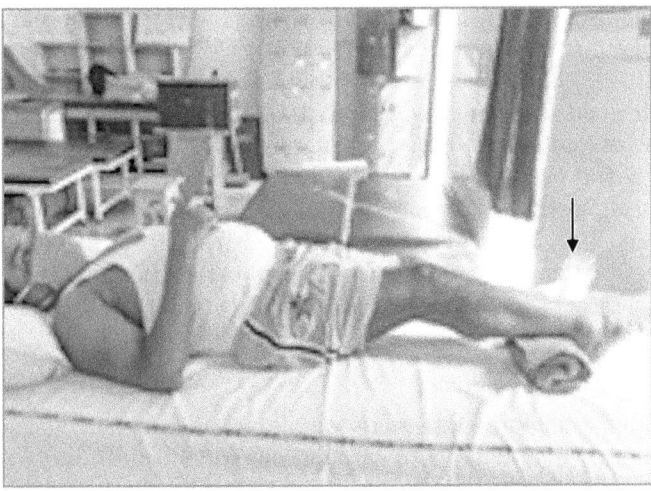

Fig. 8.48: Isometric hamstrings exercise.

the affected lower limb, agility drills are practiced and the individual is made to return to sports/activities after 4 weeks of injury.

Strengthening the quadriceps is a key factor in a successful recovery, as the quadriceps can take the place of the PCL to a certain extent to prevent the femur from moving too far forward over the tibia. Eccentric and isometric contraction of quadriceps is started first, followed by concentric contraction **(Fig. 8.49)**. Closed kinetic chain exercises such as mini squats holding on to support **(Fig. 8.50)** are used for strengthening of quadriceps.

- ❖ **Physiotherapy for grade-III PCL injuries:** Physiotherapy management during the period of immobilization include:
  – 2–4 weeks of knee immobilization, using knee immobilizer.
  – Cryotherapy/PSWD/PMWD.
  – Isometric quadriceps exercise and SLR exercises.

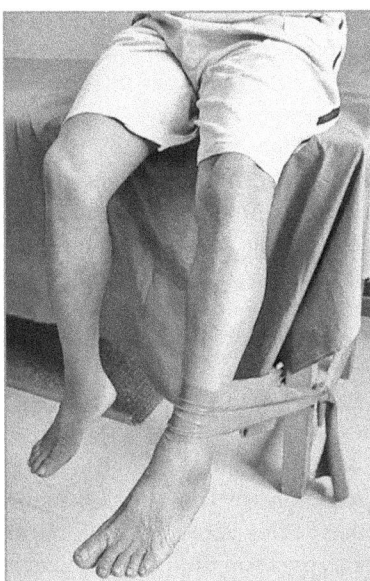

Fig. 8.49: Resisted concentric exercise to quadriceps.

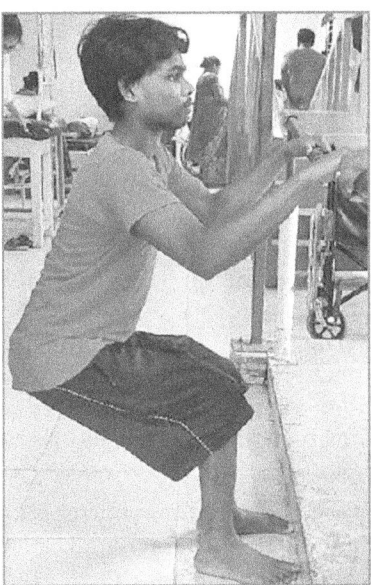

Fig. 8.50: Mini squat with support.

After 2–4 weeks of knee immobilization, physiotherapy consists of:
  – Active assisted knee flexion with in 70 degrees.
  – Multiangle isometric quadriceps exercises.
  – Surged faradic stimulation to quadriceps.
  – Progressive weight bearing from partial to full weight bearing within limits of pain.
  – Closed kinetic chain exercises, such as leg press, mini squat **(Figs. 8.43A and B)**.
  – Open kinetic chain eccentric quadriceps exercises, gradually progressing to concentric resisted quadriceps exercises.
  – Functional exercises such as static cycle exercise, stair climbing, etc.
  – Sports specific/activity specific exercises and return to sports/activity after 3 months, with and without use of a hinged knee brace.

- ❖ **Physiotherapy for chronic PCL injuries:** Chronic PCL injuries with/without knee stiffness are treated with physiotherapy and a knee brace, initially set to prevent terminal 15 degrees of extension, subsequently allowing full knee extension. The physiotherapy consists of:
  – PWB.
  – Gentle knee mobilization exercises (without producing accessory movements that may strain the injured ligament).
  – Multiangle isometric quadriceps exercise.
  – Surged faradic stimulation to quadriceps.
  – Active free knee flexion exercises, progressing gradually to active resisted knee flexion exercise.
  – Active resisted knee extension exercise using theraband/weight cuff.
  – Functional re-education, with or without a hinged knee brace/knee cap.

- ❖ **Surgical management of PCL injuries:** Surgical reconstruction of PCL in grade-III injuries, combined with other ligament injuries in the knee is performed, if there is severe posterior tibial subluxation and instability with a posterior translation greater than 10 mm. The surgery is usually performed within 2 weeks of injury.

Surgical procedures performed include:
- ❖ **Tibial inlay procedure:** Though started with diagnostic arthroscopy, but the procedure is an open surgery, where the graft is passed through the femoral tunnel and screwed to the bone. Knee immobilizing brace is applied after surgery.
- ❖ **Tibial tunnel method:** This is an arthroscopical approach, where the graft is placed either using the single bundle reconstruction, where only one tunnel is drilled or double bundle reconstruction, where two tunnels are drilled.

Postoperative physiotherapy

Following surgery, the knee immobilizer is applied, which should be removed periodically for application of cryopack to reduce pain and swelling. Postoperative PCL rehabilitation is delivered in two phases.
- ❖ **Phase-I:** Early postoperative phase (maximal protection and early rehabilitation phase): 0 to 6–8 weeks.
  The objectives include:
  – Reduce postoperative pain and swelling.
  – Restoration of knee ROM.
  – Mobilization of scar tissue.
  – Strengthening quadriceps.
  Methods followed:
  – Cryotherapy and limb elevation.
  – Patellofemoral mobilization.
  – Isometric quadriceps sets.
  – Active-assisted knee flexion (within 90 degrees) and extension exercises, with emphasis on achieving terminal knee extension.
  – Use of a dynamic PCL brace to prevent posterior sagging of tibia and elongation of graft. The brace should be used all the time for 6 months, except for periodic removal for cryotherapy, electrical stimulation, and exercises.
  – Nonweight bearing crutch gait is trained for 6 weeks followed by gradual weight-bearing exercises and ambulation
- ❖ **Phase-II:** Later postoperative rehabilitation:
  – Begins 8 weeks after surgery with the aim of preparing the patient for retraining to pre operative functional capacity by addressing all musculoskeletal deficits. The interventions given include:
    » Strengthening exercises to quadriceps and hamstrings.
    » Endurance exercises.
    » Agility drills.
    » Sports specific training and enabling the client return to sports and activities, with a dynamic knee brace (if necessary).

vii. Meniscal Lesions

The knee joint has two menisci, the lateral and medial, helpful in absorbing shock and nourishing the knee joint. The meniscus is typically an avascular structure with the primary blood supply limited to the periphery. Only the peripheral 10–25% of the meniscus is vascularized by vessels that are derived from the middle, medial, and lateral geniculate arteries. For that reason, when meniscus is damaged in the central portion, it is usually unable to undergo a normal healing process. The most peripheral portion of the meniscus has a blood supply and is more likely to heal. Medial meniscus resists more pressure during weight bearing than the lateral meniscus and therefore, it is more likely that tears occurs on the medial menisci.

Epidemiology/Etiology

Meniscal injuries are more common in males than females. Elderly people are also susceptible to meniscus injury, as the degenerated menisci get injured by minor trauma. The mean age range for meniscus injury is 28–40 years. Though children below 10 years usually do not get meniscus injury, a few children are affected with discoid meniscus, which is a rare congenital disorder, affecting the lateral meniscus, where the lateral meniscus loses its usual cupped-shape leading to instability of the lateral compartment of knee.

The injury is commonly found in athletes, where partial or total rupture of the lateral or medial meniscus is found, though medial meniscus injury is more common than lateral meniscus injury. Besides athletic activities, degenerative knee disease (osteoarthritis) can also lead to spontaneous meniscal tear through breakdown and weakening of meniscal structures.

The most common mechanism of injury is a twisting injury on a semiflexed weight-bearing knee. Medial meniscus injury may also be associated with other ligamentus injuries, typically the ACL and the MCL (Triad of O'donoghue)

Types of Meniscus Injury

Depending on severity, it could be:
- ❖ **Acute tear:** Acute tears result mostly from trauma/sports injuries and have different shapes (horizontal, vertical, radial, oblique, and complex).
- ❖ **Chronic tears:** These most often occur in elderly people, and are degenerative meniscal tears that occur after minimal trauma or stress on the knee.

Depending on pattern of injury: The tears could be of the following types (**Figs. 8.51A to F**):
- *Radial tear:* This begins at the inner edge of the meniscus and continues to the capsule. The radial cracks typically occur in the middle part of the meniscus. A radial tear of the lateral meniscus is often found together with an anterior-cruciate ligament tear.
- *Oblique tear:* Usually occurs at the height of the front or superior horn.
- *Longitudinal tear:* This type of tear can be anywhere along the meniscus. If this tear extends it may result in a bucket-handle tear.
- *Bucket handle tear:* The "bucket-handle" tear runs across nearly the entire length of the meniscus. This often causes the formation of a flap that can get caught between the intercondylar space.

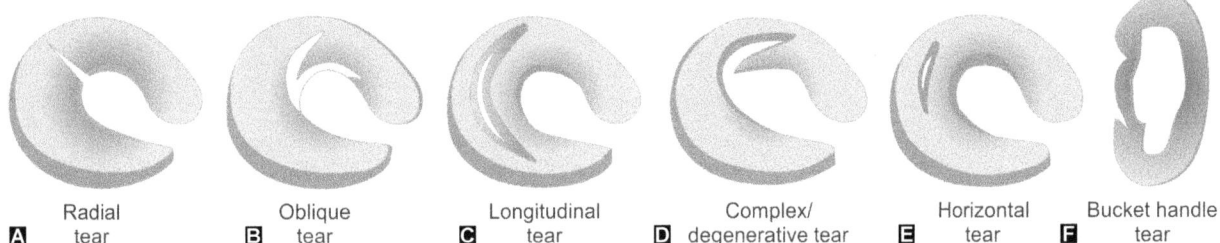

Figs. 8.51A to F: Types of meniscal tears: (A) Radial tear, (B) Oblique tear, (C) Longitudinal tear, (D) Complex degenerative tear, (E) Horizontal tear, (F) Bucket handle tear.

- *Horizontal rupture:* This tear begins at the inner edge of the meniscus and continue against the capsule.
- *Complex rupture:* These are patterns that describe tears in different planes and are seen in the degenerative meniscus.

Clinical Features

The clinical presentation of meniscal lesion (traumatic and degenerative) may be:

- Medial or lateral knee pain which is intermittent and residual in nature, depending upon the affected compartment.
- Locking of the knee (in bucket handle tears).
- Popping sound in the knee on movements.
- Marked tenderness in knee joint line as per the compartments affected.
- Apart from the above people with degenerative meniscus lesion, also show patellofemoral dysfunction, due to damage of the cartilage under patella, as well as pain on movements and loading of the of knee, such as squatting, kneeling, etc.
- The clinical tests like McMurray test, Apley's grinding test, etc., are positive.
- Discoid lateral meniscus found in children may be asymptomatic, but may produce symptoms, if tear to meniscus occurs.

Diagnostic Procedure

Diagnosis is done through:
- History of trauma/degenerative joint disease.
- Clinical features seen.
- **Clinical examinations:** Testing movement of knee, Special tests like McMurray test, Apley's grinding tests, Joint line tenderness.
- MRI/CT scan.
- Arthroscopy

Management of Meniscus Injury

Conservative treatment is usually not very successful for management of meniscal tears in young athletes, hence requiring surgical management.

Conservative management:
- **PRICE:** Immediately following injury, the knee should be immobilized in a knee immobilizing brace **(Fig. 8.38)** to prevent further injury. The player/affected individual should be off play/activity. Cold packs to be applied at regular intervals by removing knee brace, to reduce inflammation. An elastic crepe bandage may be applied along with the knee immobilizer, in case of massive swelling and the affected limb should be supported and elevated.
- **Medical management:** NSAIDs.
- **Physiotherapy:** The aim of physiotherapy in meniscus injury is to improve knee function and to reduce pain. There is strong evidence that, physiotherapy plays an important role in reducing symptoms such as pain swelling and stiffness, strengthening muscles around knee and improving physical ability/function.

As discussed earlier, during acute stage, PRICE is the initial treatment given by Physiotherapist. Cryotherapy is applied for 20 minutes at every 2 hourly intervals within the first 48–72 hours. After acute pain subsided, knee rehabilitation is started.

Knee rehabilitation

Strengthening of quadriceps, hamstrings, proprioceptive training, such as balance board exercise, mini hops on trampoline, agility drills such as figure-of-8 walking are practiced in a progressive manner as described below to improve knee stability and function.

Pulsed short-wave diathermy, pulsed ultrasound, high power laser therapy, IFT, surged faradic current stimulation to overcome quadriceps inhibition are applied judiciously after a thorough clinical reasoning and considering the evidences.

The exercises comprise of:
- **Isometric exercises for quadriceps such as:** Isometric quadriceps sets, Straight leg raises. For isometric quadriceps sets: Patient supine/long sitting. A roll of towel is placed under the knee **(Fig. 8.21A)**. He/she is asked to press the roll hold for 6–10 seconds and relax. Each set comprises of 6–10 contractions and 2–3 sets of exercise are practiced in one session.
- **Isometric hamstrings sets:** The patient in supine/long sitting. The sound leg is straight and the involved knee is kept in slight flexion with the heel on the bed/pillow **(Fig. 8.48)**. The patient is asked to push the bed/pillow with the heel, hold for 6–10 seconds and relax. Each set comprises of 6–10 contractions and 2–3 sets of exercise are practiced in one session.
- **Nonweight-bearing isotonic exercises:**
  - Short arc quadriceps exercises in supine lying/high sitting **(Fig. 8.52)**

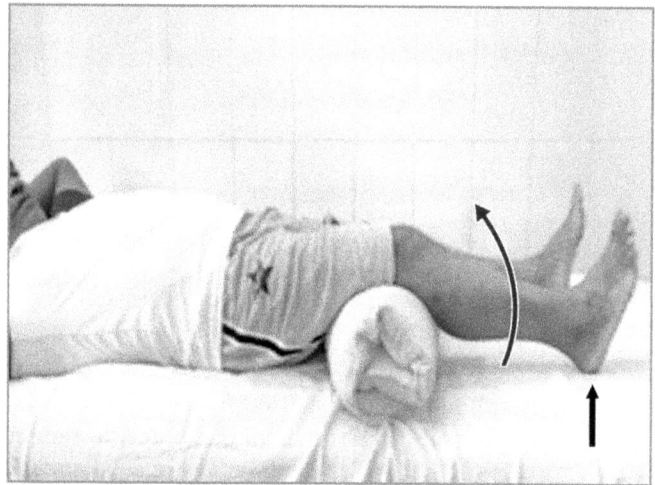

Fig. 8.52: Short arc quadriceps exercise in supine lying.

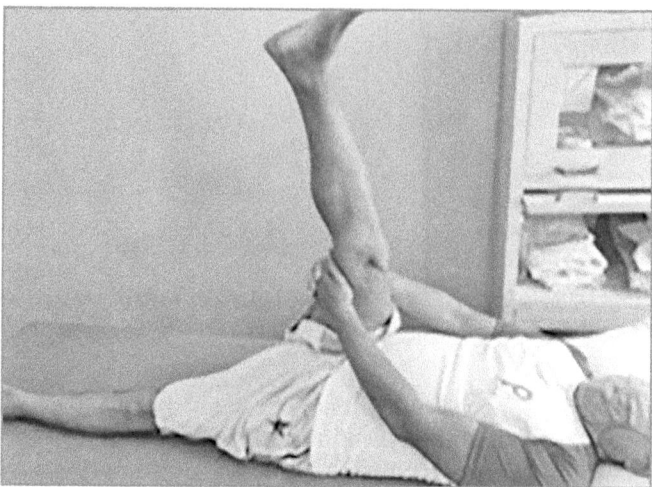

Fig. 8.54: Active stretch of knee flexors.

- Full arc quadriceps exercises in high sitting, progressing from active free to active resisted (**Figs. 8.53A and B**).
- Hamstrings curls in prone lying.

❖ **Weight-bearing resistive exercises:**
  - *Reciprocal training:* Exercising on static cycle (**Fig. 8.44**).
  - Leg press (**Fig. 8.43B**) mini-wall squats, lunges, stepping up and down, and lateral stepping.

❖ **Flexibility and joint mobilization exercises:**
  - Positional stretching of knee flexors to achieve knee extension in prone lying/long sitting. Active stretch for extension such as SLR exercises (**Fig. 8.54**) are also made to practice.
  - Prolonged flexion stretch is applied in kneel sitting/squatting as tolerated. Active stretch for flexion, such as prone knee bending is also practiced.

❖ **Joint mobilization:** In case of stiffness, following joints should be mobilized:
  - Superior tibiofibular joint.
  - Patellofemoral joint.
  - Tibiofemoral joint.

❖ **Balance and agility exercises:** Activities involving standing on both the legs, single-limb stance, etc., are practiced.

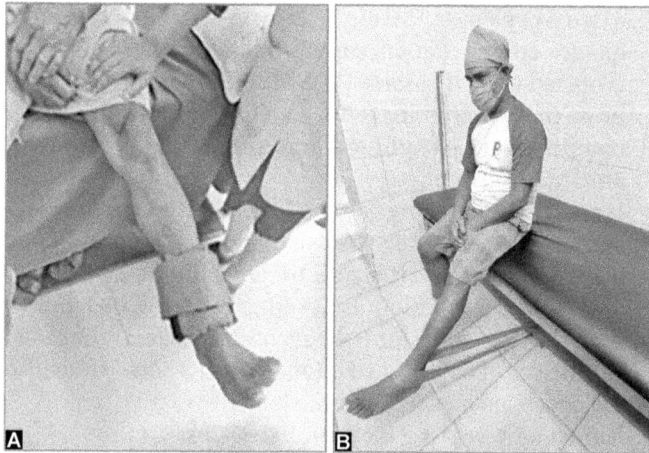

Figs. 8.53A and B: Resisted quadriceps exercise using: (A) Weight cuff, (B) Theraband.

Depending on the intensity of pain, the patient should be progressed from nonweight-bearing ambulation to partial weight-bearing ambulation using walker/Axillary/Elbow crutches and finally should be made to walk unaided. Before return to sports/activities, sports/activity specific exercises are practiced.

Surgical Management

If surgery is necessary, there are two options such as:
❖ Repair of meniscus, done arthroscopically.
❖ **Meniscectomy (Partial/full):** Partial meniscectomy is usually done arthroscopically, however, a complete meniscectomy is done through open surgery.

If a rupture can not be treated and it involves a large portion of the meniscus, or when repair failed, a significant portion of the meniscus must sometimes be removed. To avoid secondary osteoarthritis and reducing pain, meniscal transplantation may be the best solution in some cases.

Postoperative rehabilitation

After surgery the patient is advised protected weight-bearing through crutches for at least 3 weeks. Exercises and modalities used for conservative management are also used during postoperative management. Full recovery using a comprehensive rehabilitation program usually takes 3–4 months, and athletes in high level sports such as foot ball playing are expected to be in the field around 6–8 months.

viii. Medial Collateral Ligament Injury and its Management

Medial collateral ligament injury is one of the most common knee injuries, which results from a valgus force on the knee.

Epidemiology/Etiology

An impact on the outer aspect of thigh/leg with the foot on the ground results in injury to the MCL. A combined movement of flexion/valgus/external rotation results in injury to this ligament. Mostly the deep part of the ligament is damaged first, which may lead to damage of medial meniscus and/or ACL.

This injury is commonly found in athletes. Falling from height, road traffic accidents also result in injury to this ligament.

Clinical Features

Like any other ligament injury, MCL injuries are graded into grades: I, II, III. The grades and their clinical presentation are given in the **Table 8.2**.

Medial Column Injury

Besides the above three grades, a grade-IV injury is also described in literature, also called as medial column injury, to the MCL. It occurs when the injury affects more than just the medial collateral ligament (MCL).

Diagnostic Procedure

History of trauma, clinical findings such as tenderness/ pain and swelling on the medial side of knee, clinical tests such as valgus stress test, swain test, etc., help in establishing the diagnosis of MCL injury.

Magnetic resonance imaging (MRI) is also an important tool for the examination of an injury of the medial collateral ligament.

Management

The treatment of medial collateral injury is usually conservative, rarely requiring surgical intervention. Isolated grade I and II MCL injuries are managed conservatively, however, management of grade-III injury, depends on, whether the injury is an isolated MCL injury, where conservative treatment is considered, or it is MCL injury associated with other ligament injuries (grade-IV injury), where surgical reconstruction is considered.

The treatment protocols focus on early range of motion, swelling reduction, protected weight bearing, progression toward strengthening, and stability exercises.

Immediately after injury treatment consists of NSAIDs and PRICE. Physiotherapy and rehabilitation depends upon the grade of injury, which are described below.

Table 8.2: Grades of MCL injuries.

Grade	Symptoms	Signs	Translation
I	Mild, tenderness, pain and swelling in the medial aspects	Medial edema/ tenderness	0–5 mm
II	Moderate, tenderness, pain, and swelling on the medial aspect of knee with some instability (moderate joint laxity present)	Medial edema/ tenderness	6–10 mm
III	Severe medial pain, swelling, and instability (the knee gives way into valgus). A complete rupture of ligament present	Marked medial edema and tenderness	>10 mm

Grade-I: During the first 48 hours, ice, compression and elevation should be used as much as possible. These incomplete tears are treated with temporary immobilization with rest and application of elastic crepe bandage/knee cap, crutches for protected weight bearing and pain control. The degree of weight bearing depends on the intensity of pain. The crepe bandage/ knee cap should be removed periodically for application of cryo packs. After pain and swelling subsided significantly, exercises consisting of isometric, isotonic and isokinetic progressive resisted exercises are started. Modalities such as pulsed ultrasound, low intensity laser, surged faradic current stimulation to quadriceps are used to promote healing and strengthen quadriceps.

Grade-II and III injuries: The knee should be immobilized in a knee immobilizer **(Fig. 8.38)** for 3–4 weeks to allow the ligament to heal. Protected weight bearing with the knee immobilizer on, using walker/axillary crutches is followed during this period. Isometric quadriceps sets are performed at regular intervals and cryotherapy (ice packs) are applied to the knee after loosening the anterior opening of the knee immobilizer, till the swelling reduced significantly. After 4 weeks, isotonic and isokinetic progressive resisted exercises are started, preferably using a hinged knee brace **(Fig. 8.45)**/ knee cap.

Pulsed ultrasound, low intensity laser/high power laser, surged faradic current stimulation to quadriceps/Russian current stimulation to quadriceps may be used as per need to promote healing of ligament, reduce pain, and strengthen quadriceps.

The overall rehabilitation of MCL injury consists of three phases:

- **Phase-I:** The duration of this phase lasts for 1–2 weeks. During this phase, effort is to reduce swelling of the knee by applying ice 15 minutes every 2 hours (first 48 hours), and 15 minutes three times a day subsequently. Protected weight bearing through crutches are started progressing to partial weight bearing using single crutch and subsequently full weight bearing as the condition improves.

  The patient may begin with static quadriceps sets, straight leg raises, active knee range of motion exercises, sitting hip flexion exercises, side lying hip abduction exercises, standing hip extension exercises, standing hamstrings curl, etc. As soon as patient can tolerate these exercises, exercise on static cycle is advised to increase ROM of knee. Pain free stretching of hamstrings, quadriceps, and calf muscles along with upper limb workouts are performed during this phase. Use of a single crutch, and a hinged knee brace should be made till pain subsided.

  Electrotherapy modalities like pulsed ultrasound, low intensity laser, surged faradic current stimulation to quadriceps, Russian current stimulation to quadriceps, etc., should be applied as needed.

- **Phase-II:** The phase-II rehabilitation starts at the third week of injury and continues up to 5 weeks. The same exercises for gain in muscle strength and ROM as done in phase-I, are also done in this phase of rehabilitation. However, static bicycle exercises are resisted as per the patient's tolerance and the duration of the exercise may be increased up to 20 minutes. Hamstrings curls, leg press-Double leg (**Fig. 8.43B**), step up with sound leg on the ground are practiced. Heat therapy in the form of SWD (Monoplanar), MWD, high power laser may be selected to increase blood flow and promote healing. Muscle strengthening currents like surged faradic current/Russian stimulation to quadriceps may be considered.

Protected weight bearing with the hinged knee brace should be considered.

- **Phase-III:** This phase starts from week 5. The major goal in this phase is to achieve full weight bearing on the injured knee without using a brace (if possible). The exercises as done in phase –II are also done in this phase, however they may be progressed in intensity. Aerobic capacity is increased by prolonged static cycling, stepping, and exercising in hydrotherapy pool.

  Full knee range of knee motion is the expectation; any swelling present in this phase is controlled by using cryotherapy and compression bandaging.

- **Phase-IV:** This phase starts 6 weeks after injury. The hinged knee brace used during gait is now discontinued, however, for athletes participating in competitive sports the brace may be used for 3 months. Any swelling present is controlled by cold therapy and compression bandages. The intensity of the exercises is progressed from double-leg press to single-leg press using the affected leg. Running, proprioceptive training on balanced board, etc., are started, ensuring that the activity, does not require a sudden change in direction. Sports/activity specific training is imparted with the hinged brace on and gradually the athlete/worker is returned to sports/activity.

Surgical Management

Grade-III injuries, occurring at the tibial site, injuries that are unstable in 0 degree extension, and chronic MCL injuries causing significant knee instability are managed by surgical reconstruction. The postoperative management is given as per the conservative management through the four phases described earlier.

ix. Lateral Collateral Injury Management

The lateral collateral ligament (**Fig. 8.36**) is a strong connection between the lateral condyle of femur and head of fibula. This ligament is loose, when the knee is flexed to 30 degrees or more.

Epidemiology/Etiology

The ligament is injured in the same proportion in males and females. A varus stress to knee, lateral rotation of the knee, when weight bearing causes injury to the lateral collateral ligament of knee. The lateral collateral ligament can be sprained (Grade-I), partially ruptured (Grade-II), or completely ruptured (Grade-III).

Repeated varus stress to the knee as found in chronic osteoarthritis of knee can also result in injury to lateral collateral ligament.

Clinical Features

In an acute case, pain, swelling, lateral joint line tenderness, increased varus movement with varus stressing, reduced ROM of knee, knee instability, difficulty in weight bearing is the presentation. In subacute and chronic states, pain and tenderness decreases significantly, however, unspecific knee pain and knee instability persists depending on the grades of injury.

Grade-I: Mild pain and tenderness over the lateral collateral ligament. Usually no swelling and instability (< 5 mm instability).

Grade-II: Significant pain and tenderness and mild swelling on the lateral collateral ligament. The varus stress is painful with some laxity (5–10 mm instability).

Grade-III: The pain and tenderness on the lateral aspect of the knee is less as compared to grade-II injury, however the swelling may be significant with marked instability (> 10 mm laxity).

Diagnosis

The history of trauma/degenerative knee joint disease, clinical tests (varus stress test) and some times a plane radiograph (AP view) helps to diagnose the condition.

Management

Grade-I and II injuries of lateral collateral ligament are managed conservatively, however grade-III injuries requires surgical intervention to achieve a stable, well-aligned knee with normal biomechanics.

Conservative management:
- NSAIDs.
- Physiotherapy: It depends on the stage of the injury, as discussed below:
  - *Acute stage:*
    » PRICE: Protection of the knee in knee brace that allows limited knee flexion and full extension, rest, ice, compression and elevation.
    » Protected weight bearing (nonweight bearing cutch gait to partial weight bearing gait as tolerated).
    » Exercises: Active-assisted knee movements, isometric quadriceps exercises, straight leg raise exercises, are performed.
    » Pulsed ultrasound/PSWD/low intensity laser may be applied over the site of injury to promote healing.
    » Surged faradic current to the quadriceps can be applied to prevent atrophy/weakness/quadriceps inhibition.
  - *Subacute stage and chronic stage:*
    » Full weight bearing mobilization and gait as per the patient's level of pain and instability with the hinged knee brace (**Fig. 8.45**) on.
    » Resisted quadriceps (**Fig. 8.49**), hamstrings (**Fig. 8.40**) and gluteal strengthening (**Figs. 8.41 and 8.42**) exercises are performed.
    » Surged faradic current/Russian current stimulation to quadriceps may be applied to strengthen quadriceps.

» Progressive closed kinetic chain exercises, plyometric exercises, proprioceptive training are emphasized with sports/activity specific training.

Surgery

For grade-III injuries surgery is usually performed. Surgery usually involve repair of LCL using graft taken from IT band.

Postoperative management

Following surgery a knee immobilizer may be used to limit valgus/varus stress and knee flexion during gait. Early active ROM exercises are encouraged in the nonweight-bearing position and the physiotherapy program described for the conservative management are also followed postoperatively.

Nonweight bearing to partial weight bearing crutch gait is practiced during the initial 6 weeks post operatively, subsequently a full weight bearing ambulation is allowed with or without a hinged knee brace depending on the knee stability.

x. Plica Syndrome and its Management

Plica syndrome is an internal derangement of the knee caused by an inflammation or injury to the supra patellar, medial patellar or the lateral plica, or a combination of the three, and which prevents normal functioning of the knee joint. It is a painful disorder of knee, particularly seen in children and adolescents and occurs when an otherwise normal structure (plica) in the knee becomes a source of anterior or anteromedial knee pain due to injury or overuse.

A synovial plica is a shelf-like membrane between the synovium of the patella and the tibiofemoral joint, consisting of mesenchymal tissue, which is formed in the knee during the embryonic phase of development. This tissue usually starts to involute (fold inward) at 8–12 weeks of fetal growth, and is eventually resorbed, leaving a single empty area between the distal femoral and proximal tibial epiphysis. However, in many individuals the mesenchymal tissue is not fully resorbed and consequently the cavitation of the knee joint remains incomplete. In these individuals plicae can be observed, which represent inward folds of the synovial membrane in the knee joint.

Four types of plicae can be distinguished, depending on the anatomical location within the knee joint cavities: They include suprapatellar, mediopatellar, infrapatellar, and lateral plicae. The plicae in the knee joint can vary in both structure and size; they can be fibrous or fatty, longitudinal or crescent-shaped.

Epidemiology/Etiology

The disorder is commonly seen in children and adolescents. Women are affected more than men. Synovial plicae mostly are asymptomatic and of little clinical consequence. However, they can become symptomatic when they are injured or irritated. Various conditions, such as direct trauma or blow to the plica, blunt trauma, twisting injuries, repetitive flexion and extension of the knee, increased activity levels, weakness of the vastus medialis muscle, intra-articular bleeding, osteochondritis dissecans, torn meniscus, chronic, or transient synovitis, lead to development of this disorder. After the healing of initial injury, patients may remain asymptomatic for few weeks to months, and subsequently may develop anterior knee pain.

Clinical Features

The syndrome causes a series of symptoms such as pain, clicking, popping, localized swelling in knee, knee joint effusion, and reduced range of motion of knee joint, intermittent medial joint pain, instability, and locking of the patellofemoral joint.

The sufferers report sudden development of symptoms, which get worsened progressively. The pain is intermittent dull aching type, which get aggravated by performing patellofemoral loading activities such as ascending and descending stairs, squatting, kneeling etc. On flexion and extension of knee cracking noise may be heard. Sometimes the patient experiences a feeling of instability when walking up and down the stairs and walking on slopes.

Diagnostic Procedures

Diagnosis of this knee disorder is made considering the followings:
- Physical examination.
- Provocation tests: Hughston's plica test (**Fig. 8.16**), Plica stutter test (**Fig. 8.17**).
- Arthroscopy can be helpful because plica syndrome is often confused with chondromalacia or a medial meniscal tear.
- X-ray: May not be helpful in establishing plica syndrome.
- MRI: MRI is useful to evaluate the thickness and extension of synovial plicae and it can also detect a pathologic plica, particularly if an intra-articular effusion is present.

Management

The initial treatment of a plica syndrome is conservative in the form of rest, NSAIDs and physiotherapy. If no improvement results and symptoms get aggravated, intraplical or intra articular corticosteroid injections are tried by the Surgeon.

Physiotherapy

The main goal of physiotherapy in plica syndrome is to reduce pain, maximize the ROM and increase the strength of the muscles.

The therapeutic interventions consist of:
- Cryotherapy to reduce inflammation and pain.
- Relative rest (reducing activities involving repeated flexion/extension).
- Gentile stretching of hamstrings (**Fig. 8.55**) and strengthening of quadriceps isometrically.
- Modalities such as MWD/Ultrasound therapy/Phonophoresis/Iontophoresis, etc., may be considered.
- Deep transverse friction massage to mobilize scar tissue (if any).

After acute inflammation subsided, therapy is provided aiming at decreasing the compressive forces, by enhancing flexibility of hamstrings and strengthening quadriceps isometrically and concentrically (**Fig. 8.49**). Stretching of

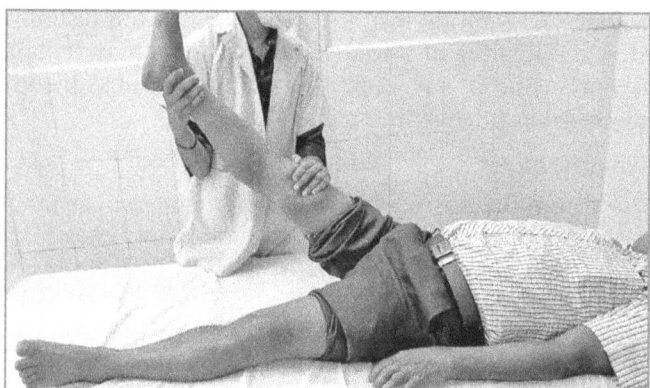

Fig. 8.55: Stretching of hamstring muscle.

hamstrings **(Fig. 8.22)** and strengthening of muscles around and adjacent to the knee such as quadriceps, hamstrings, hip adductors/abductors, and gastrosoleus are performed.

Endurance activities such as mini squats, leg press, static cycle exercises, walking up and down stairs, hydrotherapy, etc., may be advised to perform as required.

As per need modalities such as MWD/Ultrasound therapy/Phonophoresis/Iontophoresis, etc., may be considered.

After considerable reduction of pain and swelling, the individual should be given activity/sports specific training and is gradually returned to sports/activity, with the advice to continue quadriceps strengthening and to follow energy conservation measures during sports/activities.

Surgery

If nonoperative measures fail surgery should be considered.

Postoperative rehabilitation after plica resection usually goes quickly. Physiotherapy is recommended starting 48–72 hours postoperatively, to prevent intra-articular scarring, and stiffness. Physiotherapy treatment after surgery follows the same interventions as described under conservative management. Most patients can resume sporting/functional activities within 3–6 weeks.

xi. Rehabilitation After Total Knee Replacement

Total knee replacement arthroplasty (TKA), also known as total knee replacement (TKR), is an orthopedic surgical procedure, where the articular surfaces of the knee joint (femoral condyles and tibial plateau) are replaced, with or without replacement of patella **(Figs. 8.56A and B)**. The end of the femur is removed and replaced with a metal surface and the top of the tibia is removed and replaced with a plastic piece that has a metal stem. For the patella, a plastic piece may be added to the posterior surface to create a smoother joint surface. Sometimes, a partial knee replacement **(Fig. 8.57)** may be performed, as required.

Indications of Total Knee Replacement

* Disabling knee pain with functional limitation.
* Progressive arthritis of knee, i.e., Osteoarthritis/Rheumatoid arthritis.
* Ankylosis of knee joint.

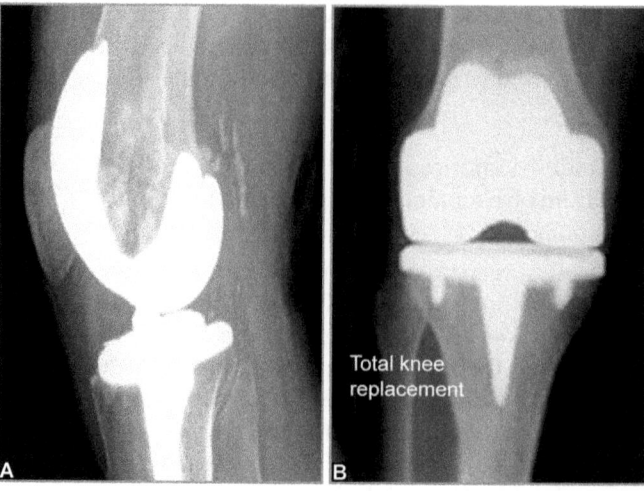

Figs. 8.56A and B: (A) TKR-Lateral view, (B) TKR-AP view.

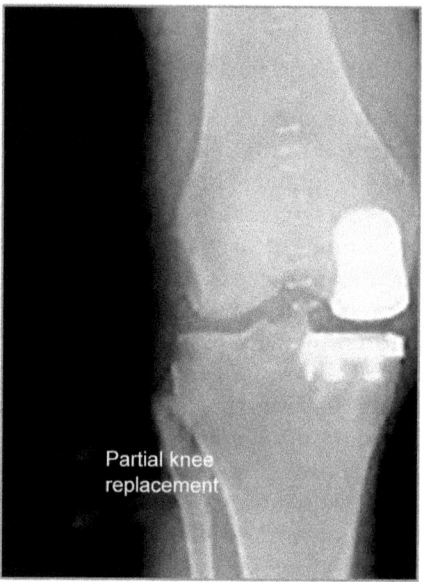

Fig. 8.57: Partial knee replacement.

Contraindications for Total Knee Replacement

* Neuropathic joints (Charcot's joint).
* Joint infection.
* Painful solid knee fusion (as a complication of reflex sympathetic dystrophy).
* Systemic infection.
* Severe osteoporosis.

Types of procedures followed:

* Cemented total knee arthroplasty **(Fig. 8.58A)**
* Noncemented total knee arthroplasty **(Fig. 8.58B)**
* Hybrid TKA: It has an uncemented femoral component and cemented tibial and/or patellar component **(Fig. 8.58C)**

The implant/prosthesis selected could be PCL retaining, PCL sacrificing, or PCL sacrificing with substitution type. The PCL retaining type achieves an increased ROM of knee, as compared to PCL substituting type. The PCL substituting type of prosthesis has higher failure rate, because of loosening.

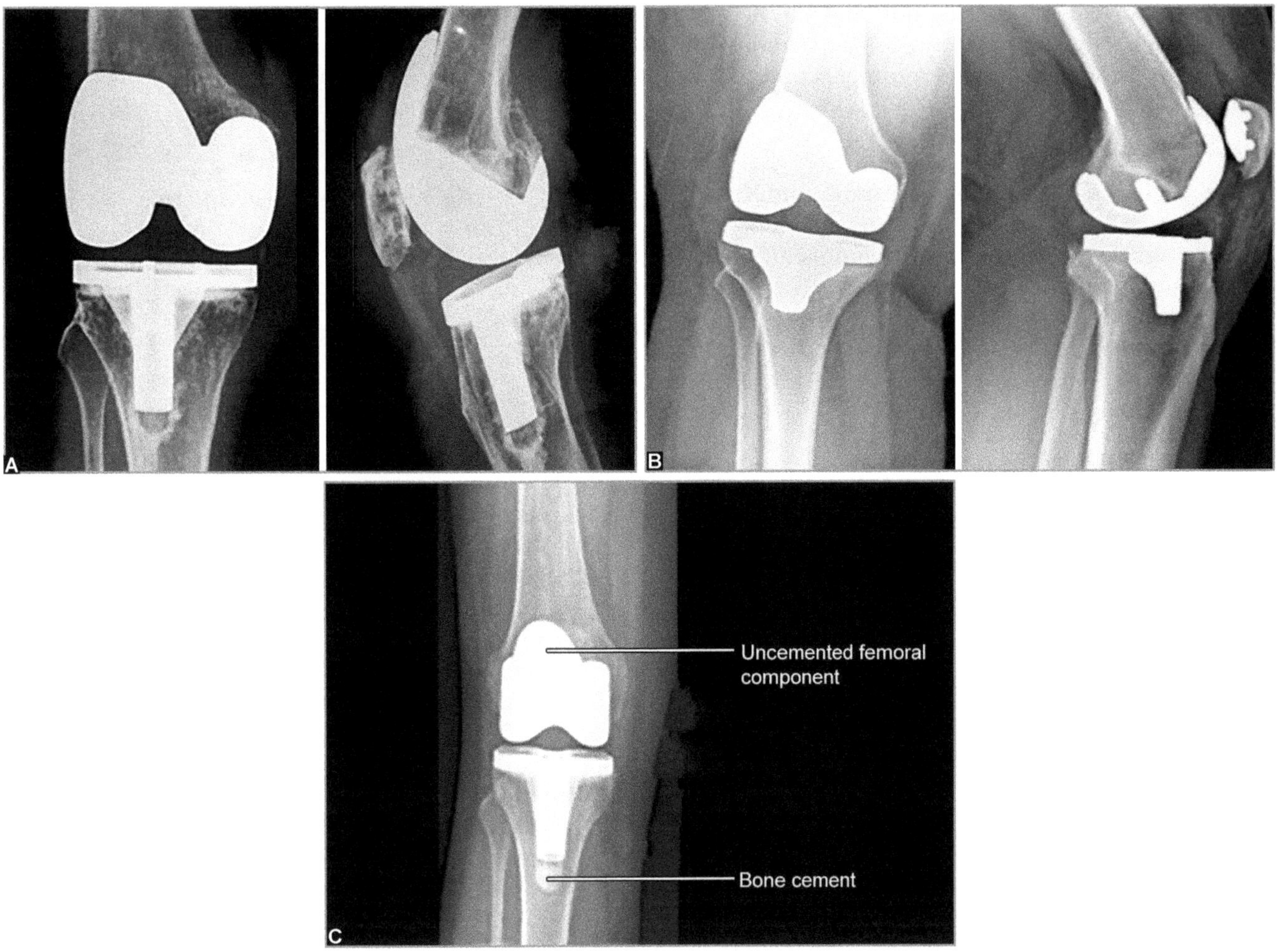

Figs. 8.58A to C: (A) Cemented TKR. (B) Uncemented TKR (C) Hybrid prosthesis.

The classical surgical approach used is the medial parapatellar approach **(Fig. 8.59)**, though other approaches include subvastus approach, mid vastus approach, and lateral approach.

Rehabilitation after Total Knee Replacement

Goals of Total Knee Replacement Rehabilitation

- Prevent bed rest complications like DVT, pulmonary embolism, pressure ulcers.
- Assist in achieving adequate functional knee range of motion.
- Strengthen knee musculature.
- Achieve 0–90 degrees of ROM in the first 2 weeks, before discharge from an inpatient setting.
- Achieve quadriceps control and strength at the earliest, enabling the patient to ambulate without knee immobilizer and walking aids.
- Achieve independent ambulation with/without an assistive device.
- Assist patient in achieving functional independence in ADL and IADL.
- Improve the overall quality of living.

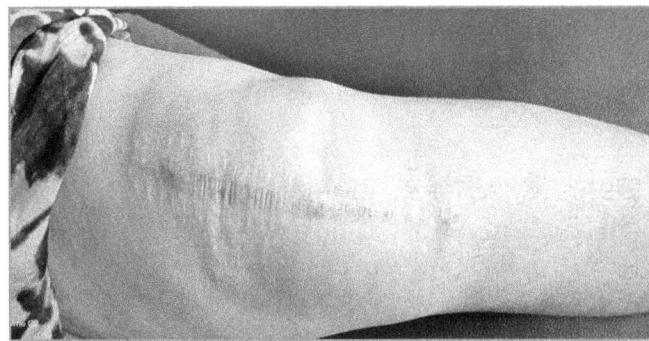

Fig. 8.59: Medial parapatellar approach for total knee arthroplasty.

Weight Bearing Schedule after Total Knee Replacement

- **Cemented total knee arthroplasty:** Weight bearing as tolerated with walker from day-1, postoperatively (or as advised by the Surgeon).
- **Hybrid (TKA with an uncemented femoral component and cemented tibial and patellar component) or in growth total knee arthroplasty (uncemented):** First 6 weeks postoperative period: touched down weight bearing with walker, next 6 weeks weight bearing as tolerated with

crutches, subsequently walking independently or walking with a stick. However, the surgeon's opinion should be sought for weight-bearing protocols and followed accordingly.

Expected Complications
- Knee stiffness is the most common complication following TKR.
- Loosening/fracture of prosthetic component.
- Joint instability.
- Infection.
- Nerve damage.
- Bone fracture.
- Swelling and joint pain.

Preoperative Physiotherapy
- Explain about the procedure and review the precautions.
- Teach preoperative strengthening exercises for quadriceps, hamstrings and glutei muscles, as well as deep breathing exercises.
- Teach postoperative exercises.
- Teach bed to chair transfers, bathroom transfers, etc.
- Teach ambulation with assistive devices for touched down weight bearing (TDWB), and weight bearing as tolerated (WBAT), to be performed postoperatively.

Postoperative Physiotherapy
Evidence indicates that, physiotherapy is always beneficial to the patient after TKR. Though level of evidence may be low, it reveals that, accelerated physiotherapy regimens can reduce acute hospital length of stay.

The most important role of physiotherapy in the management of patients after TKA is facilitation of knee mobilization within 48 hours of surgery. A continuous passive motion (CPM) exerciser **(Fig. 8.60)** may be used in the early postoperative period to maintain knee mobility. Cryotherapy may be applied in the early postoperative phase, to help reduce pain and increase knee range of motion.

Postoperative Rehabilitation Protocol

- **Days: 1–2 postoperation:**
  - Active ankle and foot exercises.
  - Isometric gluteal exercises **(Fig. 8.61)**, i.e., squeezing buttock.

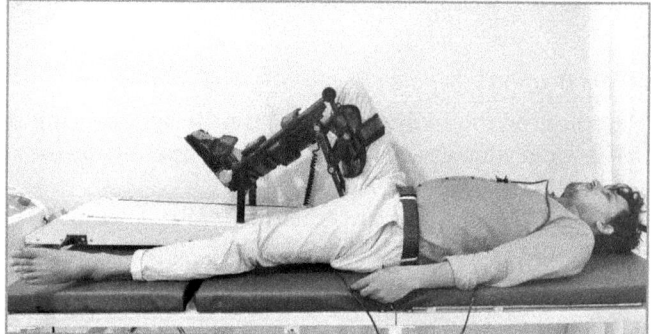

Fig. 8.60: CPM for knee mobilization.

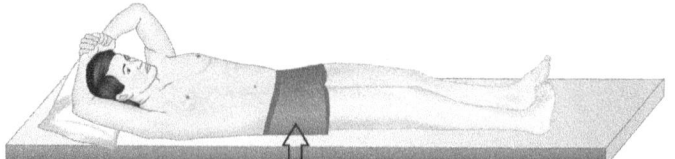

Fig. 8.61: Isometric gluteal exercise.

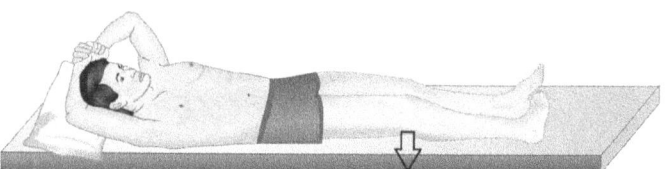

Fig. 8.62: Isometric quadriceps exercise in supine.

- **Isometric quadriceps sets:** In supine lying, the patient is asked to push the affected knee against the bed **(Fig. 8.62)** causing the muscles of front of thigh contract, hold the muscle contraction for 6 seconds and then relax for 6 seconds. The exercises are repeated for 10 times (1 set) for each leg. Total 2–3 sets of exercises are performed in each session and 3–4 sessions of exercises are performed in a day.
  - *Straight leg rises:* In supine lying the affected leg is raised 6–10 inches, keeping the knee straight, held for 6 seconds, and then slowly lowered to bed. Total 10–20 repetitions of exercises are performed in a session. If the patient does not have any difficulty, in doing the straight leg raises, gradually resistance/load is applied to the ankle to make the SLR resisted.
  - Walking with knee immobilizer applied, holding a walker twice a day:
    » Cemented prosthesis: Weight bearing as tolerated.
    » Noncemented prosthesis: Touched down weight bearing with walker.
  - Transfer training from bed to chair twice a day with the affected knee in full extension.
  - Knee mobilization using CPM machine **(Fig. 8.60)**: Till the 3rd postoperative day, knee flexion range of motion should be limited to 40 degrees of flexion. Gradually progression for gain of knee flexion should be made 5–10 degrees per day as per patient's tolerance. The rate of movement is usually maintained at 1 cycle per minute.
  - Gradually active assisted/active free ROM exercises for knee is started.
  - A pillow may be placed under the ankle to achieve passive knee extension **(Fig. 8.63)**.
  - Cryotherapy may be applied to reduce pain and swelling. A pack made from crushed ice and towel may be placed over the knee for 15–20 minutes.
- **1–2 weeks postoperation:**
  - Isometric quadriceps exercises are continued.
  - Exercise on CPM may be continued if necessary.
  - Isolated VMO strengthening is emphasized: In supine lying, a pillow or roll of towel is placed below the knee maintaining a knee flexion angle of 30–40 degrees

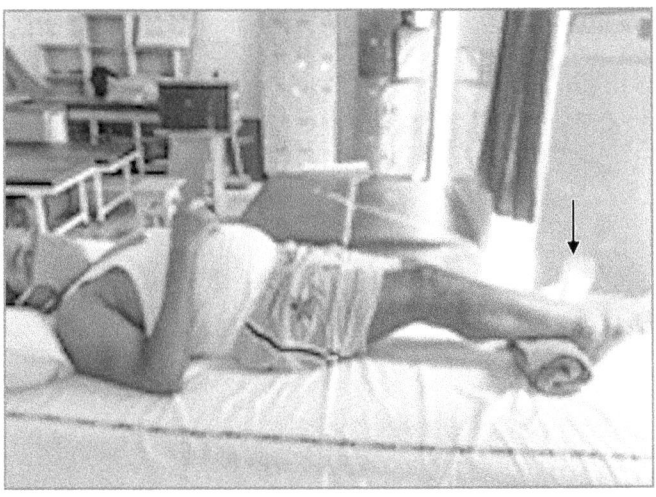

Fig. 8.63: Passive knee extension with pillow under the leg.

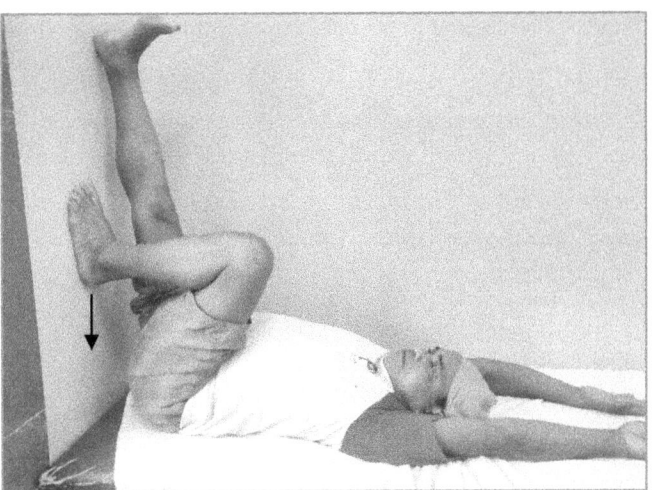

Fig. 8.65: Wall slides.

(**Fig. 8.64**). Patient is asked to tighten the quadriceps by lifting the heel off the bed, hold for 5-6 seconds, and then relax. The exercise is repeated 10-20 times in a session.
- Knee exercises such as heel slides, wall slides (**Fig. 8.65**) are gradually performed to achieve knee flexion and extension.
- Active hip abduction and adduction exercises are started gradually.
- Gentle patellar mobilization exercises can be started without damaging the incision.
- All the exercises are gradually progressed until completion of 6 weeks postoperatively.
- Walking and weight bearing to continue using the same protocol as described for day-1.
- Once the knee range of motion has increased to 0-90 degrees and the patient can do independent transfers from bed to chair, discharge can be planned to attend Physiotherapy on out patient basis.

❖ **2-3 weeks postoperation:**
- The previously described exercises are also continued during this period.

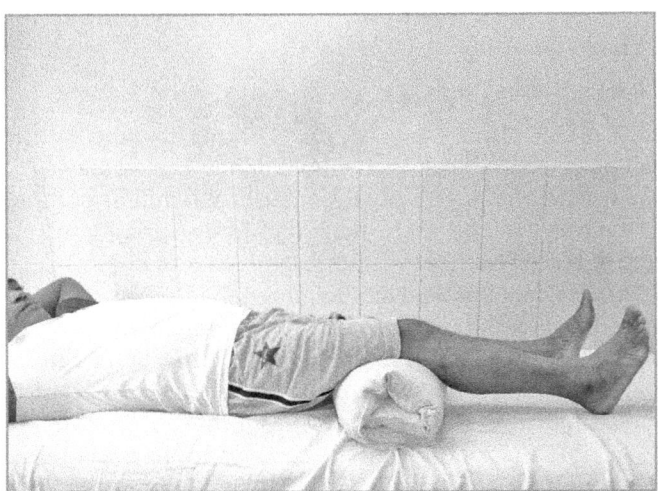

Fig. 8.64: Isolated VMO strengthening.

- Walking with a walker is continued as before.
- Driving and sexual activities putting load on the affected knee should not be performed.

❖ **3-6 weeks postoperation:**
By this time, the patient attends out patient physiotherapy clinic. The therapy involves:
- Exercises and walking are continued as before.
- For cemented procedures, walking is progressed from using the walker to using elbow crutches and finally to a walking cane. At the end of the 6th week, the patient may also be made to walk independently.
- More aggressive knee ROM exercises can be started, achieving 100-105 degrees of movement by the end of this week.
- Exercises on a static bi-cycle (**Fig. 8.44**) can be started.
- Surged faradic current stimulation to quadriceps is applied to increase strength.
- Driving and sexual activities that involve stressing the affected knee should be avoided.
- Cold pack should be applied, if swelling and pain persists.

❖ **7-8 weeks postoperation:**
- Begin weight bearing as tolerated using crutches/walking stick, progressing from touch down weight bearing for non cemented prosthesis.
- Gait training with or without a cane for cemented prosthesis.
- Emphasis is laid more on gaining strength of muscles around the knee and train proprioception and balance.
- Wall slides and lunges in short arc are performed.
- Step up and down over the affected leg is performed.
- Closed chain exercises such as leg press using both legs (**Fig. 8.43B**), are performed.
- Static cycle exercises are continued.
- Exercises on balance board are performed.

Discharge criteria after TKA:
- 0-90 degrees of movement in knee is available.
- Full weight bearing is possible.
- No pain and swelling present.

Physiotherapy for Ankle and Foot

THE ANKLE JOINT

Ankle joint **(Fig. 9.1)** also called talocrural joint is the articulation between the talus and distal tibia and fibula. The proximal joint surface is composed of the concave surfaces of distal tibia and fibular malleoli. The distal joint surface is the convex dome of the talus. The joint is a synovial hinge joint with 1 degree of freedom, i.e., dorsiflexion and plantar flexion. The joint capsule is thin and weak anteriorly and posteriorly, and the joint is reinforced by the deltoid ligament medially and anterior and posterior talofibular ligaments and calcaneofibular ligaments laterally.

Osteokinematics of Ankle Joint

The movements permitted in the ankle joint are dorsiflexion, where the foot moves up and slightly laterally, and plantar flexion, where the foot moves downward and slightly medially. The ankle is considered to be in 0° neutral position, when the foot is at right angle to the tibia.

Arthrokinematics of Ankle Joint

During dorsiflexion of ankle, the talus glides posteriorly, and the fibula moves proximally and laterally away from the tibia. During plantar flexion, the talus glides anteriorly, and the fibula moves distally, slightly anteriorly and toward the tibia.

Capsular pattern of movement limitation in ankle joint: Greater limitation of plantar flexion than dorsiflexion.
Closed pack position: Maximum dorsiflexion of ankle joint.
Ranges of motion of ankle joint are given in **Table 9.1**.

Table 9.1: Ranges of motion of ankle joint.

Movement	Range of motion
Dorsiflexion	0–20°
Plantar flexion	0–50°

The Foot

The joints of foot consist of:

Subtalar Joint

Also called as talocalcaneal joint, is composed of posterior, middle, and anterior articulations between the talus and calcaneus. This joint is reinforced by anterior, posterior, lateral, and medial talocalcaneal ligaments and the interosseous talocalcaneal ligament.

- **Osteokinematics:** It is a plane type of synovial joint having 1 degree of freedom. The motions permitted at the joint are inversion and eversion occurring around an oblique axis. Inversion has the components of adduction and supination, whereas eversion has the components of abduction and pronation.
- **Arthrokinematics:** During inversion of foot, the calcaneus slides laterally on a fixed talus, where as during eversion, the calcaneus slides medially on the talus.
- **Capsular pattern of limitation:** The capsular pattern of limitation consists of greater limitation of inversion than eversion.
- **Closed pack position:** Maximum limit of inversion (supination).

Midtarsal (Transverse Tarsal) Joints

Midtarsal joints are compound joints formed by the talonavicular and calcaneocuboid joints. The talonavicular joint, shares a capsule with the anterior and middle portions of the subtalar joint, and is reinforced by the spring, bifurcate and dorsal talonavicular ligaments.

The calcaneocuboid joint is enclosed in a capsule that is reinforced by the calcaneocuboid component of Y-shaped bifurcate/Chopart's ligament (consisting of calcaneo-navicular and calcaneocuboid ligaments).

- **Osteokinematics of midtarsal joints:** Inversion and eversion is the movement that occurs in these joints around two axes, such as one longitudinal axis and one oblique axis.

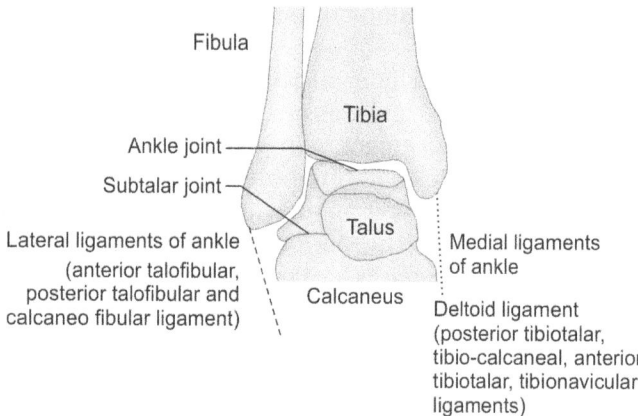

Fig. 9.1: The ankle joint.

❖ **Arthrokinematics:** During inversion, the concave navicular head slides medially and dorsally on the convex talus. During eversion, the navicular head slides laterally and towards the plantar surface on the talus.

Tarsometatarsal Joints

The tarsometatarsal joints are plane type of synovial joints that permit flexion-extension, a small degree of abduction-adduction and rotation. The arthrokinematics involve gliding of the distal joint surfaces in the same direction of movement of the shaft of the metatarsals.

Metatarsophalangeal Joints

Metatarsophalangeal joints are condyloid synovial joints with 2 degrees of freedom, permitting flexion-extension, abduction-adduction. The axis for flexion-extension is oblique and is referred to as metatarsal break. The arthrokinematics involved include during flexion, the bases of the phalanges slide in the plantar direction on the heads of metatarsals. In abduction, the concave bases of the phalanges slide on the convex heads of the metatarsals in a lateral direction away from the second toe. In adduction, the bases of the phalanges slide in a medial direction toward the second toe.

The capsular pattern of limitation at the first metatarsophalangeal joint is greater limitation of extension, than flexion. At the other joints (2nd to 5th toe) the limitation is variable.

Interphalangeal Joints

Interphalangeal joints are synovial hinge joints with 1 degree of freedom permitting flexion-extension in the sagittal plane. The arthrokinematics involve sliding of the concave base of the distal phalanx on the convex head of the proximal phalanx in the same direction as the shaft of the distal phalanx, i.e., the concave base slides toward the plantar surface of the foot during flexion and toward the dorsum of the foot during extension.

Special Test for Ankle and Foot

❖ **Anterior drawer test (Fig. 9.2):** This test is used to test for injuries to the anterior talofibular ligament.
  – *Procedure:* The patient lies supine with the foot relaxed. The examiner stabilizes the tibia and fibula, holds the patient's foot in 20° of plantar flexion, and draws the talus forward in the ankle mortise. The test is positive, if there is excessive anterior translation of the talus. Sometimes, a dimple appears over the area of the anterior talofibular ligament on anterior translation (dimple or sulcus sign), if pain and muscle spasm are minimal.

❖ **Posterior drawer test (ankle) (Fig. 9.3):** This test is performed to find injury to posterior talofibular ligament.
  – *Procedure:* The patient lies supine with the foot relaxed. With the patient's foot plantar flexed by 20°, the examiner stabilizes the tibia and fibula with one hand, and holds the calcaneus with the other hand. He/she then distracts the calcaneus from the tibia and fibula, by slowly pulling the calcaneus inferiorly. Subsequently, a posteriorly directed pressure is applied on the calcaneus and talus, with over pressure at the end of the passive range.

Excessive posterior translation of talus, with presence of a sulcus and pain is a positive sign.

❖ **Deltoid ligament stress test:**
  – *Procedure:* Patient is seated with their leg flexed at the knee and hanging over a table. The examiner stabilizes the anterior surface of the tibia and fibula proximal to the ankle (with one hand):
    » To assess the anterior fibers of deltoid ligament: The examiner uses his other hand to grasp the dorsal surface of the foot, combining eversion and plantar flexion of the foot and applying overpressure **(Fig. 9.4)**.
    » To assess the middle fibers of deltoid ligament: The examiner repositions his hand so the calcaneus is grasped (still stabilizing the anterior surface of the tibia and fibula proximal to the ankle with the other hand), patient's hind foot is taken into eversion with overpressure.

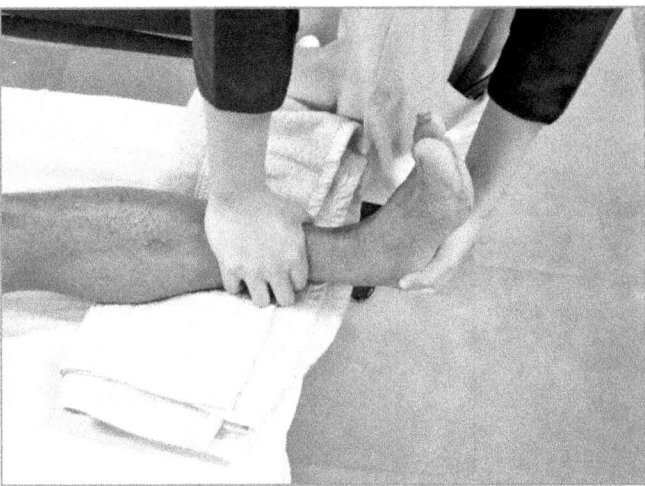

Fig. 9.2: Anterior drawer test.

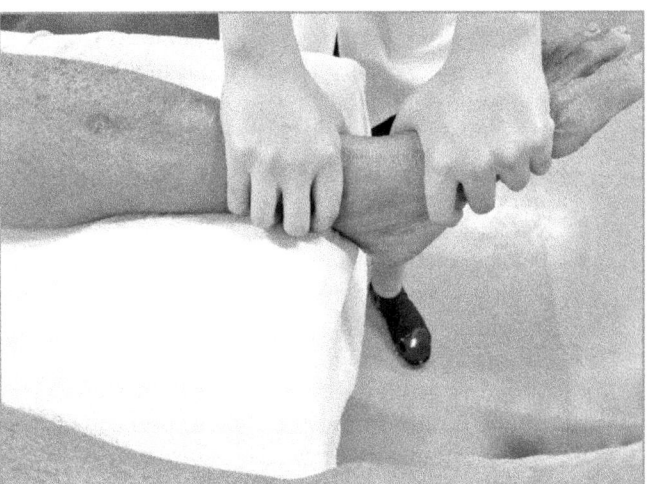

Fig. 9.3: The posterior drawer test.

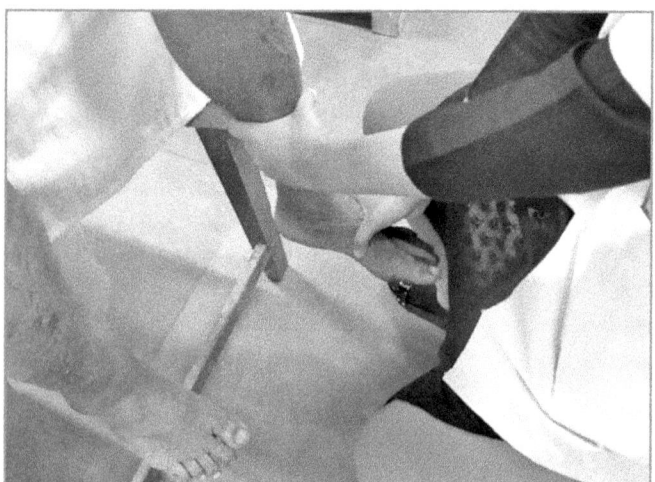

Fig. 9.4: Test for anterior fibers of deltoid ligament.

» To assess the posterior fibers of deltoid ligament: The examiner repositions his hand so the calcaneus is grasped (still stabilizing the anterior surface of the tibia and fibula proximal to the ankle with their other hand). He combines eversion and dorsiflexion of the foot with overpressure.

A positive test indicates:
  ○ Pain and hypermobility local to the ligament
  ○ Muscle spasm end feel may be present with a subacute injury.

❖ **Heel thump test:** This test is a useful screening tool for evaluating ankle injuries and for differentiating syndesmotic sprains from lateral ankle sprains. This also helps in determining presence of stress fracture of tibia.
  – *Procedure:* The patient is either in sitting or supine position. The leg of the patient is stabilized by one hand of the examiner. The examiner applies a firm thump with the fist of the other hand on the heel of the patient, so that the force is applied to the center of the heel and in line with the long axis of the tibia **(Fig. 9.5)**. The test is considered positive from the followings:

Pain in the area of the ankle indicates syndesmosis injury where as pain along with the shaft of the tibia indicates stress fracture of tibia.

❖ **Homan's sign test:** This test is performed to identify deep vein thrombosis/thrombophlebitis.
  – *Procedure:* The patient **lies** supine with the knee extended. The examiner passively dorsiflexes the patient's ankle **(Fig. 9.6)**. The test is positive, if pain is felt deeper in the calf during ankle dorsiflexion/tenderness elicited on palpation of calf.

❖ **Ramirez's test:** This test is performed to find deep vein thrombosis.
  – *Procedure:* The patient lies supine, with the affected knee flexed and foot flat on the bed. A blood pressure cuff is wrapped around the thigh and inflated to 40 mm Hg and the pressure is maintained for at least 2 minutes. Increase in pain as the cuff is inflated and inability to tolerate cuff inflation and sustained pressure for 2 minutes is a positive test.

❖ **Talar tilt test:** The test is used to assess the integrity of calcaneofibular ligament and anterior talofibular ligament on the lateral side and deltoid ligament on the medial side.
  – *Procedure-I (for calcaneofibular and anterior talofibular ligaments):* The patient in supine or side lying, with the foot relaxed. The ankle is kept in 10-20 degrees of plantar flexion. The talus is then tilted from side to side into adduction/abduction **(Fig. 9.7)**. Excessive movement on adduction is a positive test.
  – *Procedure-II (for deltoid ligament):* The eversion talar tilt test. The patient is seated comfortably on the end of the examination table. The examiner grasps the foot and places the ankle in 10-20 degrees of plantar flexion, while stabilizing the tibia and fibula. To test the deltoid ligament, the examiner abducts and everts the calcaneus into valgus position **(Fig. 9.4)**. Laxity/pain as compared to sound side indicates positive test showing laxity of deltoid ligament.

❖ **Thompson's test/ Simmond's test:** This test examines the integrity of the Achilles tendon. It is used to identify rupture of Tendo achillis (if any).

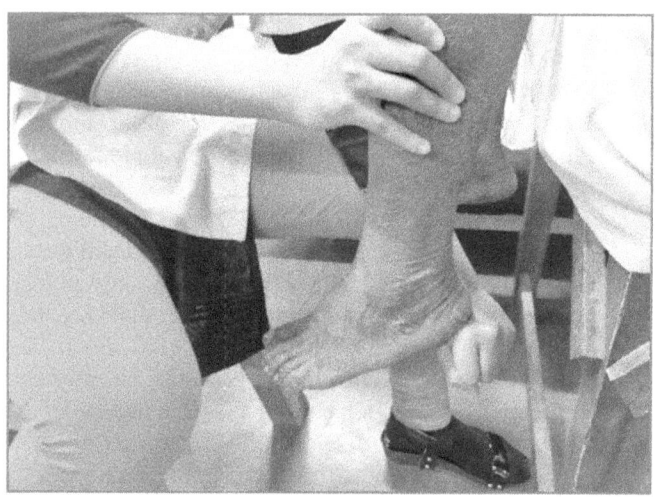

Fig. 9.5: Heel thump test.

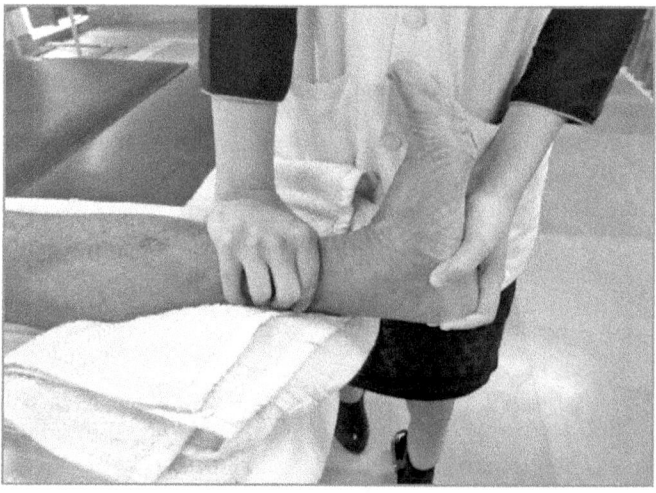

Fig. 9.6: Homan's sign test.

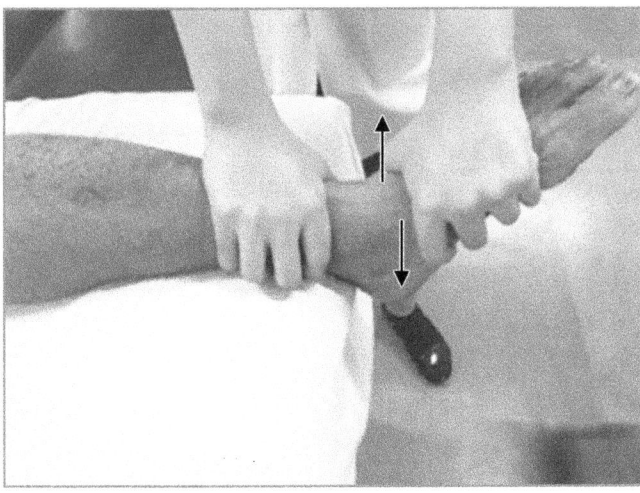

Fig. 9.7: The talar tilt test (for calcaneo fibular ligament).

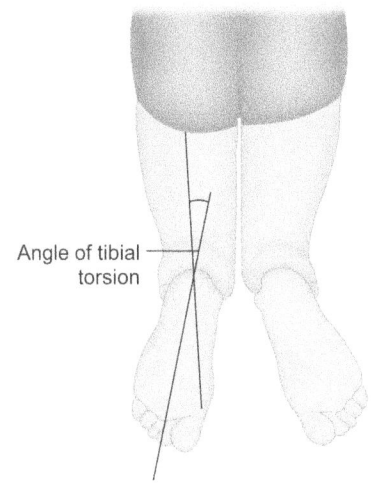

Fig. 9.9: Measurement of tibial torsion in prone.

- *Procedure:* The patient in prone lying with the feet over the edge of the table, legs relaxed. The clinician squeezes the gastro-soleus muscles **(Fig. 9.8)**.

Positive test: The test is positive, when there is no plantar flexion of the ankle, when the calf muscles are squeezed.

❖ **Tibial torsion test**: The test can be performed in sitting, supine lying, and prone lying.
   - *In sitting:* The patient sits with the knee flexed to 90° over the edge of the bed. The examiner places the thumb of one hand over the apex of one malleolus and the index finger of the same hand over the apex of the other malleolus. The examiner visualizes the axes of the knee and ankle.

Positive test: An outward angular deviation of ankle axis by more than 12–18°, with respect to the knee axis suggests excessive lateral tibial torsion.
   - *In supine lying:* The lower limbs are so aligned that, the femoral condyles are in the frontal plane (patella facing up). The examiner palpates the apex of both malleoli with one hand, and draws a line on the heel, representing a line joining the two apices. A second line is drawn on the heel parallel to the floor. The angle formed by the intersection of the two lines, indicates the amount of tibial torsion.

In prone lying: With the knee flexed to 90°, the examiner views from above, the angle formed by the foot and thigh, with the subtalar joint in the neutral position, noting the angle the foot makes with the tibia **(Fig. 9.9)**.

❖ **Kleiger's test**: This test, also known as the external rotation test, determines the rotator damage to the deltoid ligament and the distal tibiofibular syndesmosis, which is injured in ankle sprain.
   - *Procedure:* The patient sitting with the legs over the edge of the table. The examiner standing in front of the patient stabilizes the leg with one hand, not compressing the distal tibiofibular syndesmosis. The other hand of the examiner, grasps the medial aspect of the foot, while supporting the ankle in a neutral position.

The foot and talus are rotated externally: To stress the deltoid ligament the ankle is placed in neutral position **(Fig. 9.10A)**. Deltoid ligament involvement is suspected, if there is medial joint pain. To stress the syndesmosis the ankle is placed in dorsiflexion **(Fig. 9.10B)**. Syndesmosis involvement is suspected, if pain is felt at the anterolateral ankle, at the site of the distal tibiofibular syndesmosis.

❖ **Coleman block test**: This test is performed to determine, whether the cavus deformity is flexible or rigid. The test consists of supporting the lateral forefoot in order to determine, if an inverted heel is due to a forefoot issue, such as a plantar flexed first ray.
   - *Procedure:* The test is performed by having a patient stand with a 1-inch wooden block **(Fig. 9.11)** under the heel and lateral foot. This allows the first ray to be plantar flexed off the block. A rigid plantar flexed first ray can result in inversion of the heel in order to bring the lateral forefoot to the ground. If the hind foot corrects to a neutral position, the deformity is flexible. If the hind foot does not correct, the deformity is rigid.

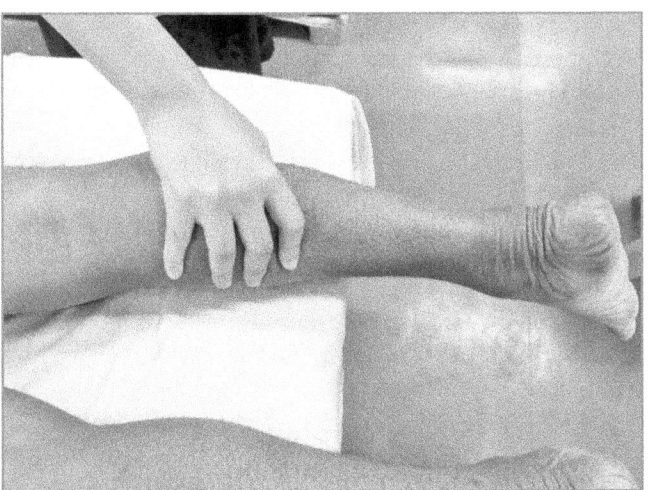

Fig. 9.8: Thompson's test.

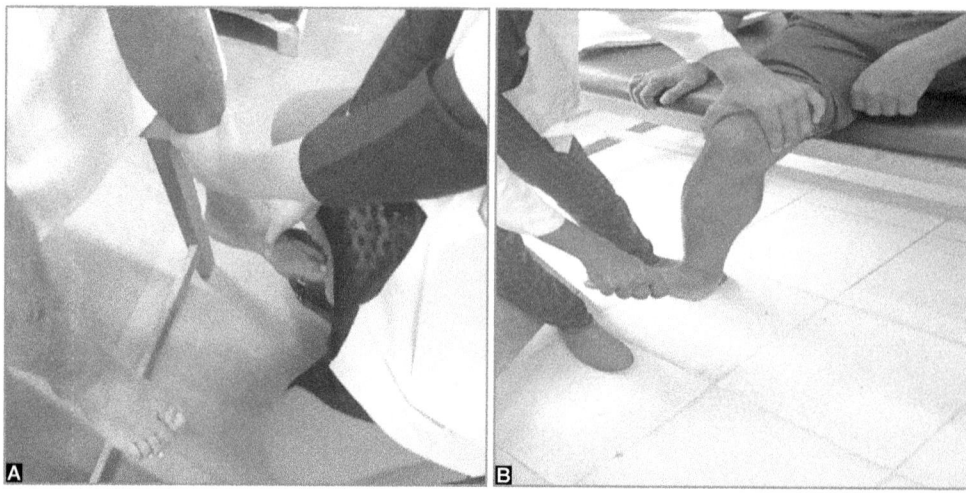

Figs. 9.10A and B: (A) Test for deltoid ligament (ankle in neutral), (B) Test for syndesmosis of ankle (ankle dorsiflexed).

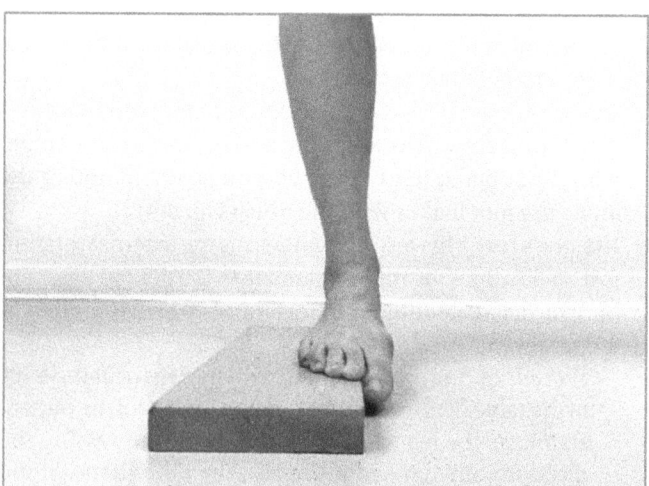

Fig. 9.11: The Coleman block test.

Table 9.2: Types and mechanism of ankle sprain.

Type of sprain	Mechanism of injury	Ligaments affected
Lateral ligament sprain	Inversion and plantar flexion	• Anterior talofibular • Posterior talofibular • Calcaneofibular
Medial ligament sprain	Eversion	• Posterior tibiotalar ligament • Anterior tibiotalar ligament • Tibiocalcaneal ligament • Tibionavicular ligament
High (Syndesmotic sprain)	Dorsiflexion and external rotation	• Anterior-inferior tibiofibular ligament • Posterior-inferior tibiofibular ligament • Transverse tibiofibular ligament • Interosseous membrane • Interosseous ligament Inferior transverse ligament

The Disorders of Ankle and Foot

i. Sprain of Ankle Ligaments

Ankle sprain is the common injury encountered by sports personnel and common men. The most common ankle sprain is lateral ligament sprain that result from inversion injury to ankle joint. Lateral ligament injuries represent approximately 85% of all ankle sprains.

Mechanism of injury

Sprains to lateral ligaments of ankle usually occur during a rapid shift of center of mass over the weight-bearing foot. This causes the ankle to roll outward, which results in the foot turning inward, causing the lateral ligaments to stretch and tear. Forceful eversion movement causes injury to the strong (medial) deltoid ligament. The **Table 9.2**, displays the different sprains in ankle and their mechanism of injuries.

Clinical features and types of ankle sprain

The patient presents with history of injury (forceful inversion injury for lateral ligaments and forceful eversion injury to medial ligaments). Pain, swelling, and bruising may be present, over medial/lateral aspects of ankle. The patient can only bear partial weight on the affected side. Passive inversion or plantar flexion with inversion, produces pain over the lateral aspect of ankle, and passive eversion produces pain on the medial aspect of ankle.

Based upon the severity of injury, the ankle ligament injury can be graded as under:
- **Grade I (mild):** Little swelling and tenderness with little impact on function.
- **Grade II (moderate):** Moderate swelling, pain and impact on function. Reduced proprioception, ROM, and stability.
- **Grade III (severe):** Complete rupture, large swelling, high tenderness loss of function and marked instability.

Diagnosis

Diagnosis of ankle ligament injury is made from history, clinical examination, and special tests. Observation of

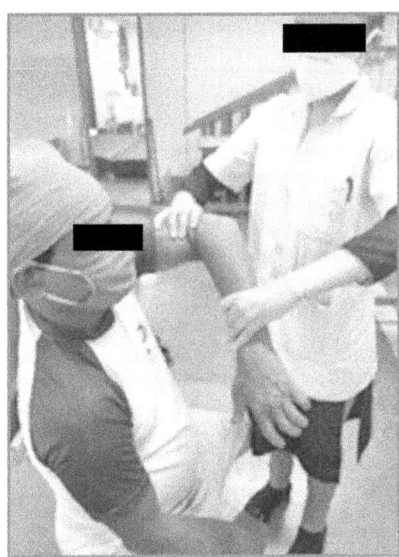

Fig. 10.3: Hawkin's Kennedy impingement test.

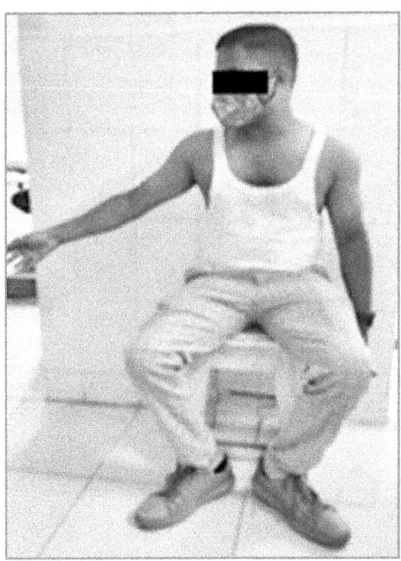

Fig. 10.5: The drop arm test.

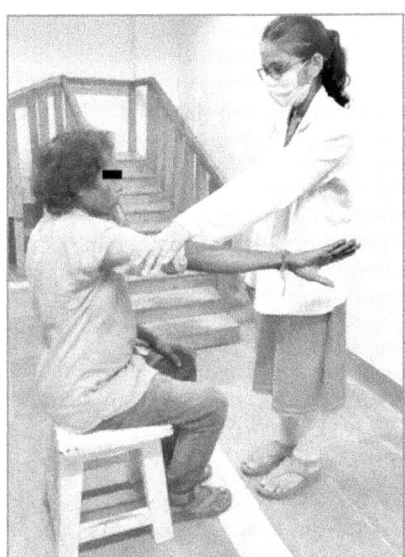

Fig. 10.4: The empty can test.

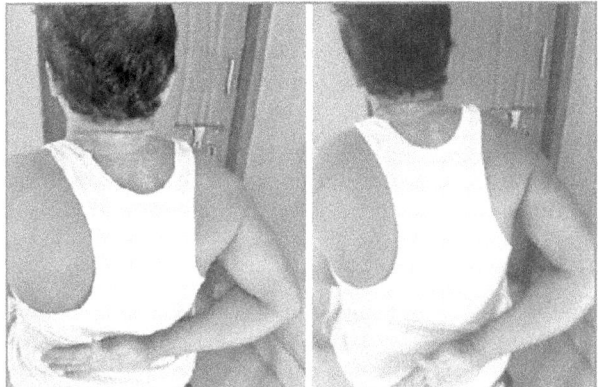

Fig. 10.6: The lift-off test.

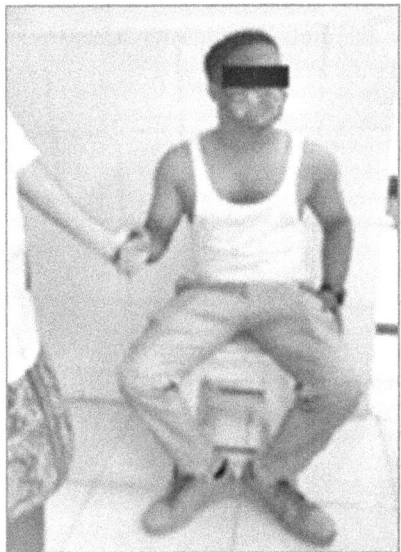

Fig. 10.7: Test for lesion to infraspinatus.

4. **Drop arm (Codman's) test (Fig. 10.5):** The patient is in sitting position. The examiner passively abducts and elevates the shoulder to approximately 120°. The patient is asked to hold the arm in this position actively, and then slowly allow the arm to drop. Difficulty in maintaining the position of the arm with or without pain, or sudden dropping of the arm suggests a supraspinatus (rotator cuff) lesion.
5. **Lift-off test (subscapularis test) (Fig. 10.6):** The patient is in a standing position. The examiner places the dorsum of the patient's hand on his/her back, and asks the patient to lift the hand away from the back. If there is a tear of subscapularis, the patient will not be able to lift the hand off in this position. If the patient is able to lift the hand off the back, the examiner then applies load pushing on the hand to check the strength of the muscle.
6. **Infraspinatus test (Fig. 10.7):** The patient sitting, the arm at the side and the elbow flexed to 90°. The examiner places his/her palm on the dorsum of patient's hand and then asks the patient to externally rotate the forearm (shoulder) against resistance of the examiner's hand. Pain

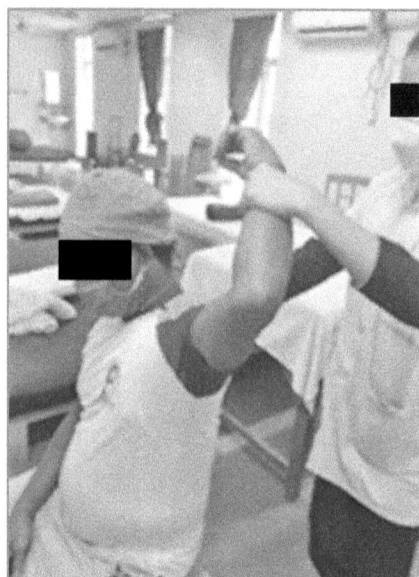

Fig. 10.8: The spring back test.

or weakness in external rotation, indicates disorder of infraspinatus. Best interpretations can be done by testing both sides of the body.

7. **Spring back test (for infraspinatus lesion) (Fig. 10.8):** The patient is either in sitting or standing position. The elbow on the tested side is flexed to 90° and is held by the side of the body. The examiner passively brings the shoulder to 90° of abduction and laterally rotates the same to the end range and asks the patient to hold the arm at that position. A positive test indicating lesion of infraspinatus is observed, when the patient fails to hold the position and the hand springs back anteriorly.

8. **Teres minor test (Fig. 10.9):** The patient lies in prone lying position and places his/her hand on the opposite posterior iliac crest. The patient is asked to extend, adduct, and medially rotate the arm against the resistance of the examiner. Pain or weakness indicates positive test.

   A positive **hornblower sign** is also indicative of pathology of teres minor/infraspinatus muscles. The test is performed with the patient in sitting/standing. The examiner brings the shoulder to 90° of abduction and full external rotation, and asks the patient to hold the position. The test is considered positive, if the patient's arm falls into internal rotation **(Fig. 10.10)**.

9. **Teres major test:** The patient is in relaxed standing position. The examiner observes the position of the patient's hands from behind. If the palm of the tested hand faces backward, as compared to the other side, there is medial rotation deformity of shoulder, suggesting contracture of teres major.

10. **Apley's scratch test (Figs. 10.11A and B):** The patient is in sitting position, and asked to touch the contralateral superior medial corner of the scapula with the index finger of the tested hand. Pain elicited in the rotator cuff and failure to reach the scapula, indicates rotator cuff pathology.

    The sitting patient is asked to touch the inferior angle of the opposite scapula. Any pain in shoulder with restriction of adduction and medial rotation indicates pathology in rotator cuff (mostly the supra spinatus muscle/tendon).

11. **Painful arc sign (Fig. 10.12):** The patient is either sitting or standing with the arm by the side. The patient is asked to actively abduct and elevate the arm sideways. Pain occurring within 140–180° of abduction suggests acromioclavicular pathology. However, pain occurring between 70 and 120° of abduction is called painful arc/impingement syndrome, resulting from impingement of supraspinatus against the acromion process of scapula.

12. **Forced adduction test (Fig. 10.13):** The patient is in sitting or standing position. The examiner forcibly adducts the affected arm across the patient's chest toward the normal shoulder. Pain over the anterior aspect of the shoulder suggests acromioclavicular joint pathology.

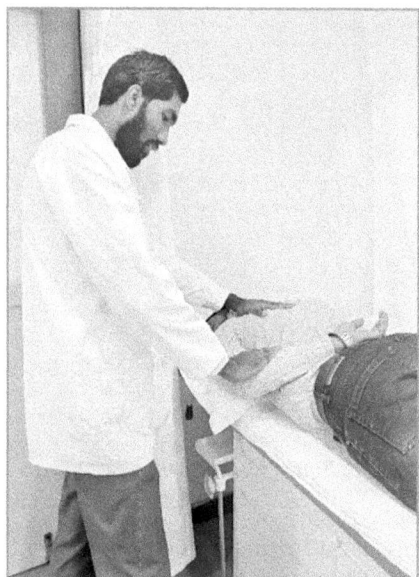

Fig. 10.9: Teres minor test.

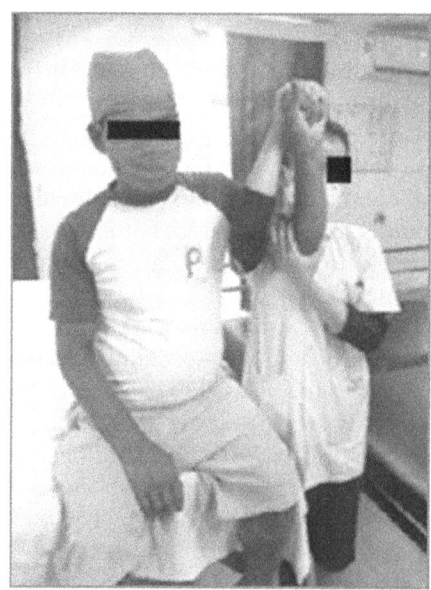

Fig. 10.10: The hornblower sign.

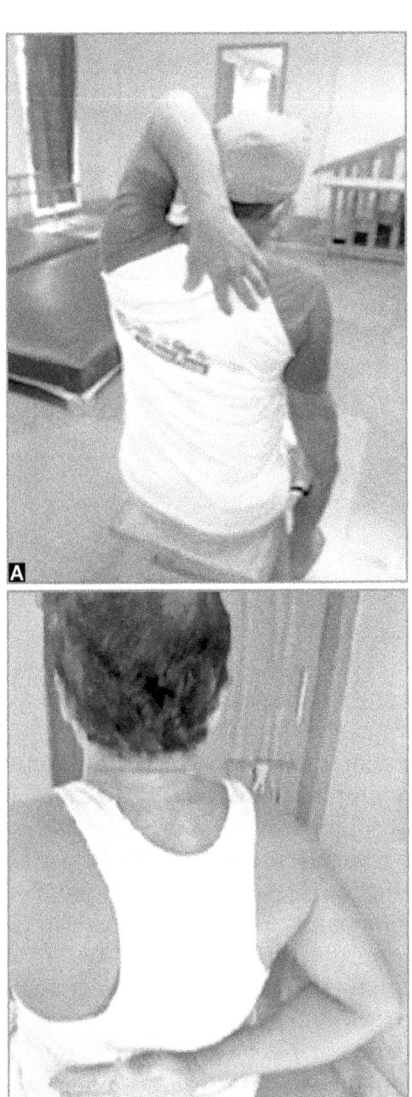

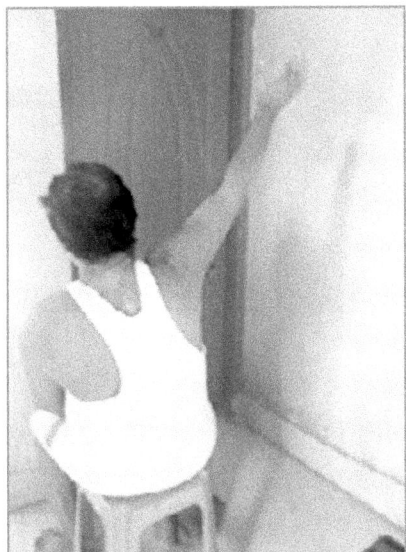

Figs. 10.11A and B: The Apley's scratch test: (A) Abduction and lateral rotating of shoulder. (B) Adduction and internal rotation of shoulder.

Fig. 10.12: The painful arc sign test.

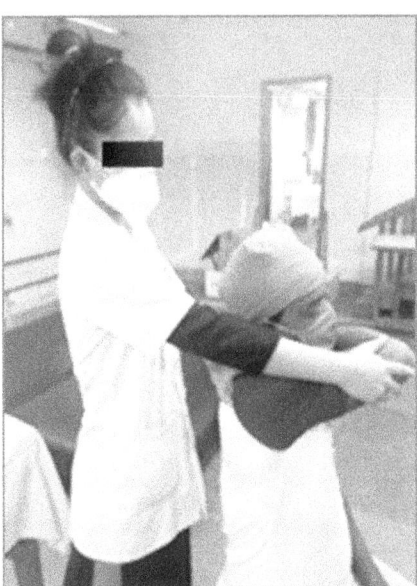

Fig. 10.13: The forced adduction test.

13. **Forced adduction test on hanging arm:** The patient standing. The examiner grasps the patient's upper arm on the affected side with one hand, while the other hand rests on the contralateral shoulder and immobilizes the shoulder girdle. Then the examiner forcibly adducts the hanging affected arm behind the patient's back against the patient's resistance. Pain over the anterior aspect of the shoulder suggests acromioclavicular joint pathology or subacromial impingement.
14. **Duga's test (Fig. 10.14):** The patient is either sitting or standing. He/she is asked to touch the opposite shoulder with the hand of the 90° flexed affected arm, and then attempts to lower the elbow toward the chest. Pain over the acromioclavicular joint suggests acromioclavicular joint pathology.

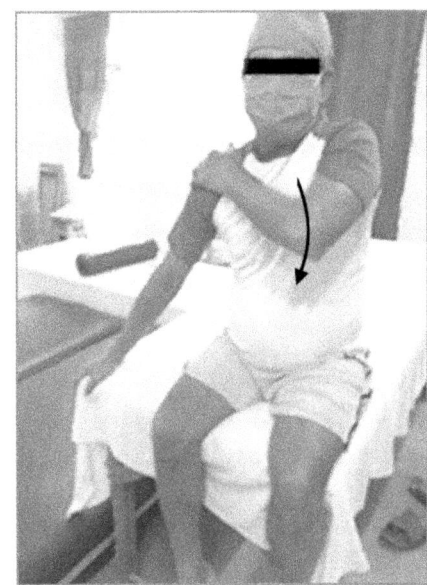

Fig. 10.14: The Duga's test.

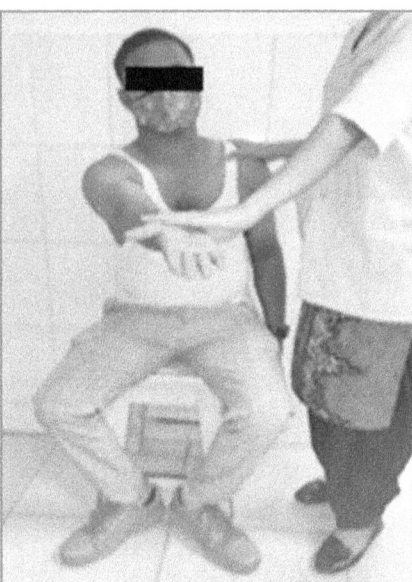

Fig. 10.15: Speed test.

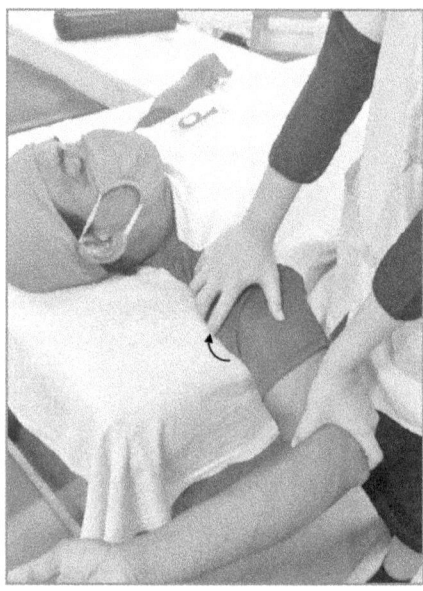

Fig. 10.17: The anterior apprehension test.

15. **Speed test (Fig. 10.15):** Patient sitting. The examiner resists patient's forward shoulder flexion, with the patient's forearm in supination. Pain in the region of the bicipital groove, suggests a disorder of the long head of biceps tendon.
16. **Yergason test (Fig. 10.16):** The patient in sitting position. With the elbow flexed to 90° and stabilized against the thorax with the forearm in pronation, the examiner resists forearm supination, while the patient laterally rotates the shoulder against resistance. Pain in the bicipital groove is a sign of lesion of the biceps tendon.
17. **Biceps tendinitis with transverse humeral ligament test:** The patient is seated with the shoulder abducted to 90°, internally rotated and extended at the elbow. From this position, the examiner externally rotates the shoulder, while palpating the bicipital groove, to verify whether the tendon snaps. In the presence of ligamentous insufficiency, this maneuver will cause biceps tendon to spontaneously displace out of the bicipital groove. Pain reported without displacement of the tendon suggests bicipital tendinitis.
18. **Anterior apprehension test (Fig. 10.17):** Patient is either in sitting/supine lying. The tested shoulder is abducted to 90° and laterally rotated slowly by the examiner. While performing the test, the patient's expressions are noted for apprehension/further resistance to rotation. The test is performed at 60°, 90°, and 120° of abduction to evaluate the superior, medial, and inferior glenohumeral ligaments. With the guiding hand, the examiner presses the humeral head in an anterior and inferior direction. Shoulder pain with reflexive muscle spasm, is a sign of an anterior instability syndrome.
19. **Posterior apprehension test (Fig. 10.18):** The patient in supine/sitting position. The examiner flexes the shoulder

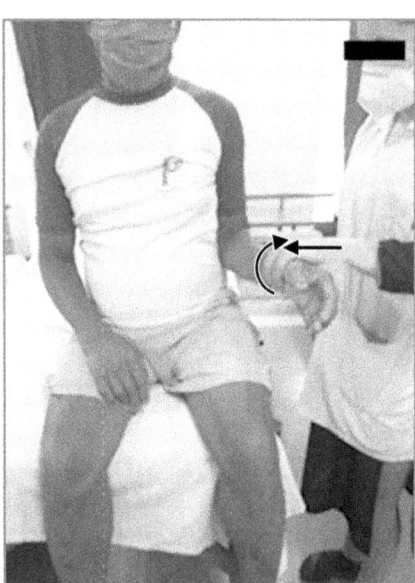

Fig. 10.16: The Yergason test.

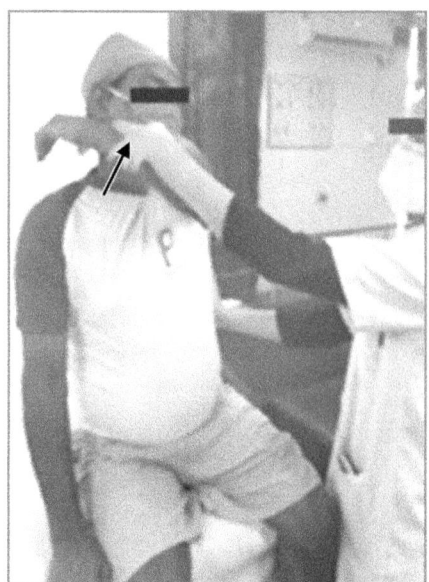

Fig. 10.18: The posterior apprehension test.

Chapter 10: Physiotherapy for Shoulder

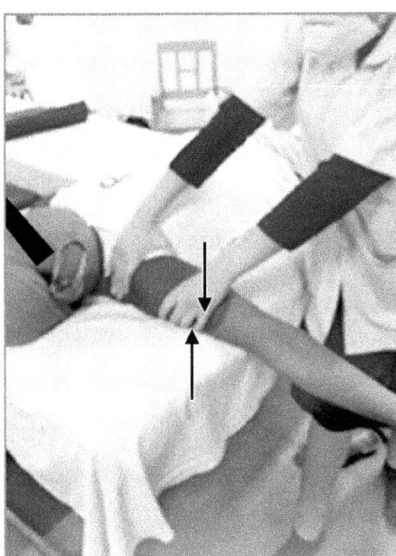

Fig. 10.19: The anterior/posterior drawer test.

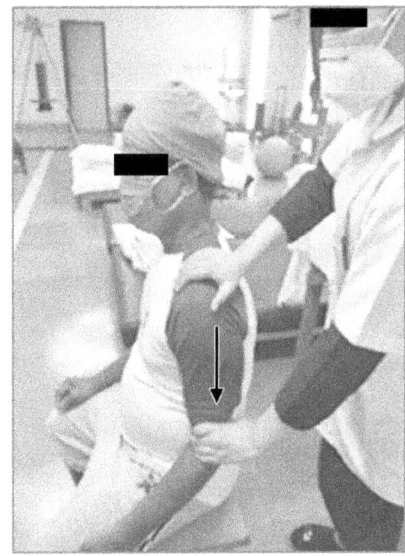

Fig. 10.21: The sulcus test.

to 90° with one hand, stabilizing the scapula with the other hand. The examiner then applies a posterior force on the flexed elbow, and moves the arm into adduction and medial rotation. Shoulder pain with reflexive muscle spasm, is a sign of posterior apprehension.

20. **Anterior and posterior drawer test (Fig. 10.19):** The patient is seated/in supine lying. The examiner stands behind the patient in sitting/stands at the side in supine lying. To examine the right shoulder, the examiner grasps the patient's shoulder with the right hand to stabilize the clavicle and superior margin of scapula, while using the left hand to move the humeral head anteriorly and posteriorly. Excessive movement of humeral head anteriorly or posteriorly indicates a positive anterior or posterior drawer test, respectively.

21. **Inferior apprehension test/Feagin test (Fig. 10.20):** The patient stands with the arm abducted to 90° and elbow extended/slightly flexed, and the hand resting on top of

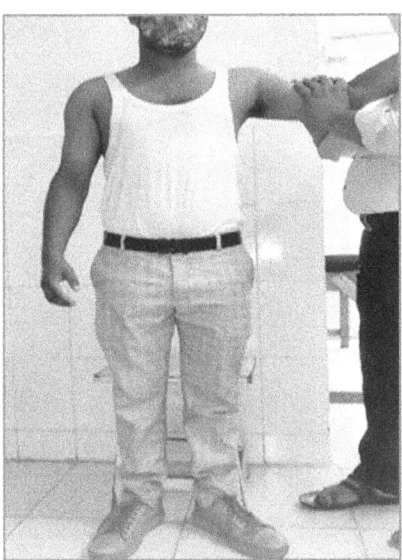

Fig. 10.20: The Feagin test.

examiner's shoulder. The examiner clasps his/her hands around the patient's upper arm and pushes the humerus down and forward **(Fig. 10.20)**. A sulcus may be seen above the coracoid process.

22. **Sulcus test (Fig. 10.21):** The sulcus test is used to assess the glenohumeral joint for inferior instability, due to laxity of the superior glenohumeral ligament and coracohumeral ligament. The patient sits with arm by the side and shoulder muscles relaxed. The examiner grasps the patient's forearm below the elbow and pulls the arm distally. The presence of sulcus/indentation inferior to acromion is the positive test.

THE COMMON SHOULDER INJURIES AND THEIR MANAGEMENT

i. Rotator Cuff Injuries

The shoulder girdle consists of five joints, such as glenohumeral, acromioclavicular, sternoclavicular, subacromial, and scapulothoracic joint. This joint allows motions in large range and has lesser passive stability. However, the primary source of stability of the joint is balanced muscular control offered by the rotator cuff muscles that consist of: supraspinatus, infraspinatus, teres minor, and subscapularis.

The rotator cuff muscles contribute significantly for shoulder stability. The subscapularis muscle makes internal rotation of shoulder, whereas the infraspinatus and teres minor produce external rotation. All muscles of rotator cuff except supraspinatus ensure that, the humeral head stays depressed in the glenoid cavity, to balance the upward pull of the deltoid, early in glenohumeral abduction. During shoulder abduction, the rotator cuff muscles act together to stabilize the humeral head within the glenoid in a process known as concavity compression.

Etiology

Rotator cuff tears are the leading cause of shoulder pain and shoulder related disabilities. The causes include:

- Violent trauma
- Degeneration
- Repetitive micro trauma
- Atraumatic injuries such as repeated steroid injections
- Secondary dysfunctions such as rheumatoid arthritis, type-1 diabetes, autoimmune pathologies, thyroid pathologies, and vascular pathologies

Clinical Features

The site of injury has an important influence on possible dysfunctions. The presentations of this disorder include:
- Severe pain at the time of injury.
- Pain at night.
- Limitation of movement (pain with overhead activities).
- Positive painful arc sign.
- Weakness of the involved muscle.
- Stiffness (frozen shoulder).

Rotator cuff tear that causes pain and instability of shoulder, involves injury/tear of one or more of the four tendons that constitute the rotator cuff, though the most common tendon affected is supraspinatus. Ladermann et al., speak of a rotator cuff tear, when at least two tendons are completely torn. Next to the number of tendons which are torn, at least one of the two tendons must be retracted beyond the top of humeral head.

Tears of rotator cuff could be of partial or full thickness types. A commonly cited classification system for full thickness rotator cuff tear, developed by Cofield (1982) is described as under:
- **Small tear:** Tear of muscle/tendon up to the length lesser than 1 cm.
- **Medium tear:** Tear of muscle/tendon up to the length of 1–3 cm.
- **Large tear:** Tear of muscle/tendon up to the length of 3–5 cm.
- **Massive tear:** Tear of muscle/tendon up to the length of more than 5 cm.

The rotator cuff tears can be divided into five categories according to Collin et al., such as:
1. **Type A:** Supraspinatus and superior subscapularis tear.
2. **Type B:** Supraspinatus and entire subscapularis tear.
3. **Type C:** Supraspinatus, superior subscapularis and infraspinatus tears.
4. **Type D:** Supraspinatus and infraspinatus tears.
5. **Type E:** Supraspinatus, infraspinatus and teres minor tears.

Assessment of Rotator Cuff Tear/Injury

Diagnosis of rotator cuff injury can be established by a careful history, structured physical examination that include inspection, palpation, range of motion (ROM) testing, strength testing, and special tests.

Active ROM (flexion/abduction, medial/lateral rotation) in acute rotator cuff injuries are usually affected, however, passive ROM is usually preserved. If prompt treatment is not started, the patient may develop passive movement limitation (periarthritis) subsequently.

Manual muscle testing, dynamometry are used to find the strength of rotator cuff muscles.

Few special tests are performed by the clinicians to find tear/injury of specific muscle/tendon, such as for subscapularis muscle—lift-off test, for supraspinatus muscle—drop arm test, etc.

Differential Diagnosis

Rotator cuff tears must be differentiated from rotator cuff tendinopathies, bursitis (subacromial bursitis), acromioclavicular joint pathologies, glenoid labrum tear, shoulder instability, adhesive capsulitis, glenohumeral ligament tear, etc.

Diagnosis

Subjective history including mechanism of injury, physical examination, diagnostic imaging (X-ray, ultrasound, CT scan, and MRI), isokinetic muscle performance test, etc., are helpful in establishing tear of rotator cuff muscles.

Management of Rotator Cuff Injury

Conservative management

Management of rotator cuff injury is mostly done conservatively through:
- Rest
- Support to shoulder, either in triangular sling or some other supportive devices **(Figs. 10.22A and B)**, that allows use of hand with the shoulder supported.

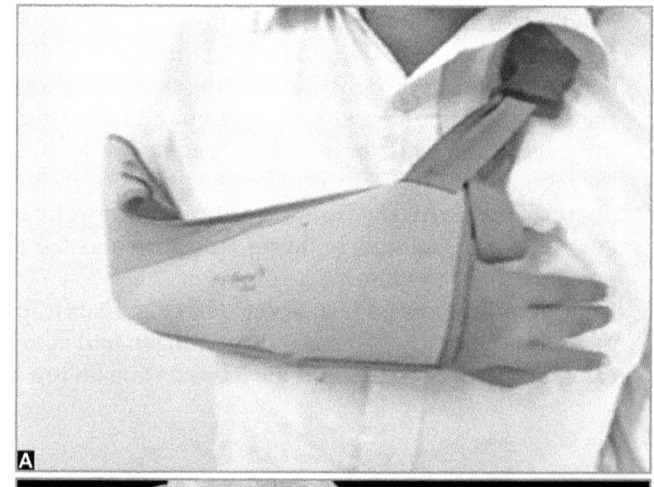

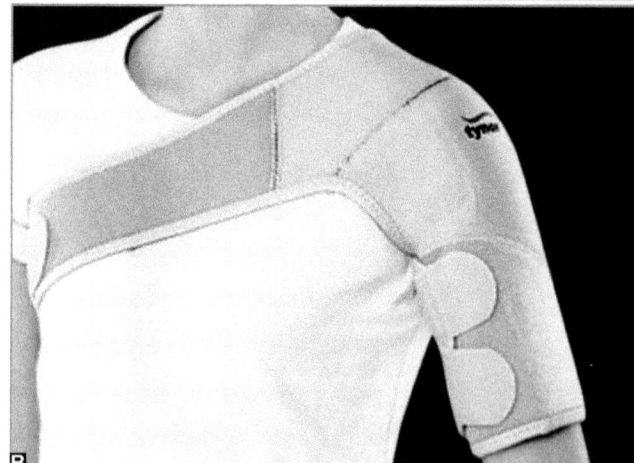

Figs. 10.22A and B: (A) Triangular sling; (B) Flexible shoulder support that allows use of hand.

- Nonsteroidal anti-inflammatory drugs (NSAIDs).
- The judicious use of not more than 3–4 steroid injections is helpful in a few cases.
- Cold/heat.
- Active physiotherapy and rehabilitation.

Physiotherapy in Rotator Cuff Tear/Injury

The goals of physiotherapy are:
- Reduction of pain and muscle spasm around shoulder and neck.
- Improvement of scapulohumeral mobility.
- Strengthening the muscles that stabilize the shoulder.
- Regaining proprioception and movement automatism through neuromotor rehabilitation.
- Improvement of function.

Techniques of Physiotherapy

Physiotherapy in the early stage (with or without surgery) consists of:
- Pulsed short wave diathermy/pulsed ultrasound/low-intensity LASER may be considered to reduce inflammation.
- Interferential therapy/TENS may be considered to reduce pain.
- Mobilization of scapulothoracic joint.
- Graduated (low to medium intensity) resistance exercises to scapular muscles (protractors and retractors in side lying position). The glenohumeral joint must be kept in slight abduction/forward flexion, while scapular movements are performed.
- Restoration of arthrokinematics of shoulder through gentile stretching of posterior joint capsule, basically to improve internal rotation.
- Restoration of osteokinematics of shoulder through active assisted exercise with manual assistance/suspension therapy **(Fig. 10.23)**.
- Promotion of muscular strength and endurance by performing open and closed kinetic chain exercises, but without stressing the injured muscles much.

Physiotherapy in the late stage (late stage rehabilitation): SWD/MWD/ultrasound therapy/high power LASER therapy

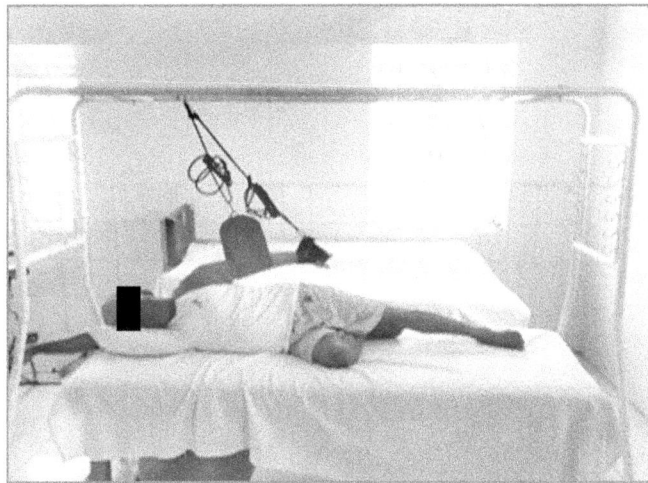

Fig. 10.23: Suspension therapy for shoulder flexion/extension.

etc, are applied as indicated to reduce pain and enhance mobility.
- Progressive resisted exercises using therabands/weight cuff/dumbbells **(Figs. 10.24A to D)**.
- Mobility exercises to shoulder through shoulder wheel exercise, shoulder pulley exercise, shoulder ladder exercises, gear shift exercises, Codman's exercises, wand exercises as tolerated **(Figs. 10.25A to D)**.
- Proprioception training through closed kinetic chain exercises **(Fig. 10.26)**
- Sports specific exercises.
- Functional re-education.

Medical and Surgical Management

In case of severe instability or when conservative management fails, surgery is performed. It includes:
- **Open repair:** This is often required for large and complex tears.
- **Arthroscopic repair:** An optical scope and a small instrument are inserted through a smaller punctured wound, instead of through a larger surgical incision. The operation is performed under visual control through video display.

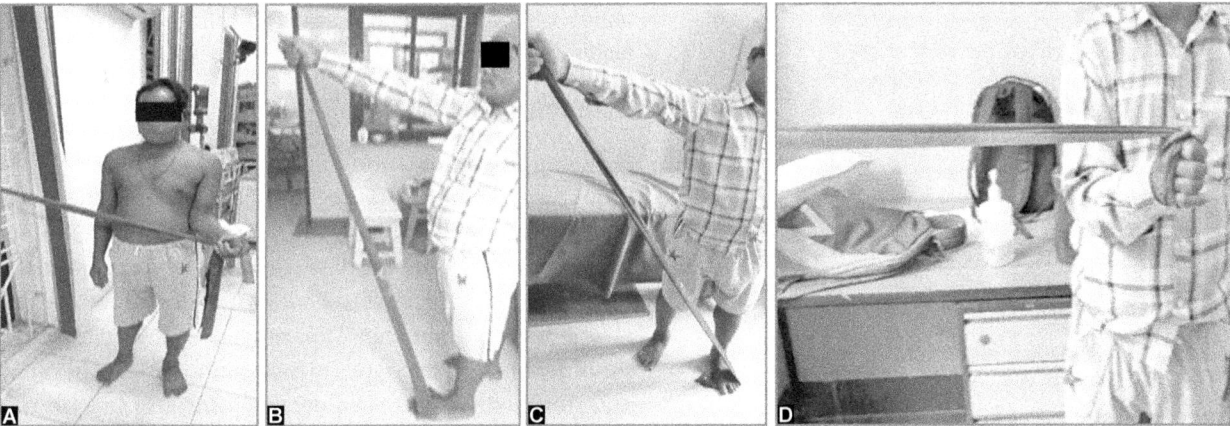

Figs. 10.24A to D: Strengthening exercises using theraband: (A) For shoulder external rotators; (B) Shoulder flexors; (C) Shoulder abductors; (D) Shoulder medial rotators.

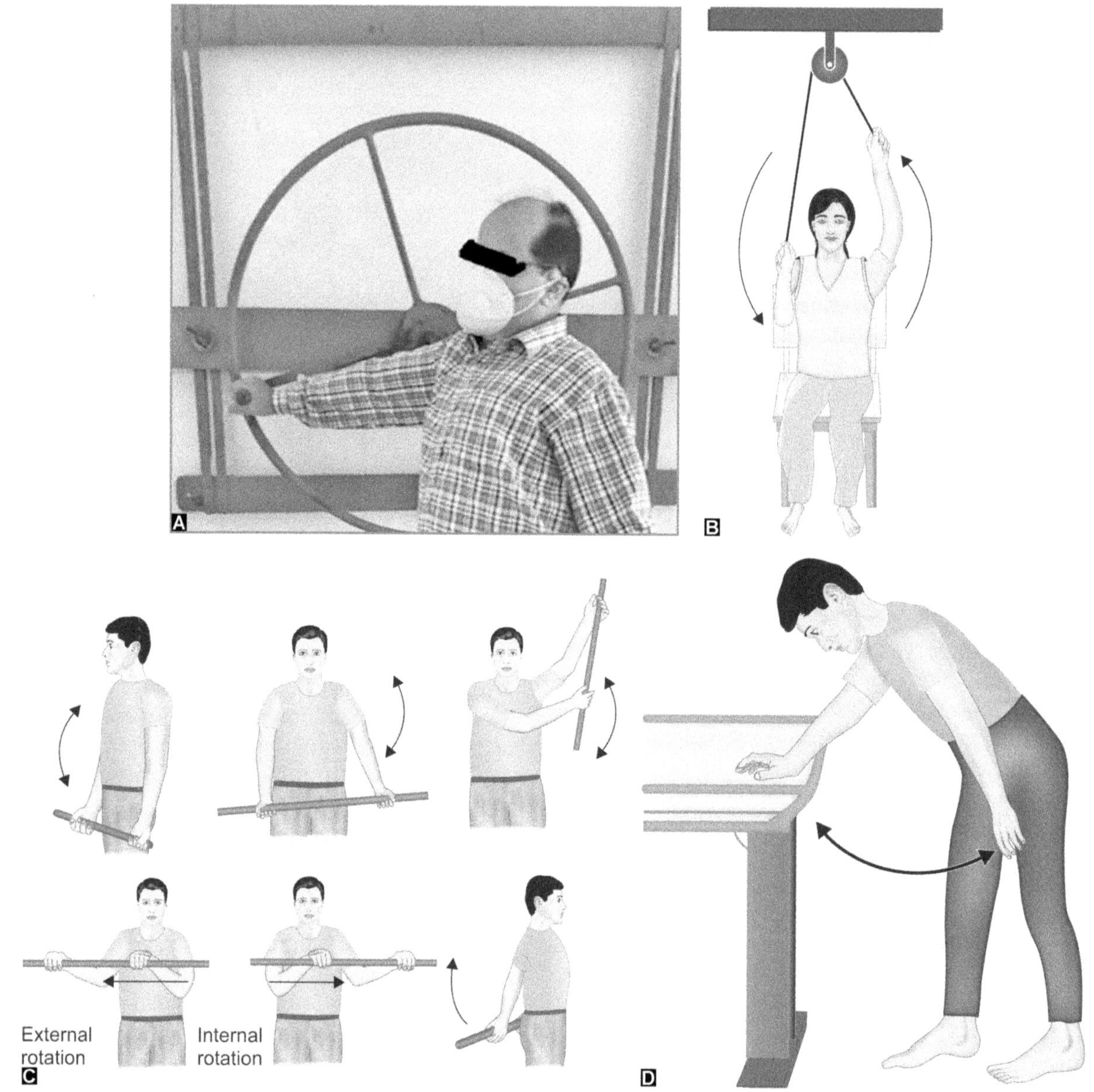

Figs. 10.25A to D: (A) Shoulder wheel exercise; (B) Shoulder pulley exercise; (C) Wand exercises; (D) Codman's exercises.

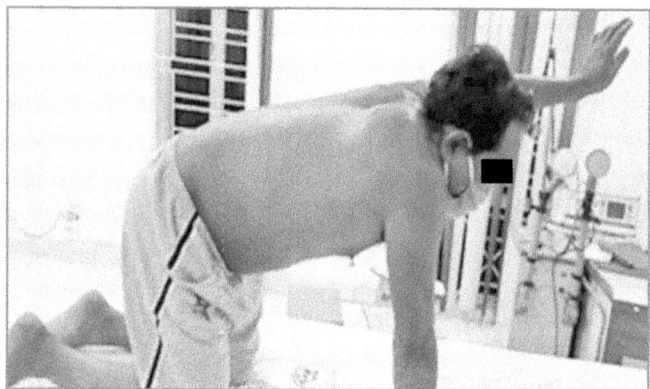

Fig. 10.26: Closed kinetic chain exercise for right shoulder.

- **Mini open repair:** New techniques and instruments allow surgeons to perform a complete recovery of the rotator cuff through a small incision of generally 4–6 cm.

The operative treatment is done mostly arthroscopically, which is less invasive than open/mini open surgery and leaves only a few small scars. The rehabilitation can start faster and the patient has less pain during recovery.

ii. Shoulder Dislocation

Dislocations of the shoulder occur when the head of the humerus is forcibly removed from its socket in the glenoid fossa. Nearly 95% of shoulder dislocations are anterior dislocations, i.e., the humeral head moves to a position in front of the shoulder joint. Posterior dislocations are those in which the humeral head has moved backward toward the shoulder blade. Other types of dislocations are luxatio erecta, an inferior dislocation below the joint and intrathoracic dislocation, in which the humeral head gets stuck between the ribs.

Etiology of Shoulder Dislocation

A great majority of patients with shoulder dislocation report with a history of trauma. But a small percentage of patients do not report a history of trauma. Such patients may have ligament laxity, a congenital abnormality of the humerus or glenoid process of the scapula, axillary nerve injury, or a neuromuscular disorder that predisposes them to shoulder dislocations. Those with a posterior dislocation may report having a seizure, suffering a blow to the front of the shoulder, or being struck by electricity. Occupations leading to frequent overhead activities, and athletes, who are involved in sports such as throwing/catching, are more prone to get shoulder dislocations.

Clinical Features

Whatever may be the type of dislocation, there is decreased ROM of shoulder. Patients with an anterior dislocation may hold the affected extremity in a position of abduction and external rotation, whereas patients with a posterior dislocation may hold the arm close to the body, adducted, and in internal rotation. In the inferior dislocation the arm is held overhead, typically with the forearm resting on the head. The patient may also experience tingling or numbness. Very rarely an axillary nerve injury/brachial plexus injury occurs in a few cases. A visible deformity of shoulder is present in all types of dislocations.

Diagnosis

Anteroposterior (AP) view of shoulder helps for identifying anterior dislocation, where the humerus is projected inferior to the coracoids process and medial to the glenoid cavity **(Fig. 10.27A)**. A Hill–Sachs lesion (fracture of the humeral head) or a Bankarts lesion (fracture to the inferior aspects of the glenoid process) if any **(Fig. 10.28)**, that are associated with anterior dislocation are found from radiographic examinations.

Posterior dislocations are difficult to diagnose and may be missed clinically and radiographically. In the AP radiograph, displacement of humeral head, combined with lack of external rotation is suggestive of posterior shoulder dislocation **(Fig. 10.27B)**. Other features in AP view suggesting a posterior dislocation include: presence of trough sign (a vertical or arch-like fracture line running parallel and lateral to the articular surface of the humeral head), positive rim sign (distance between the medial border of the humeral head and the anterior border of the glenoid rim measuring greater than 6 mm), loss of crescent sign (the crescent appearance formed by the overlapping of the humeral head and the glenoid process).

Axillary view of shoulder showing impaction of the humeral head on the posterior aspect of the glenoid process also suggests posterior dislocation. The radiographic presentation of an axillary/inferior dislocation is displacement of the humeral head, medial, and inferior to the glenoid process **(Fig. 10.27C)**.

Management of Shoulder Dislocation

Management could be conservative/surgical. The conservative management consists of:

- **Protection, Rest/Ice (PRI):** It consists of protection through application of a sling, rest to the part, ice (except for the left shoulder in the presence of cardiac pathology). The patient is not allowed to eat or drink anything, as sedations may be required to reduce the dislocation.
- **Reduction of dislocation:** The reduction is done by the physician/surgeon. There are a variety of methods of reduction of shoulder dislocation, such as closed reduction and if the same fails or not possible then open reduction is performed. However, recurrent dislocations require surgery. The various methods of reduction include:
  - *Milch maneuver:* Patient in supine lying. The clinician applies steady downward traction at the elbow, in combination with slow external rotation and abduction of shoulder.
  - *Kocher's method:* The patient in supine lying. The clinician applies traction to the shoulder with external rotation of shoulder followed by adduction and internal rotation.
  - *Cunningham method of reduction:* This is an anatomically based method that utilizes positioning (analgesic position), voluntary scapular retraction and bicipital massage. It is designed for true anterior/subcoracoid, glenohumeral dislocations in patients who can fully adduct the humerus.

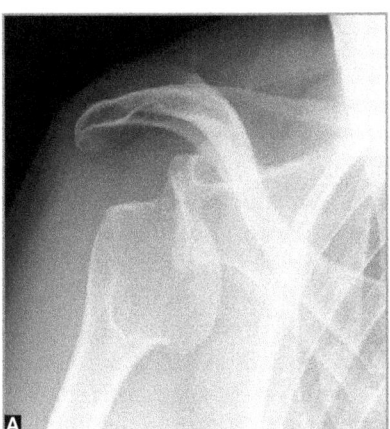 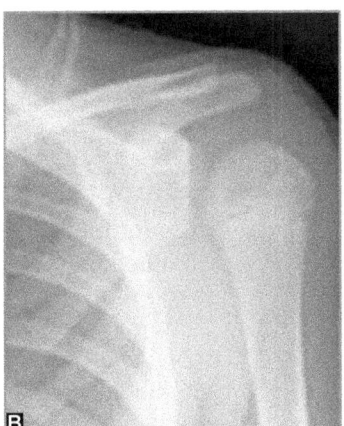 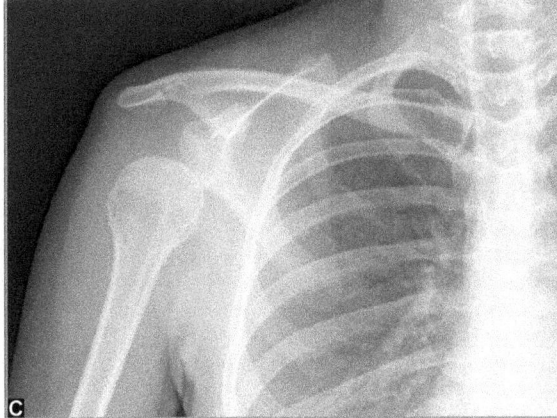

Figs. 10.27A to C: X-rays of shoulder dislocations: (A) Anterior; (B) Posterior; (C) Inferior.

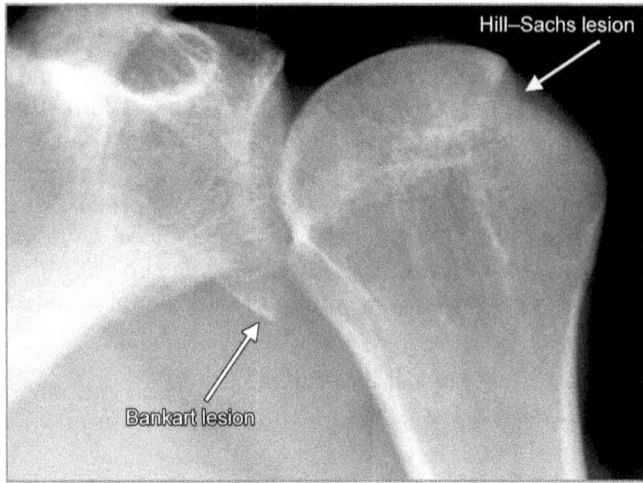

Fig. 10.28: The Hill–Sachs and Bankart's lesion.

– *Hennepin technique:* This technique uses external rotation, plus traction and abduction, if necessary. It requires only one operator, and can be done gently, sometimes without analgesia.

Immobilization After Reduction

After reduction, the shoulder is immobilized using an immobilizer **(Fig. 10.29)**.

Rehabilitation of Shoulder after Reduction of Dislocation

Physiotherapy is an important component of rehabilitation to return the shoulder joint to normal function. The therapy focuses upon:
- Teaching shoulder prophylaxis, i.e., not to perform overhead activities.
- Shoulder ROM exercises.
- Strengthening muscles of shoulder, such as rotator cuff muscles and muscles of shoulder force couple (e.g., middle deltoid-supraspinatus force couple).

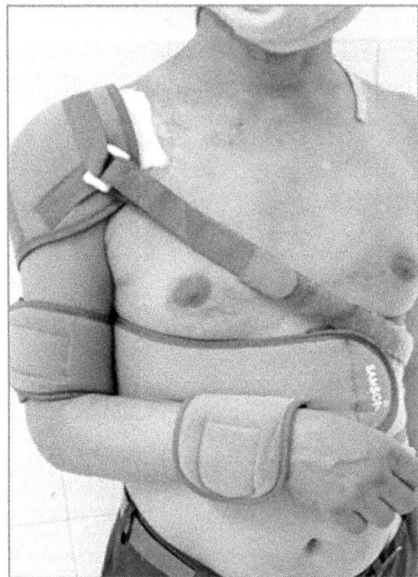

Fig. 10.29: Shoulder immobilizer applied after reduction of dislocation.

- Decreasing inflammation through heat/cold therapy (except no cold therapy to left shoulder in the presence of cardiac pathology). PSWD/SWD/MWD may be helpful for reduction of inflammation and promotion of repair.
- Reduction of pain through interferential therapy (IFT) transcutaneous electrical nerve stimulation (TENS).
- Reduction of deltoid inhibition by faradic current stimulation.

The rehabilitation of shoulder after reduction of shoulder dislocation proceeds through five phases:

1. **Phase I (0–7 days):** This starts, when the reduction has been achieved and the upper limb immobilized in sling/shoulder immobilizer. The physiotherapist tries to minimize pain/soreness by applying cold pack over the shoulder for 10–15 minutes, except to the left shoulder, when the patient has some associated cardiac pathology. Some simple exercises are recommended for practice with the sling/immobilizer or the upper limb supported by the therapist (if the same is accepted by the treating physician/surgeon), such as wrist and finger exercises. The duration of immobilization depends on the amount of pain and tenderness present, and sometimes extended upto 2-4 weeks. The most important thing to follow in this phase is not to abduct the arm sideways with palm facing up, as it may lead to further dislocation. The exercises performed are:
   - *Shoulder flexion:* Patient sitting, supports the affected upper limb with the sound hand under the elbow. The therapist removes the sling. The patient leans forward, and gently rocks the arm forward/backward producing flexion/extension of shoulder within the limit of pain.
   - *Shoulder abduction:* Patient sitting, supports the affected upper limb with the sound hand under the elbow. The therapist removes sling. The patient leans forward and gently rocks the arm sideways, producing abduction/adduction of shoulder within the limit of pain.
   - *Shoulder lateral rotation:* Patient sitting. The arm is kept by the side of body with the elbow flexed and hand supported by sound hand. The therapist removes the sling. The patient rotates the arm laterally up to a location, when the affected forearm and hand are aligned perpendicular to body and not more than this.

2. **Phase II (2-4 weeks):** When pain allows mobility exercises can begin after the sling is removed temporarily and the upper limb supported by the therapist. Simple pendulum exercises for shoulder flexion and abduction in sitting are started within the limits of pain. For shoulder lateral rotation, the patient is asked to rotate the arm laterally, with the elbow flexed and arm by the side of body to a location, when the affected forearm and hand are aligned perpendicular to the body and not more than this. Combined movements of abduction (taking the arm out to the side) and external rotation (turning the shoulder outwards), should be avoided, as this is often the position for shoulder dislocation. The exercises should be performed, if the shoulder is pain-free and wearing the sling should be continued when not performing exercises. Ice should be applied after exercise if swelling and pain occurs.

3. **Phase III (4–6 weeks):** The aim here is to begin to restore strength of the rotator cuff and scapular muscles and achieve full range of motion in the shoulder, except full range shoulder abduction with external rotation. Emphasis should be given on achievement of terminal range for shoulder internal rotation and to develop strength of the medial rotators in the inner range. The sling/support can be removed during exercises if pain allows. However a shoulder support as shown in **Figure 10.22B**, should be used during exercise (if required) and during the rest of the day. The exercises performed are:
   - *Static strengthening exercises:* These exercises are performed to strengthen the muscles around the affected shoulder without moving the joint. For all these exercises the elbow should be flexed to 90°, and arm should not move. The exercises are repeated 10 times in a session, each contraction lasting 5–10 seconds and are performed 3 times a day. The exercises are:
     » Shoulder flexor strengthening: The patient stands facing the wall, and attempts to push the fist forward into the wall **(Fig. 10.30)**.
     » Shoulder extensor strengthening: The patient stands with his back in front of the wall. He/she tries to push the elbow backward against the wall **(Fig. 10.31)**.
   - *Shoulder abductor strengthening:* Patient stands sideways in front of the wall, with the outer side of the affected arm touching the wall. He/she tries to push the wall laterally by the affected arm **(Fig. 10.32)**.
   - *Shoulder adductor strengthening:* Patient stands with the affected arm by the side of body and elbow flexed. A roll of towel placed in the arm pit is pressed inward toward the trunk by the arm **(Fig. 10.33)**.
   - *Shoulder lateral rotator strengthening:* Patient stands with the elbow flexed to 90° and the outer aspects of the affected side hand aligned against the wall. He/she pushes the hand against the wall, without moving the elbow away from the trunk **(Fig. 10.34)**.

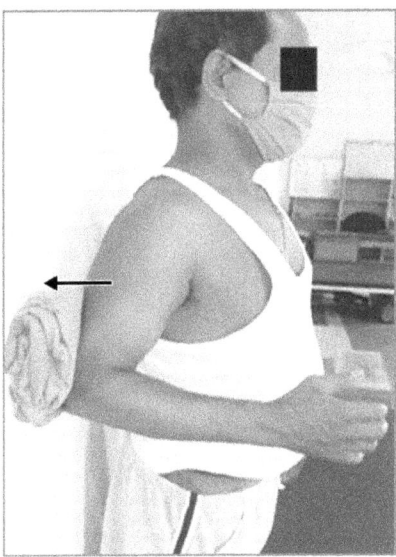

Fig. 10.31: Isometric shoulder extensor strengthening.

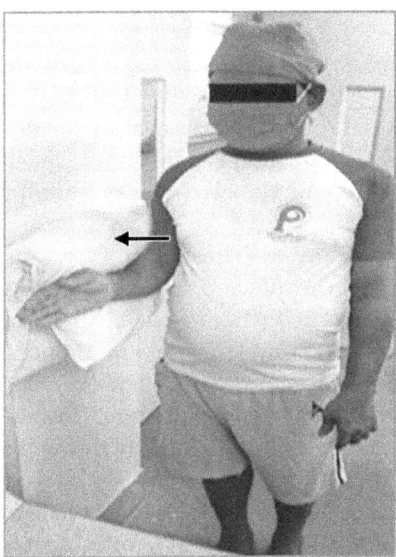

Fig. 10.32: Isometric shoulder abductor strengthening.

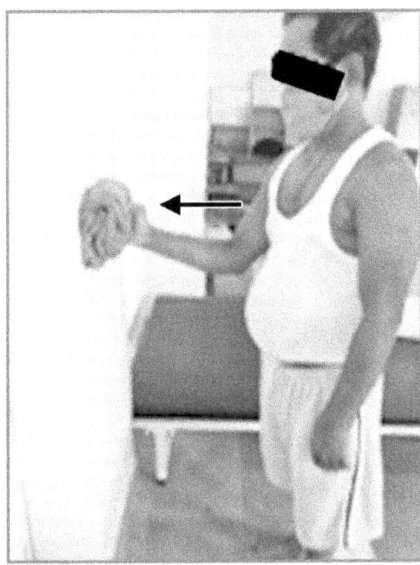

Fig. 10.30: Isometric shoulder flexor strengthening.

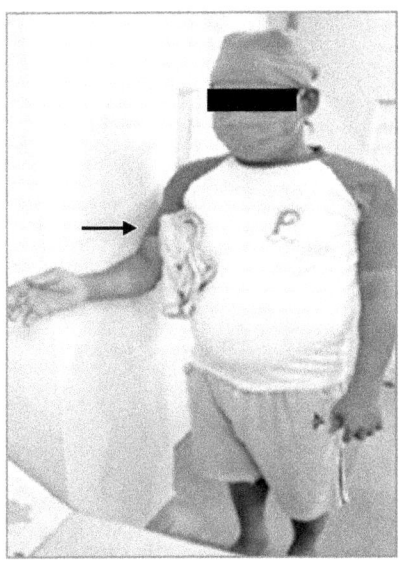

Fig. 10.33: Isometric strengthening of shoulder adductors.

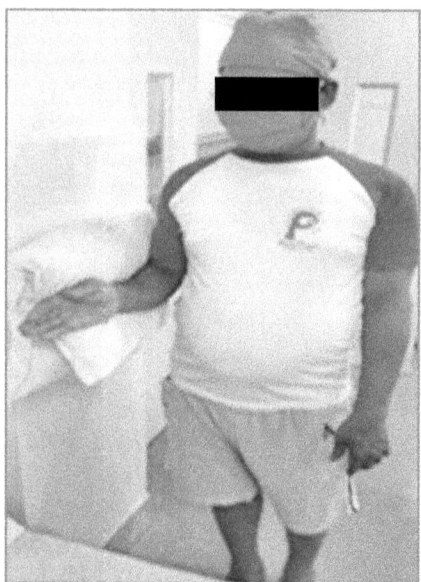

Fig. 10.34: Isometric strengthening of shoulder lateral rotators.

- *Shoulder medial rotator strengthening:* Patient stands with the elbow flexed to 90°. The inner aspect of the affected side hand is placed against the wall. The patient tries to push the wall with the inner aspect of the hand, without moving the elbow away from the body (**Fig. 10.35**).
- *Mobility exercises:* These exercises help to improve mobility of the affected shoulder. The wand exercise (*see* **Fig. 10.25C**) where a stick is held in both hands is used for the purpose. The end point of the activity is held for 5 seconds and each exercise is repeated 10 times with 4 sessions per day. However stretching the joint into terminal ranges of movement should be avoided.
- *Scapular setting exercises:* In order to achieve normal movement and function in the shoulder, it is essential that the scapulae are aligned and supported efficiently. The scapulae need to be stabilized, by strengthening two muscles, i.e., serratus anterior and lower trapezius. These exercises are done slowly, and 5–10 repetitions of exercise to be done in a session. The exercises are:
  » Lower trapezius exercise in prone: Patient in prone lying, head supported on a fold of towel and arms by the side. The patient is asked to draw the shoulder blades downward and backward with minimal effort (25%) and hold for 5–10 seconds and then lower it. 5–10 repetitions of movements are done (**Fig. 10.36**).
  » Lower trapezius exercise in prone (a progression): Patient in prone lying, head supported on a fold of towel and arms by the side. The patient is asked to draw the shoulder blades downward and backward with minimal effort (25%). Holding the shoulder blades in that position, he/she is asked to raise and lower the arm by 2 cm from the bed and repeat the same five times. Then he/she returns back to neutral position (**Fig. 10.37**).
  » Lower trapezius exercise in standing: Patient stands facing the wall, with the forearm resting on the wall. Patient pulls the shoulder blades (scapulae) backward and downward, holds the position and climbs the wall with the fingers and puts the hand down and then relaxes. Repeat the same for few times (**Fig. 10.38**).

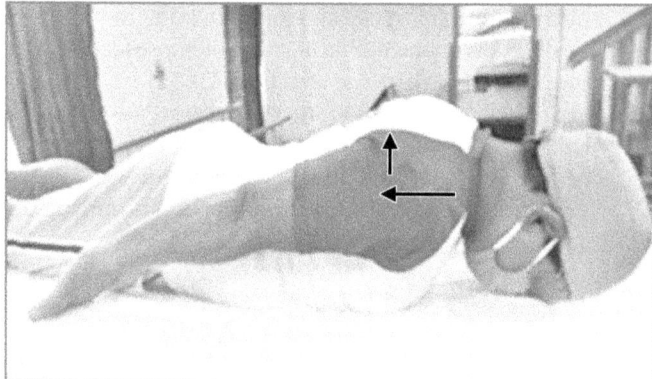

Fig. 10.36: Lower trapezius strengthening in prone.

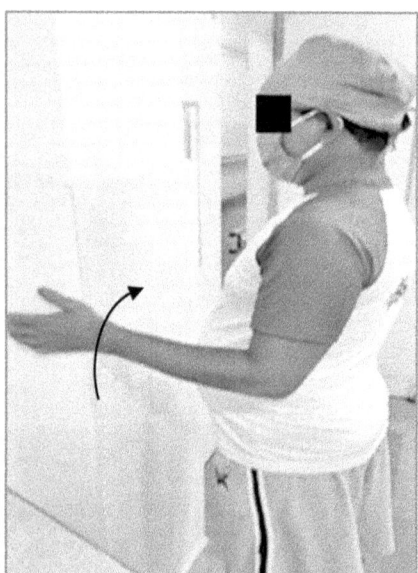

Fig. 10.35: Isometric strengthening of shoulder medial rotators.

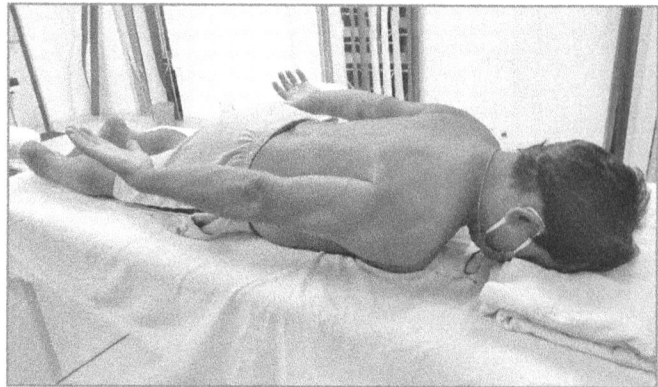

Fig. 10.37: Lower trapezius exercise in prone lying.

Chapter 10: Physiotherapy for Shoulder

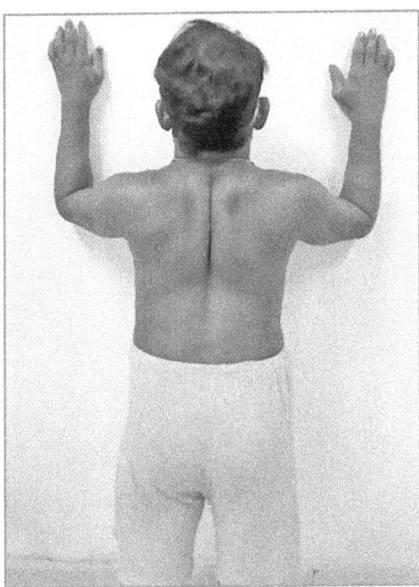

Fig. 10.38: Lower trapezius exercise in standing.

» Serratus anterior exercise in supine: Patient, lying supine, shoulder flexed to 90° with the elbow in extension. The patient lifts the arm vertically toward the ceiling **(Fig. 10.39)**, holds for 5-10 seconds and then relaxes. Repeat the same few times.

4. **Phase IV (6-10 weeks):** During weeks 6 to 10, aim is to achieve strength equal to the uninjured side, and maintain mobility. Resisted exercises within the pain free ranges are started and gradually progressed. Range of motion exercises are continued and proprioceptive training is started during this phase. The exercises performed are:
   - *Shoulder muscles strengthening exercise using theraband:* These exercises are performed to strengthen the muscles around the shoulder using a therabands. Each contraction is maintained for 3-5 seconds and 20 repetitions 3 times a day are usually performed. The following exercises are performed:
   » Strengthening of lateral rotators: Patient stands sideways to a window, elbow flexed and arm by the side of the body. One end of the theraband is tied to the railings of the window, and the other end is held tightly by the hand of the patient. The patient tries to pull the therabands out to the side, rotating the arm laterally, holds for few seconds and then relaxes **(Fig. 10.40)**. A few repetitions of exercise are performed.
   » Strengthening the shoulder internal rotators: Patient stands sideways, to a window, elbow flexed. One end of the theraband is tied to the railings of the window, and the other end is held in the patient's hand. The patient pulls the theraband and moves the hand across the body rotates the arm inward and then relaxes. A few repetitions of exercise are performed **(Fig. 10.41)**.

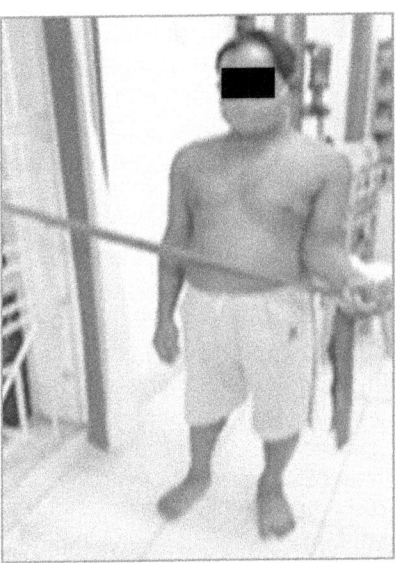

Fig. 10.40: Shoulder external rotator strengthening using theraband.

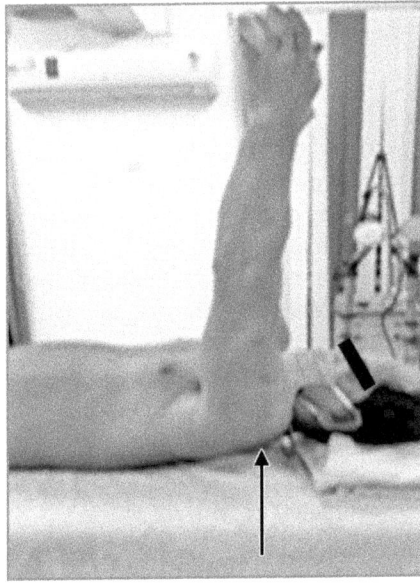

Fig. 10.39: Serratus anterior strengthening in supine.

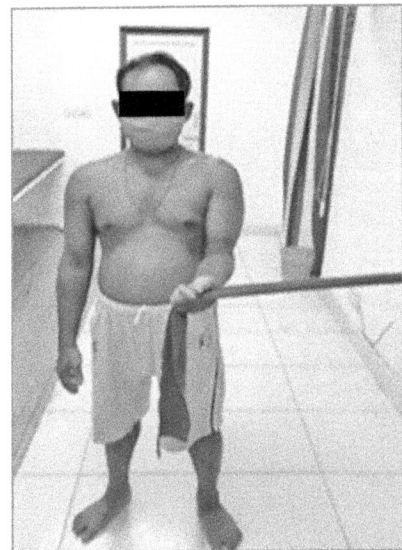

Fig. 10.41: Shoulder internal rotator strengthening using theraband.

» Strengthening of shoulder extensors: Patient stands facing the window. One end of the theraband is tied to the railing of the window. The patient holds the other end and pulls it backwards holds for few seconds and then relaxes. A few repetitions of exercise are performed **(Fig. 10.42)**.
» Strengthening of shoulder flexors: Patient standing. One end of therabands tied to a railing at the back of the patient. The patient holds the other end of the theraband and pulls it forwards in a punching motion, holds it for few seconds and then relaxes. A few repetitions of exercise are performed **(Fig. 10.43)**.
» Strengthening of shoulder abductors: The patient standing. One end of theraband is pressed under foot on the affected side of body. Keeping the shoulder at 45° of abduction and holding the other end of the therabands in hand, the patient pulls the theraband laterally and upwards, holds the position for few seconds and then relaxes. A few repetitions of the exercise are performed **(Fig. 10.44)**.
» Proprioceptive training: Sitting, weight bearing on the affected hand, four point kneeling (prone kneeling), controlled weight bearing on the affected hand are started in this phase.

5. **Phase V (10–16 weeks):** Aim of therapy in this stage is to make the client return to normal sports and function. Resistance used for strengthening, progress from advanced theraband exercises to exercises with dumbbells and body weight exercises. Functional activities such as throwing and catching are gradually progressed. Non contact games are started initially and load on the affected shoulder is gradually increased. A flexible shoulder support may be used in this stage if required.
The exercises performed are:
   – The phase-V of rehabilitation after shoulder dislocation consists of high resistance progressive exercises to shoulder performed in full range. The exercises are:

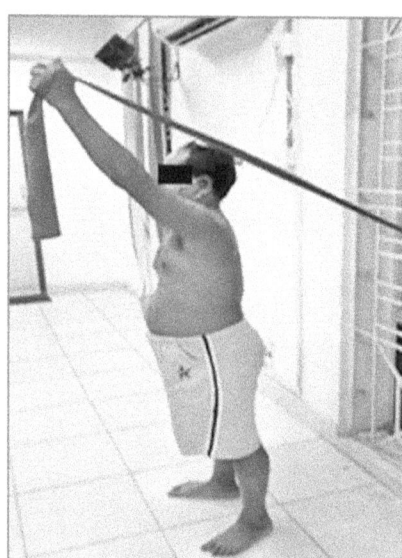

Fig. 10.43: Shoulder flexor strengthening using theraband.

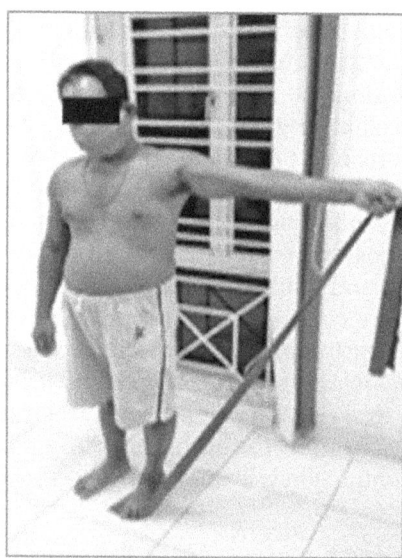

Fig. 10.44: Shoulder abductor strengthening using theraband.

   – *Advanced theraband exercise for shoulder external rotators:* The patient sits facing a table, elbow flexed at 90°, resting on table. One end of theraband is held in hand and the other end is securely tied to the leg of the table. The patient pulls the therabands outwardly, producing external rotation, holds the contraction of muscles for a few seconds, then relaxes **(Fig. 10.45A)**. A few repetitions of the exercise are performed.
   – *Advanced therabands exercise for shoulder internal rotators:* The patient sits facing a table/bed, with elbow flexed to 90° and placed on the table. One end of the theraband is tied securely to a fixed support on the leg of the chair/table. The other end of the theraband is held in the hand and the theraband is pulled forward rotating the arm inward **(Fig. 10.45B)**. The muscle contraction is held for few seconds and then the patient relaxes. A few repetitions of the exercise are performed.

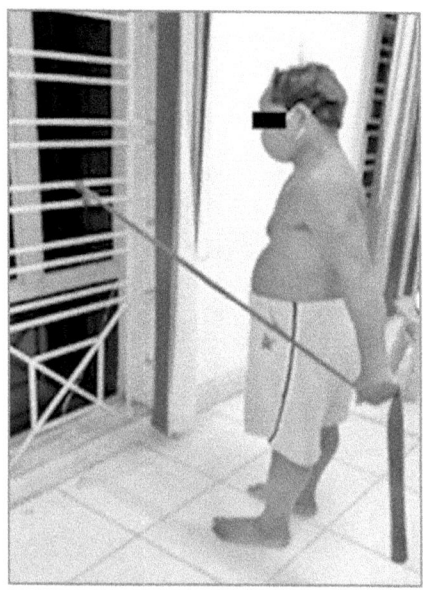

Fig. 10.42: Strengthening of shoulder extensors using theraband.

Chapter 10: Physiotherapy for Shoulder 225

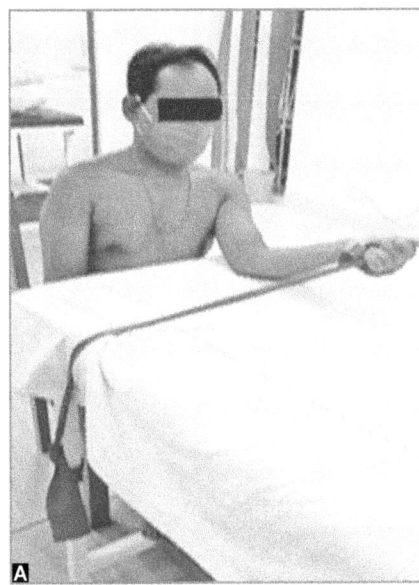

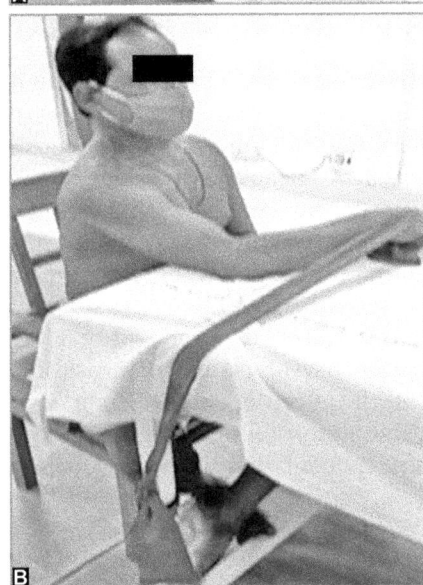

Figs. 10.45A and B: (A) Strengthening of shoulder external rotators; (B) Strengthening of shoulder medial rotators.

- *Scapular setting exercises:*
  » Lower trapezius exercise in prone: Patient in prone, forehead resting on a pad of towel. The hands placed at the back of the head, with the elbows bent. The patient is asked to set the shoulder blades by pulling the scapulae backwards and downwards. Maintaining the position, the patient is asked to lift both the arms off the bed, hold the position for 5–10 seconds and then relaxes. A few repetitions of the exercise are performed **(Fig. 10.46A)**.
  » Serratus anterior exercises in four points kneeling: Patient in prone keeling position. He/she is asked to push the chest and upper back upwards and pull the shoulder blades backwards. Maintaining this position, he/she is asked to lift the sound hand off the floor, without letting the shoulder dip down. The position is held for 5–10 seconds, and after that the

hand is put down **(Fig. 10.46B)**. A few repetitions of the exercise are performed.
- *Weight-bearing exercises/proprioceptive training:*
  » Push ups against the wall: The patient stands facing the wall at a distance of 2 feet from the wall. He/she places both the hands on the wall and leans on to it. Then he/she lowers the body toward the wall and returns back to the initial position. The exercise is repeated 10 times **(Fig. 10.47A)**.
  » Push ups in four points kneeling: The patient kneels on the hands and knees. Keeping the head and trunk straight, he/she is asked to lower the upper body toward the floor, and again return back to the initial position. The exercise is repeated 5–10 times **(Fig. 10.47B)**.
- *Electrotherapy:* Shortwave diathermy (SWD), Microwave diathermy (MWD), High power laser, pulsed/continuous ultrasound, Faradic current stimulation to muscles of shoulder force couples **(Fig. 10.48)** may be applied as required.

Surgery

Indications for surgery:
- Initial dislocation in a patient (athlete/mountain climber/construction worker), who participates in high-risk/high-demand activities, in whom recurrent dislocation would be dangerous.
- Recurrent dislocation after conservative treatment failed.

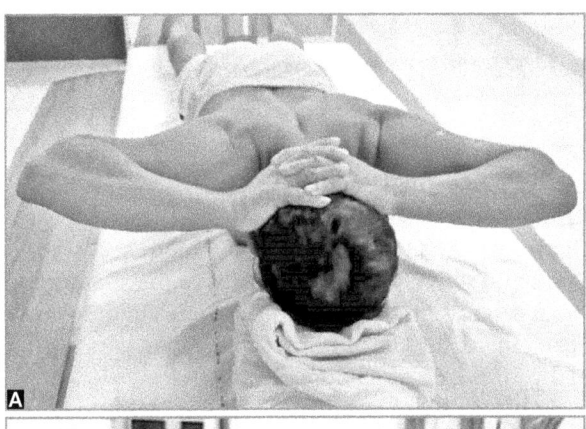

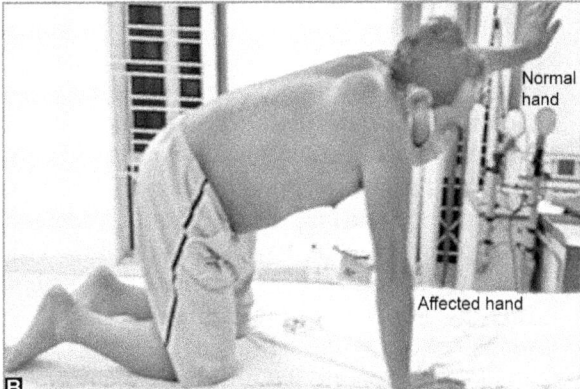

Figs. 10.46A and B: (A) Lower trapezius exercise in prone; (B) Serratus anterior exercise in prone kneeling.

Section 2: Physiotherapy for Musculoskeletal Conditions

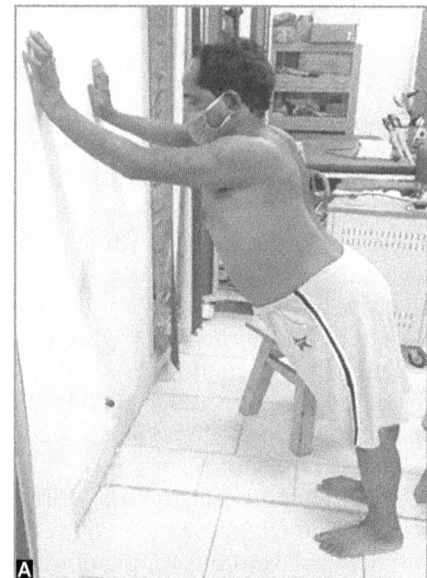

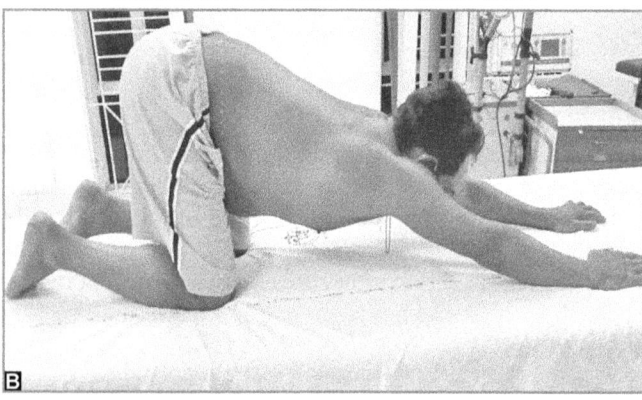

Figs. 10.47A and B: Weight-bearing exercises; (A) Push up against the wall; (B) Push ups in prone kneeling.

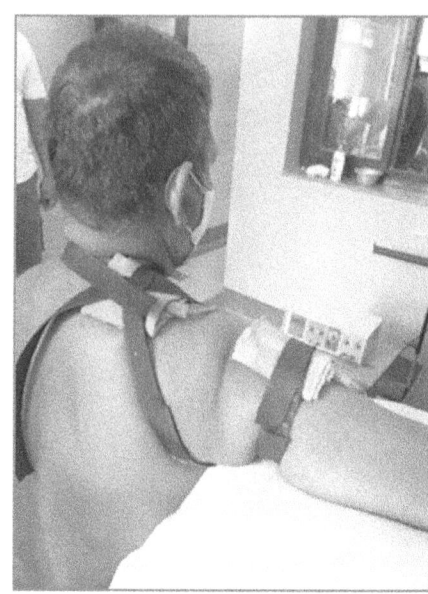

Fig. 10.48: Faradic stimulation to deltoid-supraspinatus force couple.

Surgeries performed could be:
- Arthroscopic surgery.
- **Open surgery:** Open means, the surgeons access the joint through a single incision made above the shoulder joint. Open surgery may be performed to repair injured tendons, ligaments, or the labrum, or to address damage to the bones of the joint. The procedures involved are:
  - **Bankart's procedure:** A Bankart shoulder repair procedure is a surgical technique for the repair of recurrent shoulder joint dislocations. Within the procedure, the worn out ligaments/capsule are re-attached to the proper place in the shoulder joint, using the objective of rebuilding normal function.
  - **Putti-Platt procedure:** Putti-Platt is one of the surgical treatment options for anterior shoulder instability. In this procedure, the flexible cord (tendon) of the subscapularis muscle is cut and then reattached to the head of the upper arm bone (humerus).
  - **Capsular shift:** A capsular shift tightens the ligaments that become lax, after multiple dislocations. The procedure involves tightening the ligaments to eliminate loose tissue.
  - **Latarjet procedure (Bristow procedure):** This procedure involves, transferring bone from the coracoid process and attaching the same to the conjoint tendon at the front edge of glenoid cavity. This bone augmentation helps in restoring stability of shoulder.
  - **Remplissage procedure:** It may be done in tandem with the Latarjet procedure, where the humeral head has been damaged due to a Hill–Sachs lesion. The procedure involves resurfacing the head and/or filling the defect, by fixing it to part of rotator cuff muscles.
  - **Shoulder joint replacement:** Hemi arthroplasty/or total arthroplasty of shoulder is performed some times in selected patients, having severe shoulder instability.

Postoperative Physiotherapy

Postoperatively physiotherapy is applied as per the protocols.

Prophylactic advises

The patients with shoulder dislocations, whether managed conservatively/surgically, should be advised on prophylactic measures to be taken to prevent recurrent dislocations. The measures to be taken include:
- Doing regular exercises to strengthen muscles of affected shoulder.
- Avoiding overhead activities.
- Using dynamic shoulder supports, while engaged in repetitive activities.
- Avoiding lying over the affected shoulder for few weeks, if pain and instability persists.

iii. Frozen Shoulder (Adhesive Capsulitis) and its Management

Frozen shoulder, also known as adhesive capsulitis, is a condition of uncertain etiology, characterized by stiffness, and pain in the shoulder joint. Signs and symptoms typically begin gradually, worsen over time and then resolve, usually within 1–3 years.

Causes of Frozen Shoulder

The causes of adhesive capsulitis are incompletely understood. The risk factors for primary/idiopathic adhesive capsulitis include many systemic diseases such as diabetes mellitus, stroke, lung disease, heart disease, connective tissue diseases, autoimmune diseases, thyroid disease, etc. Risk factors for secondary adhesive capsulitis include trauma or surgery that lead to prolonged immobility.

Classification of Frozen Shoulder

Frozen shoulder is classified as:
- **Primary/idiopathic frozen shoulder**: Primary or idiopathic frozen shoulder, though does not have a definite cause, is often associated with other diseases and conditions, such as diabetes mellitus, and may be the first presentation of a diabetic patient. Patients with systemic diseases such as thyroid diseases and Parkinson's disease are at higher risk of developing this type of disorder.
- **Secondary frozen shoulder:** Secondary adhesive capsulitis can occur after shoulder injuries or immobilization (e.g., rotator cuff tendon tear, subacromial impingement, biceps tenosynovitis, and calcific tendinitis). These patients develop pain from the shoulder pathology, leading to reduced movement in that shoulder, and thus developing frozen shoulder.

Pathophysiology of Adhesive Capsulitis (Frozen Shoulder)

Though the underlying pathophysiology of adhesive capsulitis is not fully understood, it is generally accepted to have both inflammatory and fibrotic components. The inflammation and subsequent tightness (fibrosis) of the shoulder joint capsule is central to the disease process. There may be reduction in synovial fluid, affecting mobility of the shoulder joint. In the early stage, there is evidence of inflammatory cytokines in the joint fluid. Later stages are characterized by dense collagenous tissue in the joint capsule.

Clinical Features of Adhesive Capsulitis (Frozen Shoulder)

Patients with frozen shoulder typically experience insidious shoulder pain and stiffness that usually worsen at night. Though all movements of shoulder are limited, movement limitation in the capsular pattern of restriction, i.e., more limitation of abduction, lateral rotation and less limitation of internal rotation of shoulder is found. The pain is usually dull aching in nature. Due to pain and stiffness of shoulder, the individual is not able to perform activities of daily living (ADLs) and instrumental activities of daily living (IADLs), qualitatively as well as quantitatively, affecting the quality of life.

Stages of Frozen Shoulder

Frozen shoulder usually progresses through three stages such as:
1. Freezing (painful)
2. Frozen (adhesive)
3. Thawing (gradual recovery)

A summary of the three stages of frozen shoulder are given in **Table 10.4**.

Although adhesive capsulitis is self-limiting, usually resolving in 1-3 years, mild pain may persist for long time affecting the patient's function.

Diagnosis of Adhesive Capsulitis (Frozen Shoulder)

Adhesive capsulitis (frozen shoulder) can be diagnosed by history of onset and physical examination. On physical examination, this condition presents with limitation of both active and passive ROM. Abduction and external rotation of shoulder is significantly limited as compared to internal rotation and flexion.

Imaging studies are not usually required to diagnose the condition. Radiographs are usually normal in this condition.

Management of Adhesive Capsulitis (Frozen Shoulder)

Management of this disorder focuses on reduction of pain and restoration of mobility of shoulder subsequently leading to restoration of lost function. The methods of management are:
1. **Medical management**: NSAIDs are prescribed by the physician/surgeon for reduction of pain. In case of nonremitting acute pain, corticosteroids are prescribed by physician/surgeon for some patients, which are applied

Table 10.4: Stages of frozen shoulder.

Stages	Freezing	Frozen	Thawing
Duration	2–9 months	4–12 months	5–26 months
Signs and symptoms	Gradual onset of diffuse, severe shoulder pain that worsen at night	Pain begins to subside, but there is characteristic progressive loss of joint range of motion (glenohumeral flexion, abduction, external rotation, and internal rotation)	Gradual return of range of motion and relief of pain
Medical management	NSAIDs, oral or intra-articular glucocorticoids (if intractable pain persists)	Usually not required	Usually not required
Physiotherapy	Gentile active and passive exercises, ice/heat therapy, PSWD/PMWD/pulsed ultrasound. IFT/TENS, LILT	Stretching/strengthening exercises, SWD/MWD/infrared/ultrasound/faradism under tension/cryokinematics/hot pack IFT/TENS	Stretching/strengthening exercises, SWD/MWD/infrared/ultrasound/faradism under tension/cryokinematics/hot pack/IFT/TENS

NSAIDs: nonsteroidal anti-inflammatory drugs; PSWD: pulsed shortwave diathermy; PMWD: pulsed microwave diathermy IFT: interferential therapy; TENS: transcutaneous electrical nerve stimulation; LILT: low-intensity laser therapy; SWD: shortwave diathermy; MWD: microwave diathermy

orally or through local injection. It must be remembered that the benefits of steroid injections are usually short-term and not free from complications, hence selection of such injections should be judiciously made for the patient.

2. **Physiotherapy:** Timely referral of a patient with adhesive capsulitis (frozen shoulder) to physiotherapists and judicious selection of therapeutic modalities, along with advice on activity modifications and observation of energy conservation techniques help the patient to live a pain-free life with participation in family, community and job activities maintaining an enhanced quality of living. The physiotherapy treatment depends on the stage of the disorder, when the patient reports the physiotherapist. The components of physiotherapy in different stages of the disorder are described below:
   - *Physiotherapy in freezing (acute) stage:* Pain is the most dominating feature in this stage leading to movement limitation and loss of function. Gentle active and passive exercises, ice (except for left shoulder in the presence of cardiac pathology)/superficial heat therapy, PSWD/PMWD/pulsed ultrasound. IFT/TENS, low-intensity laser therapy (LILT), etc., may be used by the physiotherapist in this stage. Ice therapy to left shoulder in presence of cardiac disease is contraindicated, as it may affect functioning of the heart (as left shoulder and heart has the same parasympathetic supply). The selection of therapeutic modalities depends on the tissues affected and the evidences available regarding the selection of modalities and their parameters. However, when selecting SWD/MWD/ultrasound, the pulsed mode at lower intensities and for shorter duration is selected, which can gradually be progressed, as the condition changes, subsequently requiring the application of these modalities in the continuous mode in the frozen state. The use of IFT/TENS is made to modulate pain. Iontophoresis using NSAIDs, as well as steroidal drugs may be used to reduce inflammation and pain.

   As this stage lasts for months, once significant pain reduction and mobility is achieved, the patient should be advised to continue the exercises at home and report to the physiotherapist periodically for evaluation and further advice. The exercises should be performed within the pain-free range. The exercises advised in this stage are:
   » Wand exercises using a stick/towel (**Figs. 10.49A to D**).
   » Shoulder pulley exercises.
   » Shoulder ladder exercises (**Figs. 10.50A to C**)
   » Shoulder wheel exercises (**Fig. 10.51**)
   » Gear shift exercises (**Fig. 10.52**)
   » Codman's pendular exercises (**Fig. 10.25D**)

   While doing the exercises, it should be kept in mind that energy conservation is strictly followed, and the number of repetitions of exercise in a session and number of sessions per day should be decided depending upon the tolerance and responses of the patient. In the very acute stage, when pain severely limits function, cryokinematics, application of analgesic gel may used when performing the exercises. Use of moist heat in conjunction with passive stretching has been found to increase flexibility of tight muscles.

   - *Physiotherapy in the frozen stage:* In this stage, the pain reduces considerably; however, there is significant stiffness in the joints affecting the individual's self care and occupational activities. The aims of physiotherapy in stage are:
   » Reduction of stiffness
   » Reduction of pain
   » Increase of function

     The exercises continued in the freezing (acute) stage are also continued in this stage. In addition to above, interventions for stiffness and pain described below are also performed.
   » Maitland mobilization in grade-III/grade-IV to increase arthrokinematic motion/joint play such as: AP glide for increasing medial rotation and flexion, PA glide for increasing lateral rotation and extension, superoinferior glide for increasing abduction.
   » Kaltenborn technique, where traction and mobilization is used to reduce pain and increase mobility of hypomobile joints. A Kaltenborn grade of II and III is used for the mobilization.
   » Mulligan's mobilization with movement (**Fig. 10.53A**).
   » Passive stretching of the joint capsule and tight muscles/ligaments: Towel stretch (**Fig. 10.53B**), corner stretch.

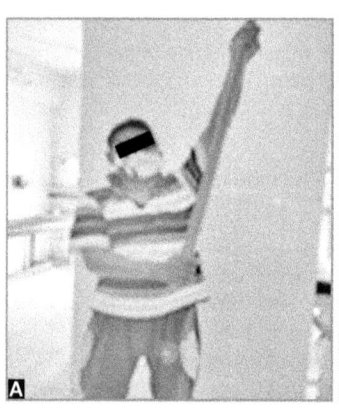 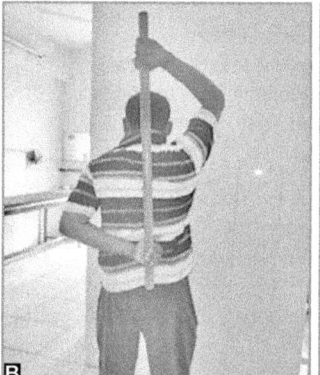 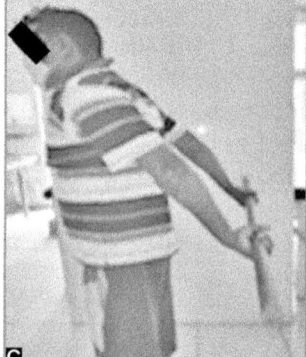 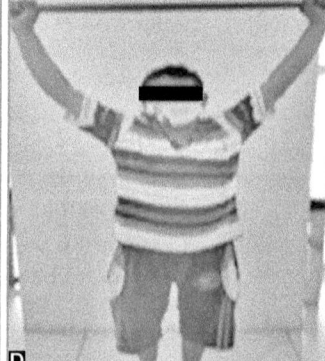

Figs. 10.49A to D: The wand exercises.

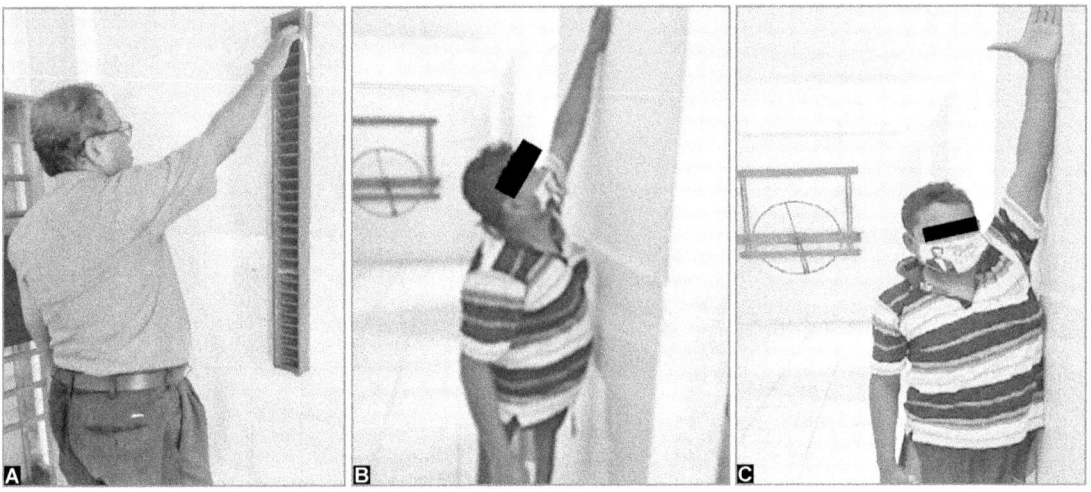

Figs. 10.50A to C: (A) The shoulder ladder; (B and C) Wall ladder exercise.

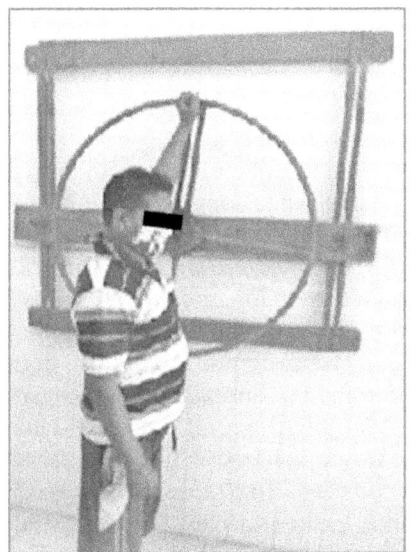

Fig. 10.51: The shoulder wheel exercise.

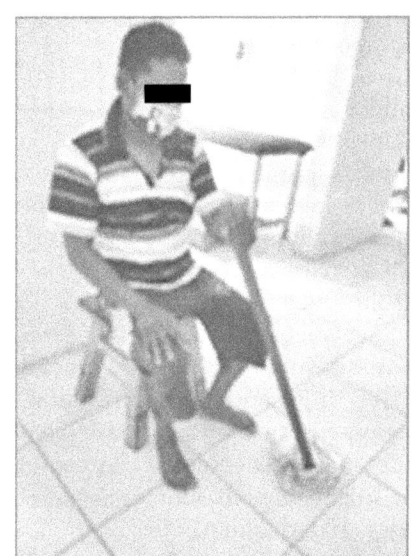

Fig. 10.52: The gear shift exercise for shoulder.

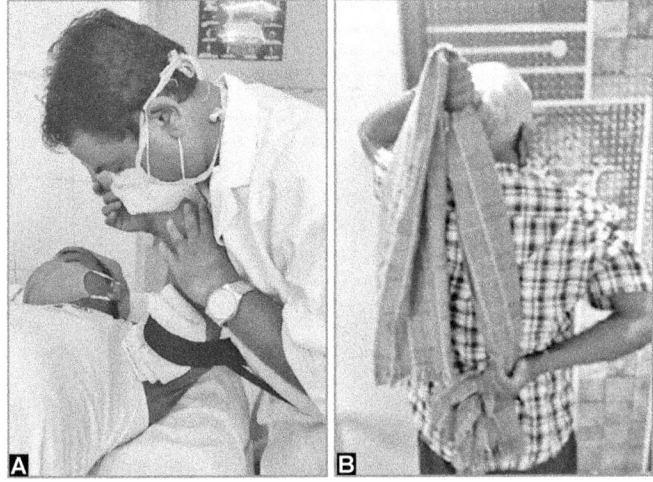

Figs. 10.53A and B: (A) Mulligan mobilization exercise; (B) Towel stretch exercise to improve shoulder internal rotation.

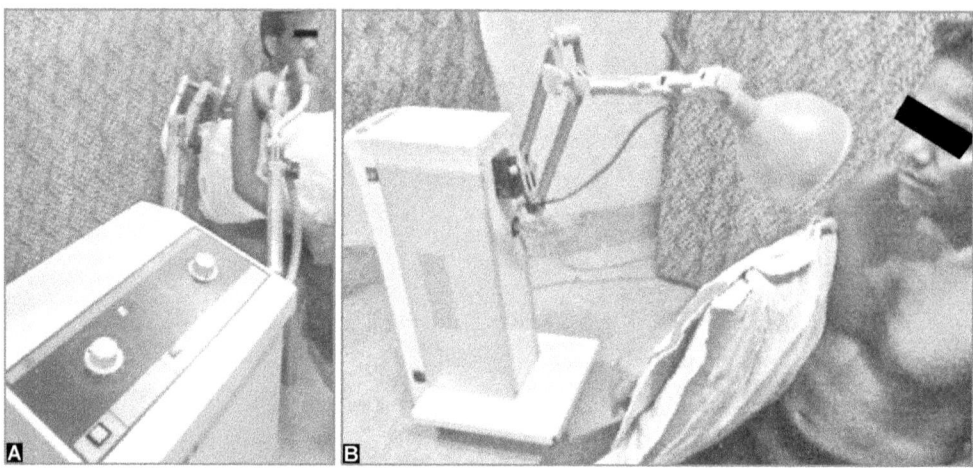

Figs. 10.54A and B: (A) SWD to shoulder joint; (B) MWD to shoulder joint with anterior shoulder pain.

- Active exercises, including the followings are emphasized, with increased amplitude and repetitions as compared to freezing stage:
  » Active assisted/free exercises
  » Shoulder pulley exercises
  » Shoulder ladder exercises
  » Codman's pendular exercises **(Fig. 10.25D)**: A weight as tolerated may be held in the hand while doing pendular exercises.
  » Wand exercises
  » Gear shift exercise
  » Shoulder wheel exercise

Before mobilization certain heat modalities such as SWD/MWD/IRR/continuous ultrasound, high power laser therapy etc., are used to increase extensibility of the tight collagenous tissues such as joint capsule, ligaments, muscles, making mobilization easier and causing pain relief **(Figs. 10.54A and B)**.

Specific techniques such as faradism under tension to tight muscles, say supraspinatus **(Fig. 10.55)** may be applied to lengthen tight muscles, causing gain in range of motion (say medial rotation in this example).

For relief of pain IFT **(Fig. 10.56)**/TENS/iontophoresis using NSAIDs, as well as steroids (hydrocortisone) may be used as indicated.

Strengthening exercises in the form of concentric/eccentric exercises can be started in this stage, as the pain gradually subsides.

Once considerable range is gained by the patient, he/she should be advised to continue home exercise program, and gradually return to occupational activities.

- *Physiotherapy in the thawing stage:* Gradual reduction of pain and return to function occurs in this stage. In this stage, the emphasis should be laid on more and more home exercise program in the form active exercises and self stretching. Strengthening exercises for muscles of shoulder and postural muscles to maintain erect posture are emphasized in this stage. Use of therabands, weight cuff **(Figs. 10.57A and B)** can be made to apply resistance to the muscles, that are usually weak due to lack movement and functional activities during the previous stages of the disorder. If considerable pain persists, the patient should be advised to attend the physiotherapy clinic for a short course of therapy,

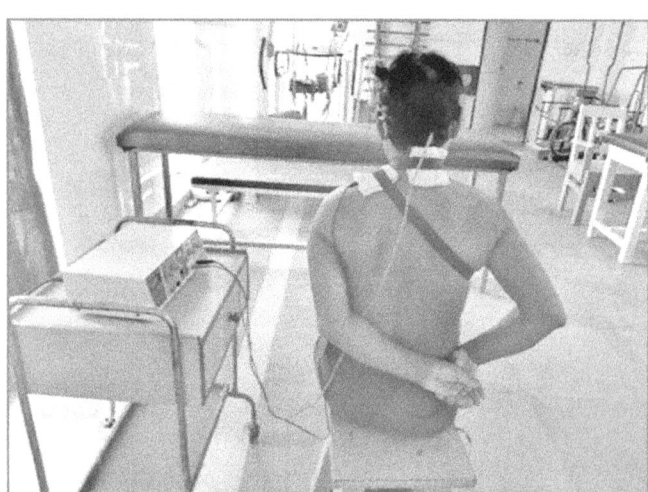

Fig. 10.55 : Faradism under tension to supraspinatus.

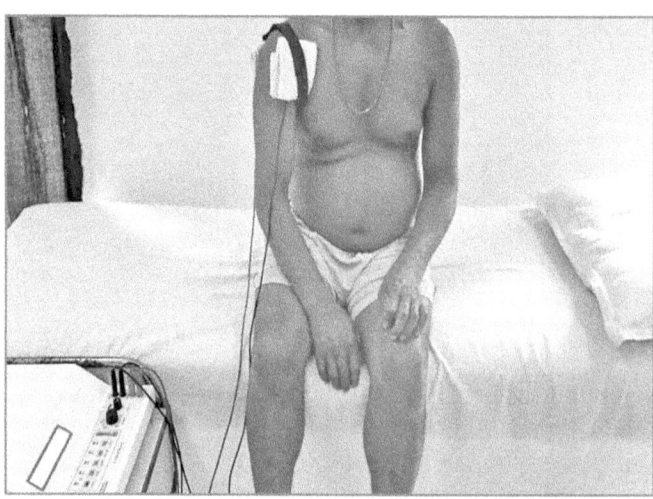

Fig. 10.56: IFT (Premodulated mode) application to shoulder.

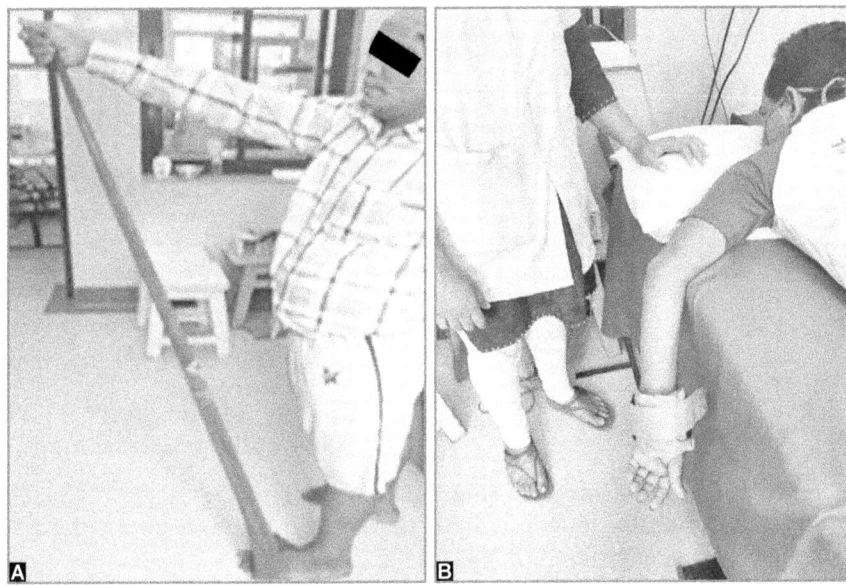

Figs. 10.57A and B: (A) Strengthening the shoulder flexors using theraband; (B) Strengthening the rotator cuff muscles using weight cuff.

where modalities such as SWD/MWD/US/High power LASER therapy etc., are applied before stretching and mobilization exercises. After the exercises if pain persists, modalities such as IFT/TENS may be used to reduce pain. The patient should be advised to continue the occupational activities with observation of energy conservation and joint protection.

Surgical management and manipulation under anesthesia is considered in those cases, where, the conservative treatment is unsuccessful. However, manipulation of shoulder carries a risk of shoulder dislocation, hence should be decided and performed judiciously.

Physiotherapy for Disorders of Elbow

THE ELBOW JOINT

The elbow joint is a hinged compound synovial joint (**Fig. 11.1**) that consists of the humeroulnar and the humeroradial joints. It is also known as trochleogingylomoid joint, as it can flex and extend like a hinge (ginglymoid). The joint is extremely congruent and stable and because of this after injury, it is more prone to stiffness rather than instability.

The proximal joint surface of the humeroulnar joint consists of the convex trochlea, located on the anteromedial surface of the distal humerus. The distal joint surface is the concave trochlear notch on the proximal ulna.

The proximal joint surface of the humeroradial joint is the convex capitulum located on the anterolateral surface of the distal humerus. The concave radial head on the proximal end of the radius is the opposing joint surface.

The joints are enclosed in a large, loose, and weak joint capsule, which also encloses the superior radioulnar joint. The mediolateral stability is obtained by the medial and lateral collateral ligaments that reinforce the joint capsule.

In the normal anatomical position, the long axes of the humerus and forearm form an acute angle at the elbow, called carrying angle, which is about 5° in males and 15° in females.

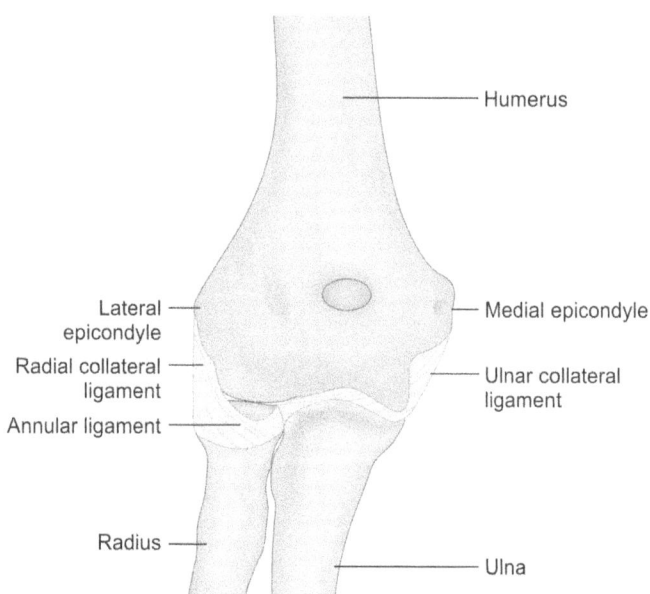

Fig. 11.1: The elbow joint.

Osteokinematics of Elbow Joint

The elbow joint has 1 degree of freedom, flexion-extension in the sagittal plane and around the coronal axis.

Arthrokinematics of the Elbow Joint

* **At the humeroulnar joint:**
  - *During flexion* of elbow, the trochlear edge of ulna slides along the trochlear groove, until the ulnar coronoid process reaches the floor of the coronoid fossa of the humerus.
  - *During extension*, sliding of the ulna on the trochlea continues, until the ulnar olecranon process, enters the humeral olecranon fossa.
* **At the humeroradial joint:**
  - *During flexion:* The rim of the radial head slides anteriorly in the capitulotrochlear groove to enter the radial fossa.
  - *During extension:* The concave radial head slides posteriorly on the convex surface of the capitulum.

Capsular pattern of limitation of elbow joint: Flexion is more limited than extension.

THE SUPERIOR AND INFERIOR RADIOULNAR JOINTS

* **Superior radioulnar joint:** The radial notch of the ulna and the annular ligament at the upper end of radius, form the concave joint surface that articulates with the convex head of the radius.
* **Inferior radioulnar joint:** The convex ulnar head articulates with the ulnar notch of the radius and the articular disc.

Osteokinematics of the Radioulnar Joint

The superior and inferior radioulnar joints are mechanically linked; therefore motion at one joint is always accompanied by motion at the other joint. The mechanically linked joint is a synovial pivot joint with 1 degree of freedom. The movement of pronation and supination that take place in this joint occur around the longitudinal axis extending from radial head to ulnar head.

Arthrokinematics of Radioulnar Joints

- **At the superior radioulnar joint**: During supination and pronation, the convex rim of the head of radius spins within the annular ligament and the concave radial notch. The spin is posterior during pronation and anterior during supination.
- **At the inferior radioulnar joint:** The concave articular surface of the radius slides anteriorly over the ulnar head during pronation, and posteriorly during supination.

Capsular Pattern of Limitation of Radioulnar Joint

As per Cyriax and Magee, the capsular pattern is equal limitation of supination and pronation. According to Hertling and Kessler, a greater limitation of supination than pronation occurs at the superior radioulnar joint, whereas involvement of the inferior radioulnar joint produces little loss of movement.

Ranges of motion of elbow and forearm are given in **Table 11.1**.

Table 11.1: Ranges of motion of elbow and forearm.

Movement	Range of motion
Flexion	0–150°
Extension	0
Pronation	0–80°
Supination	0–80°

FACTORS CONTRIBUTING TO ELBOW PAIN AND SPECIAL TESTS FOR ELBOW DISORDERS

Elbow pain does not occur in isolation. Many proximal structures can refer pain to the elbow and certain local structures can contribute to the elbow pain and dysfunction. For example, cervical dysfunction such as cervical spondylosis can refer pain to the elbow. The cervical and thoracic spines have been found to influence elbow pain. In a study by Berglund et al., (2008), 70% of subjects with lateral elbow plain also experienced pain in the cervical and thoracic spine.

The disorders that cause elbow pain are discussed below:

i. Tennis Elbow

Tennis elbow called lateral epicondylitis is the most common overuse syndrome/cumulative trauma disorder of the upper limb. It is a tendinopathy involving the extensor muscles of the forearm, at their origin on the lateral epicondyle of the humerus.

Etiology/Epidemiology

Tennis elbow occurs in persons between the age of 30 and 50 years, affecting males and females equally. Though the name tennis elbow is given to the disorder, only 5% of sufferers have the history of playing tennis, and a great majority of sufferers present with a history of chronic activity involving flexion/extension of the wrists, or pronation/supination of the forearm. Besides tennis players, the disorder also seen in other sporting activities, such as badminton, baseball, swimming, and other throwing games/activities. People with repetitive movements in their job such as, carpenters, electricians, gardeners, computer operators, manual laborers, and household workers frequently develop this condition. In many cases no predisposing cause is established, and attributed to cumulative trauma disorder (CTD), due to repeated daily activities.

Pathophysiology

Lateral epicondylitis is an overuse injury that may result in hyaline degeneration of the origin of the extensor tendons, most commonly the origin of extensor carpi radialis brevis (ECRB). There is an inflammatory lesion with degeneration occurring at the origin of extensor tendons, most commonly ECRB, and other tendons such as extensor carpi radialis longus, extensor digitorum, and extensor carpi ulnaris. Along with these, the origin of superficial part of supinator, which is in closer proximity to origin of ECRB, is also involved. This may lead to maladaptations of tendon structures that cause pain over lateral epicondyle, mostly over distal and anterior part of lateral epicondyle. Continued inflammation and fraying occur at the origin of the common extensors of wrist **(Fig. 11.2)**. Hypovascularity and fibrosis in the extensor aponeurosis and the subaponeurotic space may develop, along with contracture of anterolateral elbow capsule.

Clinical Features

The onset of the condition may be sudden or gradual. The patient complains maximum tenderness over an area distal to the origin of common extensors of wrist. There is pain in activities involving movement of wrist and fingers and twisting of forearm.

The pain sometimes radiate upward along the upper arm and downward along the outside of the forearm and in rare cases even to the third and fourth fingers. Sometimes, there is decreased strength and flexibility of wrist extensors, forearm supinator and patients report weakness in grip strength and difficulty in carrying objects in their hands.

According to Warren, there are four stages on the development of this injury with regard to the intensity of the symptoms, such as:

1. **Stage 1:** Faint pain a couple of hours after the provoking activity.
2. **Stage 2:** Pain at the end or immediately after the provoking activity.

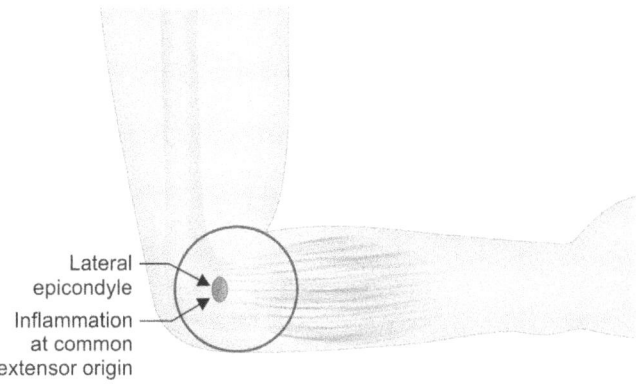

Fig. 11.2: Inflammation at common extensor origin.

3. **Stage 3:** Pain during the provoking activity, which intensifies after ceasing that activity.
4. **Stage 4:** Constant pain, which prohibits any activity.

Symptoms last, on an average, from 2 weeks to 2 years and many patients recover spontaneously.

Diagnostic Procedure

Diagnosis of lateral epicondylitis is done by history (mostly occupation), physical examination/clinical tests. Physical examination reveals strong tenderness over the origin of common extensors (mostly ECRB).

By the following methods (tests), the physiotherapist/clinician may be able to reproduce the typical pain, confirming the diagnosis:

- **Cozen's test**: Cozen's test is also known as the resisted wrist extension test. The elbow is stabilized in 90° flexion resting on a table/over pillows. The therapist aligns the patient's wrist in extension and asks the patient to extend the wrist against therapist's resistance. The test is positive if the patient experiences a sharp, sudden, severe pain over the lateral epicondyle **(Fig. 11.3)**.
- **Chair test**: The patient grasps the back of the chair while standing behind it and attempts to lift the chair by using a three finger pinch (thumb, index and middle fingers) with the elbow fully extended. The test is positive when pain occurs at the lateral epicondyle **(Fig. 11.4)**.
- **Mill's Test**: The patient is seated with the upper extremity relaxed at side and the elbow extended. The examiner passively stretches the wrist into flexion with forearm in pronation **(Fig. 11.5)**. Pain at the lateral epicondyle or proximal musculotendinous junction of wrist extensors is positive for lateral epicondylitis.
- **Maudsley's test**: The examiner resists extension of the third digit of the hand (middle finger), while palpating the lateral epicondyle. A positive test is indicated by pain over the lateral epicondyle **(Fig. 11.6)**.
- **The coffee cup test (by Coonrad and Hooper)**: While doing a specific activity such as picking up a full cup of coffee or a milk bottle, patient feels pain over lateral epicondyle **(Fig. 11.7)**.

Investigations

- Investigations are usually not performed in the straightforward case of lateral elbow pain. However, in longstanding cases, plain X-ray (AP and lateral views) of the

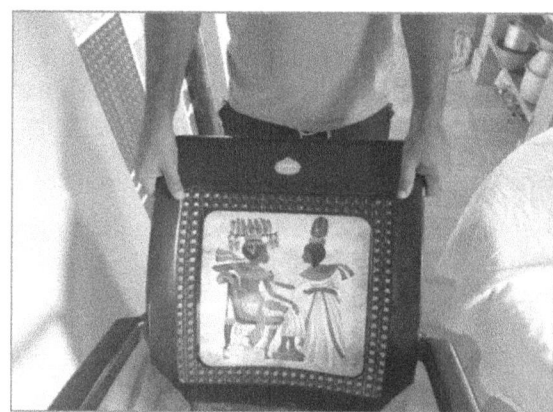

Fig. 11.4: The chair test.

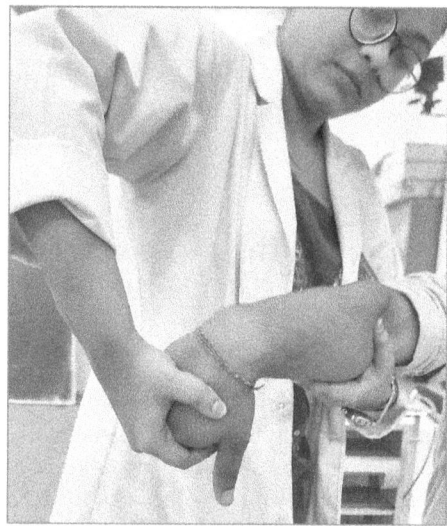

Fig. 11.5: The Mill's test.

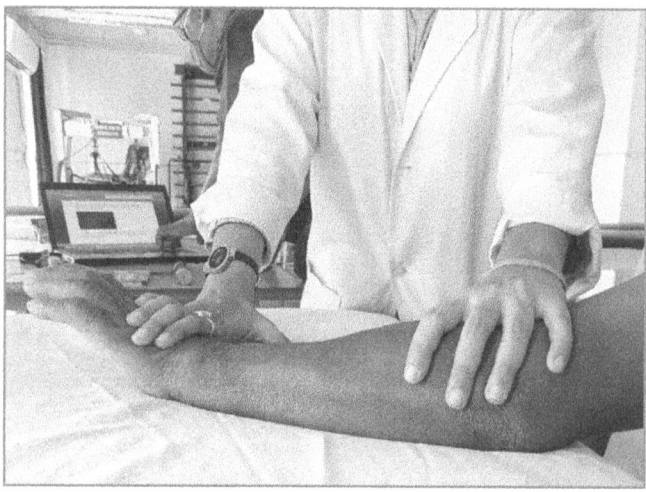

Fig. 11.3: The Cozen's test.

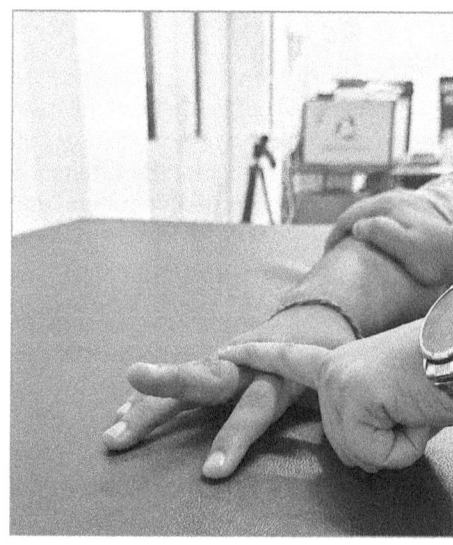

Fig. 11.6: The Maudsley's test.

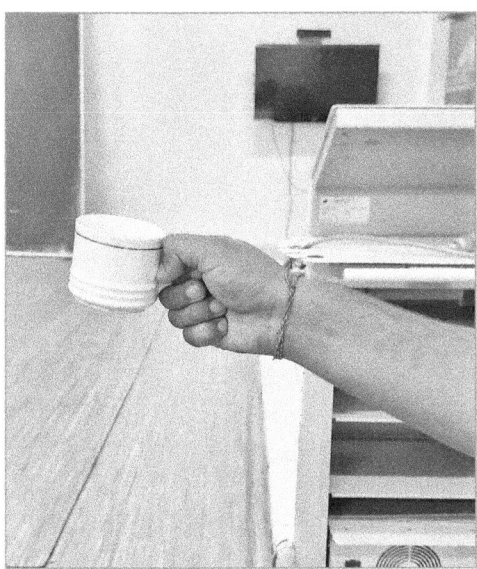

Fig. 11.7: The coffee cup test.

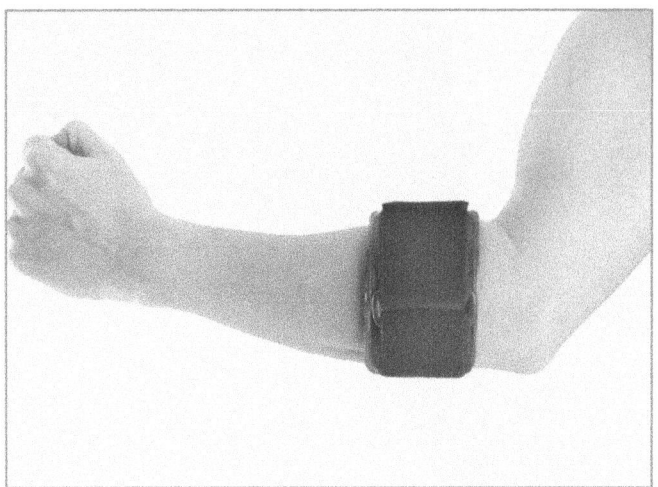

Fig. 11.8: The tennis elbow splint.

elbow may show osteochondritis dissecans, degenerative joint changes, or evidence of heterotopic calcification.
- **Ultrasound** examination may prove to be a useful diagnostic tool in the investigation of patients with lateral elbow pain. Ultrasound may demonstrate the degree of tendon damage as well as the presence of a bursa.
- **Magnetic resonance imaging (MRI):** If the symptoms are related to neck problems, MRI of cervical spine can be recommended.
- **Electromyography (EMG):** An EMG is used to rule out nerve compression, such as compression of radial nerve in supinator teres syndrome.

Management of Lateral Epicondylitis
- **Medical management:** It consists of use of NSAIDs to reduce pain and inflammation in the acute stage. In case of nonremittance of pain with NSAIDs, local injection of steroids may be considered (a steroid injection should be followed by 1–2 weeks rest and should not be repeated more than 2 times).
- **Physiotherapy:** Physiotherapists are associated largely in the assessment and treatment of tennis elbow. The interventions used by physiotherapists include the followings:
  - *Physiotherapy in acute/subacute stage:* The objectives of physiotherapy in the acute/subacute stages are reduction of inflammation and pain. The interventions include:
    » Ice therapy for 10–15 minutes, three times a day.
    » Use of tennis elbow splint **(Fig. 11.8)**, to reduce pressure at the common extensor origin, as the splint acts as a secondary muscle attachment. The splint is applied around the upper forearm (below the head of radius) and tightened as tolerated.
    » Modalities like low-intensity laser therapy, pulsed ultrasound **(Fig. 11.9)**, interferential therapy (IFT), transcutaneous electrical nerve stimulation (TENS) can be applied in the acute stage for reduction of inflammation and pain.

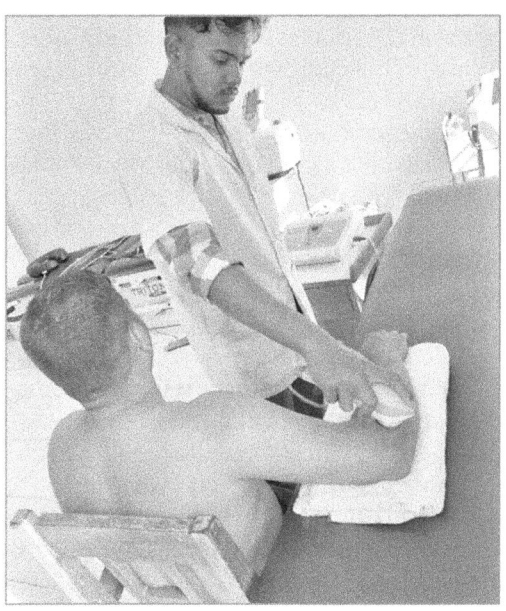

Fig. 11.9: Application of pulsed ultrasound for acute tennis elbow.

  - *Physiotherapy in the chronic stage:* The objectives of physiotherapy in this stage are:
    » To reduce inflammation and pain.
    » To stretch the scar over the common extensor origin.
    » To strengthen the common extensors.
    » To improve function.
    » To educate the patient on activity modification and pain control.
    » To promote activity/sports-specific training.

Methods of physiotherapy:
- **Electrotherapy:** The modalities of treatment in this stage are discussed below. The therapist should decide the modality needed through clinical reasoning considering the available evidence for selection of the modality and treatment parameters.
  - *Extracorporeal shockwave therapy:* The use of radial shockwave therapy (RSWT) **(Fig. 11.10)** produces a

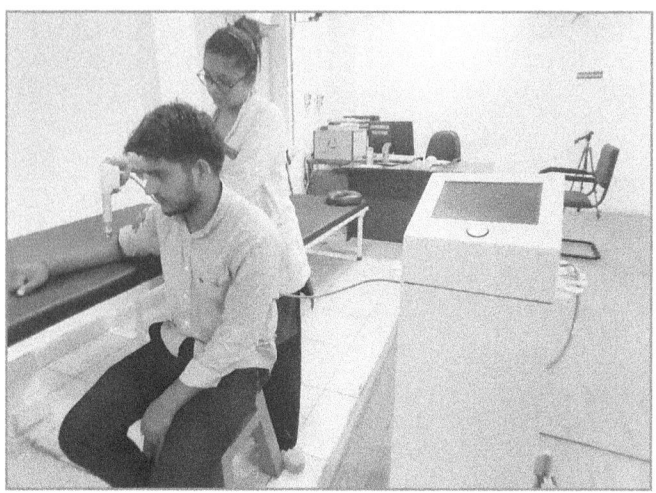

Fig. 11.10: Shockwave therapy for tennis elbow.

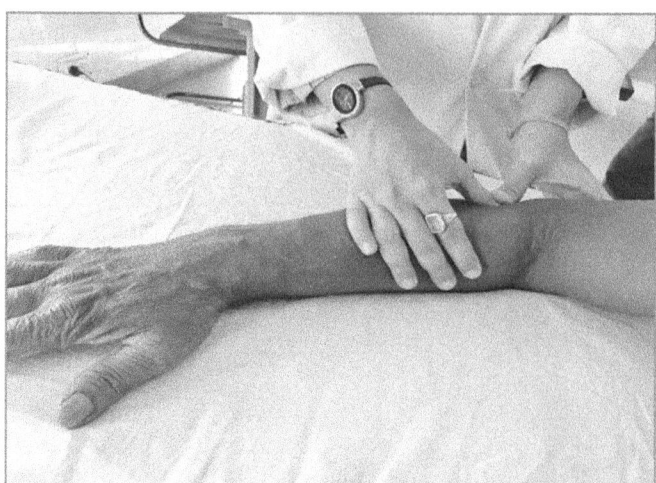

Fig. 11.11: DTFM to common extensor origin in tennis elbow.

decrease of pain, and functional impairment, and an increase of the pain-free grip strength test, in patients with tennis elbow.
- *Continuous ultrasound therapy:* Ultrasound therapy over the musculotendinous junction helps in mobilizing scar tissue and reduces pain.
- *High power laser therapy:* The modality when applied reduces inflammation and pain.
- *Faradism under tension* to wrist extensors helps in breaking adhesions at the common extensor origin.
- *SWD (monoplanar method)/MWD/PWB:* These modalities, as indicated can be selected in some patients before stretching and mobilization exercise.
- *Iontophoresis/phonophoresis:* Drugs such as diclofenac, salicylates, hydrocortisone, etc., when applied through iontophoresis/phonophoresis are helpful for reduction of inflammation and pain and to improve flexibility of scar tissue.
- *IFT:* IFT (premodulated mode), helps in modulating pain.

❖ **Exercise therapy and massage:**
  - *Exercises and mobilization/manipulation:* Exercises in the form of stretching and strengthening of the extensor muscles in the forearm, mobilization and manipulation of elbow joint, deep transverse friction massage etc., all help in reducing pain and improving function and prevent further damage: The exercise therapy and massage include:
    » Cyriax deep transverse friction (DTF): Cyriax deep transverse friction **(Fig. 11.11)** combined with Mill's manipulation performed three times a week for 4 weeks found to be beneficial in reducing pain and improving function in patients with tennis elbow. The therapist must try to reach an analgesic effect applying the DTFM at the point of the lesion for 10 minutes till a numbing effect has been reached. An interval of 48 hours between two sessions of massage should be maintained.
    » Mill's manipulation: It is a small-amplitude high-velocity thrust performed at the end of elbow extension while the wrist and hand are held flexed **(Fig. 11.12)**. The aim of this technique is to elongate the scar tissue by rupturing adhesions within the teno-osseous junction, making the area mobile and pain free.

The procedure involves, patient seated with the affected shoulder in 90° abduction and internal rotation (olecranon faced up). Therapist stands behind the patient, stabilizes the patient's wrist, in flexion with forearm in pronation, while the other hand is placed on the olecranon. The high-velocity low amplitude (HVLA) thrust at the end range of elbow extension, is applied as quick movement. This manipulation may produce mild discomfort at the instant of its performance. The clinician applies this procedure 2–3 times a week, and 4–12 sessions may be required.

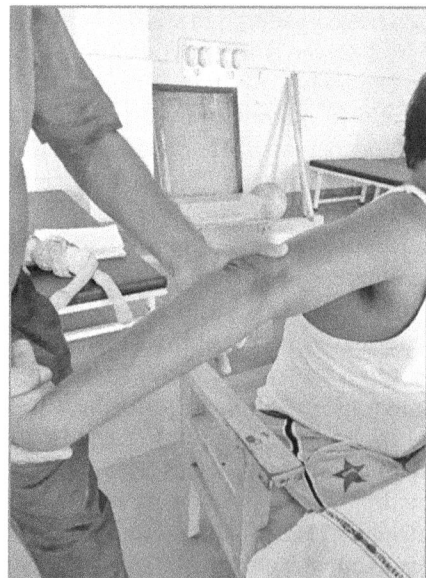

Fig. 11.12: The Mill's manipulation.

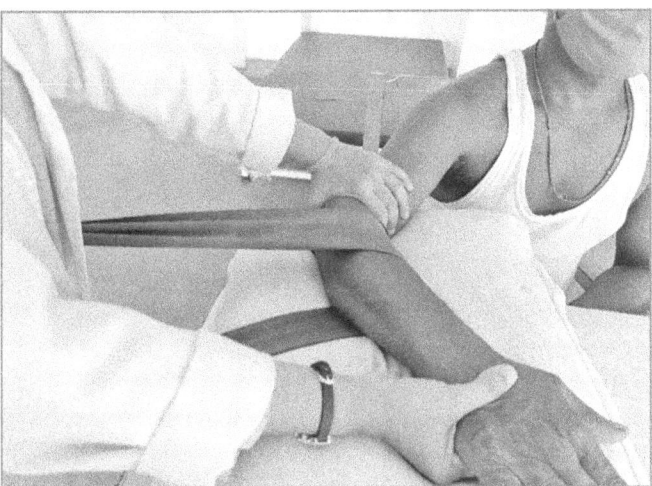

Fig. 11.13: Mulligan's mobilization with movements.

- Besides stretching by therapist **(Fig. 11.14A)**, the sufferer should also be taught stretching exercise as home exercise program **(Figs. 11.14B and C)**.
  - Eccentric strengthening exercises: The three principles of eccentric exercise, i.e., progressive loading, low speed to avoid pain and frequency of 3 sets 10 each are beneficial for lateral epicondylitis **(Fig. 11.15)**.
- **Strengthening exercises using therabands/small weight** in the hand **(Figs. 11.16A and B)**. These exercises are performed each day at 3 sets of 10 each. One end of therabands is held under the foot, and other is held in the hand, while pulling the band up to get resistance.
- **Flexbar exercise:** The flexbar exercise is **(Fig. 11.17)** an effective and beneficial eccentric exercise for patients with lateral epicondylitis. This resistance device is easy for home use.

The steps for this exercise are:
- Hold flexbar in the affected hand with wrist in full extension.
- Hold the other end of this device in the unaffected hand.
- Twist the flexbar with the unaffected hand while holding **(Fig. 11.18)**.

The flexbar exercise is performed each day for 3 sets of 15. It takes 4 seconds to complete each repetition and between each set of 15 repetitions there is 30 seconds of rest. Once the patients can perform 3 sets of 15, they progress to another color flexbar with a higher intensity of eccentric resistance. The treatment should continue until the patient has a resolution of symptoms.

- **Taping:** Taping **(Fig. 11.19)** may be applied in the acute stage and/or, when the individual is discharged to resume activity/sports for reducing pain and improving grip strength and functional performance.
- **Training sports specific exercises:** Before discharge, sports/activities similar to the sporting activities/functional activities, the individual was performing before onset of pain, that involve throwing and catching are performed under the supervision of the therapist. Once he/she is

» Mulligan's mobilization exercise: Mobilization with movement (MWM) is a modern technique developed by Mulligan for treating lateral epicondylitis. MWM is a form of manual therapy that includes a sustained lateral glide to the elbow joint with concurrent physiological movement. Mobilization of the elbow joint by laterally distracting the upper part of radius and ulna with a belt, helps in reducing pain **(Fig. 11.13)**.

» Conventional exercise therapy: The literature on the treatment of a lateral epicondylitis suggests that strengthening and stretching exercises are the most important components of exercise programs, for enhancing the strength and flexibility of the extensor tendons. The exercises performed in tennis elbow are:
  - Stretching exercise: ECRB can be stretched by holding the elbow in extension, forearm in pronation, wrist in flexion and ulnar deviation **(Figs. 11.14A to C)**. The stretch should be held for 30–45 seconds and performed for 3 times before and after eccentric exercises during each treatment session with 30 seconds rest interval.

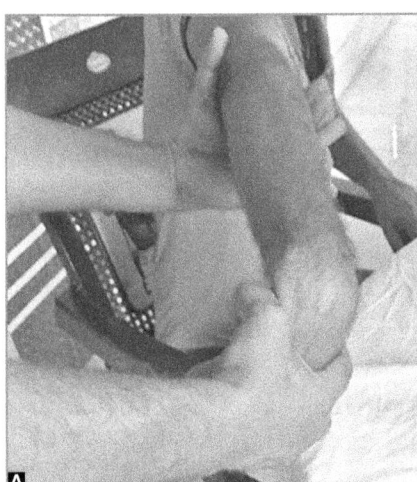 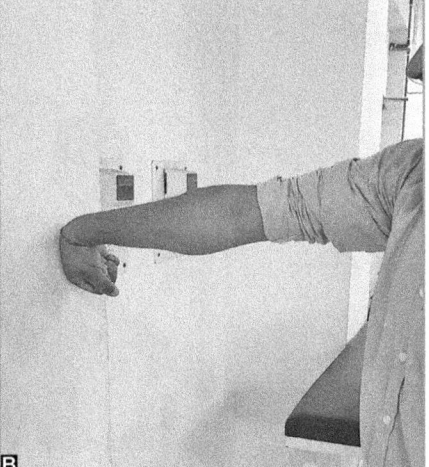 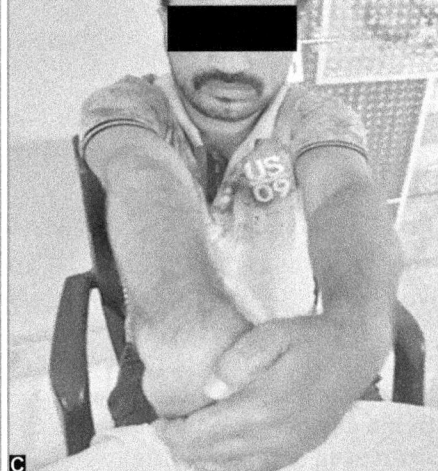

Figs. 11.14A to C: (A) Stretching of ECRB by therapist; (B and C) Self-stretching as home exercise program.

Section 2: Physiotherapy for Musculoskeletal Conditions

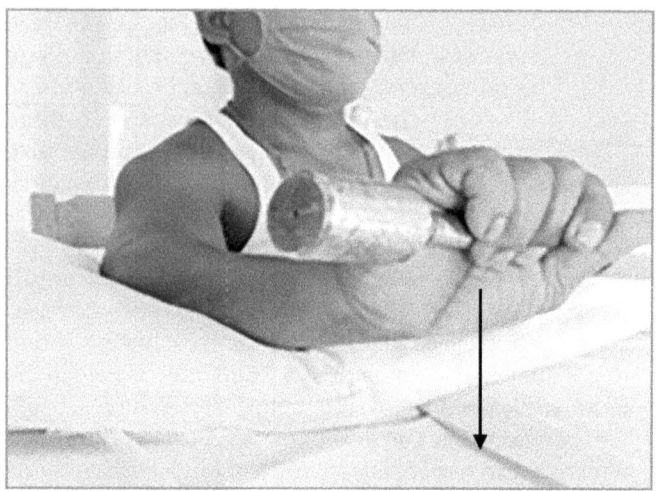

Fig. 11.15: Eccentric exercise for wrist extensors.

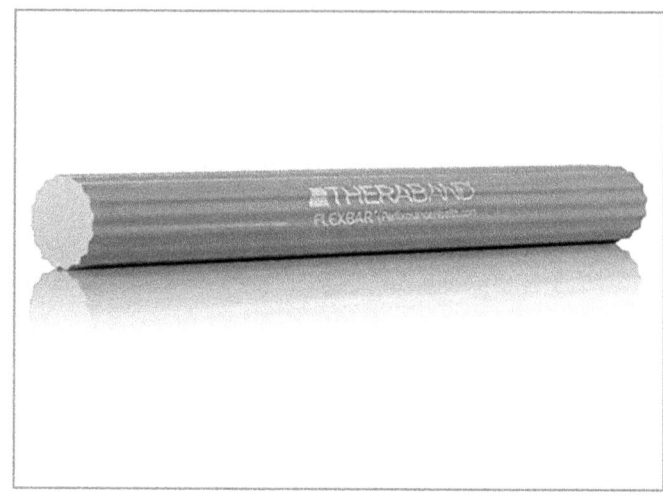

Fig. 11.17: The flexbar.

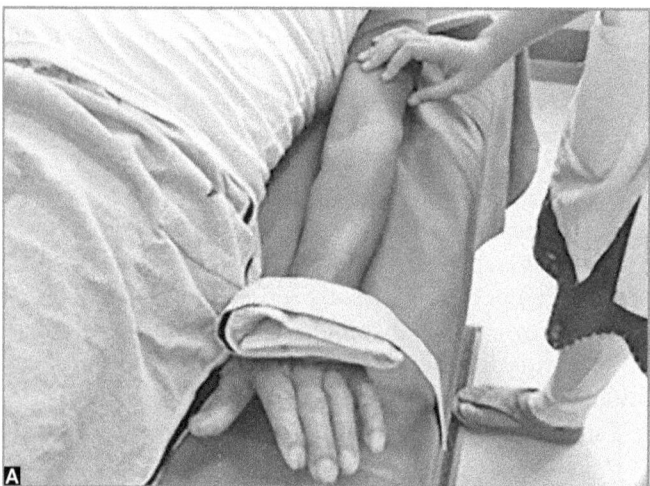

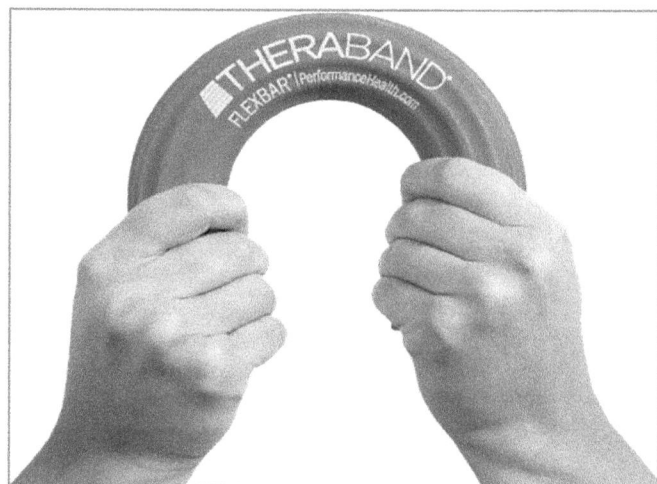

Fig. 11.18: Flexbar exercise.

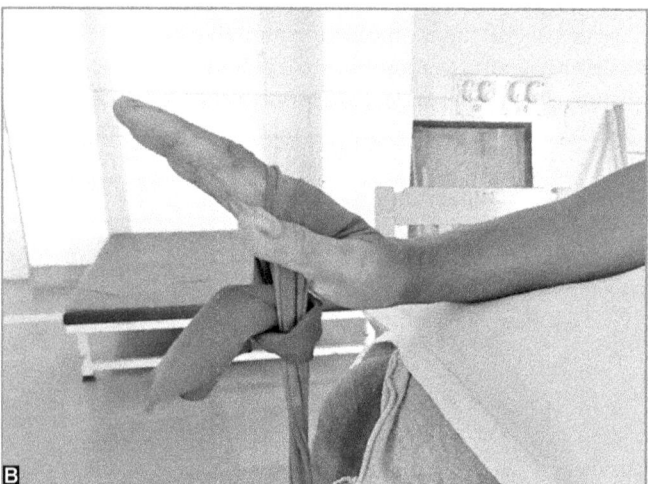

Figs. 11.16A and B: Strengthening of wrist extensors using: (A) Weight cuff; (B) Theraband.

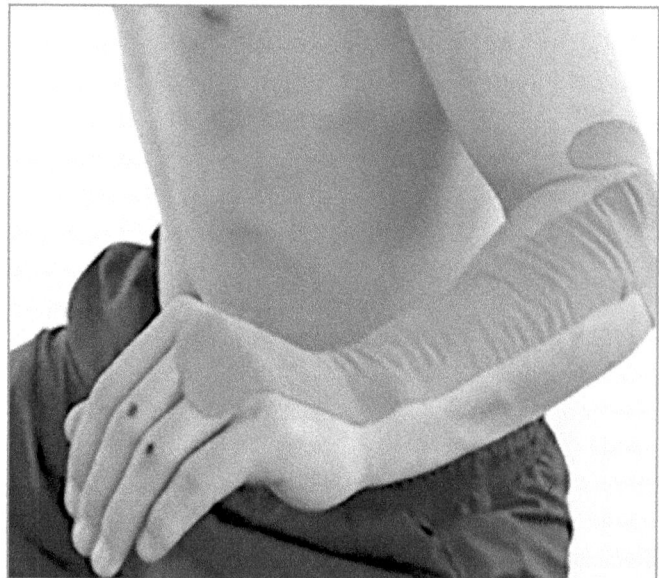

Fig. 11.19: Taping for tennis elbow.

able to perform the sports/activities specific exercises, uncomplicated, discharge is planned.

❖ **Home advice:** The sufferer is advised to continue home stretching/strengthening exercises as advised. The activities/sports are to be performed with observation of energy conservation and use of tennis elbow splint (if required).

Surgical Management of Lateral Epicondylitis

After a failed conservative treatment for more than 6 months, surgery may be considered. Most surgical procedures for tennis elbow involve removing diseased muscle and reattaching healthy muscle back to bone. Surgery considered can be open surgery (most common), or arthroscopic surgery.

ii. Medial Epicondylitis (Golfer's Elbow)

Golfer's elbow, known as medial epicondylitis or pitcher's elbow causes pain, inflammation, and tenderness over the medial aspect of elbow and forearm. It develops due to stress overload on the flexor muscles of hand and the medial collateral ligament of the elbow.

Etiology/Epidemiology

Golfer's elbow has a lower incidence than Tennis elbow. Chronic repetitive concentric or eccentric contractile loading of the wrist flexors and pronator are the most common etiology. Though commonly found in golf players, 90-95% of individuals from other occupations such as carpentry, plumbing, and meat cutting also suffer from this condition. Smokers and sufferers of type-II diabetes carry the risk factors for medial epicondylitis.

Pathophysiology

Besides inflammatory pathologies, problems in the cells of the tendons are the pathology found in sufferers of this condition. Wear and tear in the tendinous origin of the flexor muscles of wrist, leads to tissue degeneration, resulting in abnormal arrangement of collagen fibers, and increased mucoid ground substance deposition between fibers. Focal necrosis and calcification may be found at the origin of the flexors of the wrist and hand. The collagen fibers lose the strength, which become fragile and break easily. Each time, the collagen breaks down, the body responds by producing inflammation, forming scar tissue on resolution of inflammation in the tendon. The extra scar tissue formed causes thickening of the tendons. The tendon changes from a white, glistening firm structure to a dull appearing, slightly brown, and soft structure. The resulting inflammation and binding of soft tissues due to tight scar in the medial aspect of elbow causes pain.

Clinical Features

The onset may be sudden or gradual. The patient usually complains about pain of the elbow distal to the medial epicondyle of the humerus **(Fig. 11.20)** with radiation up and down the arm, most common on the ulnar side of the forearm, the wrist and occasionally in the fingers.

Tenderness over the medial epicondyle of humerus and the conjoined tendon of the flexors of wrist is a common feature. Stiffness of the elbow, weakness in the hand and the wrist and tingling numbness in the fingers (mostly ring and little finger) is sometimes present.

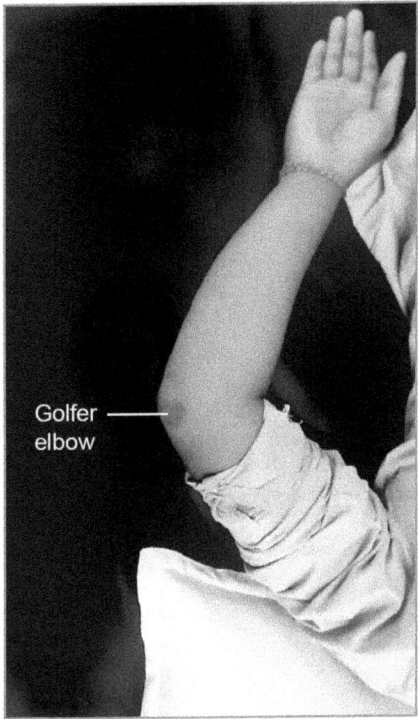

Fig. 11.20: Site of medial elbow pain in Golfer's elbow.

The pain is evoked by resisted flexion of the wrist and pronation of forearm. Hand grip weakness is very often present.

Diagnosis

Besides local tenderness over medial epicondyle of humerus, pain on resisted isometric flexion of wrist and pain on repetitive flexion of wrist and pronation of forearm are suggestive of the condition. Confirmatory tests such as Golfer elbow test described below are performed to establish the condition.

Golfer elbow test:

The tests include:

- **Passive test:** The patient sitting on bed/chair and should have the fingers flexed to a fist position. The examiner passively supinates the forearm and extends the elbow and wrist. If pain or discomfort is reproduced in the medial aspect of the elbow, in the region of the medial epicondyle, the test is positive **(Fig. 11.21)**.
- **Active test:** The seated patient is asked to flex the elbow and supinate the forearm. The examiner grasps the patient's wrist and elbow and asks the patient to flex the wrist against the clinician's resistance **(Fig. 11.22)**. If pain or discomfort is produced in the medial aspect of the elbow, in the region of the medial epicondyle, the test is positive.

Management

Conservative management

The nonsurgical treatment can be divided into three phases: **Phase I:** "PRICEMM", which starts for prevention/protection, rest, ice, compression, elevation, modalities, and medication. The procedure involves:

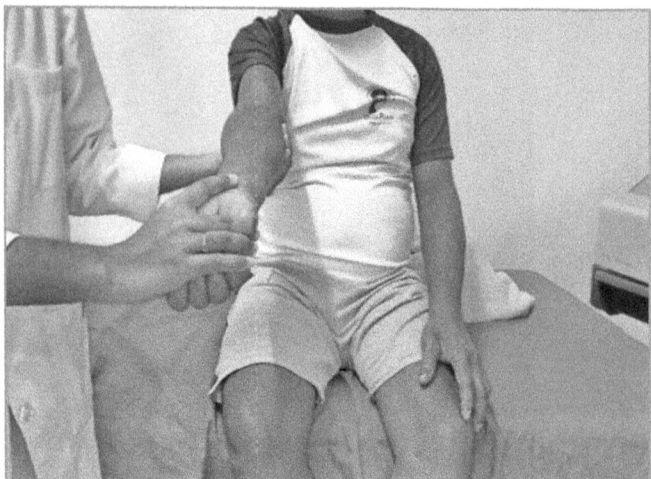

Fig. 11.21: The passive test.

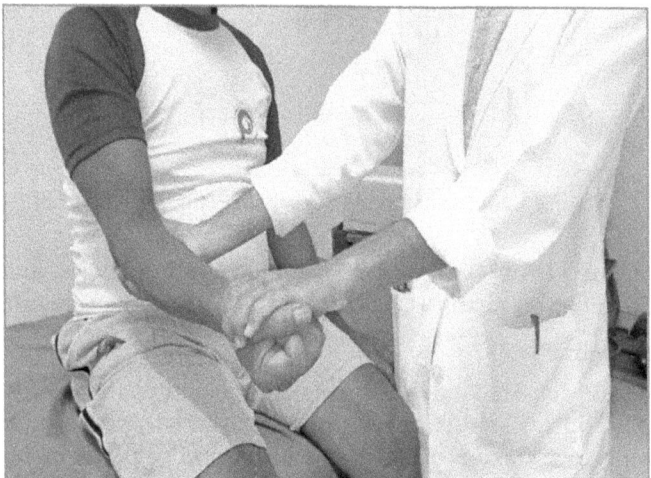

Fig. 11.22: Active test for medial epicondylitis (Golfer's elbow).

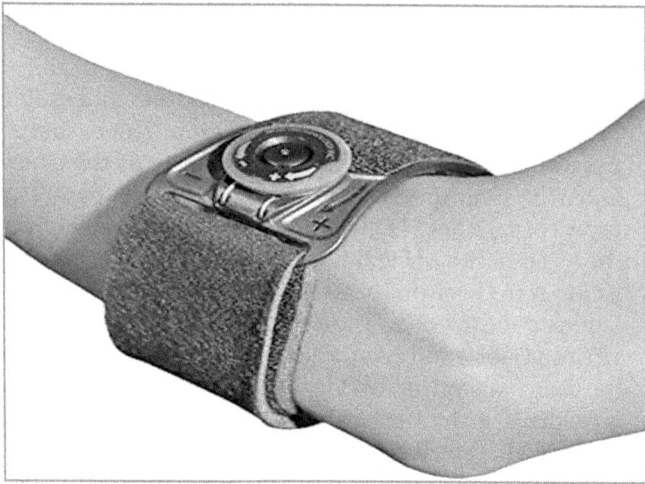

Fig. 11.23: The Golfer elbow splint.

- Stopping the offending activities.
- Rest to the elbow by using golfer elbow splint **(Fig. 11.23)**.
- Ice to the painful site, applied for 10–15 minutes, 3–4 times a day.
- NSAIDs as advised by the Physician.

- Modalities, such as pulsed ultrasound, PSWD/ HVPGC, TENS/IFT, iontophoresis using analgesic/anti-inflammatory medications, should be selected and applied as per the available evidences.

Phase II: The goal of this phase is to develop full, painless motion in elbow and wrist. The procedure involves:
- Stretching of the flexor group of muscles and progressive isometric exercises **(Figs. 11.24A and B)** to the flexor groups are started.
- Concentric and eccentric exercises to the wrist flexor muscles **(Figs. 11.25A and B)**.
- Muscle energy techniques (METs) to improve ROM, at the elbow and wrist.
- Modalities like PWB to elbow, extracorporeal shockwave therapy, pulsed ultrasound, high power laser, IFT, etc., can be considered as per the need to improve muscle flexibility and to reduce pain.

The final part of this phase-III is a simulation of sport or occupational activities of the patient.

Phase III: The exercises performed in phase-II, are also continued in this phase. The client is made to perform catching, throwing, striking activities in a gradually progressive manner using the Golfer elbow splint. Any inflammation,

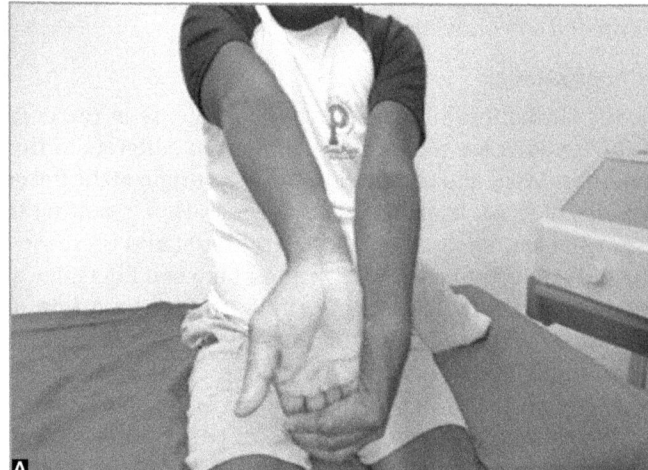

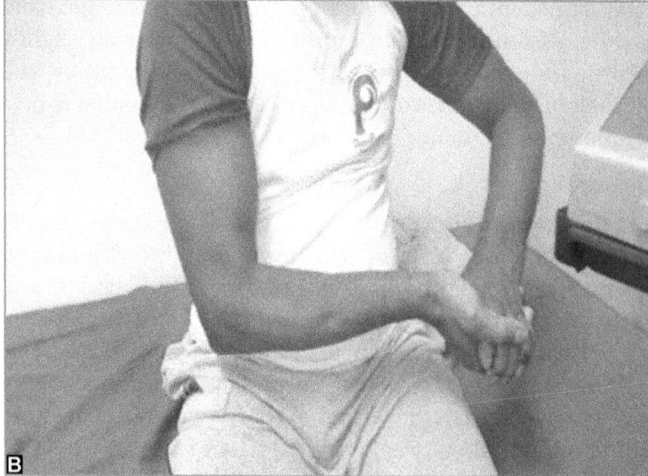

Figs. 11.24A and B: (A) Stretching of flexor muscles of hand; (B) Isometric strengthening of flexor muscles of hand.

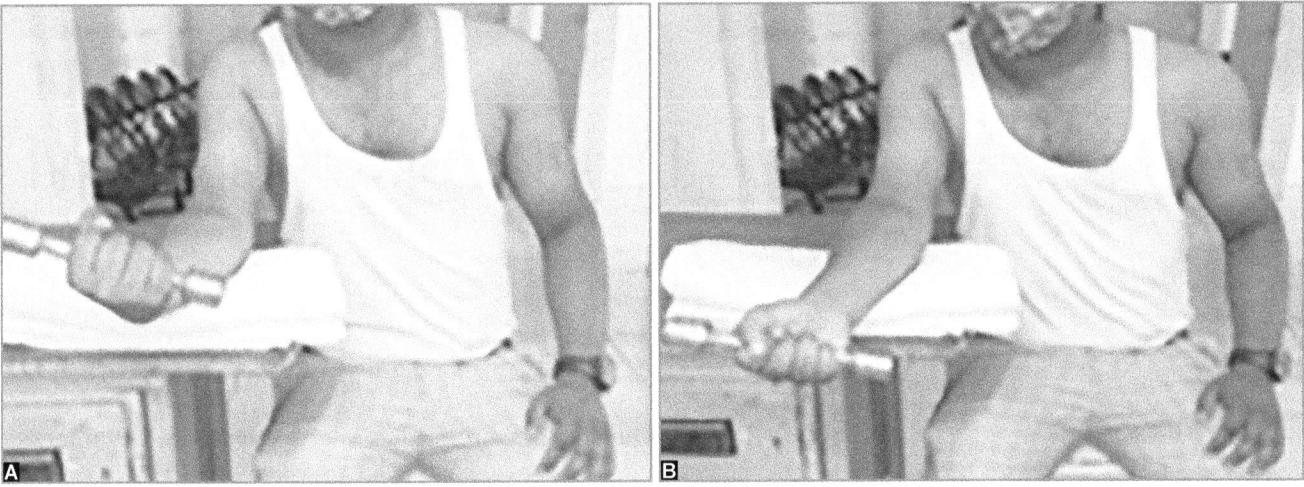

Figs. 11.25A and B: (A) Concentric exercise to wrist flexors; (B) Eccentric exercise to wrist flexors.

produced during this phase is managed by application of cold pack. Gradually, the activities/sports are performed and progressed. The use of the splint is weaned, once activities could be performed unhurted. When the patient is able to return to his sport/occupational activities, it is necessary to take a look at his equipment and/or technique for a safe return to activities.

Surgical management

Surgery is reserved for individuals (mostly athletes) who do not benefit from conservative management, and pain significantly affects their function.

The surgeries performed are:

- **Mini-open muscle resection procedure:** In this procedure, performed under local anesthesia, the degenerative tissue at the origin of flexor carpi radialis is removed. This procedure produces low levels of postoperative pain, a short hospital stay and rehabilitation period and early return to daily activities.
- Fascial elevation and tendon origin resection.

Postoperative management

After suture removal (7-10 days after surgery), therapy is started in the form of:

- Gentle passive and active elbow, wrist, and hand exercises.
- Gentle isometric exercise to the flexor muscles of hand at 3-4 weeks.
  - Resisted exercise to the flexor muscles of hand is started at 6 weeks postoperation.
  - Pulsed ultrasound, SWD/MWD/laser therapy, etc., can be selected to reduce pain and inflammation and promote healing.
  - Making the patient return to activities 3-6 months after surgery.

Physiotherapy for Disorders of Wrist and Hand

INTRODUCTION

The wrist joint is a condyloid type of synovial joint (**Fig. 12.1**) having two degrees of freedom, i.e., flexion/extension in the sagittal plane and radial deviation/ulnar deviation in the frontal plane. Though the joint is mostly formed by the concave articulating surface of the radius, articulating with the convex articulating surface made by three carpal bones such as scaphoid, lunate, and triquetrum, joined together by the interosseous ligament, the wrist complex includes, inferior radioulnar joint, radiocarpal joint, ulno menisco carpal joint, and the midcarpal joints.

The inferior radioulnar joint is considered unique, because between it lies the triangular fibrocartilaginous complex (TFCC) (**Fig. 12.1**), which is very often injured causing significant functional impairment. The TFCC is an important complex structure, made up of soft tissue that includes a disc, meniscus, and ligaments. It acts to protect, cushion and stabilize the wrist, when weight bearing through the hand takes place.

The ulnar side of the wrist (ulnocarpal joint), is not formed through a direct articulation between the ulna and carpal bones, rather it has the TFCC in between, which acts as the meniscus for the joint.

The midcarpal joint is considered as a functional, rather than an anatomical joint. It has a joint capsule that is continuous with the intercarpal joints. The joint surfaces are reciprocally convex and concave, and consists of the scaphoid, lunate, triquetrum and pisiform proximally, and trapezium, trapezoid, capitates, and hamate bones distally.

Osteokinematics of Wrist Joint

The wrist joint has two degrees of freedom, i.e., it permits flexion-extension in the sagittal plane around a mediolateral axis, radial, and ulnar deviation (abduction-adduction) in the frontal plane around the anteroposterior axis.

Arthrokinematics of Wrist Joint

Motion at the radiocarpal joint occurs, because the convex surface of the proximal row of carpals slide on the concave surface of the radius and the radioulnar disc. The proximal row of carpals slides in a direction opposite to the movement of the hand, i.e., during wrist flexion, the carpals move dorsally, and during wrist extension, the carpals move ventrally.

During ulnar deviation, the carpals slide in a radial direction, and during radial deviation, they slide in an ulnar direction.

At the midcarpal joints, motion occurs due to sliding of the distal row of carpals on the proximal row. During flexion, the convex surfaces of capitates and hamate slide dorsally on the concave surfaces of portions of the scaphoid, lunate, and triquetrum. The surfaces of trapezium and trapezoid are concave and slide volarly on the convex surface of the scaphoid.

During extension, the capitate and hamate slide volarly on the scaphoid, lunate, and triquetrum, the trapezium and the trapezoid slide dorsally on the scaphoid.

During radial deviation, the capitates and hamate slide ulnarly, and the trapezium and trapezoid slide dorsally. In ulnar deviation, the capitates and hamate slide radially, the trapezium and trapezoid slide volarly.

Capsular Pattern

The capsular pattern of limitation at the wrist is an equal limitation of flexion and extension. There occurs slight limitation of both radial and ulnar deviation.

Special Tests for Wrist and Hand

Various special tests for wrist and hand are described in **Table 12.1**.

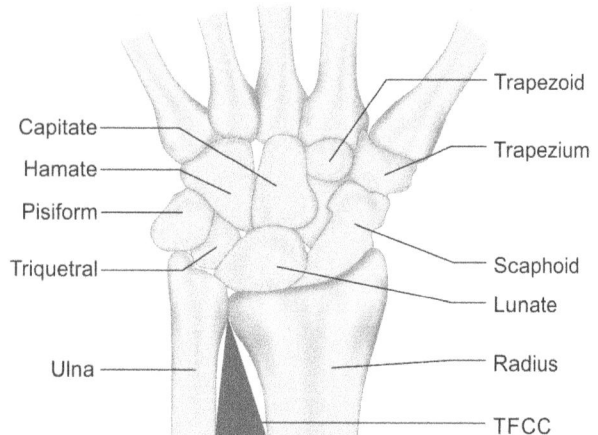

Fig. 12.1: The wrist joint showing triangular fibrocartilage complex (TFCC).

Table 12.1: Special test for wrist and hand.

Name of test	Procedure	Result
Valgus stress test (**Fig. 12.2A**)	Patient sitting, the supinated forearm and hand supported. The examiner stabilizes the lower forearm with one hand and proximal hand with other hand. A valgus force is applied to the wrist.	Excessive gapping/pain in the medial side of the wrist suggest tear/sprain of medial collateral ligament.
Varus stress test (**Fig. 12.2B**)	Patient sitting, the supinated forearm and hand supported. The examiner stabilizes the lower forearm with one hand and proximal hand with other hand. A varus force is applied to the wrist.	Excessive gapping/pain in the lateral side of the wrist suggest tear/sprain of lateral collateral ligament.
Phalen's test (**Fig. 12.3A**)	The patient either in sitting/standing. He/she is asked to flex both the wrists maximally, so that the distal aspects of dorsum of both hands are in contact with each other. The wrist flexion is maintained for 1 minute.	Numbness and tingling in the lateral aspects of hand and fingers (three and half fingers) suggests carpal tunnel syndrome, producing compression of median nerve.
Reverse Phalen test (**Fig. 12.3B**)	The patient either in sitting/standing. He/she is asked to extend both the wrists maximally, so that the distal aspects of palm of both hands are in contact with each other. The wrist extension is maintained for 1 minute.	Numbness and tingling in the lateral aspects of hand and fingers (three and half fingers) suggests carpal tunnel syndrome, producing compression of median nerve.
Finkelstein test (**Fig. 12.4**).	The patient sits or stands. The forearm is pronated and the thumb is held in palm. The patient is asked to curl the fingers around the thumb and makes a fist. The examiner stabilizes the lower forearm with one hand, and flexes and ulnar deviates the wrist maintaining the fist with other hand.	Pain at the region of the anatomical snuff box, over the tendons of abductor pollicis longus and extensor pollicis brevis suggests teno synovitis/De Quervain's disease.
Murphy's sign (**Fig. 12.5**)	The patient is either in sitting/standing. He/she is asked to make a fist of the painful hand. The examiner notes the position of the third metacarpal.	If the third metacarpal is in level with the second and fourth metacarpal, a dislocated lunate is indicated.
Froment's sign (**Fig. 12.6**)	The patient sitting/standing. He/she is asked to grasp a small piece of paper between the thumb and index finger. The examiner tries to pull the paper out.	If the patient tries to grasp the paper producing flexion of DIP joint of thumb, it suggests paralysis/weakness of adductor pollicis due to ulnar nerve injury.
Digital Allen's test (**Fig. 12.7**)	The patient is instructed to make a fist several times in succession in order to "pump" the blood out of the hand and fingers. He/she is then instructed to maintain a fist while the examiner compresses the radial and ulnar artery with the fingers. The examiner then releases pressure from one artery at a time and observes the color of the hand and fingers.	A delay in or absence of flushing of the radial or ulnar half of the hand and fingers is indicative of partial or complete occlusion of the radial or ulnar arteries.
Tinel's sign test in carpal tunnel syndrome (CTS) (**Fig. 12.8**)	Patient sitting, hand resting on a flat surface with palm facing up. The examiner taps along the median nerve over the carpal tunnel.	Complaints of tingling, paresthesia, or pain by the subject in the area of the thumb, index finger, middle finger, and radial one-half of the ring finger signal a positive sign. This may be indicative of a compression of the median nerve in the carpal tunnel syndrome (CTS).

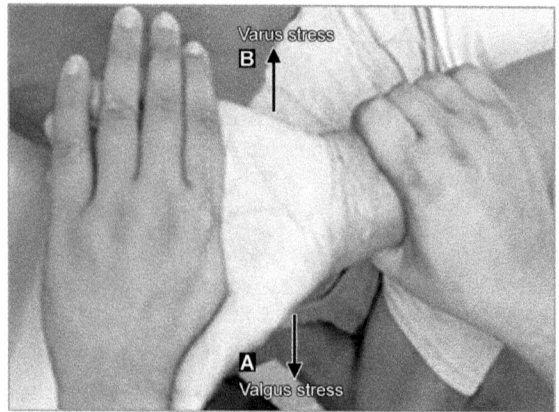

Figs. 12.2A and B: (A) Valgus stress test; (B) Varus stress test.

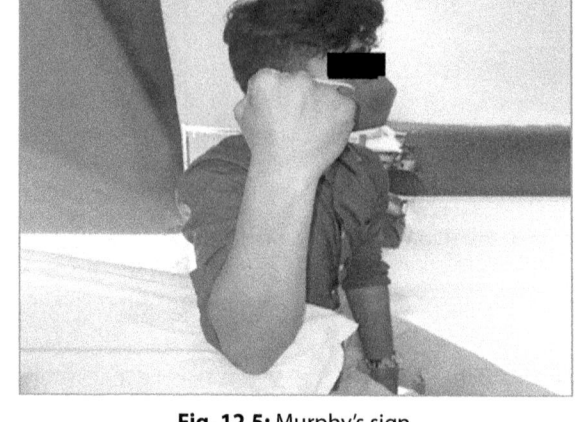

Fig. 12.5: Murphy's sign.

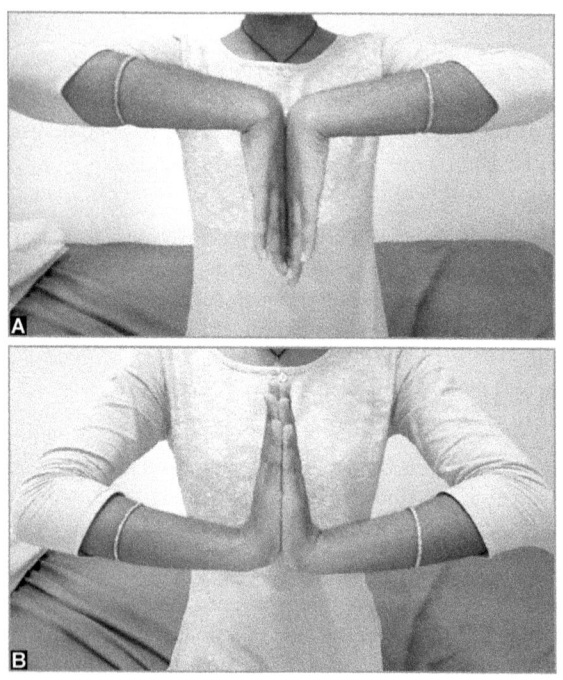

Figs. 12.3A and B: (A) Phalen's test; (B) Reverse Phalen's test.

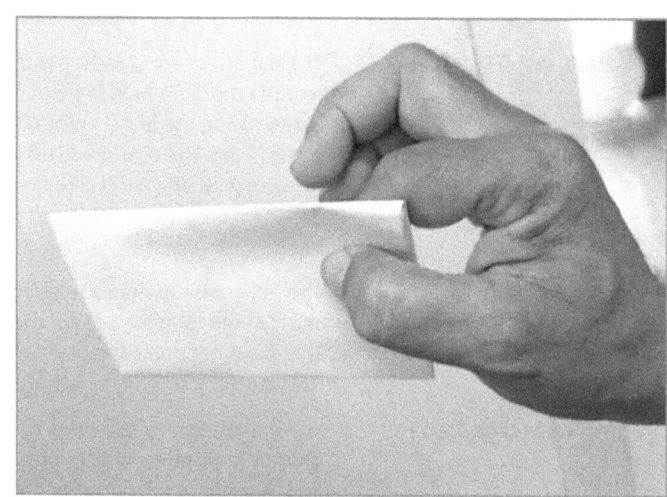

Fig. 12.6: Froment's sign.

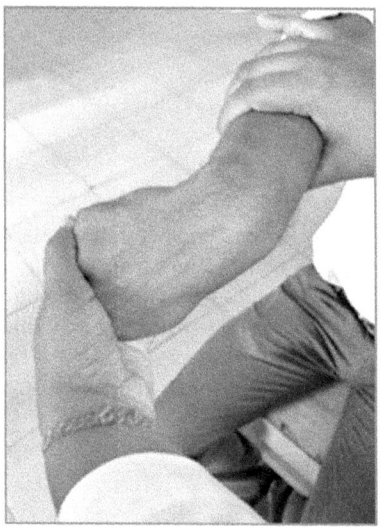

Fig. 12.4: Finkelstein test.

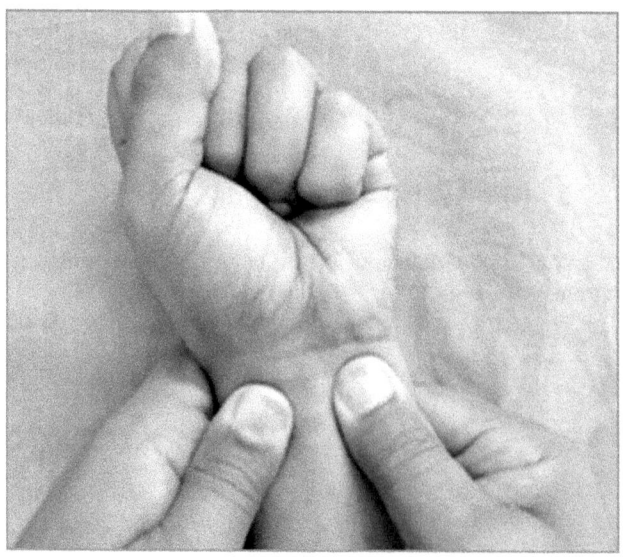

Fig. 12.7: Digital Allen's test.

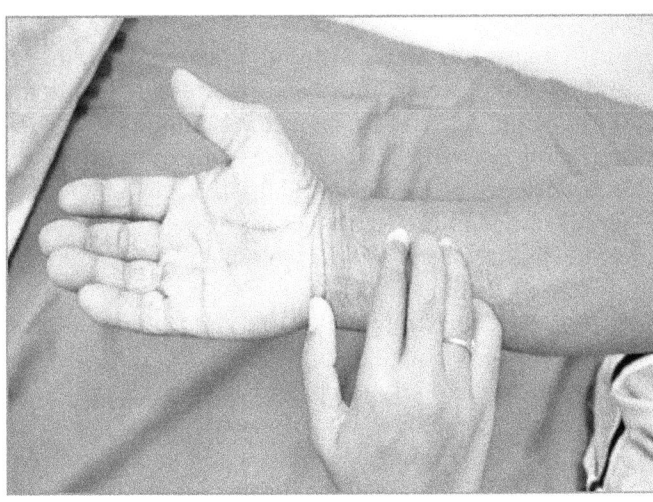

Fig. 12.8: Tinel's sign test in CTS.

DISORDERS OF THE WRIST AND HAND

The disorders of the wrist and hand requiring physiotherapist's intervention are:

i. Carpal Tunnel Syndrome

Carpal tunnel syndrome (CTS) is an entrapment neuropathy caused by compression of the median nerve as it travels through the wrist's carpal tunnel (CT).

The CT is formed by a nonextendable osteofibrous wall that forms a tunnel protecting the median nerve and flexor tendons. The transverse carpal ligament (flexor retinaculum) makes up the superior boundary, and the carpal bones form the inferior border. The CT contains the median nerve and nine flexor tendons, such as four tendons of flexor digitorum profundus, four tendons from the flexor digitorum superficialis, and one tendon of flexor pollicis longus **(Fig. 12.9)**.

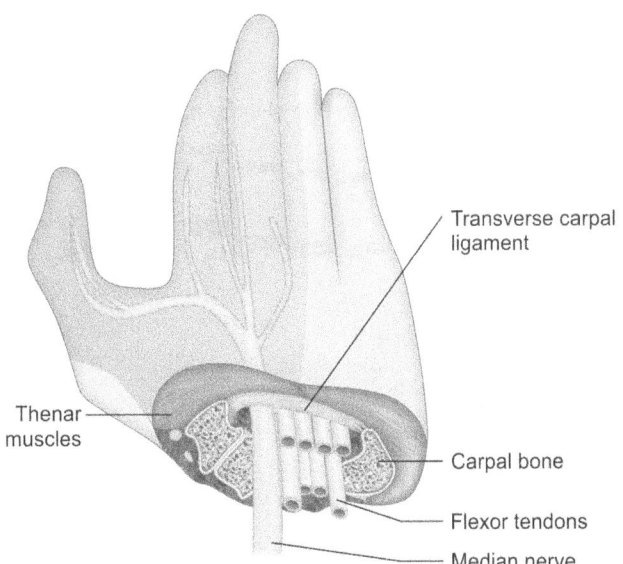

Fig. 12.9: Carpal tunnel and its structures.

Epidemiology/Etiology

Carpal tunnel syndrome usually occurs in adults and is more common in women than men with a female to male ratio of 2–5:1.

It results from the increased pressure in the CT causing compression of the median nerve. The most common causes of CTS include:
- Genetic predisposition
- History of repetitive wrist movements such as typing or machine works
- Obesity
- Autoimmune disorders such as rheumatoid arthritis
- Pregnancy
- Idiopathic

Pathophysiology

The combination of compression and traction mechanisms result in the development of symptoms. Compression of structures in the CT leads to obstruction of venous return, increasing local edema and compromising median nerve's intraneural microcirculation, resulting in compromise of structural integrity of the nerve, such as damage to myelin sheath and axons. The surrounding connective tissues become inflamed and lose normal physiologic and supportive function.

Repetitive traction due to wrist motion exacerbates the negative environment, further injuring the nerve. In addition, any of the nine flexor tendons traveling through the CT can become inflamed and compress the median nerve.

Clinical Features

The onset is usually gradual, with the sufferer presenting sensory and motor features:
- **Sensory features:** The sensory features are first to develop, starting with tingling numbness in the hand in the distribution of median nerve. The sensory symptoms get aggravated while grasping objects, such as a glass of water. The symptoms may also get aggravated during night or early in the morning. As the disorder progresses, the tingling and numbness may become constant, and burning pain may be felt. Complete anesthesia in the lateral part of palmar aspect of hand is not found, as the palmar cutaneous nerve that supplies sensation to the lateral part of palmar aspect of hand is spared, as it passes over the flexor retinaculum.
- **Motor features:** Motor features that develop in progressive cases include, weakness and atrophy of muscles of thenar eminence. The combined effect of sensory and motor impairment, result in complaint of clumsiness in hand, loss of grip, and pinch strength and subsequently dropping of objects from the hand.

Differential Diagnosis

The condition should be differentiated from:
- Pronator teres syndrome
- Anterior interosseous nerve syndrome
- Cervicobrachial syndrome

Diagnostic Procedure

These include:
- **Clinical tests:** The clinical tests to establish diagnosis are:
  - *Carpal compression test:* This test is done by applying firm pressure over the CT for 30 seconds. The test is positive when pain, paresthesia is reproduced.
  - *Square sign test:* This test determines the risk to develop CTS. The test is positive, if the ratio of thickness of the wrist to the width of the wrist is greater than 0.7.
  - *Phalen's test:* Also called reverse prayer test. The test is positive, when the wrist flexion in both hands, maintaining the dorsum of hands in close contact, held for 1 minute, reproduces, tingling, numbness, and pain **(Fig. 12.3A)**.
  - *Reverse Phalen's test:* Also called the prayer test. The test is positive, if extension of both wrists maintaining the prayer position for 1 minute reproduces symptoms **(Fig. 12.3B)**.
  - *Hoffmann-Tinel sign:* In this test, the clinician taps over the median nerve in the CT to produce symptoms.
- Ultrasound imaging and MRI studies.
- X-ray of wrist.
- EMG and nerve conduction velocity (NCV) for median nerve, where, the sensory and motor conduction velocities of median nerve in the hand is significantly reduced.

Management of Carpal Tunnel Syndrome

Management of CTS is usually conservative that consists of:
- **Medical management:** It consists of NSAIDs/local steroid injection (to be considered, if no improvement occurs with NSAIDs and physiotherapy.
- **Orthotic management:** Customized volar or dorsal splints are provided with neutral position of wrist joint. Dorsal-based splint **(Fig. 12.10)** is preferred, as there is no contact pressure on the CT, as occurs in volar splints.
- **Physiotherapy:** It is started along with medical management. It consists of pulsed ultrasound therapy, pulsed short-wave diathermy (PSWD), contrast bath, to reduce inflammation/edema in the CT. Heat therapy in the form of paraffin wax bath (PWB), continuous ultrasound therapy, SWD, microwave diathermy (MWD), etc., should not be considered as the vasodilatation and resulting edema, may increase pressure inside the CT causing increase of symptoms. Though evidence regarding use of TENS to reduce pain is limited, still it is worth to advise this modality to reduce pain after mobilization and stretching exercises.

As the condition becomes less acute, mobilization exercises are started, that include:
- Mobilization/stretching of CT and the long flexors that passes through the CT.
- Mobilization of intercarpal joints **(Fig. 12.11)**.
- Passive stretching/auto-assisted stretching **(Fig. 12.12)** of the thumb flexor and adductor to prevent adhesion formation along the palmar cutaneous and motor branch of median nerve.
- The exercises advised to glide the median nerve and long flexors in the CT called nerve/tendon gliding exercises **(Fig. 12.13)**. These exercises are performed three sets of 10 repetitions, once daily.

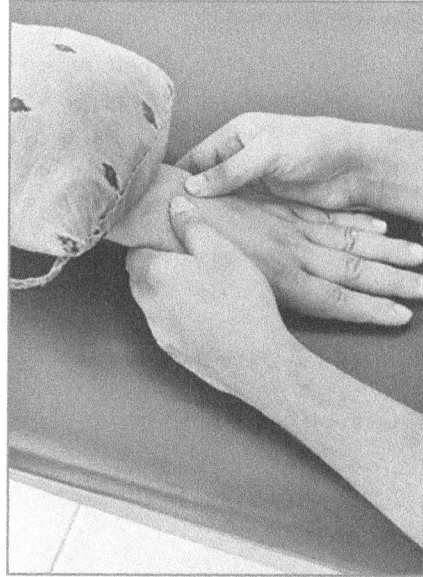

Fig. 12.11: Mobilization of intercarpal joints.

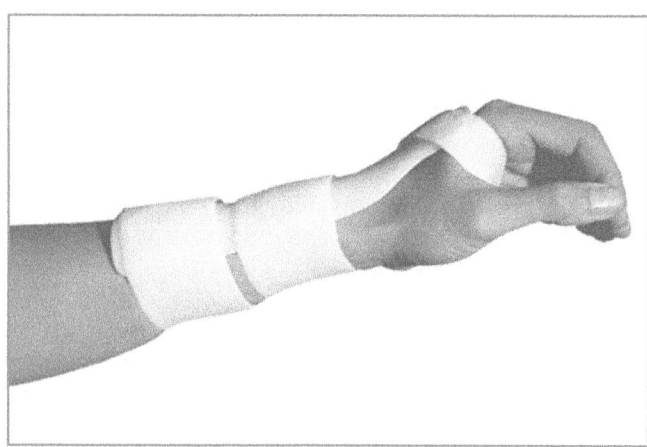

Fig. 12.10: Splint for carpal tunnel syndrome.

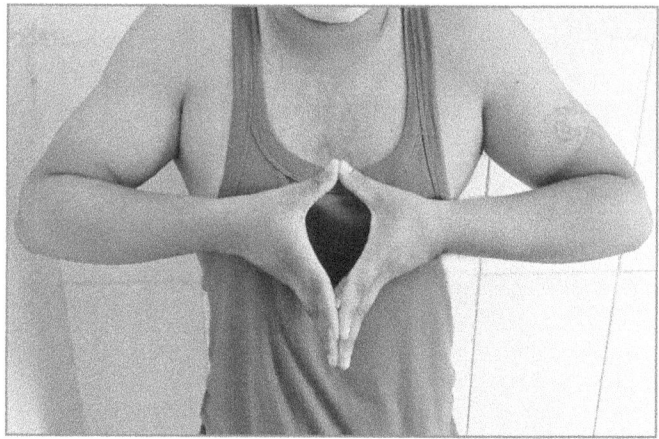

Fig. 12.12: Self-stretching of thumb flexor and adductor.

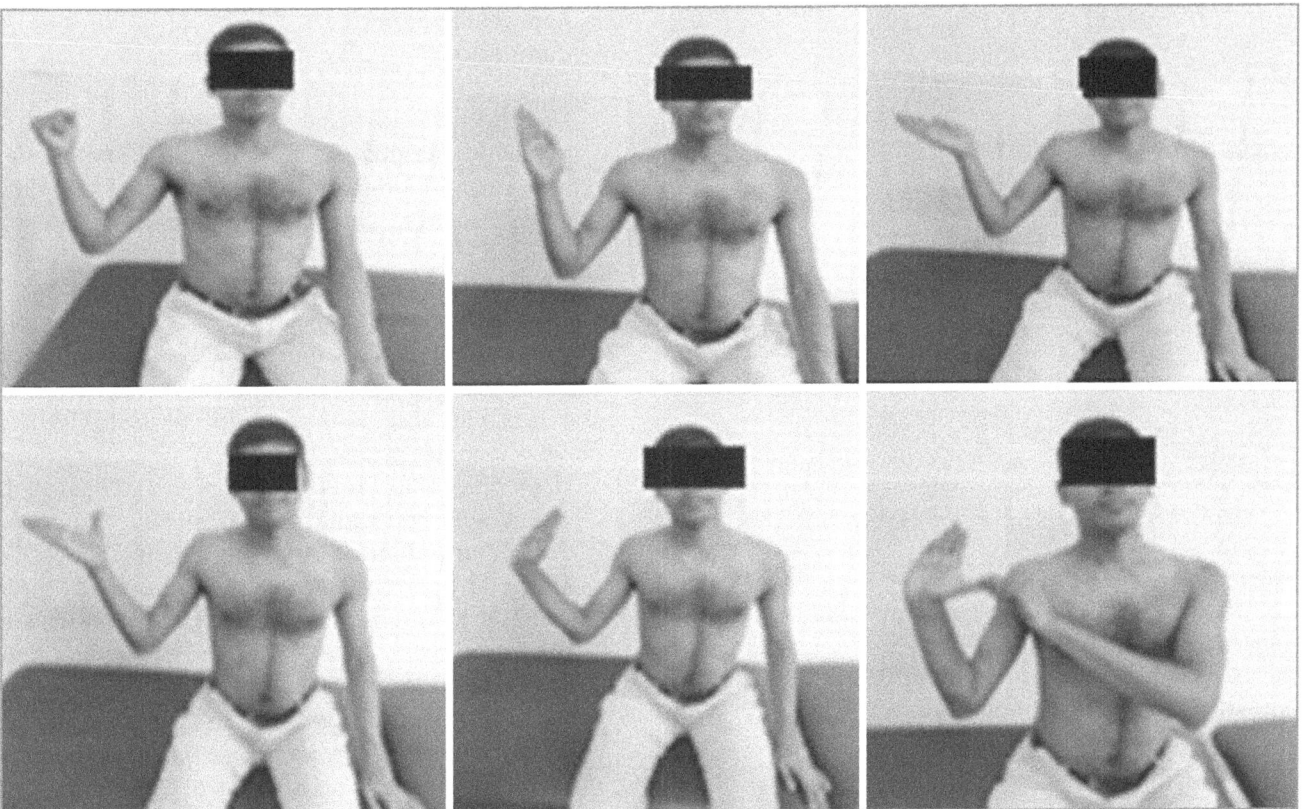

Fig. 12.13: Tendon gliding exercises.

- Advice on ergonomic measures and energy conservation/joint protection techniques.
- **Surgical management:** The surgical procedure may be open/endoscopic. Postoperative physiotherapy is started after stitch removal with an objective to:
  - Mobilize the wrist and hand.
  - Enhance flexibility of soft tissues of wrist and hand.
  - Mobilize the median nerve.
  - Reduce pain (if any).
  - Improve function.
  - Prevent recurrence, through activity modification.

ii. De Quervain's Disease

De Quervain's disease is a painful condition, affecting the tendons at the base of the thumb. In 1895, De Quervain noted a condition of stenosing tenosynovitis, resulting in pain and swelling of tendon sheaths of abductor pollicis longus and extensor pollicis brevis muscles near the area of radial styloid process of the wrist over the lateral boundary of anatomical snuff box. The pain, which is the main complaint, is associated with abduction of thumb, grasping of objects in the hand, and ulnar deviation of wrist.

Epidemiology/Etiology

- The condition is most commonly found in women than men.
- Repeated use of the hand for functional activities (over use) is considered as the main cause of this condition.
- Myxoid degeneration (the process in which the connective tissues are replaced by a gelatinous substance) with fibrous tissue deposits and increased vascularity rather than acute inflammation of the synovial lining is also considered as one cause of this condition. This deposition results in thickening of the tendon sheath, painfully entrapping the abductor pollicis longus and extensor pollicis brevis tendons.

Pathophysiology

Repetitive gripping, grasping, clenching, pinching, or wringing of objects can cause inflammation of the tendons and tendon sheaths and narrows the first dorsal compartment and causes limitation of motion of the tendons. The inflammation and progressive narrowing (stenosis) can lead to scarring that further limits thumb motion.

The fibrous tissue deposition from myxoid degeneration results in thickening of the tendon sheath, painfully entrapping the abductor pollicis longus, and extensor pollicis brevis tendons **(Fig. 12.14)**.

Clinical Features

The patient may present with the following features.
- Pain (constant aching, burning, pulling type) near the base of the thumb, which gets aggravated by repetitive lifting, gripping, and twisting motions of hand. The pain may sometimes radiate up the forearm.
- Swelling near the base of the thumb (anatomical snuff box).
- Tenderness at the radial styloid process.

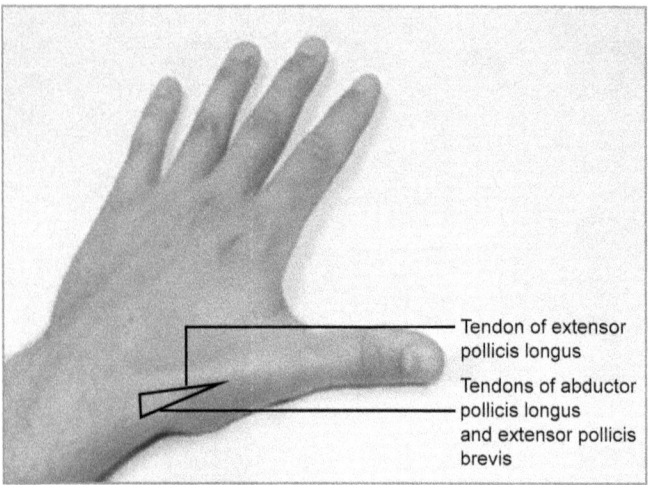

Fig. 12.14: Tendon's affected in De Quervain's disease.

- Decreased ROM of thumb.
- A "sticking" or "stop-and-go" sensation/crepitus on movement of thumb.
- Resisted isometric contraction of APL/EPB, is painful, and the Finkelstein test **(Fig. 12.4)** is positive, provoking symptoms.
- Weakness and paresthesia in the hand is felt sometimes.

Diagnosis

Diagnosis of this condition is confirmed by eliciting localized tenderness and by a positive Finkelstein's test.

Management

De Quervain's tenosynovitis is sometimes self-limiting, does not requiring any treatment. However, in those with persisting pain that affects function, treatment is advocated, which consists of:
- **PRICEM:** It consists of:
  - Protection to the inflamed tendon in a thumb spica splint **(Fig. 12.15)**.
  - Relative rest and immobility of thumb (advice on energy conservation techniques).
  - Application of cold pack.
  - Compression to the inflamed site by making proper use of the splint.
  - Keeping the hand elevated.
  - Modalities like pulsed ultrasound, LILT, iontophoresis using anti-inflammatory agents such as salicylates, diclofenac, hydrocortisone, contrast bath etc., can be selected.
- NSAIDs/local steroids (if no remission with conservative methods)
- **Physiotherapy:** Besides, the modalities used in the acute stage, physiotherapy in the subacute and chronic stage, aimed at reducing pain and improving strength and mobility include:
  - Deep transverse friction massage (DTFM) to the affected tendons within the limit of pain tolerance.
  - Graston technique of manual soft tissue mobilization along with the eccentric exercise is also helpful. Graston technique includes breaking down fascia restriction, stretching connective tissue, and promoting better healing environment.
  - Mobilization with movement has shown effectiveness in decreasing the pain, improving range of motion and improving the function of a patient with De-Quervain tenosynovitis. The therapist provides a manual radial glide of the proximal row of carpals, and then asks the patient to move the thumb into radial abduction-adduction. Mobilization with movement is performed for 3 sets of 10 repetitions.
  - Ultrasound therapy for the mechanical/thermal effects helps in reducing pain and improving function.
  - High power laser therapy may be applied to reduce pain and improve function.
  - Stretching and strengthening exercises, such as grip strengthening exercises, finger spring exercises **(Fig. 12.16A)**, wrist extension/radial deviation exercises, wrist flexion exercise, wrist flexion/extension stretching exercise **(Fig. 12.16B)**, opposition stretch exercise **(Fig. 12.16C)**, strengthening using elastic band **(Fig. 12.16D)**.
  - *Kinesiotaping:* When applied during functional activities help in reducing pain and improving function.
  - Energy conservation techniques to provide rest to the affected tendons and prevent recurrence.
- **Surgical management:** Surgery is indicated for those who do not improve with conservative treatments and persistent pain significantly affects function. The goal of surgery is to open the dorsal compartment covering to make more room for the irritated tendons. The opening allows pressure relief of the tendons, to ultimately restore free tendon gliding. Postoperative therapy is directed in improving, mobility, strength, and function.

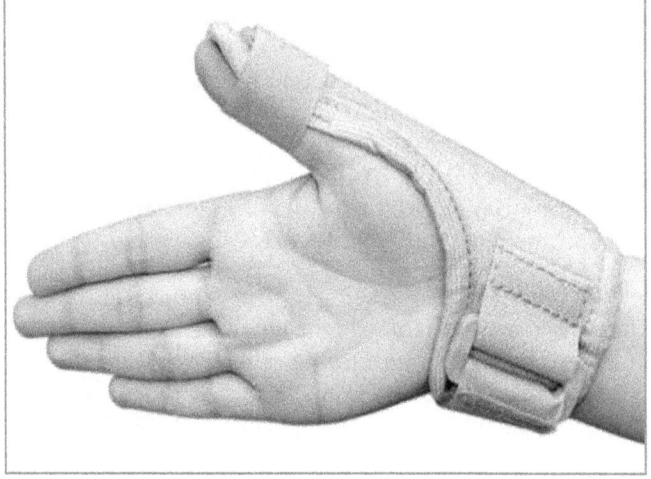

Fig. 12.15: The thumb spica splint.

iii. Trigger Finger/Trigger Thumb

Trigger finger/trigger thumb is a condition that causes pain, stiffness, and a sensation of locking or catching when fingers and thumbs are moved in the direction of flexion and extension. The ring finger is most commonly affected.

This condition also called as stenosing tenovaginitis, results from flexor tendinitis, leading to a disproportion between the flexor tendon and its sheath. This is further aggravated by constriction of the pulley near the metacarpal head, causing painful snapping of the flexor tendons. The finger/thumb gets stuck in the bent position and snaps straight **(Figs. 12.17A and B)**.

Epidemiology/Etiology

Women between 50 and 60 years of life are more likely to be affected by trigger finger, as compared to men. Diabetics, patients with CTS, DQ disease, hypothyroidism, and rheumatoid arthritis, renal disease, amyloidosis are more prone to be affected with the condition, as compared to general population. The disorder also develops due to overuse of hand.

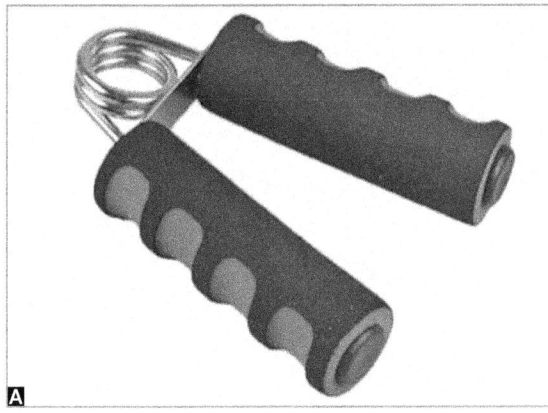
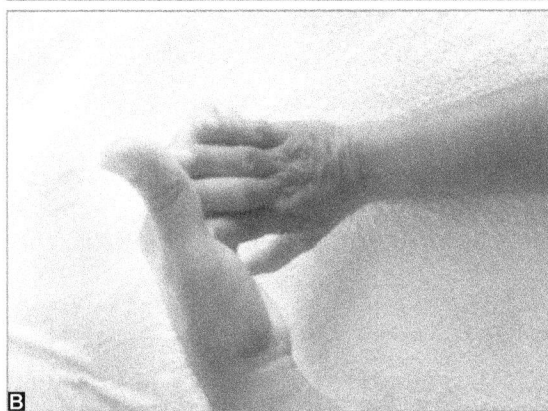
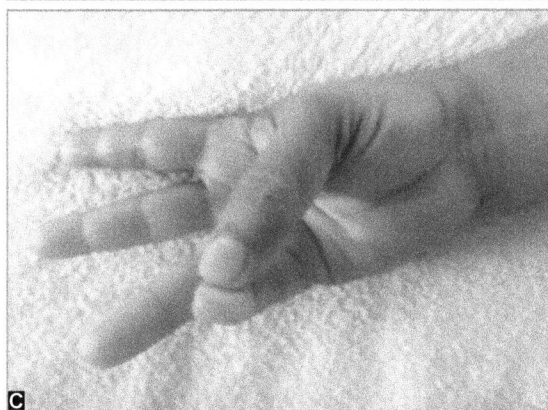
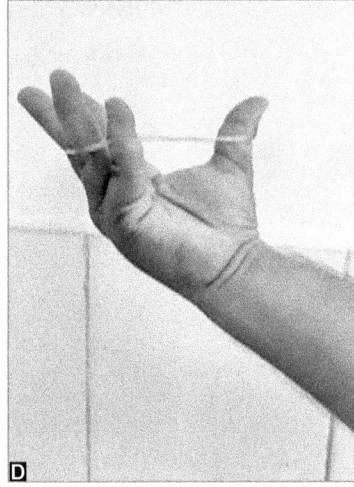

Figs. 12.16A to D: (A) Finger spring; (B) Wrist flexor/extensor stretching; (C) Opposition stretch exercise; (D) Strengthening using elastic band.

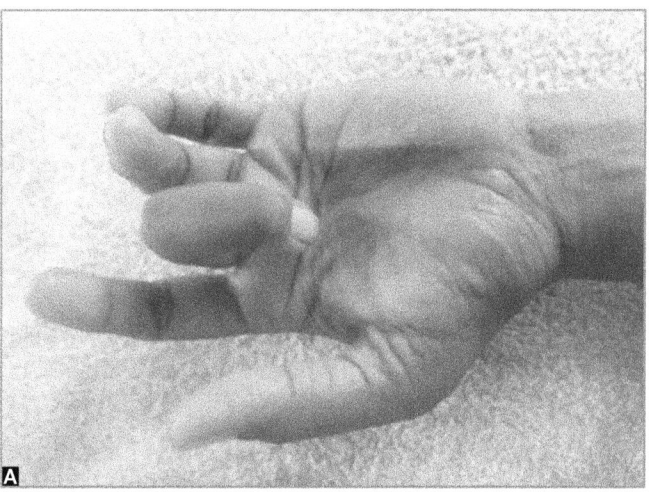
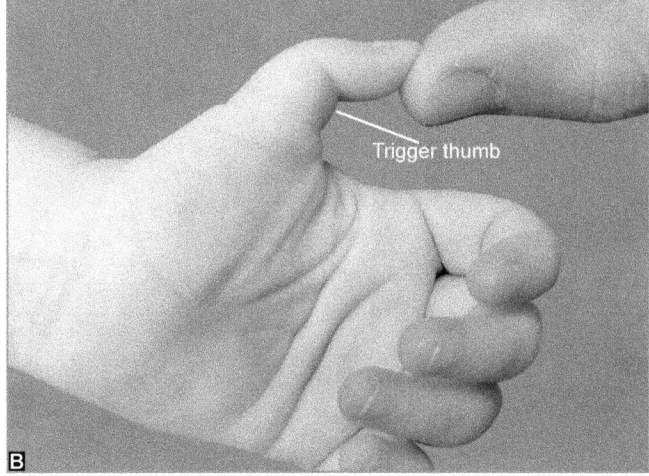

Figs. 12.17A and B: (A) Trigger finger; (B) Trigger thumb.

Clinical Features

Initially, patients may present with painless clicking/popping with movement of the digit that can progress to painful catching or popping, typically at the MCP or PIP joints. The pain and stiffness is more in the morning. Swelling of finger/thumb and loss of full flexion/extension with palpable and painful nodule at the base of finger/thumb may be present. Locking of finger/thumb into a flexed position is the common presentation.

Management

It includes:

- **Medical management:** NSAIDs/local steroids (if required)
- **Physiotherapy and orthotic management:** It consists of:
  - A splint for finger/thumb to provide rest to the tendon and prevent shortening (**Fig. 12.18**).
  - Patient education regarding use of splint and minimize use of the affected hand/modification of activities/making use of special tools with observation of energy conservation.
  - Exercises and modalities such as the followings may be selected and used as needed:
    » Ice to reduce inflammation in acute stage.
    » Ultrasound therapy to mobilize the adherent tendon inside the sheath.
    » Deep transverse friction massage to mobilize tight structures.
    » Heat in the form of PWB, hydrocollator pack, infrared, and MWD can be applied before stretching to enhance blood flow and extensibility of the tendons.
    » Stretching exercises such as weight bearing on hand, hold relax exercises, active stretch using theraband/elastic loop (**Fig. 12.19**).
    » Mobilization exercise to MCP and IP joints of finger/thumb.
    » Faradic stimulation to promote tendon glide.
    » Iontophoresis using calcium ions.
    » Extracorporeal shock wave therapy: This modality has been found to be beneficial for trigger finger.

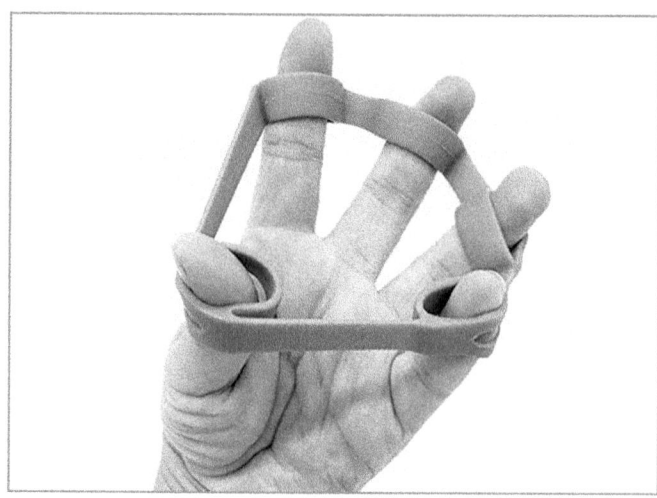

Fig. 12.19: Active stretching of finger and thumb flexors using elastic loops.

- **Surgical management:** Surgery may be required, if conservative management fails. After stitch removal, postoperative therapy is applied to mobilize joints and improve function.

iv. Dupuytren's Contracture

Dupuytren's contracture is a condition found in the hand due to thickening of the palmar fascia (palmar aponeurosis), leading to flexion contracture of fingers (**Fig. 12.20**). The condition was originally described by Clive in 1808. It was subsequently known as Dupuytren's contracture after the name of the Surgeon, who first described an operation for its treatment.

Etiology/Epidemiology

This condition is more prevalent in men than women, and is seen mostly in fifth to seventh decades. The cause of this condition is not known.

Pathophysiology

The condition, frequently resulting in flexion deformity of the fourth and fifth digit is usually unilateral, but bilateral cases

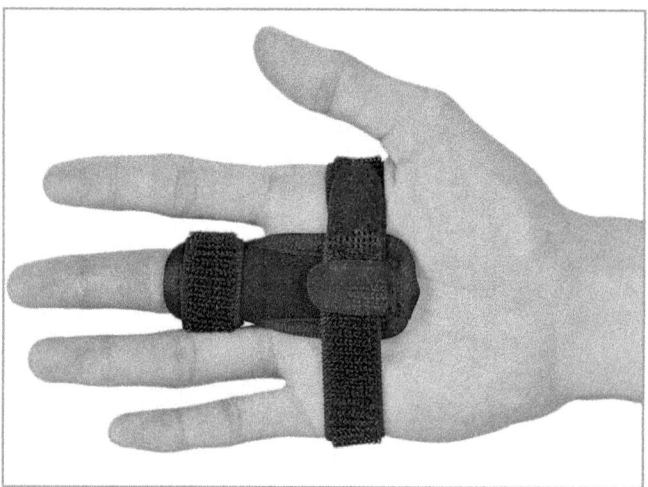

Fig. 12.18: Splint for trigger finger.

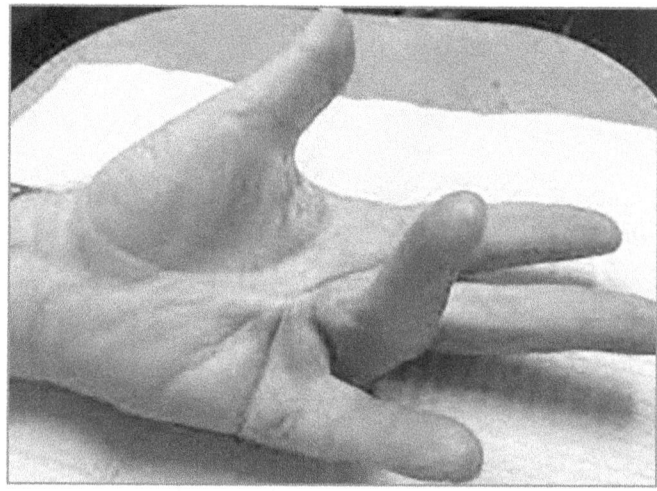

Fig. 12.20: Dupuytren's contracture.

Table 12.2: Stages of Dupuytren's contracture.	
Stage	**Criteria**
Stage-1	Development of nodule in palmar fascia
Stage-2	Involvement of skin along with the development of nodule
Stage-3	Development of flexion contracture of one or more fingers
Stage-4	Fixed contracture of tendon and joint structures

are also seen. There is progressive thickening of the palmar fascia, leading to compromise of the penetrating nutrient arteries, and subsequent thickening, contracture of the fascia and atrophy of the overlying skin. Though the ring finger is most commonly affected, the fifth, third, second fingers, and thumb are then affected in decreasing order of frequency. However, the thumb and the index fingers are rarely affected.

The condition can be classified into four stages, as per the classification system proposed by Shaw **(Table 12.2)**.

Management

Initially, a course of conservative treatment can be tried. If the same fails, surgery is the treatment of choice. The conservative treatment includes:
- **Medical management.**
- **Physiotherapy:** It includes:
  - Iontophoresis over the nodule using Iodex (Iodine with methyl salicylate) using the negative pole.
  - Ultrasound therapy.
  - Passive stretching.
  - Moist heat before stretching followed by application of cold after stretching.
  - Advising for use of a posterior extension splint **(Fig. 12.21)**.

Surgery

If severe contracture/deformity of affected finger persists even after conservative treatment, surgical release is the choice.

Postoperatively, stretching/mobilization and strengthening exercises are applied to improve hand function. A hand splint as required should be used during the early postoperative period.

v. Hand Injury

Hand injuries are very common in people, working in industries, as well as in those who sustain trauma due to road traffic accidents. The injuries caused could be simple fractures, tendon cuts or crush injuries. Management of hand after tendon injuries is challenging, requiring intervention of orthopedic surgeons, therapists, and orthotists. A brief description of flexor and extensor tendon injuries and their management are discussed below.

Flexor tendon injuries are traumatic injuries to the flexor digitorum superficialis and flexor digitorum profundus tendons that are usually caused by laceration or trauma. Extensor tendon injuries are traumatic injuries to the extensor tendons that are usually caused by laceration, trauma, or overuse.

The injuries occur in different locations in the hand called zones of hand **(Figs. 12.22A and B)**.

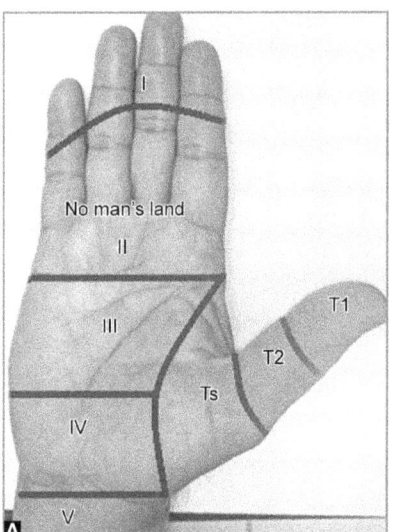

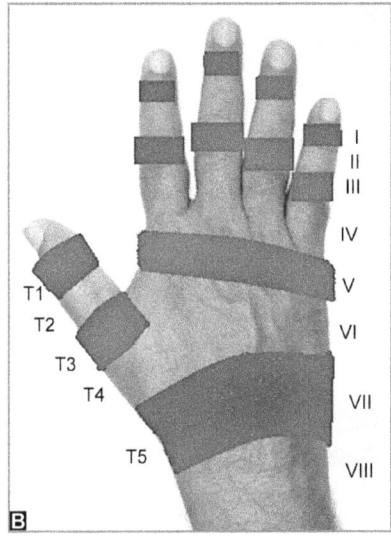

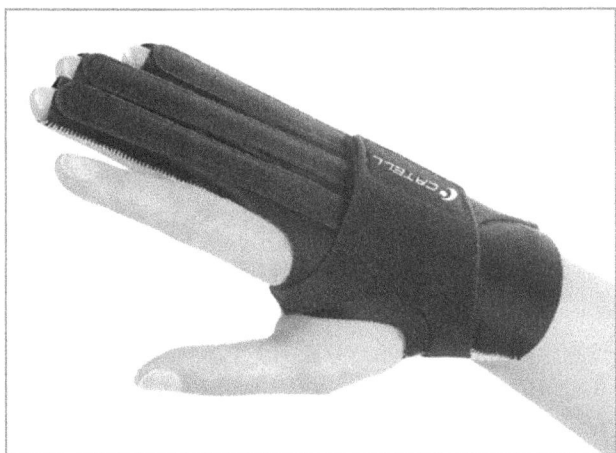

Fig. 12.21: Splint for Dupuytren's contracture.

Figs. 12.22A and B: (A) Flexor zones of hand; (B) Extensor zones of hand.

The Finger Pulleys

Digits 2 to 5 contain five annular pulleys (A1–A5), which are thicker and stiffer than the cruciate pulleys (**Fig. 12.23**).

The five annular pulleys are thicker and stiffer than the cruciate pulleys. A2 and A4 pulleys arise from the periosteum and are the most important pulleys to prevent flexor tendon bowstringing. Pulleys A1, A3, and A5 arise from the volar plates. The cruciate pulleys C1, C2, and C3, are collapsible and flexible, which allow the annular pulleys to approximate each other during digital flexion.

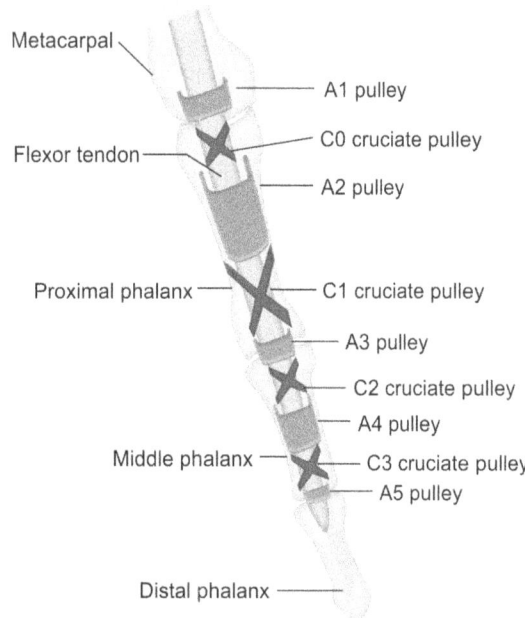

Fig. 12.23: The finger pulleys.

Zones of Hand and Injuries of Tendons with their Management

- Injuries to tendons in different flexor zones of hand are described in **Table 12.3**.
- Zones of extensor tendon injuries are described briefly in the **Table 12.4**.
- Phases of tendon healing (**Table 12.5**).

Assessment of Tendon Injury

History of trauma with absence/reduced (weakness) active flexion and extension of the digits. Absence of tenodesis effect such as, passive/active wrist extension not producing finger flexion (suggesting tear of flexor tendons), passive/active wrist flexion not producing finger extension (suggesting tear of extensor tendons) is suggestive of tendon rupture. Electrical tests such as faradic stimulation of the suspected muscle, if fails to produce movements of the digits, indicates tear of the tendons of the concerned muscles.

Management of Tendon Injuries in Hand

For minor injuries (where loss of continuity is less than 50%), conservative treatment is usually instituted. However, for injuries with less than 50% continuity of tendon, conservative treatment may not help.

The conservative treatment depends on the stage, when the patient reports for therapy. For acute injuries, PRICEM, i.e., protection and rest using a proper hand splint, compression to prevent swelling through crepe bandaging, and observing limb elevation and application of modalities like pulsed ultrasound/pulsed SWD, LILT etc., are the methods of choice.

After acute symptoms subsided, PWB/contrast bath, ultrasound therapy, high power laser therapy, etc., are applied to promote healing and facilitate mobilization.

Table 12.3: Injuries to tendons in different flexor zones of hand.

Zone	Definition	Characteristics	Treatment
I	Distal to insertion of FDS	Jersey finger: A Jersey finger is a traumatic rupture of the flexor digitorum profundus (FDP) tendon at its point of attachment to the distal phalanx	Direct tendon repair
II (no man's land)	FDS insertion to distal palmar crease (up to proximal part of A1 pulley)	This is the unique zone, where FDS and FDP tendons are in the same sheath. Tendons retract, if vinculae are disrupted	• Direct tendon repair, followed by early ROM exercises • Tendon repair in this zone yields poor results. However, advanced, postoperative protocol followed currently yields better results
III	Palm (A1 pulley to distal aspect of carpal ligament)	Often associated with neurovascular injury, which carries a worse prognosis	Direct tendon repair gives a good result, if there is no neurovascular injury
IV	Region of flexor retinaculum		
V	Carpal tunnel to forearm	Often associated with neurovascular injury, which carries a worse prognosis	Direct tendon repair
Thumb	TI, TII, TIII	Outcome different than fingers. Early motion protocols do not improve long-term results and there is higher possibilities of re-rupture, as compared to flexor tendon repairs in fingers	Direct end to end repair of FPL is advocated

Table 12.4: Zones of extensor tendon injuries.

Zone	Characteristics
I	Disruption of terminal extensor tendon, distal to or at the DIP joint of the fingers and IP joint of thumb (EPL injury). Mallet finger deformity results
II	Disruption of tendons over middle phalanx of fingers and proximal phalanx of thumb
III	Disruption of tendons over the PIP joint of fingers, or MCP joint of thumb. Boutonniere deformity is common
IV	Disruption of tendons over the proximal phalanx of fingers, or metacarpal of thumb
V	Disruption of tendons over the MCP joint of fingers, or CMC joint of thumb
VI	Disruption of tendons over the metacarpals of fingers. Nerve and vessel damage is likely
VII	Disruption of extensor tendons of fingers at the wrist joint. Repair of retinaculum may be required to prevent bowstringing. Tendon repair is followed by immobilization with wrist in 40 degree extension and MCP joint in 20° flexion for 3–4 weeks
VIII	Disruption of the tendons at the distal forearm. Extensor muscle belly is cut. Often have associated neurologic injury. Tendon repair followed by immobilization with elbow in flexion and wrist in extension

Table 12.5: Phases of tendon healing.

Phase	Days	Histology	Strength
Inflammatory	0–5	Cellular proliferation	Nil
Fibroblastic	5–28	Fibroblastic proliferation with disorganized collagen	Increasing
Remodeling	>28	Linear collagen organization	Tolerates active range of motion

Gentle passive ROM, exercises without stretching the injured tendon are started as early as possible. Active exercises are usually started in the remodeling phase (usually after 4 weeks), which includes gentle eccentric exercises gradually progressing to concentric free and resisted exercises with elastic bands.

In case of development of adhesion/tight scar, gentle massage without affecting the integrity of the tendon is instituted. Gradually, the client should be made to perform light functional activities with the affected hand.

Tendon Repair

When the tendons of the fingers and thumb are cut or damaged and clinical and electrical tests reveal less than 50% (for which conservative treatment cannot be followed) continuity of the tendon exist, resulting in loss of function of hand, surgical repair of the tendons are performed. Tendon repair surgery is an invasive surgery and healing times are subsequently affected. Full recovery following extensor and flexor tendon repairs is approximately 12 weeks. Surgery is usually undertaken immediately following tendon rupture. Sometimes surgery can be delayed up to 2 to 3 weeks, but not later that, as tendon retraction restricts end-to-end repair.

Two types of surgeries are performed:
1. Attachment of tendon to bone.
2. Attachment of tendon to tendon.

Physiotherapy After Flexor Tendon Repair

After flexor tendon repair casts/splints are applied with the wrist and MCP joints positioned in flexion and the IP joints in extension, e.g., using the dorsal blocking splint. **(Fig. 12.24)**.

Full recovery after a tendon repair is expected to occur within 12 weeks. Physiotherapy is started as early as possible with the following aims:
- To decrease swelling.
- To decrease pain.
- To increase ROM and muscle strength.
- To improve sensory perception in the hand.
- To restore function.

Week wise protocols of physiotherapy are discussed below. However, the consent of the operating surgeon should be taken for start of therapy.

Weeks 1–3: The aim of physiotherapy is to reduce swelling and pain and restore controlled mobility of hand and to promote healing of tendon. The modalities used include:
- Cryotherapy.
- Electrotherapy (pulsed ultrasound/low intensity laser therapy)
- Hand splinting
- Dorsal blocking splint **(Fig. 12.24)**.
- Controlled passive movements of wrist and fingers.
- Active movements of elbow and shoulder to prevent stiffness, loss of movement and muscle strength.

Weeks 4–6: The aims of physiotherapy during this period are to achieve range of motion of fingers and to restore strength in the repaired tendons. The procedures involved are:
- Pulsed ultrasound/LILT for pain and wound management.
- Scar mobilization through gentle friction/kneading massage without affecting the integrity of the tendon.
- Hand splinting.
- Increased passive movements of wrist and hand.
- Active and active assisted of movement of affected tendon, starting with eccentric contractions, gradually progressing to concentric exercises.

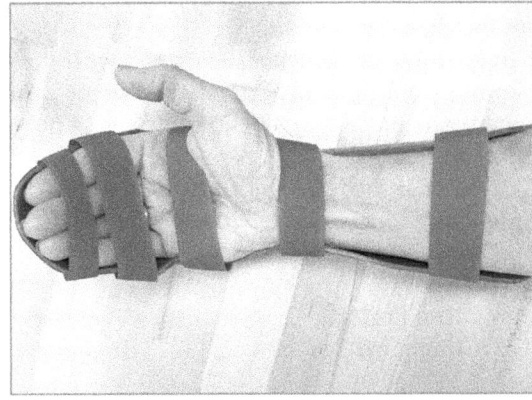

Fig. 12.24: The dorsal blocking splint.

Weeks 7–12: The aims of physiotherapy during this period are to increase full range of motion of hand, increase strength of the repaired tendon and to encourage functional use of the hand. The procedures involved are:
- Initiation of strengthening exercises.
- Full passive range of movement exercises.
- Increased active range of movement exercises.
- Progressive wrist and finger strengthening exercises.
- Isolated strengthening of repaired tendon.
- Hand dexterity training.
- Soft tissue massage.
- Functional activity exercises.

After 12 weeks, the patient is advised home exercises and asked to continue lighter functional activities using the affected hand till the completion of 6 months, after which he/she is advised to use the hand for heavier activities.

Management of Extensor Tendon Injury

Patients with an extensor tendon injury can be treated in two ways, surgically or conservatively. The choice of treatment depends on the degree of the injury. In general, open injuries and complete ruptures demand surgical treatment. Closed injuries and partially lacerated tendons require conservative management with pulsed ultrasound, active exercises (eccentric followed by concentric exercises) and splinting. Surgery for extensor tendon injury is preferably performed on the same day.

- **Physiotherapy after repair of extensor tendon injury of fingers (EDC tendon injury):** Therapy after extensor tendon injury repair should start as early as 1–5 days postoperatively for better result. The aim of physiotherapy after extensor tendon repair are:
  - Promotion of healing of surgical wound, using pulsed ultrasound, PSWD, LILT, etc.
  - Scar management using pulsed ultrasound.
  - Edema relief using pulsed ultrasound, exercises, contrast bath, after the surgical wound is healed.
  - Restoration of mobility and strength in the hand performing exercises within and without the splint.
  - Restoration of function, performing functional activities after the splint is removed after 6–8 weeks postoperatively.

Immediately after surgery, the patient is fitted with a resting hand splint that keeps the wrist in 20–30° of extension, MCP joint in 20–30° of flexion, and IP joints in neutral position **(Fig. 12.25)**.

The following exercises are performed with the splint on, upto 6 weeks postoperatively at 5 times a day and 10 repetitions in each time. The exercises as per Merrit protocol are:
  - Active MCP flexion. The flexion of the MCP joint produces gliding of the tendons preventing formation of adhesion.
  - Hook fist.
  - Composite flexion.
  - Active finger extension.

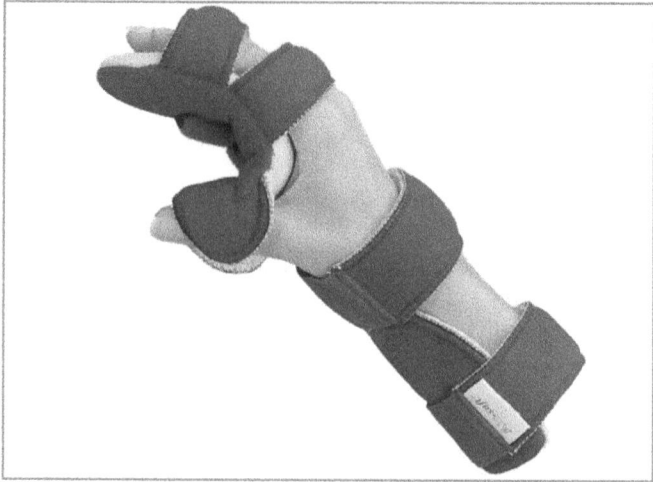

Fig. 12.25: The resting hand splint.

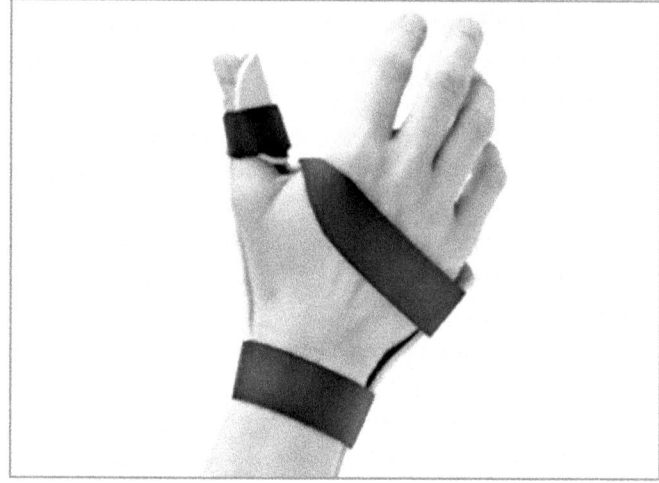

Fig. 12.26: Thermoplastic splint for wrist and thumb.

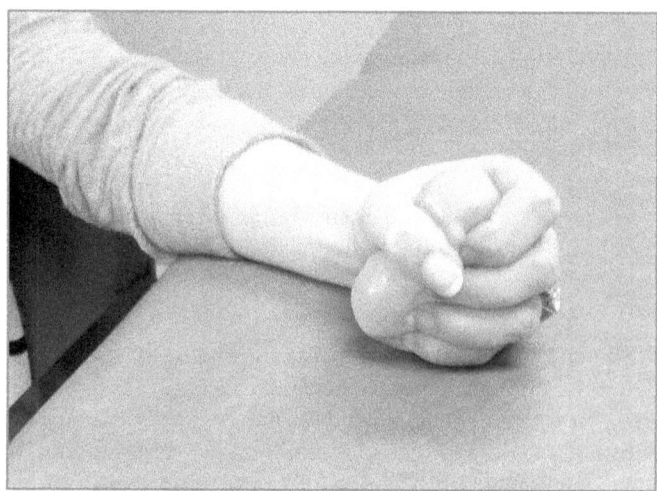

Fig. 12.27: Thumb muscle strengthening using therapy putty.

At 6 weeks postoperatively, splints can be removed while doing active exercises, and at 7 weeks gentle passive stretching of fingers are started. Strengthening of the muscles of hand including grip strengthening is started from 8 weeks postoperatively. At 8 weeks postoperatively, full passive flexion stretches can be commenced, if full finger flexion has not yet been regained. The patient is then advised to use the hand for light functional activities.

- ❖ **Physiotherapy after EPL injury/repair:** Immediately after surgery/injury, the patient is fitted with a thermoplastic splint **(Fig. 12.26)**, that keeps the wrist and thumb in extension, which is worn for 6 weeks. The patient is instructed to perform active extension of thumb with the splint on and the strap loosened. With the splint on and the thumb strap released, he/she is advised to perform isolated IP and MCP flexion of thumb. The patient may be allowed to perform thumb opposition in a progressive manner, i.e., opposition to index finger at 1st week, middle finger at 2nd week, and so on, after releasing the thumb off the splint.

After 6 weeks, the patient is encouraged to use the hand for lighter functional activities and strengthening the muscles of thumb are started after 8 weeks, using therapy putty **(Fig. 12.27)**/elastic bands **(Fig. 12.19)**.

Physiotherapy in Scoliosis

INTRODUCTION

Scoliosis is a deformity of spine, where the spine is bent laterally. This is the most common deformity of spine, causing significant cosmetic issues and functional problems.

Epidemiology/Etiology

Scoliosis is about two times more common in girls than boys. It can be seen at any age, but it is most common in those over 10 years of age. The etiologies of scoliosis are:
- **Idiopathic:** This is the most common type of scoliosis, constituting nearly 90% of cases, where no cause is established.
- **Congenital:** This is mostly due to one or more hemivertebrae **(Fig. 13.1)**, present in the baby by birth.
- **Paralytic/neuromuscular:** This is caused by paralyzed/ weak muscles of lower limbs and/or spine, as found in post-polio patients, cerebral palsy, myopathies, etc.
- **Sciatic:** This is caused due to compression of nerve roots in lumbar region, and seen in prolapsed intervertebral disc (PIVD), lumbar spondylosis, etc.
- **Bony cause:** This is caused in individuals with shortening of the lower limb.
- **Pulmonary cause:** This occurs in individuals who suffer from pleurisy, or those who have undergone surgery on the chest wall on one side.

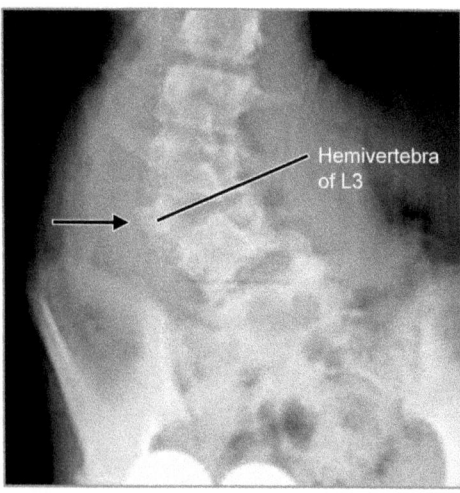

Fig. 13.1: Congenital scoliosis due to hemivertebrae.

Clinical Features

The individual with scoliosis presents with the following features:
- Body bent to one side with uneven shoulders and pelvis.
- Presence of rib humps on the convex side of the curve.
- Reduction of height of the individual when compared with the left to right middle finger distance, when both arms are stretched laterally, as this distance is equal to the standing height of the individual.
- Asymmetric chest expansion.
- Back pain.
- Neuromuscular problem in trunk and lower limbs in progressive conditions that affect the spinal cord.

Assessment of Scoliosis

The clinician should perform different tests discussed below, to assess the scoliosis that helps for understanding, whether the scoliosis is structural/functional and for planning the management accordingly. The tests performed include:
- X-ray examination/inspection of back to ascertain the side (the side of convexity is the side of scoliosis) and apex of the scoliosis—pont of maximum bending/the peak of the curve **(Fig. 13.2A)**. X-ray of the pelvis should be done to grade the Risser sign **(Fig. 13.2B)**. The Risser sign is an indirect measure of skeletal maturity, whereby the degree of ossification of the iliac apophysis by X-ray evaluation is used to judge overall skeletal development. It proceeds from grade: 0 (no ossification to grade: IV (where all the four quadrants/parts show ossification of the iliac apophysis). When the ossified apophysis is completely fused with the ilium, it is graded as-V. A Risser scale of 0 corresponds to an immature skeleton of someone with a lot of growing left to do, and no ossification is observed along the ilium **(Fig. 13.2C)**.
- Examination of the ROM of the spine.
- **Adam's forward bending test:** The test is performed in sitting or standing to establish, whether the scoliosis is structural/functional (flexible). The **Figures 13.3A and B** shows a structural scoliosis, as the curve is not corrected on forward bending.
- **Cobb's angle measurement:** Cobb suggested that the angle of curvature be measured by drawing lines parallel to the upper border of the upper vertebral body and the lower border of the lowest vertebra of the structural

Chapter 13: Physiotherapy in Scoliosis

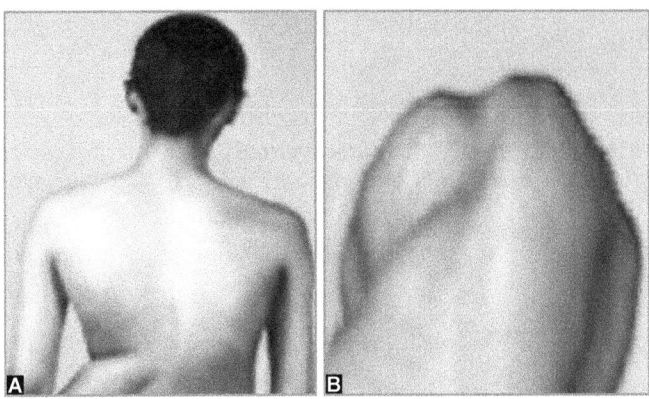

Figs. 13.3A and B: (A) Scoliosis in standing; (B) Scoliosis persisting after forward bending.

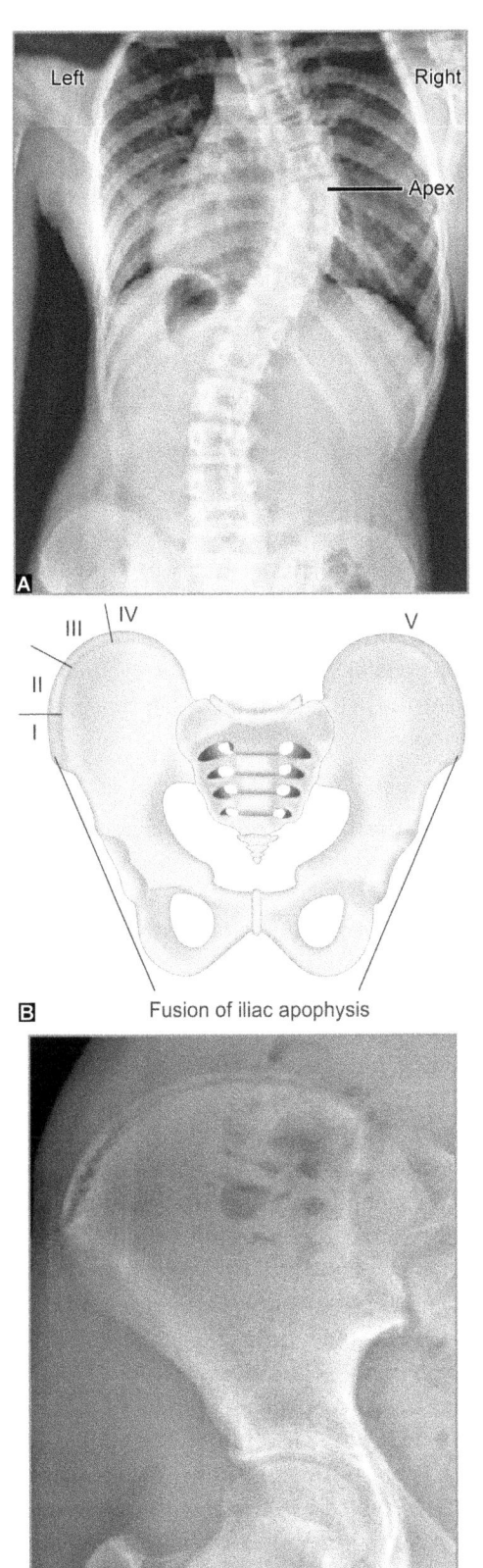

Figs. 13.2A to C: (A) X-ray of D-L spine showing right-sided T-L scoliosis with apex at T8; (B) Risser sign; (C) Risser grade: 0, where, no ossification of iliac apophysis is seen.

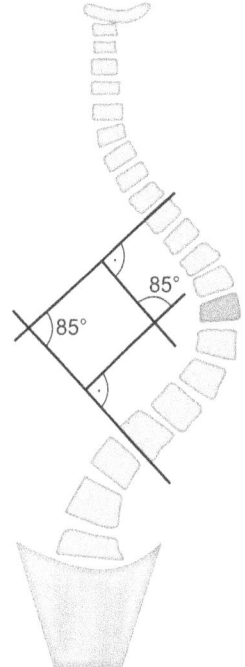

Fig. 13.4: Measurement of Cobb's angle.

- **Measurement of trunk asymmetry:** Measurement of trunk asymmetry and axial trunk rotation using inclinometer.
- **Measurement of height loss:** Measurement of distance between tip of middle fingers of both hands, with both arms stretched laterally, gives the standing height of the sufferer, which should be compared with the height of the individual taken in standing. The difference between the arm span length and actual height of the individual gives the loss of height due to scoliosis.
- **Measurement of chest expansion and lung function:** Chest expansion at the nipple level, measurement of FVC (provides information about lung volume) and FEV_1 (provides information about flow function) should be performed.

Management of Scoliosis

Management of scoliosis is mostly done conservatively basing on the Cobb's angle, and fusion of the iliac apophysis (Risser sign). Complete fusion of iliac apophysis indicates

curve, then erecting perpendiculars from these lines to cross each other. The angle between these perpendiculars being the "angle of curvature" **(Fig. 13.4)**.

Section 2: Physiotherapy for Musculoskeletal Conditions

Table 13.1: Schedule of scoliosis management.

Cobb's angle in degrees	Risser grade	Treatment followed
10–19	0–1, with very high growth potential	Observation/monitoring at every 6 month interval and home based physiotherapy
10–19	2–4, with limited growth potential	Observation/monitoring at every 6 month interval and home based physiotherapy
20–29	2–4, with limited groth potential	Bracing, physiotherapy and intensive scoliosis rehabilitation
20–29	0–1, with high growth potential	Bracing, physiotherapy and intensive scoliosis rehabilitation
29–40	0–1, with high growth potential	Bracing, physiotherapy and intensive scoliosis rehabilitation
29–40	2–4, with limited growth potential	Bracing, physiotherapy and intensive scoliosis rehabilitation
>40	0–4	Surgery

completion of growth of the adolescent. If the iliac apophysis is not completely ossified, it indicates skeletal growth is continuing, necessitating deferral of surgical intervention. For a Cobb's angle of 20° or less, only exercises are followed, without any bracing/surgery. The schedule of treatment followed is indicated in the **Table 13.1**.

In children before completion of growth and adolescents and adults with Cobb's angle <40°, physiotherapy combined with or without bracing **(Fig. 13.5)** is the treatment of choice. It is seen that, those having a Cobb's angle of equal to or less than 20°, are managed by ergonomic advice and therapeutic exercises. Individuals with Cobb's angle between 20 and 40 degrees, are managed with exercises and spinal brace. If the Cobb's angle is more than 40°, and the individual has, neuromuscular and pulmonary complications surgery should be undertaken.

Physiotherapy in Scoliosis

The aims of physiotherapy are:
- To teach the individual about auto correction of deformity and ergonomic measures.

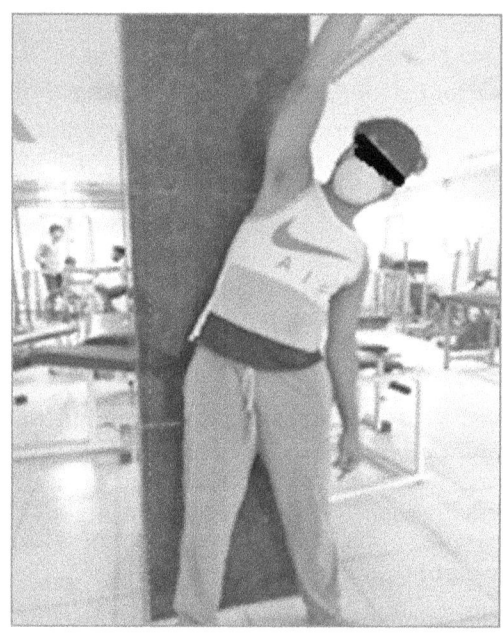

Fig. 13.5: Trunk lateral flexor stretching (right) in standing.

- To teach posture correction.
- To improve ROM of spine.
- To improve strength and endurance of spinal muscles.
- To improve chest expansion and lungs function.
- To reduce pain (if any).
- To provide postoperative care in the event of surgery.
- To educate the patient about the deformity and possibility of recurrence.

Methods/Techniques of Physiotherapy

- **Auto correction of deformity and ergonomic measures:** The patient should be taught self-stretching exercises, such as:
  - Standing, trunk bending toward the convex side **(Fig. 13.5)**.
  - Stretching of spine in chair sitting, standing, and side lying **(Figs. 13.6A to C)**.
  - Stretching the spine through hanging, holding a bar over head **(Fig. 13.7)**.
  - *Advanced lateral spine movements:* Stretching the spine holding a stick in hands, with convex side hip abducted and resting on bed. Arms with the sticks are made to move towards the convex side **(Fig. 13.8)**.
  - Sitting on a chair with proper back and neck support, with a pad of cloth under the concave side buttock and a firm pillow under the axilla on the concave side.
- **Posture correction exercises:** For scoliosis like functional T-L scoliosis, sciatic scoliosis, the patient should be taught self-correction of the postural dysfunction, preferably in standing. For example, for a right-sided T-L scoliosis, with trunk bent to left side, the patient is advised to perform frequent correction of posture, by keeping one hand on pelvis and other hand on the opposite side thorax and pushing the pelvis toward left, and thorax toward right (for a right-sided scoliosis in the said example) **(Fig. 13.9)**. A postural mirror is of great help in auto correction.
- **To improve ROM of thoracolumbar spine:** Spinal flexion exercises in supine **(Fig. 13.10A)**/long-sitting, spinal lateral flexion exercise toward the convex side, thoracic rotation

Chapter 13: Physiotherapy in Scoliosis

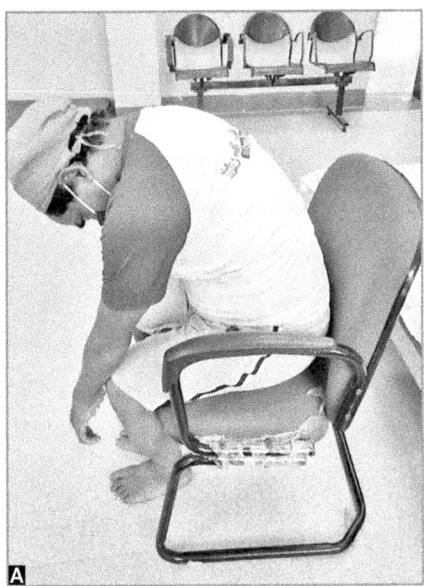

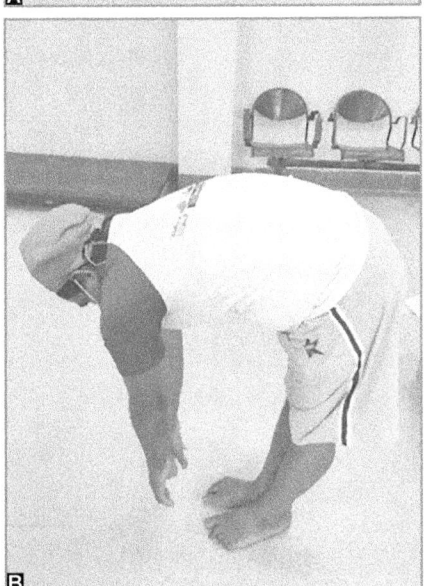

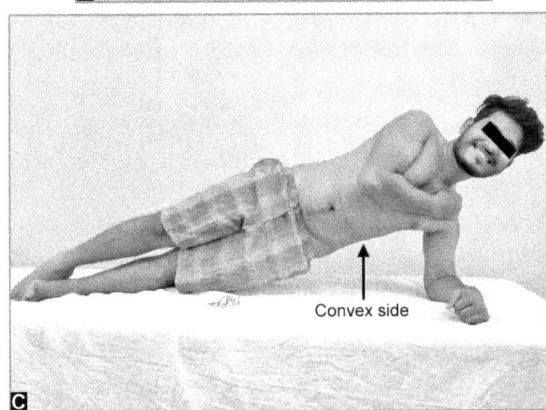

Figs. 13.6A to C: (A) Stretching of spine in sitting; (B) standing; (C) side lying.

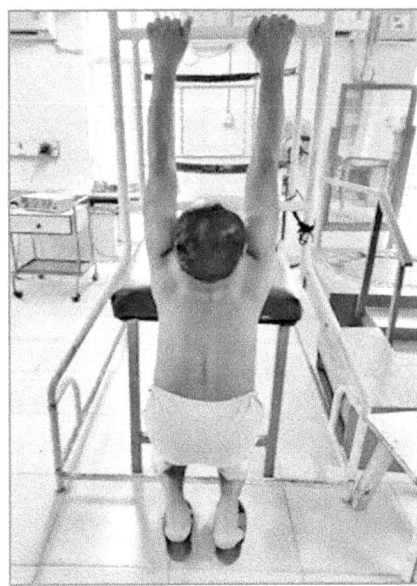

Fig. 13.7: Hanging from overhead to stretch spine.

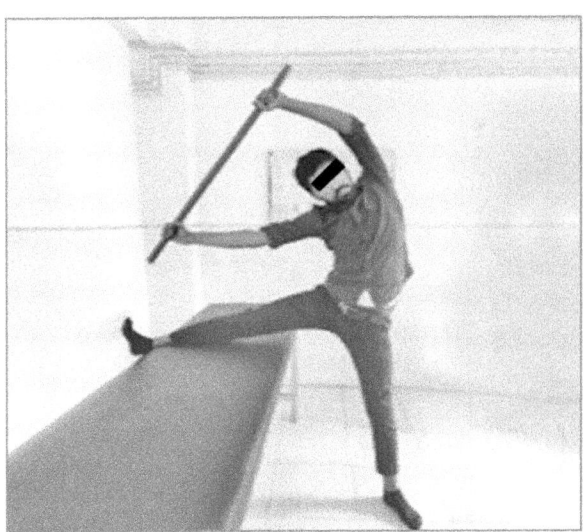

Fig. 13.8: Advanced lateral spine movements.

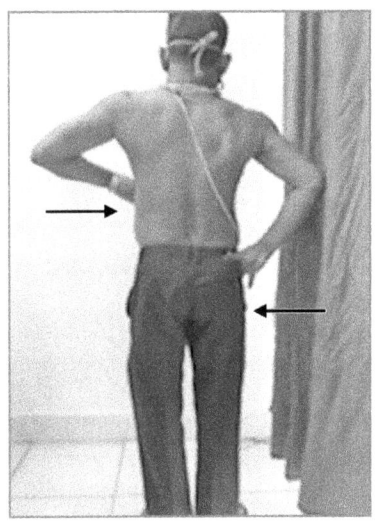

Fig. 13.9: Auto correction of scoliosis in standing.

exercises, followed by spinal extension exercises **(Fig. 13.10B)** should be taught.
- **To improve strength and endurance of spinal muscles:** Spinal extension exercise in prone lying and quadruped

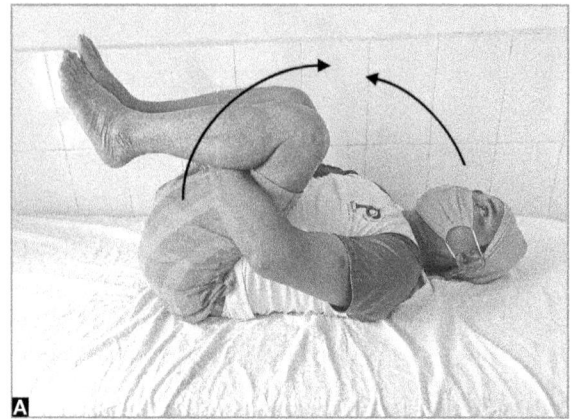
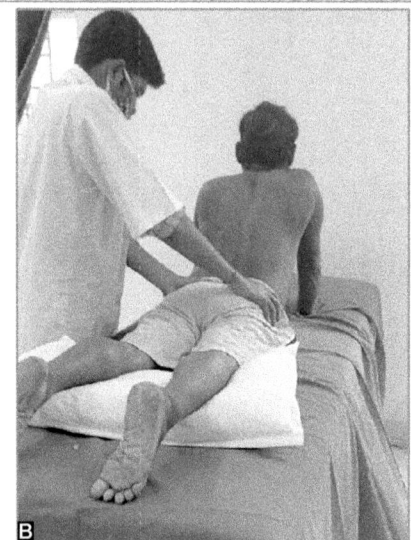

Figs. 13.10A and B: (A) Spinal flexion exercise; (B) Spinal extension exercise.

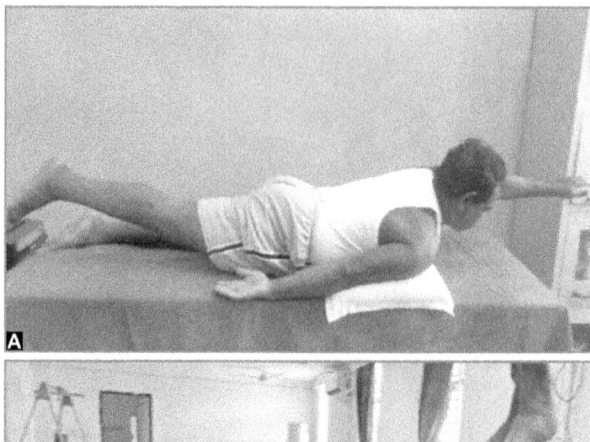
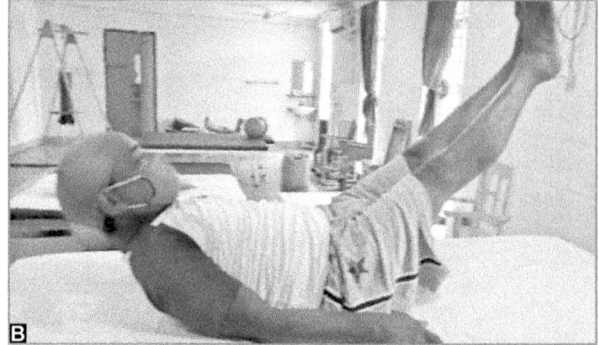
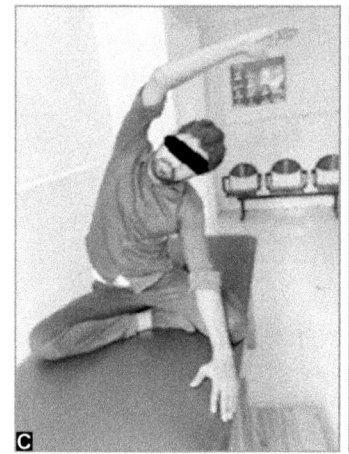
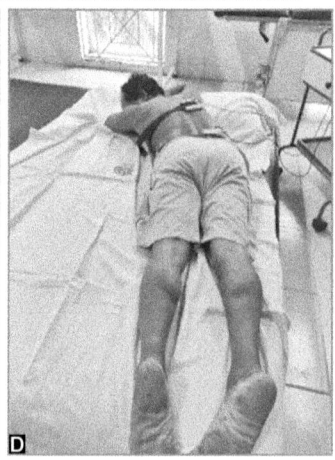

Figs. 13.11A to D: (A) Spinal extension exercise; (B) Core muscle strengthening exercise; (C) Pilate exercise; (D) Faradic stimulation.

posture (**Fig. 13.11A**), pelvic bridging exercise core muscle strengthening exercises (**Fig. 13.11B**), and pilates (**Fig. 13.11C**) are taught. Faradic stimulation of muscles on the convex side (**Fig. 13.11D**), which suffers from stretch weakness, helps to improve the strength, and endurance of the paraspinals on convex side.

- **Schroth therapy:** Schroth therapy that helps to correct the deformity by stretching the curvature and improving strength and endurance of the spinal muscles is an effective method of correcting the deformity. The methods include:
  – Keeping the body as straight as possible in lying/sitting/standing.
  – Hanging, holding on with hands from overhead bar (**Fig. 13.7**).
  – Exercise on therapy ball (**Fig. 13.12A**).
  – Practicing breathing exercises.
  – Stretching trunk lateral flexors, placing a bolster under thigh (**Fig. 13.12B**), under the convex side of trunk (**Fig. 13.12C**).
- **Klapp exercise:** Klapp's method also known as Kriechmethode (crawling method) was developed in Germany in the beginning of the 20th century as a method for treating idiopathic scoliosis. This concept was created by orthopedist Bernhard Klapp and soon after it was developed by his son Rudolf Klapp. It was a nonsurgical method established with the aim of correcting the spinal curvature by stretching and strengthening the back muscles (**Figs. 13.13A to E**).
- **To improve chest expansion and lung function:** Deep breathing exercises, i.e., inspiration combined with upper limb elevation, expiration combined with upper limb lowering (**Figs. 13.14A and B**) are taught.
- Incentive spirometry is also a very effective method of improving chest expansion and lung function (**Fig. 13.15**).
- **To reduce pain:** Mechanical lumbar traction, positional traction with pillows/bolster placed on the convex side (**Fig. 13.12C**), myofascial release to tight paraspinals on the concave side (**Fig. 13.16**), moist hot packs,

Chapter 13: Physiotherapy in Scoliosis 261

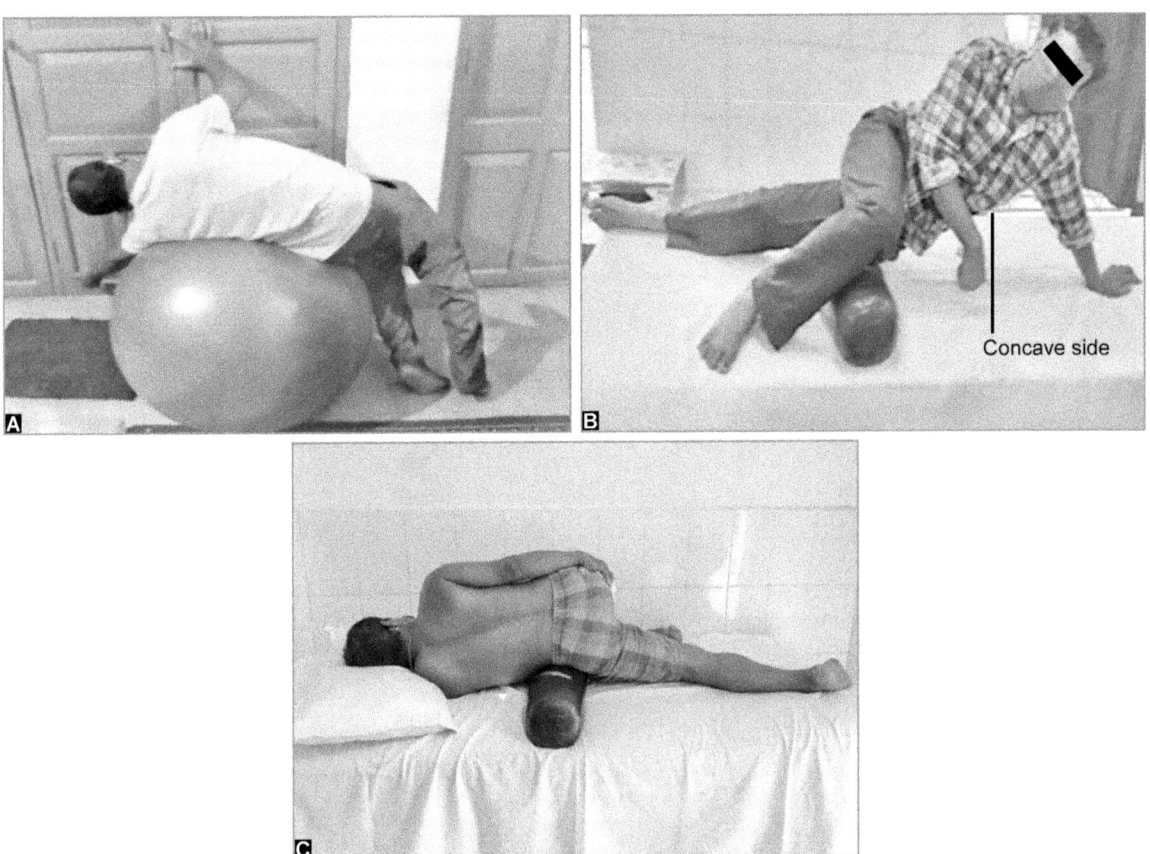

Figs. 13.12A and B: (A) Stretching of spine on Swiss ball; (B) Stretching of trunk lateral flexors by placing bolster under thigh; (C) Stretching of trunk lateral flexors by placing pillow/bolster under the convex side.

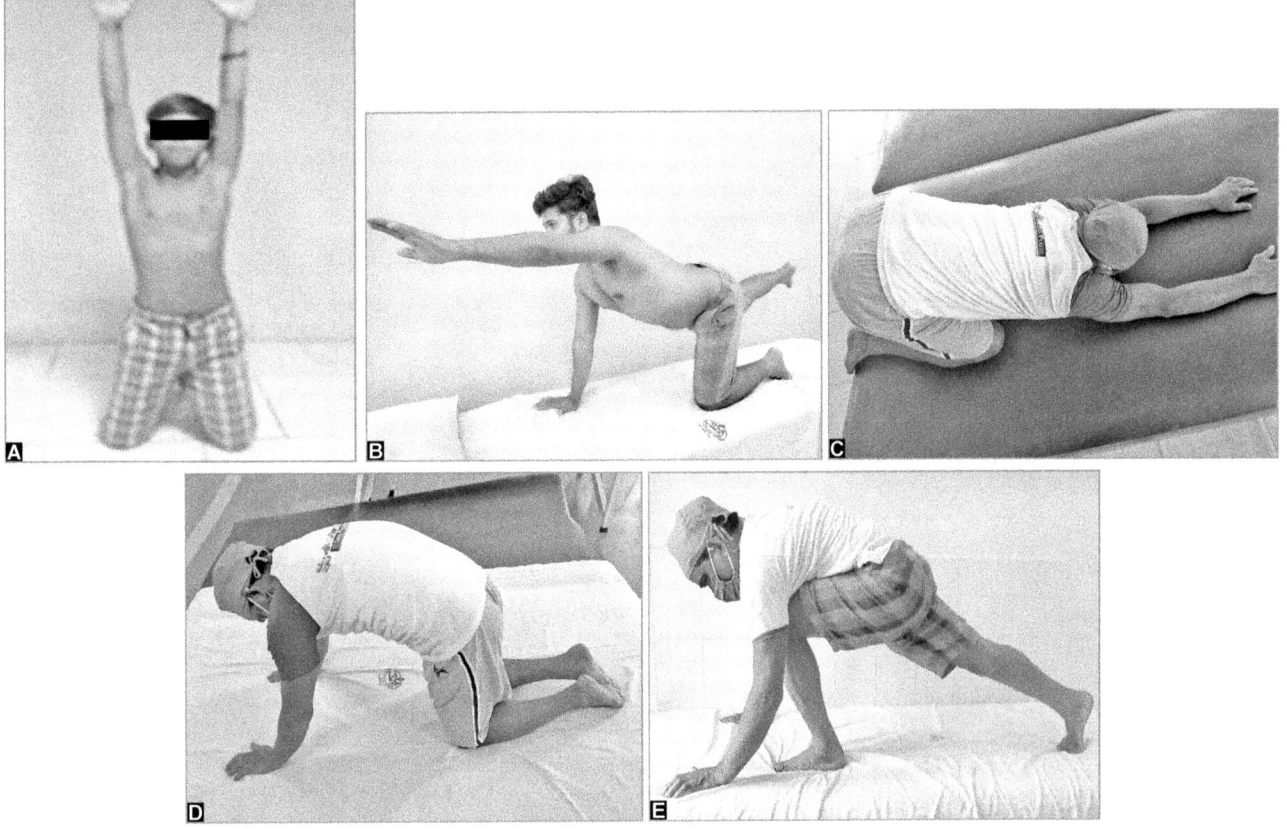

Figs. 13.13A to E: Klapp exercises for scoliosis.

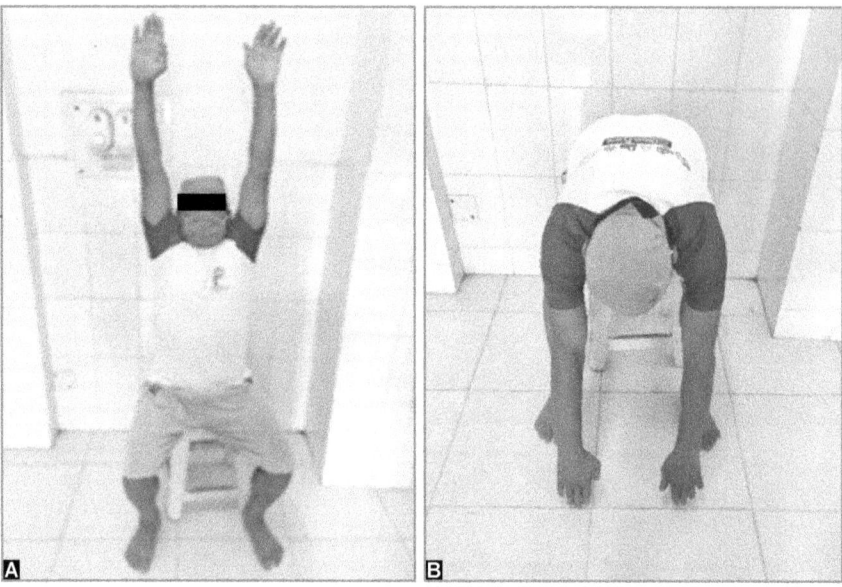

Figs. 13.14A and B: (A) Inspiration with upper limbs elevation; (B) Expiration with upper limb lowering.

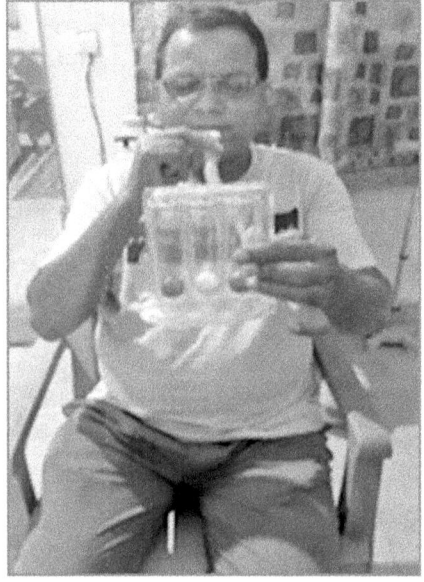

Fig. 13.15: Incentive spirometry to improve chest expansion.

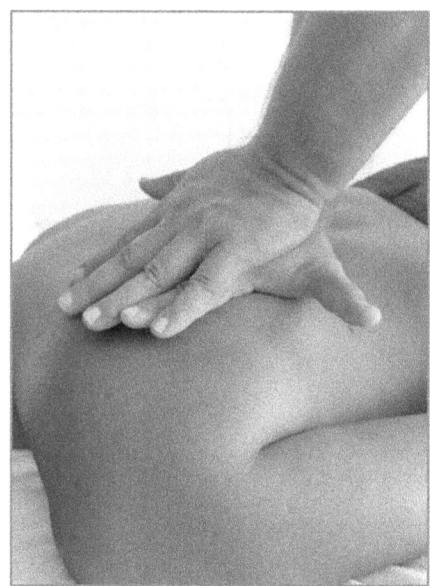

Fig. 13.16: Myofascial release to paraspinals on the concave side.

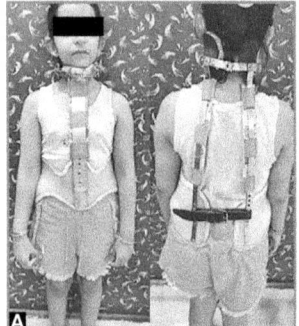
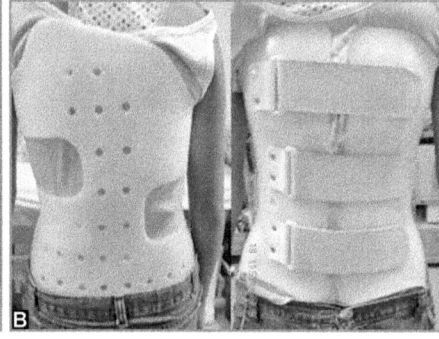
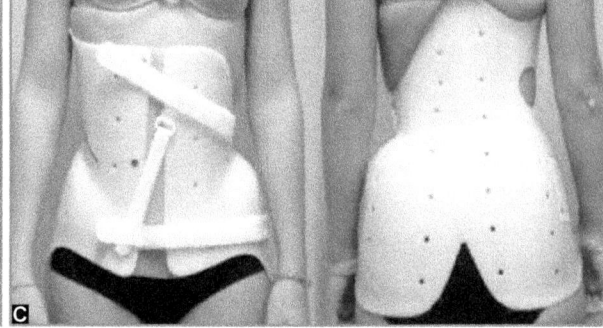

Figs. 13.17A to C: (A) Milwaukee brace; (B) Miami brace; (C) Boston brace.

interferential therapy (IFT)/transcutaneous electrical nerve stimulation (TENS) over the painful site of back are applied.
* **Orthosis for scoliosis**: The orthoses selected for patients with scoliosis, depends on the parts of spine affected, which are as follows:
    – For scoliosis affecting the whole spine, CTLSO (Milwaukee brace) **(Fig. 13.17A)** is considered.
    – For scoliosis affecting the T-L spine, a Miami brace (Apex of curve below T6) **(Fig. 13.17B)**/Boston brace (Apex of curve below T8) **(Fig. 13.17C)** can be considered.

Surgery for Scoliosis

Most spine surgeons agree that, adolescents who have very severe curve with Cobb's angle above 40°, and in whom growth is completed as ascertained from the Risser sign discussed above, surgery should be undertaken. Surgery is needed to lessen the curve and prevent it from getting worse. The surgery for scoliosis is spinal fusion **(Fig. 13.18)**. A complementary surgical procedure a surgeon may recommend is called thoracoplasty (also called costoplasty). This is a procedure to reduce the rib hump that affects most scoliosis patients with a thoracic curve.

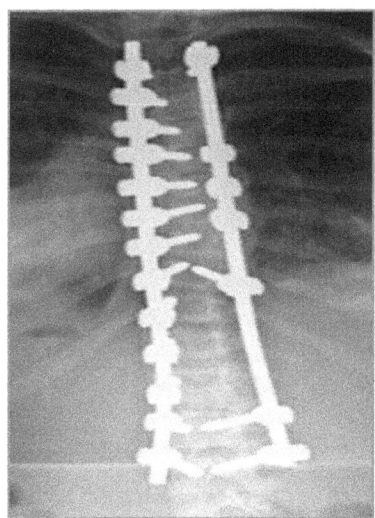

Fig. 13.18: Spinal fusion surgery using implants.

Postoperative Management

Postoperatively emphasis is given for:
* Healing of surgical wound
* Scar mobilization
* Chest expansion/breathing exercises
* Pain reduction using IFT/TENS

Physiotherapy for Amputees

INTRODUCTION

Amputation is the intentional surgical removal of a limb or part of a limb/part of body. For limb, it is done through the bone(s) or through a joint. When amputation surgery is done through a joint, it is called disarticulation. It can either be planned or performed as an emergency procedure. Sometimes autoamputation occurs as a result of direct trauma or from the presence of constriction bands.

INCIDENCE OF AMPUTATION

Common age groups affected are individuals between 50 and 70 years of age, though amputation due to trauma is common in young adults. Approximately 75% of males and 25% of females are subjected to this condition. It is performed more in the lower limbs (85%), as compared to upper limbs (15%).

CAUSES/INDICATIONS OF AMPUTATION

- **The most common causes include:**
  - Injury (< 50 years).
  - Peripheral vascular disease (> 50 years).

- **Less common causes include:**
  - Infection (gas gangrene).
  - Malignancy.
  - Nerve injury (e.g., complete preganglionic brachial plexus injury).
  - *Congenital anomalies:* Phocomelia (partial absence of the limb)/amelia (complete absence of limb).
  - Miscellaneous.

Three D's for amputation: Limb is Dead, Deadly, causing Dam nuisance are the indications of amputation.

Site of Limb Amputation/Types of Amputation (Fig. 14.1)

- **Upper limb:**
  - Forequarter
  - Shoulder disarticulation (SD)
  - Transhumeral [above elbow (AE)]
  - Elbow disarticulation (ED)
  - Transradial [below elbow (BE)]
  - Hand/wrist disarticulation
  - Transcarpal [partial hand (PH) amputation]

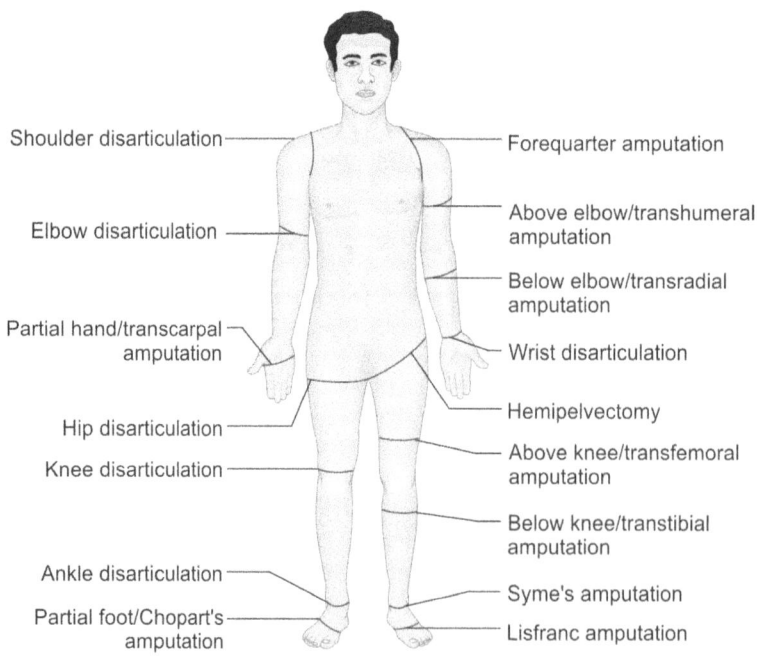

Fig. 14.1: Levels and types of limb amputation.

- **Lower limb:**
  - Hemipelvectomy
  - Hip disarticulation (HD)
  - Transfemoral (above knee) amputation.
  - Knee disarticulation (KD)
  - Transtibial (below knee) amputation.
  - Ankle disarticulation
  - Symes amputation.
  - Partial foot/Choparts amputation—amputation at mid-tarsal level.
  - Toe amputation (Lisfranc amputation). Amputation at tarsometatarsal level.

  The **Figure 14.1** shows the levels of limb amputation.

Some Special Types of Amputations

- **Duputryen's amputation:** Amputation of the arm at the shoulder joint.
- **Gritti-Stoke's amputation:** Amputation of the leg through the knee, using an oval anterior flap.
- **Hey's amputation:** Amputation of the foot between the tarsus and metatarsus.
- **Interpelviabdominal amputation:** Amputation of the thigh, with excision of the lateral half of the pelvis.
- **Interscapulothoracic amputation:** Amputation of the arm, with excision of the lateral portion of the shoulder girdle.
- **Larrey's amputation:** Amputation at the shoulder joint.
- **Spontaneous amputation:** Loss of a part without surgical intervention (commonly found in diabetes mellitus).
- **Sarmiento's amputation/modified Syme's amputation:** Amputation at 1.3 cm proximal to the ankle joint line.
- **Syme's amputation:** Disarticulation of the foot with removal of both malleoli, 0.6 cm proximal to the ankle joint line.
- **Pirogoff amputation:** Amputation of the foot at the ankle, part of the calcaneus being left in the stump.
- **Krukenberg amputation:** In this procedure, the forearm stump is converted into a pincer that is motorized by the pronator teres muscle **(Fig. 14.2)**.

- **Boyd's amputation:** Boyd's amputation refers to amputation at the level of the ankle, with preservation of the calcaneus and heel pad and consequent fixation of the calcaneus to tibia. It allows for complete weight bearing and provides both stabilization of the heel pad and suspension of the prosthesis.

Ideal Stump and Stump Length

A stump is considered ideal, if it exhibits the following qualities:
- It has no wound.
- Its shape is either conical or cylindrical.
- It has no bony projections and the stump end has enough padding of muscles.
- It should have sufficient length to hold the prosthesis.
- It should not have a neuroma or phantom pain **(Phantom limb pain:** It is the pain that feels like coming from a body part that is no longer there. It is not a psychological problem, but a real sensation, that originate in the brain and spinal cord. In contrast, **phantom limb sensation** is the feeling of the presence of the amputated limb, even though the same has been removed. This sensation is advantageous for gait training with the prosthesis, as utilizing the sensation, the amputee fitted with the prosthesis is able to walk in a better manner. This sensation, has the disadvantage that, when not using prosthesis, the patient may try to take load on the imaginary limb, which may result in a fall).
- It should have adequate movement and muscle strength in the proximal joints.

The ideal length of the stumps (**Figs. 14.3A to D**):
- **Above knee stump length (Fig. 14.3A):** 23–27 cm from greater trochanter of femur.
- **Below knee stump length is (Fig. 14.3C):** 12–17 cm from the knee.
- **Above elbow stump length (Fig. 14.3B):** 20 cm from the shoulder.
- **Below elbow stump length (Fig. 14.3D):** 18 cm from the olecranon process of ulna.

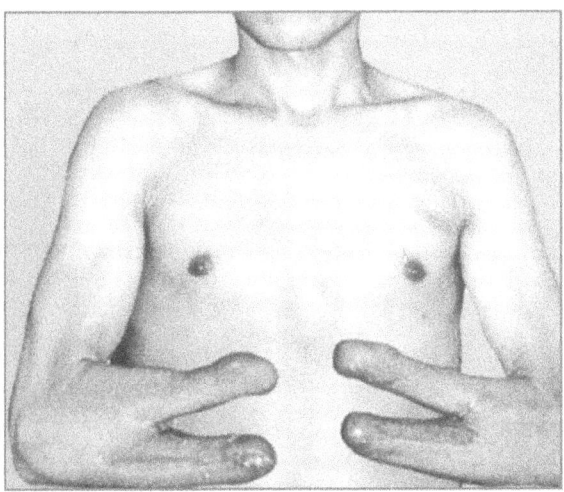

Fig. 14.2: Krukenberg's amputation.

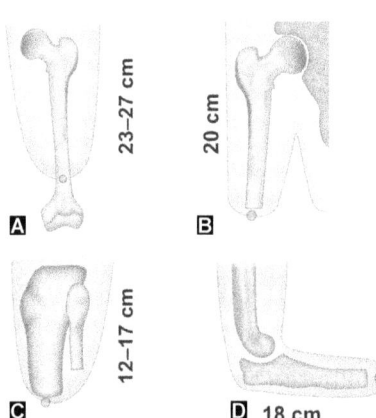

Figs. 14.3A to D: The ideal length of stumps. (A) Above knee stump; (B) Above elbow stump; (C) Below knee stump; (D) Below elbow stump.

Goals of Postoperative Management

The goals of postoperative management include:
- Prompt and uncomplicated wound healing.
- Control of edema.
- Control of postoperative pain (including phantom limb pain).
- Prevention of joint stiffness, soft tissue tightness/contracture.
- Prevention of muscle weakness.
- Reduction of deconditioning effects.
- Rapid rehabilitation (early return to function and participation in society/community and achieving a productive vocation).

PHASES OF AMPUTEE REHABILITATION

Rehabilitation of the amputees is carried out through the following phases:
- **Preoperative**: Assessment of body condition that includes ROM and muscle power over the proximal joints as well as cardiorespiratory fitness, patient education, surgical level discussion, and postoperative prosthetic plans.
- **Amputation surgery:** It focuses on length of stump, [myoplastic (muscle-muscle suturing)/myodesis (muscle-bone suturing)] procedure of wound closure as well as application of rigid dressing.
- **Acute postsurgical:** It focuses on wound healing, pain control, exercises to proximal joints/segments, breathing exercises, and emotional support.
- **Preprosthetic:** It focuses on shaping and shrinking of the stump through application of elastic crepe bandage/shrinker socks, strengthening of proximal muscles, reduction of phantom limb pain and pain due to neuroma, and increase of endurance.
- **Prosthetic prescription**: A team of professionals including the orthopedics surgeon and prosthetists take the decision regarding prosthetic prescription and fabrication.
- **Prosthetic training:** Training on donning and doffing of the prosthesis and its functional use done by the prosthetists, physiotherapist, and occupational therapist.
- **Community integration:** Enabling the patient to resume life roles in community and society, teaching the coping strategies, and promotion of recreational activities are emphasized in this phase.
- **Vocational rehabilitation:** Vocational assessment, training, and placement are emphasized during this phase.
- **Follow-up:** Periodic follow-up for repair/change of the prosthesis, emotional support for lifelong use of prosthesis are emphasized during this phase.

ROLE OF PHYSIOTHERAPY IN AMPUTEE REHABILITATION

Preoperative Physiotherapy

Focuses on the objective assessment looking at ROM and muscle power and provides the patient appropriate exercises and education to assist postamputation mobility. The preoperative assessment also helps the surgeon to decide the level of amputation to achieve an ideal length of stump described in **Figure 14.3**.

Acute Postoperative Physiotherapy

In this phase, rigid dressing using rigid material such as plaster of Paris is applied immediately after surgery, which is kept in place for 5–7 days **(Fig. 14.4)**. Chest physiotherapy in the form of deep breathing exercises, postural drainage (if required) are applied. Transfer practice from bed to wheel chair and from wheel chair to commode and specific exercises to increase muscle strength and ROM over the proximal joints of the stump are the emphasis.

Preprosthetic Rehabilitation

It focuses on:
- **Positioning of the stump**: After amputation, positioning the residual limb is very important to prevent tightness/contracture/deformity in the proximal joints. Use of pillows under the thigh/knee/arm/forearm should be restricted to prevent development of flexion deformities in hip, knee, shoulder, and elbow, respectively. As tolerated the patient with lower limb amputation is encouraged lie in prone, a few hours in a day.
- **Ambulation with temporary prosthesis and/or using a pair of axillary crutches:** The amputee should be made to remain engaged in light activities as soon as possible with the help of a temporary prosthesis, which should be taken off when the patient sleeps. However in bilateral transfemoral amputees, stubbies **(Fig. 14.5A)** can be used as temporary prosthesis. When not using the temporary prosthesis, he/she should be taught to walk using a pair of axillary crutches **(Fig. 14.5B)**.

Ambulation with a temporary prosthesis offers the following benefits:
- The patient is made active.
- Stump shrinkage is further accelerated.
- Flexion contracture of hip/knee is prevented.
- Phantom limb pain is reduced

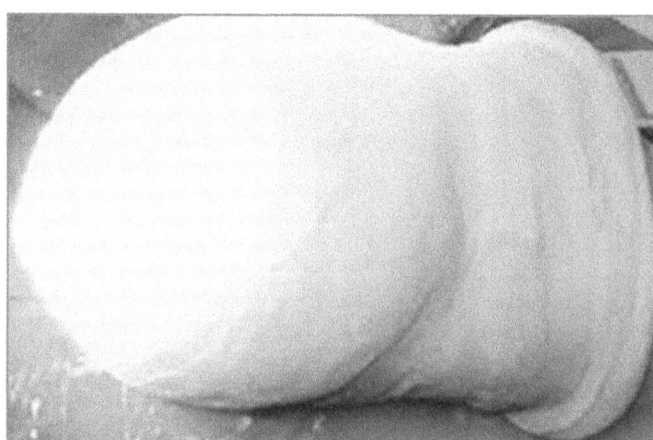

Fig. 14.4: Plaster of Paris bandage applied postoperatively.

Chapter 14: Physiotherapy for Amputees

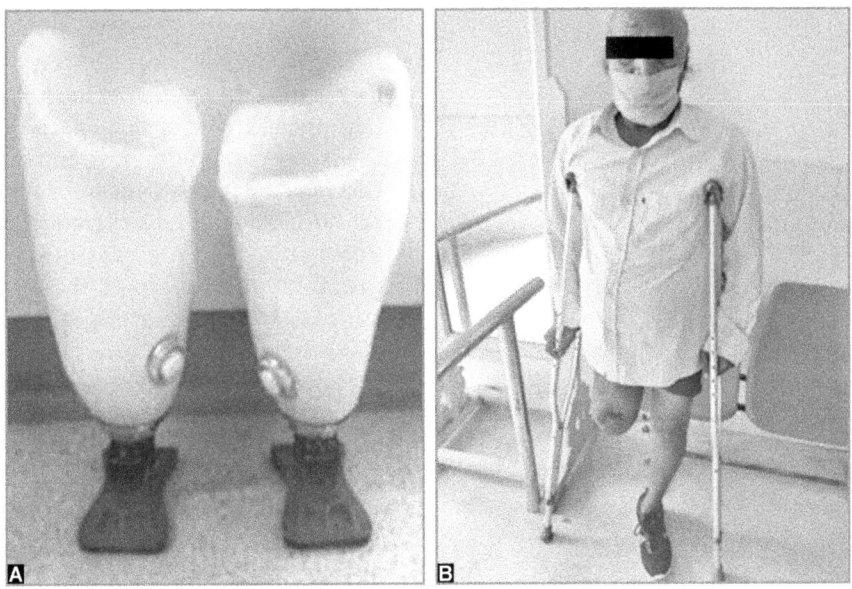

Figs. 14.5A and B: (A) Stubbies for bilateral transfemoral amputees; (B) Amputee walking with axillary crutches.

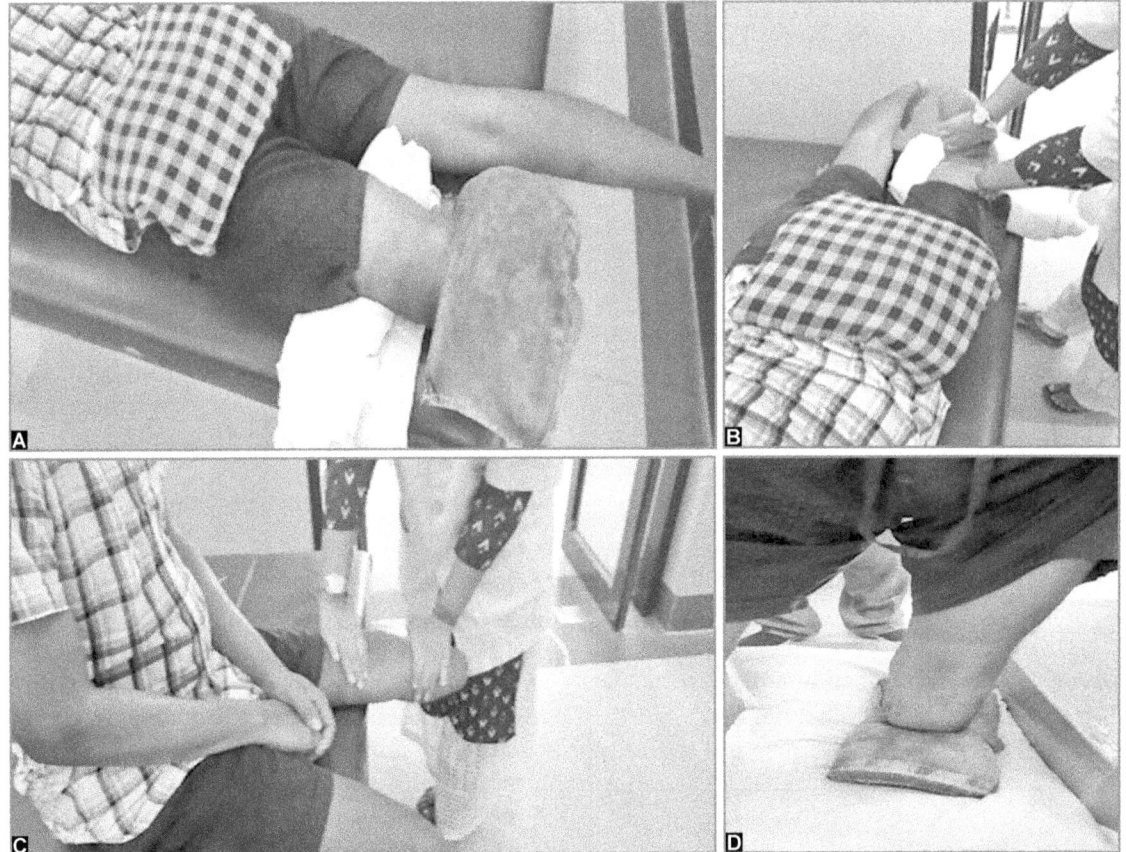

Figs. 14.6A to D: (A) Positional stretching to correct tightness/deformity in hip and knee; (B) Strengthening of hamstrings; (C) Strengthening of quadriceps; (D) Weight bearing on end of stump.

- Stump exercises, i.e., stretching of tight muscles and strengthening of weak muscles of stump **(Figs. 14.6A to C)**, crepe bandaging **(Figs. 14.7A to D)**, hydrotherapy for stump, weight bearing on stump **(Fig. 14.6D)** are performed to prepare the stump for the fitment of prosthesis.

- Stump conditioning is very much essential during this preprosthetic rehabilitation phase. It is the process of accelerating the rate at which the stump shrinks after an amputation. With proper conditioning, the stump should shrink naturally in the first few days postsurgery. Shrinkers

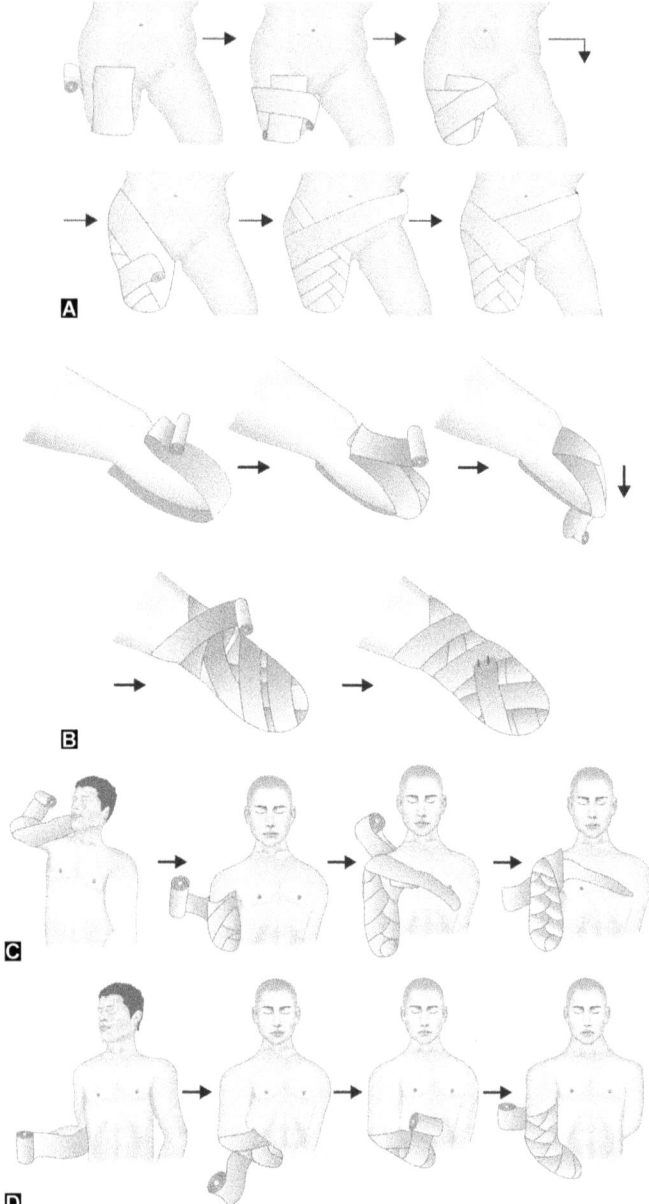

Figs. 14.7A to D: (A) AK stump bandaging; (B) BK stump bandaging; (C) AE stump bandaging; (D) BE stump bandaging.

or elastic bandages are used to taper the stump in order to speed up this process.
* Neuroma (if any) is managed by ultrasound therapy, friction massage, tapping to desensitize, weight bearing on the end of stump, TENS, etc.
* Phantom pain (if any) is managed by application of TENS and counseling to patient.
* Liaisoning with the prosthetist and other members of the rehabilitation team are done for the fitment of prosthesis.

Prosthetic Prescription/Fabrication and Fitment

This is done by the prosthetists. However, the physiotherapist may assist in the cast appointment and cast taking.

Use of Prosthesis and Prosthetic Training

* Before training on uses of prosthesis, for both the upper and lower limbs, the physiotherapist makes a complete checkout (alignment, fit, and functioning) of the prosthesis and teaches the patient about donning and doffing of the prosthesis. Gait rehabilitation, upper limb functional training using the prosthesis are started and gradually progressed.
* Before donning the prosthesis for the checkout, the therapist should check the stump for any wounds, abrasions, blisters, areas of redness, or discoloration, presence of bony protuberances or scars, as well as presence of any tightness of muscles in the proximal joints.
* The prosthesis should be checked, before it is donned, as well after donning. The check out of the prosthesis before donning (**Figs. 14.8A to D**) consists of:
  - Checking, whether, the prosthesis has been made of the components as prescribed.
  - Checking the tightness of all screws and adaptors, to rule out any hazards due to loose component fixation.
  - Checking the movement of the components without any noise.
  - Checking the interior of the socket for any roughness/ridges. For quadrilateral socket, it should be checked to find that, the posterior brim of the prosthesis is parallel to the ground.
  - Checking the foot wear for proper fitting into the prosthetic foot.
  - A rough guide to check the alignment of the transtibial prosthesis is that, when placed on the ground, it can stand unsupported.
* Checking the prosthesis after donning (**Figs. 14.9A to D**), the following points need to be checked:
  - Whether it is easy to don the prosthesis?
  - Whether, the prosthesis is properly fitting into the stump?
  - Whether, the alignment of the prosthesis over the stump seems proper?
  - Whether, the patient has any pain/discomfort with the prosthesis on?

Training on the Use of Prosthesis

Gait assessment and gait training: While assessing amputee gait it is important to be aware of normal gait and how normal gait in the amputee is affected. Furthermore, there may be deviations which an amputee will adopt to compensate for the prosthesis, muscle weakness or tightening, lack of balance and fear. These deviations create an altered gait pattern and it is important that these are recognized, as rehabilitation of the gait will need to encompass corrections of these deviations. The gait deviations can be found through observational gait analysis, as well as analyzing the gait in gait laboratory, where the prosthetist and the physiotherapist work together to find such deviations and make necessary modifications in prosthesis and train gait with or without walking aids. Visual biofeedback in the form of use of postural mirror is a very good method for training gait with prosthesis. The following gait deviations are found in transfemoral and transtibial amputees.

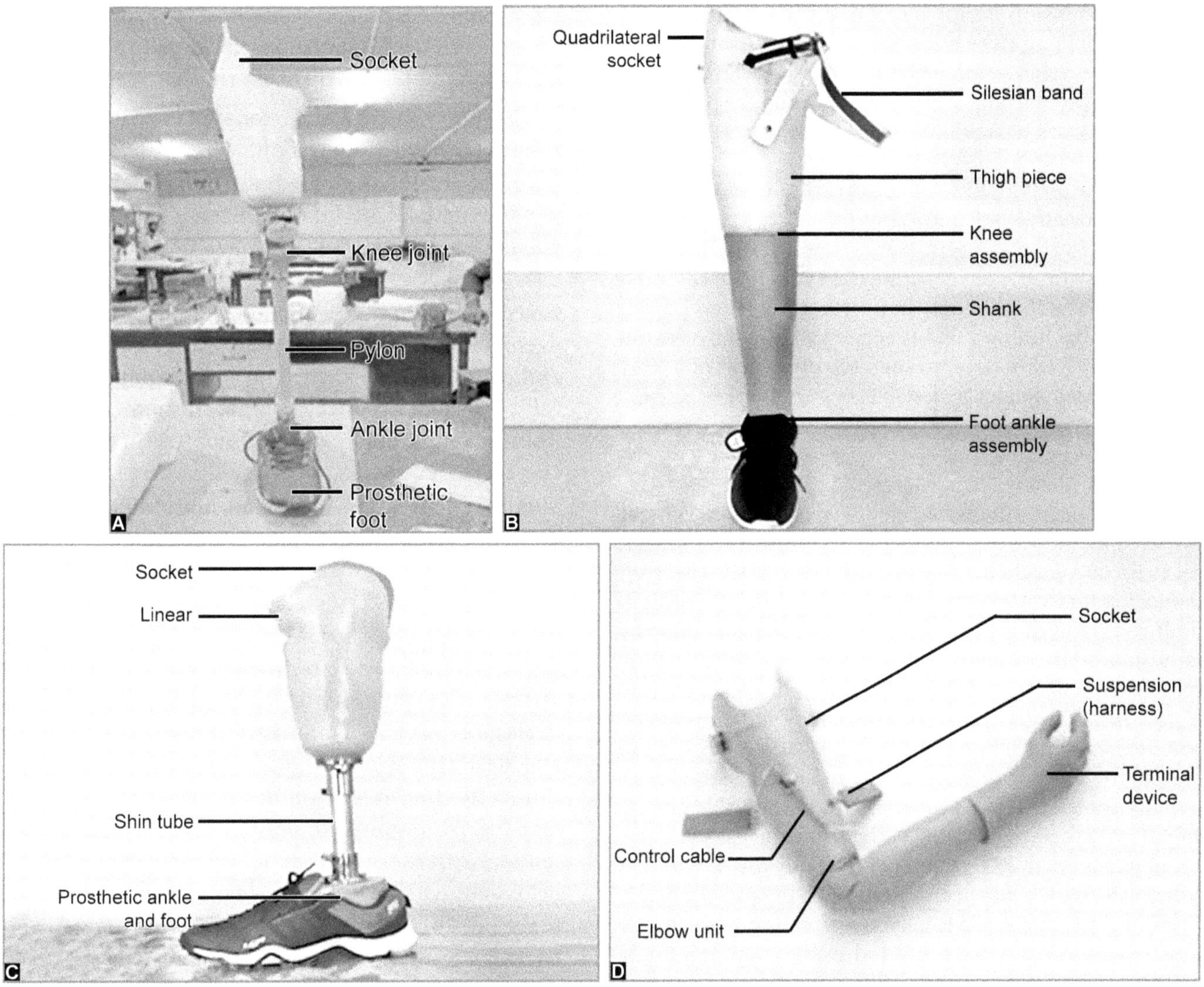

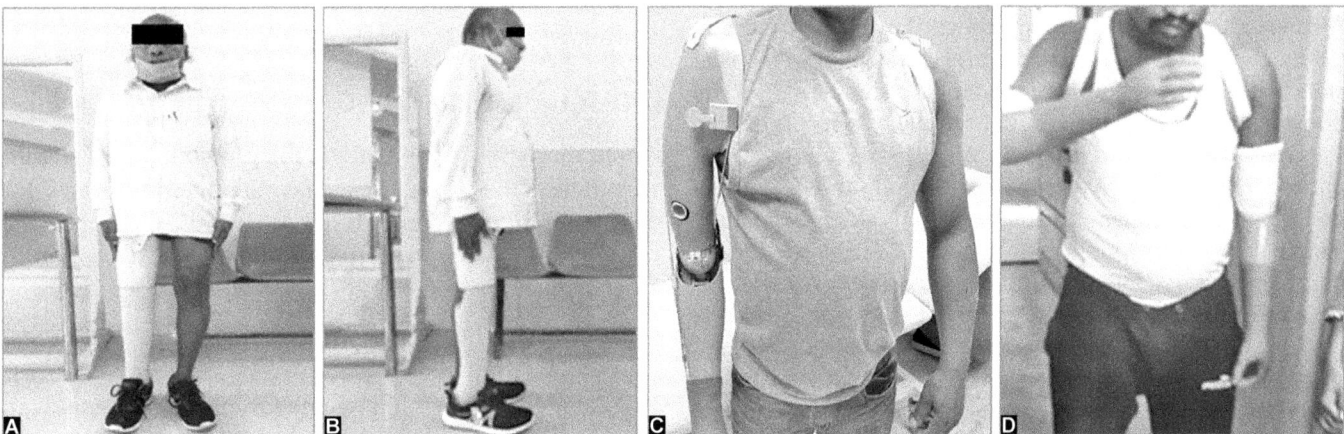

Figs. 14.8A to D: (A) AK prosthesis (endoskeletal design); (B) AK prosthesis (final design); (C) BK prosthesis (endoskeletal design); (D) AE prosthesis.

Figs. 14.9A to D: (A) Right AK prosthesis (front view); (B) Right AK prosthesis (side view); (C) Right AE prosthesis; (D) Bilateral below elbow prosthesis.

For Transfemoral Amputees

A person with a transfemoral amputation using AK prosthesis has to compensate for the loss of both the knee and ankle joint. The main focus of the gait cycle is to prevent the knee from buckling during stance phase. When a free knee joint, that allows movement in the knee is used, the knee need to remain in extension for longer time during stance phase, to ensure buckling does not occur. This extension causes prolonged heel strike and the body moves forward over the prosthetic leg as one unit. The hip extensors on the prosthetic side need to work to stabilize the limb in prosthetic weight bearing.

During the swing phase of the prosthetic limb, the hip extensors and calf muscles on the sound side help to generate force for the prosthetic limb to swing forward. Hip flexors on the prosthetic limb must generate the same force required during normal gait. Although the prosthesis is generally 30% lighter than the limb would be, speed generated by the hip flexors is required in order to snap the prosthesis of a "free knee" into extension for heel strike.

For Transtibial Amputees

During stance phase
The ankle of the prosthesis has a reduced range of movement compared to the anatomical ankle. This results in prolonged heel strike and weight bearing through the heel with delayed forefoot loading. The energy generated by the prosthetic limb is reduced significantly to that which would be generated by the normal limb, which is compensated by greater energy expenditure in muscles higher up the limb. The rocker effect of the prosthesis results in increased instability and the reduced knee flexion achieved on the prosthetic side requiring hip muscles to generate greater energy to ensure stability. As the body transfers weight in a forward motion this energy generation is then transmitted to the trunk muscles in order to generate enough force to propel the body forward and to compensate for the loss of energy through the prosthesis.

Due to the reduced ankle movement of the prosthesis the range of extension at the hip is reduced to approximately half of that of the opposite limb. The stance time on the non-prosthetic side is also increased compared to the prosthetic side.

During swing phase
During swing phase of the nonprosthetic limb the body weight begins to move forward over the prosthetic limb, which is in stance phase. In order to gain adequate step length of the nonprosthetic limb, heel rise on the prosthesis occurs earlier. The heel rise achieved is greater than that of a normal gait pattern. This creates an elevation of the body and results in a greater loading force on the nonprosthetic side, as the body weight drops more rapidly onto the limb. Greater quadriceps contraction is needed to absorb the force. The "toe off" force generated from the prosthetic limb is reduced, which is compensated for by the hip flexors. Flexion of the knee on the prosthetic limb occurs with some hamstring with maximum eccentric contraction of the quadriceps.

Training on Functional Use of Upper Limb Prosthesis

The prosthesis is either body powered or motorized (myoelectric). If a myoelectric prosthesis is being considered, this is an appropriate time to utilize a myotester to gauge the electric potential generated by various muscles. The myotester results should be discussed with a prosthetist, particularly for the proximal levels of amputation. This helps to determine the best positions for placement of electrodes.

The following body control motions are used to operate the prosthesis powered by body for functional use.

- **Scapular abduction:** Spreading the shoulder blades apart in combination with humeral flexion, or alone, provide tension on the figure-of-8 harness in order to open the terminal device.
- **Chest expansion:** This motion should be practiced by deeply inhaling, expanding the chest as much as possible, and then relaxing slowly. The chest expansion may be utilized in a variety of ways for the transhumeral, shoulder disarticulation, or forequarter amputee, through a cross-chest strap harness.
- **Shoulder depression, extension, and abduction:** This is the combined movement necessary to operate the body-powered, internal-locking elbow of the transhumeral prosthesis.
- **Humeral flexion:** The amputee is instructed to raise his residual limb forward to shoulder level and to push his arm forward while sliding the shoulder blades apart as far as possible. This motion applies pressure on the cable and allows the terminal device to open.
- **Elbow flexion/extension:** It is critical to instruct the transradial amputee to maintain full elbow range of motion. This range will enable him to reach many areas of his body without undue strain or special modifications to the prosthesis.
- **Forearm pronation/supination:** In the long transradial amputee, it is equally important to maintain as much forearm pronation and supination as possible. This will enable the amputee to position the terminal device where he chooses without manually prepositioning the wrist unit.

DISCHARGE PLANNING

Before discharge of the patient, the physiotherapist should ensure that, the patient has been adequately educated for ongoing management with the prosthesis, has learnt the strategies for coping and has been adequately trained to resume functional/vocational activities.

Follow-up Management

The patients are advised to come for follow up regularly to the rehabilitation center. The physiotherapist along with the other members of the team, reviews the patient and establishes, whether the patient's mobility has increased or decreased at follow up. Any modification of the prosthesis and exercise regime, required to maintain/enhance mobility are recommended, and done at follow up.

Physiotherapy in Arthritis

ARTHRITIS

The term arthritis is derived from arthr (meaning joint) and itis (meaning inflammation)

Arthritis is the destructive inflammatory lesion of joint(s) leading to joint pain, joint stiffness, swelling, redness, deformity of joints, abnormal gait, and loss of function. In some types of arthritis such as rheumatoid arthritis, systemic lupus erythematosus apart from joints other organs of the body are also affected, leading to malaise, weight loss, fatigue, poor sleep, etc. Arthritis can have a gradual or sudden onset.

Pain, which can vary in severity, is a common symptom in all types of arthritis. Besides joint symptoms, secondary effects such as muscle weakness, loss of flexibility and decreased aerobic fitness are also found in the sufferers.

Though different types of arthritis exist, the most common types described in this chapter include Osteoarthritis (OA), Rheumatoid arthritis (RA), Psoriatic arthritis, Syphilitic arthritis, Gouty arthritis, Ankylosing spondylitis (AS).

Whatever may be the type of arthritis, treatments including physiotherapy are instituted as per the stages of the International classification of function (ICF) model, i.e., Impairment→Activity limitation→Participation limitation, so that the patient lives a painless life with maintenance and restoration of function and overall improved quality of life.

Physiotherapy for arthritis focuses upon:
- Assessment of patients, goal settings and management planning.
- Reduction of inflammation, so that pain, swelling will subside and function will be maintained/restored.
- Maintenance and restoration of joint range of motion.
- Prevention of muscle atrophy and weakness and improving muscle strength and endurance.
- Prevention of deconditioning effects and maintain and restores fitness.
- Improvement of functional mobility, self-care skills, gait and skills for instrumental activities of daily living.
- Teaching joint protection and energy conservation techniques for better living (Described under Rheumatoid arthritis).
- Recommending appropriate splints, orthosis, modified footwear, adaptive devices/equipment, walking aids for making living comfortable.
- Providing postoperative therapy as and when surgical management is performed.

It should be understood tha, there is no cure for arthritis. Medical, therapeutic, orthotic, and surgical managements are performed through a coordinated approach of members of arthritic clinic to make living of the patient comfortable.

The common arthritic conditions and their managements are discussed below:

Osteoarthritis (OA)

Osteoarthritis is also called, degenerative arthritis, is a most common type of arthritis. Though it mostly affects the weight-bearing joints of the body, it can also affect any large and small joints such as hip, knee, ankle, vertebral column, wrist, small joints of hands, and feet. OA is now recognized as a disease involving the entire joint, including progressive destruction of articular cartilage, formation of bone spurs (osteophytes) at the margins of joints and involvement of the periarticular soft tissues.

Epidemiology and Etiology

Osteoarthritis is the most common type of arthritis. It is the main cause of chronic musculoskeletal pain and disability among the elderly population. It affects men more than women, under the age of 50 years, however, women over the age of 50 years are more affected than men. Overall, women are more affected than men for this disorder. More than 30% of women have some degree of OA by age 65 years. The population suffered from OA increases with age.

Risk factors for osteoarthritis include prior joint trauma, obesity, and a sedentary lifestyle.

The disorder is categorized into:
1. Primary OA (acquired from day-to-day wear and tear of joints).
2. Secondary OA (acquired as a result of injury to joint).

Though osteoarthritis affects many joints, the most common type, i.e., OA of knee is described here. When the spine is affected, it is called spondylosis. Sometimes Heberden's nodes (small pea sized bony growths) occur on the joints, closest to the tip of fingers), found in patients with OA of the hand.

Osteoarthritis of knee

Degenerative arthritis of knee joint is a common joint disorder affecting more or less every individual over the age of 40 years. Though the most common cause of OA is degeneration due to aging, significant other factors increase the risk of developing significant arthritis at an earlier age.

Common causes/risk factors for OA knee:
- **Age:** The ability of cartilage to heal decreases as a person gets older, hence results in progression of damage and subsequent changes in joint.
- **Weight:** Weight increases pressure on all the joints, especially the knees. Every pound (nearly 0.5 kg) of weight the person gains, adds 3–4 pounds (nearly 1.5 to 2 kg) of extra weight on the knees.
- **Heredity:** This includes genetic mutations that might make a person more likely to develop OA of the knee. It may also be due to inherited abnormalities in the shape of the bones that surround the knee joint.
- **Gender:** Women aged 55 years and older are more likely than men to develop OA of the knee.
- **Repetitive stress injuries:** These are usually a result of the type of job a person has. People with certain occupations that include a lot of activity that can stress the joint, such as kneeling, squatting, or lifting heavy weights (55 pounds/25 kilogram or more), are more likely to develop OA of the knee because of the constant pressure on the joint.
- **Athletics:** Athletes involved in soccer, tennis, or long-distance running may be at higher risk for developing OA of the knee, as very often they injure their menisci, ligaments, etc., making the knee joints unstable, which cause more wear and tear in the joint leading to arthritis.
- **Other illnesses:** People with rheumatoid arthritis/psoriatic arthritis/syphilitic arthritis are prone to develop OA knee. People with certain metabolic disorders, such as excess growth hormone, also run a higher risk of OA knee.

Pathophysiology

Osteoarthritis begins in the cartilage and eventually causes the two opposing bones to erode into each other. At first, there occurs increased water content of the articular cartilage.

The proteoglycans in articular cartilage swells with water far beyond normal. This process, together with disruption of other components of the extracellular matrix, decreases the stiffness of the matrix and leads to further mechanical damage. In later stages of disease progression, proteoglycans are lost, which diminishes the water content of cartilage. As proteoglycans are lost, articular cartilage loses its compressive stiffness and elasticity, which, in turn, results in the transmission of compressive forces to underlying bone. As the articular cartilage is destroyed, the joint space narrows. The early phases of cartilage degeneration are

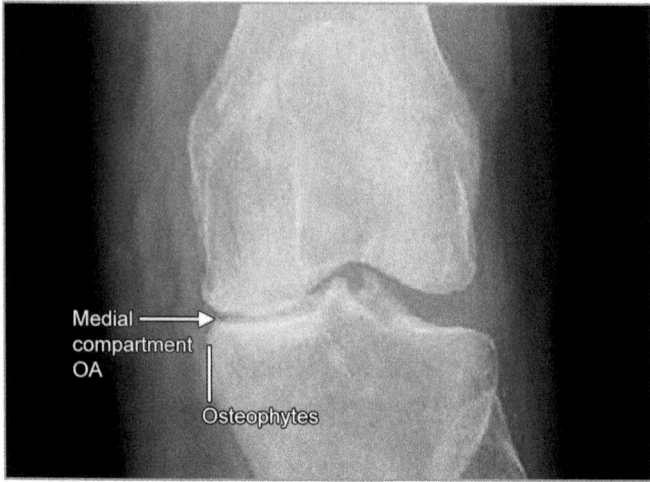

Fig. 15.1: X-ray showing osteoarthritis involving the medial compartment of knee joint with formation of osteophytes.

characterized by biosynthesis and repair as the chondrocytes attempt to restore the damaged matrix, while the later phase is degradative in nature as catabolic enzyme activity digests the matrix and erodes the cartilage.

As the cartilage degenerates, there are accompanying changes in the subchondral bone including increased bone density or subchondral sclerosis, creation of cyst-like bone cavities, and formation of marginal osteophytes **(Fig. 15.1)**. The cartilage may degenerate to the point that, the exposed subchondral bone becomes necrotic and eburnated (polished or ivory-like).

The condition starts with minor pain during physical activity, but soon the pain can be continuous and even occur while in a state of rest. Its progression usually occurs through the following four stages **(Figs. 15.2A to D)**:

Stage-1: At this stage, there occurs very minor wear and tear of the components of joints, resulting in minor growth of bone spurs.

Stage-2: At this stage, the cartilage of joint is still at a healthy size with sufficient amount of synovial fluid to facilitate joint motion. But there is greater bone spur growth, resulting in pain in joints after long-distance walking, kneeling, etc.

Stage-3: This is the moderate type of OA, in which the articular cartilage shows obvious damage and the joint space begins to decrease. The sufferers at this stage experience significant pain while walking, running, kneeling, squatting, as well as pain on prolonged sitting including morning stiffness.

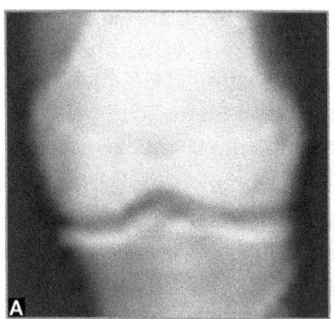 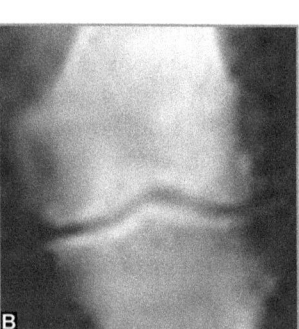 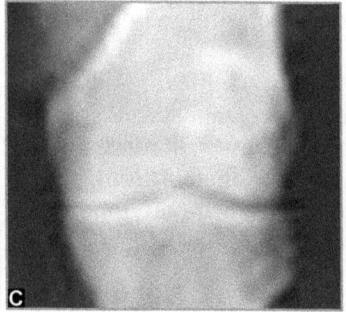 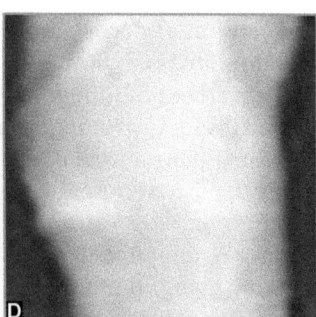

Figs. 15.2A to D: (A) Stage-1 OA knee; (B) Stage-2 OA knee; (C) Stage-3 OA knee; (D) Stage-4 OA knee.

Stage-4: This is the most severe type of OA, where the joint space is drastically reduced and the articular cartilage is completely lost. The joint becomes stiff, and the subject gets significant pain and discomfort, when walks or moves the joint.

Clinical Features

Although traditionally OA is viewed as a noninflammatory disease, inflammatory reactions occur in the joint in response to cartilage fragments in the synovial cavity and results in low grade synovitis. The following presentations are commonly seen:

- Pain that increases when the patient is active, but gets a little better with rest.
- Swelling.
- Presence of Baker's cyst (**Fig. 15.3**).
- Feeling of warmth in the joint.
- Stiffness in the knee, especially in the morning or when the patient is standing for a while. Limitation of patellofemoral and tibiofemoral range of motion (ROM) is usually seen.
- Tracking of patella laterally resulting in tightness of lateral patellar retinacular ligaments.
- Decrease in mobility of the knee, making it difficult to get in and out of chairs or cars, climb the stairs, or walk.
- Creaking/crepitus sound that is heard when the knee moves.
- Deformity in the form of genu varum (most common deformity due to involvement of medial compartment of knee) (**Fig. 15.4**), genu valgum, pes varum/pes valgus and knee flexion deformity due to tightness of posterior capsule of knee may be present in isolation or in combination. For example genu varum deformity is commonly associated with pes varum foot, and genu valgum is commonly associated with pes valgum foot.

The condition starts with minor pain during physical activities involving weight bearing on the affected leg such as climbing steps and squatting, but soon the pain can be continuous and even occur while in a state of rest, such as prolonged sitting. The medial compartment of the knee is commonly affected first due to higher weight bearing on

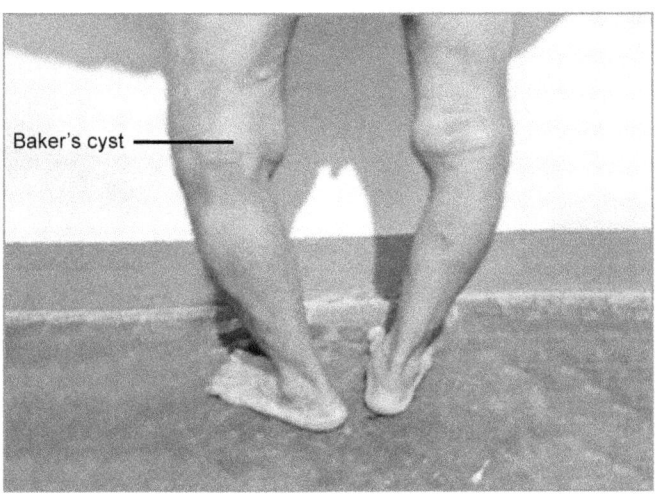

Fig. 15.3: Patient of OA knee with Baker's cyst.

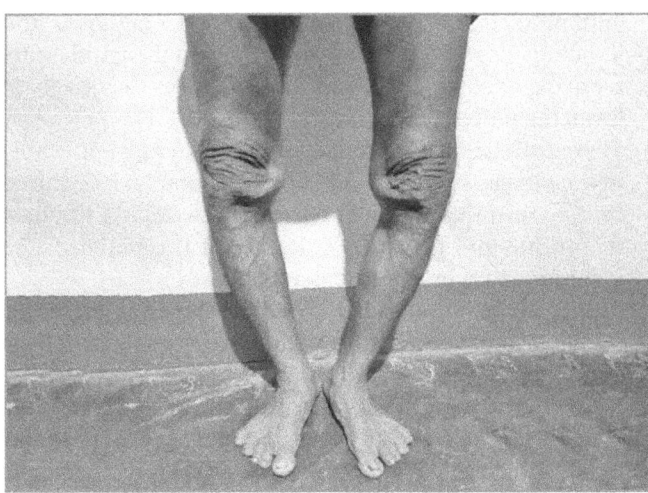

Fig. 15.4: OA knee with genu varum.

this compartment. Due to a decrease in medial joint space, there occurs laxity of medial collateral ligament, resulting in stretching of the lateral collateral ligament resulting in genu varum deformity. Symptoms of joint locking and buckling may also occur due to damage to stabilizing menisci and ligaments. Less commonly genu valgum deformity is seen due to involvement of the lateral compartment of the knee. Flexion deformity of the knee commonly develops due to the prolonged desire to keep the knee flexed (as it is the loose-packed position, giving more comfort), resulting in apparent shortening of the affected lower limb, producing limping on the affected side. Limping may also develop due to pain called antalgic gait.

Pain in the anterior aspect of the knee is due to involvement of patellofemoral joint and lateral tracking of patella.

Investigations

Radiology (X-ray): Reveals a decrease in joint space in medial compartment in the early stage with osteosclerosis of articular margin. Subsequently as the condition progresses, osteophytes form at the articular margin of femur, tibia, and patella and development of subchondral cysts occur. A varus or valgus deformity is also visible in the late stage of the disease.

Laboratory tests: Usually not required.

Management

A. **Medical management:** The medical management consists of NSAIDs, and sometimes injection of corticosteroids or hyaluronic acid into the knee.
B. **Physiotherapy:** Physiotherapy helps to reduce the pain, swelling, and stiffness of knee, and it can help improve knee joint function. It can also make it easier for the patient to walk, bend, kneel, squat, and sit. In fact, a 2000 study found that a combination of manual physical therapy and supervised exercise has functional benefits for patients with knee osteoarthritis and may delay or prevent the need for surgery.

The author is with the strong opinion that, physiotherapy started from the beginning, combined with weight control, joint protection and energy conservation techniques and judicious use of foot/knee orthosis help in significantly reducing pain and deformity and enhances the quality of life of the individual.

There are a multitude of therapeutic techniques applicable in the management of OA knee. The therapist is required to do a thorough clinical reasoning to decide the best technique and modality suitable for the patient. The techniques are briefly discussed below:

- **Advice on weight loss:** For patients, who are overweight, exercises and diet control advice are very essential to have a pain-free living.
- **Cold therapy:** Cold therapy is applied in acute stage, when severe pain and swelling persists. Cryopacks are also applied during active ROM exercises, when movement is grossly limited due to pain (Cryo-kinematics).
- **Heat therapy:** Heat therapy in the form of Paraffin wax bath, moist packs are applied before mobilization, when significant stiffness persists.
- **Deep transverse friction massage and patellofemoral mobilization:** Deep transverse friction massage (DTFM) to lateral patellar retinacular ligaments, stretching the lateral structures in patellafemoral joint and patellofemoral mobilization/gliding for patellofemoral joint pain/lateral tracking of patella.
- **Manual therapy:** Friction massage to lateral patellar retinacular ligaments to correct patellar alignment due to lateral tracking, patellofemoral mobilization and low-grade tibiofemoral mobilization (both accessory and physiological) in the presence of significant stiffness, help in reducing pain and increasing mobility and function.
- **Flexibility exercises:** Because knee OA often makes joint hard to move, flexibility exercises such as passive stretching of iliotibial band, quadriceps, hamstrings **(Fig. 15.5)**, tendo-Achilles, posterior capsule of knee, lateral patellar retinacular ligaments are very important. Doing them regularly can help increase range of motion, and restore normal knee joint function. Both strengthening and flexibility exercises are important to do because they can help take strain off the knee.
- **Traction:** Traction to the knee either manually or by using weight and pulley system is found to be helpful, in the chronic stage, particularly in stage-3 and stage-4, where significant joint space reduction and deformity like varus/valgus is present. However, studies required to be done to establish long-standing effects and load to be applied. The author successfully treats patients with OA knee by using ankle traction combined with Faradic type current stimulation with a load that gives comfort to the patient. **Figures 15.6A and B** show application of traction to knee using ankle strap for a patient of OA knee.
- **Strengthening exercises:** Isometric quadriceps sets **(Fig. 15.7)**. Nonweight-bearing concentric and eccentric exercises without increasing much joint pressure can be taught as per need and condition of knee joint.
- Prioceptive training as tolerated.
- **LASER therapy:** Low-level laser therapy (LLLT) is thought to have an analgesic effect as well as a

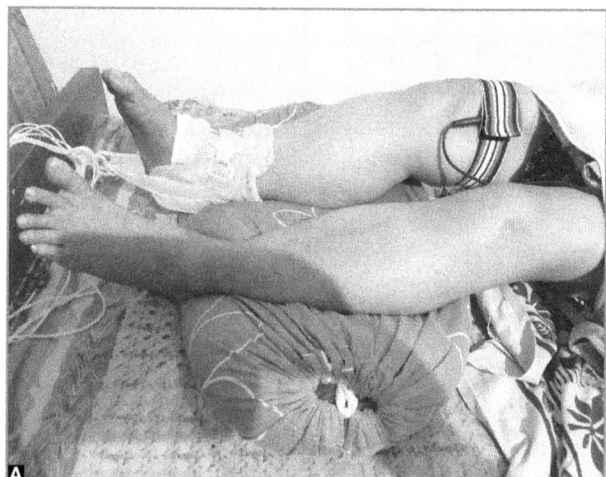

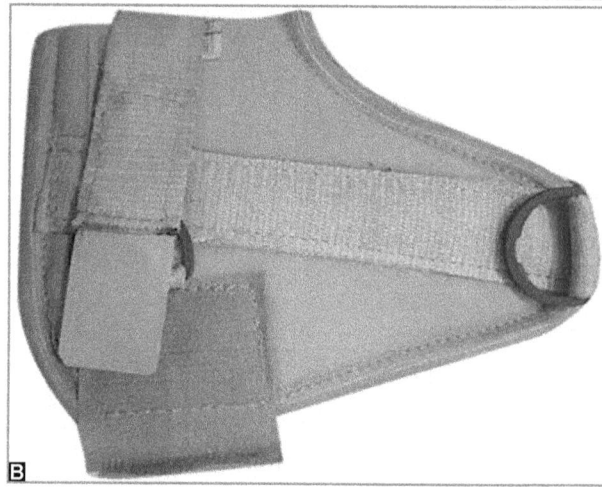

Fig. 15.5: Self-stretching of hamstrings and tendo achilles (TA).

Figs. 15.6A and B: (A) Patient of OA knee treated with ankle traction; (B) Ankle traction strap.

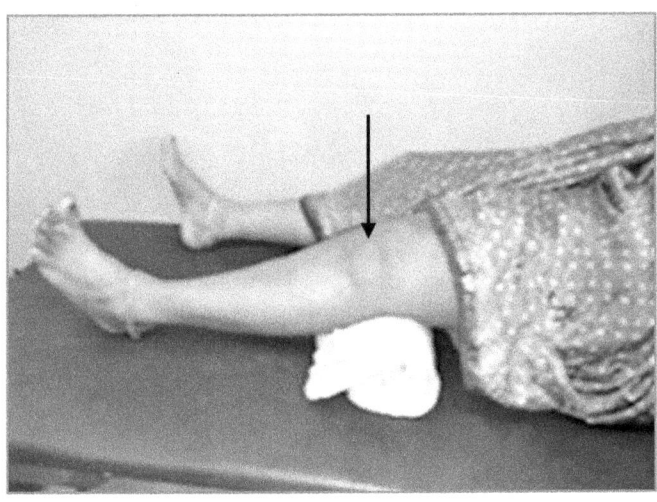

Fig. 15.7: Isometric quadriceps exercise.

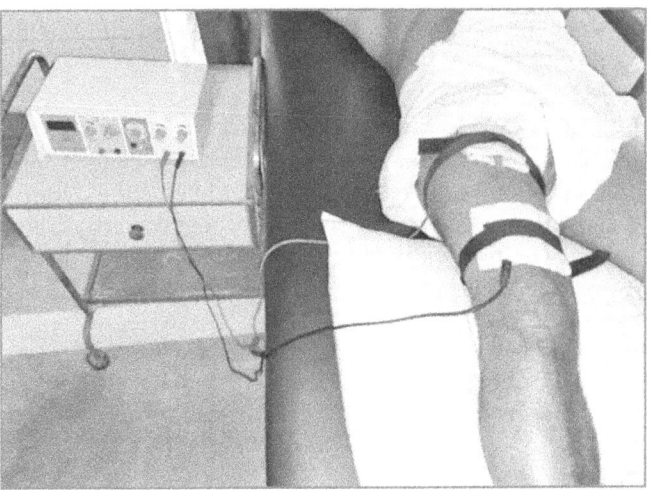

Fig. 15.8: Faradic stimulation to quadriceps.

biomodulatory effect on microcirculation. A study showed, patients with mild to moderate knee OA when delivered LLLT twice a week over a period of 4 weeks with a diode laser (wavelength 830 nm, continuous wave, power 50 mW) in skin contact at a dose of 6 J/point, resulted in improvement of pain (confirmed by VAS) and microcirculation (confirmed by thermographic measurements).

* **Low-intensity pulsed ultrasound (LIPUS):** Many researches have reported that LIPUS could induce extracellular matrix synthesis and increase rates of chondrocyte migration and proliferation, supporting that LIPUS has a chondroprotective effect in cellular experiments. In addition, data from animal experiments also showed that LIPUS could increase the synthesis of type II collagen in articular cartilage and exhibited the ability to attenuate the progression of cartilage degeneration in OA in different animal models. The intervention of LIPUS was suggested as early as possible by Gurkan et al.

In one study, the effect of therapeutic ultrasound on the pain, joint mobility, muscle strength, physical function, and quality of life of people with knee OA (Grade II or III tibiofemoral OA) was evaluated using 10 therapeutic ultrasound sessions using parameters such as (duty cycle = 20%, ERA = 10 cm², BNR = 6:1, SATP = 2.2 W/cm², SATA = 0.44 W/cm², frequency = 1 MHz, time = 4 minutes). It was found that therapeutic ultrasound applied in accordance with the parameters used, could decrease the intensity of pain after the 5th session, and this reduction was maintained until the end of the intervention.

12. **Neuromuscular electrical stimulation (NMES):** Various rehabilitation methods have been proposed to reverse the muscle weakness process. Among these, NMES such as stimulation with Faradic type current **(Fig. 15.8)** or Russian current treatment has been used to reduce the risk factors associated with the development and aggravation of the degenerative processes of OA. Its

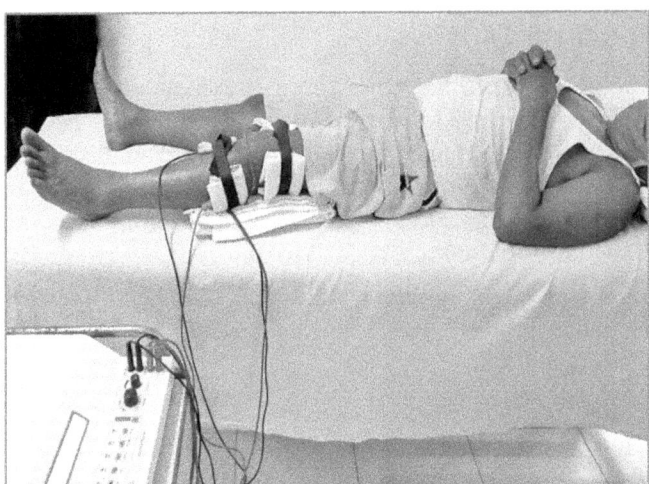

Fig. 15.9: IFT to knee joint.

main objective is to increase the musculature force that is inhibited due to joint pain (minimizing quadriceps inhibition), through the artificial generation of muscle contractions.

13. **Interferential therapy (IFT):** IFT to the knee can be selected to reduce pain and swelling. A quadripolar application is preferred over bipolar/premodular application **(Fig. 15.9)**.
14. **Hi-tone therapy:** It is an effective electrotherapy for OA of hip and knee and evidence exists for its efficacy.
15. **Hydrotherapy:** The warmth of water in hydrotherapy helps in facilitation of movement of painful joint; therefore helps in reduction of pain and restoration of ROM. The hydrostatic pressure helps in reducing swelling (if any) and gives proprioceptive stimulus to the knee. The buoyancy of water helps in strengthening of weak quadriceps, therefore improves strength and stability.
16. **Advice on joint protection and energy conservation:** The patient should be advised, not to stand for long time, not to sit on floor with legs crossed, to avoid frequent stair

climbing, not to carry heavy load on head and shoulders and to take frequent rest while engaged in physical/occupational activities.

Orthotic and assistive mobility devices:
- **Shoe modification:** Patients who develop genu varum/genu valgum are provided with modified shoe. **Figures 15.10A and B** show use of lateral border raised shoes with medial arch support in a patient of OA knee.
- Unloading knee brace/knee cap **(Figs. 15.11A and B)** with opening for patella.
- A walking stick should be advised to reduce load on the affected knee, if possible.

Surgery

Patients suffering from grade-4 OA knee are usually subjected to total knee replacement surgery, discussed in detail under physiotherapy for knee.

Rheumatoid Arthritis

Rheumatoid arthritis (RA) is a chronic inflammatory disease characterized by joint swelling, joint tenderness, and destruction of synovial joints, leading to severe disability, fatigue on activities, and premature mortality, due to involvement of various systems (such as cardiovascular, respiratory, gastrointestinal, etc.) of the body.

It is a systemic inflammatory polyarthritis, which is usually symmetrical, though a few (even a single joint)

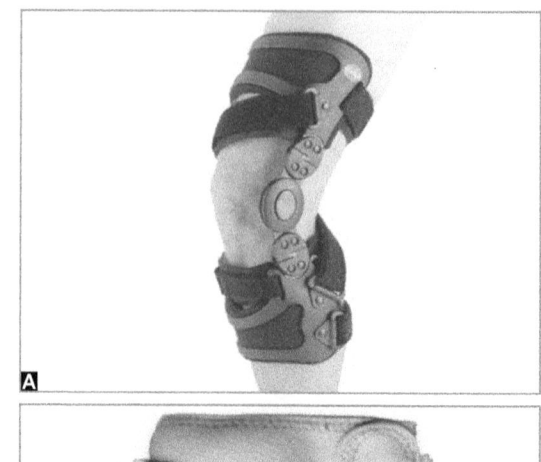
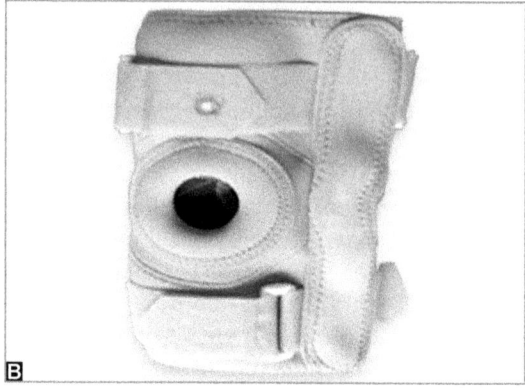

Figs. 15.11A and B: (A) Joint unloading knee brace; (B) Hinged knee cap.

joint affection is also seen. It is primarily a disease of the synovium. It is a disease in which the body's own immune system starts to attack body tissues. The attack is not only directed at the joint but at many other parts of the body. In RA, most damage occurs to the joint lining and cartilage, which eventually results in erosion of two opposing bones. RA often affects joints in the fingers, wrists, knees, and elbows, is symmetrical (appears on both sides of the body), and can lead to severe deformity in a few years, if not treated.

Epidemiology

The disease commonly occurs in women as compared to men at a female to male ratio of 3:1. Individuals between 35 and 55 years are commonly affected. In children, the disorder can present with a skin rash, fever, pain, disability, and limitations in daily activities. With earlier diagnosis and aggressive treatment, many individuals can lead a better quality of life.

Etiology

Rheumatoid arthritis is basically an autoimmune disease. Current theory and research on the cellular basis of autoimmunity suggest that aberrant functioning of cell-mediated immunity and defective T lymphocytes may trigger the autoimmune response that underlies RA.

Pathophysiology

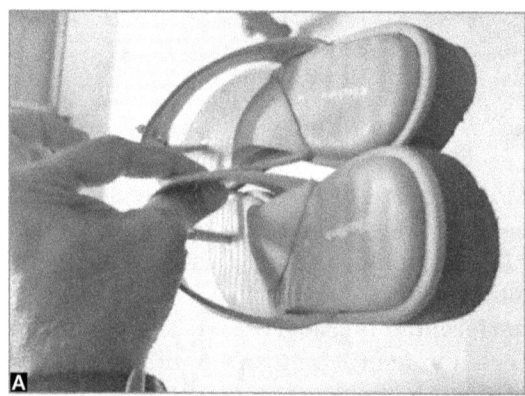
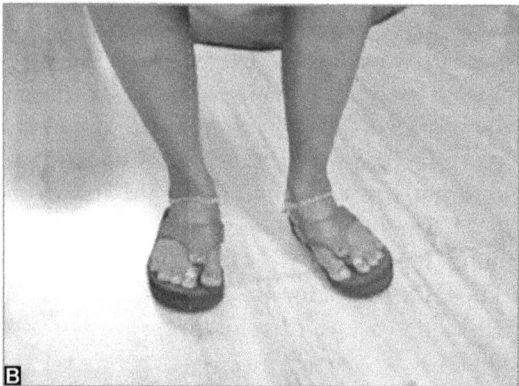

Figs. 15.10A and B: (A) A pair of shoes with lateral border raised and medial arch support; (B) Patient with OA knee and genu varum walking with modified (lateral border raised) shoe.

The condition starts with synovial inflammation that leads to pain, stiffness and restricted ROM. Subsequently, the joint capsule is inflamed and cartilage degradation occurs by immune cells. The synovium in long-standing arthritis, grossly becomes edematous causing slender villous projections into the joint cavity. With established synovitis, polymorphonuclear (PMN) leukocytes are drawn into the joint cavity and coupled with lysosomal enzyme activity contribute to destruction of synovial tissues, synovial proliferation of vascular granulation tissue called pannus, dissolves collagen as it extends over the joint cartilage. With progression of the disease the granulation tissue leads to adhesion, fibrosis of capsule, or bony ankylosis in some cases. Fraying of tendon sheaths and rupture of tendons lead to musculoskeletal deformities.

Classification of Progression of Rheumatoid Arthritis

Table 15.1 Briefly describes the stages of progression of the disease.

Table 15.1: Stages of progression of rheumatoid arthritis.			
Stage-I: Early (Stage of Synovitis)	**Stage-II: Moderate (Development of pannus)**	**Stage-III: Severe (Stage of fibrous ankylosis)**	**Stage-IV: Terminal (Stage of bony ankylosis)**
• No destructive changes on radiographic examination • Radiographic evidence of osteoporosis may be present • Synovitis is present	• Radiographic evidence of osteoporosis, with or without subchondral bone destruction. Slight cartilage destruction may be seen • Synovial proliferation of vascular granulation tissue (pannus) develops. • No joint deformity, although limitation of joint mobility may be seen • Adjacent muscle atrophy • Extra-articular soft tissue lesion such as nodules or synovitis may be seen	• Radiological evidence of cartilage and bone destruction, in addition to osteoporosis • Joint deformity such as subluxation, ulnar deviation, hyperextension with or without fibrous ankylosis • Extensive muscle atrophy • Extra-articular soft tissue lesion such as nodules or tenosynovitis may be present	• Fibrous or bony ankylosis • Criteria of stage-III

Diagnostic Criteria for Rheumatoid Arthritis

The American Rheumatism Association 1987, revised criteria help clinicians to diagnose rheumatoid arthritis. At least three joint areas (out of 14 possible areas, such as right or left PIP, MCP, wrist, elbow, knee, ankle, MTP joints) simultaneously have had soft tissue swelling or fluid (not bony overgrowth alone) as observed by a Physician. At least one area swollen (as defined above) in a wrist, MCP or PIP joint. Criteria 1–4 must be present for minimum 6 weeks. Confirmation of 4 or more of these 7 criteria, establishes rheumatoid arthitis.

The 1987 ARA revised criteria for the diagnosis of RA are given in **Table 15.2**.

Table 15.2: Criteria for diagnosis of RA.	
Criterion	**Definition**
1. Morning stiffness	Morning stiffness in and around the joints, lasting at least one hour before maximal improvement
2. Arthritis of three or more joints	At least three joint areas have had soft tissue swelling or fluid. The 14 possible areas are right or left PIP, MCP, wrist, elbow, knee, ankle, and MTP joints
3. Arthritis of hand joints	At least one area swollen in wrist, MCP or PIP joints
4. Symmetrical arthritis	Simultaneous involvement of same joint areas on both sides of the body
5. Rheumatoid nodules	Subcutaneous nodules over bony prominences, extensor surfaces or over juxta-articular regions
6. Serum rheumatoid factor	Demonstration of abnormal amount of serum rheumatoid factor by any method for which the result has been positive in less than 5% normal control subjects
7. Radiographic changes	Radiographic changes typical of rheumatoid arthritis on postero-anterior hand, wrist radiographs, which must include erosion or unequivocal bony decalcification, localized in or most marked adjacent to the involved joint

Clinical Features

❖ Tender, warm, swollen joints usually bilateral and symmetrical **(Fig. 15.12A)**.
❖ Early RA tends to affect the smaller joints first. As the disease progresses, symptoms often spread to the wrists, knees, ankles, elbows, hips, and shoulders.
❖ Joint stiffness that is usually worse in the mornings and after inactivity.
❖ Deformities, such as flexion deformities in hips, knees, elbows, and flexion and radial deviation deformities in wrist with dorsal subluxation of the ulnar head, with ulnar drift of fingers at the MCP joints, are commonly seen. Swan neck

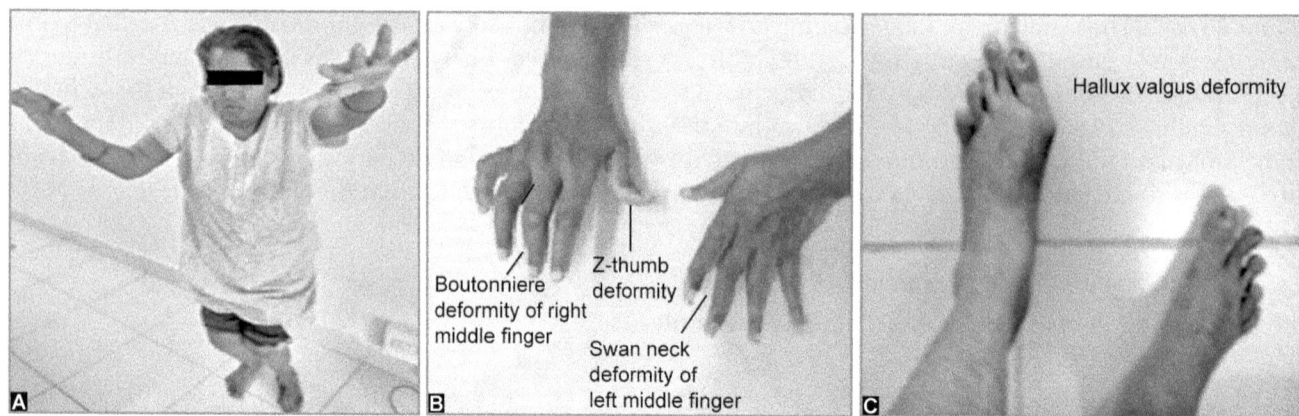

Figs. 15.12A to C: (A) Symmetrical involvement of joints; (B) Deformities in hand in RA; (C) Deformities in foot in RA.

deformity, boutonniere deformity, mallet finger deformity in fingers, and Z-thumb deformity of thumb **(Fig. 15.12B)** is found in progressive conditions. Deformities in foot, such as valgus foot deformities, hallux valgus deformities are found in most sufferers **(Fig. 15.12C)**.
- Muscle weakness and decreased endurance.
- Involvement of the ligaments of the cervical spine may produce subluxation and pain in cervical spine.
- Fatigue, fever, and weight loss.
- Other nonjoint structures affected are skin, eyes, lungs, heart, kidneys, blood vessels, nerves, etc.

Associated complications

Rheumatoid arthritis increases the risk of developing:
- **Osteoporosis:** The disease combined with the medications used for treating the same can increase the risk of osteoporosis.
- **Rheumatoid nodules:** These firm bumps of tissue most commonly form around pressure points, such as the elbows. However, these nodules can form anywhere in the body, including the lungs.
- **Sjogren's syndrome:** People who have RA are much more likely to experience this syndrome, where there is dryness of eyes and mouth.
- **Infections:** The patient is likely to get infections due to the disease process as well as medications used to treat the same.
- **Soft tissue problems:** Carpal tunnel syndrome, plantar fasciitis, etc., are commonly found in this disease.
- **Heart problems:** RA can lead to arteritis, pericarditis, etc.
- **Lung disease:** Inflammation and scarring of the lungs, leading to progressive dyspnea are the complications found in the lungs.
- **Lymphoma:** RA increases the risk of lymphoma, a group of blood cancers that develop in the lymphatic system.

Diagnosis

Blood tests to find the presence of the abnormal protein called rheumatoid factor (found positive in 85% of sufferers), helps in establishing the diagnosis when combined with clinical and radiological findings. Other blood tests such as ESR, CRP, which are usually elevated also help in establishing the diagnosis.

Management

There is no cure for the disease. Early identification, medical management, therapeutic interventions, orthotic management, joint protection, and energy conservation strategies, patient education, surgical intervention play a great role in controlling the disease and improving the quality of life of the patient.

Physiotherapy

The aims of physiotherapy are:
- Relief of pain and inflammation.
- Maintain joint range of motion and mobilize stiff joints.
- Prevention/correction of deformity.
- Prevention of muscle atrophy and weakness and strengthen inhibited/weak muscles.
- Improving endurance.
- Improving function and overall quality of life.

Procedure of physiotherapy:
- **In acute phase**: When pain swelling, erythema are significant, the below mentioned procedures are followed:
  - Positioning the affected joints in positions of ease, taking care that such positioning does not precipitate deformities.
  - Splints and casts to rest the affected joints.
  - Deep breathing exercise.
  - Low-intensity isometric exercises to muscles over inflamed joints.
  - Few repetitions of relaxed passive/active assisted/free exercises to the affected joints in the pain-free range.
  - Cryo packs/contrast bath to affected joints.
  - Faradic current stimulation to large postural muscle groups to overcome muscle inhibition due to pain.
  - Pulsed ultrasound/low-intensity LASER/TENS/IFT to be selected as indicated.
  - Hydrotherapy helps in resolution of joint symptoms and improves endurance.
- **In chronic arthritis:** In this state, the aims of therapy are:
  - Reduce pain and swelling.
  - Mobilize stiff joints and correct deformities.
  - Strengthen weak muscles.
  - To minimize cardiorespiratiory complications, if any.

- To improve endurance.
- To improve function.
- To make recommendation for appropriate splints, walking aids and adaptive devices to improve function.
- To improve the quality of life.

Strategies of physiotherapy in chronic arthritis:
- PWB to stiff joints.
- Contrast bath to reduce swelling.
- Low-grade mobilization exercises in the presence of joint stiffness.
- Gentle stretching/positional stretching exercises to stretch tight soft tissues and correct deformities.
- Active assisted/free exercises.
- Isometric exercise to postural muscles, like glutei, quadriceps, etc.
- Faradic stimulation to inhibited muscles.
- Pulsed ultrasound/LLLT/IFT/TENS.
- Splinting/serial casting for correction of deformities. A silver ring splint/gutter splint **(Figs. 15.13A to C)** is used to correct swan neck/boutonniere and mallet finger deformity. A ring splint can also be used to correct deformities in thumb.
- Hydrotherapy.
- Advice on use of assistive and adapted devices such as use of a gutter crutch, adapted spoon/adapted comb **(Figs. 15.14A and B)**, etc., to perform functional activities without damaging joints.
- *Advice on joint protection and energy conservation:* Energy conservation and joint protection techniques are suggested for persons with RA, OA, or any other joint-compromising disorder.

Joint protection and energy conservation techniques

Some tips to reduce joint pain and deformity are:
- Identify and respect **pain** as a warning signal of joint damage needing to **stop** the activity.
- Make a **schedule** of daily activities. Find out when pain and fatigue develops during activity and accordingly schedule rest breaks.
- Avoid **positions of deformity,** for example, when getting up from a chair, with hand pushing, use the palm, instead of the knuckles.

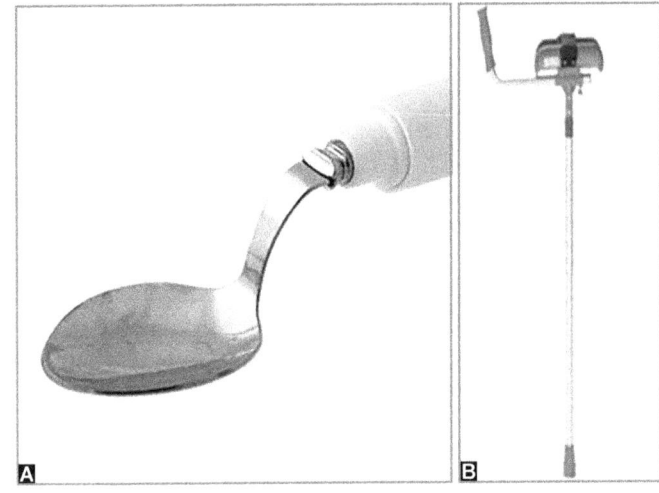

Figs. 15.14A and B: (A) Adapted spoon with handle; (B) Gutter crutch.

- Use the **largest** and **strongest** joints available for an activity. For example, carry bags on the shoulder instead of at the elbow, wrist, or fingers.
- Avoid staying in **one position** for a **long period of time.**
- Don't give the joints the **chance to become stiff**. When writing or doing handwork, release the grip every 10-15 minutes. On long car trips, get out of the car, stretch and move around at least every hour. While watching television get up and move around every 30 minutes. While doing official works, in one position, say working in the cash counter of a bank, use money counting machine, follow ergonomic measures and take rest breaks as much as possible.
- Use a **cart** to carry heavy items. If no cart is available, make several trips to get the job done, rather than lifting and carrying in one trip. **Slide** or **push** items whenever possible.
- Avoid making a **tight fist/tight pinch.** Use utensils with thick handle to make a grasp that places the **knuckles parallel** to the handle of the tool or utensil being used.
- **Do not** start an activity that cannot be **stopped immediately**, if pain or fatigue should occur.
- Follow **ergonomic** measures, for a commode in toilet, place kitchen sink up to the level of the waist, computer and key board should be placed within a distance of reach, and a revolving chair should be used to avoid repeated twisting of the spine.
- Do not climb stairs frequently. While climbing stairs hold railings.
- Reduce weight.

Surgery in RA

Sometimes, the patient with severe painful deformities in hands require surgery in the form of:
- Joint replacement surgery (including that of fingers).
- Arthrodesis (mostly for deformed wrist and foot).

Postoperative physiotherapy is instituted as per protocol to improve function.

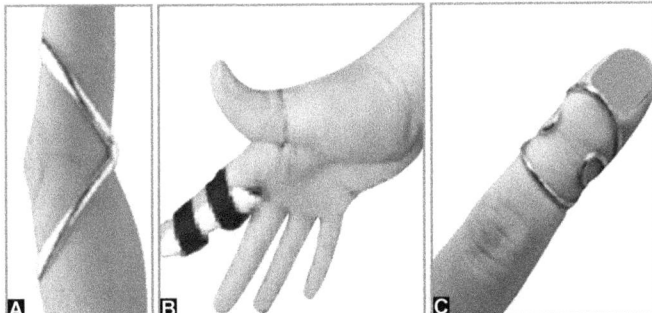

Figs. 15.13A to C: (A) A silver ring splint over PIP joint to correct swan neck/boutonniere deformity; (B) A volar gutter splint for deformities of finger; (C) A ring splint over DIP joint to correct mallet finger deformity.

Psoriatic Arthritis

Psoriatic arthritis (PsA) (also called as arthritis psoriatica, arthropathic psoriasis, or psoriatic arthropathy) is a type of inflammatory arthritis that develops in between 6 and 42% of people who have the chronic skin condition psoriasis. Psoriatic arthritis is classified as a seronegative spondyloarthropathy and therefore occurs more commonly in patients with tissue type HLA-B27 (predominantly spinal involvement). Those linked with HLADR4 demonstrate polyarthritis.

It is a form of arthritis that affects some people who have psoriasis—a condition that features red patches of skin topped with silvery scales **(Fig. 15.15)**. Most people develop psoriasis first and are later diagnosed with psoriatic arthritis, but the joint problems can sometimes begin before skin lesions appear.

Epidemiology/Etiology

Psoriatic arthritis usually shows up between ages 30 and 50 years, but it may start in childhood. Both men and women are equally affected.

Psoriatic arthritis occurs when the body's immune system begins to attack healthy cells and tissue. The abnormal immune response causes inflammation in the joints as well as overproduction of skin cells.

It is not entirely clear why the immune system turns on healthy tissue, but it seems likely that both genetic and environmental factors play a role. Many people with psoriatic arthritis have a family history of either psoriasis or psoriatic arthritis. Researchers have discovered certain genetic markers that appear to be associated with psoriatic arthritis.

Types of Psoriatic Arthritis

- **Symmetric psoriatic arthritis** affects several joints in pairs on both sides of the body, like both elbows and knees. It can be mild to severe. This type accounts for around 15% of cases, and affects joints on both sides of the body simultaneously. This type is most similar to rheumatoid arthritis and is disabling in around 50% of all cases. It destroys the joints over time, and they may stop working.

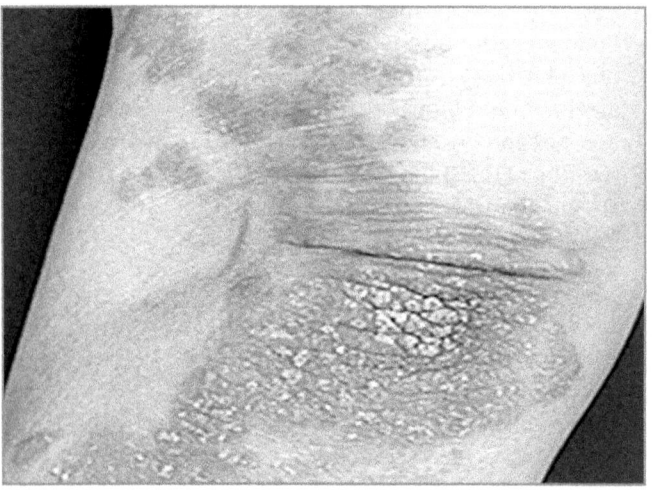

Fig. 15.15: Psoriasis.

- **Asymmetrical oligoarthritis:** This type affects around 70% of patients and is generally mild. This type does not occur in the same joints on both sides of the body and usually only involves fewer than three joints. It typically affects only a few joints. They can be large or small and anywhere in the body. Fingers and toes may swell-like sausages.
- **Distal interphalangeal predominant (DIP) psoriatic arthritis:** This type of psoriatic arthritis is found in about 5% of patients. It mainly affects small joints at the ends of the fingers and toes, as well as the nails. Sometimes it is confused with OA, what most people think of when they hear "arthritis", when the cartilage and bone in the joints wears away.
- **Psoriatic spondylitis:** It affects the spine. It is found up to 5% of cases. It can cause inflammation and stiffness between the vertebrae—the bones of the neck, spine, and lower back, and pelvis. Spondylitis can also attack ligaments that connect muscles to bones and other connective tissue (enthesitis). This type is characterized by stiffness of the spine, but can also affect the hands and feet, in a similar fashion to symmetric arthritis. The ankylosis in spine is patchy in nature, which differentiates it from ankylosing spondylitis.
- **Arthritis mutilans:** Arthritis mutilans affects less than 5% of patients and is a severe, deforming, and destructive arthritis. This condition can progress over months or years causing severe joint damage. Arthritis mutilans has also been called chronic absorptive arthritis, and may be seen in RA as well. It is the most severe and destructive form of psoriatic arthritis. Fortunately, it's rare. It damages the small joints in the fingers and toes so badly that they become deformed.

Clinical Features

Pain, swelling, or stiffness in one or more joints is commonly present in psoriatic arthritis. Psoriatic arthritis is inflammatory, and affected joints are generally red or warm to the touch. Asymmetrical oligoarthritis, defined as inflammation affecting 1–3 joints during the first 6 months of disease, is present in 70% of cases. However, in 15% of cases the arthritis is symmetrical. The joints of the hand that are involved in psoriasis are the proximal interphalangeal (PIP), the DIP, the metacarpophalangeal (MCP), and the wrist. Involvement of the DIP is a characteristic feature and is present in 5% of cases.

In addition to affecting the joints of the hands and wrists, psoriatic arthritis may affect the fingers, nails, and skin. Sausage-like swelling in the fingers **(Fig. 15.16)** or toes, known as dactylitis, may occur. The nail changes include pitting or separation from the nail bed (onycholysis), hyperkeratosis under the nails, and horizontal ridging. Psoriasis classically presents with scaly skin lesions, which are most commonly seen over extensor surfaces such as the scalp, posterior trunk, natal cleft and umbilicus.

Along with the above noted pain and inflammation, there is extreme exhaustion that does not go away with adequate rest. The exhaustion may last for days or weeks without remission.

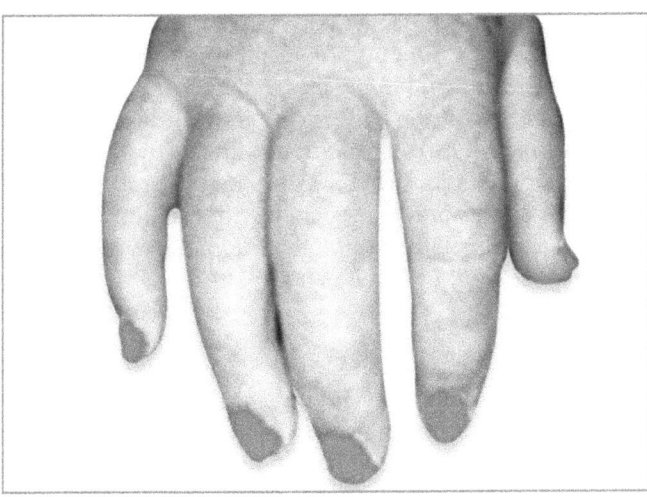

Fig. 15.16: Sausage finger.

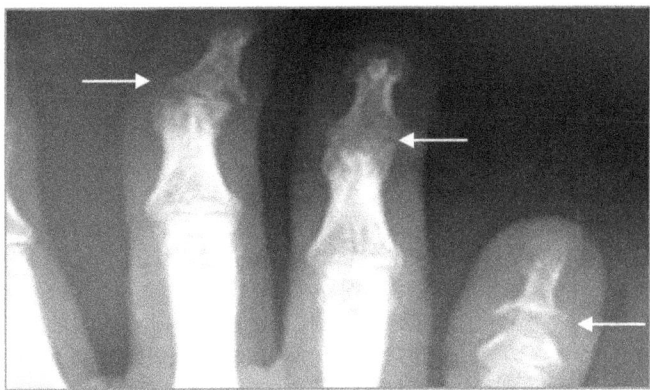

Fig. 15.17: X-ray shows pencil-in-cup deformity (typical in PsA).

Psoriatic arthritis may remain mild, or may progress to more destructive joint disease. Periods of active disease, or flares, will typically alternate with periods of remission.

Diagnosis

There is no definitive test to diagnose psoriatic arthritis. Physical examinations, health history, blood tests, and X-rays (pencil in cup deformity) **(Fig. 15.17)**, help to diagnose psoriatic arthritis, differentiating it from other similar conditions like RA.

Factors that contribute to a diagnosis of psoriatic arthritis include:
- Psoriasis in the patient, or a family history of psoriasis or psoriatic arthritis.
- A negative test result for rheumatoid factor, a blood factor associated with RA.

Management

The disease is managed in the same lines as rheumatoid arthritis, except the additional factor psoriasis (if present) needing separate consideration. The components of management include:
- **Medical management:** NSAIDs, Disease-modifying antirheumatic drugs (DMARDs), immunosuppressants, biologic agents, enzyme inhibitors, etc. are prescribed by the rheumatologist/physician.
- **Physiotherapy:** Therapeutic exercises/cryotherapy/ heat therapy/ultrasound therapy/laser therapy/Faradic current stimulation/IFT/TENS/Energy conservation and joint protection techniques are applied thorough clinical reasoning in the same lines of management of rheumatoid arthritis. Breathing exercise and endurance training are also important components of management. Hydrotherapy in the absence of psoriasis is an effective method to improve mobility and reduce pain. PUVA (Psoralen UVA) is applied for treatment of psoriasis.
- Orthosis and splints such as a Bunion splint for great toe **(Fig. 15.18A)**, thumb spica splint **(Fig. 15.18B)**, gutter splint **(Fig. 15.18C)**, etc., should be considered as applicable. Walking aids such as a gutter crutch is recommended, if the patient needs such devices for ambulation.

Surgery

In psoriatic arthritis patients with severe joint damage, orthopedic surgery may be implemented to correct joint destruction, usually with use of a joint replacement. Joints that have been severely damaged by psoriatic arthritis can be replaced with artificial prostheses made of metal and plastic. In the absence of joint replacement, arthrodesis of the joints in functional position can be considered.

Postoperatively physiotherapy is instituted as per the protocol.

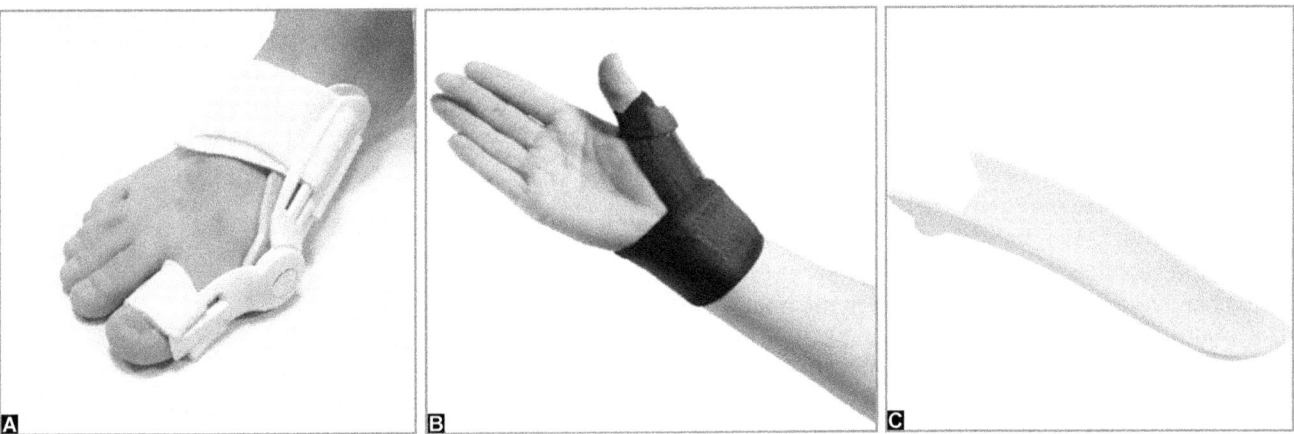

Figs. 15.18A to C: (A) Bunion splint; (B) Thumb spica splint; (C) Finger gutter splint.

Syphilitic Arthritis

Syphilis is a sexually transmitted infection caused by the bacterium *Treponema pallidum*. The disease could be of two types such as:
1. Acquired syphilis;
2. Congenital syphilis.

- **Aquired syphilis:** The signs and symptoms of acquired syphilis vary depending on which of the four stages it presents (primary, secondary, latent, and tertiary).
  - **Primary stage:** The primary stage (3–30 days) classically presents with single/multiple chancres (a firm, painless, non-itchy ulceration) in skin, mouth and genital organs. There is no arthritis in this stage.
  - **Secondary stage:** In the secondary stage (4–12 weeks), diffuse rash develops, which frequently involves the palms of the hands and soles of the feet. There may also be sores in the mouth or vagina. Lymphadenopathy, arthritis, malaise, fever are also the presentations in this stage.
  - **Latent syphilis:** In latent syphilis, which is dormant for 1–2 years, there are a few or no symptoms present.
  - **Tertiary syphilis:** In tertiary syphilis (noninfectious), there are gummas (soft noncancerous growths), neurological, or heart symptoms.
- **Congenital syphilis:** This disease is transmitted during pregnancy or during birth. Two-thirds of syphilitic infants are born without symptoms. Common symptoms that develop over the first couple of years of life include enlargement of the liver and spleen (70%), skin rash (70%), fever (40%), neurosyphilis (20%), and lung inflammation (20%). If untreated, late congenital syphilis may occur in 40%, cases, causing saddle nose deformation, Higoumenakis sign (unilateral enlargement of the sternoclavicular portion of the clavicle), saber shin (malformation of the tibia, resulting in anterior bowing), or Clutton's joints (painless swelling of joints, most commonly knee joints on both sides), etc.
  - **Syphilitic arthritis:** Arthritis occurring in secondary and tertiary stages of acquired syphilis and in congenital syphilis, with or without tenderness, swelling and limitation of motion of joints is termed as syphilitic arthritis.

Joint involvement in acquired secondary syphilis leads to arthralgia in which the pain is never severe and is felt like an ache. It usually affects one or more of the larger joints and the pain felt mostly at night. There is no joint inflammation and deformity found. However, joint involvement in tertiary syphilis leads to painless joints called "Charcot's joints".

Joint lesions in congenital syphilis leads to:
- **Parrot's syphilitic osteochondritis:** Within the first 8 months of life, osteochondritis especially of the long bones and ribs may cause pseudoparalysis of the limbs with characteristic radiologic changes in the bones. This is an epiphysitis, or a juxtaepiphyseal inflammation, which occurs during the first few months of life in children with inherited syphilis. It affects the upper limbs more frequently than the lower, and is often associated with an effusion into the adjacent joint.
- **Clutton's joint:** It occurs between 5 and 20 years of age in both sexes. This condition results in symmetrical joint swelling. It is also known as symmetrical hydrarthrosis of childhood. Knees are most commonly affected by synovitis and joint effusions followed by the ankles, elbows, wrists and fingers. It is usually painless and usually no disability associated with the joint swelling. Recovery is usually complete. The patients are able to walk quite well.

Diagnosis

Syphilis is difficult to diagnose clinically early in its presentation. Confirmation is either via blood tests or direct visual inspection using microscopy.

Blood tests are divided into nontreponemal [veneral disease research laboratory test (VDRL), rapid plasma regain (RPR) test] and treponemal tests [*Treponema pallidum hemagglutination* (TPHA) test, or fluorescent treponemal antibody absorption test (FTA-Abs)]. Dark ground microscopy of serous fluid from a chancre may be used to make an immediate diagnosis.

Management

Treatment is most unsatisfactory and disappointing. Penicillin is the drug of choice for the condition.

Physiotherapy

Cold packs to reduce inflammation and swelling, relaxed passive exercises, isometric exercise to major muscle groups (quadriceps, glutei, hamstrings), proprioceptive training, joint protection and energy conservation techniques, use of modalities like IFT/TENS to reduce pain (if any).

Orthotic management

For anesthetic joints like Charcot's joints, Clutton's joint a functional orthosis is recommended to prevent injury to joints.

Surgery

It consists of arthrodesis of unstable painless joints in functional position to improve function.

Gouty Arthritis

Gouty arthritis is a form of arthritis characterized by severe pain, redness, and tenderness in joints, caused due to accumulation of too much uric acid in joints. When the body has extra uric acid, sharp crystals (Sodium biurate crystal) may form in the big toe **(Fig. 15.19)** or other joints, called gouty tophi, causing episodes of swelling and pain called gout attacks.

Pathophysiology

It is caused by a build-up of uric acid crystals in the joints. Uric acid is a breakdown product of purines that are part of many foods. An abnormality in handling uric acid and crystallization of these compounds in joints can cause attacks of painful arthritis.

Clinical Features

Acute gout attacks are characterized by a rapid onset of pain in the affected joint followed by warmth, swelling, erythema,

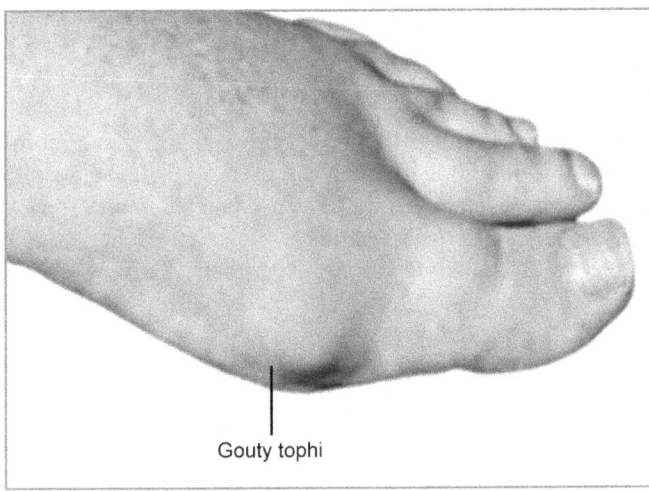

Fig. 15.19: Gouty tophi (Deposit of sodium biurate crystals) on metatarsophalangeal joint of great toe.

and marked tenderness. The small joint at the base of the big toe is the most common site for an attack. Other joints that are affected include the ankles, knees, wrists, fingers, and elbows. In some people, the acute pain is so intense that even a bedsheet touching the toe causes severe pain. These painful attacks usually subside in hours to days, with or without medication. In rare instances, an attack can last for weeks. Most people with gout will experience repeated bouts over the years.

Diagnosis

Diagnosis of gouty arthritis is mostly done from the appearances of the affected joint, i.e., pain and swelling, erythema, and deposition of uric acid crystals over the affected joints. However, the following diagnostic tests help in confirming diagnosis:
- Joint fluid examination to find biurate crystals.
- Blood tests, indicating raised uric acid level [Normal uric acid levels are 2.4–6.0 mg/dL (female) and 3.4–7.0 mg/dL (male)].
- X-ray showing crystal deposits over joints and features of arthritis **(Fig. 15.20)**.
- Ultrasonography to detect uric acid crystals.

Management
- **Medical management:** It consists of drugs to reduce pain and inflammation as well as levels of uric acid. Dietary advice is an important component of management. Foods and drinks that often trigger gout attacks include organ meats, game meats (flesh of wild animals/birds), some types of fish, fruit juice, sugary sodas and alcohol. On the other hand, fruits, vegetables, whole grains, soy products and low-fat dairy products may help prevent gout attacks by lowering uric acid levels.
- **Physiotherapy:** It consists of:
  - Cryotherapy to reduce inflammation during acute stage.
  - Isometric exercises.
  - PWB/Contrast bath as indicated.

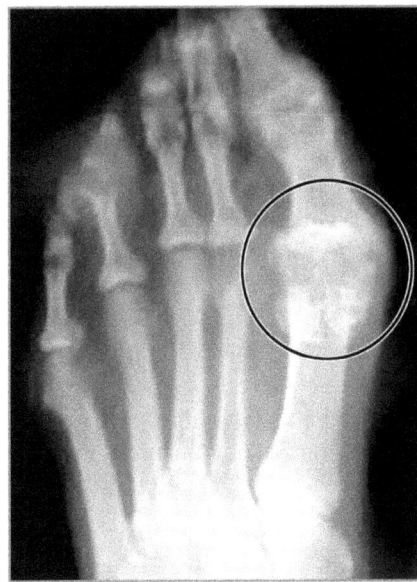

Fig. 15.20: X-ray showing gouty arthritis of first MTP joint.

- Relaxed passive exercises, active assisted/free exercises.
- Iontophoresis with lithium ion to reduce gouty tophi.
- Recommendation for appropriate splints, such as a Bunion splint to prevent development of hallux valgus deformity.
- Advice on energy conservation and joint protection techniques.

Ankylosing Spondylitis

Ankylosing spondylitis (AS) is a seronegative chronic inflammatory autoimmune disease of the spine and sacroiliac joints with or without involvement of the peripheral joints. It may be associated with pathology involving a number of extra-articular structures, such as the eye, gastrointestinal (GI) tract, skin, lungs, kidneys, and heart.

Etiology/Epidemiology

Ankylosing spondylitis usually begins in the second or third decade with a male-to-female prevalence between 2:1 and 3:1. The etiology of the disease remains unclear, but appears to be immune-mediated, and associated with a strong inheritable component: human leukocyte antigen (HLA) B27. HLA-B27 is found in 90–95% of patients with AS, compared to a 6–9% incidence in the normal population.

A strong link has been established of complex interactions between genetic background and environmental factors. Studies have shown factors such as genetic background, microbial infection, endocrine abnormalities, etc., are related to the occurrence of the disease.

Types of Ankylosing Spondylitis

The disease is classified into the following types:
- Classification depending upon the areas affected. As per the pattern of affection, it is classified into the following two types:
  - *Marie-Strumpell disease:* Named for the French neurologist Pierre Marie (1853–1940) and the German

neurologist whose full name was Ernst Adolf Gustav Gottfried von Strumpell (1853–1925). This is the axial spondyloarthritis, typically affecting, the thoracic cage, spine, and sacroiliac joints and hips. The onset of this disease is usually insidious. In this type, the patient presents with dull pain in the lower lumbar region or gluteal region. He/she complains of morning stiffness of the lower back that lasts for a few hours and improves with activity. The pain tends to persist for more than 3 months, and is notably worsened by rest and improved by exercise. Nocturnal exacerbations of the pain will often force the patient to rise, and move around. Enthesitis (inflammation at tendinous and ligamentous attachments) is one of the central features of the disease, and results in many of the presenting symptoms of pain.

- *Bechterew's disease:* This is a spondyloarthritis, affecting spine and the large joints. The symptoms typically appear in the early adulthood, which include reduced flexibility and pain in the spine, as well as pain in the peripheral joints such as hip joint, shoulder joint, ankle/foot etc. It is a chronic rheumatic disorder mostly found in young male adults aged between 20 and 30 years.

❖ **Classification as per radiographical changes:** It is classified into the following two types such as:
- *Nonradiographic axial spondyloarthritis (nr-axSpA):* This is the less severe form of spondyloarthritis. "Nonradiographic" means that something is not easily visible on an X-ray, suggesting AS. Other sensitive tests such as MRI, serological tests, etc., may be required to diagnose the condition.
- *Radiographic axial spondyloarthritis:* This is the last phase of AS. It happens when nr-axSpA gradually gets worse and affects the sacroiliac joints and the joints of the spine. Noticeable changes in the X-ray, in the SI joints and spine suggests about this disease.

Pathophysiology

The primary pathology of the spondyloarthropathies is enthesitis with chronic inflammation, including CD4+ and CD8+ T-lymphocytes and macrophages. Cytokines, particularly tumor necrosis factor-α (TNF-α) and transforming growth factor-β (TGF-β), are also important in the inflammatory process leading to inflammation, fibrosis, and ossification at sites of enthesitis. The pathology mainly affects the entheses, where ligaments, tendons and capsules are attached to the bone. Three processes are observed at the entheses: inflammation, bone erosion and syndesmophyte (spur) formation. Tumor necrosis factor is an important mediator of the inflammatory processes, but this proinflammatory cytokine is not closely involved in bone erosion or syndesmophyte formation.

Calcification of the ligaments and the syndesmophytes that form, leads to fusion of the vertebrae, resulting in the appearance of bamboo spine. Progressive erosion of anterior margin of vertebrae (called Romanus lesion), leads to kyphotic deformity of spine.

Clinical Features

The disease starts insidiously, with presentation of symptoms of low back pain, due to involvement of sacroiliac joints and lumbar spine (in Marie Strumpell type—most common). There is decreased lumbar lordosis and painful limitation of movements of spine **(Fig. 15.21A)**. Gradually, the thoracic spine, costochondral/costovertebral joints, along with shoulders and hips are affected. However, in Bechterew's type, the peripheral joints are affected predominantly, along with involvement of spine.

The individual, usually a young adult male complains of pain more during rest (mostly at night), with significant morning stiffness. There is gradual remission on activities/exercises.

As the disease progresses, the joints become stiff, initially due to fibrous ankylosis, progressing to bony ankylosis. Ankylosis is mostly seen in the spines and hips making the patient disabled with a reduced quality of life. The individual develops kyphotic deformity in spine and has significantly reduced chest excursion/vital capacity. He/she may also have other extra-articular features like involvement of GI system, lungs, kidney, heart, eyes, etc.

The individual develops postural and gait abnormalities **(Fig. 15.21B)**, and subsequently, has difficulty in self-care and occupational activities. The disease sometimes worsens progressively, or the symptoms sometimes have a remitting and relapsing course. If the disease could not be arrested, sometimes it turns fatal mostly due to respiratory complications.

Diagnosis

X-ray, clinical features, blood tests help in the diagnosis of the disease.

❖ **X-ray:** Initially shows involvement of sacroiliac joints in the form of sclerosis and reduction of joint space. Subsequently, the patient develops fusion of SI joints, inter-vertebral joints due to calcification of the ligaments and formation of syndesmophytes **(Figs. 15.22A and B)**.

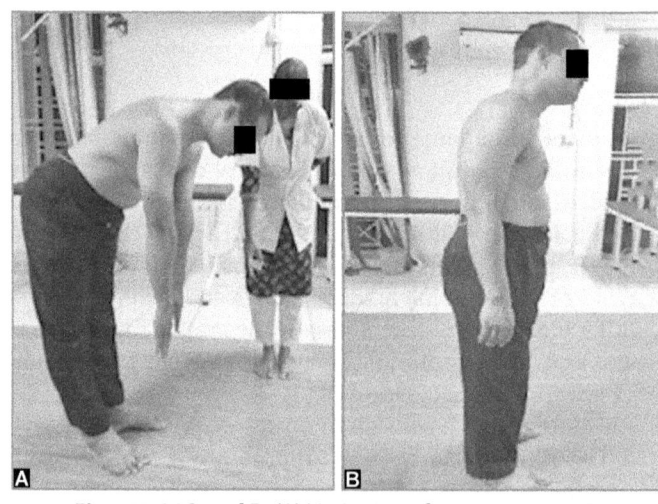

Figs. 15.21A and B: (A) Limitation of movement in AS; (B) Postural abnormalities in AS.

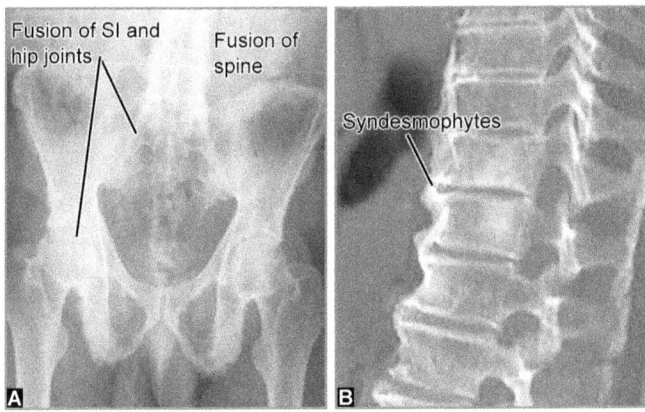

Figs. 15.22A and B: (A) X-ray showing fusion of spine, SI joints and hips; (B) X-ray shows syndesmophytes.

There is squaring of vertebral body with erosion of the anterior margin of the vertebral bodies (Romanus lesion).
- *MRI:* MRI scans can reveal evidence of AS earlier in the disease process, but are much more expensive.
- *Blood tests:* The ESR may be slightly elevated, with elevation of CRP in serum, however, in some sufferers ESR and CRP may be found normal. HLAB27 may be positive in nearly 90% of sufferers.

The Modified New York Criteria for diagnosis of ankylosing spondylitis

The criteria proposed in 1984 help in diagnosing the condition.
- Low back pain for at least 3 months' duration that is improved by exercise, and not relieved by rest.
- Limitation of the lumbar spine motion in the sagittal and frontal planes.
- Chest expansion that is decreased relative to normal values for age and sex.
- Radiographic unilateral sacroiliitis grade 3–4.
- Radiographic bilateral sacroiliitis grade 2–4.

Sacroiliitis grading can be achieved using plain radiographs according to the New York criteria. The grades are:
- **Grade 0:** Normal **(Fig. 15.23A)**
- **Grade 1:** Suspicious changes (some blurring of the joint margins) **(Fig. 15.23B)**.
- **Grade 2:** Minimum abnormality (small localized areas with erosion or sclerosis, with no alteration in the joint width) **(Fig. 15.23C)**.
- **Grade 3:** Unequivocal abnormality (moderate or advanced sacroiliitis with erosions, evidence of sclerosis, narrowing of width, or partial ankylosis) **(Fig. 15.23D)**.

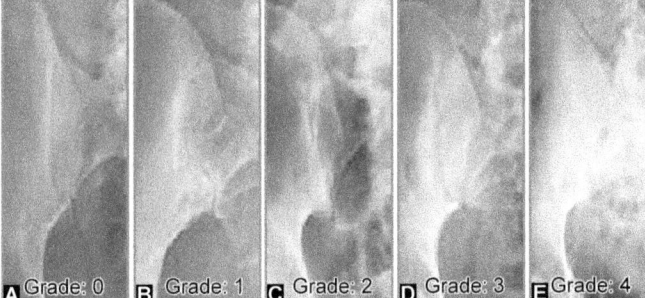

Figs. 15.23A to E: Grades of sacroiliitis.

- **Grade 4:** Severe abnormality (complete ankylosis) **(Fig. 15.23E)**.

Management of Ankylosing Spondylitis
- Medical management
  - Nonsteroidal anti-inflammatory drugs (NSAIDs) prescribed by physician.
  - Disease-modifying antirheumatic drugs are sometimes prescribed by the physician, to prevent progression of the disease.
  - Intra-articular corticosteroids to SI joints sometimes help to reduce pain.

Physiotherapy
Physiotherapy is an essential part of the treatment of AS. As the disease runs through a long course, home exercise program is more emphasized. The aims of physiotherapy are:
- To decrease pain.
- To increase mobility of spine, sacroiliac joints and peripheral joints.
- To correct posture.
- To improve chest expansion and lung capacities.
- To improve strength and endurance.
- To improve function and gait.
- To enhance quality of life.

Methods of physiotherapy
The methods/techniques of physiotherapy depend on the stage (early/late) at which the patient reports to the therapist. Once the patient reports, the therapist should do a brief assessment with special emphasis on:
- ROM of spine (modified Schober's test), mobility of SI joints, ROM of hips, knees, ankles, shoulders, elbows, forearms, and hands.
- Examination of posture.
- Level of pain using VAS.
- Chest expansion.
- Gait and function.

After the assessment, the therapist should make a problem list and decide the techniques of therapy after a thorough clinical reasoning. Brief guideline of therapy procedures are discussed below. However, the therapist is required to modify/design therapeutic strategies to meet the clinical needs of the individual patient.
- **For pain reduction:** Pulsed ultrasound over site of enthesitis, hydrotherapy, moist hot packs, IFT/TENS may be selected as appropriate.
- **To increase mobility of spine and SI joint and peripheral joints:** Mobilization with movement as described by Mulligan's **(Figs. 15.24A and B)**, McKenzie methods of mobilization of spine for dysfunction **(Fig. 15.24C)**, rocking in supine **(Fig. 15.24D)**, auto-assisted SI mobilization exercises, assisted-knee rolls **(Fig. 15.24E)** are performed. The patient is demonstrated home exercise program to maintain and increase mobility.
- Shoulder wheel exercises **(Fig. 15.25)**, shoulder pulley exercises, static cycle exercises, heel drag exercise, active free exercises to upper and lower limbs help in maintaining and improving the ROM of upper and lower limbs.

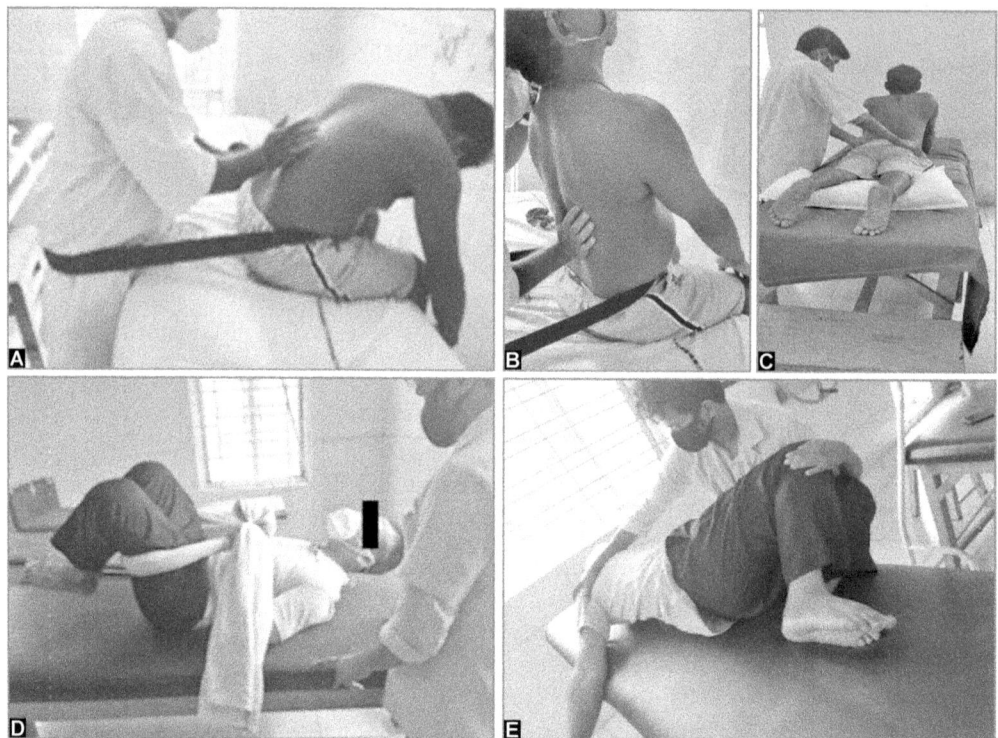

Figs. 15.24A to E: (A) Mulligan's mobilization to improve spinal flexion; (B) Mulligan's mobilization to improve spinal extension; (C) McKenzie extension exercise for thoracolumbar spine; (D) Auto-assisted rocking in supine lying; (E) Assisted knee roll.

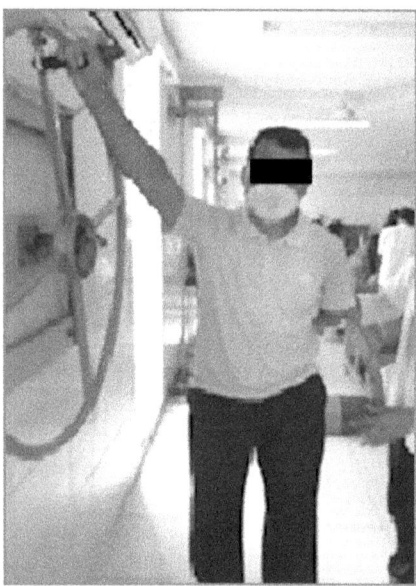

Fig. 15.25: Shoulder wheel exercise.

- **To correct posture:** Frequent periods of prone lying without/with pillow under the head and chest **(Fig. 15.26A)**, using chairs with proper back and neck support, avoiding the use of thick pillow while lying in supine, performing frequent corner stretch **(Fig. 15.26B)** exercises, wall slide exercise **(Fig. 15.26C)**, etc., are to be advised to the patient.
- **To improve chest expansion and vital capacity:** Deep breathing exercises with a strap **(Fig. 15.27)**, incentive spirometry are taught to the patient.

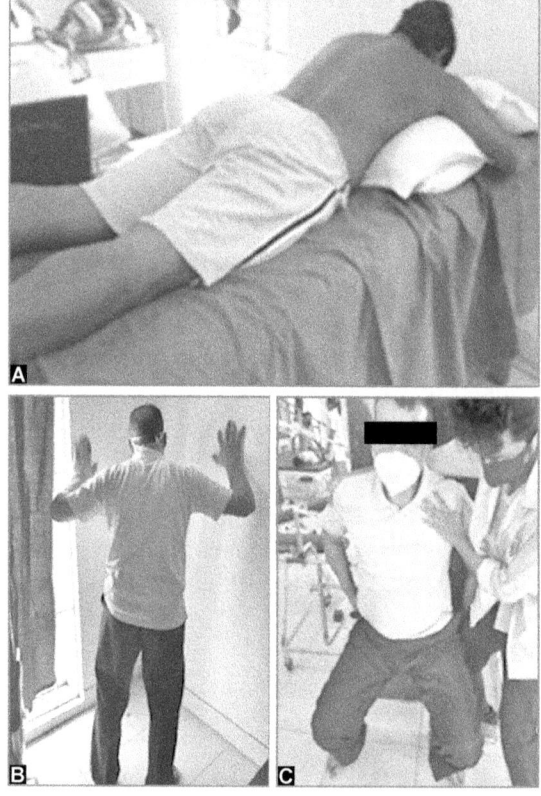

Figs. 15.26A to C: (A) Prone lying; (B) Corner stretch exercise; (C) Wall slides.

- **To improve strength and end endurance:** Low-intensity strength training without inducing fatigue, brisk walking, static cycle exercises **(Fig. 15.28A)**, hydrotherapy **(Fig. 15.28B)** indoor and outdoor sports are advised to the patient.

❖ **To improve gait:** Gait training in front of a postural mirror is emphasized. Functional activities respecting pain and observing energy conservation and joint protection are advised.

Surgery

Untreated AS can cause spinal deformity, with more than 30% of patients suffering from thoracolumbar kyphosis. Corrective osteotomy and stabilization are very common surgical procedures and are recommended under certain conditions, such as adult patients suffering from severe kyphosis. Hip arthroplasty may be considered for advanced hip arthritis with ankylosis.

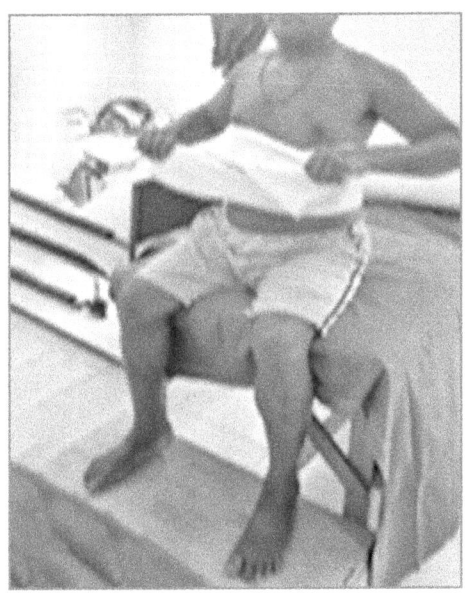

Fig. 15.27: Deep breathing exercises with strap.

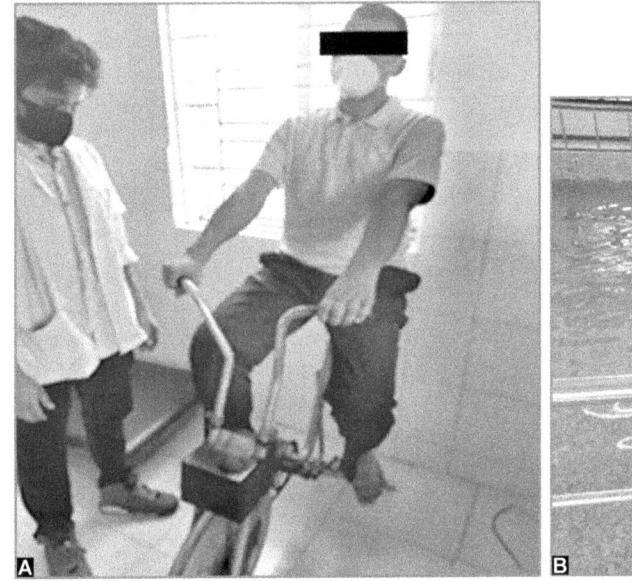
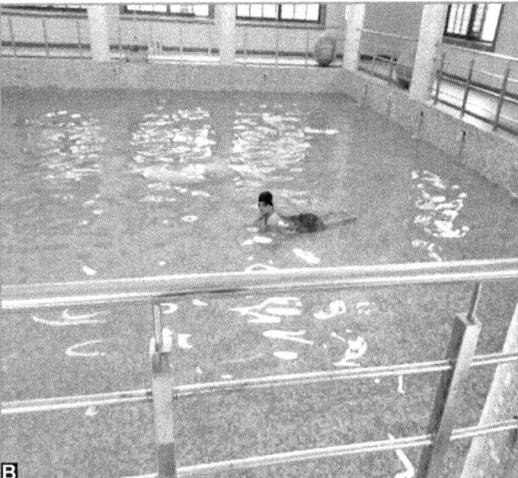

Figs. 15.28A and B: (A) Static cycle exercise; (B) Hydrotherapy.

16. Physiotherapy in Fractures

FRACTURE

The break in the continuity of bones is called fracture. This condition may lead either to a temporary impairment of function for a few weeks (4-6 weeks for upper limb and 6-12 weeks for lower limb and spine), or permanent disability (activity limitation) or handicap (participation limitation) due to stiffness of adjoining joints, nonunion, deformity, infections of bone such as osteomyelitis, arthritis (most commonly septic arthritis and osteoarthritis), paralysis of muscles from nerve injuries, etc.

A fracture could be of the following types:
1. **Simple fracture/closed fracture:** Fracture without breaking of skin.
2. **Compound fracture/open fracture:** The bone breaks through the skin causing open wound.
3. **Nondisplaced fracture:** The bones break, but alignment is maintained.
4. **Displaced fracture:** The bone breaks into two or more pieces and moves out of alignment.
5. **Comminuted fracture:** The bone breaks into several pieces.
6. **Pathological fracture:** Fracture caused by diseases that weaken the bone.
7. **Stress fracture:** Hair lines cracks that develop due to repetitive activities such as found in Army, who marches.
8. **Avulsion fracture:** In this a bone fragment is separated from the main mass of bone.
9. **Buckled fracture/impacted fracture:** The fracture ends are driven into each other, which are commonly seen in children.
10. **Greenstick fracture:** An incomplete fracture, where the bones are bent.
11. **Oblique fracture:** The break of bone has a curved or sloped pattern.
12. **Spiral fracture:** In this one part of bone remains twisted at the break point.
13. **Compression/wedge fracture:** Here body of a vertebra is compressed.
14. **Transverse fracture:** The broken piece of bone remains at right angle to the bone's axis.

A physiotherapist should have adequate knowledge in management of fracture, particularly how to manage the complications arising after fracture immobilizations and surgery, so that early restoration of function could be achieved.

Brief information on common fractures of limbs and spine are discussed below.

FRACTURE OF SPINE

A fracture of spine mostly results from trauma, such as fall from heights or road traffic accident (RTA). Depending on the region affected, it may cause simple dysfunctions to severe spinal cord injury resulting in quadriplegia/quadriparesis (for cervical injuries) or paraplegia/paraparesis (thoracic/lumbosacral injuries). Very rarely a hemiplegia also develops due to cervical spinal cord injury (called Brown-Séquard syndrome). The different types of spinal cord injuries and their management have already been described in detail in Chapter 20. A general outline of management of fractures of vertebrae is briefly discussed below:

Cervical Spine Fracture (Fig. 16.1)

Fracture/injuries involving the cervical spine, could be a common fracture of vertebral body **(Fig. 16.1)**, or its complicated events like: Hangman fracture, Whiplash injuries etc. Hangman fracture, also known as traumatic spondylolisthesis of the axis, is a fracture which involves the

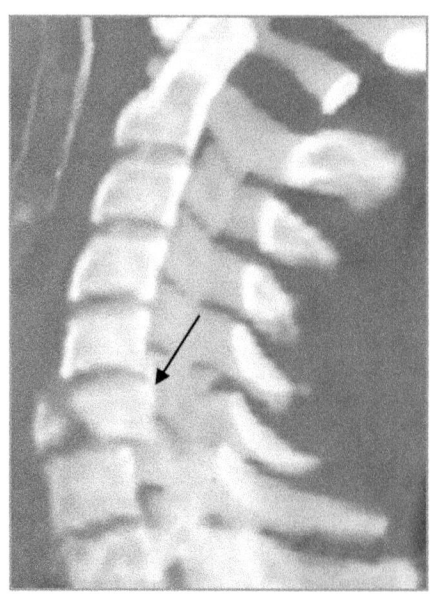

Fig. 16.1: Fracture of C6, vertebra with posterior displacement.

pars interarticularis of C2 on both sides, and is a result of hyperextension and distraction.

Whiplash is a neck injury due to forceful, rapid back-and-forth movement of the neck, like the cracking of a whip.

Whiplash injury is commonly caused by rear-end car accidents. But whiplash can also result from sports accidents, physical abuse and other types of traumas, such as a fall. Whiplash may be called a neck sprain or strain,
The overall goals of treatment are to preserve or improve neurologic function, provide stability, and decrease pain. If these goals can be accomplished with conservative means, then that is generally preferred. However, because many cervical fractures and dislocations are highly unstable and will not adequately heal on their own, surgical stabilization is routinely performed.

- **Conservative management:** Conservative treatment is indicated in all fractures which are not dislocated and show no other signs of instability. Conservative treatment includes a cervical spine immobilization in a cervical collar for around 6–8 weeks, NSAIDs.

However, management of severe cervical fractures and dislocations may involve skeletal traction and closed reduction, with metal pins placed in the skull connected to a pulley, rope, and weights. This is followed by use of cervical orthoses. There are a wide range of cervical orthoses, which range from soft collars to hard plastic cervicothoracic orthoses such as Minerva jacket brace, Philadelphia collar, four-poster orthoses to halo vest immobilization (using pins anchored into the skull stabilized by a padded plastic vest) **(Figs. 16.2A to D)**.

Surgical Management

Surgical treatments frequently involve posterior (back of the neck incision) cervical fusion (mending the spine bones together) and instrumentation (small metal screws and rods stabilizing the spine). Other options include anterior (front of the neck incision) decompression and fusion, with or without instrumentation (metal plate and screws). Severely unstable fractures may require anterior and posterior neck surgery.

Thoracolumbar Spine

The three major types of thoracolumbar spine fracture patterns are:

- **Flexion pattern:** These are compression fractures **(Fig. 16.3)** in which the front (anterior) of the vertebra breaks and loses height, the back (posterior) part of it remains intact. This type of fracture is usually stable (the bones have not moved out of place) and is rarely associated with neurologic problems.
- **Extension pattern:** This type of fracture can occur in a head-on car collision when the upper body is thrown forward while the pelvis is stabilized by a lap seat belt. This is typically an unstable fracture.
- **Rotation pattern:** This could be:
  - *Transverse process fracture:* This uncommon fracture results from rotation or extreme sideways (lateral) bending. It does not usually affect stability.
  - *Fracture-dislocation:* This is an unstable injury involving bone and/or soft tissue in which a vertebra moves off an adjacent vertebra (displacement). These injuries frequently cause serious spinal cord compression.

Management

Most flexion injuries including stable burst fractures and osteoporotic compression fractures can be treated with bracing for 6–12 weeks. Extension fractures are usually treated conservatively by Plaster of Paris (POP) jacket or spinal brace for 12 weeks. This should be followed by physiotherapy. Fractures involving the transverse processes are managed conservatively by rest/bracing and gradual mobilization exercises.

Surgery is typically required for:
- Unstable burst fractures that have:
  - Significant comminution (multiple bone fragments)
  - Severe loss of vertebral body height
  - Excessive forward bending or angulation at the injury site
  - Significant nerve injury due to parts of the vertebral body or disc pinching the spinal cord
  - Ligament damage that makes the spine unstable

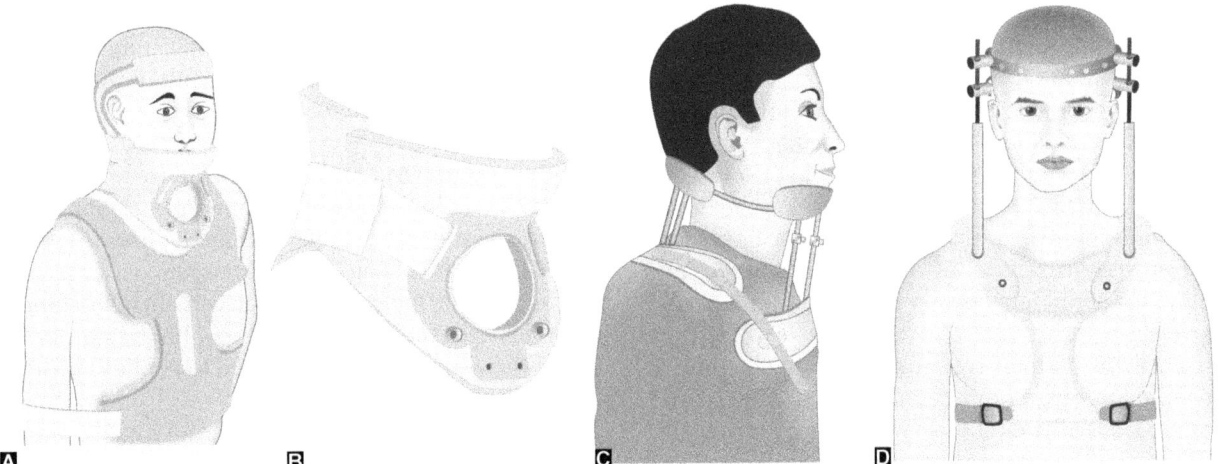

Figs. 16.2A to D: (A) Minerva jacket; (B) Philadelphia collar; (C) Four-poster brace; (D) The halo vest immobilization.

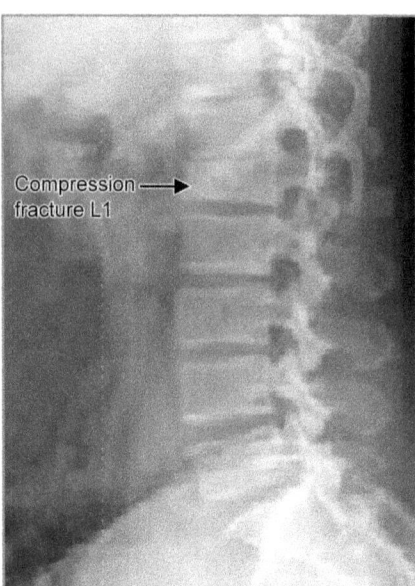

Fig. 16.3: Wedge compression fracture of L1.

These fractures should be treated surgically through laminectomy and decompression of the spinal canal (if there is nerve damage) and stabilization of the fracture by screw fixation.
* Extension fractures that occur only through the vertebral body can typically be treated without surgery. However, if there is an associated posterior ligament injury, surgery may be required.
* Rotational fractures: Fracture dislocations of thoracolumbar spine always require surgical stabilization.
  Postoperatively, the patient is nursed in bed for 3–4 weeks, and is then mobilized with a spinal brace.

Physiotherapy for Spinal Fractures Managed Conservatively

Cervical Spine Fractures

* **For stable fractures managed conservatively:** Ergonomic advice to maintain proper neck posture during immobilization is very important. As soon as immobilization period is completed, SWD/MWD/Moist hot packs are applied and graduated mobilization of cervical spine is started.
* **For unstable fractures managed by skeletal traction/ surgery:** During immobilization, bed side physiotherapy in the form of relaxed passive movements (in the presence of cord injury), active assisted/free exercises to the limbs, isometric gluteal, and quadriceps exercise, deep breathing/ assisted-breathing exercises are performed, without fully abducting the shoulders beyond 90 degrees for a period of 3–4 weeks.
  As soon as the skeletal traction is removed/spine is stable with surgery, a hard cervical collar is fitted and the patient is mobilized. If the patient has quadriplegia/ quadriparesis, the same are managed accordingly as discussed in Chapter 20.

Thoracic and Lumbar Spine Fractures

* For stable fractures, during immobilization with or without spinal brace/plaster jacket:
  – Proper position maintenance on a firm bed.
  – Isometric abdominal (achieved by resisting cervical flexion), isometric spinal extensor (achieved by resisting cervical extension) exercises are performed to prevent atrophy and weakness of trunk.
  – Passive ROM exercises are performed for lower limbs. However, hip flexion beyond 70 degrees and SLR exercises should not be performed during the first 3–4 weeks after injury to lumbosacral spine.
  – Deep breathing exercises to expand chest are performed, as chest expansion is reduced during immobilization.
* After 4 weeks of immobilization, the patient is gradually mobilized. The interventions include:
  – Correct method of turning on bed (log rolling) and transition from lying to sitting, avoiding undue strain on the fracture site such as flexion and rotation of spine in flexion injuries, and hyperextension of spine in extension injuries.
  – Those treated with POP jacket can be made to sit and ambulate earlier, as tolerated.
  – Modalities such as SWD/MWD/Hot packs should be applied to the fracture/painful site, provided, if the patient has the ability to perceive heat at the site.
  – Graded extension exercises with auto assistance should be started for those having flexion injuries such as wedge compression fracture. Side flexion and rotation of spine should be gradually added as tolerated. Flexion exercises (for young adults) are the last to be taught and practiced.
  – Ergonomic training while doing activities of daily living is emphasized to prevent exacerbation of symptoms and the patient is gradually returned to activities with use of appropriate braces.

Physiotherapy for Thoracolumbar Spine Fractures Treated by Surgery

The physiotherapy intervention includes:
* **During days 1–2:** Emphasis on eliminating postsurgical complications like DVT, chest complications, etc.
* **From 3rd day onward:** The interventions include:
  – Deep breathing exercises.
  – Log rolling.
  – Relaxed passive/active assisted/active free exercises to the lower limbs taking precautions for not moving the hips beyond 70 degrees, during the first 3–4 weeks for fractures involving the lumbar spine.
  – Supported/inclined sitting on bed, tilt table standing as tolerated, standing and walking holding on to walker with/without spinal brace and lower limb orthoses (if required) are practiced.
  – If the patient has spinal cord injury with paraplegia/ paraparesis, the same should be managed as described in Chapter 20.

FRACTURES OF UPPER LIMB

Fracture of Clavicle

This is the most common fracture **(Figs. 16.4A and B)** found in children and elderly resulting from indirect injuries such as fall on out stretched hands and direct injuries such as road traffic accidents.

Management

This fracture rarely requires open reduction and surgical fixation, and in most cases requires conservative management in the form of:
- Figure of 8 straps **(Fig. 16.5)** for mid shaft fracture and a shoulder sling for fracture involving lateral 1/3rd of the clavicle.
- Surgical management (plate and screw fixation) **(Fig. 16.6)**, is considered if there is nonunion, neurovascular involvement, fracture of distal end of the clavicle with torn coracoclavicular ligaments, soft tissue interposition, and floating shoulder (fracture involving mid shaft of clavicle, and neck of the glenoid).

Physiotherapy

After immobilization period (4–6 weeks), physiotherapy is started with an aim of:

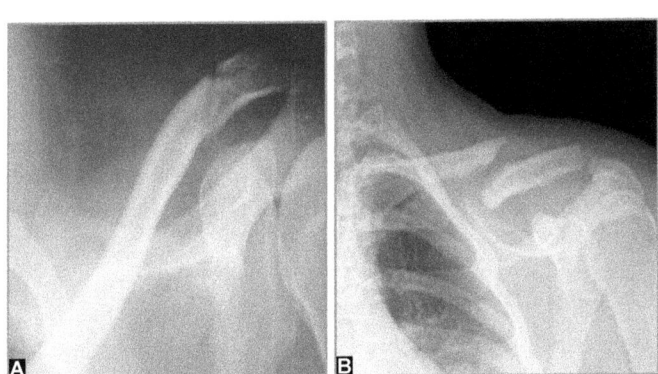

Figs. 16.4A and B: (A) Fracture of lateral 1/3rd of clavicle; (B) Fracture mid shaft of clavicle.

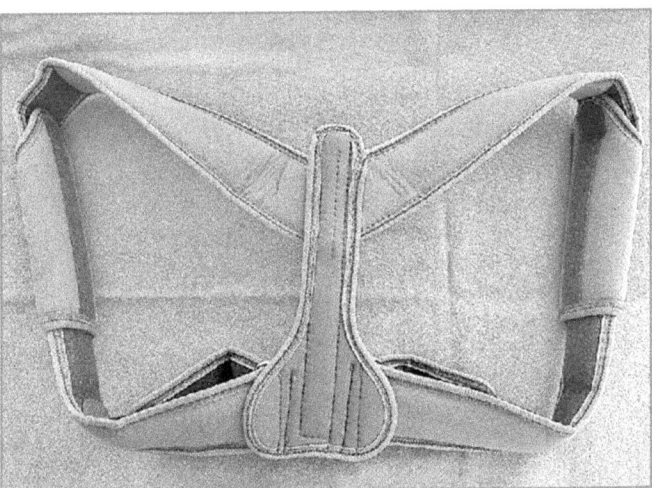

Fig. 16.5: Figure-8 strap.

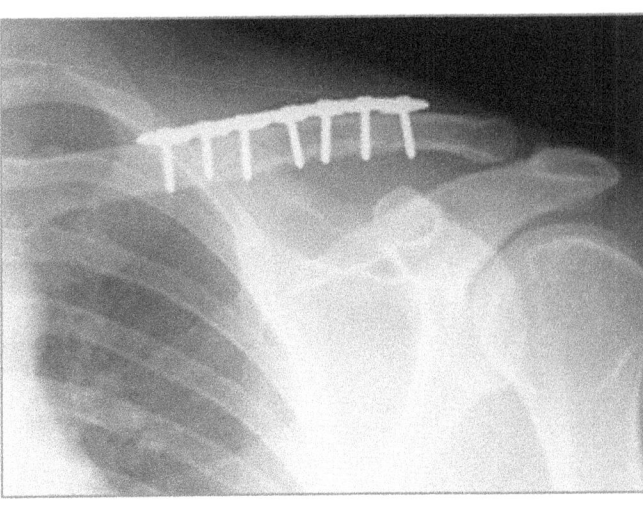

Fig. 16.6: Plate and screw fixation for fracture mid shaft of clavicle.

- **Reduction of stiffness**: Gentile passive and active shoulder mobilization exercises are helpful. The active mobilization exercises include: Wand exercises, shoulder pulley exercises, shoulder ladder exercises, gear shift exercises, shoulder wheel exercises, shoulder circumduction exercises **(Fig. 16.7)**, etc.
- **Reduction of pain**: Pain, basically develops from soft tissue inflammation in acromioclavicular, or glenohumeral joints. SWD/MWD (except for cases where ORIF has been done)/Ultrasound therapy/moist heat/IFT/TENS, Laser therapy, etc., may be applied in conjunction with exercises to reduce pain and improve function.
- **Strengthening of muscles**: Any muscle weakness that has resulted from immobilization, pain, nerve injuries, etc., should be strengthened by active assisted/free/resisted exercises and electrical stimulation.

Fracture of Scapula

This fracture is less commonly seen and is caused by trauma such as road traffic accidents **(Fig. 16.8)**.

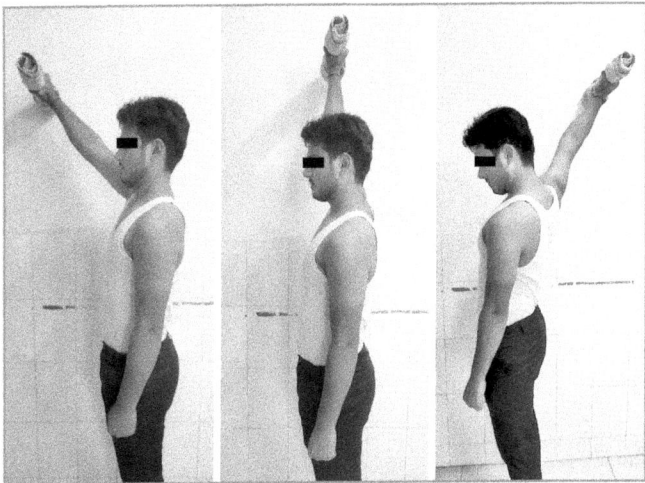

Fig. 16.7: Shoulder circumduction exercise.

Section 2: Physiotherapy for Musculoskeletal Conditions

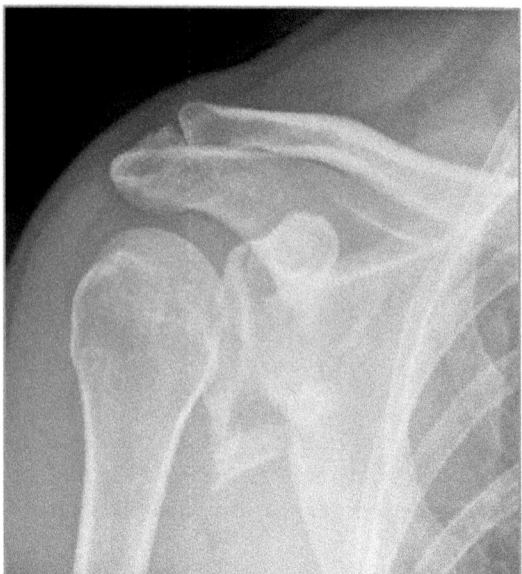

Fig. 16.8: Shows fracture of scapula.

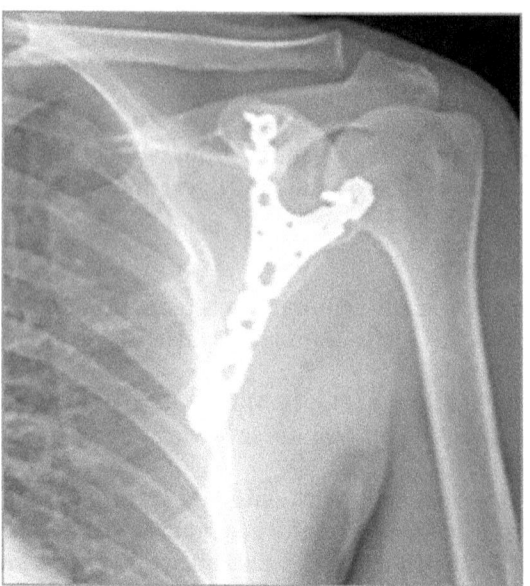

Fig. 16.10: ORIF for fracture scapula.

Management

Conservative management

Most fractures of the scapula can be treated conservatively without surgery. Treatment involves immobilization with a sling or a shoulder immobilizer **(Fig. 16.9)**, icing and pain medications. The sling is usually kept for the first 4 weeks followed by shoulder mobilization exercises.

Physiotherapy

It consists of active movements of the affected side upper limb as well as breathing exercises.

Modalities such as PSWD, pulsed ultrasound, TENS, etc., can be applied over the site of fracture to reduce pain promote healing of the fracture.

Surgery

Surgery **(Fig. 16.10)** is rarely needed for this fracture. The indications of surgery include:

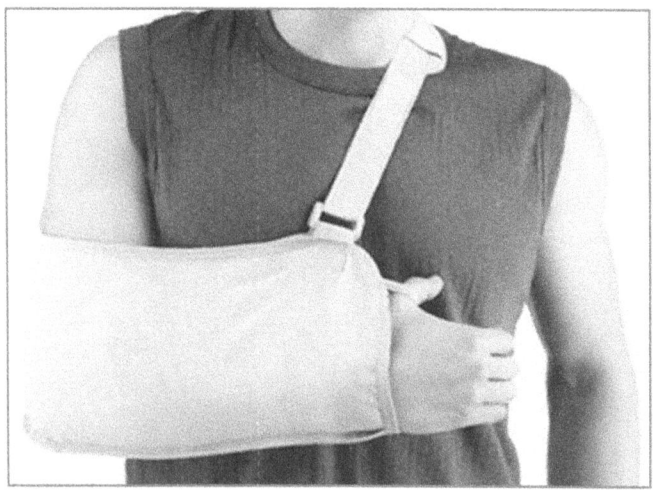

Fig. 16.9: Shoulder sling.

- Significantly displaced fracture of the acromion with retraction of the fracture fragment and encroachment on the subacromial space.
- Fractures of the coracoid process with acromioclavicular separation.
- Glenoid rim fracture.

Postoperative Management

Physiotherapy in the form of shoulder mobilization exercises, breathing exercises, strengthening exercises to upper limb muscles, moist heat/IFT/TENS, etc., are applied to increase mobility of shoulder and muscle strength and to reduce pain (if any).

Fracture of Humerus

Fracture of humerus occurs as a result of high velocity trauma, especially in young people. In old people osteoporotic bones predispose to such fractures when the individuals sustain a fall. The common fractures that occur include:

Fracture of Proximal Humerus

This includes:

Fracture of the tuberosities: Most often, these types of fractures are avulsion type **(Fig. 16.11)**, occurring as a result of seizures leading to fall, direct trauma and secondary to glenohumeral dislocations.

Management: Treatment is usually conservative with application of a U-cast **(Fig. 16.12A)**. If displacement is more than 1 cm then open reduction and internal fixation (ORIF) **(Fig. 16.12B)** may be considered.

Physiotherapy: Whether managed conservatively or surgically, the aims of physiotherapy are:
- **To mobilize shoulder:** Graded passive and active shoulder mobilization exercises, without causing violent stretching/contraction of the supraspinatus muscle.

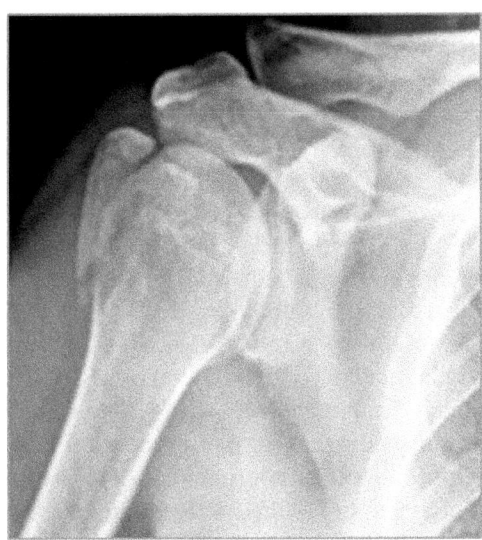

Fig. 16.11: Fracture of greater tuberosity of humerus (avulsion type).

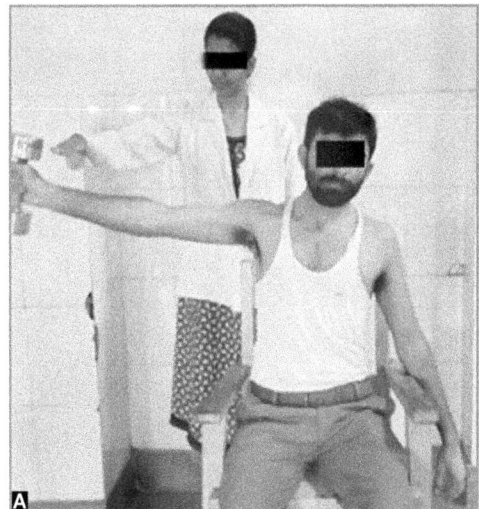

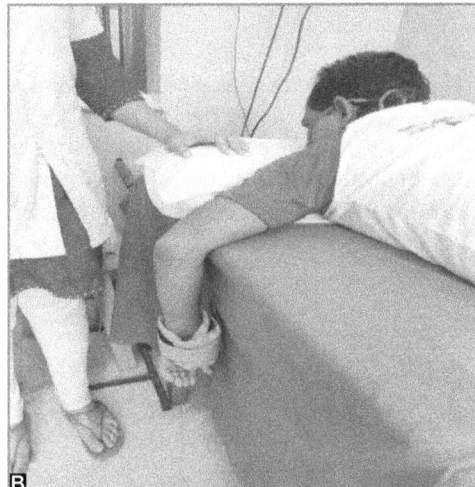

Figs. 16.13A and B: (A) Strengthening of middle deltoid using dumbbell; (B) Strengthening of rotator cuff muscles using weight cuff.

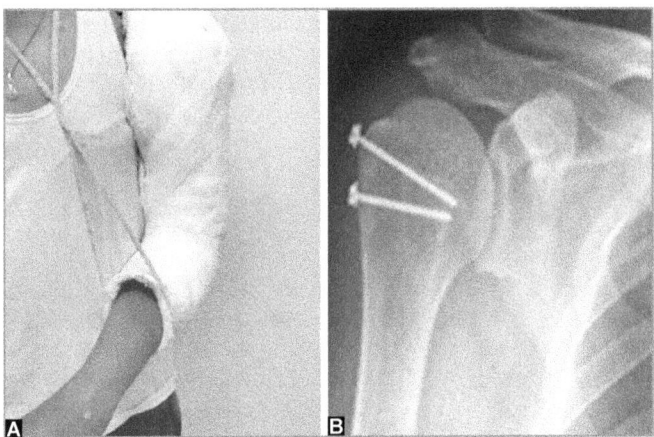

Figs. 16.12A and B: (A) U-cast; (B) ORIF for fracture greater tuberosity.

- **Tendinitis of rotator cuff muscles can be managed by:** Pulsed ultrasound, LASER, PSWD, SWD/MWD (If no metallic implant used for fixation), iontophoresis using drugs that have a sclerolytic effect.
- Strengthening of deltoid rotator cuff muscles are done progressing from low-intensity eccentric exercises to multi-angle isometrics and concentric free and resisted exercises **(Figs. 16.13A and B)**.
- Any pain affecting movement and function can be managed by TENS/IFT **(Fig. 16.14)**.

Fracture of the surgical/anatomical neck of humerus (Fig. 16.15): Results from high impact trauma, such as motor vehicle accidents.

Management: If impacted, managed by conservative means with U-cast followed by a course of physiotherapy to improve mobility, pain, and function, in the same manners as described for fracture of greater tuberosity.

If, the fracture is displaced type, ORIF are done followed by a course of physiotherapy to improve mobility, strength and

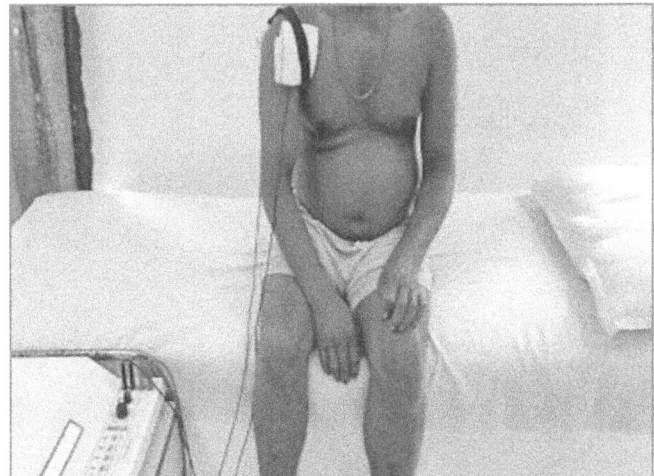

Fig. 16.14: IFT to shoulder joint.

reduce pain and restore function. The physiotherapy methods followed are same as described for physiotherapy Treatment of fracture of greater tuberosity.

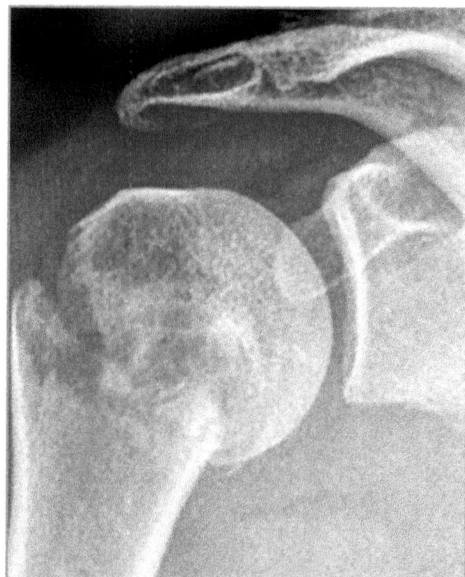

Fig. 16.15: Fracture surgical neck of humerus.

Injury to axillary nerve (a common complication of fracture surgical neck of humerus), is managed either conservatively (neuropraxia/axonotmesis) or surgically (neurotmesis).

Fracture shaft and lower end of humerus (Figs. 16.16A to E): Mostly caused by trauma due to RTA. Fall from height, domestic and communal violence, war injuries are also some of the causes.

Management: Closed fracture of shaft of humerus is usually managed by closed reduction and immobilization in a POP cast for 6 weeks. Injury to radial nerve (mostly axonotmesis) if develops resulting in wrist drop, are managed after the fracture has united and POP removed. Open and displaced fractures are usually managed by ORIF.

Fractures of lower end of humerus, i.e., intercondylar/supracondylar/medial condyle/lateral condyle fractures are either managed conservatively with closed reduction and POP cast immobilization, or open reduction and internal fixation with immobilization in a POP slab. Complications like radial nerve injury (stated above), gun stuck deformity (with supracondylar fractures), cubitus valgus/cubitus varus deformities, Volkman's ischemic contracture (VIC), stiffness of elbow and forearm develop, which requires management by a team of professionals.

Physiotherapy: After the immobilization completed and fracture found to have healed, the patient reports to the physiotherapist for managements of complications.

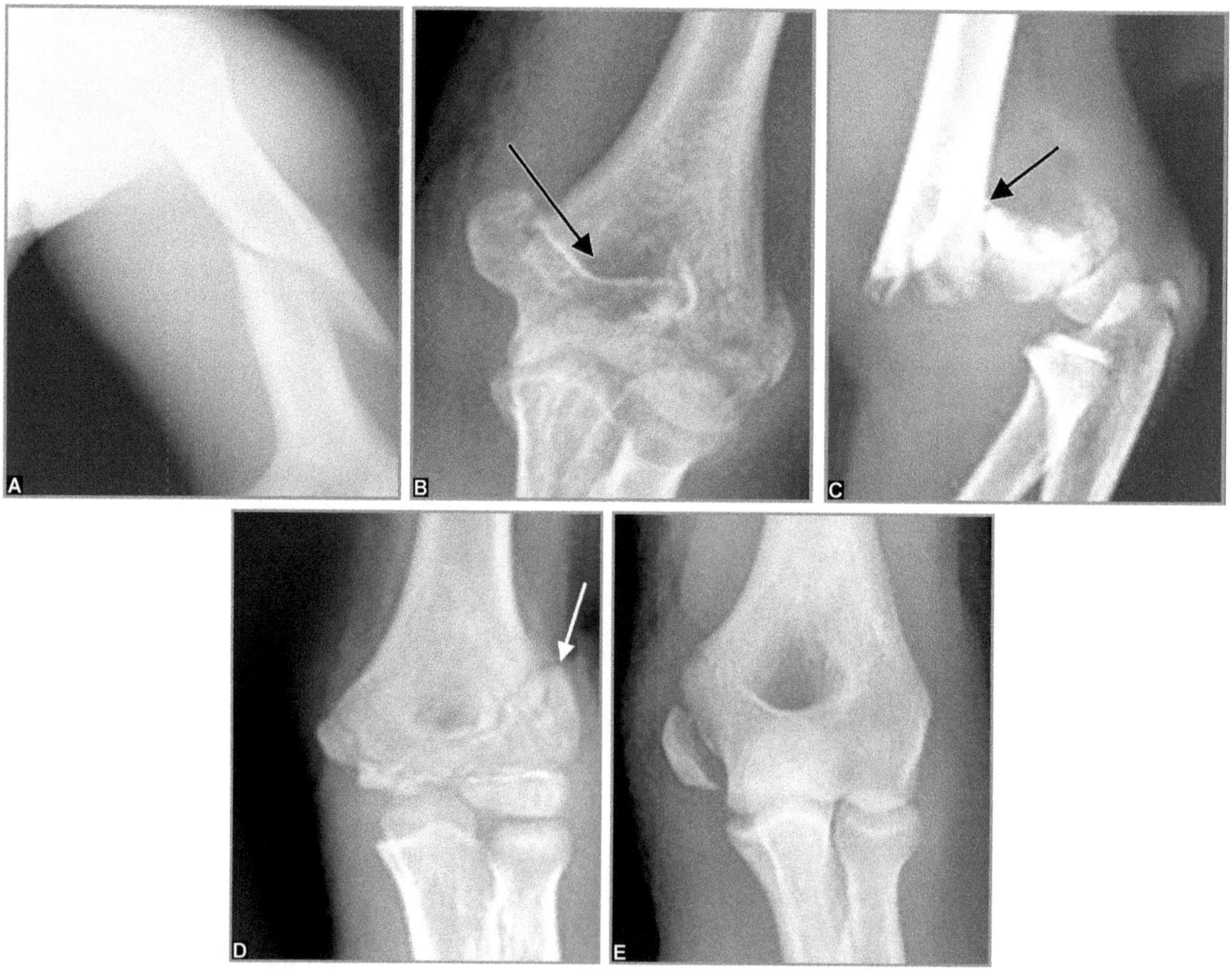

Figs. 16.16A to E: (A) Fracture shaft of humerus; (B) Intercondylar fracture; (C) Supracondylar fracture (extension type); (D) Lateral condyle fracture; (E) Medial epicondyle fracture.

The physiotherapist examines the ROM of shoulder, elbow, and forearm using the universal goniometer. Motor and sensory examination along with examination of function are done and documented.

The aims of physiotherapy for management of post-immobilization complications are:
- To reduce pain and swelling.
- To mobilize stiff joints.
- To strengthen weak muscles.
- To re-educate sensation.
- To correct deformities.
- To improve function.

Physiotherapy methods:
- Contrast bath to hand (for swelling, if any)
- PWB to elbow/forearm (pouring/brushing method)
- Manual mobilization exercises (Maitland/Mulligan/Kaltenborn), PNF hold-relax techniques.
- Self-mobilization exercise using hand skater (**Figs. 16.22B and C**), dumbbell in hand, theraband, re-education board, forearm exerciser.
- Faradism under tension in the presence of elbow flexion deformities (**Fig. 16.17**)
- **Splints for VIC:** Turn buckle splint (**Fig. 16.18**)
- For elbow flexion deformity, turn buckle splints (**Fig. 16.19A**), adjustable ROM elbow orthosis (**Fig. 16.19B**) may be considered along with exercises to maintain correction.
- Electrical stimulation to paralyzed muscles after conducting Faradic/IDC test.
- Mobilization of shoulder using shoulder wheel/shoulder pulley.
- Exercise using forearm exerciser.

Fracture of Forearm Bones

- Fracture of head of radius (**Fig. 16.20A**).
- Fracture of both bones of forearm (**Fig. 16.20B**).
- **Monteggia fracture-dislocation:** Fracture, shaft of ulna with dislocation of head of radius (**Fig. 16.20C**).
- **Galeazzi fracture (Fig. 16.20D):** The Galeazzi fracture is a fracture of the middle to distal one-third of the radius associated with dislocation or subluxation of the distal radioulnar joint.

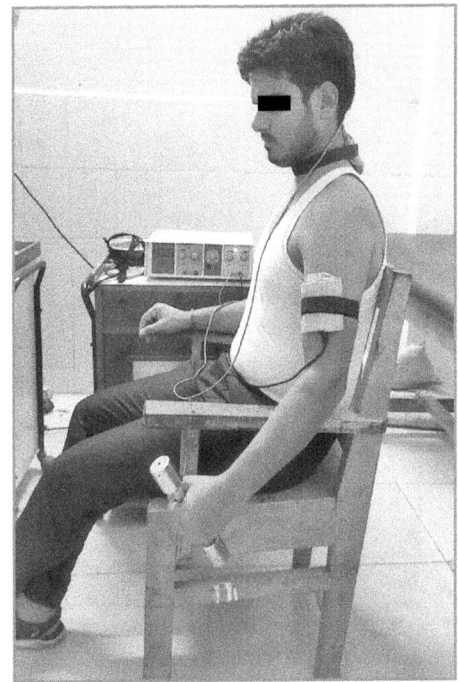

Fig. 16.17: Faradism under tension to elbow flexor for correction of flexion deformity of elbow.

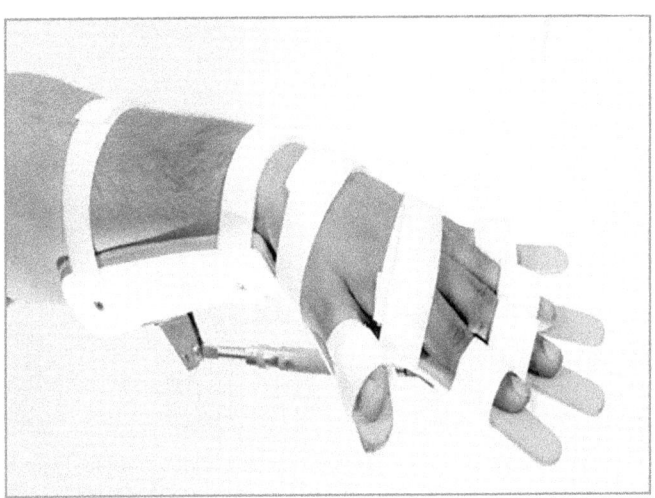

Fig. 16.18: Turn buckle splint for Volkman's ischemic contracture (VIC).

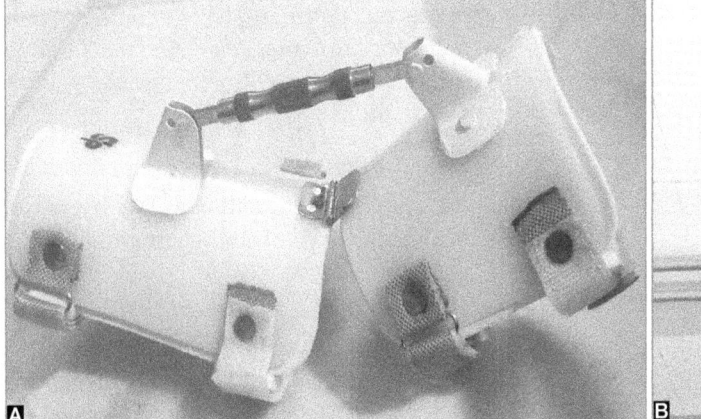
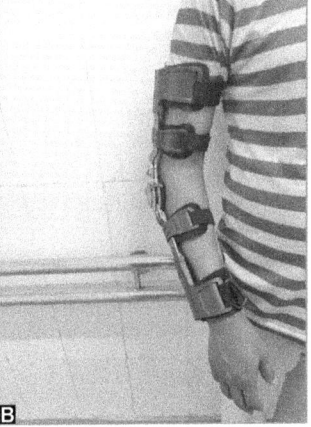

Figs. 16.19A and B: (A) Turn buckle splints for elbow flexion deformity; (B) Adjustable ROM elbow orthosis.

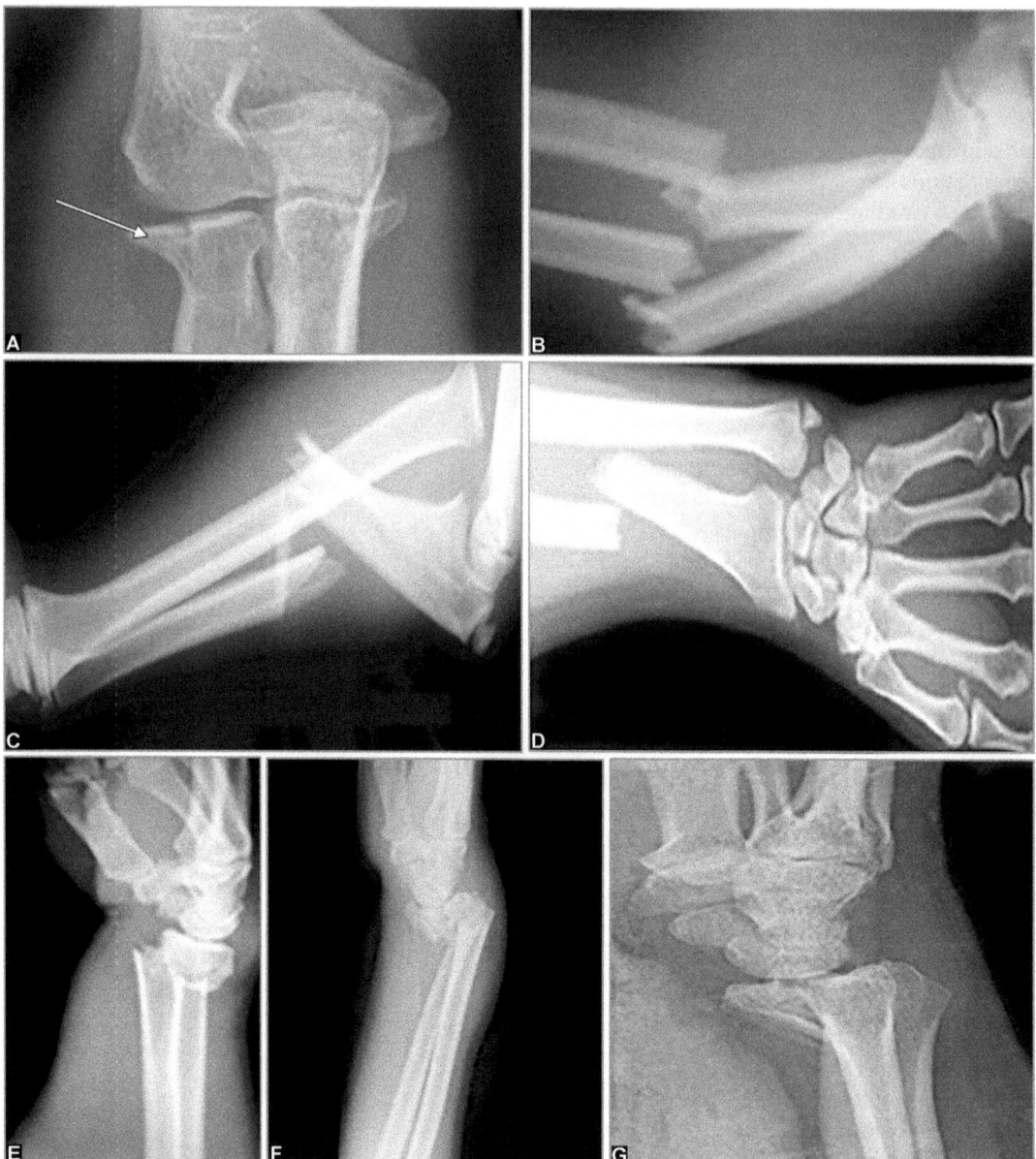

Figs. 16.20A to G: (A) Fracture head of radius; (B) Fracture both bones of forearm; (C) Monteggia fracture-dislocation; (D) Galeazzi fracture; (E) Colles fracture; (F) Smith's fracture; (G) Barton's fracture.

- **Colles fracture (Fig. 16.20E):** Colles fractures are very common extra-articular fractures of the distal radius that occur as the result of a fall onto an outstretched hand. They consist of a fracture of the distal radial metaphyseal region with dorsal angulation and impaction, but without the involvement of the articular surface.
- **Smith's fracture (Fig. 16.20F):** It is an extra-articular fracture of the distal radius featuring a volar displacement or angulation of the distal fragment.
- **Barton's fracture (Fig. 16.20G):** It is an intra articular fracture involving the lower end of radius with dislocation of radiocarpal joints.

Management of Fracture of Bones of Forearm

Closed fractures with minimal displacement are managed with closed reduction and immobilization in a POP cast for 4–6 weeks. However, open fractures and closed fractures with severe displacement, which could not be reduced by closed reduction are managed by open reduction and internal fixation. After ORIF, above elbow/below elbow POP slab is applied for 4–6 weeks.

Complications of Fracture of Both Bones of Forearm

The complications following fracture of bones of forearm are:
- Osteoarthritis of elbow/superior radioulnar joint and wrist joint.
- Radioulnar synostosis.
- Nonunion/malunion/delayed union.
- Deformity (dinner fork deformity in Colles fracture).
- Stiffness of shoulder, elbow, forearm and hand.
- Nerve injuries (median/ulnar nerve injuries).

- Sudeck's osteodystrophy (complex regional pain syndrome/shoulder hand syndrome): Found as a complication in fractures of wrist.

Physiotherapy after Fracture of Both Bones of Forearm

After immobilization is completed and fracture found to have healed completely, physiotherapy is started, which focuses on:
- Mobilization of stiff joints.
- Strengthening of weak muscles.
- Reduction of pain and swelling as found in Sudeck's osteodystrophy.
- Reduction of pain due to osteoarthritic changes in elbow and wrist.
- Treatment of nerve injuries (if any).

Methods of physiotherapy:
- PWB to elbow and wrist **(Fig. 16.21)**
- Contrast bath to hand for control of edema.
- Mobilization of shoulder, elbow hand using Maitland/Mulligan/Kaltenborn techniques.
- Mobilization using hold-relax technique of PNF.
- Use of shoulder wheel/shoulder pulley/forearm exerciser/skater/Nirmal Hand apparatus, etc. **(Figs. 16.22A to C)**.
- Strengthening of hand muscles using therapy putty, squeeze ball.
- IFT/TENS.

Fracture of Bones of Hand

Scaphoid fracture: A scaphoid fracture is a break in one of the small bones of the wrist. This type of fracture occurs most often after a fall onto an outstretched hand. Symptoms of a scaphoid fracture typically include pain and tenderness in the area just below the base of the thumb **(Fig. 16.23A)**.

Bennett's fracture: Intra-articular fracture of the base of the first metacarpal **(Fig. 16.23B)**. It may be associated with dislocation of the first carpometacarpal joint. The fracture is unstable, and with inadequate treatment leads to osteoarthritis, weakness and/or loss of function of the thumb.

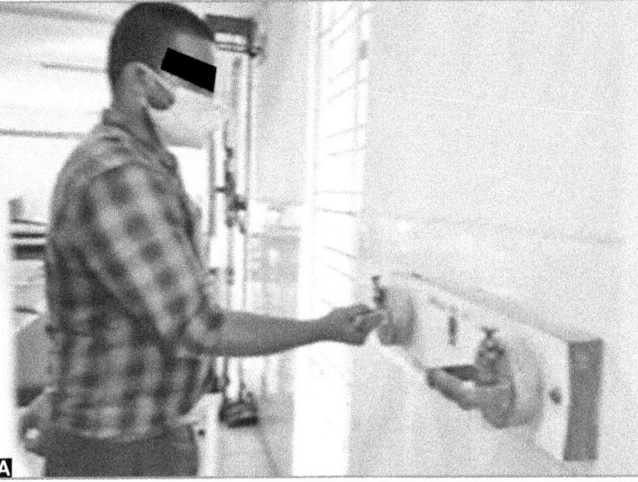

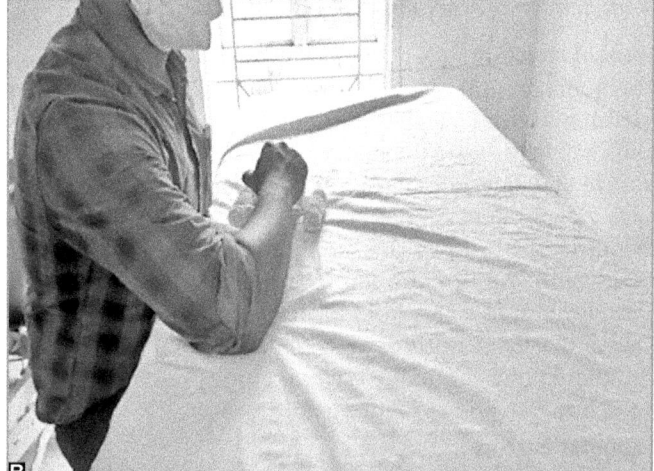

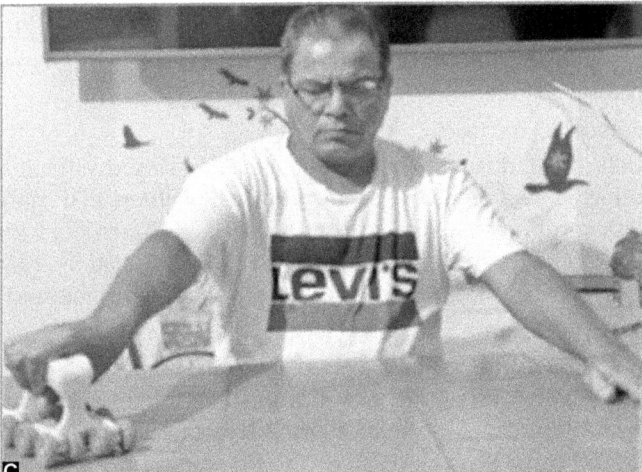

Figs. 16.22A to C: (A) Supination/pronation using forearm exerciser; (B) Skater for elbow flexion; (C) Skater for elbow extension.

Metacarpal fractures (Fig. 16.23C): Metacarpal fractures are the most common hand injury, and are divided into fractures of head, neck and shaft of the bone.

Phalanx fracture: Phalanx fractures can be intra or extra-articular and can occur at the base, neck, shaft or head of the phalanx. They often result from direct trauma to the finger such as in sports, where a ball may directly hit the finger causing fracture **(Fig. 16.23D)**.

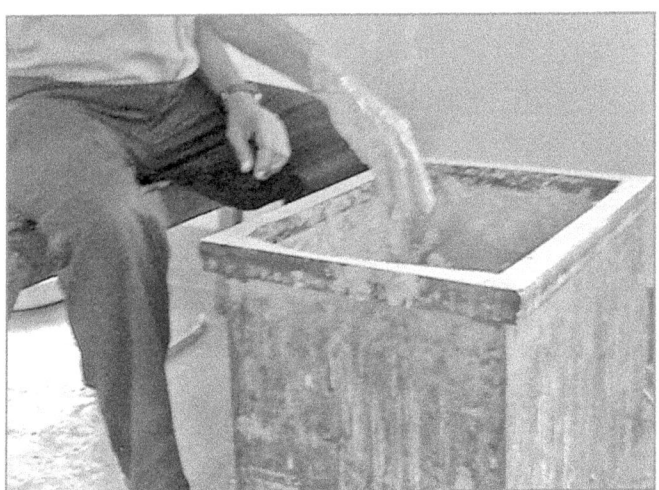

Fig. 16.21: PWB to wrist and hand.

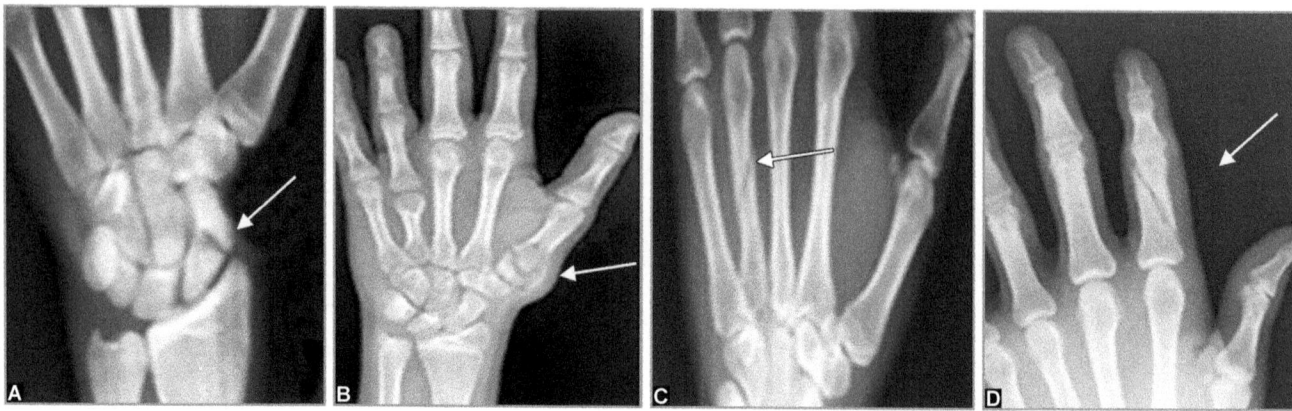

Figs.16.23A to D: (A) Scaphoid fracture; (B) Bennett's fracture; (C) Metacarpal fracture; (D) Phalanx fracture.

Management of Fractures of Hand

Scaphoid fracture
The management of acute fractures includes conservative treatment with cast (below elbow cast/scaphoid cast) in minimally displaced to open reduction and internal fixation in case of displaced ones. Because portions of the scaphoid have a poor blood supply, and a fracture can further disrupt the flow of blood to the bone, complications with the healing process are common. Avascular necrosis is common complication of a scaphoid fracture resulting in nonunion, pain and osteoarthritis of wrist joint. After immobilization is completed physiotherapy is started to restore mobility and hand function and to reduce pain.

Bennett's fracture
Nonoperative treatment in a thumb spica cast for 3–4 weeks is considered in stable, nondisplaced fractures. However, for displaced and unstable fractures ORIF with K-wire/screw fixation is done.

Metacarpal fractures
Metacarpal fractures are mostly managed by closed reduction followed by a forearm based splint/below elbow POP slab, with cotton wrap/wrap with crepe bandage. Fractures with displacement are managed by ORIF with K-wire fixation. After removal of immobilization/K-wire, physiotherapy is started.

Phalanx fracture
Stable fractures can be successfully treated nonoperatively, whereas unstable injuries benefit from surgery. Immobilization in an "intrinsic-plus" position through metacarpophalangeal (MCP) joint flexion reduces the displacing force of the interossei and also shifts the extensor tendon distally so that two-thirds of the proximal phalanx is embraced by the extensor mechanism, adding to the overall fracture stabilization. After immobilization physiotherapy is started to reduce pain and improve mobility and function.

LOWER LIMB FRACTURES

Lower limb fractures result from high-impact trauma, affecting mostly old people (due to loss of balance) and young men/women due to involvement in high risk jobs and out of home mobility that may lead to road traffic accidents. Fractures in the lower limbs involve pelvis, femur, tibia, fibula and bones of foot. The lower limb fractures are briefly discussed below:

Fracture of Pelvis

A pelvic fracture (**Fig. 16.24**) is a disruption of the bony structures of the pelvis that constitutes ilium, ischium, and pubis, which in combination with sacrum forms the bony pelvis. This fracture mostly results from high impact trauma and sometimes leads to fatal complications.

Management
Stable pelvic fractures are usually treated conservatively with heavy skeletal traction to reduce displacement, if any. The traction is maintained for 6 weeks, after which the patient is gradually mobilized. However, unstable fractures of pelvis need surgical management, in the form of application of external fixator. Surgical management of an unstable pelvic ring injury allows earlier mobilization, preferably after 3 weeks, and thereby diminishes the complications of immobilization.

Physiotherapy
The goals of the physiotherapy are an optimal return of function by reducing pain, increasing flexibility of spine, and hips, increasing strength of muscles of the pelvic floor and

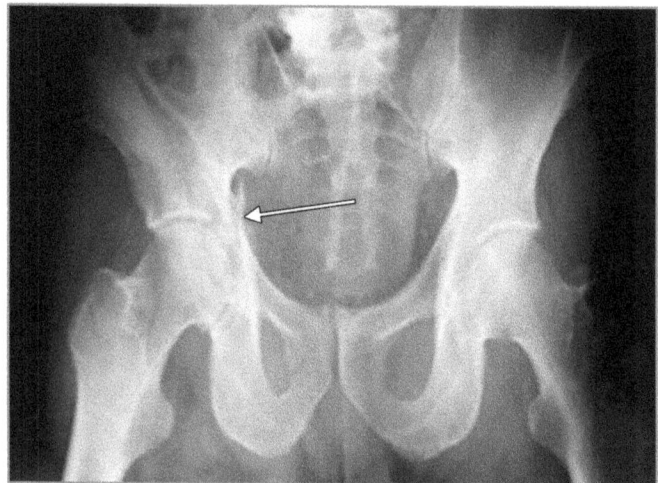

Fig. 16.24: Fracture of pelvis.

hips, improving functional skills, self-care skills and safety awareness.

During the non-weight-bearing state, the patient is made to perform isometric glutei, isometric quadriceps, ankle, foot exercises as well as exercises for the upper limbs.

Initial weight-bearing and ambulation starts in parallel bar, followed by walker and crutches, gradually progressing to independent ambulation with or without walking stick. During the period of weight bearing, resisted exercises for lower limbs, spinal exercises, and endurance exercises such as hydrotherapy, treadmill exercises, static cycle exercises, exercise on rowing machine, balance and proprioceptive training are started.

Modalities such as PSWD (mean power output of <5 watt), in the presence of any metal implant, TENS to reduce pain may be applied as required.

Fracture Neck of Femur

Femur fracture commonly occurs in elderly people, mostly women, following trauma due to fall, mostly in bathroom or on slippery surface. The fracture results are of two types:
- **Intracapsular fracture:** This extends from the subcapital area to the middle of the neck **(Fig. 16.25)**, which are of the following types:
  - Subcapital
  - Trans cervical
  - Basal (at the junction of neck of shaft)

The intracapsular fracture is classified into:
- **Abduction type fracture:** It is impacted and may unite with conservative management.
- **Adduction type fracture:** It is unimpacted type of fracture needing surgical management. This commonly results into avascular necrosis and nonunion.
- **Extracapsular fractures:** These are mostly the trochanteric fractures **(Fig. 16.26)** of various types **(Fig. 16.27)**.

Management

The fracture can be managed by:
- **Conservative methods (weight bearing starts at 10–12 weeks):** It includes:

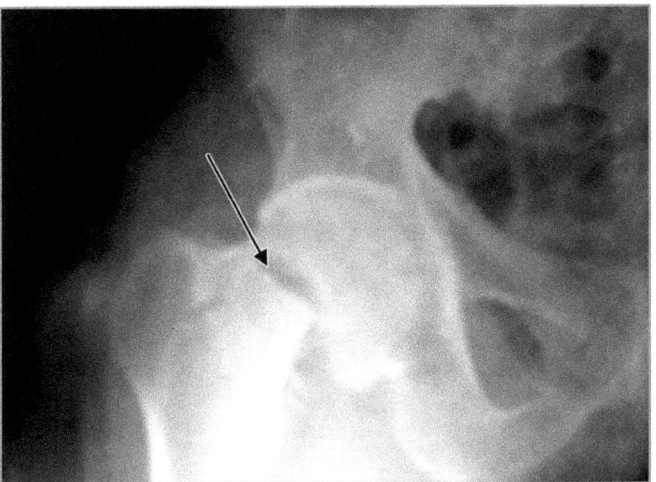

Fig. 16.25: Intracapsular fracture of neck of femur.

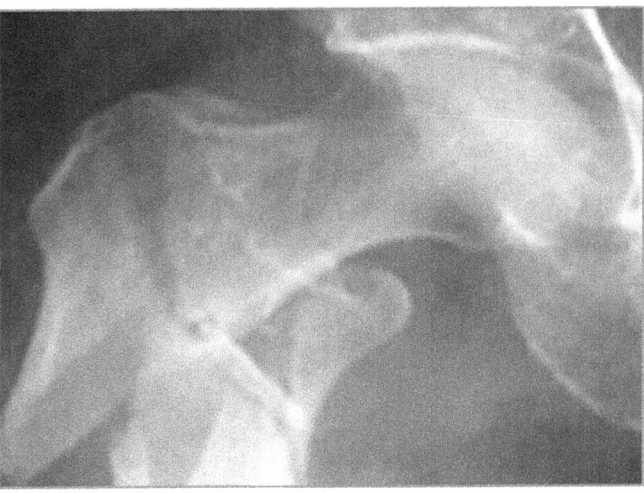

Fig. 16.26: Extracapsular (intertrochanteric) fracture.

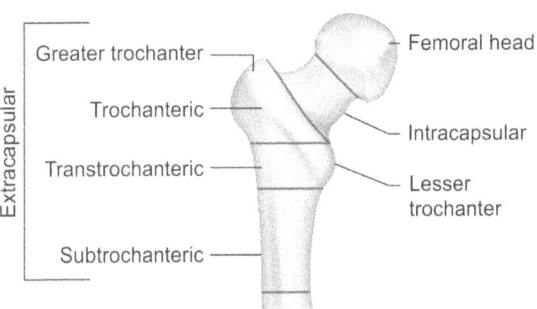

Fig. 16.27: Shows both intracapsular and extracapsular femoral neck fractures.

- Plaster of paris boot and bar with/without skin traction for 4 to 6 weeks **(Fig. 16.28)**.
- POP hip spica (for children only) for 6 weeks.
- *Painless pseudarthrosis (Early mobilization as pain permits):* Indicated for people who are not fit for any treatment (conservative/surgery).
- **Surgical methods:** It consists of the followings:
  - Internal fixation by Knowle's/Moore's pins **(Fig. 16.29A)**
  - S-P (Smith-Petersen) nailing **(Fig. 16.29B)**
  - A-O screw fixation **(Fig. 16.29C)**

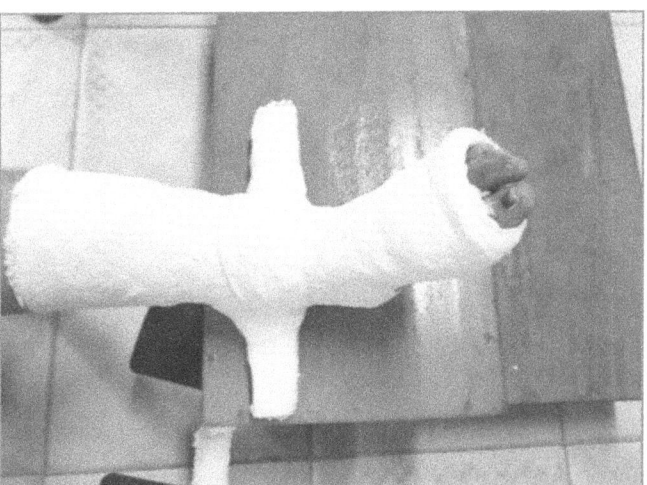

Fig. 16.28: POP boot and bar.

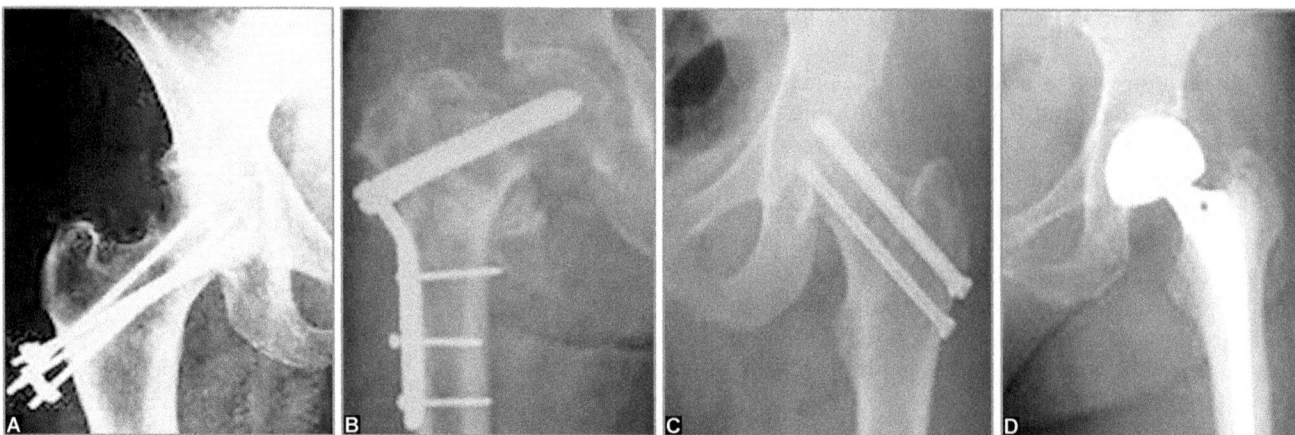

Figs. 16.29A to D: Management of fracture neck with: (A) Moore's pin; (B) S-P nailing; (C) A-O screw; (D) Hemiarthroplasty.

- Replacement arthroplasty (partial/total-usually partial-hemiarthroplasty) **(Fig. 16.29D)**.

Physiotherapy

It consists of the followings:
- **When fracture managed by conservative methods (skin traction/derotation boot bar application, etc.), physiotherapy consists of:**
  - Breathing exercises in lying/half lying.
  - *Isometric exercises:* Quadriceps sets, hamstrings sets, glutei sets.
  - Ankle and foot exercises.
  - Knee mobilization (when lying on split bed, after traction removed).
  - Initiation of sitting with back supported.
  - After pain subsided, active mobilization of hip and knee are started, if allowed by the Surgeon.
  - Pre weight-bearing exercises in the form of four-point kneeling **(Fig. 16.30)** can be started, before making the patient stand with walker/crutches (by 10–12 weeks).
  - Supported squatting in front of wall can be started as tolerated.
- Resisted exercises to hip abductors, extensors, quadriceps, and hamstrings are started using theraband **(Fig. 16.31)**.
- Partial weight-bearing gait with walker **(Fig. 16.32)**, crutches, walking sticks as tolerated to be started by 10–12 weeks, progressing to full weight-bearing by 16 weeks.
- For patients treated by pseudoarthrosis, movement should be started with ice (cryokinematics)/TENS. Isometric strengthening of muscles of hip should be emphasized, rather than isotonics. Graduated weight-bearing should be started with the help of walker/crutches/sticks.
- **When fracture is treated surgically:** The advantages of fractures managed surgically are early mobilization of hip and knee and early ambulation (mostly after arthroplasty), avoiding complications of bed rest. Management of a patient after arthroplasty of hip has been described separately under physiotherapy for hip disorders. However, physiotherapy after ORIF of hip is discussed below:
  - Physiotherapy during the initial 1 week-10 days:
    » Deep breathing exercises and chest clearance techniques.

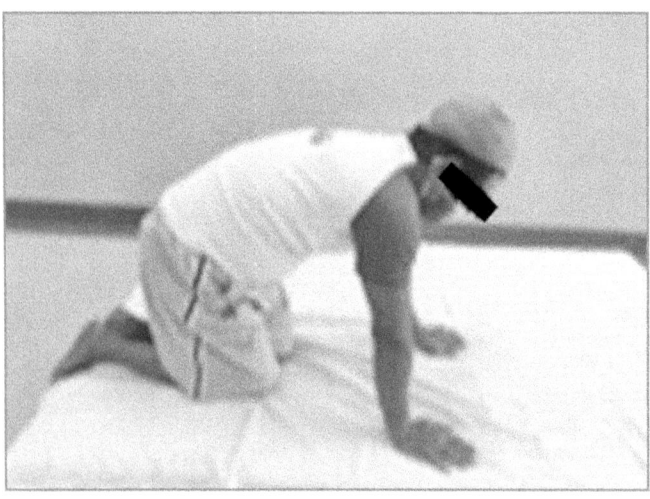

Fig. 16.30: Four-point kneeling.

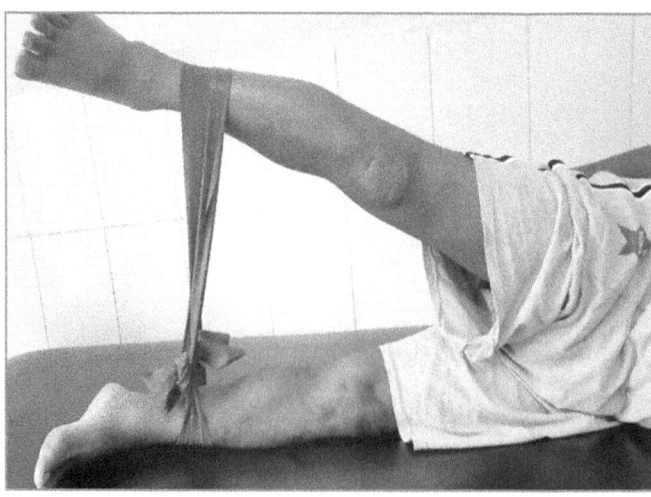

Fig. 16.31: Resisted exercise to hip abductors with theraband.

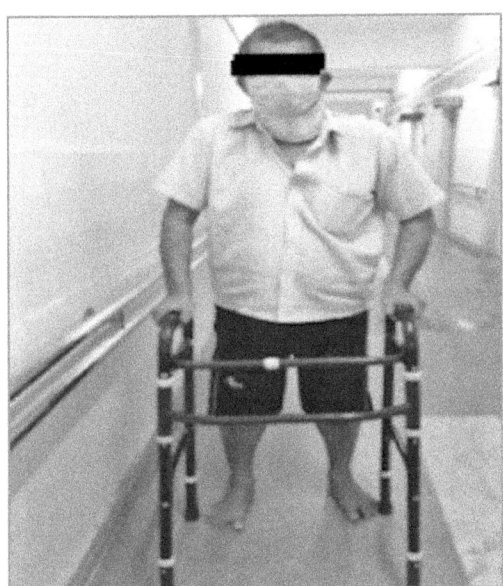

Fig. 16.32: Partial weight-bearing ambulation with walker.

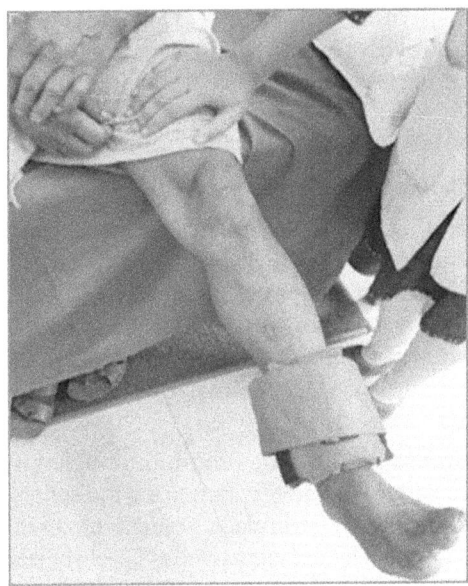

Fig. 16.34: Resisted knee extension with weight cuff.

- » Active ankle/foot exercises, isometric quadriceps, hamstrings and glutei exercises.
- Physiotherapy after 1 week-10 days:
  - » Relaxed passive movement to the hip with leg fully supported with utmost care.
  - » Auto assisted hip and knee flexion exercises in the form of heel drag **(Fig. 16.33)**.
  - » Assisted SLR exercise.
  - » Suspension therapy to enhance hip movements, particularly hip abduction.
  - » Resisted knee extension in high sitting with theraband/weight cuff **(Fig. 16.34)**.
  - » Partial weight-bearing ambulation with walker/crutches is started after 6–8 weeks and full weight-bearing ambulation is started after 12 weeks.

Fracture of Trochanters (Greater Trochanter/Lesser Trochanter/Intertrochanteric) (Fig. 16.26)

Mostly common in elderly people and in people having osteoporotic bones. These fractures generally unite readily, as they occur readily in the region of cancellous bone.

Management

- ❖ **Conservative:** Management is mostly conservative in the form of:
  - Plaster of paris boot and bar with/without skin traction for 6–8 weeks.

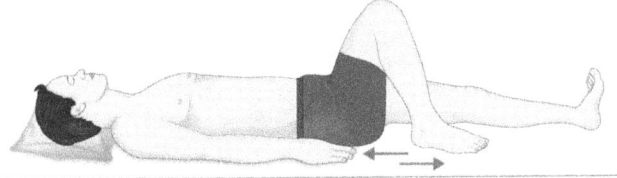

Fig. 16.33: Heel drag to increase hip and knee flexion.

- POP hip spica (mostly for young individuals maintained for 6–8 weeks).

Physiotherapy

This is done in the same lines of management of fracture neck of femur. However, after immobilization (after 6–8 weeks), active mobilization of hip is started. Weight-bearing is gradually started after 3 months.

- ❖ **Surgery:** Mostly performed in elderly people and has the advantage of minimizing the complications of prolonged immobilization. The techniques involve:
  - Reduction under X-ray and immobilization by S-P nail/Ender's nail **(Fig. 16.35)**.

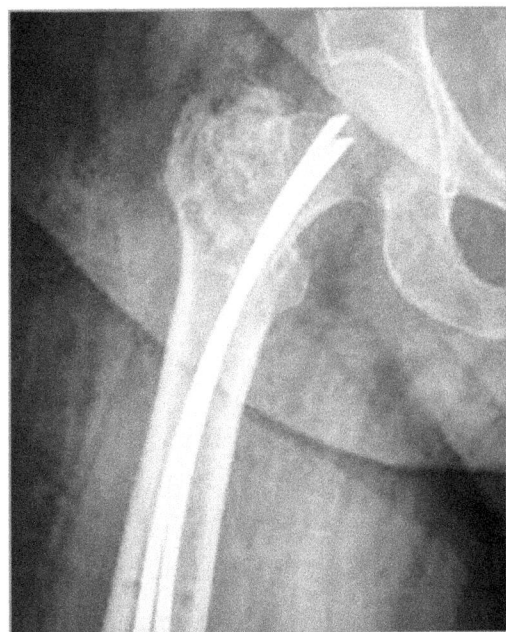

Fig. 16.35: ORIF with Ender's nail for intertrochanteric fracture.

This is done in the same manner as fracture in neck of femur. However, the patient is made to sit on bed on the next day and weight-bearing is gradually started after about 3 months.

Fracture Shaft and Condyles of Femur

Fracture Shaft of Femur

This fracture **(Fig. 16.36)** can be managed by both conservatively and surgically, which are briefly discussed below.

- **Conservative management:** It includes:
  - Gallow's traction for 3–4 weeks for children below 2 years.
  - Traction in Thomas splint for 6–8 weeks/immobilization in POP hip spica/AK POP cast in old children and adults for 12–14 weeks.

  Physiotherapy: With the limb immobilized in skeletal traction, early knee mobilization using the split bed can be started with the traction in place. Isometric glutei, quadriceps, and dynamic ankle, and foot exercises should be started. After immobilization is completed, patient should be made to walk with walker/crutches, initially after 12 weeks with minimum load, progressing to full weight-bearing by 16 weeks.

- **Surgical management:** ORIF with Kuntscher intramedullary nail or plate and screw fixation **(Fig. 16.37)** is performed in those cases, where conservative management is not possible or fails.

  Physiotherapy: After surgery no external immobilization is usually needed. Isometric glutei/quadriceps (low-intensity) exercises and active ankle and foot exercises are started on the next day. Knee mobilization using split bed/aligning the knee at the edge of the bed can be started after 2 weeks. Weight bearing progressing from partial to full weight-bearing is started between 2 and 3 months.

  Physiotherapy for complications: Knee stiffness is one important complication associated with fractures managed by conservative/surgical methods. Intensive mobilization of knee taking fracture into consideration should be started at the earliest to prevent joint fibrosis.

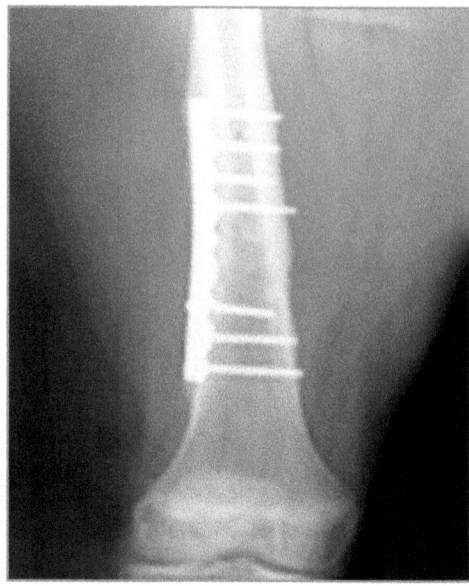

Fig. 16.37: Plate and screw fixation for fracture shaft of femur.

The methods used for knee mobilization after fractures in the lower limb are:
- PWB to knee **(Fig. 16.38)**.
- Accessory movements (gliding of patella, tibiofemoral joints using Maitland/Kaltenborn's principles).
- Mulligan's mobilization exercises **(Fig. 16.39)**.
- PNF stretching (hold-relax).
- Faradism under tension to quadriceps **(Fig. 16.40)**.
- Weight-bearing exercises [4-point kneeling to kneel sitting **(Fig. 16.41)**, squatting (wall supported/holding on to support)].
- Exercise on rowing machine/leg press device **(Fig. 16.42)**, static cycle, CPM (if necessary).

Fractures at and around Condyles of Femur

- **Supracondylar fracture:** The fracture is just proximal to the femoral condyles **(Fig. 16.43)**.
- Intercondylar and condylar fractures **(Figs. 16.44A and B)**

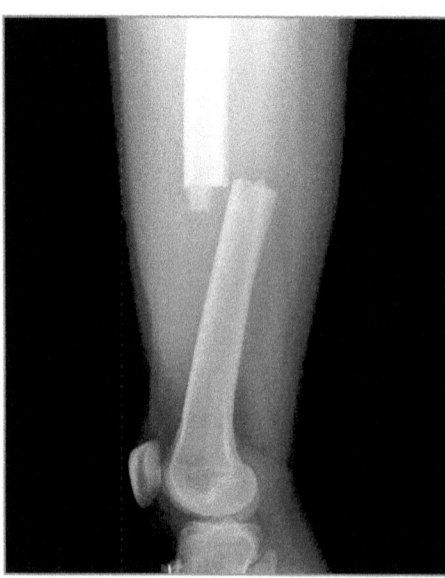

Fig. 16.36: Fracture shaft of femur.

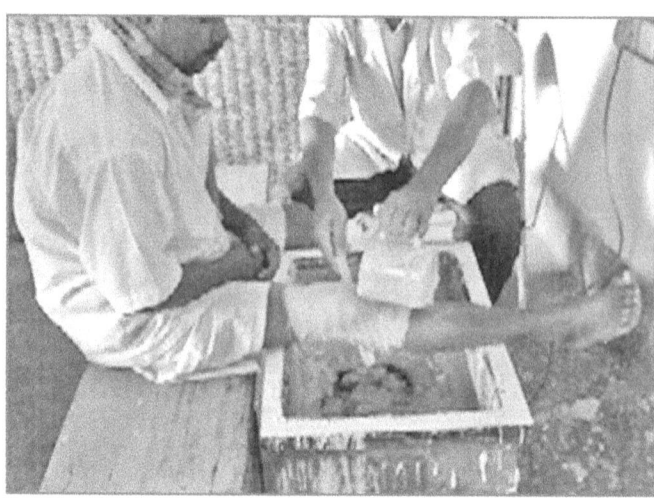

Fig. 16.38: PWB to knee.

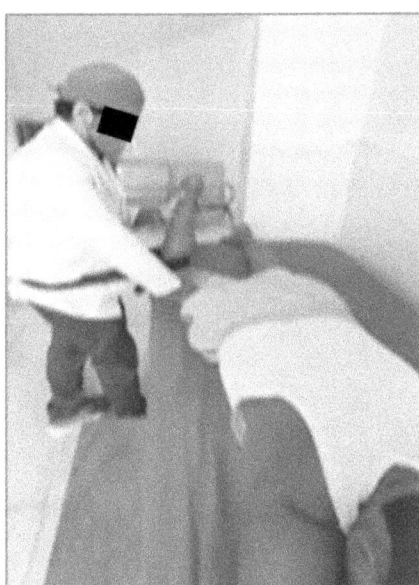

Fig. 16.39: Mulligan's MWM (lateral distraction with belt combined with active knee flexion).

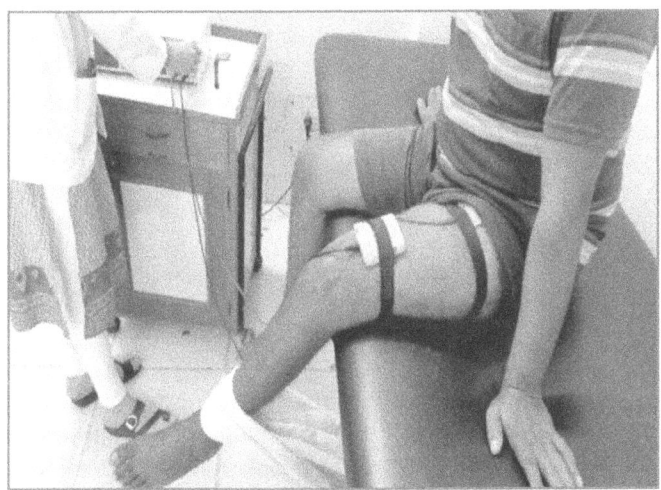

Fig. 16.40: Faradism under tension to quadriceps.

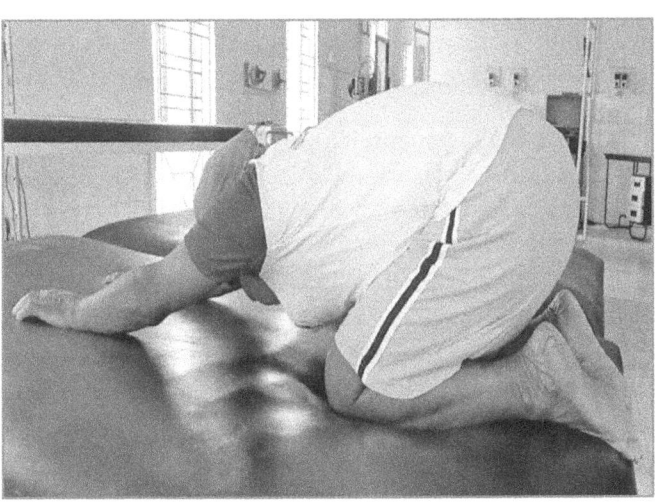

Fig. 16.41: 4-point kneeling to knee sitting.

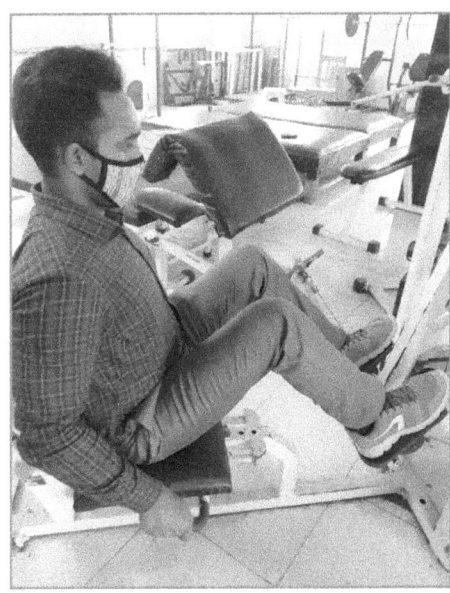

Fig. 16.42: Exercise on leg press device.

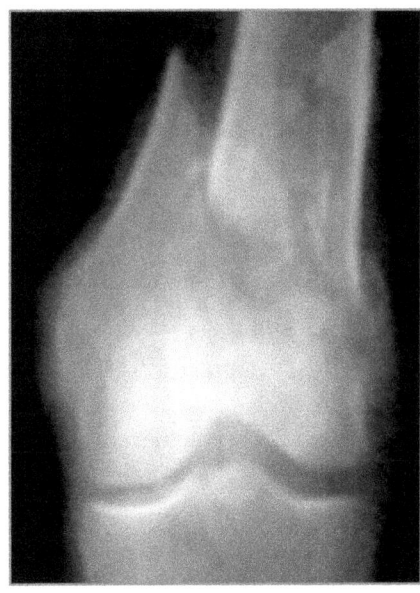

Fig. 16.43: Supracondylar fracture of femur.

Management of Fractures around the Femoral Condyles

The management of all these fractures is done by:

- **Conservative methods:**
  - *Supra condylar fractures:* Reduction under GA and immobilization of the limb is done in a Thomas splint, with skeletal traction applied to the upper end of tibia with knee in 30 degrees of flexion. After traction removed, patient remains immobilized for 8–12 weeks.
  - *Intercondylar fractures:* Skeletal traction to upper end of tibia is applied for 6–8 weeks.
  - *Condylar fractures (Medial/lateral femoral condyles):* Usually managed by surgery (ORIF).

Physiotherapy: During immobilization in traction, therapy consists of:

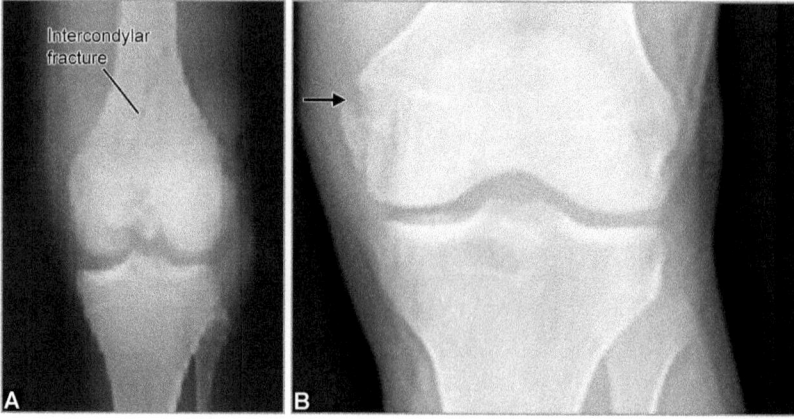

Figs. 16.44A and B: (A) Intercondylar fracture, (B) Medial condyle fracture.

- Active ankle and foot exercises.
- Isometric glutei, quadriceps, hamstrings.
- After reduction achieved, AK POP cast (cast brace) is applied and the patient is allowed for nonweight-bearing crutch gait. The cast brace with polycentric hinges are applied for 3–6 weeks.
- Mobilization of knee with the cast brace should be started.
- Partial weight-bearing is started by 12 weeks, gradually progressing to full weight-bearing.
- Complications like knee stiffness is managed as described above.
❖ **Surgery:**
  - *Supracondylar fracture:* ORIF by condylar blade-plate.
  - *Intercondylar/condylar fractures:* ORIF through multiple screws, Kirschner wires, and blade-plates.

  Physiotherapy: After ORIF for supracondylar/intercondylar/condylar fractures, nonweight-bearing knee mobilization is done after 2 weeks and by 4–6 weeks, 90 degrees of knee flexion is achieved and partial weight-bearing is started after 9 weeks, gradually progressing to full weight-bearing by 12 weeks. Complications like knee stiffness is managed as discussed earlier.

Fracture of Patella (Fig. 16.45)

A patellar fracture is a break in the patella/knee cap, which usually results from trauma. It could be a stable (non displaced), displaced, transverse (where the bone breaks into two pieces), comminuted (where the bone breaks into three or more pieces), or open types (where the skin over the bone is also broken along with fracture of patella).

Management: It could be:
❖ **Conservative:** This is mostly followed for undisplaced (crack/stellate type) fractures, managed through POP cylindrical cast maintained for 4 to 6 weeks followed by physiotherapy.
  Physiotherapy:
  - Static quadriceps exercise in the plaster, isometric glutei, active ankle and foot exercise.
  - SLR exercise.

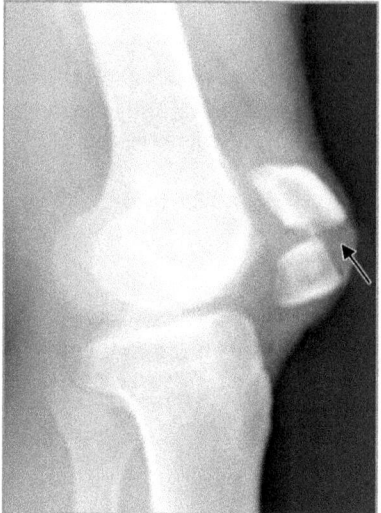

Fig. 16.45: Fracture of patella.

- Partial weight-bearing crutch gait is started on the next day with the cast if tolerated with the consent of the Orthopedic surgeon.
- After POP cylindrical cast removed by 4–6 weeks, mobilization of knee as described earlier is performed with/without CPM **(Fig. 16.46)**. Active free exercises to the lower limb in the form of heel drag, knee flexion in prone lying, knee extension in high sitting are performed.
- Full weight bearing and function is achieved by 8–12 weeks.
❖ **Surgical management:** It includes:
  - Tension band wiring (TBW) **(Fig. 16.47)**, or screw fixation for fractures with 2–3 fragments.
  - Patellectomy (removal of patella) for comminuted fracture.

Physiotherapy after internal fixation: After surgery the knee is immobilized in a POP slab or pressure bandage. Physiotherapy in the postoperative period is applied as discussed below:

❖ Early postoperative period (1–10 days postoperatively): The therapy with POP slab/pressure bandage on consists of:
  - PSWD (mean power output < 5W)

Chapter 16: Physiotherapy in Fractures

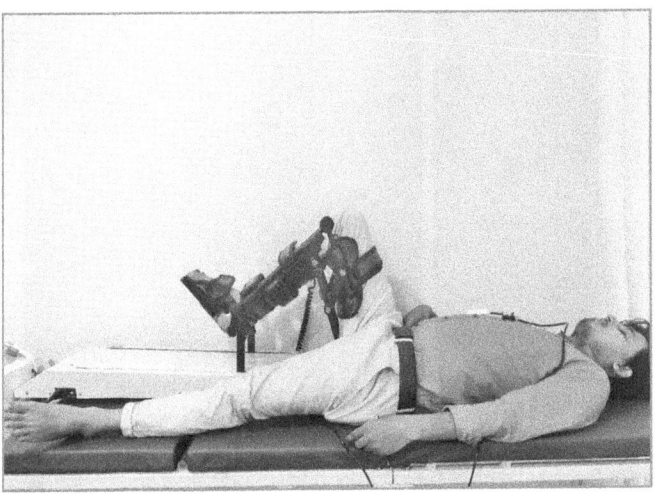

Fig. 16.46: CPM for knee mobilization.

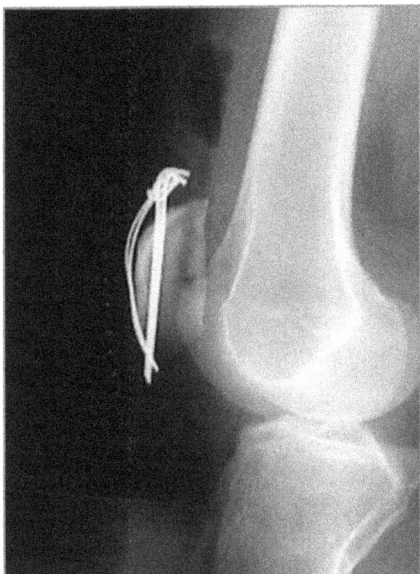

Fig. 16.47: TBW for fracture patella.

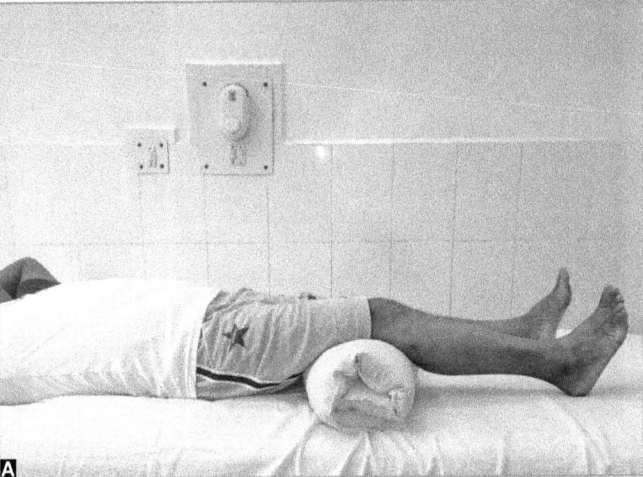

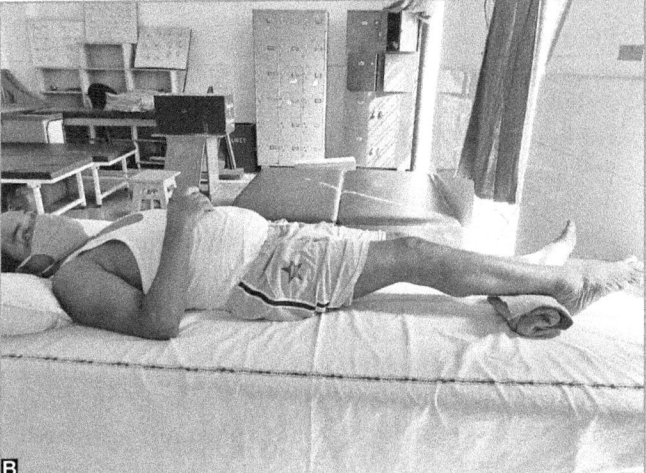

Figs. 16.48A and B: (A) Short arc knee flexion/extension exercise; (B) Isometric hamstring exercise.

- Limb elevation and active ankle/foot exercises.
- Isometric quadriceps exercise, SLR exercise at 3–4 days postoperatively.
- Nonweight-bearing crutch gait as pain permits.
❖ **Therapy after 10 days:** By this time the stitches are removed and emphasis is laid on:
  - Graduated knee flexion with or without CPM.
  - Self-assisted knee flexion such as heel drag.
  - Strong isomeric quadriceps, Short arc knee flexion/extension exercises and Isometric hamstring exercises (Figs. 16.48A and B)
  - PRE to quadriceps, prone kneeling to kneel sitting should be started after 6 weeks if the fracture has united.
  - Quadriceps lag (if any) should be managed by faradic type current stimulation to VMO.
  - Partial weight-bearing is started in parallel bar/walker/crutches at 6 weeks, gradually progressing to walking with a stick and subsequently full weight-bearing by 12 weeks.

Physiotherapy after patellectomy: Intensive physiotherapy should be started after patellectomy to achieve full knee flexion and to minimize/correct quadriceps lag. Physiotherapy after patellectomy is applied as discussed below:

Physiotherapy in the first week: It consists of:
- Ankle and foot exercises.
- Isometric quadriceps exercise (low-intensity), isometric glutei and hamstrings exercise.
- Faradic stimulation to quadriceps.
- Assisted SLR exercise.
- PSWD to promote healing and reduce swelling.

Physiotherapy in the second week: The exercises performed in the first week are continued in the second week also. Partial weight-bearing gait with walker/crutches are started during this time, with the POP posterior splint applied with. However, for knee flexion exercises, the splint should be removed temporarily. The therapy consists of:
- Short arc knee flexion exercises, maintaining the integrity of incisional wound.
- CPM in controlled manner.

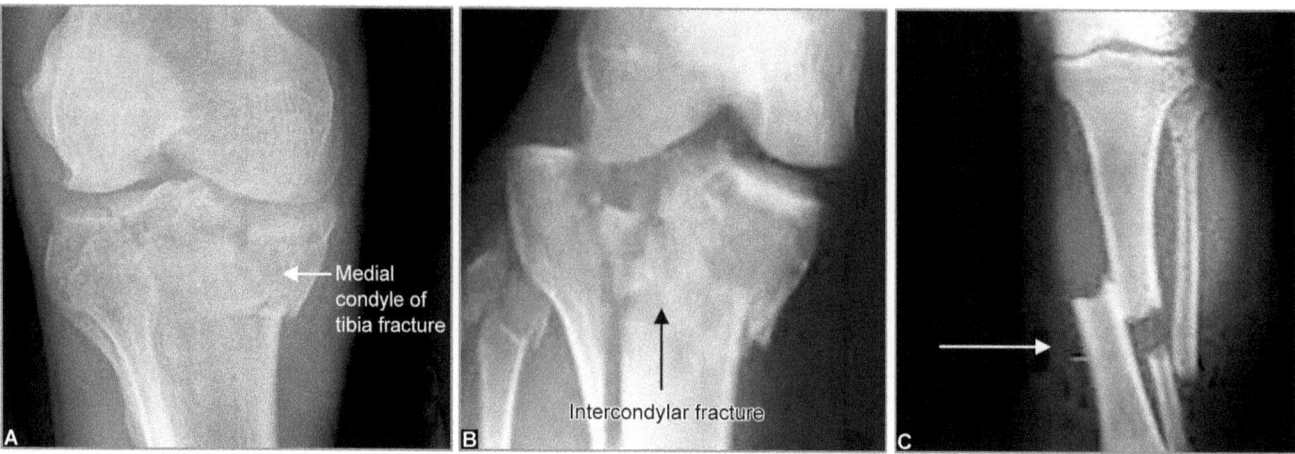

Figs. 16.49A to C: (A) Fracture medial condyle of tibia; (B) Intercondylar fracture of tibia; (C) Fracture both bones (tibia and fibula).

Physiotherapy after third week: The stitches are removed by this time, but the POP posterior splint is still in place, which is continued for 6 weeks. Active physiotherapy and graduated weight-bearing ambulation are emphasized during this period. The POP splint should be removed during knee flexion exercises and reapplied till the completion of periods of immobilization, i.e., 6 weeks. After 6 weeks of immobilization, therapy consists of:
- Vigorous knee mobilization exercises including use of CPM, static cycle exercises etc.
- Resisted isometric quadriceps exercise. PRE for quadriceps and hamstrings, with weight cuff/theraband.
- Hydrotherapy to increase ROM and muscle strength.
- Strong faradic stimulation to quadriceps helps in correcting quadriceps lag.
- Gait training with/without walking aids.
- Integration to family and social life: By about 8–12 weeks postoperatively, the patient is expected to have achieved adequate ROM, and muscle strength and can walk independently and is able to return to function.
- Any pain persisting is managed by Ultrasound/IFT.

Fracture of Tibia

It includes the following fractures:
- **Fracture of tibial condyles (Fig. 16.49A):** Lateral condyle fractures also called bumper fracture is more common as compared to medial condyle fractures. Injury to the collateral ligaments is sometimes associated with the respective condylar fractures.
- **Intercondylar fracture of tibia (Fig. 16.49B):** It is a fracture through the lateral and medial condyles of tibia.
- Fracture both bones (tibia and fibula) of leg **(Fig. 16.49C)**.

Management
- **Tibial condyle fractures:** It depends on, whether the fracture is displaced (needs surgical management) or undisplaced (managed conservatively).
  - *Conservative:* AK POP cast (for undisplaced fractures) **(Fig. 16.50)** and skeletal/skin traction for minimally

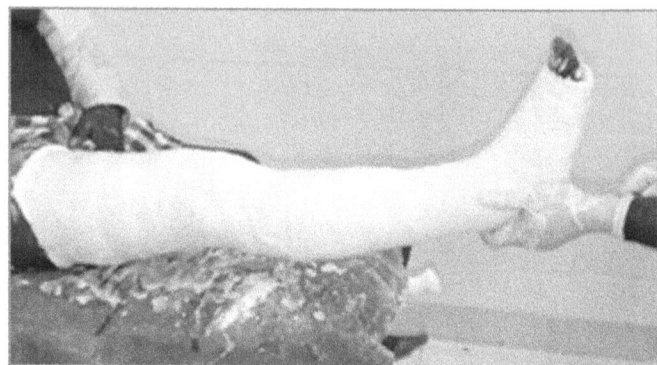

Fig. 16.50: Application of AK POP cast.

displaced fractures. The AK POP cast is maintained for 6–8 weeks and if traction is applied for minimally displaced fractures, traction is maintained for 3 weeks followed by application of AK POP cast. However, maintaining immobilization (with POP slab/crepe bandage) nonweight-bearing knee mobilization is started after POP removal. Weight-bearing is started after 12 weeks.
- *Surgery:* ORIF is performed for highly displaced fractures. For fractures with depression of tibial plateau, bone grafting and elevation of tibial plateau and fixation by a special type of plate is performed **(Fig. 16.51)**. Minimally displaced fractures are fixed with screws. Postoperatively nonweight-bearing crutch gait is performed after 3–4 days, and knee mobilization is started after 1 week and partial weight bearing is allowed after 6 weeks, progressing to full weight bearing by 3 months.

Physiotherapy:
» Isometric quadriceps, glutei exercises.
» Active toe movements.
» Nonweight-bearing crutch gait with axillary crutches as permissible usually started after 3–4 days.
» Gentle knee mobilization exercises during immobilization.
» After fracture united, vigorous knee mobilization exercises using thermotherapy (PWB), manual

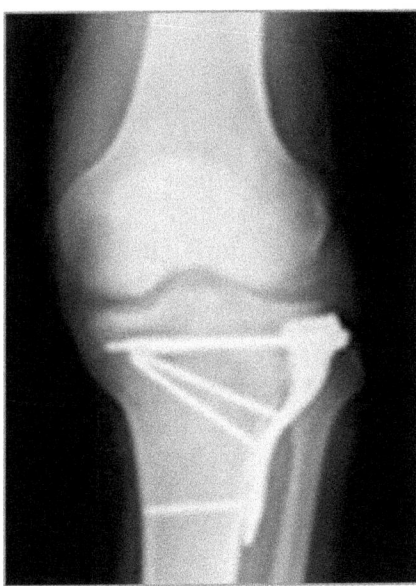

Fig. 16.51: Elevation of tibial plateau by ORIF.

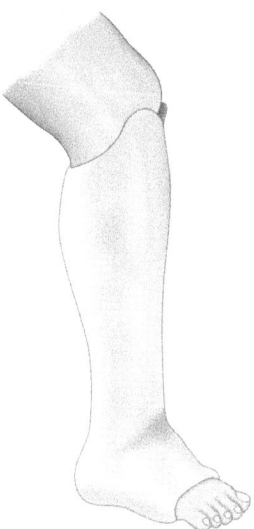

Fig. 16.52: Shows the PTB cast.

mobilization techniques, electrotherapy, CPM, etc., are done as described earlier.
» Strengthening of quadriceps and hamstrings are performed.
» Partial weight-bearing crutch gait with crutches is usually started by 6 weeks (considering fracture union) and progressed to full weight bearing by 12 weeks.

❖ **Intercondylar fractures of tibia:**
  – This fracture occurs more commonly in children than adults. In children the fracture is divided into three types, such as:
    » Type-I (fracture without dislodgement), Type-II (fracture segment is dislodged partially), Type-III (fracture fragment is completely dislodged).
    » Type-I, fractures are managed by POP immobilization for 4 to 6 weeks, and Type-II fractures require closed reduction with or without skeletal traction, and the reduction is maintained by POP cast. After 6 weeks when POP cast is removed, POP slab/knee immobilizer or a hinged knee brace is used.
  – *Conservative:* Nonweight-bearing knee mobilization is started after POP removal and weight bearing progressing from partial to full weight bearing started by 12 weeks.
  – *Surgical:* ORIF with screw and plates is performed for grossly displaced fractures (Type-III fractures). Postoperatively nonweight bearing knee mobilization is started after 1 week and weight bearing progressing from partial (usually starting at 6 weeks) to full weight-bearing starting by 12 weeks is allowed.
    Physiotherapy: It is applied using the same guidelines as described for condylar fractures.

❖ **Fracture of both bones of leg:** The following methods of management is followed:

  – AK POP cast is the commonly adopted method of treatment. Nonweight-bearing crutch gait (after 2 weeks of immobilization), isometric quadriceps exercises in POP cast, active toe movements are performed. POP is removed by 8 weeks and nonweight-bearing knee mobilization is started. Partial weight-bearing crutch gait is started after 8 weeks (considering fracture union), gradually progressing to full weight bearing after 12 weeks.
  – Functional cast bracing that involves AK POP cast for 3–4 weeks followed by PTB cast **(Fig. 16.52)** application, that allows early knee mobilization and weight-bearing, is followed, particularly, when there is delayed union.
  – ORIF with plate and screw fixation **(Fig. 16.53)**/intramedullary nail application is followed for displaced fractures. Postoperatively knee mobilization is started after 1 week and partial weight-bearing using walker/crutches are allowed after 8 weeks and full weight bearing is allowed after 12 weeks.

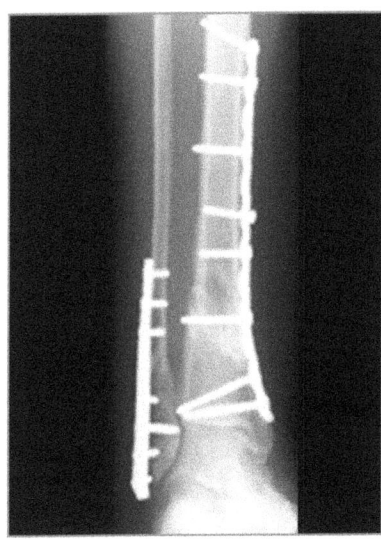

Fig. 16.53: Plate and screw fixation for fracture both bones of leg.

- *External fixator application:* Done for severely comminuted fractures with marked soft tissue damage. Patient is made to walk with partial weight bearing crutch gait till complete union of the fracture.

FRACTURES AROUND THE ANKLE AND FOOT

It includes:
- **Pott's fracture (Fig. 16.54A):** A Pott's fracture also called as Dupuytren's fracture involves fracture to one or both malleoli (lateral and medial).
- **Trimalleolar fracture (Fig. 16.54B):** A trimalleolar fracture in ankle involves fracture of three bones, such as: medial, lateral malleoli and posterior malleolus (The posterior aspect of tibial plafond).
- Fracture of tarsals (calcaneus/talus/navicular) **(Figs. 16.54C to E)**.
- Metatarsal and phalangeal fractures **(Fig. 16.54F)**.

Management

a. **Pott's and trimalleolar fractures:** The management of the fracture could be:
   - *Conservative:* Manipulative reduction followed by BK POP cast for 6-8 weeks.
   - For severely displaced fragments, where closed reduction is not possible, ORIF with plate and screws **(Fig. 16.55)**/TBW (tension band wiring) is performed. 3-4 weeks of immobilization in POP cast is followed after surgery.

Physiotherapy

- **During immobilization:**
  - Limb elevation, toe movements, exercises for hip and knee are performed.
  - PSWD (mean power output < 5W) may be applied over the cast to promote healing.
  - Nonweight-bearing crutch gait is promoted.
- **After POP cast removal** (after 6-8 weeks for conservative management and 3-4 weeks for operative management), the followings are performed.
  - Relaxed passive movements/active assisted/free exercises to ankle and foot after 8 weeks in case of conservative management and after 4 weeks in case of surgery performed.
  - Contrast bath for management of swelling and pain.
  - PWB.
  - Ultrasound therapy for associated ligament injury (for conservative treatment only).
  - Gentle stretching of TA is performed, when there is tightness of the same.
  - Exercise in ankle exerciser **(Fig. 16.56)**.
  - Partial weight bearing on walker/crutches to start after 8 weeks when there is satisfactory union of the fracture. Full weight bearing should be allowed after 12 weeks.
  - TENS/IFT can be used to manage pain.

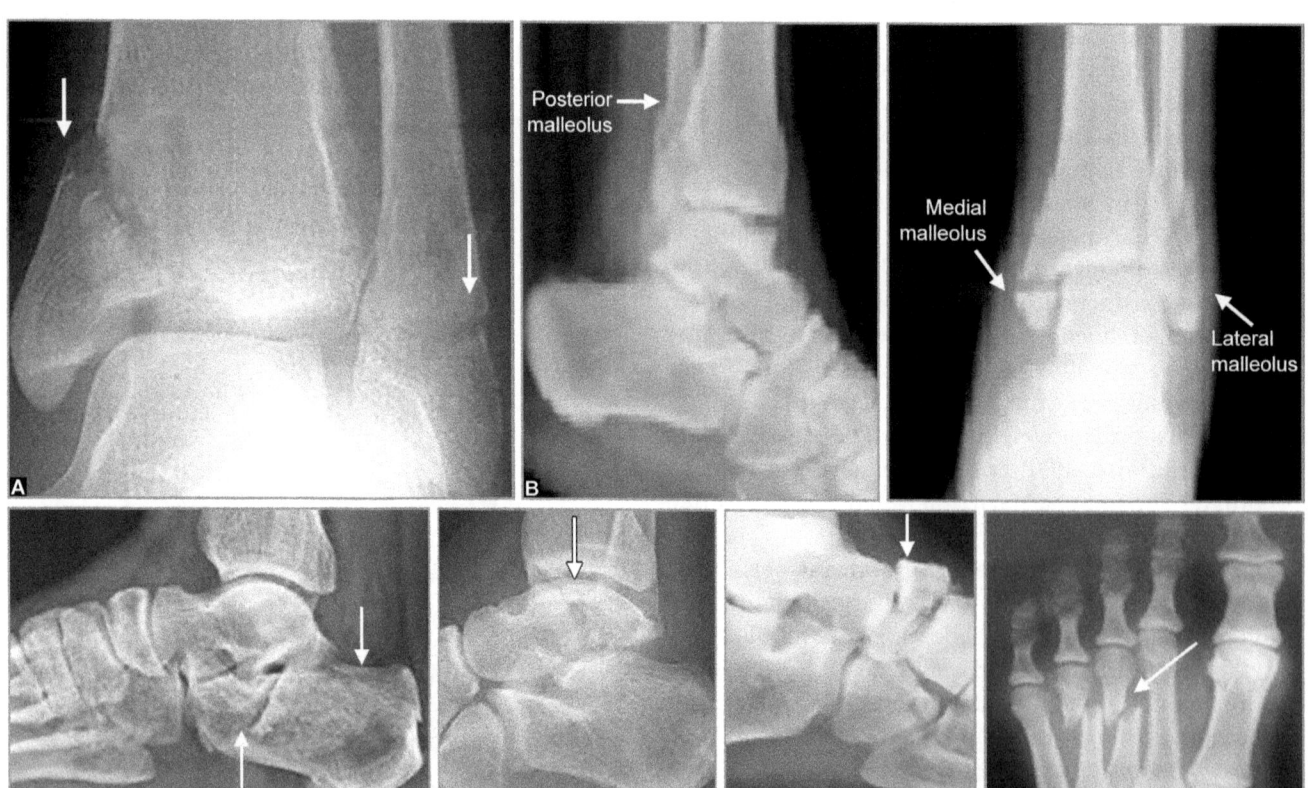

Figs. 16.54A to F: (A) Pott's fracture; (B) Trimalleolar fracture; (C) Calcaneus fracture; (D) Talus fracture; (E) Navicular fracture; (F) Metatarsal fracture.

Chapter 16: Physiotherapy in Fractures

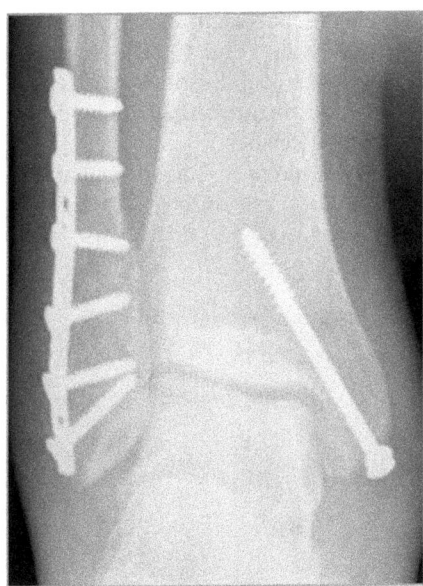

Fig. 16.55: ORIF for Pott's fracture.

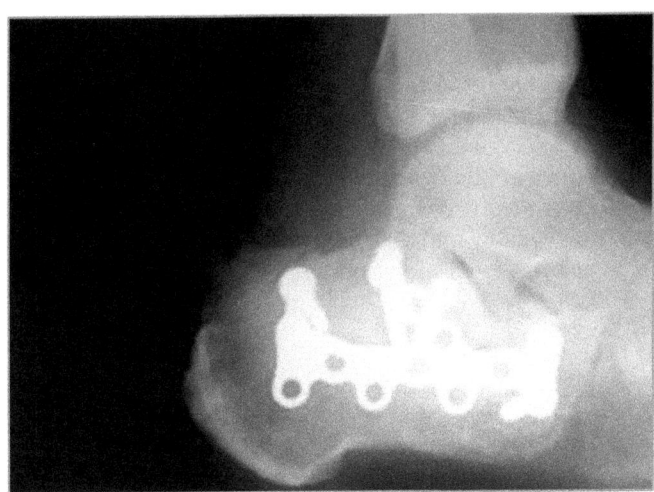

Fig. 16.57: ORIF for calcaneal fracture.

(except when subtalar arthrodesis performed where the foot is not mobilized) are done in the same lines discussed under physiotherapy for ankle fractures.

Partial weight-bearing gait is started after 8 weeks and full weight bearing should be gradually progressed considering the intensity of pain, which is generally possible after 3–4 months.

Pain (if any) is managed by TENS/IFT.

FRACTURE OF TALUS/NAVICULAR AND OTHER TARSAL BONES

- **Talus fracture:** Closed reduction and BK POP casting for 6–8 weeks, followed by physiotherapy as described under ankle fracture. Nonweight-bearing crutch gait is allowed as tolerated. Weight-bearing is allowed after 3 months.

  If the fracture needs surgical intervention, ORIF with K-wire fixation is performed, followed by BK POP casting

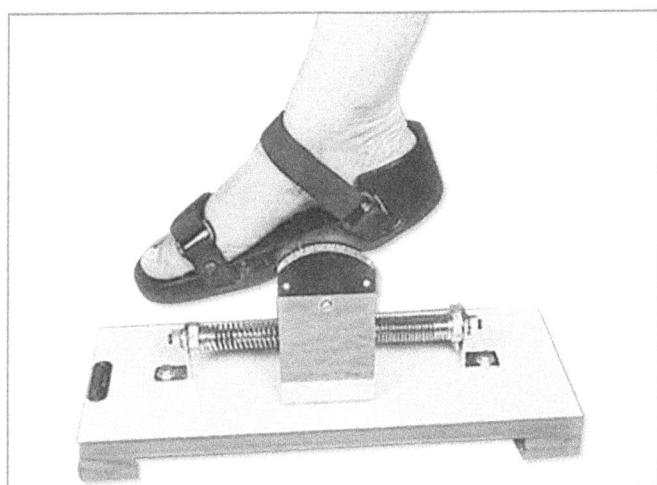

Fig. 16.56: Exercise on ankle exerciser.

FRACTURES OF TARSALS, METATARSALS, AND PHALANGES

Calcaneus Fracture

Treatment of the fracture is mostly conservative, by BK POP casting for 6–8 weeks, followed by physiotherapy. In case of displaced and comminuted fractures ORIF with K-wire (**Fig. 16.57**)/plate and screws is performed. Arthrodesis of subtalar joint is sometimes performed.

Physiotherapy

- **During immobilization:** Isometric quadriceps/hamstrings/glutei exercises, and active movement of toes are emphasized. PSWD (mean power output<5W) may be considered with the cast to promote healing.
- **After cast/POP slab removal:** Besides exercises performed during immobilization, mobilization of ankle and foot

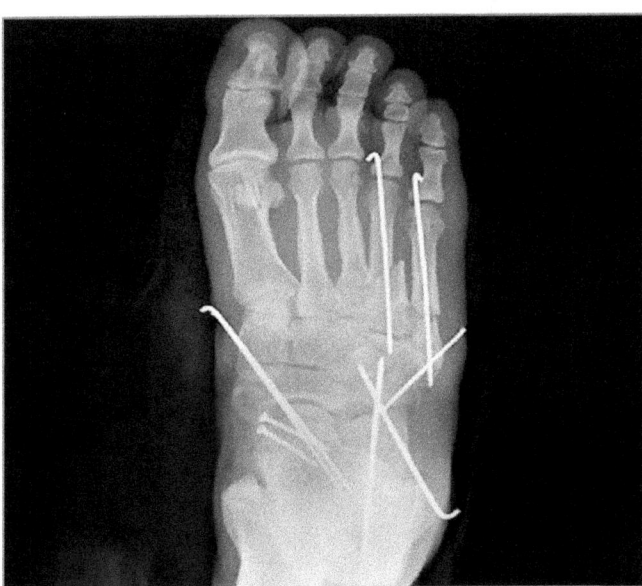

Fig. 16.58: X-ray showing K-wire fixation for tarsals and medial 2 metatarsals.

for 8–10 weeks and physiotherapy after cast removal is as described under ankle fracture.

- ❖ **Fracture of other tarsal bones:** Managed conservatively by BK POP cast for 3–4 weeks, followed by mobilization of ankle and foot and graduated weight bearing.
- ❖ **Fracture of metatarsals:**
  - *Conservative management:* BK POP cast for 3–4 weeks followed by mobilization exercises and gradual weight bearing.
  - *Surgery:* Reserved for fractures with displacement. ORIF with K-wire fixation **(Fig. 16.58)**, followed by BK POP slab for 3–4 weeks. Mobilization exercises are performed after 4 weeks of immobilization. Weight-bearing is allowed after 4–6 weeks.
- ❖ **Fracture of phalanges:** Managed conservatively by soft strapping with adjacent digit for 2 weeks, followed by mobilization exercises.

Physiotherapy for Burn

INTRODUCTION

Burns are injuries to skin and underlying tissues, caused by materials that produce heat, chemicals, electricity, friction, prolong cold, radiation, etc.

CAUSES OF BURN

The causes include:
- **Breakout of fire:** As occurs in domestic kitchen accidents, short circuiting, industries, motor vehicles, etc.
- Exposure to hot metals and steam.
- Exposure to chemicals such as accidents in industries, acid attacks, etc.
- **Electrocution:** Mostly found in electricians, however, electric burn may also occur in patients who receive low and medium frequency current treatments.
- **Exposure to radiation:** Sun burn, burns developing due to prolonged exposure to higher grade erythema dose of ultraviolet radiation (UVR), etc., are caused due to exposure to radiations.
- **Prolonged exposure to ice (frost bite):** That may develop due to prolong application of cryo pack, walking on bare foot on snow, etc.
- **Prolong friction:** As found in individuals treated with deep transverse friction massage (DTFM).
- Abuse due to domestic and communal violences.

TYPES OF BURN INJURIES

Burn injuries can be classified into various types, which are as follows:
- Depending upon the causes, burns can be classified into:
  - Thermal burn
  - Chemical burn
  - Electrical burn
  - Ice burn
- As per the depth of tissue affection, burns can be classified into several degrees such as:
  - First degree burn
  - Second degree burn
  - Third degree burn
  - Fourth degree burn

Table 17.1 discusses the various degrees of burn.

Further, the burns are classified into the following types, depending on the depth of tissues affected:
1. **Superficial burns:** They involve only the epidermal layer of the skin.
2. **Partial thickness burn:** This is the burn involving the epidermis and portions of dermis. It involves damage to capillaries and free nerve endings in the dermis. It could be superficial partial thickness burn, that forms blister between epidermis and dermis OR the deep partial thickness burn, that extends into deeper dermis, damaging hair follicles and glandular tissues.

Table 17.1: Degrees of burn.

Degrees of burn	First degree/ superficial burn	Second degree/ partial thickness burns (superficial)	Second degree/ partial thickness burns (deep)	Third degree/full thickness burns	Fourth degree/deep full thickness burn
Layer of skin involved	Epidermis	Dermis Superficial layer	Dermis: Deep layer	Subcutaneous fat	Muscles, tendons, and bones
Signs and symptoms	Redness, pain, and swelling	Pink/red, blister, moist, sore	Dry, white and nonblanching	Leathery, dry, white/red with thrombosed vessels	Black, charred with eschar, dry
Healing time	3–7 days	10–14 days	17–21 days/requires skin graft	Requires skin graft	Requires reconstruction

3. **Full thickness burn:** Full thickness burns extend through and destroy all layers of the dermis. They involve all layers of the skin and may involve the structures beneath, such as muscles and bone. These burns are usually anesthetic/hypoesthetic.
4. **Deeper fourth degree burn:** Deeper (fourth degree) burns extend through the skin into underlying soft tissues, such as fascia, muscle and/or bone.

PERCENTAGE OF BURN

The rule of nines is a method that clinicians use to easily calculate the treatment needs for a person who has been burnt. Depending on the area of body surface affected, burns are given percentage **(Table 17.2** and **Fig. 17.1)**.

Rule of Nine in Children

The same calculation, as done in case of adult to document the percentage of burn are not followed for children, as children have proportionately larger head and small extremities. The **Table 17.3** gives the percentage calculation for burns in children, generated with few adjustments.

CLINICAL FEATURES OF BURN

The features of burn depend on the degree and nature of offending agent. Sometimes, complete features due to damage are not seen immediately, after burn takes place, and for a severe burn, it may take 1–2 days for the features to develop. The common features of burn are:
- Blisters
- Pain
- Swelling
- White or charred (black) skin
- Peeling of skin

Table 17.1 gives the features of different degrees of burn. However, the features of burns caused by different agents are discussed below.

- **Electric burn:** Direct contact, high-voltage injury causes a painless, full-thickness, indented, yellowish-gray skin burn that is sometimes accompanied by central necrosis **(Fig. 17.2)**. Flashing high-voltage injury can cause a superficial burn, a partial thickness burn, or devastating full-thickness injury brought about by an electric arc.

  In high-voltage electric burns, a contact and a ground point can often be identified. The contact point is characterized by charred, centrally depressed, and leathery wounds, while the ground point is more likely to explode as the charge exits.

- **Heat (thermal) burn:** Thermal burns **(Fig. 17.3)** cause both local injuries and, if severe (>20% of body surface area), a systemic response. The local injuries can be roughly separated into three zones of injury analogous to a circular target pattern. The innermost injury is the zone of coagulation or necrosis, representing the area of irreversible cell death. Surrounding this is the zone of ischemia or

Table 17.3: Percentage of burn in children.

Portion/area of body	Percentage
Head and neck (front and back)	18%
Each upper limb (front and back)	9%
Anterior trunk	18%
Posterior trunk	18%
Each lower limb (front and back)	14%

Table 17.2: Percentage of burn as per body area affected.

Portion/area of body	Percentage
Head and neck	9%
Anterior trunk (front of body)	18%
Posterior trunk (back of body)	18%
Each upper limb (front/back)	9% (total)
Groin	1%
Each lower limb (front/back)	18% each

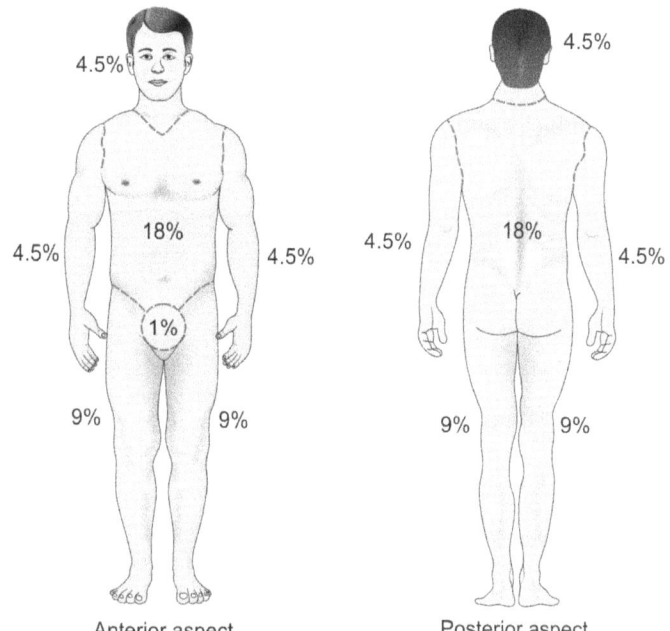

Fig. 17.1: Body chart showing percentage of burn.

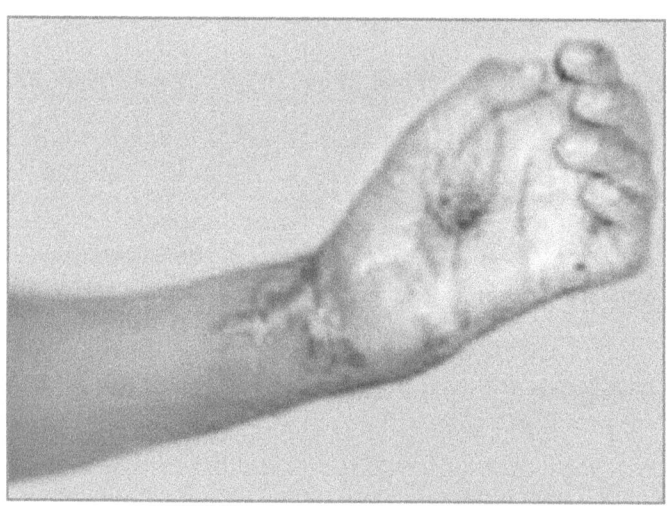

Fig. 17.2: Electric burn in hand.

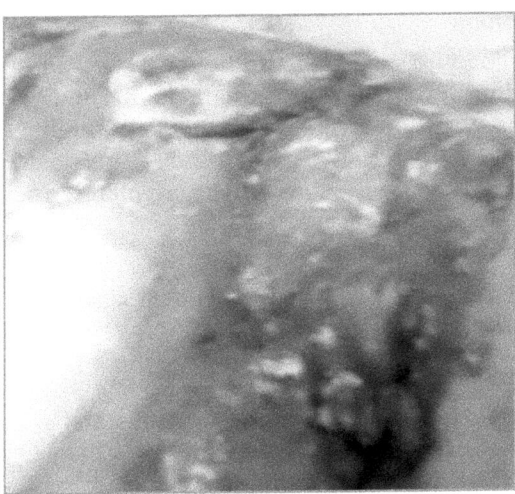

Fig. 17.3: Thermal burn to trunk.

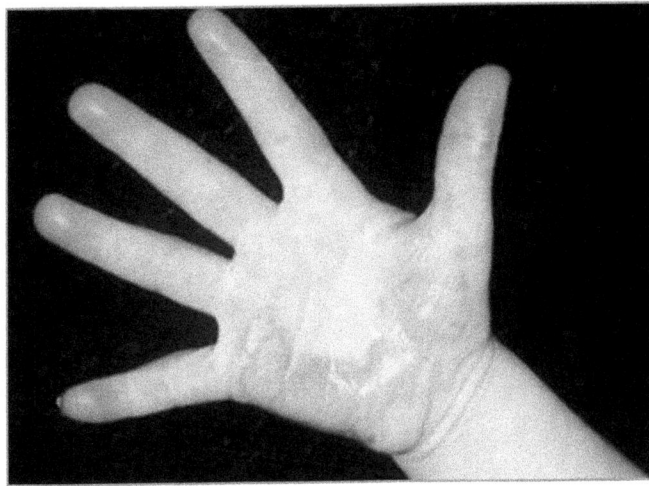

Fig. 17.5: Cold burn.

stasis, representing an area of decreased circulation and an area at increased risk of progression to necrosis due to hypoperfusion or infection. The outermost area is the zone of hyperemia, representing an area of reversible vasodilation and an area that usually returns to normal.

- **Chemical burn:** These burns occur in the face, eyes, arms, and legs. Usually, they are smaller in size. Signs and symptoms of chemical burns **(Fig. 17.4)** include the following:
  - Redness, irritation, or burning at the site of contact
  - Pain or numbness at the site of contact
  - Formation of blisters or black dead skin at the contact site
  - Vision changes, if the chemical gets into eyes
  - Cough or shortness of breath, due to irritating smell of the chemicals
- **Cold burn (frost bite):** The symptoms of an ice burn **(Fig. 17.5)** can include:
  - Red, white, dark, or gray skin
  - Pain
  - Blisters
  - Numbness
  - Tingling

- Itchiness
- Hard or waxy skin

Besides the typical features unique to the type of burn, hypovolemic shock (in extensive burn injuries), respiratory complications, formation of hypertrophied scar/keloids, tightness/contracture deformity, bone loss (4th degree burn), disfiguring of body and disability, etc., are the features of burn. A keloid is a scar, where, the extra connective tissue that forms, extends beyond the original wound area **(Fig. 17.6A)**, where in for hypertrophic scars, the extra connective tissue remains confined to the original wound area **(Fig. 17.6B)**.

MANAGEMENT OF BURN

A systematic approach to burn care focuses on the six "Cs": clothing (clothes should be removed from the burnt site), cooling (cool water should be applied and the patient should be nursed in an air conditioned room), cleaning (the burn wound should be dressed), chemoprophylaxis (silver containing antibiotic creams should be applied), covering (patient should be kept inside a mosquito net), and comforting (i.e., pain relief).

Most minor burns can be treated at home with medicines, wound dressing. They usually heal within a couple of weeks. For full thickness burns, the patient is admitted to a specialized burn care center. After appropriate first aid and wound assessment, treatment may involve medications, wound dressings, therapy, splinting, and surgery (skin grafting). The goals of treatment are to control pain, remove dead tissue, prevent infection, reduce scarring risk, and regain function, which are achieved by proper medical and therapeutic interventions.

Medical management: It consists of:
- Tetanus toxoid injection and IV fluid delivery
- Pain and anxiety medications/antibiotics
- Wound dressing
- Burn cream and lotion application

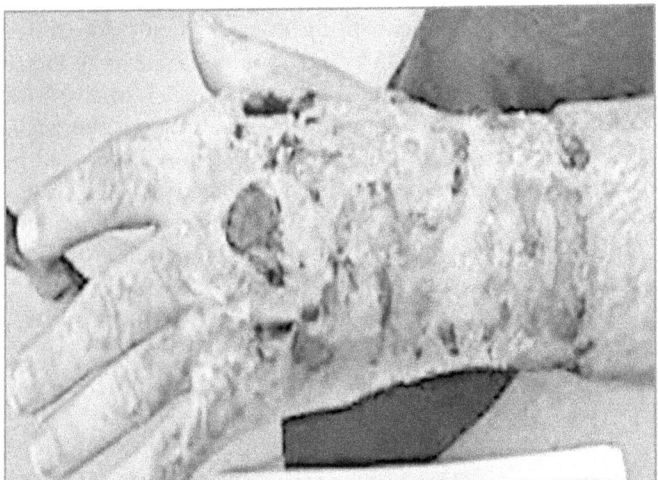

Fig. 17.4: A chemical burn in hand.

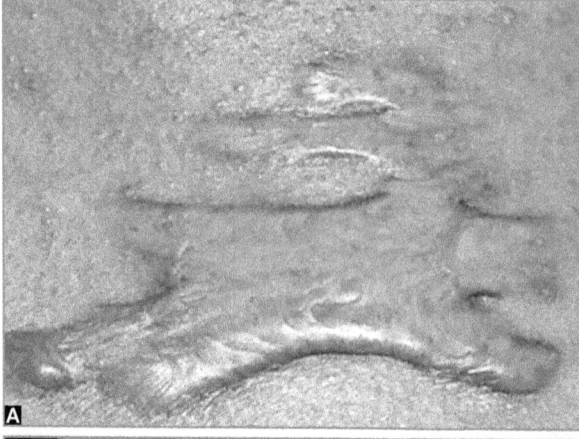

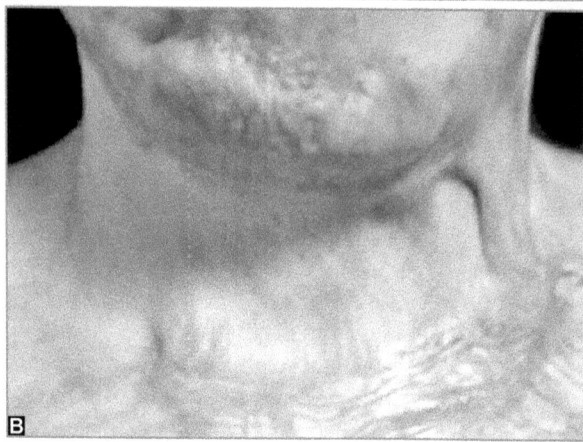

Figs. 17.6A and B: (A) Shows keloid; (B) Shows hypertrophied scar.

REHABILITATION OF BURN INJURY

It involves a team of professionals, including physician, plastic surgeon, physiotherapist, occupational therapist, orthotist, social worker, etc. A thorough assessment to find the patient's functional status should be done prior to the commencement of rehabilitation. This helps to develop a customized treatment plan for individual patients. The aims of post-burn rehabilitation are geared toward the reintegration of the individuals back to society. Before active rehabilitation is started, it is essential to cause healing of the burn wound through medical and surgical procedures. The common surgeries performed (skin grafting and escharotomy) are briefly discussed below.

Skin Grafting for Burns

Skin grafting is a term used to describe the process of transferring skin from one part of the body (the donor site) to another area, known as the recipient site, which has been damaged by burns, mostly deep second degree, third degree burns. Common donor sites for grafting are the upper arm and thighs. Other areas may include the back, buttocks, or abdomen. A protection period of 5–7 days is required, for the graft to survive by taking nutrition from the recipient site. During this time movement is not allowed in the grafted areas, but the neighboring parts of the body can be moved.

Escharotomy

Escharotomy is a surgical procedure used to treat full thickness (third/fourth degree) burns, where dermis and epidermis are destroyed along with the sensory nerve endings in the dermis. The tough leathery scar tissue called eschar need to be released surgically, to allow free movements to occur.

Physiotherapy for Burn

The aims of physiotherapy depend on the stage (early stage/late stage) when patient reports.

i. *Physiotherapy in Early Stage*

The aims of physiotherapy in the early stage are:
- To maintain chest expansion (for burns involving trunk and chemical burns).
- To maintain range of motion (ROM).
- To prevent development of strong scar/keloids and, tightness/contracture/deformity.
- To maximize social integration and psychological well being.
- To maximize functional ability and recovery.
- To enhance quality of life.

Physiotherapy techniques in this stage include:
- **Respiratory care:** Respiratory care is very important especially for cases of inhalation injury and burns to the, neck, chest and abdomen. Chest physiotherapy in the form of the followings points are given to improve lungs function.
  – Breathing exercises
  – Active cycle of breathing technique (ACBT)
  – Manual techniques such as chest percussion/vibration (however, percussion/vibration should be avoided in individuals having burn to the chest wall)
  – Postural drainage or modified postural drainage
  – Suction (if necessary)
  – Thoracic mobility exercises
  – Incentive spirometry
- **Positioning to the joints affected by burn:** The correct position is opposite to the positions of comfort and common contractures develop in patients. The hip should be positioned in abduction, neutral extension and rotation; knee should be kept in extension and ankle in plantigrade using a resting splint **(Fig. 17.7A)**. The shoulder should be abducted (as adduction contracture is common after a burn involving axilla), elbow extended and hand in neutral position using a proper hand splint **(Fig. 17.7B)**. The neck should be positioned in extension using a cervical roll **(Fig. 17.7C)**. Positioning is performed on the first day of the patients admitted to hospital until the scars mature. Joints involved are positioned correctly to achieve the following goals:
  – Prevent development of tightness/contracture/deformity.
  – Reduce swelling.
  – Prevent deep vein thrombosis (DVT).
  – Prevent further damage to the joints or exposed tendons.
  – Avoid damage to new skin graft/reconstructed soft tissues.

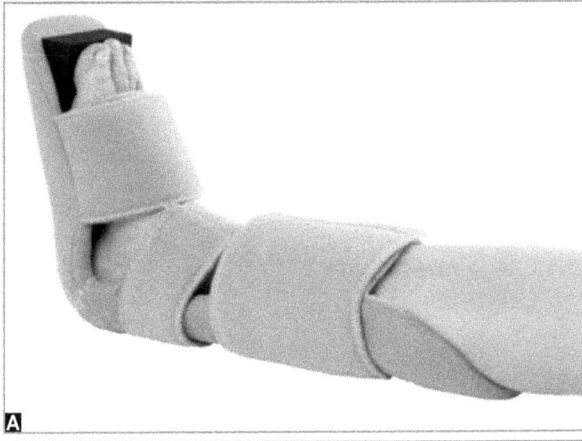
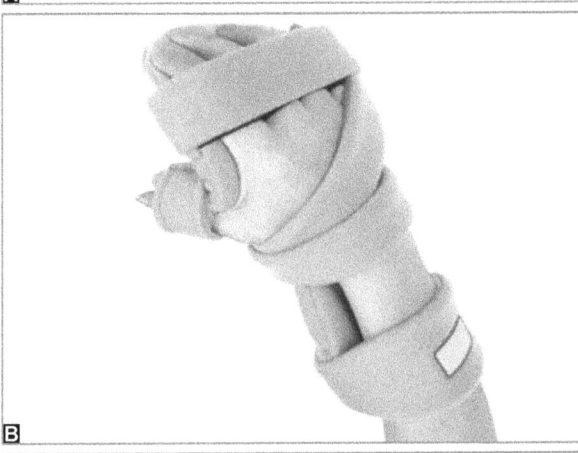
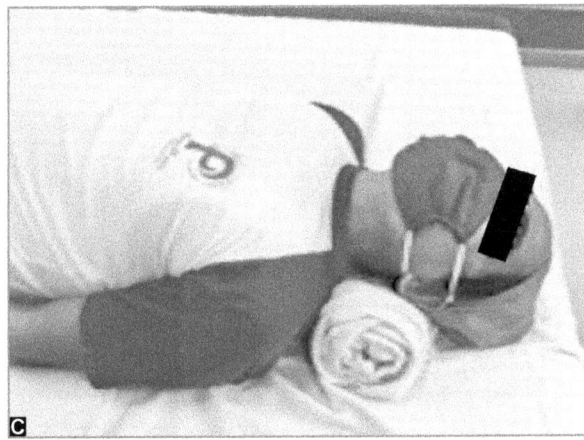

Figs. 17.7A to C: (A) Night splint for ankle; (B) Night splint for hand; (C) Cervical roll.

- Avoiding pressure sores on bony areas such as the heel, olecranon process, etc.
- **Regular passive movements:** As the skin allows, regular passive movements should be performed at frequent intervals to maintain ROM and prevent DVT.
- Pain (if any) should be managed by TENS, where electrodes are placed over the areas, where the skin is intact.
- Regular change of position should be made to prevent development of pressure ulcer.

ii. Physiotherapy in Late (Post healing) Stage

The aims of physiotherapy in this stage are:
- To improve muscle strength, endurance, balance, coordination.
- Mobilize scar tissue.
- Improve chest mobility and ventilation.
- Improve function and gait.
- To integrate in family and society.

Physiotherapy techniques in this stage include:
- **Therapeutic exercises:** Exercise should be done on the first day of admission. Once the wound has healed, it is ideal to soak the hand/foot in warm water before doing exercises. The purposes are to:
  - Maintain joint integrity.
  - Maintain muscle flexibility and elasticity of the skin.
  - Maintain joint range of motion and prevent contractures.
  - Increase muscle strength and endurance.
  - Restore the musculoskeletal function to optimal level.

  Therapeutic exercises performed include:
  - Stretching exercises.
  - Muscle strengthening exercises using theraband/dumbbell.
  - Aerobic exercises in the form of circuit training, stair climbing, static cycle exercises, etc.
  - PNF techniques.
- **Hydrotherapy:** If wounds have completely healed and movements are grossly limited due to pain, weakness etc., hydrotherapy with controlled temperature of water may be beneficial.
- **Chest care:** Active cycle of breathing techniques (ACBT), postural drainage, and incentive spirometry are performed as per need.
- **TENS** to reduce pain.
- **Pulsed ultrasound therapy** to mobilize tight scar.
- **Scar massage:** Scars are to be applied with lotions, and massaged 3–4 sessions in a day.
- **Low temperature PWB:** Low temperature paraffin wax bath can be used to supple soft tissues (in the absence of hypertrophic scar/keloids) over stiff joints, before mobilization exercises.
- **LASER therapy:** Willows et al., (2017) recommend the use of laser therapy, especially ablative fractional lasers in the management of burns to improve the pliability, vascularity and overall burn scar appearance.
- **Extracorporeal shock wave therapy:** Low energy, extracorporeal shock wave therapy, along with traditional physiotherapy has been found to be effective for management of burn scar.
- **Posture care**: Balance and proprioceptive training to improve posture are given on wobble board/trampoline etc.
- **Cognitive behavioral therapy:** To reduce pain and anxiety.

Home Advice and Exercise Program

The patient should be advised to apply lotions regularly, wear loose garments, avoid exposure to sunlight and perform exercises regularly. He/she should be advised to use gloves/adaptive devices for activities like cooking (if there is no sensation in hands due to full thickness burns). If he/she has sensory loss in feet, should be given MCR-lined sandals for walking.

SECTION 3

Physiotherapy for Neurological Conditions

Section Outline

- Chapter 18: Cerebral Palsy
- Chapter 19: Stroke/Cerebrovascular Accident
- Chapter 20: Physiotherapy for Spinal Cord Injury
- Chapter 21: Parkinson's Disease
- Chapter 22: Traumatic Brain Injury
- Chapter 23: Physiotherapy in Multiple Sclerosis
- Chapter 24: Physiotherapy for Muscular Dystrophies, Motor Neuron Disease and Spinal Muscular Atrophies
- Chapter 25: Physiotherapy for Peripheral Nerve Injuries
- Chapter 26: Physiotherapy in Guillain-Barre Syndrome: Acute Inflammatory Demyelinating Polyneuropathy and Chronic Inflammatory Demyelinating Polyneuropathy
- Chapter 27: Physiotherapy in Ataxias (Ataxic Disorders)

Cerebral Palsy

INTRODUCTION

Cerebral palsy (CP) is the most chronic childhood disease today. It occurs all-around the world. In spite of improved obstetrical and perinatal care, the condition is very much prevalent. The condition was first described by an English physician Sir Francis William Little in 1861, and is known as Little's disease.

As per the PWD Act 2016, "cerebral palsy" means a group of nonprogressive neurological conditions affecting body movements and muscle coordination, caused by damage to one or more specific areas of the brain, usually occurring before, during, or shortly after birth.

Though, posture and movement are the primary impairments in CP, the child may also present with other problems such as speech problem, visual problem, hearing problem, intellectual problem (low IQ), perceptual and cognitive problem, etc.

Considering the above facts, CP is defined as a nonprogressive but not unchanging disorder of posture and movement caused by a damage to the developing brain during prenatal, perinatal and postnatal periods of life, which may or may not be associated with other handicaps, such as speech problem, hearing problem, visual problem, intellectual deficits, cognitive and perceptual problem, gastrointestinal problem, epilepsy, etc.

Most children with CP lead a normal life span. The condition is not contagious and not progressive.

Epidemiology

This is the most common physical disability of childhood. The incidence has increased since the 60s, which may be due to survival of very low-birth-weight infants. The incidence in Western societies is 2–2.5/1,000 live births. In India, the estimated incidence is around 3/1,000 live births. Nearly 15–20% of physically disabled children in India are affected by CP.

Etiology/Risk Factors

Variety of prenatal, perinatal and postnatal factors contribute either in single or in combination for the causation of cerebral palsy. Earlier, birth asphyxia was thought to be the most common cause of cerebral palsy, however presently, prenatal brain injury is considered as the dominant cause of the disorder. Premature birth, though is the most important factor for causation of cerebral palsy, postnatal factors also contribute significantly for the causation of the disorder.

The risk factors/etiology of CP are categorized into the followings:

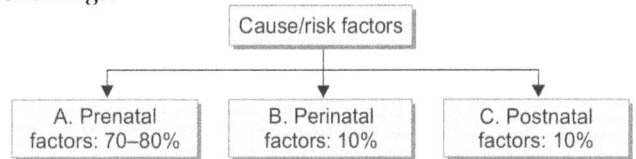

A. **Prenatal (conception to onset of labor) factors (70–80%):**
   - Prematurity (gestational age less than 32 weeks).
   - Low birth weight (less than 2.5 kg).
   - Maternal epilepsy.
   - Infection: TORCH [Toxoplasmosis, Other infection such as Hepatitis-B, Rubella (German measles, Cytomegalovirus, Herpes simplex].
   - Hyperthyroidism.
   - Bleeding in the third trimester.
   - Incompetent cervix.
   - Severe toxemia.
   - Eclampsia.
   - Drug abuse.
   - Trauma.
   - Maternal overage.
   - Multiple pregnancies.
   - Maternal diabetes.
   - Placental insufficiency.

B. **Perinatal (onset of labor to 1st week following birth) factors (10%):**
   - Prolonged and difficult labor.
   - Premature rupture of membrane.
   - Presentation anomalies (breech presentation)
   - Forceps delivery.
   - Vaginal bleeding at the time of admission for labor.
   - Birth asphyxia due to knotting of umbilical cord round the neck.
   - Birth hypoxia (Delayed birth cry).
   - Cesarean section delivery.
   - Severe jaundice.

C. Postnatal (1st week of birth to 2 years) factors (10%):
- CNS infection (encephalitis, meningitis)
- Trauma.
- Neonatal hyperbilirubinemia.
- Drowning.
- Seizure disorders.
- Coagulopathies.

Pathology of CNS in Cerebral Palsy

The lesions occur in the regions of CNS that are sensitive to the disturbance of blood supply and are grouped under the term hypoxic ischemic encephalopathy.

Five types of hypoxic ischemic encephalopathy, such as parasagittal cerebral injury, periventricular leukomalacia, focal and multifocal ischemic brain necrosis, status marmoratus, and selective neuronal necrosis have been recognized.

The location of injury and the clinical findings of different lesions in CNS are briefly discussed in **Table. 18.1**.

Classification of Cerebral Palsy

- **Physiological classification:**
  - *Spastic CP:* It is the most common form of CP. Approximately, 70–80% of children with CP are spastic. It is characterized by hyper-reflexia, hypertonicity, clonus, extensor plantar responses, and primitive reflexes with poor postural control **(Fig. 18.1)**. The lesion is located to cerebral cortex or the descending tracts.
  - *Dyskinetic cerebral palsy:* Dyskinetic CP accounts for approximately 10–15% of all cases of CP. Hyperbilirubinemia or severe anoxia causes basal ganglia dysfunction and results in dyskinetic CP. Abnormal movements (worm-like writhing, rapid jerky,

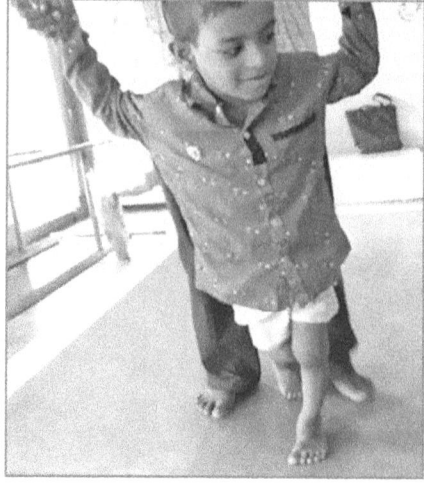

Fig. 18.1: Spastic cerebral palsy.

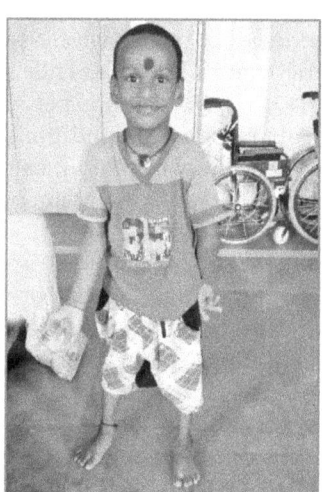

Fig. 18.2: Dyskinetic cerebral palsy.

rapid flinging) **(Fig. 18.2)**, that occur when the patient initiates movement are termed dyskinesias. Dysarthria, dysphagia, and drooling accompany the movement problem. Mental status is generally normal, however, severe dysarthria makes communication difficult. The lesion lies with the basal ganglia or the extrapyramidal system.

- *Ataxic cerebral palsy:* Ataxia is loss of balance, coordination, and fine motor control. Ataxic children cannot coordinate their movements. They are hypotonic during the first 2 years of life. Muscle tone becomes normal and ataxia becomes apparent toward the age of 2–3 years. Children who can walk have a wide-based gait and a mild intention tremor (dysmetria) **(Fig. 18.3)**. Dexterity and fine motor control is poor. Ataxia is associated with cerebellar lesions.
- *Mixed cerebral palsy:* Children with a mixed type of CP commonly have mild spasticity, dystonia, and/or athetoid movements. Ataxia may be a component of the motor dysfunction in patients in this group. Ataxia and spasticity often occur together. Spastic ataxic diplegia

Table 18.1: The location and clinical findings of different lesions.		
Lesion	Location	Clinical findings
Parasagittal cerebral injury	Bilateral superior or medial and posterior portion of the cortex	Upper extremities are more severely affected than the lower extremities
Periventricular leukomalacia	Bilateral white matter necrosis near lateral ventricles, descending fibers of the motor cortex, optic and acoustic radiations	Spastic diplegia and quadriplegia with visual and cognitive deficits
Focal and multi-focal ischemic brain necrosis	Infarction in a specific vascular distribution (most commonly left MCA)	Hemiplegia and seizures
Status marmoratus	Neuronal injury in basal ganglia	Choreoathetosis or mixed CP
Selective neuronal necrosis	Lateral geniculate body, thalamus and basal ganglia	Mental retardation and seizures

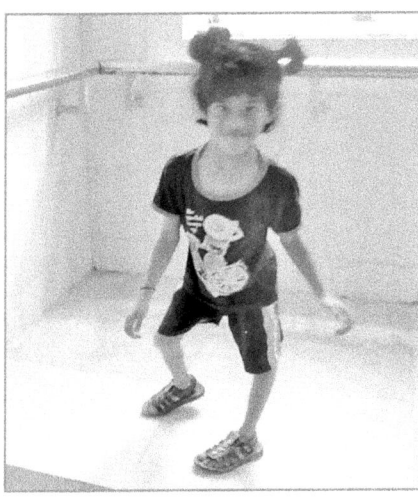

Fig. 18.3: Ataxic cerebral palsy.

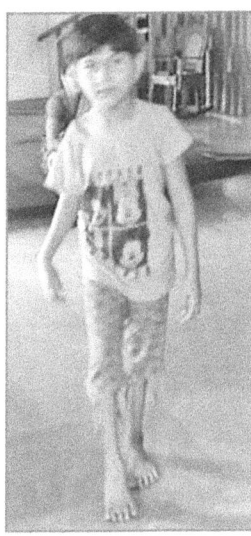

Fig. 18.5: Spastic hemiplegic cerebral palsy.

is a common mixed type that often is associated with hydrocephalus. In this type of CP, the lesion in the brain is diffuse.
- Atonic/hypotonic cerebral palsy: In this type of CP, the child presents with hypotonicity and has difficulty in maintaining erect posture **(Fig. 18.4)**. This type is also called as floppy baby syndrome. The exact site of lesion of this type of CP, which carries a poor prognosis, is not known.

❖ **Topographical types of CP:** This classification is based upon the area/part of the body that are affected as a result of damage to different parts in the brain. The types include:
1. *Hemiplegia:* Upper and lower extremity on one side of body are affected **(Fig. 18.5)**.
2. *Diplegia:* All four limbs affected, but lower limbs affected more than upper limbs **(Fig. 18.6)**.
3. *Quadriplegia:* All four extremities are affected, the upper limbs are either affected equally, or affected more than the lower limbs **(Fig. 18.7A)**.

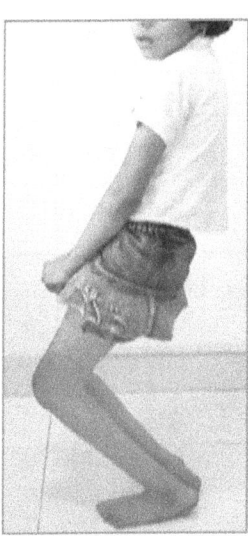

Fig. 18.6: Spastic diplegic cerebral palsy.

4. *Triplegia:* Both lower extremities and one upper extremity are affected.
5. *Monoplegia:* One extremity is usually affected, and this type is rare.
6. *Double hemiplegia:* All four extremities are affected; one side is affected more than the other.
7. *Pentaplegia:* A form of spastic CP affecting all four limbs with paralysis/paresis of neck and face, often accompanied by eating and breathing complications **(Fig. 18.7B)**.

❖ **Gross motor function classification:**
The gross motor skills (e.g., sitting and walking) of children and young people with CP can be categorized into five different levels using a tool called the Gross Motor Function Classification System (GMFCS).
- *GMFCS Level-I:* Can walk indoors and outdoors and climb stairs without using hands for support **(Fig. 18.8)**. Can perform usual activities such as running and jumping. Has decreased speed, balance, and coordination.

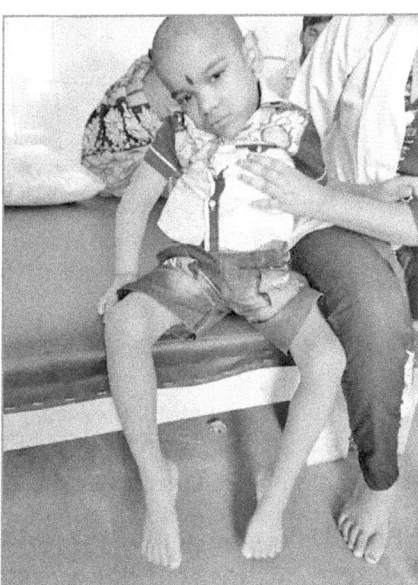

Fig. 18.4: Hypotonic cerebral palsy.

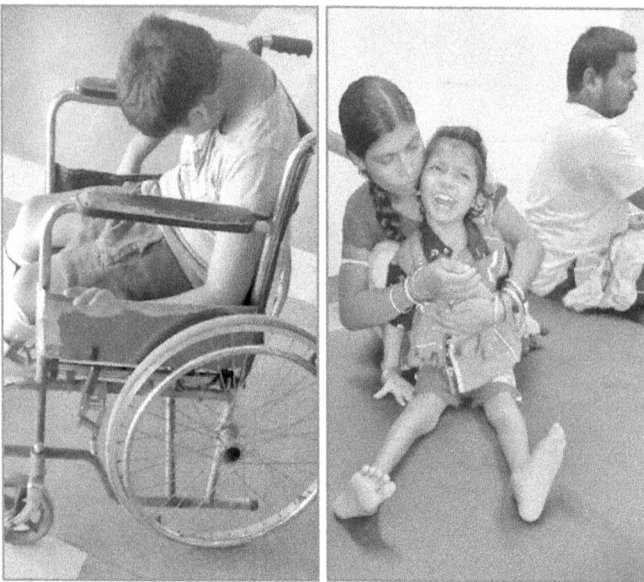

Figs. 18.7A and B: (A) pentaplegic cerebral palsy; (B) Spastic quadriplegic cerebral palsy.

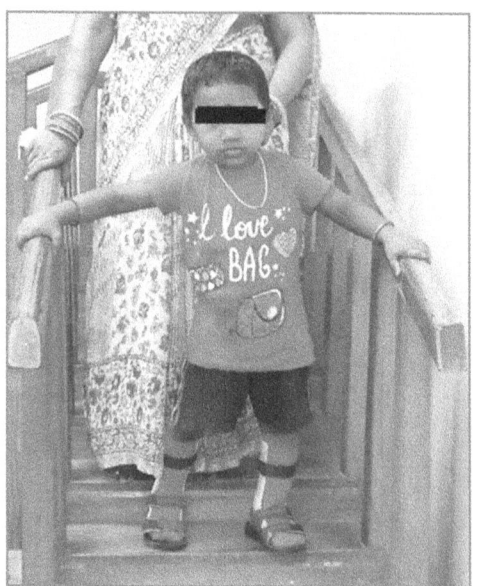

Fig. 18.9: GMFCS level-II.

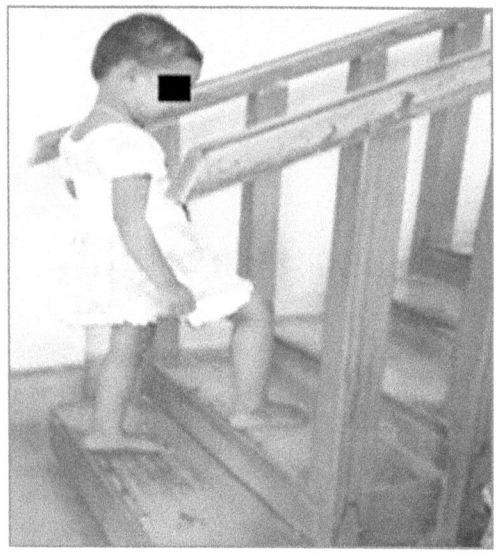

Fig. 18.8: GMFCS level-I.

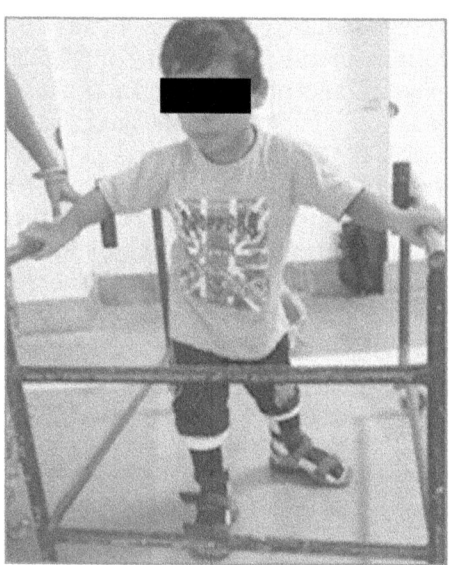

Fig. 18.10: GMFCS level-III.

- *GMFCS Level-II:* Has the ability to walk indoors and outdoors and climbs stairs with a railing **(Fig. 18.9)**. Has difficulty with uneven surfaces, inclines or in crowds. Has only minimal ability to run or jump.
- *GMFCS Level-III:* Walks with assistive mobility devices indoors and outdoors on level surfaces **(Fig. 18.10)**. May be able to climb stairs using a railing. May propel a manual wheelchair (may require assistance for long distances or uneven surfaces).
- *GMFCS Level-IV:* Walking ability severely limited **(Fig. 18.11)** even with assistive devices. Uses wheelchairs most of the time and may propel their own power wheelchair. May participate in standing transfers.
- *GMFCS Level-V:* Has physical impairments that restrict voluntary control of movement and the ability to maintain head and neck position against gravity.

The child is impaired in all areas of motor function. Cannot sit or stand independently, even with adaptive equipment **(Fig. 18.12)**. Cannot independently walk, though may be able to use powered mobility.

- **Depending upon the degree of severity, CP is classified into:**
  - *Mild CP—20% of cases:* They are usually independent.
  - *Moderate CP—50% of cases:* Requires self-help for assisting their impaired ambulation capacity.
  - *Severe CP—30% of cases:* Totally incapacitated and bed-ridden. They always need care from others.

Clinical Features of Cerebral Palsy

The clinical features of CP can be typed into: (a) Early features, (b) Late features. **Table 18.2** gives the features of CP.

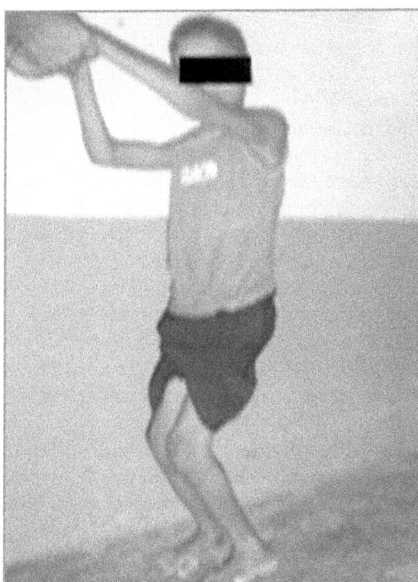

Fig. 18.11: GMFCS level-IV.

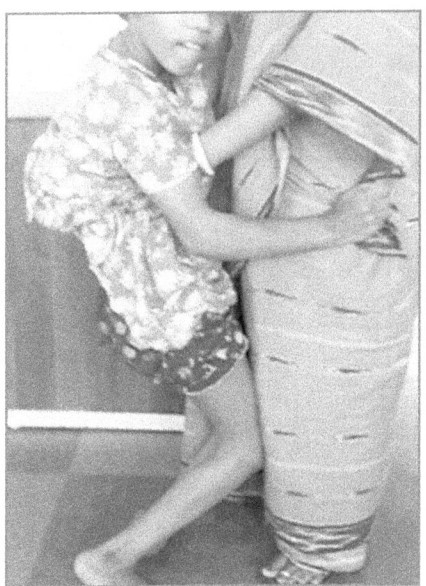

Fig. 18.12: GMFCS level-V.

Table 18.2: Clinical features of cerebral palsy.

Early features of cerebral palsy	Late features of cerebral palsy (Depend on the physiological and topographical types to which the child fits)
Infant is irritable and has poor sleep	**Features of spastic cerebral palsy:** Hypertonia, which is velocity dependent, hyperactive deep tendon reflexes, and positive Babinski sign and clonus. Poor voluntary movements/muscle weakness, synergistic/spastic pattern of movements, contractures and deformities in extremities and spine. Abnormal gait (Scissoring gait/crouch gait/stiff knee gait/jump knee gait/equinus gait, etc.) Low intelligence and loss of memory. Epilepsy may be present
Infant has feeding difficulties	**Features of dyskinetic cerebral palsy:** Fluctuation of muscle tone from high to low, presence of athetosis (slow writhing/worm-like movements in distal parts of body)/chorea (rapid involuntary jerks affecting the proximal and axial parts of body)/dystonia (fluctuation of muscle tone with transient posturing)/ballismus (rapid flinging movements of body), postural instability, normal/diminished deep tendon reflexes, emotional lability, delayed head and trunk control, feeding/sucking difficulties
Infant exhibits low muscle tone	**Features of ataxic cerebral palsy:** Hypotonia, incoordination. Intention tremor diminished deep tendon reflexes, speech/vision/hearing/perceptual problems, nystagmus, dysmetria, joint hyper-mobility, asthenia (muscle weakness), poor posture and balance, unsteady/ataxic/waddling gait, etc
Infant exhibits delayed disappearance of the primitive reflexes, e.g., the ATNR, which normally disappears by 4–6 months, may persist beyond 6 months and the STNR, which usually disappears by 8–12 months may persist in the child	**Features of mixed cerebral palsy:** The child has combination of features from spastic and dyskinetic types such as spastic athetoid/spastic athetoid-dystonic
Infant exhibits delayed development of righting reactions that help for maintenance of posture and balance, e.g., delayed development of righting reactions, say neck righting (mature), which develops in a healthy baby by 6–7 months is delayed in a cerebral palsy child. The Landau reaction **(Figs. 18.13A and B)** normally presents between 3–4 months and 2 years may also remain absent and develops late in the child with cerebral palsy. The neonatal reflexes and reactions found normally and affected in the cerebral palsy child are given in the **Table. 18.3**	**Features of atonic/hypotonic cerebral palsy:** The muscle tone of such children are very low (floppy baby syndrome) with significant postural instability and delayed motor milestones

Contd...

Contd...

Early features of cerebral palsy	Late features of cerebral palsy (Depend on the physiological and topographical types to which the child fits)
Infant/child shows delayed development of motor milestones **(Table. 18.4)**, delayed development of speech and language as well as perceptual/cognitive function **(Table. 18.5)**	The affected child may have involvement of one or both limbs as well as spine. The common deformities in cerebral palsy children are: Hip adduction flexion/internal rotation deformity, knee flexion/recurvatum deformity, ankle equinus deformity, kyphoscoliosis deformity in spine **(Fig. 18.14)**, hip subluxation/dislocation, etc. The deformities develop may be of primary type resulting from spasticity/tightness such as dynamic ankle equinus, or secondary type resulting from the primary tightness, such as fixed equinus deformity, and tertiary type resulting from secondary, such as genu recurvatum developing from secondary ankle equinus. **Figures 18.15A and B** show the secondary and tertiary deformities in the lower limbs in the cerebral palsy child
	The child may also have gait abnormalities such as scissoring gait (walking with both the hips adducted and medially rotated), crouch gait (walking with both hips and knees flexed and ankle dorsi flexed), jump knee gait (walking with hips and knees flexed and ankles plantar flexed), lurching gait (walking with a limp on either side, also called as waddling gait), athetoid dance gait (walking with head turning from side to side), ataxic gait (walking with unsteadiness). The cerebral palsy gait is described separately below

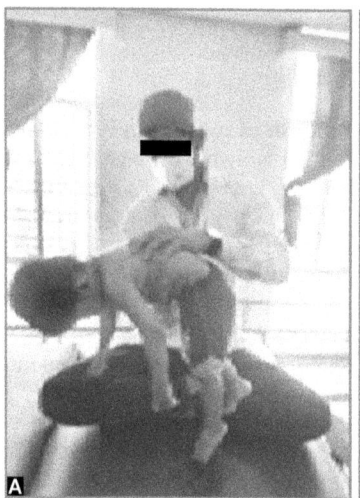 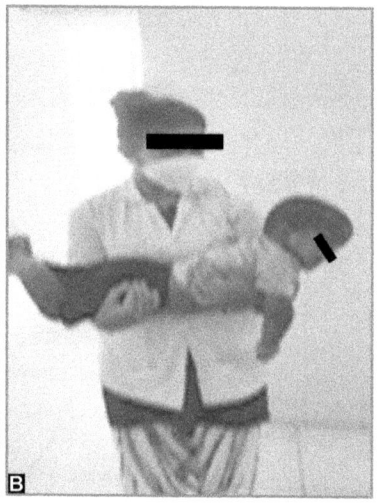

Figs. 18.13A and B: (A) Absence of Landau reaction; (B) Presence of Landau reaction.

Table.18.3: Neonatal reflexes and reactions.

Reflex/reaction	Age range	Test position	Test stimulus	Response	Clinical significance
I. Innate Primary Reactions:					
Rooting reflex: (Fig. 18.16)	28 weeks of gestation–3–4 months	With the infant supine, the head in midline and hands on chest	Gently stroke the infant from the lips to the cheek	The infant turns his/her head toward the stimulated side with the mouth opening and a trial of sucking the finger	Presence of the reflex helps in locating the food source in early infancy. Absence of this reflex suggests significant neurological impairment
Sucking reflex	28 weeks of gestation–2–5 months	Infant supine with the head in midline	Place a finger or nipple of feeding bottle into the infant's mouth	Rhythmical sucking	Presence of the reflex helps in locating the food source and suck food in early infancy. Absence suggests significant neurological impairment and persistence beyond period of integration may impair voluntary sucking.

Contd...

Contd...

Reflex/reaction	Age range	Test position	Test stimulus	Response	Clinical significance
Palmar grasp reflex	32 weeks of gestation–4–6 months	Infant supine, head midline, arms and hands free	Place a finger in infant's hand from the ulnar to the palmar surface	Infant's fingers will flex around the Clinician's finger	Following the development of grasp, the infant begins to reach for objects and utilizes a crude palmar grasp to hold them. Persistent beyond 6 months results in failure to release objects from the hands.
Plantar grasp reflex	32 weeks of gestation–9–12 months	Child supine, head midline, legs relaxed	Apply firm pressure to the plantar surface of the child's foot at the base of toes	Plantar flexion of all of the toes	This reflex is referred to as the "readiness tester". Integrates at the same time that independent gait first becomes possible
Walking/stepping reflex: (Fig. 18.17)	37 weeks of gestation–2–4 months	Infant is supported in the vertical position	Support the infant upright with the feet touching a hard surface. Incline the infant forward and gently move the infant forward to accompany any stepping	Alternating, rhythmical, and coordinated steps	Premature infants will tend to walk in a toe-heel fashion while more mature infants will walk in a heel-toe pattern
Limb placement reflex	Birth–Early infancy	Infant held vertically with the leg below the knee, hand below the elbow at the undersurface/edge of table	Gently rub the dorsum of foot/hand at the edge of table	Infant places the foot/hand over the surface of table	The reflex is readily demonstrable in a normal infant. Absence of the reflex in infancy suggests neurological impairment
II. Spinal Level Reflexes:					
Flexion withdrawal	28 weeks of gestation–2 months	Child supine, head midline, lower extremities extended	Apply a noxious stimulus to the sole of the foot	Withdrawal of the foot from the stimulus employing hip and knee flexion	Failure to attain and integrate this reflex may indicate sensorimotor delay and/or CNS depression
Extension thrust	28 weeks of gestation–4 months	Child supine, head neutral, one leg flexed and other extended	Apply a noxious stimulus such as stroking to the sole of the foot of the flexed leg	Sudden extension, adduction and medial rotation of the flexed leg with ankle plantar flexion	Failure to attain and integrate this reflex may indicate sensorimotor delay and/or CNS depression
Crossed extension	28 weeks of gestation–1–2 months	Child in supine, head in midline, one leg flexed and other extended	The clinician flexes the extended leg passively	There is sudden extension of the flexed leg	This reflex promotes reciprocal movements of lower limbs
III. Lower Brainstem Level Reflexes:					
Asymmetrical tonic neck reflex (ATNR) (Fig. 18.18)	Birth to 4–6 months	Supine lying	Rotation of the head to one side	Flexion of skull limbs, extension of the jaw limbs, "bow and arrow" or "fencing" posture	• Helps in initiation of rolling. • Persistence of this reflex beyond period of integration may indicate CNS damage, which may impair rolling.
Symmetrical tonic neck reflex (STNR) - (Figs. 18.19A and B)	Onset: 4–6 months. Integrates: 8–12 months	Supine lying/Sitting/Quadruped	Passive flexion or extension of the neck	With neck flexion: flexion of UEs, extension of LEs; with neck extension: extension of UEs, flexion of LEs	Necessary to achieve quadruped crawling. If positive response persists, it causes difficulty with crawling, rolling over, transfers and walking.

Contd...

Contd...

Reflex/reaction	Age range	Test position	Test stimulus	Response	Clinical significance
Tonic labyrinthine reflex (TLR) (Figs. 18.20A and B)	Onset: Birth. Integrated: 6 months	Supine/ Prone lying	Prone or supine position	• With prone position: Increased flexor tone/flexion of all limbs • With supine: Increased extensor tone/extension of all limbs	Persistence of TLR will impede activities which require graded coactivation of flexor and extensor muscles, such as sitting. The supine TLR if persists also prevents rolling.
Positive supporting reaction (PSR)	Onset: Birth. Integrated: 6–8 months	Child held vertically at the axillae	Contact of the ball of the foot to ground/bed in upright standing position	Rigid extension (co-contraction) of the LEs	Persistence beyond period of integration indicates damage to CNS
Negative supporting reaction (NSR)	After 8 months presence of pos. supporting (+) is abnormal. Also excessive flexion (–) is abnormal after 4 months	Child held vertically at the axillae	Contact of the ball of the foot to ground/bed in upright standing position	• Negative: No release of extensor tone. Positive supporting persists • Positive: Release of extensor tone allows flexion.	Persistence of PSR and absence of NSR suggests damage to CNS
Associated reactions	Onset: Birth-3 months, Integration: 8–9 years	Sitting	Grasping an object for younger children, rapid arm movements in older children	Overflow of movement to the contralateral side	Excessive build-up of movement or tonal increases in the opposite extremity indicates brain damage
IV. Midbrain Level Reactions:					
Neck righting (immature)	Birth-6 months	Supine, arms and legs extended	Rotate the neck to one side and maintain	Body rotates as a whole, in a direction of head rotation	Helps in initiation of rolling. Persistence after 6 months may suggest damage to CNS
Neck righting (mature) reaction (NOB reaction) (Fig. 18.21)	Onset: 4–6 months, Integration: 5 years	Supine lying	Flex the child's neck and rotate to one side	Child will segmentally roll in the direction of the head rotation	Helps for mature rolling and gait rotation
Body righting acting on head: (Fig. 18.22)	Onset: 6 months. Integration: 5 years	Leg prone lying on table/bed, eyes blindfolded	Asymmetrical stimulation of pressure sense organs on anterior aspect of the body	Head is brought to a face vertical position	Helps in controlling the head in relation to the body in all positions
Body righting acting on body: (Fig. 18.23)	Onset: 4–6 months. Integrates: 5 years	Supine with head in midline	Flex one leg and rotate it across the pelvis to the opposite side	Child will roll sideways segmentally	Working with NOB, promotes segmental rolling and is important for sitting, quadruped and standing positions
Labyrinthine righting reaction: (Fig. 18.24)	Onset: Birth-2 months Integration: Persists throughout life	Child is held vertically, eyes blind folded	Child is tilted anteriorly/posteriorly/laterally from vertical	The head orients to the vertical position and is maintained steady	In order to move around in space, this reflex is necessary to allow the body to turn freely around the head
V. Automatic Movement Reflexes/Reactions:					
1. More reflex: (Figs. 18.25A and B)	Onset: Birth. Integration: 5–6 months	Child in supine with head in midline: Support the child's head while pulling the child to a position halfway between supine and upright sitting	Support the infant's head and shoulders with one hand. Allow the head to drop back to allow the anterior neck muscles to stretch	The shoulders abduct, the elbows, wrists and fingers extend. Subsequently, the shoulders adduct, and the elbows and fingers flex (Embracing)	Asymmetry of the response within 6 months and persistence of the same beyond 6 months suggest damage to CNS

Contd...

Chapter 18: Cerebral Palsy 327

Contd...

Reflex/reaction	Age range	Test position	Test stimulus	Response	Clinical significance
2. Landau reflex/reaction: (Fig. 18.26)	Onset: 3–4 months. Integration: 12–24 months	Child is supported under chest and abdomen in prone position	Wait for response after placement	The head will extend and the back and hips will extend in sequence ("superman" appearance)	Breaks up the total flexion pattern seen at birth. Helps in development of erect posture
3. Protective extensor thrusts					
a. Protective extension forward: (Fig. 18.27)	Onset: 6–7 months Integration: Persists throughout life	Child vertically supported/long sitting	Plunge the child downward, head first	The child should extend and abduct the arms with the fingers extended and spread as if to break a fall.	Necessary for prop sitting
b. Protective extension downward (leg parachute)	Onset: 4 months Integration: Persists throughout life	Child vertically suspended in air	Plunge the child downward	The legs externally rotate and abduct with the feet dorsiflexion in preparation for weight-bearing	Preparation for standing and breaks a fall
c. Protective extension sideways: (Fig. 18.28)	Onset: 7 months Integration: Persists throughout life	Child is placed in long sitting	Apply a laterally directed force to the shoulder to displace the center of gravity	The arms should abduct and extend on the side toward the fall with weight borne on the open palm and fingers	Needed for independent sitting
d. Protective extension backward (Fig. 18.29)	Onset: 9–10 months Integration: Persists throughout life	Child is placed in long sitting with the legs extended	Push the child backward with enough force to displace the center of gravity	The child will extend the arms backwards and take support on the hands	Necessary for independent sitting
e. Staggering reaction	Onset: 15–18 months Integration: Persists throughout life	Standing	Push the child in all directions	The child will make corrective movements such as stepping side ways in order to restore the position of COG	Protects upright standing
VI. Cortical Level Reactions:					
Optical righting: (Fig. 18.30).	Onset: Birth to 2 months Integration: Persists throughout life	The child is held vertically	Tilt the child anteriorly, posteriorly, and laterally from the vertical	The head orients to the vertical position and is maintained vertically oriented in the environment	Helps in upright alignment of the head and body
Equilibrium reaction	Onset: Depends on test position Integration: Persists throughout life	Prone (5 months), Supine (7–8 months), Sitting (6–7 months), Quadruped (9–12 months), Kneel standing (15 months), Standing (15 months) (Figs. 18.31A and B)	Rock the client/supporting surface to disturb balance sufficiently	Right head and body and perform movements to maintain balance	Helps to maintain body stability while performing gross and fine motor activities
Postural fixation reaction	Onset: Depends on test position Integration: Persists throughout life	Prone on bed (6 months), Supine on bed (7–8 months), Sitting on a stool (7–8 months)	• For prone: Encourage the child to support on one extremity while reaching for an object. For supine: Encourage the child to reach at object, exert a minimal force on the shoulder of the reaching arm	• For prone: The child will not lose balance when reaching • For supine: The child will lose his balance in response to the push and demonstrate a slight curving of the spine	Necessary for preservation of center of gravity and maintain balance

Contd...

Contd...

Reflex/reaction	Age range	Test position	Test stimulus	Response	Clinical significance
		Quadruped on floor (9–12 months), Standing one legged/ both legged (12–21 months)	• For sitting: Encourage the child to reach while exerting a minimal force to the opposite shoulder or trunk • For quadruped: Apply force to the shoulder and observe to the extremities. • For standing: Exert minimal force to the pelvis in all four directions	• For sitting: The child will not lose balance. • For quadruped: Rotation of the body in the plane of the applied force is observed • For standing: The lower extremities become rigid to prevent tipping/ falling	

Table 18.4: Gross motor developments.

Age of development of skill	Skill	What happens in cerebral palsy
0–12 months		
2 Months	Lifts head in prone	Delayed
4 Months	Bears weight on forearms in prone, brings hands to midline, achieves neck control (Head is kept in line with the trunk when pulled to sitting)	Delayed
5 Months	Lifts head in supine, bridges pelvis, rolls to side	Delayed
6 Months	Sits with hands in front for support, rolls supine to prone, takes both feet to mouth, helps pull self to sitting	Delayed
7 Months	Pivots and pushes self backwards in prone	Delayed
8 Months	Creeps forward on forearms, sits unsupported with straight back, can reach in sitting	Delayed
8–10 months	Crawls on all fours, pulls to standing	Delayed
10–12 Months	Gets down from standing, walks with one or both hands held	Delayed
12 Months	Most children walk independently	Delayed
13 months–5 years.		
13 months	Walks	Delayed
15 months	Independent rise to stand, kneels up holding on	Delayed
18 months	Kneels up without support, squats to play	Delayed
18–30 months	Goes upstairs—holding on, both feet on each step	Delayed
24–30 months	Jumps off floor, both feet together	Delayed
30–36 months	Goes upstairs—alternate feet up- and down-stairs	Delayed
3 years	Stands momentary on one leg	Delayed
4 years	Stands on one leg for 3–5 seconds	Delayed
5 years	Jumps over knee high cord, feet together	Delayed

Table 18.5: Development of speech/hearing/perception/cognition.

Age of development	Skill	What happens in CP
2 Months	Smiles at the sound of the voice of mother/ closed relative, and follows the mother with the eyes as she moves	Usually delayed
3 Months	Smiles at other people	Usually delayed
4 Months	Babbles, laughs and tries to imitate sounds	Usually delayed
6 Months	Moves objects from one hand to other	Usually delayed
7 Months	Responds to own name. Finds partially hidden objects	Usually delayed
9 Months	Babbles " mama", "dada"	Usually delayed

Contd...

Contd...

Age of development	Skill	What happens in CP
12 Months	Says at least one word. Enjoys imitating people	Usually delayed
18 Months	Says at least 15 words, points to body parts	Usually delayed
2 years	Follows simple instructions, speaks two word sentences, and begins to play	Usually delayed
3 years	Sorts objects by shape and color, speaks multiword sentences	Usually delayed
4 years	Draws circles and squares, rides a tricycle	Usually delayed
5 years	Tells name and address, counts 10 or more objects, puts on dresses	Usually delayed

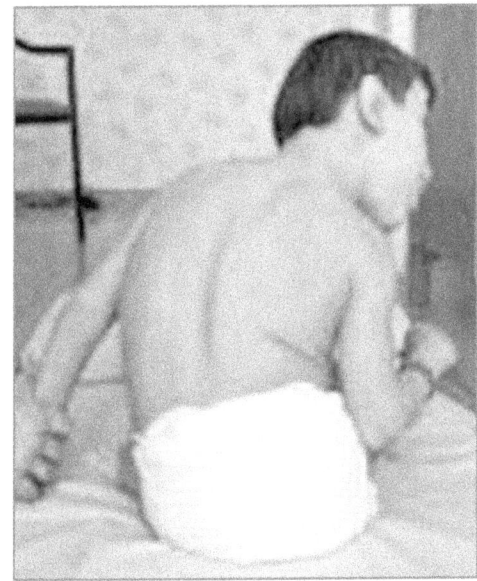

Fig. 18.14: Kyphoscoliosis deformity—Kyphoscoliosis deformity in cerebral palsy.

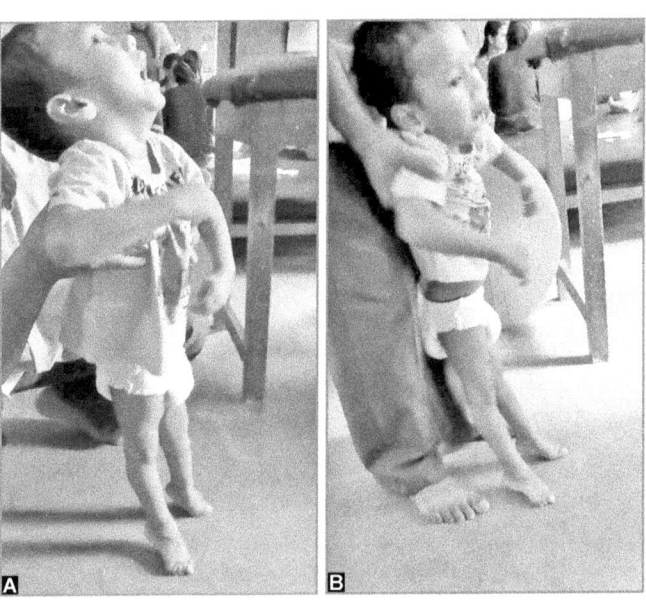

Figs. 18.15A and B: (A) Secondary ankle equinus; (B) Tertiary genu recurvatum.

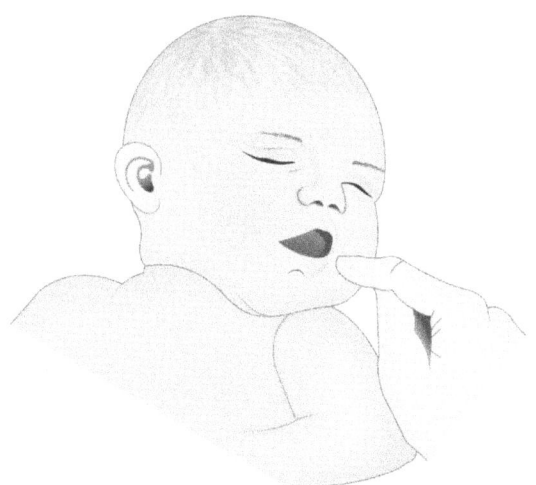

Fig. 18.16: Rooting reflex.

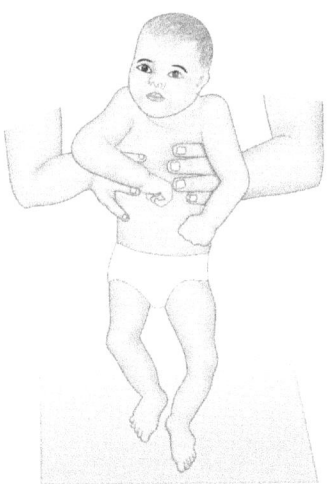

Fig. 18.17: Stepping reflex.

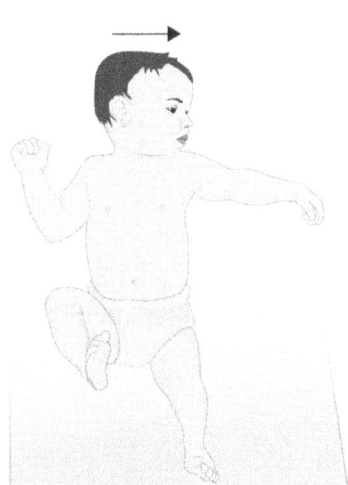

Fig. 18.18: ATNR.

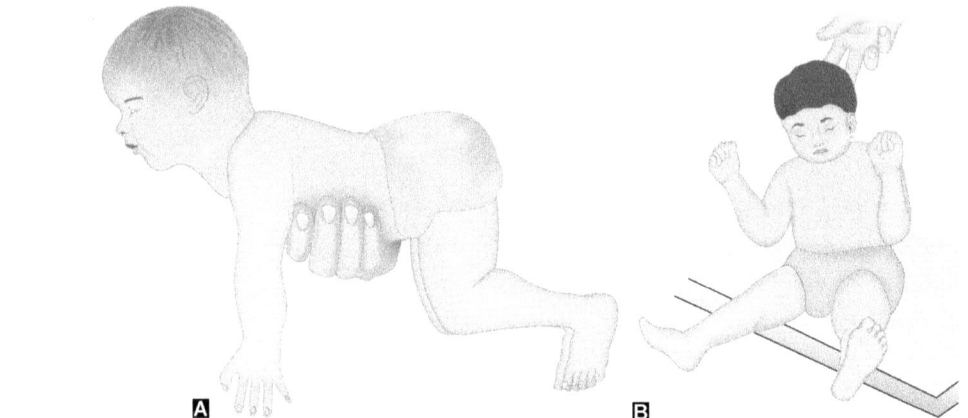

Figs. 18.19A and B: STNR: (A) Quadruped; (B) Sitting.

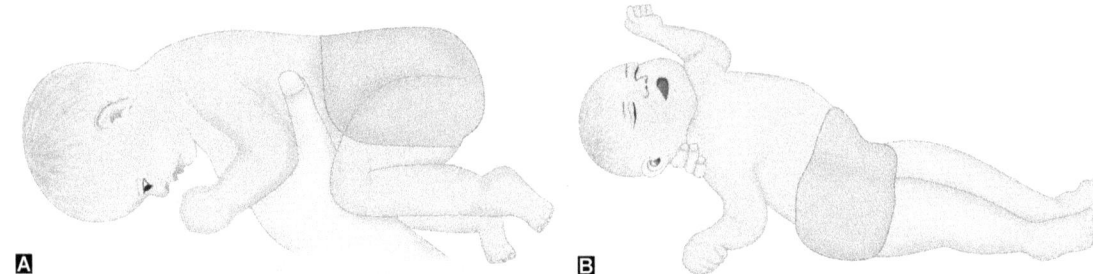

Figs. 18.20A and B: TLR (A) Prone; (B) Supine.

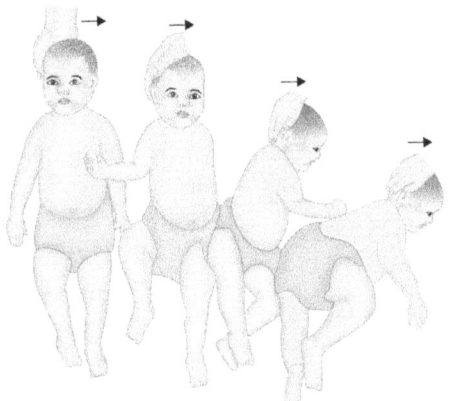

Fig. 18.21: Neck righting reaction.

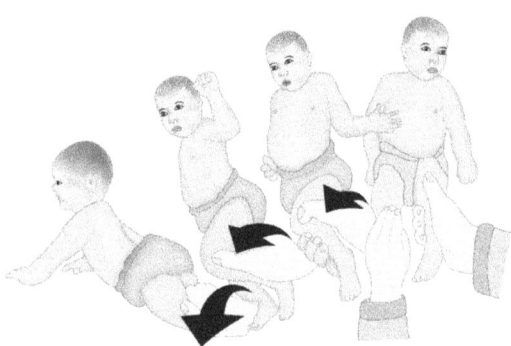

Fig. 18.23: Body righting acting on body.

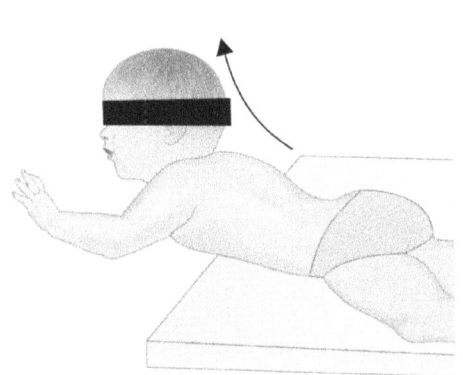

Fig. 18.22: Body righting acting on head.

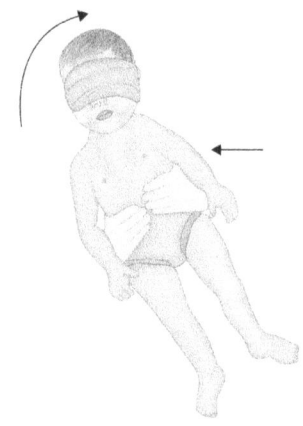

Fig. 18.24: Labyrinthine righting.

Chapter 18: Cerebral Palsy

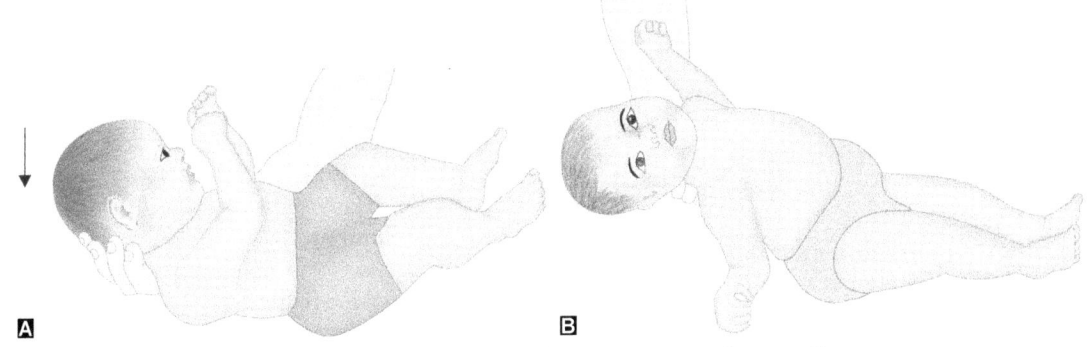

Figs. 18.25A and B: Moro reflex: part-I; Moro reflex: part-II.

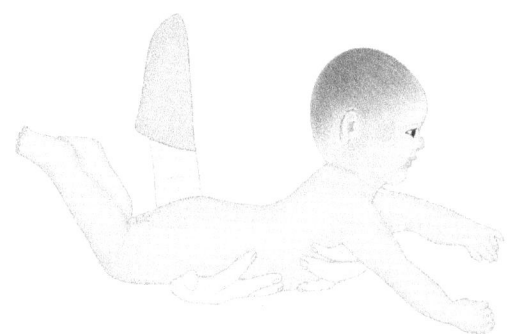

Fig. 18.26: Landau reflex/reaction.

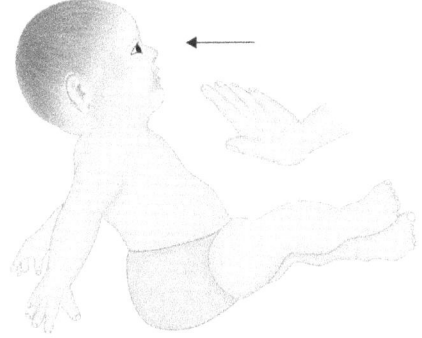

Fig. 18.29: Protective extension: Backwards.

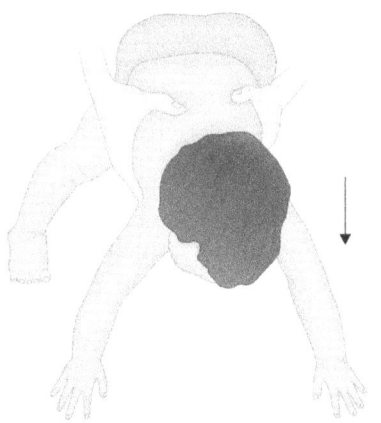

Fig. 18.27: Protective extension (parachute reaction): Forward.

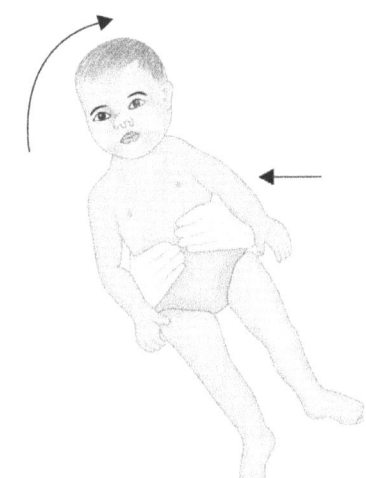

Fig. 18.30: Optical righting reaction.

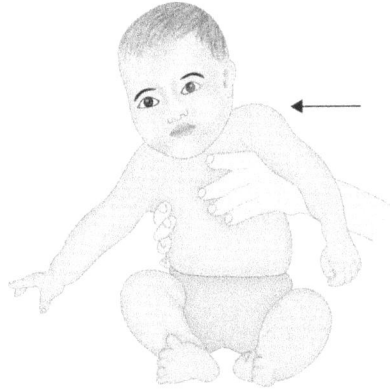

Fig. 18.28: Protective extension: Sideways.

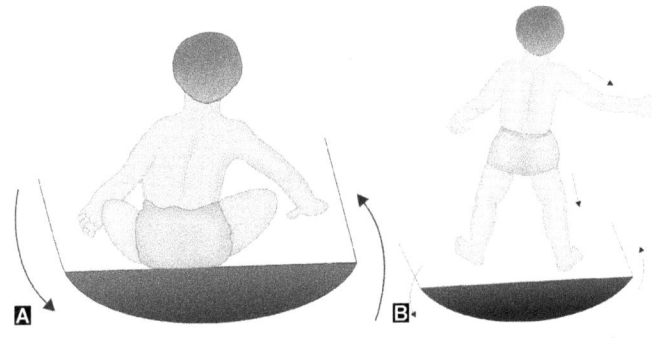

Figs. 18.31A and B: Equilibrium reaction: (A) Sitting, (B) Standing.

Cerebral Palsy Gait

Children who are ambulatory walk in abnormal patterns. The abnormal gaits found in such children are:

Jump Knee Gait

The child walks with hips in flexion, knees in flexion and ankles in plantar flexion as if getting ready to jump **(Fig. 18.32)**.

This is typical for diplegic and ambulatory total body involved children when they begin to walk. The reason is spasticity of hip and knee flexors and ankle plantar flexors.

Crouch Gait

Increased knee flexion and ankle hyperdorsiflexion occur during stance phase **(Fig. 18.33)**. They occur in older children and after isolated triceps surae lengthenings that have been performed without addressing the spastic hamstrings.

Hip flexors and hamstrings are tight, and quadriceps and gastro-soleus are weak.

Stiff Knee Gait

- Decreased knee flexion occurs during swing phase.
- The rectus femoris muscle is spastic and does not allow the knee to flex in initial and midswing phases.
- Limitation of knee flexion causes difficulty in foot clearance and stair climbing.
- These sagittal plane gait patterns coexist with frontal and transverse plane pathologies.

Scissoring Gait

Scissoring gait is defined as crossing over of the legs during gait **(Fig. 18.34)**. The cause is hip adductor and medial hamstring spasticity combined with excessive femoral antiversion.

Lurching Gait/Waddling gait

Lurching gait is the side bending of the trunk while walking. When bending of trunk occurs from side to side, it is called waddling gait. This gait is the result of weakness of hip abductors (unilateral hip abductor weakness produces lurching, and bilateral hip abductor weakness produces waddling gait). It is also caused by deficiency of balance.

Circumductory Gait

Found in children with spastic hemiplegia. Such children walk with excessive pelvic hiking and forward rotation to clear the ground in swing phase due to lack of activity in hip and knee flexors and ankle dorsi flexors **(Fig. 18.35)**.

Vaulting gait: This is found in cerebral palsy children with unilateral ankle equinus, where the child walks with raising of the heel on the contralateral side to clear the ground.

Ataxic Gait

Found in children with cerebellar lesion. Such children walk with lots of incoordination and suffer from frequent falls due to loss of balance.

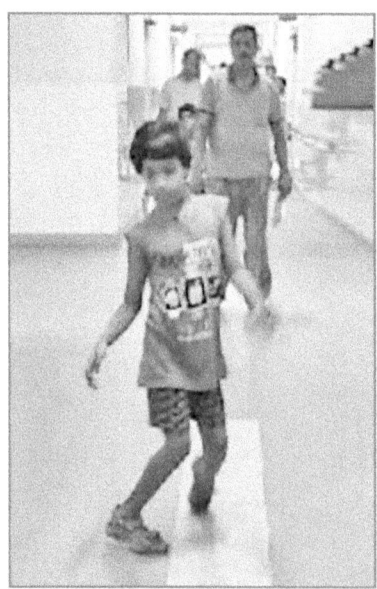

Fig. 18.32: Jump knee gait.

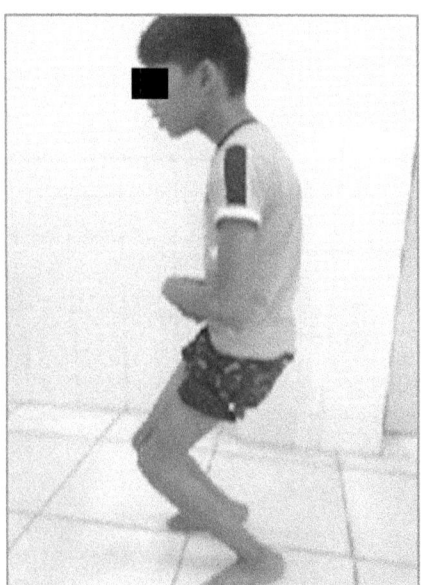

Fig. 18.33: Crouch gait.

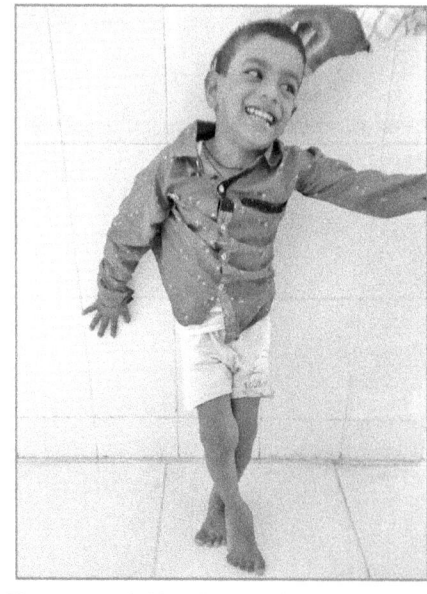

Fig. 18.34: Child walking with scissoring gait.

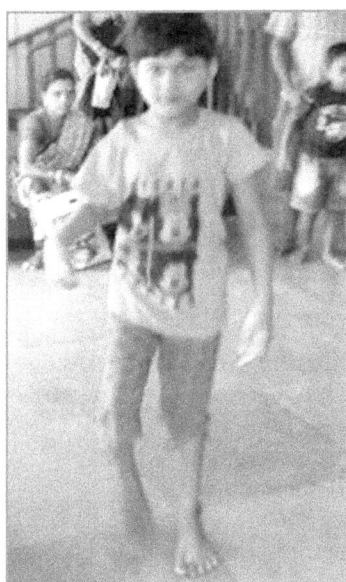

Fig. 18.35: Child walking with circumductory gait.

Athetoid Dance Gait

The child walks with alternate turning of face toward the stance limb to increase the extensor tone on the stance side to take load and to increase flexor tone on the other side to produce flexion of hip and knee for ground clearance.

Associated Problems in Cerebral Palsy Children

Besides the motor problems, the child may have associated problems such as speech and language problem, visual problem (strabismus/blindness), mental retardation, gastrointestinal problem, epilepsy, dental problems, etc.

Signs Suggestive of Cerebral Palsy in an Infant

- Poor eye contact.
- Excessive irritability.
- Poor sleep.
- Abnormal behavior.
- Poor head control.
- Poor mobility.
- Oromotor problem.
- Frequent vomiting.
- Poor sucking.
- Abnormal muscle tone.
- Facial grimacing.

Cerebral palsy is likely if there is no:
- Head control by 3–4 months
- Sitting by 6–8 months
- Rolling over by 6–7 months
- Walking by 18 months.

Assessment of a Child with Cerebral Palsy

Cerebral palsy is a heterogeneous disorder of posture and movement, and is one of the most important causes of disability affecting children. The child exhibits a plethora of neuromusculoskeletal manifestations, such as spasticity, poor muscle function, rigidity, muscle weakness, poor selective motor control, soft tissue tightness/contracture/deformities, hip dislocation, torsional deformities, etc., which need to be identified so that the diagnosis can be established and appropriate management can be planned. A comprehensive assessment that includes a combination of detailed medical history, functional assessment, clinical examination, analysis of gait, and radiological assessment is required to provide a favorable treatment outcome in these children. A close surveillance is essential so as to identify risk factors for the development and progression of musculoskeletal problems so that early interventions can be carried out to minimize the disabilities. After a thorough assessment, the therapist/clinician should set the goal, which is realistic and achievable. For a child with cerebral palsy, the time set to achieve the short-term goal is 3 months and the time set to achieve long-term goal is 1 year. The **Flowcharts 18.1** and **18.2** highlight the assessment process for CP.

The assessment process is discussed in detail as under:

a. **Initial contact:** Receiving the patient taking demographic data, such as: Name, age, sex, address, etc., and noting the complaint.

b. **Subjective examination:** Obtained from parents especially mother, or from relatives and through case sheet.

A. Developmental History:

Review of complications of pregnancy and delivery, birth weight, any neonatal and perinatal difficulties, feeding problems, etc. The developmental histories included are:

- **Prenatal History:**
  - Age of mother.
  - Consanguinity (marriage among blood-related individuals, if any)
  - Any drug taken during pregnancy.
  - Any trauma/stress.
  - Any addiction—smoking/alcohol.
  - History of TORCH infection.
  - History of previous abortions, stillbirth, etc.
  - Multiple pregnancies.

Flowchart 18.1: The cerebral palsy assessment process.

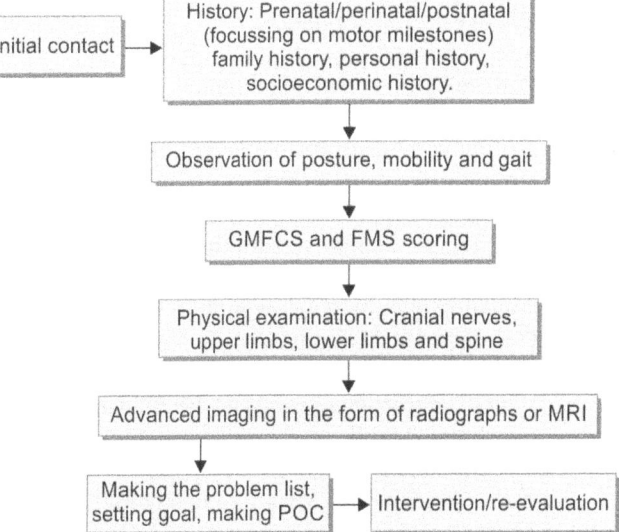

Flowchart 18.2: Cerebral palsy assessment process using NDT principles.

Initial contact → Data collection → Evaluation Analysis → Plan of care Goals Objectives → Intervention plan → Re-examination Re-evaluation

- ❖ **Perinatal History:**
  - Place of delivery.
  - History of preterm or postterm delivery.
    » History of hypoxia/asphyxia at birth, such as delayed birth cry/knotting of umbilical cord round the neck.
    » Weight of the child at birth.
  - History of prolonged labor pain.
  - Type of delivery.
    » Presentation of the child (Breech, i.e., caudal-cephal as against cephalocaudal)
    » Condition of the mother at the time of delivery.
- ❖ **Postnatal History:**
  - History of trauma to brain such as fall, drowning in water, etc., between 1 week of birth and 2 years of life.
  - History of neonatal jaundice, meningitis, hypoglycemia, hydrocephalus, and microcephaly.
  - Nutritional habits of the child (malnutrition, feeding difficulties, etc.).
  - History of developmental milestones.
- B. **Family history.**
- C. **Personal history of child.**
- D. **Socioeconomic history of family.**
- ❖ **On Observation**
  - Behavior of the child.
    » Communication of the child.
    » Posture.
    » Involuntary movements.
    » Contracture and deformities (such as windswept deformity of hip, flexion deformity of knee, etc.)
    » Scar/trophic changes.
    » Gait abnormalities.
    » Use of external appliances.
    » Attention span.
    » Postural control and alignment.
    » Use of limbs and hands.
    » Attitude of the limb during playing and in all positions.
    » Drooling of saliva (if any).
    » Wetting of pant (if any).
  - Observation of sensory functions such as speech, hearing, vision, touch, and smell
  - *Observation of form of locomotion:*
    » How the child brought carried.
    » Any use of wheelchair/walking aids.
    » Which daily activities motivate the child to roll, creep, crawl, stand, walk, etc.
  - *Observation of involuntary movements:*
    » Athetoid posturing/dystonic posturing/ballismus, chorea, tremor, etc.

- ❖ **On Examination:**
  - *Higher function:*
    Speech, hearing, vision, higher cognitive function (memory, intelligence, attention span, etc.).
  - *Cranial nerve integrity:*
    » Strabismus or squint (3rd, 6th).
    » Visual defects (Optic nerve)
    » Auditory defects (8th nerve)
    » Feeding and swallowing problems (Lower cranial nerves).
  - *Sensory assessment:* Assessment of superficial, deep, and cortical sensation as much as possible.
  - *Motor integrity:*
    » Abnormalities of muscle tone: Tone grading scale **(Table 18.6)**
    » Spasticity: Spasticity is graded by using, modified modified Ashworth scale **(Table 18.7)** and Tardieu scale.

The Tardieu scale (Tables 18.8 and 18.9): It assesses spasticity by passively moving the joint at three specified velocities (slow, under gravity and fast), while the intensity and muscle reaction to stretch is rated on a 6-point scale, with the joint angle recorded at where the muscle reaction is first felt. Velocities of joint movement used in Tardieu scale are given in **Table 18.8**.

Table 18.6: Tone grading scale.	
Grade	Criteria
0	Flaccid
1+	Hypotonia
2+	Normal
3+	Mild hypertonia
4+	Severe hypertonia

Table 18.7: Modified modified Ashworth scale.	
Grade	Criteria
0	No increase in muscle tone
1	Slight increase in muscle tone, manifested by a catch followed by release, or minimal resistance at the end of the ROM, when the joint over which the muscle works is moved passively in the direction of action of the antagonist
2	Increase in muscle tone with resistance throughout the range of motion when the joint over which the muscle works is moved passively in the direction of action of the antagonist. Passive movement is possible.
3	Considerable increase in muscle tone, passive movement in the direction of antagonist is difficult
4	Very high muscle tone, and the limb is rigid

Table 18.8: Velocities of joint movement used in Tardieu scale.	
Velocity	Criteria
V1	As slow as possible (slower than the natural drop of the limb segment under gravity)
V2	Speed of the limb segment falling under gravity
V3	As fast as possible (faster than the rate of the natural drop of the limb segment under gravity)

Table 18.9: The Tardieu scale.	
Grade	Criteria
0	No resistance throughout the course of the passive movement.
1	Slight resistance throughout the course of the passive movement with no clear catch at a precise angle.
2	Clear catch at precise angle, interrupting the passive movement followed by release.
3	Unsustained clonus (less than 10 seconds when maintaining the pressure) occurring at a precise angle, followed by release.
4	Sustained clonus (more than 10 seconds when maintaining the pressure) occurring at a precise angle
5	Joint is immobile.

(Angle of muscle action is measured relative to the position of minimal stretch of the muscle (corresponding to angle zero) for all joints except the hip where it is relative to the resting anatomical position).

The Modified Tardieu Scale: Due to the large amount of time required to perform the full Tardieu scale, the Modified Tardieu scale was developed. It records the joint angle during fast and slow movements only. The angle of catch at the most rapid velocity (R1) and the joint angle when the muscle length is at its maximum (R2) is assessed by moving the joint through full ROM, using slow passive movements **(Figs. 18.36A and B)**. The difference in degrees between the angles R2 and R1 is referred to as the dynamic components of spasticity.

Muscular weakness: The Medical Research Council (MRC) scale for manual muscle testing is the widely accepted clinical assessment tool to grade the muscle strength in a child with cerebral palsy. However, if the muscle tone increases when test movement is attempted or resistance to muscle work is provided, or if the child does not cooperate, voluntary control grading should be followed **(Table 18.10)**. A hand dynamometer may be used to assess the grip strength.

- **Reflex Integrity:**
  - *Deep tendon reflexes (DTR):* DTR grading scale **(Table 18.11)**
  - *Superficial reflexes:* Plantar response is commonly checked. An extensor plantar response up to the age of 2 years is considered normal as CNS myelination continues up to 2 years following birth.
  - *Primitive reflexes:* The innate primary reactions (palmar grasp, plantar grasp, rooting reflex, sucking reflex, etc.), spinal level reflexes (flexion withdrawal, extensor thrust, crossed extension reflex), lower brain-stem level reflexes

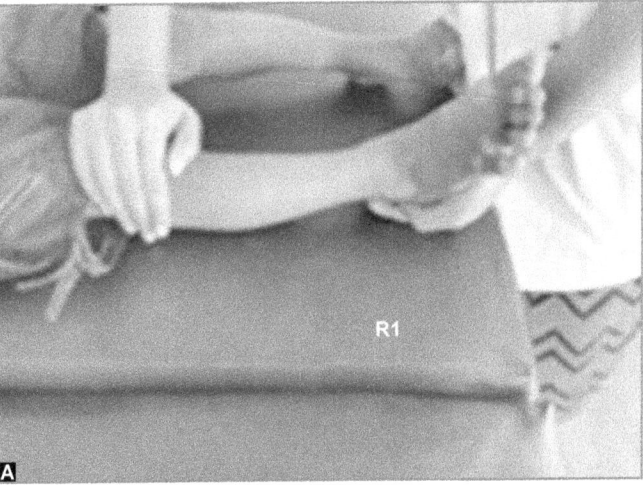
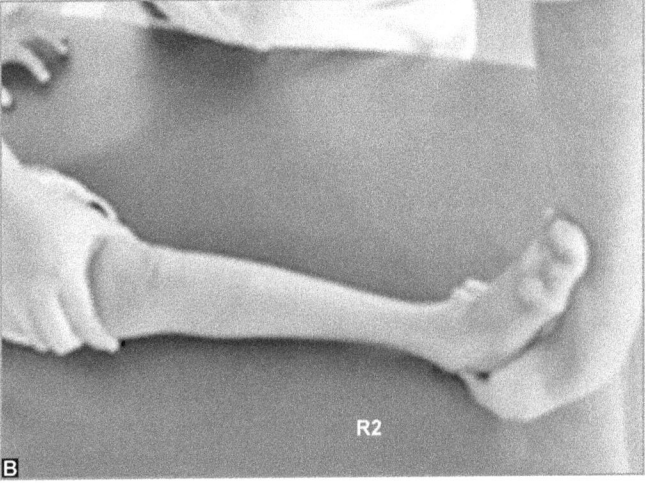

Figs. 18.36A and B: Showing procedure of grading spasticity using the modified Tardieu scale.

Table. 18.10: Voluntary motor control grading in cerebral palsy.	
Grade	Criteria
0	No movement is possible.
1	Able to move partially in the direction of desired movement.
2	Able to move fully in the direction of desired movement

Table 18.11: Grading of deep tendon reflexes.	
Grade	Criteria
0	Absent
1+	Diminished
2+	Normal
3+	Brisk (mild hyperreflexes)
4+	Exaggerated (moderate to severe hyperreflexes with clonus)

(ATNR, STNR, TLR, PSR, NSR, associated reaction) are to be tested as per **Table 18.2**, and interpreted with normal parameters regarding delayed integration **(Figs. 18.37A to C)**.

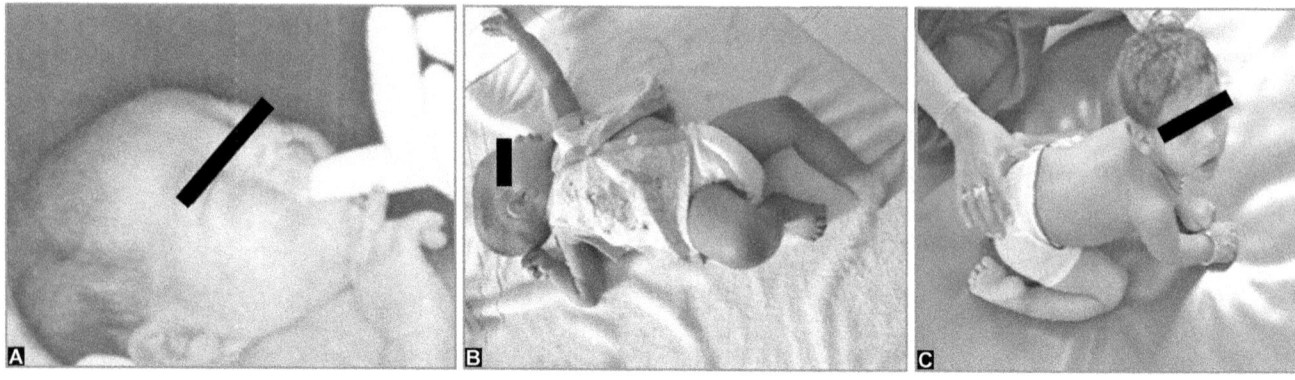

Figs. 18.37A to C: (A) Sucking reflex; (B) ATNR; (C) STNR.

- ❖ **Automatic movement reactions:** Moro reflex, Landau reaction, protective extension reactions (hand parachute reaction, leg parachute reaction, staggering reaction) are to be tested for their appearance/integration.
- ❖ **Righting and equilibrium reactions:** Neck righting, body righting acting on body/head, labyrinthine righting, optical righting reactions and balance/equilibrium reactions are to be tested for their development, as these reactions will help the child to maintain an upright posture and to move.
- ❖ **ROM and flexibility:** Range of motion of the joints where movements are limited, is measured by using a goniometer. Muscles that cross more than one joint, such as hip flexor, long adductor of hips (gracilis and medial hamstrings), hamstrings, gastrocnemius, which are more prone to be tight, are tested for their flexibility. The following figures show testing the flexibility of some important muscles of hip, knee and ankle.
  - – *Hip joint:*
    - » For the hip flexor tightness:
      - ○ Thomas test **(Figs. 18.38A and B)**.
      - ○ Staheli's prone extension test for bilateral hip flexion deformities: Staheli described the prone extension test to assess hip flexion contracture, especially for children with CP having bilateral hip pathologies. The test is performed with the patient prone on the edge of the couch, one hand of the examiner stabilizes the pelvis and the other extends the thigh while observing the lumbar lordosis. The point at which the pelvis rises indicates the end point and the angle between the long axis of thigh and the horizontal line measures the flexion deformity **(Fig. 18.39)**.
    - » For tightness of rectus femoris: Eley's test **(Fig. 18.40)**.
    - » For tightness of hip adductors: Phelps test **(Figs. 18.41A and B)**.
      a. In prone lying **(Figs. 18.41A and B)**
      b. In supine lying **(Figs. 18.41C and D)**
    - » For femoral anteversion: The Craig's test/Trochanteric prominence test: The patient in prone lying and the knee is flexed to 90 degrees. The hip is rotated so that the greater trochanter is fully horizontal (mostly prominent). The angle between the vertical line and long axis of the leg, at the greatest prominence of the greater trochanter palpated laterally, measures the amount of femoral anteversion **(Fig. 18.42)**.
  - – *Knee joint and leg:*
    - » Popliteal angle measurement for hamstrings tightness/spasticity **(Fig. 18.43)**: The tested leg is kept in 90–90 position of knee and hip with the other limb extended. The knee of the tested limb is quickly

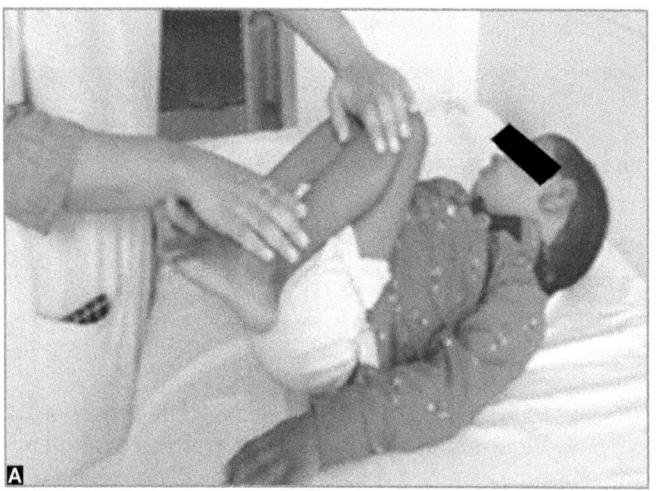
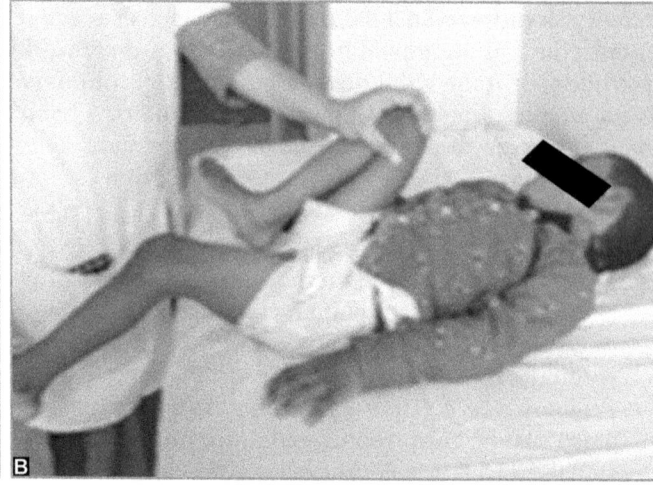

Figs. 18.38A and B: Thomas test for testing tightness of hip flexors: (A) Starting phase; (B) Ending phase.

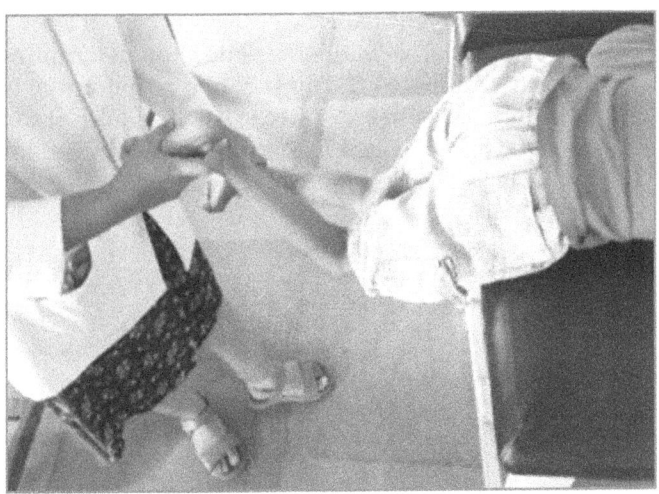

Fig. 18.39: Staheli's prone extension test.

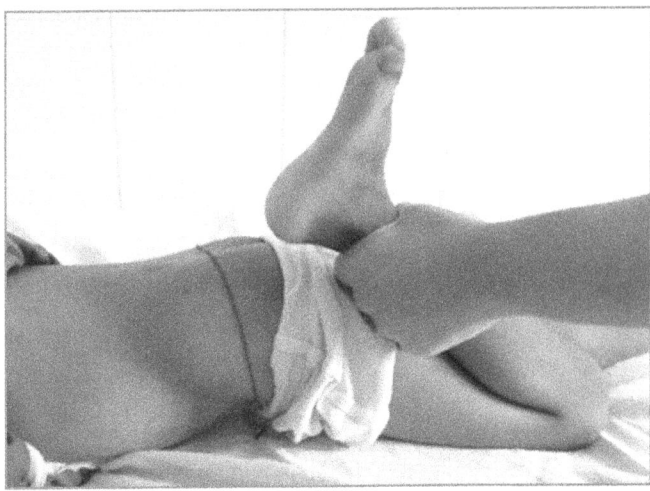

Fig. 18.40: Eley's test for rectus femoris.

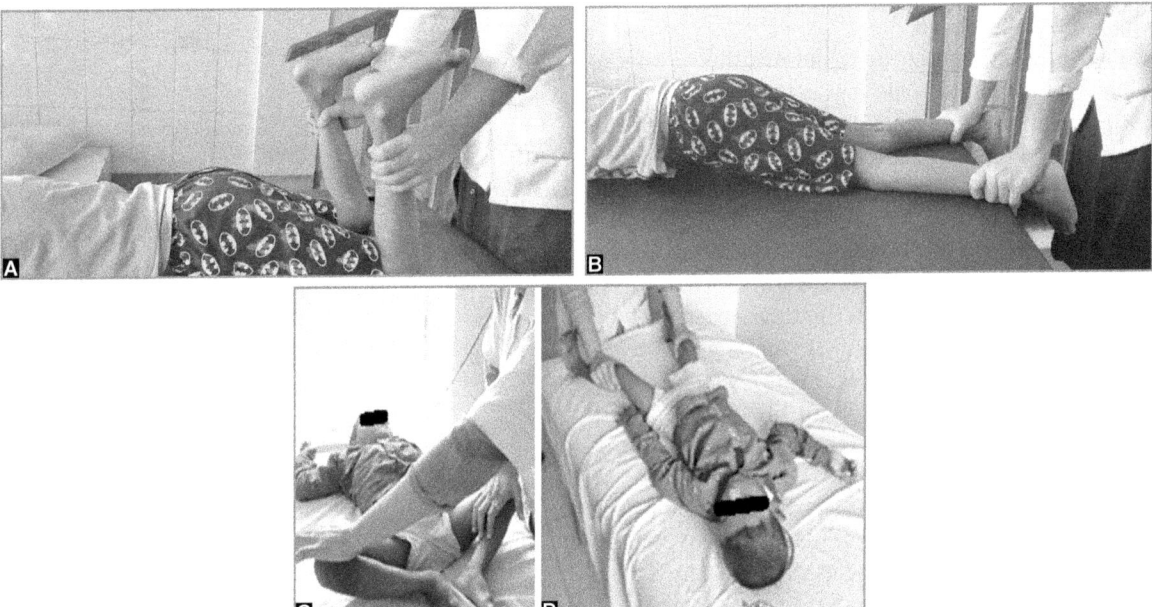

Figs. 18.41A to D: In prone lying: (A) Short adductors; (B) For long adductor (gracilis and medial hamstrings); In supine lying: (C) For short adductors; (D) For long adductors (gracilis and medial hamstrings).

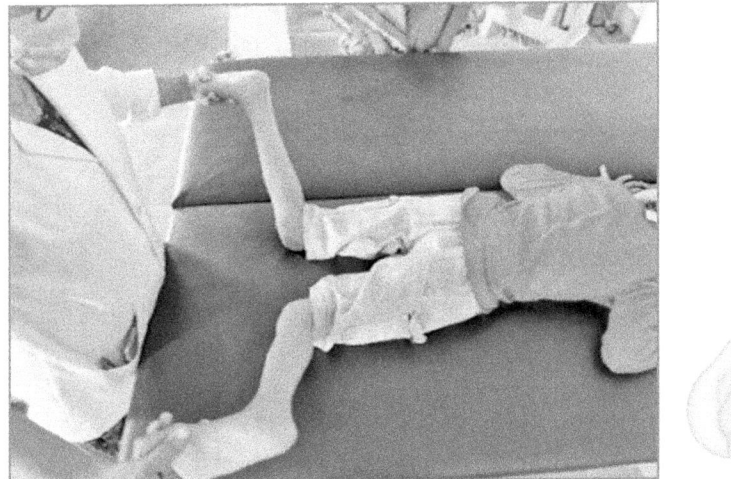

Fig. 18.42: Test for femoral anteversion.

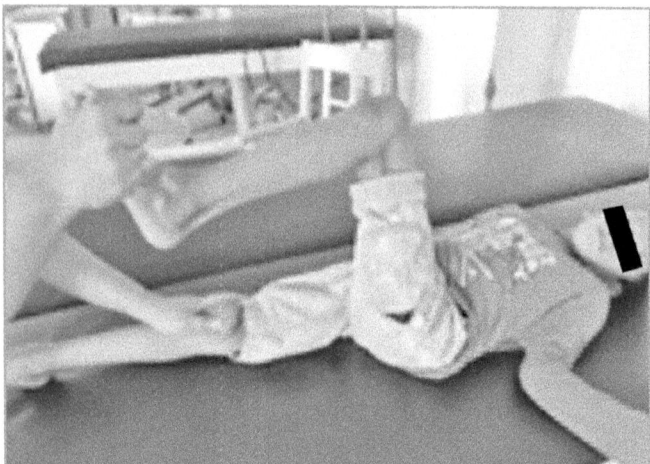

Fig. 18.43: Assessment of popliteal angle.

extended until resistance and further loss of knee extension is measured.

In case of bilateral tightness/deformities of knees, a bilateral popliteal angle test is performed, where both the limbs are kept in 90-90 position of hip and knee joints, and the popliteal angle is measured one by one with the assistance from an assistant.

» Measurement of tibial torsion (The thigh foot angle): The patient is laid in prone position with the knees flexed to 90 degrees and the ankle and foot in neutral position. The angle between the thigh axis and foot axis (axis between the 2nd and 3rd metatarsals) gives the angle of tibial torsion **(Fig. 18.44)**.

- *Ankle joint/foot:* The Silfverskiold test for finding spasticity/tightness in soleus (A) and/or gastrocnemius (B) **(Figs. 18.45A and B)**.

Planovalgus feet: Many CP children, who are ambulatory, develop hypermobility in the midfoot due to spastic gastro-soleus muscle, resulting in planovalgus/rocker bottom foot **(Fig. 18.46)**. The ROM of ankle and foot and the shape of foot should be assessed for planning management effectively.

- *Examination of the spine:*
  » Cerebral palsy children also develop deformities in the spine and the most common deformity is kyphoscoliosis **(Fig. 18.14)**. The flexibility of the curve, loss of height in the client and the need for bracing and surgery should be evaluated.

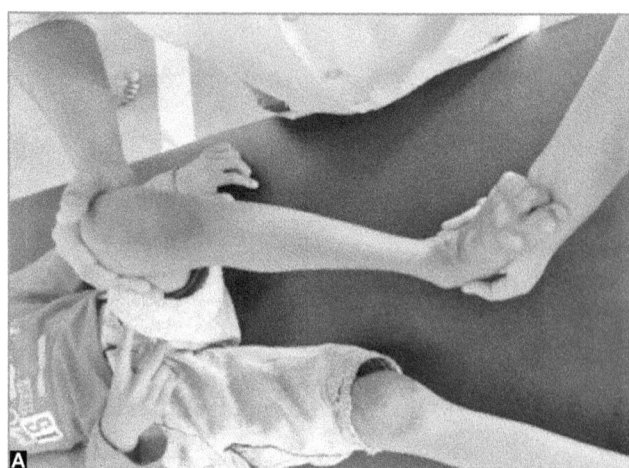
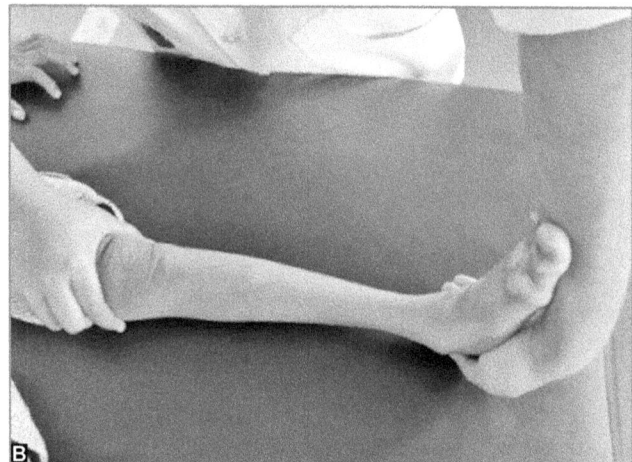

Figs. 18.45A and B: Silfverskiold test: (A) First phase to find soleus spasticity/tightness; (B) Second phase to find tightness/spasticity of gastrocnemius.

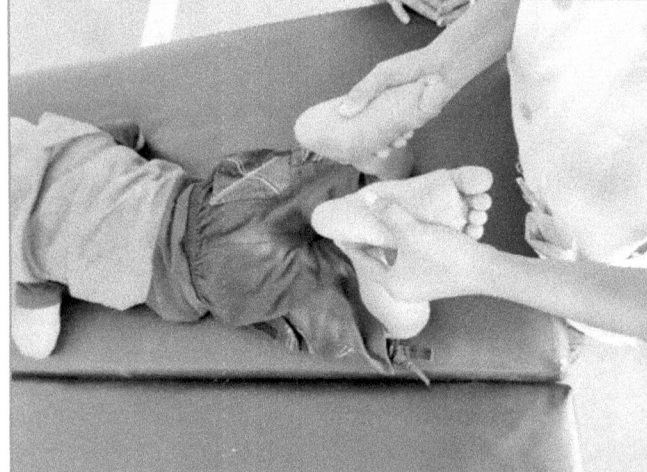

Fig. 18.44: Measurement of tibial torsion.

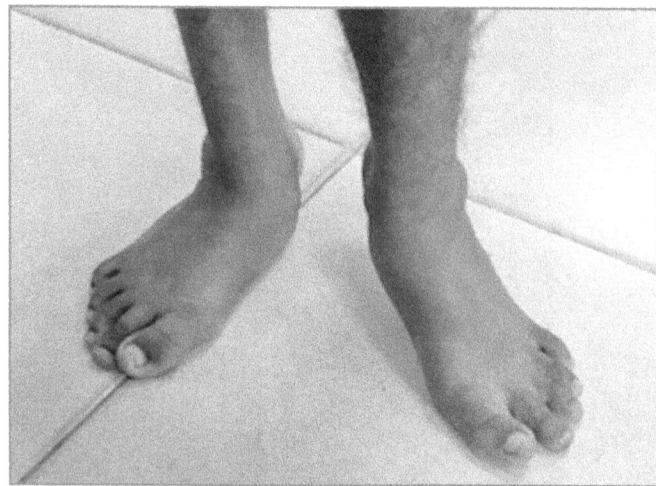

Fig. 18.46: The planovalgus feet.

- *Examination of the upper limbs:* The upper limbs should be examined for any tightness/contracture/deformities such as tightness of shoulder adductors and medial rotators, elbow flexors, forearm pronators, wrist and finger flexors and thumb adductors. In the hands tightness of the short and long flexors of the wrist should be differentiated and documented.
  The Manual Ability Classification System describes how children with CP use their hands to manipulate relevant and appropriate objects for activity of daily living, classifying them into five levels:
  » Level-I—indicates the ability to handle objects easily and successfully.
  » Level-II—handles most objects, but with somewhat reduced quality or speed of achievement.
  » Level-III—handles objects with difficulty, needs help to prepare or modify activities.
  » Level-IV—handles a limited selection of easily managed objects, in adapted situations.
  » Level-V—indicates inability to handle objects and requires total assistance.
- *Involuntary movements:* Tremor, athetosis, dystonia, ballismus, etc., if any, should be identified and recorded.
- *Coordination:* To find dysmetria (if any)—Finger to nose test, heel to shin test. Dysdiadochokinesia (inability to produce rapid alternating movements) is assessed by making the patient perform rapid alternating movements such as: supination and pronation of forearm.
- *Posture and balance assessment:* Balance and equilibrium reactions are prerequisites for walking. Both static posture and dynamic balance in lying, sitting and standing should be assessed. A balance board can be used to test balance in different body postures. A standing child may be pushed gently from the front, back, and side to see whether he or she can promptly regain balance. A deficiency of balance and equilibrium can be assessed using the Romberg sign, unilateral standing balance test, and the hop test.
  » Romberg sign: Shows whether the child can maintain balance. If the child sways and cannot keep his balance with feet held together and eyes closed, indicates positive Romberg's sign.
  » Unilateral standing balance test: Reveals inability to maintain balance in less severely involved children. A 5-year-old child should be able to stand on one foot for 10 seconds. Failure in the unilateral standing balance test explains why children sometimes show excessive trunk leaning when walking.
  » Hop test: Boys can hop on one leg for 5–10 times from age 5 years and girls from age 4 years onward. Inability to perform single-leg hop is another sign of poor balance and neuromuscular control.
- *Anthropometric measurements:*
  » Measurement of limb length discrepancies: Both the apparent and true limb lengths of the lower limbs should be assessed using the measuring tape.

Table 18.12: Weight chart.

Age of the child	Weight (in kilograms)
At birth	2.5–3.5 kg
At 3–6 months	Age in months + 9/2 kg.
At 1–6 years	Age in years × 2 + 8 kg.
At 7–12 years	[(Age in years × 7) + 5]/2 kg.

  » Measurement of height using inch tape and establishing loss of height (if any) due to a spinal deformity. The distance between tips of middle fingers when the upper limbs are fully abducted in the coronal plane, gives the actual height of the child, which should be compared with the height measured in standing and any loss of height, if there is established.
  » Measurement of weight: The weight of the child in kilograms should be taken on a standard weighing machine and compared with the age-appropriate weights using **Table 18.12**.
- *Measurement of chest circumference:* Chest circumference at birth at the level of nipple is 32–34 cm. **Table 18.13** gives the chest circumference of infants and children of varying ages.

Table 18.13: Chest circumference.

Babies/children	Age	Chest circumference
Infants	0–6 months	At birth: 32–34 cm, monthly gain: 2 cm
Infants	6–12 months	Monthly gain: 0.5 cm
Children	1–10 years	Yearly gain: 1.5 cm
Children	11–15 years	Yearly gain: 3 cm

- *Head circumference measurement:* The measuring tape is used to measure occipitofrontal head circumference from external occipital protuberance to glabella. **Table 18.14** gives the head circumferences from birth to 2 years.

Table 18.14: Head circumference.

Age	Head circumference (in cm)
Birth	34–35
2 months	38
3 months	40
4 months	41
6 months	42–43
1 year	45–46
2 years	47–48

- *Assessment of function:* Functional skills should be examined in line with developments in prone, supine, sitting, and standing. Bed mobility, out of bed mobility, self-care, and instrumental activities of daily living (IADL) as per age of the child are identified and documented. The gross motor function classification system can be applied to document functional abilities of the child. The

ambulation capacity of the child is assessed by using the functional mobility scale, having 6 levels, such as:
» 0—indicating full activity.
» 1—walking with assistance.
» 2—walking with assistance for short periods.
» 3—walking with assistance for activities of daily living.
» 4—confined to a wheel chair.
» 5—indicating bedridden.
- *Assessment of sitting ability:* Sitting function/ability of the child should be assessed and typed into the following categories:
  » Hands-free sitter (Independent sitter): The child can independently come to a sitting position, does not need hands to sit up and can sit in a normal chair without losing his balance.
  » Hand-dependent sitter: The child uses hands for support when sitting, needs a chair with side supports to be able to use his hands for eating or writing.
  » Propped sitter: The child has to be brought to a sitting position by someone else, needs external support and sits in a reclining position when strapped into the seat.
- *Assessment of gait:* The different methods used are:
  » Observational analysis.
  » Motion laboratory analysis **(Fig. 18.47)** that uses motion capture systems, force plates, and electromyography.
  » Biochemical analysis, i.e., analysis of energy consumption.

Diagnosis of Cerebral Palsy

History (Developmental history including motor milestones—usually delayed significantly—**Table 18.4**), Apgar scores (assesses muscle tone/activity, pulse, grimace/reflex irritability, appearance/skin color and respiration, and getting a score of 0–3, indicating severe depression or 4–6, indicating

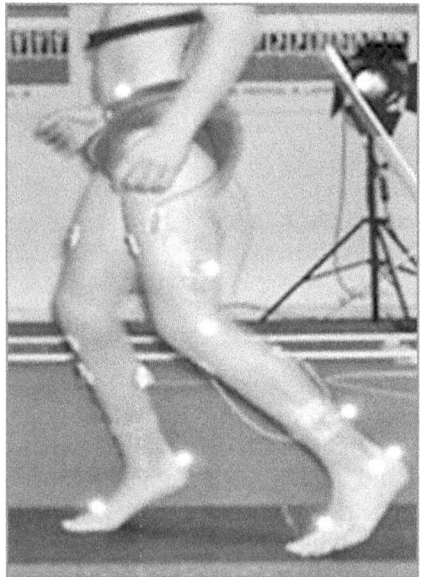

Fig. 18.47: Gait analysis in motion laboratory.

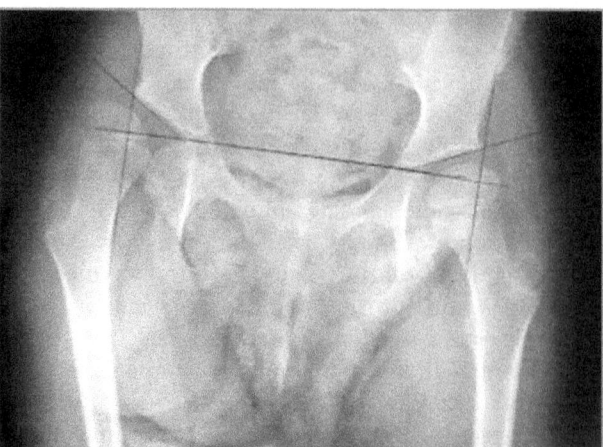

Fig. 18.48: X-ray of pelvis showing dislocation of hip joint.

moderate depression, when combined with history and physical examination, helps in establishing the diagnosis), physical examination help the clinician establishing the diagnosis of CP and differentiate this condition from myopathies, spina bifida, spinal cord tumor, spinal muscular atrophies, etc. In a few cases, where, diagnostic confusion arises, EEG, CT/MRI scan, etc., may be recommended. An X-ray of pelvis **(Fig. 18.48)** may be taken to identify pelvic obliquity and hip dislocation, if any.

Management of Cerebral Palsy

A comprehensive management comprising medical, therapeutic (physiotherapy/occupational therapy/speech therapy), psychological, orthotic, surgical, educational, and vocational measures required through an interactive and cooperative contribution from different professionals, is essential for the complete habilitation of the client, so that, he/she can be a meaningful citizen of the country. Those with GMFCS level-IV/V, can also be provided guardianship as per the norms of the particular country. In India, the National Trust Act has a provision of appointing guardians to those CP children, who are dependent after the death of their parents/guardians.

"Inclusive education" for CP children means a system of education wherein students with and without disability learn together and the system of teaching and learning is suitably adapted to meet the learning needs of different types of students with disabilities.

Medical, therapeutic, surgical, and orthotic treatment strategies selected are age-specific and should include the followings:
- **Infancy:** Supportive measures for prolonging and optimizing physical status and life, nutritional support, exercise/early intervention.
- **Childhood:** Maximum independent mobility, medication, exercise, botulinum toxin, bracing.
- **Preschooler:** Maximum independent mobility, medication, exercise, botulinum toxin, bracing, surgery.
- **Adolescence:** Education, vocational training and integration into the community, schooling, sports, psychosocial support.

A CP child is managed efficiently by a team of professionals (the CP habilitation team). The team comprises the followings—physician, pediatric neurologist, pediatric orthopedic surgeon, physiotherapist, occupational therapist, orthotist, speech therapist and audiologist, clinical psychologist, pediatric neurosurgeon (as and when required), ophthalmologist (as and when required), dentist (as and when required), gastroenterologist (as and when required), nutrition specialist (as and when required).

Medical Management

It consists of drugs to reduce spasticity and dystonia and management of other complications like epilepsy, gastrointestinal disorders, etc. For the management of spasticity, the therapist should take the help of physician as and when needed as per the following requirements. **Table 18.15** indicates the schedule of medical management that may be required for the CP child, which is decided by the physician/surgeon.

Table 18.15: Schedule of medical management for CP child.

Agent	Age-group	Indications
Oral medications	Any age, 2–5 years are most common group of CP children.	Severe generalized spasticity.
Botulinum toxin-A	Any age, 2–10 years are most common group of CP children.	Focal spasticity.
Intrathecal baclofen	Above 3 years, abdomen should be large enough for pump insertion	Severe spasticity interfering with function.

Physiotherapy

It consists of generating the problem list after a thorough assessment, deciding the short-term goal (set to be achieved within 3 months, say achieving neck control), as well as the long-term goal (set to be achieved within 1 year, say standing with support). The therapist should be able to decide the plan of care (therapeutic strategies) with an aim to maintain and increase the joint range of motion, maintain and increase soft tissue flexibility, such as stretching a tight gastrocsoleus muscle, and establish a stable posture such as sitting with head held vertically, and achieve posture and movement skills one after the other to make the child as independent as possible. During the process the physiotherapist may take help from other team members as per need, say help from a physician to prescribe oral antispastic drugs, help from a pediatric orthopedic surgeon to lengthen a spastic/ tight tendo-Achilles, or help from an orthotist to provide antirecurvatum ankle foot orthosis (AFO) for the child who walks with knee in hyperextension. A physiotherapist tries to improve the followings:

- Postural control.
- Muscle strength.
- Range of motion.
- Decreasing spasticity and involuntary movements.
- Increasing soft tissue flexibility.
- Joint alignment.
- Motor control.
- Muscular/cardiovascular endurance and mobility skills.
- Increasing coordination/agility.
- Balance.
- Transitions.
- Use of assistive devices.
- Mobility/gait/function.

The physiotherapist designs a set of exercises to improve motor control in the child through motor learning. Therapeutic exercises help the child learn how to sit, stand, walk and use his upper extremity for function. The child also learns how to use his remaining potential to compensate for the movements he cannot perform. Decreasing spasticity, gaining muscle strength and improving joint alignment decrease deformity. The education of caregivers involves training them to set reasonable expectations for their children, and teaching them to follow their children's exercises at home. Parents should encourage their children to participate in daily living activities by using the functional skills they learned during therapy. Community and social support is very much essential to provide environmental stimuli for acceleration of development of the child.

Physiotherapy begins in early infancy and continues throughout adolescence. The primary purpose is to facilitate normal neuromotor development. With the help of correct positioning, appropriate stimulation and intensive exercise, the therapist tries to gain head control, postural stability and good mobility in the child. Besides stretching of tight/spastic muscles and mobilizing stiff joints, a therapist tries to improve motor control through motor learning procedures. Once a child's movements are facilitated, strengthening exercises are applied to develop strength and endurance, provided the child's muscle tone does not increase with such exercises. This is possible only to the extent of the child's neurological capacity.

The therapist works with the kid in supine and prone postures during physiotherapy sessions to enhance head and trunk control as well as rolling.

He/She assists the child in developing weight shifting and sitting tolerance while he or she is seated. The therapist progresses to prone kneeling, standing with support/ independently, and eventually walking once the child has adapted to sitting. During these procedures, any abnormal reflexes and reactions that dominate the child's motor behavior are inhibited by designing appropriate strategies. The child when placed in a particular position is encouraged to use the upper limb for manipulation of different toys, which later on is carried over into different self-care activities, such as taking food to mouth. The therapist uses different positional devices like CP chair with lap board, corner chair, prone stander, supine stander, walker, elbow crutches, etc., to improve posture and movements. Different gadgets like Swiss ball, wedge-board trampoline, peg board, etc., are used by therapists to improve posture and movement. Positional devices such as knee gaiters, hip abduction orthoses, hand splints, etc., are used by therapists to maintain normal postural requirements to accomplish functional movements.

Methods of physiotherapy:

a. **Conventional exercises:** Conventional exercises consist of active and passive range of motion exercises, stretching, strengthening exercises, balance training, etc. It also includes facilitation of muscle action using Faradic type currents, static cycling, hydrotherapy and calisthenics to improve cardiovascular fitness. A few conventional methods of management are discussed below:
   - Stretching exercises **(Figs. 18.49A to E):** (a) Hip flexors, (b) Short adductors of hip, (c) Long adductors of hips, (d) Hamstrings, (e) Tendo-Achilles.
   - Strengthening exercises: **(Figs. 18.50A to E):** (a) Glutei through pelvic bridging, (b) Back extensors, (c and d) Abdominals, (e) Quadriceps.
   - Mat exercises **(Figs. 18.51A to E):** (a) Quadruped weight shifting, (b) Kneel standing, (c) Half-kneeling, (d) Kneel sitting to kneel standing, (e) Sit to standing.
   - Body weight-supported walking **(Fig. 18.52).**
   - Faradic type current stimulation **(Fig. 18.53).**
   - Balancing exercises **(Figs. 18.54A to C):** (a) Sitting balance on rocking horse, (b) Sitting balance on Swiss ball, (c) Standing balance on trampoline.
   - Functional training **(Figs. 18.55A to C)** (a) Training of hand function, (b) Walking on staircase, (c) Gait training with/without walking aids.

b. **Specific treatment approaches:**
   - **Muscle education and bracing of WM Phelps:** WM Phelp, an orthopedic surgeon in Baltimore recommended the use of the followings for treatment of CP children:

» He recommended the use of passive exercises, active assisted, free and resisted exercises as per the child's capacity for enhancing posture and movement.

» He recommended the use of massage for hypotonic muscles.

» He recommended the use of special braces to correct deformity and to obtain the upright position and to control athetosis.

» He recommended that children with spasticity should be given muscle education based on an analysis of whether muscles are spastic, weak, normal or zero cerebral (being unable to act), or atonic. Muscles antagonistic to spastic muscles need to be activated, which is to obtain muscle balance between spastic muscles and their antagonists.

» He recommended that athetoids should be trained to control simple joint motion and not muscle education. Ataxic children should be given strengthening exercises for weak muscle groups.

» He recommended for the use of conditioned motion for babies, small children, and mentally retarded children.

» The use of confused motion/synergistic motion, where the stronger muscles in the pattern are resisted to activate the weaker muscles, were emphasized in the technique.

» Relaxation techniques such as Jacobson's method of tensing and relaxing are recommended for children with involuntary movements such as athetosis.

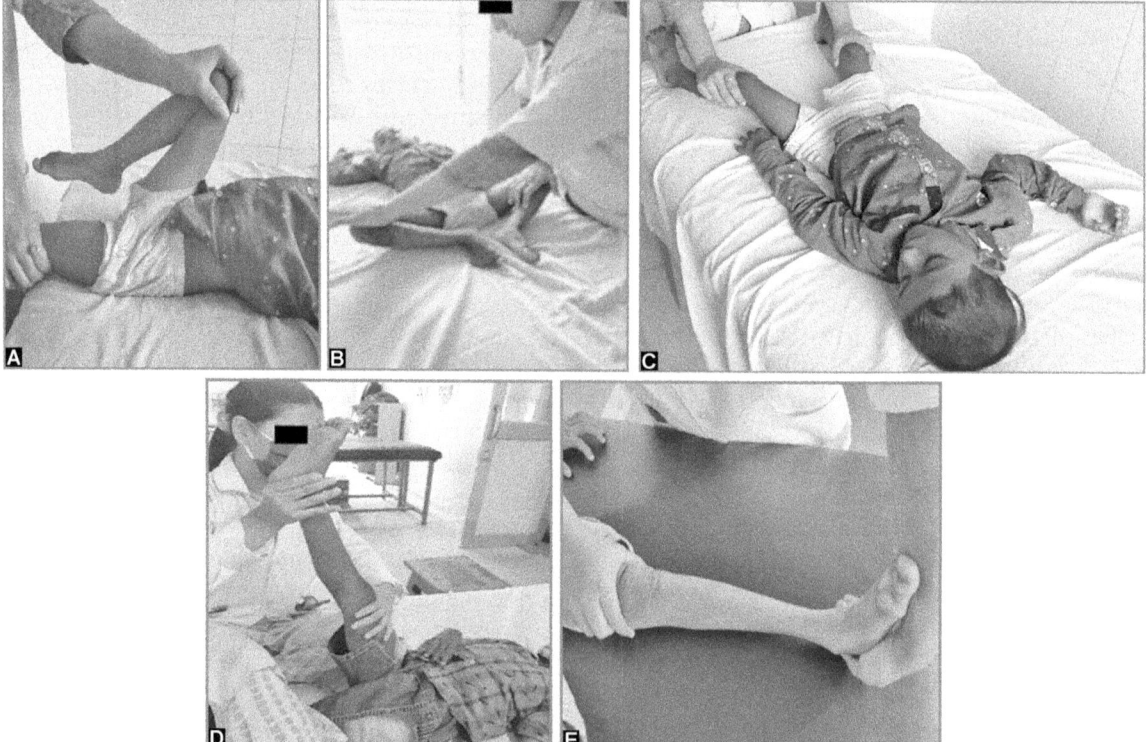

Figs. 18.49A to E: Stretching exercises: (A) Hip flexors; (B) Short adductors of hip; (C) Long adductors of hips; (D) Hamstrings; (E) Tendo-Achilles.

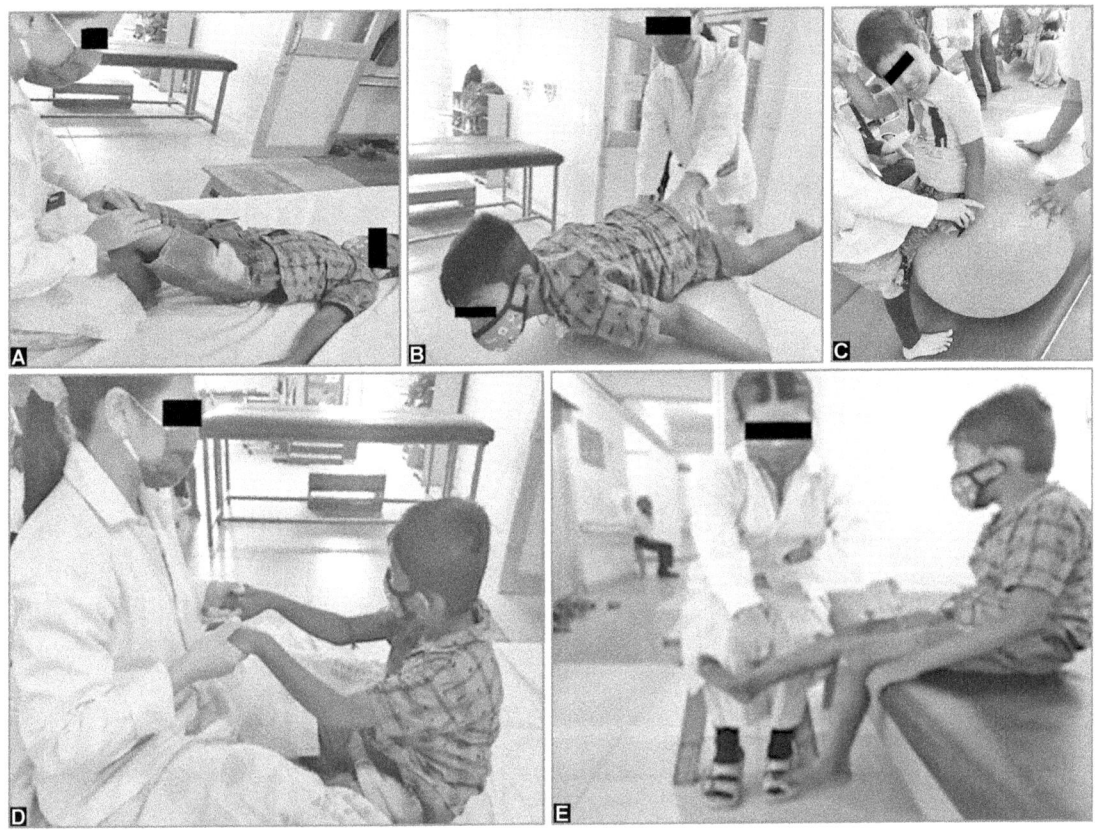

Figs. 18.50A to E: Strengthening exercises: (A) Glutei through pelvic bridging; (B) Back extensors; (C and D) Abdominals; (E) Quadriceps.

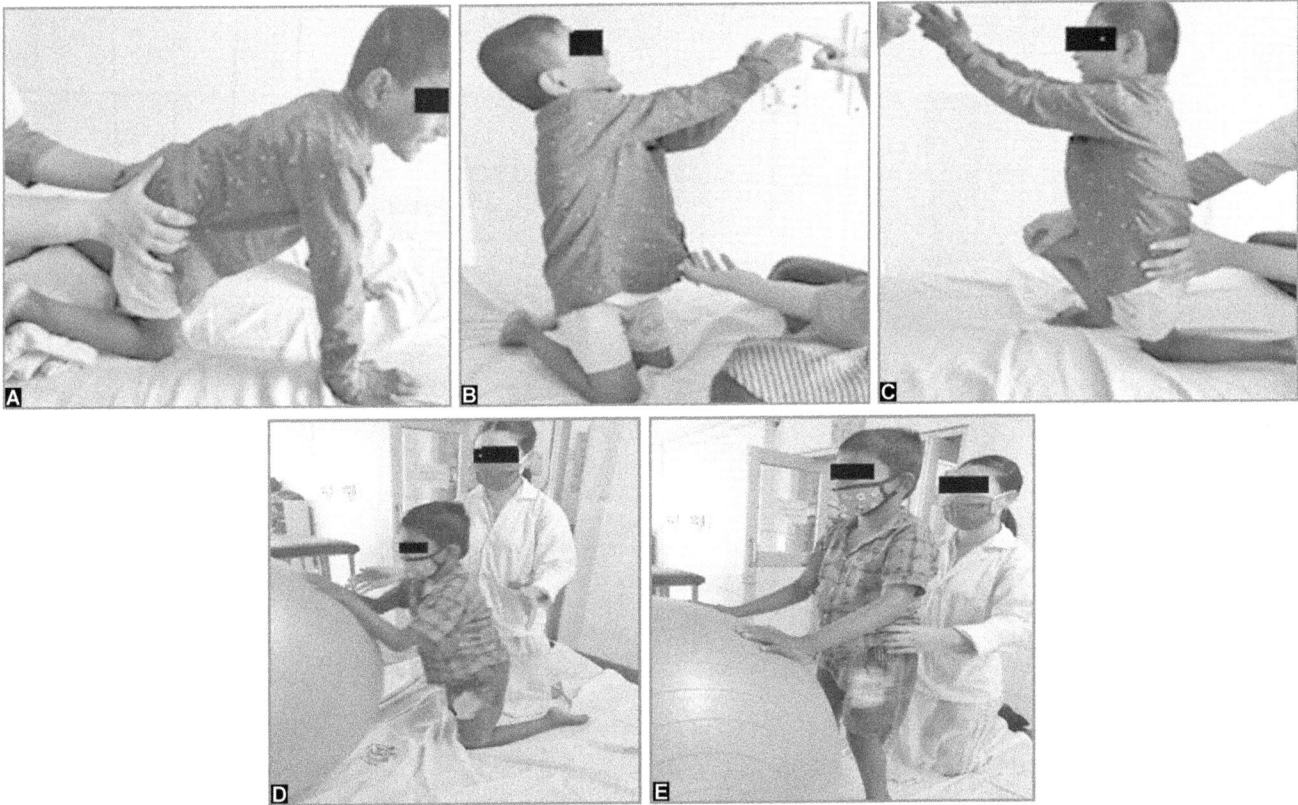

Figs. 18.51A to E: Mat exercises: (A) Quadruped weight shifting; (B) Kneel standing; (C) Half-kneeling; (D) Kneel sitting to kneel standing; (E) Siting to standing.

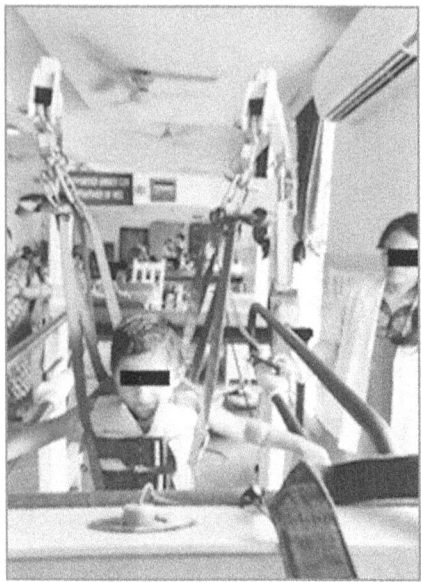

Fig. 18.52: Body weight-supported walking.

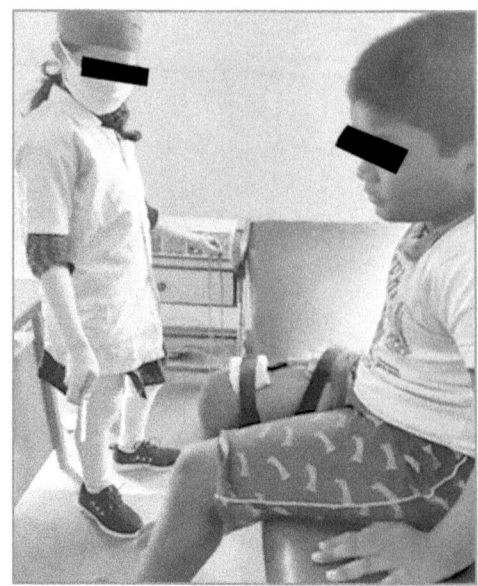

Fig. 18.53: Faradic stimulation for facilitation/strengthening of quadriceps.

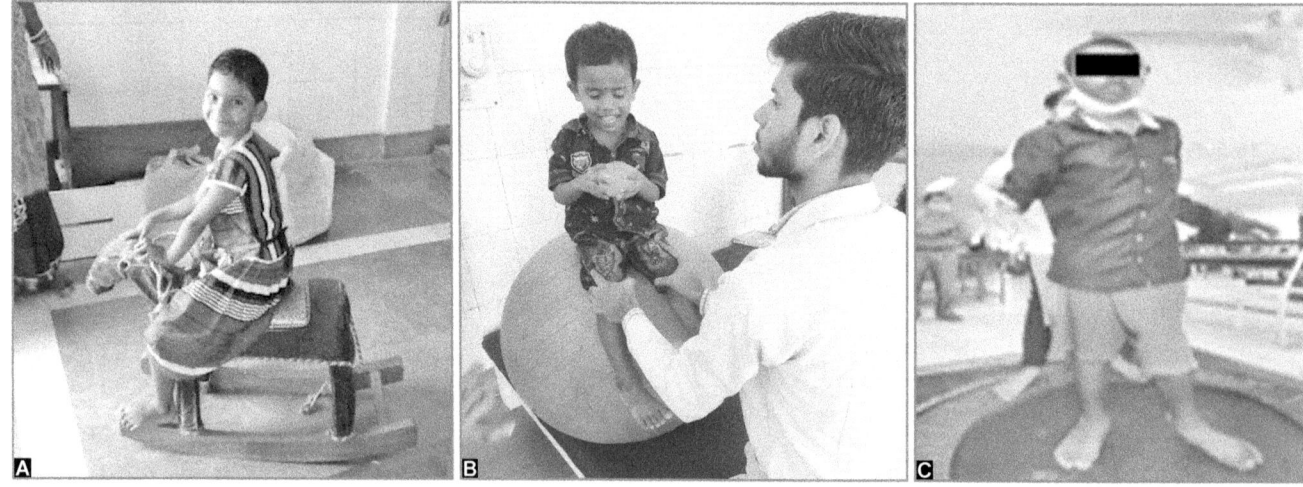

Figs. 18.54A to C: Balance training on: (A) Rocking horse; (B) Swiss ball; (C) Trampoline.

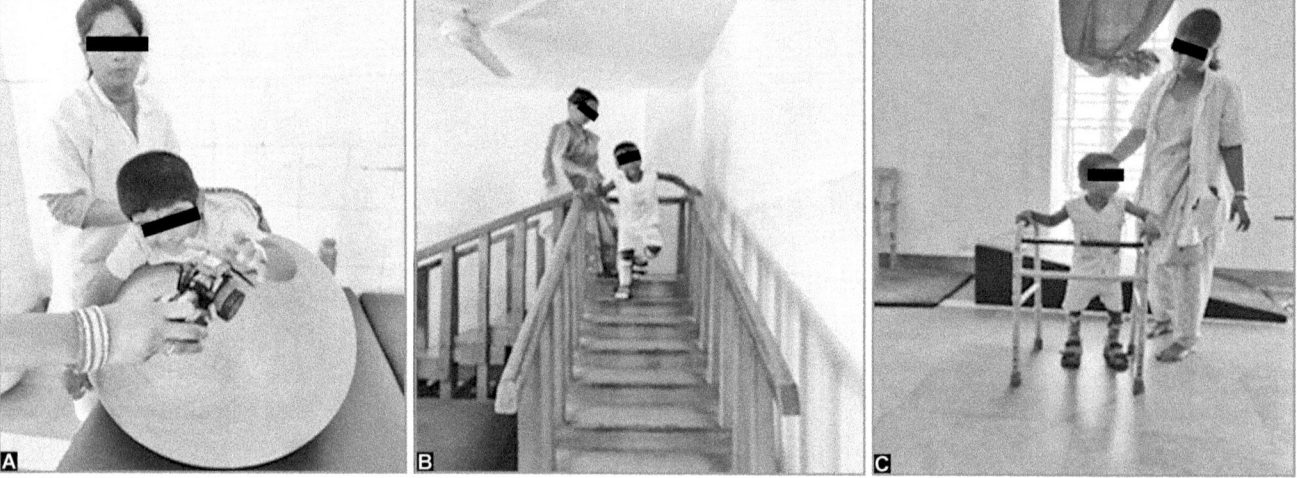

Figs. 18.55A to C: (A) Hand function training; (B) Walking training on staircase; (C) Gait training with walker.

» Balance training with or without braces, reciprocal movements of the limbs, reaching and grasping for hand function are emphasized in the technique.
- **Progressive pattern of movement by Temple Fay:**
  » This technique of treatment was developed by Temple Fay, a neurosurgeon in Philadelphia.
  » He recommended that the CP children be taught motion according to its development in evolution.
  » He regarded ontogenetic development (in humans) as a recapitulation of phylogenetic development (in evolution of the species).
  » He suggested building up motion from reptilian squirming to amphibian creeping, through mammalian reciprocal motion "on all fours" to the primate erect walking. Fay also described "unlocking reflexes" which reduces hypertonus.
  » He developed progressive pattern movements based on above ideas which consist of five stages:

Stage 1 – Prone lying:
Head and trunk rotation from side to side

Stage 2 – Homolateral stage:
» Prone lying, head turned to side
» Arm on the face side in abduction—external rotation, elbow semiflexed, hand open, and thumb out towards the mouth.
» Leg on the face side in abduction, knee flexion opposite stomach, and foot dorsiflexion—Arm on the occiput side is extended, internally rotated, hand open at the side of the child or on the lumbar area of his back.
» Leg on occiput side is extended.
» Movements involve head turning from side to side with the face, arm and leg sweeping down to the extended position and the opposite occiput arm and leg flexing up to the position near the face as the head turns round.

Stage 3 – Contralateral stage:
» Prone lying: Head turned to side, arm on the face side as in stage 2.
» Leg on the face side is extended.
» Other leg on the side of occiput is flexed.
» As the head turns this contralateral pattern changes from side to side.

Stage 4 – On hands and knees:
Reciprocal crawling and on hands and feet stepping in the bear walk or elephant walk.

Stage 5 – Walking pattern:
» This is sailor's walk called by Fay "reciprocal progression on lower extremities synchronized with the contralateral swing of the arms and trunk".
» A wide base is used and the child flexes one hip and knee into external rotation and then places his foot on the ground, still in external rotation.
» As the foot is being placed on the ground the opposite arm and shoulder are rotating towards it.
» As weight is taken on the straight leg, the other leg flexes up.

- **Synergistic movement pattern by Signe Brunnstrom:** The technique was developed by Signe Brunnstrom, a female physiotherapist.

  She emphasized upon movement production through provocation of primitive movement patterns or synergistic movement patterns. Reflex responses are used initially and later voluntary control of these reflex patterns are trained. Control of head and trunk is attempted trough stimulation of the attitudinal reflexes, such as tonic labyrinthine reflex, tonic lumbar reflex, etc., which is followed by stimulation of righting reflexes for training of balance.

  Associated reactions and hand reactions such as hyperextension of the thumb resulting in finger relaxation are used in therapy.

- **Proprioceptive neuromuscular facilitation (PNF):** This technique of treatment was designed by Herman Kabat, Margaret Knott, and Dorothy Voss. It emphasizes upon practice of movement patterns (mass movement patterns) based on patterns observed with functional activities such as spiral and diagonal with synergy of muscle groups.

  The movement patterns consist of the following components:
  » Flexion or extension.
  » Abduction or adduction.
  » Internal rotation or external rotation.

  Sensory stimuli, such as touch, pressure, traction and compression, stretch, proprioceptive effect of muscle contraction against resistance, auditory and visual are skillfully applied to facilitate movement.

  Various techniques such as rhythmic stabilization, Hold-Relax, Contract-Relax, Rhythmic Initiation, Slow-Reversal, etc., are used in a developmental context to facilitate movement such as rolling **(Figs. 18.56A and B)**, creeping, crawling, walking, etc., and to enhance function in children with cerebral palsy.

- **Neuromotor development by Eirene Collis:** This technique of treatment for cerebral palsy was developed by Eirene Collis, a therapist and pioneer in CP in Britain. According to her, the mental capacity of the child determines results, and the term management should be used instead of treatment while caring for CP

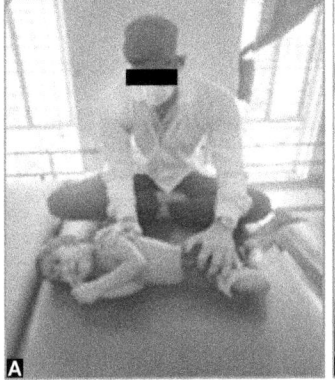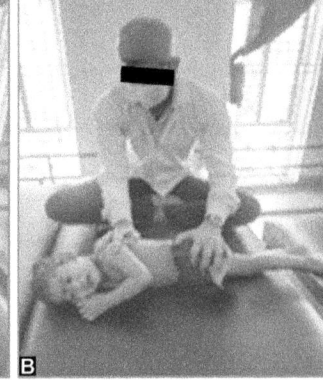

Figs. 18.56A and B: PNF to facilitate rolling.

children, where feeding, dressing, toileting, and other activities of the day should be planned for the child.

Strict developmental sequence was followed in the technique. The child was not permitted to use motor skills beyond his level of development.

The child was placed in normal postures, in order to stimulate normal tone. Once postural security was obtained, achievements were facilitated and developmental sequences were followed throughout this training. She said, the therapists (PT/OT/Speech therapists) should be called as CP therapists, as they all work with the aim of managing the child.

– **Neurodevelopmental treatment:** Neurodevelopmental treatment (NDT) is a problem-solving approach, which states that identifying and targeting the system impairments that underlie the functional limitations of an individual with neuropathology is the most effective way to improve the individual's ability to carry out meaningful life skills.

The technique was developed by Karl Bobath and his wife Berta Bobath, which was earlier based upon Reflex Hierarchical theory of motor control, and subsequently was modified in the basis of Dynamic systems theory and Neuronal group selection theory [NGST: incorporates the knowledge that brain development or recovery from brain damage is aided (having helped) when the individual engages in activities that occur in functionally or develop mentally appropriate environment context].

Neurodevelopmental treatment as a neuromuscular and functional re-education technique now includes neuroplasticity as a basis, how the brain can change and reorganize itself and its processes based on practice and experience.

In NDT practice, the clinician looks very specifically and carefully at each domain and the relationships among the domains presented in the ICF model. Hypotheses about these relationships are made during information gathering, examination, evaluation, and intervention planning, and within every intervention session. The NDT clinician also looks at the body structure and function domain and further discriminates general issues of posture and movement (multisystem functions) from issues of single system function. In addition, the therapist carefully analyzes the impact of the environmental and personal contextual factors on each of the domains.

Therapeutic handling (techniques of inhibition, techniques of facilitation and key point stimulation) is done in a developmental and task contexted manner to improve posture and functional movements. The proximal key points such as head, trunk, pelvic girdle, shoulder girdle, as well as the distal key points, such as, hands, feet are manipulated to inhibit abnormal tone and facilitate more normal pattern of movements.

Three stages of inhibition and facilitation, such as stage of sensation, stage of cognition, and stage of fading of control are used in the technique.

Developmental sequence is followed in the technique, but not in a rigid manner.

Sensory motor experience is emphasized in the technique that is the abnormal movement patterns are to be inhibited, giving the child the feeling of normal postural tone and movement.

A few techniques of NDT are shown below:
A. Development (facilitation of neck and trunk control) (**Figs. 18.57A to C**).
B. Development of rolling (**Figs. 18.58A to D**).
C. Development of sitting (**Figs. 18.59A and B**).
D. Development of creeping and crawling (**Figs. 18.60A and B**).
E. Development of kneel standing, half kneeling, and standing balance (**Figs. 18.61A to C**).
F. Development of hand function (**Figs. 18.62A and B**).

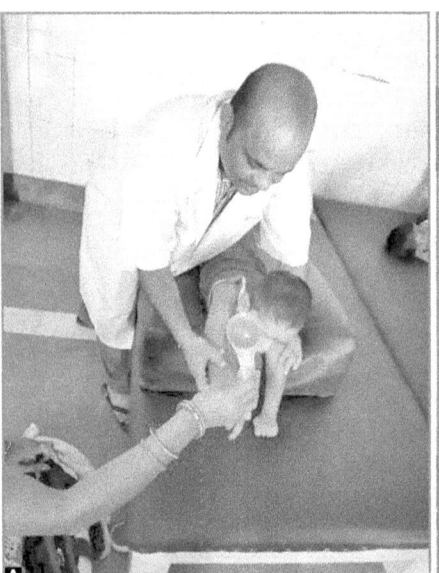 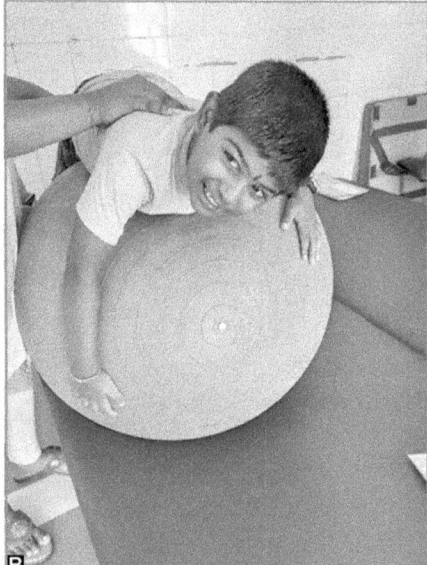 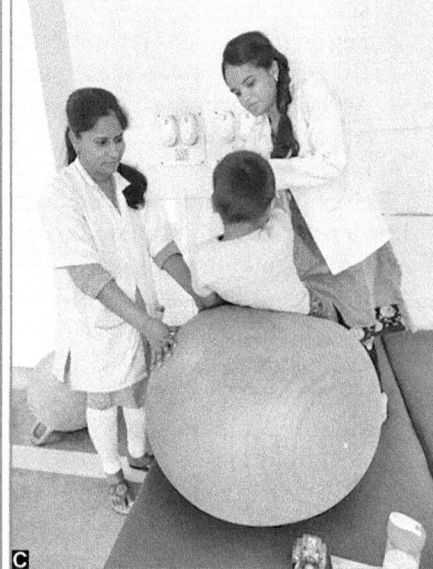

Figs. 18.57A to C: Strategies to improve neck and trunk control.

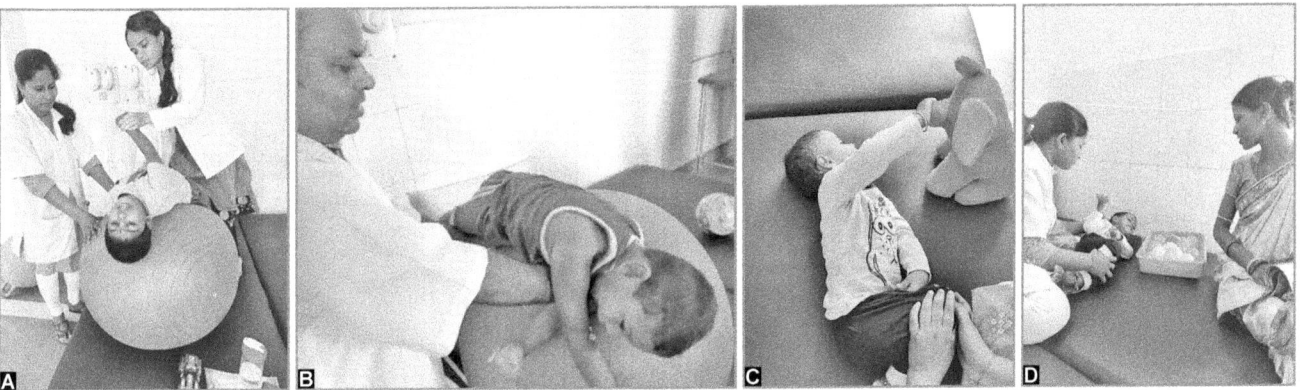

Figs. 18.58A to D: Strategies to develop rolling.

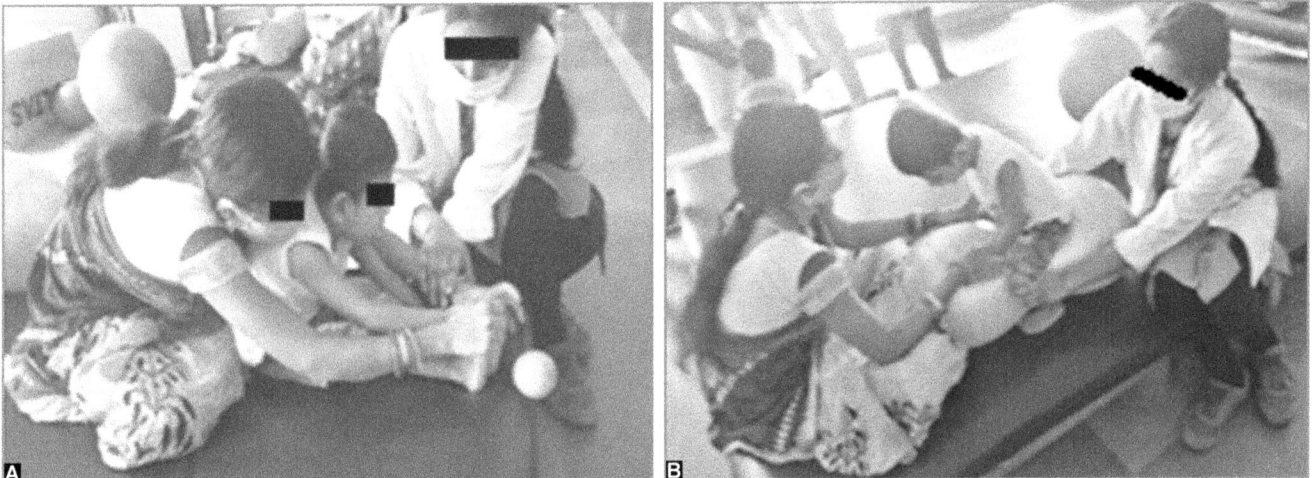

Figs. 18.59A and B: Development of sitting.

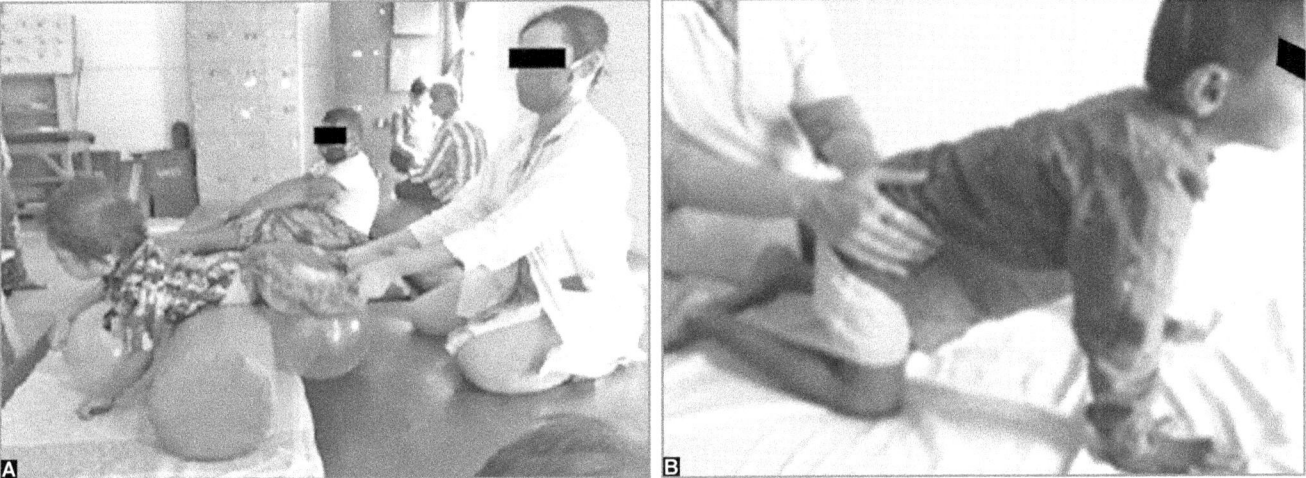

Figs. 18.60A and B: (A) Creeping; (B) Crawling.

- **Sensory stimulation for activation and inhibition (Rood's approach):** This technique was developed by Margaret Rood, Physiotherapist and Occupational Therapist, who used techniques of stimulation, such as stroking, brushing, icing, heating, bone pounding, slow and quick muscle stretch, joint traction and approximation, muscle contraction (proprioception) to activate, facilitate or inhibit motor response in children with CP.

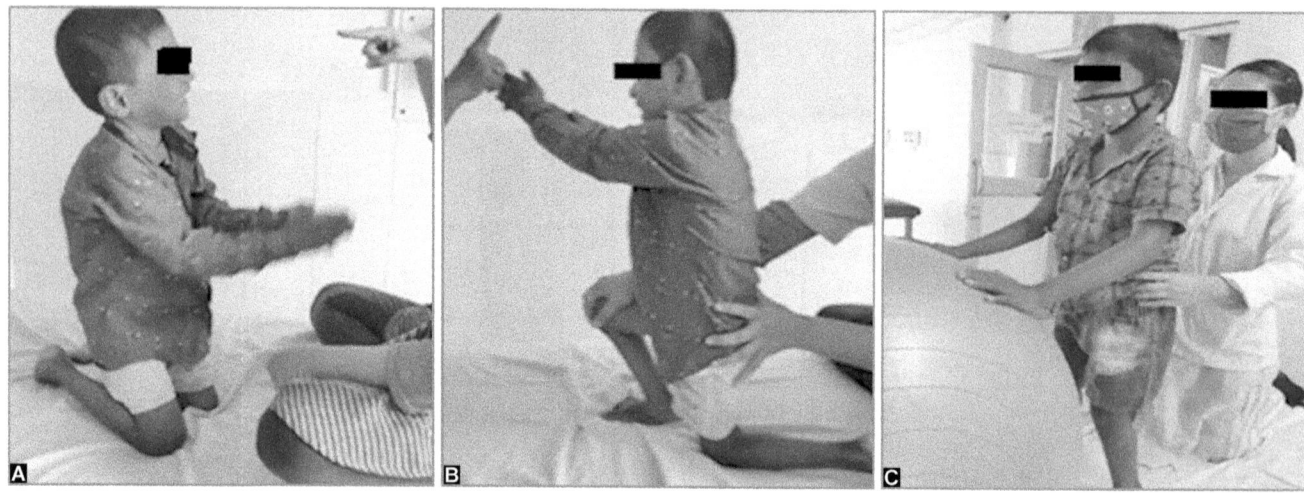

Figs. 18.61A to C: (A) Kneel standing; (B) Half kneeling; (C) Standing.

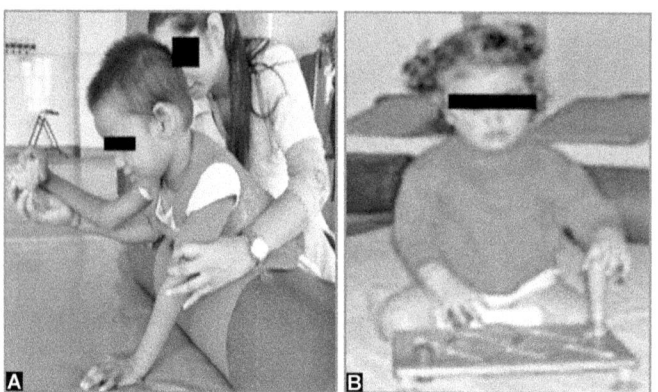

Figs. 18.62A and B: Development of hand function.

Ontogenetic developmental sequences were strictly followed in the application of stimuli, such as:
- Total flexion or withdrawal pattern (in supine).
- Rollover (flexion of arm and leg on the same side and rollover).
- Pivot prone (prone with hyperextension of neck, trunk and legs).
- Co-contraction of neck (prone head over edge for co-contraction of vertebral muscles).
- On elbows (prone and push backward).
- All fours (static weight shift and crawl).
- Standing upright (static weight shift).
- Walking (stance, push off, pick up, heel strike).

A developmental sequence for respiration, sucking, swallowing, phonation, chewing, and speech was followed in the treatment through sensory stimulation techniques such as icing, brushing, pressure, etc.

- **Reflex locomotion through trigger point stimulation:** Vaclov Vojta, a Neurologist, developed his approach from the work of Temple Fay. The basic treatment is to use proprioceptive trigger points on the trunk and extremities to initiate reflex movement, which produces rolling, crawling, and other specific functions. Vojta established 18 points in the body for stimulation and used the positions of reflex crawling and reflex rolling (**Figs. 18.63A to D**). He proposed that placing the child in these positions and stimulation of the trigger points in the body would enhance CNS development. In this way the child is presumed to learn normal movement patterns in place of abnormal motion. These stimulations have to be done every day by the family at home at least 4–5 times daily. The treatment is believed to be of most benefit in the first or second year of life.

  The main features are: (1) Reflex creeping: The creeping patterns involving head, trunk and limbs are facilitated in prone through trigger point stimulation. (2) Reflex rolling: Rolling patterns are stimulated in supine through trigger point stimulation. (3) Sensory stimulation: Touch, pressure, stretch and muscle action against resistance are used in facilitation of reflex locomotion. Besides the 18 main trigger points (9 on left, 9 on right such as tip of acromion process of scapula, root of spine of scapula, medial epicondyle of humerus, just above the styloid process of radius, 7th intercostals space, gluteus medius muscle, ASIS, medial condyle of femur, lateral border of calcaneum) there is an auxillary trigger point under the chin, which is used to stimulate movement of jaw and swallowing.

- **Sensory integration therapy:** Jean Ayers, who is trained as an occupational therapist has developed this treatment approach. She recognized that some children with CP have difficulties with attention, behavior and visual perception. These difficulties are related to sensory integration, the basic goal of this therapy technique is to teach children how to integrate their sensory feedback and then produce useful and purposeful motor responses. The sensory integration approach tries to have these children access and integrate all their sensory input to use for functional gain.

  Activities such as catching a ball in different positions may be used as a way of stimulating and requiring integration of visual, vestibular, and joint

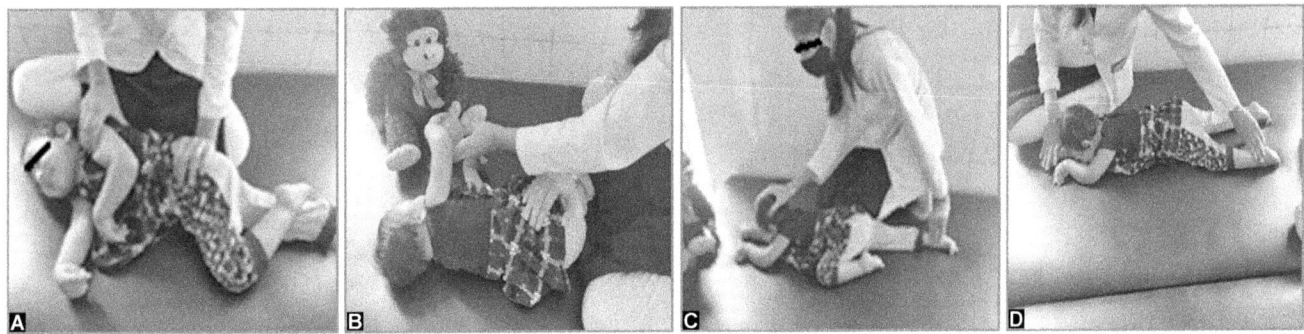

Figs. 18.63A to D: Vojta's trigger point stimulation for: (A) Rolling; (B) Rolling; (C) Creeping and uprighting; (D) Creeping.

proprioception feedback systems at the same time. Typical stimulations include vestibular stimulation and tactile stimulation by brushing, rubbing, joint compression and traction. Educating the parents is recognized as an important aspect of the treatment. The theory underlying this system is that sensory input followed by appropriate motor function will contribute to the improved development of higher cortical motor and sensory function. **Figures 18.64A to C** demonstrate some of the sensory integration approaches used by therapists.

- **Conductive education:** Andreas Peto developed conductive education as an educational technique for children with CP. The children are treated by conductors in a facility where they lived full time. The main features of this system are the integration of therapy and education by having:
  » A conductor acting as a mother, nurse, teacher, therapist. The conductor is trained in the habilitation of motor-disabled children, and has one or two assistants.
  » Group of children; about 15-20 children work together in groups **(Figs. 18.65A and B)**, which is a fundamental part in this training system.
  » An all-day program; a fixed time-table is planned. It includes: getting out of bed in the morning, dressing, feeding, toileting, movement training, speech, reading, writing, and other school work.
  » The movements form the elements of a task or motor skill. The tasks are carefully analyzed for each group of children. They include activities of daily living, motor skills including hand function, balance and locomotion.
  » The purpose of each movement is explained to the children and the movements were repeated throughout the day.
  » Rhythmic intention is used for training the elements or movements. The conductor and the children state the intended motion, e.g., **"1 touch my mouth with my hands"**
  » Individual sessions are conducted for some children to help them to participate more adequately in the work of the group.
- **Hippo therapy:** This therapy is performed with the child sitting on the horse back over a thin soft saddle. Three people, one individual for leading the horse, the therapist standing alongside the horse, working with the child and the third, the assistant stands on the opposite side of therapist helps in preventing the child from falling and assists the child to change positions.

  This therapy gives them a platform (hairy, olfactory stimulating, warm, four-legged Bobath ball platform) on which a trained therapist can capitalize on motor control, stretching and equilibrium.

  Benefits of Hippo therapy:
  » Improves joint co-contraction.

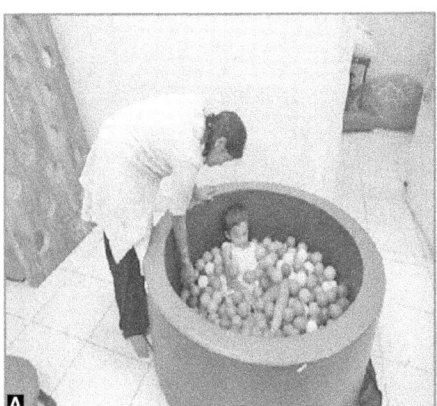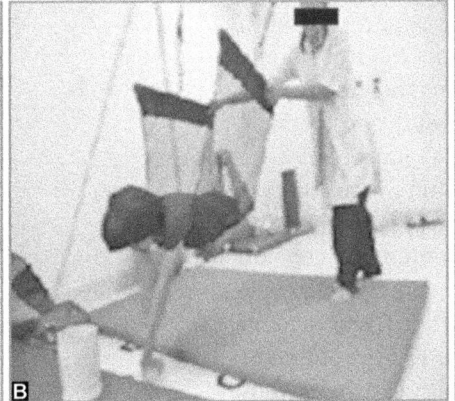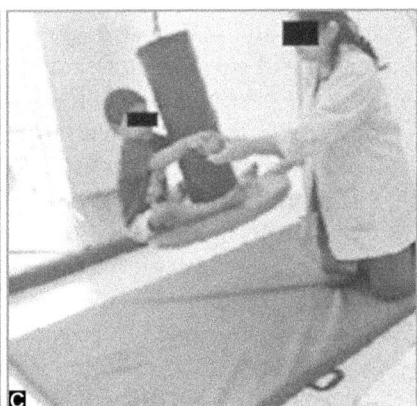

Figs. 18.64A to C: Sensory integration therapy: (A) In ball pool; (B) On hammock; (C) On disk.

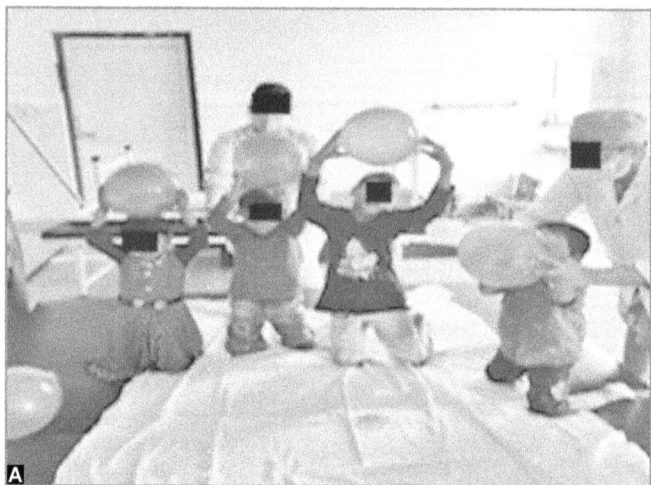 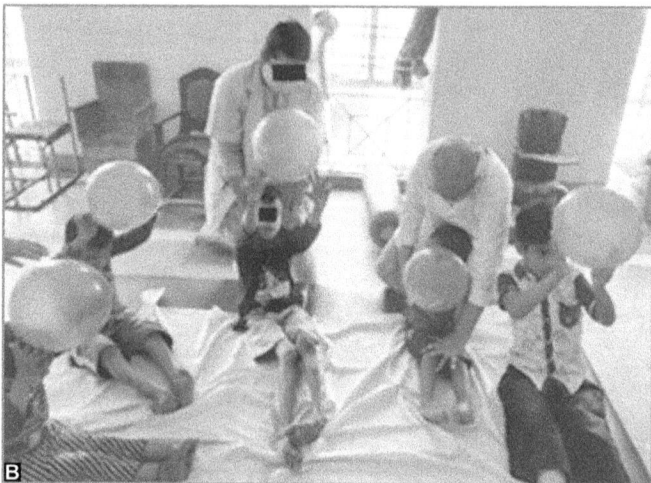

Figs. 18.65A and B: Group therapy (conductive education in progress).

- » Normalizes muscle tone.
- » Decreases energy expenditure with movement.
- » Improves stability.
- » Facilitates weight shifting.
- » Facilitates postural and equilibrium responses.
- » Increases visual perception.
- » Increases self-confidence.
- » Improves respiration.
- » Increases co-ordination.
- » Increases attention span.
- » Mobilizes, pelvis, hips and spine.
- » Improves posture and balance.
- » Improves speech and language.
- » Improves gait.
- » Improves relationships of one with other.

– **Hydrotherapy/aquatic therapy:** Hydrotherapy/aquatic therapy when applied cautiously provides opportunities to the child to learn and enjoy new movement skills, which leads to increase in functional skills, mobility and self-confidence. The temperature of warm water (92–96°F) causes increase of core temperature of the body, causing reduction of the gamma fiber activity, which in turn reduces muscle spindle activity, causing a decrease in muscle tone/spasticity. The buoyancy of water assists weaker muscles and resists stronger muscles, resulting in increase of strength and endurance. The hydrostatic pressure exerted helps in stabilizing unstable/ataxic body parts, thereby increasing stability and balance. The **Figure 18.66A** shows the hydrotherapy pool.

– **Targeted training:** Targeted training is promising treatment technique and is based on the principle that the normal child achieves motor control in a cephalo to caudal direction. The training program uses specially designed equipment to provide the correct level of support so that the child can learn to control one or two joints at a time, rather than being overwhelmed by too many control demands. After careful assessment, the highest body segment lacking in control is targeted (often the neck and head in children with cerebral palsy). By using the program for some periods every day, it is possible to progress motor control learning in a downward direction. Encouraging results are being achieved with the technique.

– **Virtual reality training:** This advanced method of training helps to improve motor control, posture and balance in children with cerebral palsy. Studies suggests that, using virtual reality games in therapy, improves motor function for children with cerebral palsy. The virtual reality games as a part of physiotherapy, can increase motor performance in children with cerebral palsy.

– **Robotic therapy:** The use of robotic trainers for neurorehabilitation application has increased in the last decades for children with severe motor diseases. The exoskeleton gait trainers, helps in rehabilitation of gait function in children with cerebral palsy (**Fig. 18.66B**). Robotic therapy is also claimed to be helpful for improvement of upper limb function in children with cerebral palsy.

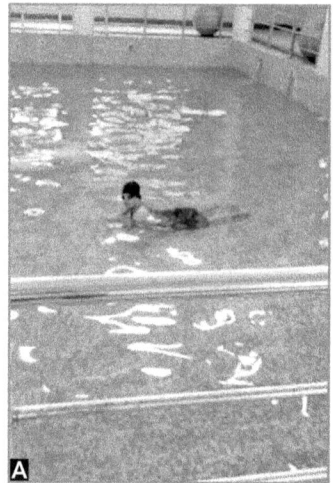 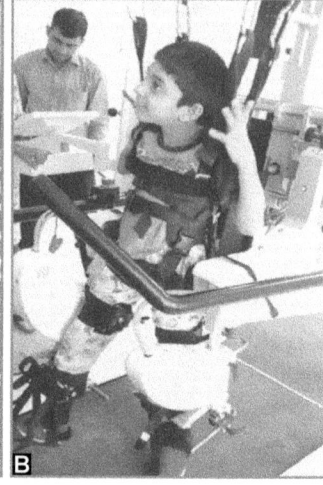

Figs. 18.66A and B: (A) The hydrotherapy pool; (B) Robotic therapy for gait training in a child with cerebral palsy.

Orthotic Management and Assistive Devices for Cerebral Palsy

Various orthotic and assistive devices are recommended for CP children for maintenance of posture and accomplishment of function. The goals of the orthotics in CP are:
- To increase function
- To prevent deformity
- To keep joint in a functional position
- To stabilize the trunk and extremities for function
- To facilitate selective motor control
- To decrease spasticity
- To protect extremity from injury in the postoperative phase.

The orthosis should be custom-made for each child, and should be simple, light, and strong allowing functional independence. Long leg braces such as hip, knee, ankle foot orthosis, (HKAFO), knee, ankle foot orthosis (KAFO) should be avoided as these are heavy and impose more functional restrictions. Ankle foot orthosis, mostly articulated/hinged type should be the choice, as besides stabilizing effects, it also promotes function, by allowing joint movements.

The brace should be simple, light but strong. It should be easy to use. Most importantly, it should provide and increase functional independence. The braces used are:
- **Ankle foot orthoses (Figs. 18.67A to F):**
  - Solid type AFO (mostly used as positional device).
  - Hinged AFO (used for function).
  - *Floor/Ground reaction AFO:* Used for ankle and knee stability mostly for children with a crouch gait, where the hip and knee remain flexed and ankle dorsiflexed.
  - *Antirecurvatum AFO:* Used for children with spastic ankle plantar flexors causing knee hyperextension.
  - Leaf spring AFO.

The ground/floor reaction AFO that aligns the ankle in few degrees of plantar flexion has the anterior restraint, which prevents the tibia from moving forward to cause knee flexion. Alignment of the ankle at around 5-7 degrees of plantar flexion shifts the line of gravity that is in line with the ground reaction force vector, anterior to the knee causing knee extension and also prevents excessive ankle dorsiflexion and crouch gait. The antirecurvatum AFO that aligns the ankle in 5 degrees of dorsiflexion is recommended for spastic CP children with knee hyperextension. This may be solid or hinged as per the child's tolerance. The initial contact occurs with the ankle in dorsiflexion, preventing equinus. The back of the AFO pushes the tibia forward and the ground reaction force vector slides behind the knee joint creating a flexion moment at the knee. A leaf spring AFO, that is very light and flexible, is sometimes used for support and function.

Knee Orthosis

- Knee orthoses are used as resting splints in the early postoperative period and during therapeutic ambulation. The use of such orthoses protects the knee joint, prevents recurrence after multilevel lengthening, and enables a safer start to weight-bearing and ambulation after surgery.

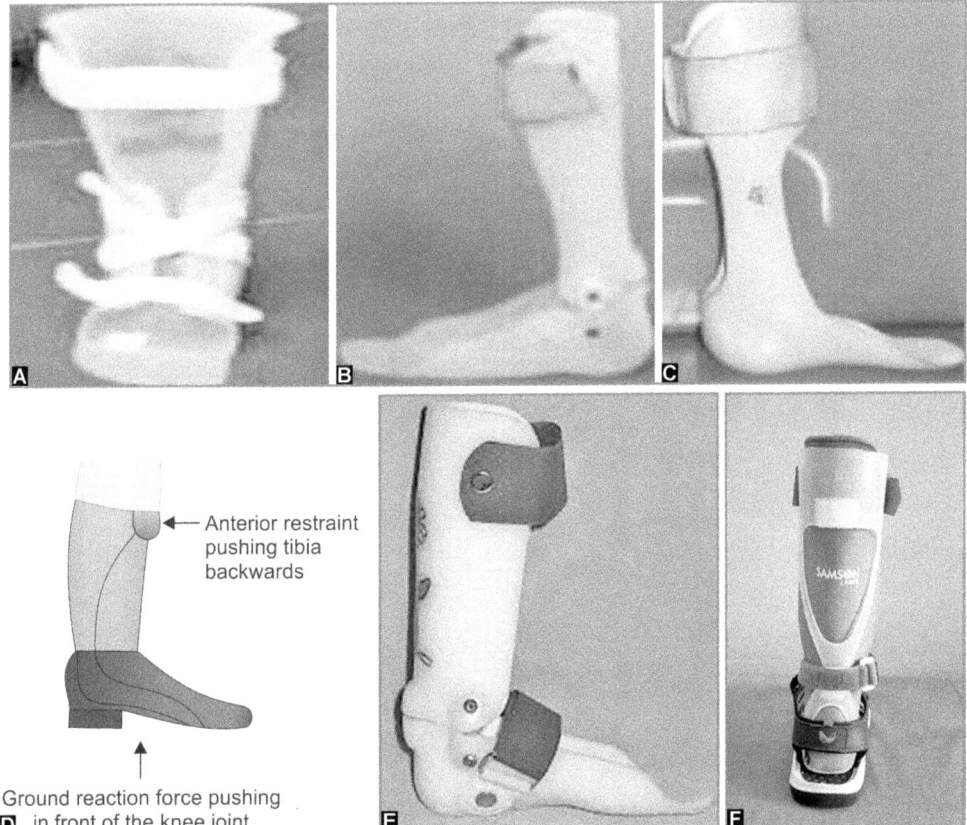

Figs. 18.67A to E: (A) Solid AFO; (B) Hinged AFO; (D) Ground/floor reaction AFO; (E) Antirecurvatum AFO; (F) Posterior leaf spring AFO.

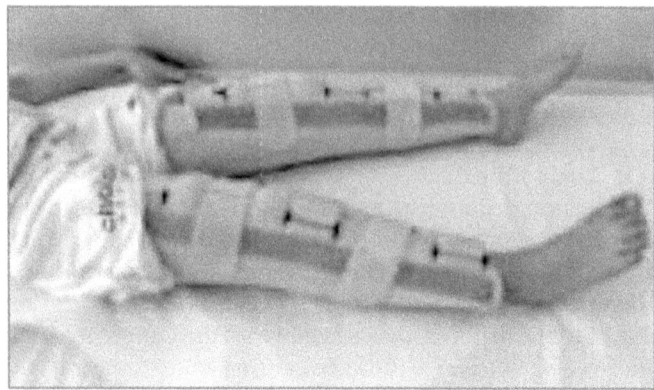

Fig. 18.68: The knee immobilizer/gaiter.

There are three types of knee orthoses, such as:

- The knee immobilizer (knee gaiter) **(Fig. 18.68)**. This is a therapeutic orthosis, made of canvas cloth and aluminum/plastic bars. It is lighter in weight, and is selected by the therapist to develop standing tolerance, as well as for use as night splint.
- The polypropylene KAFO **(Fig. 18.69)**: This orthosis is rarely selected by the clinicians, as it is motion-limiting in knee and ankles. However, in the early phase of habilitation training, this orthosis may be used to develop standing posture. However, for gait training, this orthosis should not be selected, as walking with such orthosis is very much energy-consuming and it also makes learned nonuse of knee and ankle. For these reasons, KAFOs for functional ambulation have disappeared from use in children with CP. Instead, antirecurvatum AFOs or ground reaction AFOs (GRAFOs) are used for knee problems in ambulatory children.
- The supracondylar knee-ankle-foot orthosis (SKAFO): This is the orthosis of choice in CP children walking with knee hyperextension **(Fig. 18.70)**. This is a functional orthosis that allows full knee flexion and prevents knee hyperextension.

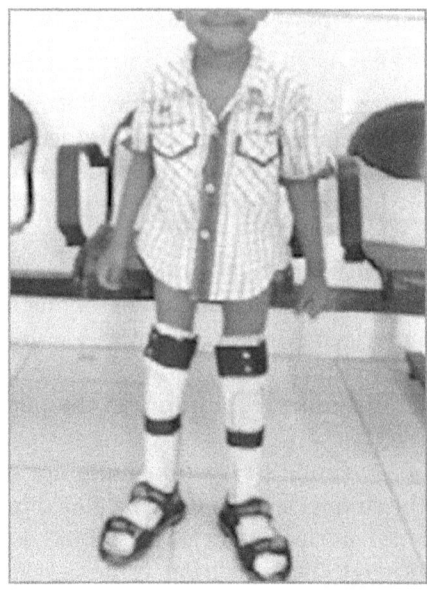

Fig. 18.70: Cerebral palsy child with SKAFO.

Hip Abduction Orthosis

Hip abduction orthosis **(Fig. 18.71)** is recommended in children with hip adductor tightness to protect hip range of motion and prevent the development of subluxation. An abduction pillow is a simple and cheap hip abduction orthosis, which is recommended for use as a night splint, as well as in the early period after adductor lengthening.

Foot Orthosis

Supramalleolar orthosis (SMO) **(Fig. 18.72)**: This orthosis extends to just above the malleoli and to the toes. Mild dynamic equinus, varus, and valgus instability are all factors to consider.

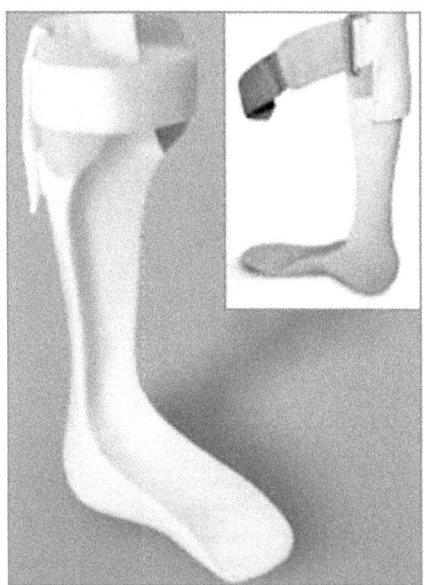

Fig. 18.69: The polypropylene KAFO.

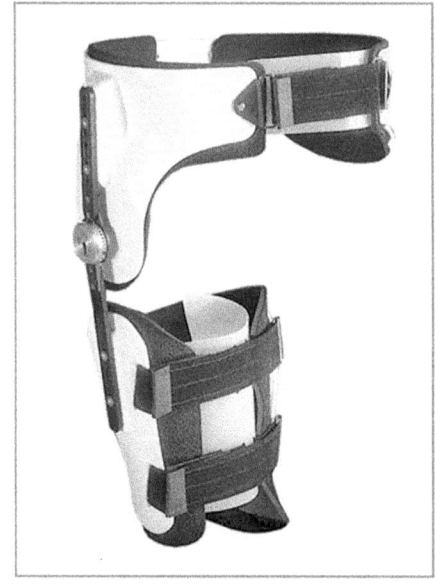

Fig. 18.71: Hip abduction orthosis.

Chapter 18: Cerebral Palsy

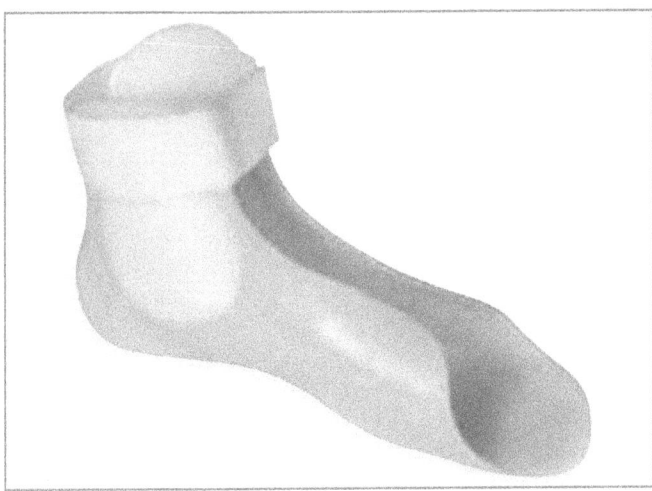

Fig. 18.72: The supramalleolar orthosis.

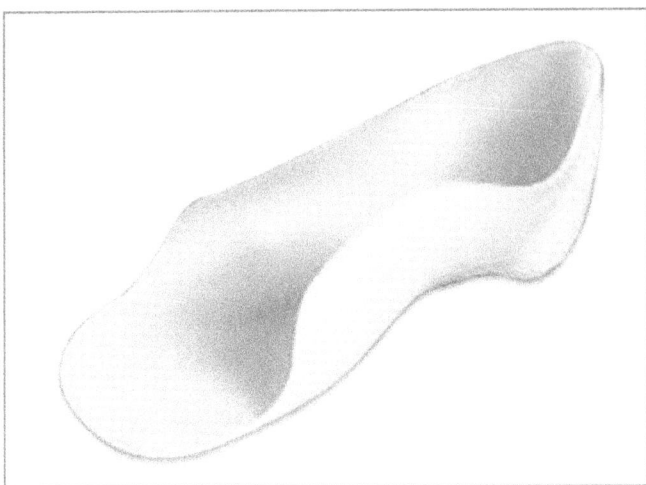

Fig. 18.73: The UCBL orthosis.

University of California Biomechanics Laboratory (UCBL) Orthosis

Medial side of this orthosis is higher than the lateral side. It holds the calcaneus more firmly and supports the medial longitudinal arch (Fig. 18.73). This is usually recommended for CP children with hind and midfoot instability. This orthosis is used inside the shoe.

Spinal Orthosis

There are various types of braces used for spinal deformity, even though they cannot reverse the deformity. The Boston brace (Fig. 18.74), is a commonly used spinal brace for scoliosis in children with cerebral palsy. As most children with scoliosis need spinal surgery to establish and maintain sitting balance in the long run, spinal brace is recommended for use, for the time period until surgery to enable the child to grow as much as possible.

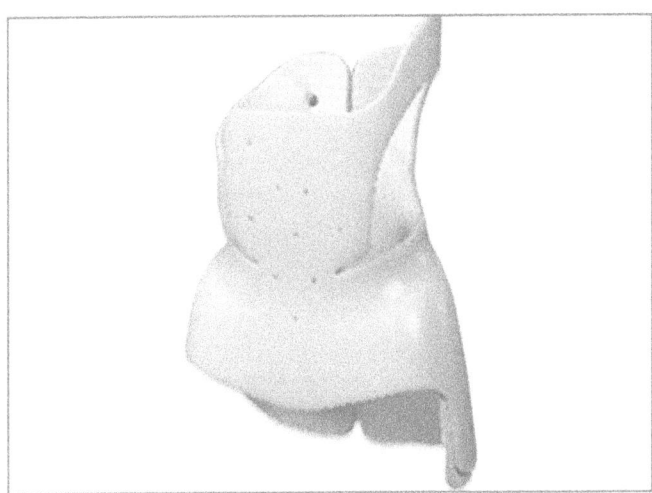

Fig. 18.74: The Boston brace for scoliosis.

Hand Splints

Different types of hand splints are used in children having spastic/dystonic hands. The splint used could be a static resting hand splint (Fig. 18.75A) to maintain the hand in functional position. A twister splint (Fig. 18.75B) that keeps the forearm in supination and thumb in opposition to perform hand function may be selected to improve function. A short cock-up splint (Fig. 18.75C), may be recommended to align the wrist in functional position and allow functional use of the hand.

Adjunct Devices

As per need of the child with CP, different chairs such as corner chair, chair with lap board (Fig. 18.76), prone and supine standers and vertical standing units (Figs. 18.77A to C), walkers (anterior opening type/posterior opening type (Fig. 18.78A), elbow crutches, etc., are to be used to develop as normal a posture as possible and to make the child ambulatory. If a child does not have the potential for walking, an appropriate wheelchair with modifications such as abdominal belt should be recommended. If there is persistent absence of neck control,

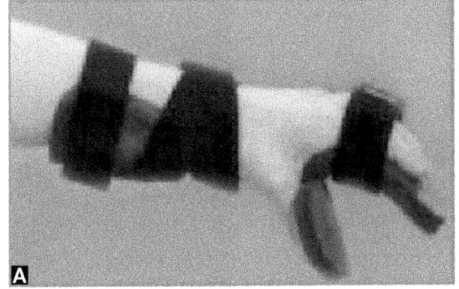
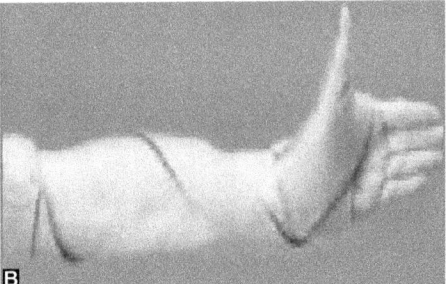
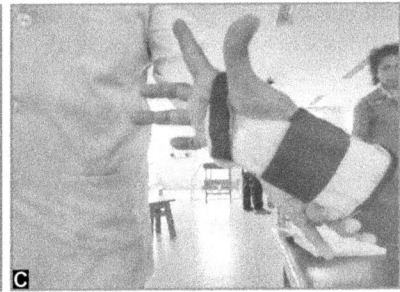

Figs. 18.75A to C: (A) The resting hand splint (pancake splint); (B) The twister splint; (C) Short cock-up splint.

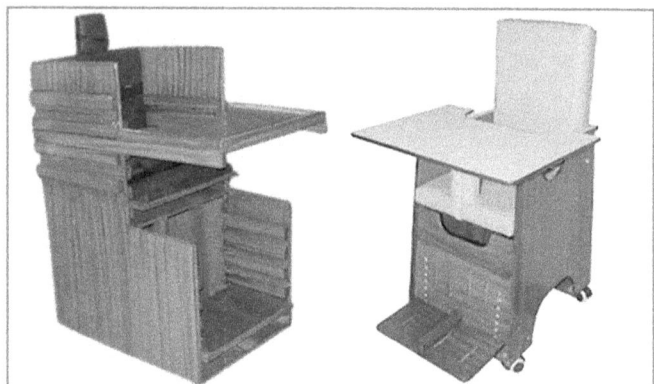

Fig. 18.76: Cerebral palsy chairs with lap boards.

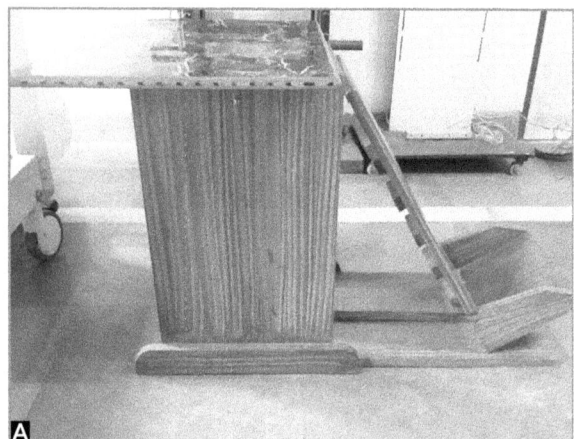

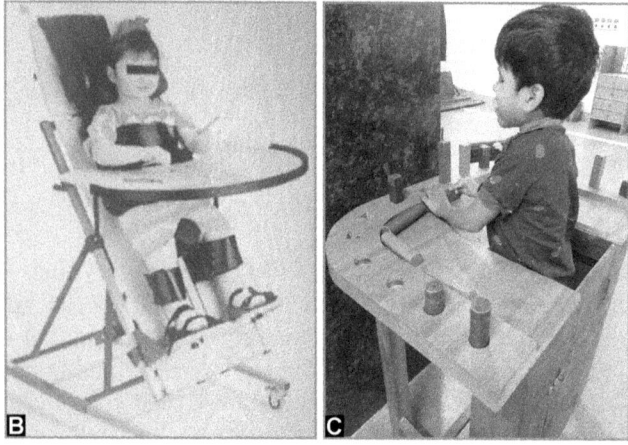

Figs. 18.77A to C: (A) Prone stander; (B) Supine stander with lap board; (C) Vertical standing unit.

a soft cervical collar, that allows minimal neck movements should be considered **(Fig.18.78B)**.

Surgery in Cerebral Palsy

A physiotherapist/occupational therapist should have the knowledge of different surgeries performed in children with CP, as it will help them to select children who need surgery and refer them to orthopedic surgeon/neurosurgeon and to provide postoperative therapy. The surgeries performed could be:

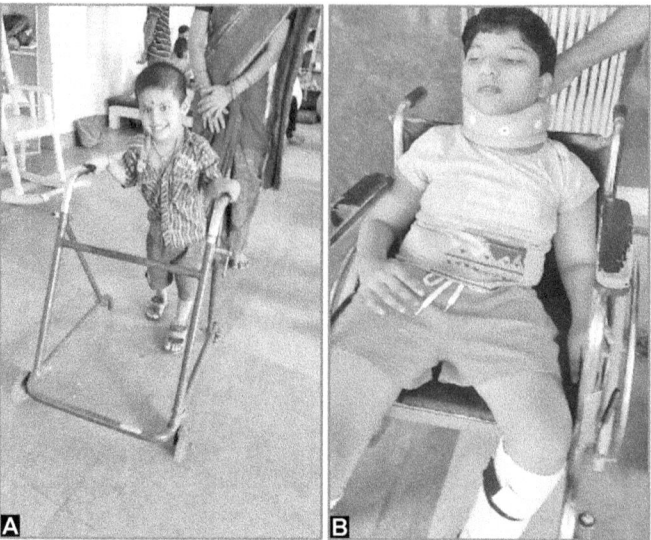

Figs. 18.78A and B: (A) Walker (posterior opening); (B) Use of a soft cervical collar to promote neck control.

Orthopedic Surgery

- Soft tissue procedures: 4–7 years.
- Hand surgery: 6–12 years.
- Bony procedures: After puberty.

Decisions for surgery are made with the observations on gait analysis and physical examination. The surgical intervention consists of lengthening of short muscle-tendon units, shortening of long muscles, and correction of osseous deformities.

The choice for orthopedic surgery **(Fig. 18.79)** nowadays is single-event multilevel surgery (SEMLS), where all necessary surgical interventions are planned to be performed at the same time to avoid birthday syndrome (the child celebrated last birth day in the hospital as he was operated, and this birth day will also be celebrated in the hospital due to the present surgery planned). Single-event

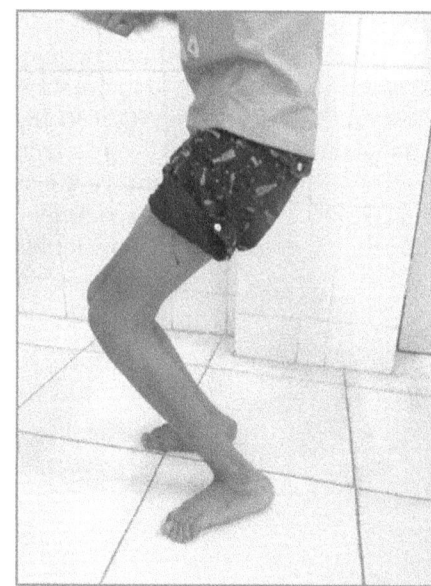

Fig. 18.79: A child with flexion deformity of hip and knee (a candidate for orthopedic surgery).

multilevel surgery refers to the correction of the secondary musculoskeletal problems, by performing between 4 and 20 separate orthopedic procedures, during one operative session, requiring one hospital admission, and one period of rehabilitation. The optimum time for SEMLS is between the age of 6 and 10 years. Very few younger children, except those with hip displacement, require SEMLS before age 6 years.

As per the recommendations of Royal Children's Hospital Melbourne, the surgical intervention for knee flexion deformity (KFD) is done as follows:
* <5 degree KFD: Medial hamstring lengthening (MHL)
* 5–15 degree KFD: MHL + Semi-T to adductor tubercle
* 15–25 degree KFD: Semi-T transfer + Growth plate surgery
* 25 degree KFD: Supracondylar extension osteotomy with patellar tendon shortening.

Types of orthopedic surgeries:
* **Tendon lengthening:** Weakens spastic and shortened muscles, balance muscle forces.
* **Split transfer/tendon transfer:** Balances deforming forces (e.g., split transfer of tibialis posterior muscle to correct dynamic equino varus deformity). Tendon transfer in the form of Sutherland procedure, Egger's procedure, Rectus transfer etc are performed to correct deforming forces in the lower limbs and improve function. Tendon transfer is also considered for improving function in spastic hand.
* **Simple tenotomy:** Balances deforming forces.
* **Angular osteotomy:** Corrects varus and valgus deformities of the knee and flexion deformities in the knee joint (e.g., posterior angulation osteotomy to correct flexion deformity of knee joint).
* **Hip surgery:** Stabilizes the subluxated or dislocated hip.
* **Rotational osteotomy:** Corrects torsional deformities of the tibia or femur
* **Arthrodesis:** Corrects deformity and stabilizes joints
* **Spine surgery:** Corrects spinal deformity

Postoperative physiotherapy after SEMLS:
Physiotherapy is aimed at gaining independent or assisted transfer ability, initiation of weight-bearing as allowed and tolerated and safe wheelchair mobility prior to discharge. It is important to communicate with community therapists with regard to surgeries performed, weight-bearing status, and home program to be continued until return to hospital for outpatient review.

A significant change in all the primary impairments is expected after surgery. Immediate postoperative physiotherapy reintroduces movement and the new alignment. There is a need for gentle return to function. The therapist should try to regain range of motion and strength as early as possible after surgery. Mobilization should be started as soon as the child is comfortable and painless, usually on the second to fourth day after soft tissue procedures. Weight-bearing should not be allowed for 3 weeks after osteotomies, which should gradually progress to partial weight-bearing and full weight-bearing.

The therapist should begin training with range of motion exercises and gradually progress to strengthening as healing allows. It usually takes approximately 3 months to regain the preoperative muscle strength after multilevel surgery. Physiotherapy ends when the child has no more change in strength, function, and skill level.

SEMLS (single event multi level surgery) rehabilitation is performed under the following headings:
* Preoperative planning.
* Postoperative positioning.
* The first 3 weeks
* Weeks 4–6
* Weeks 7–12
* Weeks 13–24
* Months 6–12
* The 12-month gait laboratory reassessment

Preoperative planning: The important components of the preoperative planning which can be very helpful for certain children and families include a preoperative visit to the hospital, anesthetic preassessments, a visit to the inpatient facility and to the rehabilitation facility and to meet the inpatient team. It can be difficult for children and families to understand the complexity and duration of the rehabilitation despite detailed explanations. Discussion with another child and family who have recently been through the surgery and rehabilitation may be helpful.

Postoperative positioning: After SEMLS, a below knee plaster(pop cast/slab), or a above knee plaster **(Fig. 18.80)** (pop cast/slab) or a knee immobilizer, that allows early knee motion into flexion may be considered. All of the surgery below the knee, including gastrocsoleus lengthening, rotational osteotomy of the tibia, and stabilization of the mid-foot, are maintained in satisfactory alignment in below-knee casts. The casts must be well padded and split to accommodate postoperative swelling. The plantar flexors of the ankles are maintained in the lengthened position by the below knee-plaster casts. The knee flexors (hamstrings) are looked after by the knee immobilizers, reinforced by long sitting with knee extension. Following femoral derotation osteotomy, the lower limbs tend to roll into excessive external rotation, particularly under the relaxation of

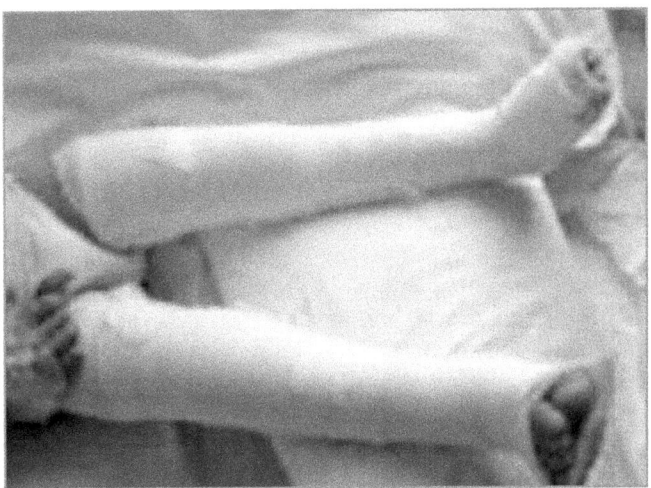

Fig. 18.80: A K POP cast after patellar tendon shortening procedure.

the epidural analgesia. Excessive external rotation can quickly progress to an external rotation contracture at the hip level. Most commonly sandbags and pillows are positioned laterally at the level of the foot and the knee. Pillows or a foam abduction wedge placed between the lower legs/thighs may be used to maintain abduction range as well.

It is essential, following psoas lengthening at the brim of the pelvis, to have a period in prone each day, for a minimum of 1 hour, to stretch the iliopsoas across the front of the pelvis. It is best, if this can be combined with some enjoyable leisure activity such as watching a favorite television program, or DVD, listening to music, or reading a book, which may further encourage extension of the trunk.

Transfer of the rectus femoris is typically done through a nonanatomic region to one of the hamstring tendons. As such, early motion is required to prevent the formation of adhesions, which may mature into scar tissue and prevent the transfer working which may result in an extension contracture at the knee. Patients who have had a rectus transfer must have removal of the knee immobilizer and early ranging into flexion to achieve at least 30 degree of knee flexion at the end of the first week, 60 degree at the end of week 2 and 90 degree at the end of week 3. If significant problems are noted in achieving these flexion ranges, it is sometimes appropriate to use continuous passive motion to improve the ranging of the knee and the rectus femoris transfers.

The first 3 weeks: Most patients are discharged from hospital 5-7 days after SEMLS and spend the next 2 weeks at home for healing, recovering from surgery and commencing rehabilitation. Soft-tissue surgery is designed to be stable and, if there has been no bony surgery, full weight-bearing in the plaster casts without restriction is advised from day 2-3 postoperatively.

When bony surgery has been performed there may be a short delay until full weight-bearing is allowed but this interval is becoming shorter and shorter. Almost all femoral osteotomies are sufficiently stable to allow full weight-bearing within days of surgery but the usual recommendation is a delay of 1-2 weeks for tibial osteotomies and for midfoot stabilization by os calcis (lateral column) lengthening or subtalar fusion. At the 3-week visit, the below-knee casts are removed and moulds are taken for new AFOs. Full weight-bearing can be safely achieved at a maximum of 3 weeks after surgery.

Weeks 4-6: This is a very important period of rehabilitation during which the priorities are maintenance of muscle length, regaining muscle strength, maintenance of lower-limb alignment, encouragement of weight-bearing, standing, and reintroduction of walking. This involves activities in prone lying and long sitting, strengthening exercises for the hip and knee.

The level of assistive device depends on the child's age, cognitive level, and baseline gross motor function. Most children start either on parallel bars in the physiotherapy gym or using a posterior walker. A posterior walker encourages trunk and hip extension, which is the desired sagittal alignment. Progression of walking is important and should be encouraged.

Weeks 7-12: The removal of plaster casts and fitting of AFOs allows for a change in the rehabilitation program to include both formal hydrotherapy and recreational activities. Weight-bearing in the supportive environment of a hydrotherapy pool can be a major confidence booster for many children. At this early stage, the only time unprotected weight-bearing (i.e., without AFOs) is permitted is within the hydrotherapy pool. In terms of assistive devices, the majority of children will progress from parallel bars to the use of a posterior walker or forearm crutches at this stage of recovery.

Weeks 13-24: An assessment in the gait laboratory using videographic analysis-VDA is essential during this phase to assess sagittal alignment, knee coupling, transverse plane alignment, and to check on the fit of orthoses and the appropriate use of assistive devices. The intensity of rehabilitation is usually reduced (compared to weeks 7-12) between two and four 1-hour sessions per week, including both land-based sessions and hydrotherapy sessions.

The majority of children will be back at school and co-ordination with classroom aids and school authorities is very important to ensure that children are given the opportunity to practice their walking in safe surroundings.

Months 6-12: The frequency of physiotherapy sessions, can be reduced for the majority of children and replaced with recreational activities including family walks, bicycle riding (often a tricycle or modified bicycle), and swimming. Older children and teenagers may benefit from a formal strengthening program. Adolescent boys readily identify with gym-based activities using a variety of standard equipment designed to strengthen the muscles which contribute to the body-support moment, the hip extensors, quadriceps, and ankle plantar flexors.

At 12 months: The majority of children are ready for a full instrumented gait analysis (IGA) at 12 months after surgery. The majority of children are scheduled for removal of the implants between 12 and 18 months after surgery.

Neurosurgery

Various neurosurgical procedures, such as selective obturator neurectomy to reduce spasticity of hip adductors, selective dorsal rhizotomy (for spastic diplegic children), and stereotaxic surgery (for dystonia, epilepsy, etc.) are recommended as per need.

Selective dorsal rhizotomy

Disinhibition of the spinal reflex arc resulting from an upper motor neuron lesion is thought to be the basis of spasticity in the child with CP. Selectively dividing portions of the dorsal lumbosacral roots of the spinal cord (**Figs. 18.81A and B**), and thus interrupting the spinal reflex arc on the sensory side leads to reduction in spasticity without causing paralysis.

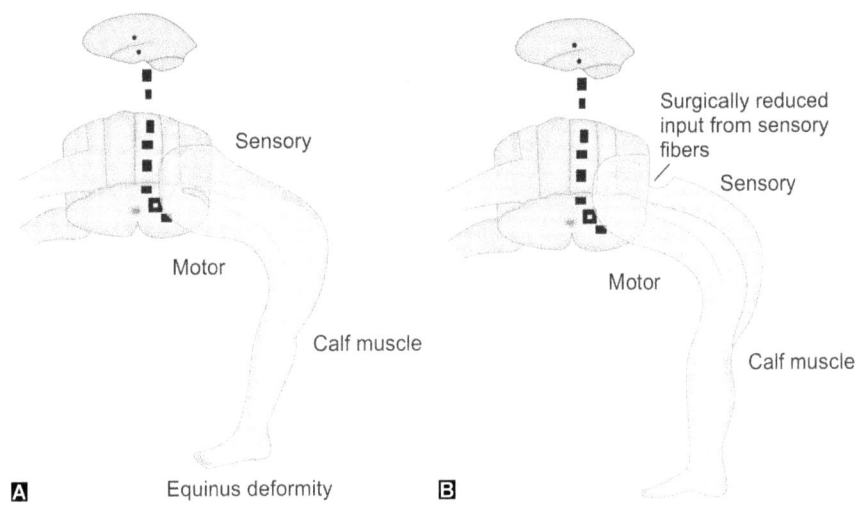

Figs. 18.81A and B: Selective dorsal rhizotomy: (A) Before surgery; (B) After surgery.

Postoperative physiotherapy after selective dorsal rhizotomy: Though the muscle tone after the surgical procedure reduces significantly, causing temporary regression of postural and movement skills, intensive therapy after surgery is helpful in normalizing, postural tone and movements.

Selective obturator neurectomy

The procedure involves cutting the anterior branch of the obturator nerve to reduce spasticity of the hip adductors.

Stereotaxic surgery: These procedures involve introduction of a probe into deep brain and performing surgeries, mostly for dystonia, epilepsy etc.

Stem Cell Therapy

This method of treatment in CP is in the developmental stage and as far as the knowledge of this author, no significant result on stem cell therapy in CP has yet been established.

Stroke/Cerebrovascular Accident

DEFINITION

According to WHO, stroke is defined as "acute onset of neurological dysfunction due to abnormality in cerebral circulation with resultant signs and symptoms that correspond to involvement of focal area of brain lasting more than 24 hours". Stroke is also known as "cerebral vascular accident (CVA)", "brain attack", or "apoplexy".

Epidemiology and Etiology

Stroke is one of the most common neurological conditions affecting very young to very old subjects creating a challenge to healthcare professionals in the present time. Stroke is the fourth leading cause of death and the leading cause of long-term disability among adults in the United States. In India, stroke is also a leading cause of death and disability. According to WHO (16th November, 2011), the incidence of stroke in India was 130/100,000 individuals every year. Women have a lower age-adjusted stroke incidence than men. However, this is reversed in older ages; women over 85 years of age have an elevated risk compared to men.

The incidence of stroke increases dramatically with age, doubling in the decade after 65 years of age. Twenty-eight percent of strokes occur in individuals younger than 65 years of age. Between 5 and 14% of persons who survive an initial stroke may experience another one within 1 year. Within 5 years stroke may recur in 24% of women and 42% of men. A few of the affected individuals suffering from hemorrhagic stroke resulting in massive hemorrhage, die immediately, if no medical care is available immediately. The type of stroke is significant in determining survival of patients with stroke, hemorrhagic stroke accounts for the largest number of deaths, with mortality rates of 37–38% at 1 month, whereas ischemic strokes have a mortality rate of only 8–12% at 1 month. Survival rates are dramatically lessened by increased age, hypertension, heart disease, and diabetes.

Loss of consciousness at stroke onset, lesion size, persistent severe hemiplegia, multiple neurological deficits, and history of previous stroke are also important predictors of mortality. However, majority of the affected individuals survive with significant neurological impairment, which sometimes leads to disability or handicap, if no proper medical and therapeutic intervention is provided timely. It must be understood by all clinicians that "time is brain". Once the patient is medically stable, active physiotherapy should be started immediately. However, if the patient is medically unstable or in the state of coma, passive therapy in the form of positioning, joint range of motion (ROM) exercises should be started without delay to prevent development of stiffness of joints, and tightness, contracture and deformities, as in many instances, it has been found that patients report to physiotherapists with deformity in hand and foot, which becomes a challenging complication for achieving successful rehabilitation.

Classification of Stroke

Stroke is classified into ischemic and hemorrhagic types depending upon the pathology involved. It can also be classified into anterior cerebral artery (ACA) stroke, middle cerebral artery (MCA) stroke, posterior cerebral artery (PCA) stroke, depending upon the vascular territory affected.

A. Classification of stroke depending upon the pathology.
- *Ischemic stroke:* This is the most common type of stroke, which accounts to about 60 to 70 % of stroke population. These are the result of a thrombosis, embolism, or conditions that produce low systemic perfusion pressures.

    An ischemic stroke or "brain attack" occurs when brain cells die because of inadequate blood flow. When blood flow is interrupted, brain cells are robbed of vital supplies of oxygen and nutrients. The lack of cerebral blood flow deprives the brain of needed oxygen and glucose, disrupts cellular metabolism, and leads to injury and death of tissues. Thrombi lead to ischemia, or occlusion of an artery with resulting cerebral infarction or tissue death. Thrombi can also become dislodged and travel to a more distal site in the form of an intra-artery embolus. The most common source of cerebral embolism is disease of the cardiovascular system. Occasionally systemic disorders may produce septic, fat, amniotic fluid, or air emboli that affect the cerebral circulation. Ischemic strokes may also result from low systemic perfusion, the result of cardiac failure or significant blood loss with resulting systemic hypotension. Hypertension may also lead to ischemia

due to vasospasm as a result of increased pressure on the wall of arteries leading to reduction of blood flow distally. The neurological deficits produced with systemic failure are global in nature with bilateral neurological deficits.
- *Hemorrhagic strokes:* The incidence of this type of stroke is less as compared to the ischemic stroke. It accounts for about 30–40% of the total stroke population. There occurs bleeding into the extravascular areas of the brain, as a result of rupture of a cerebral vessels.

  A hemorrhagic stroke is caused by a burst blood vessel in the brain that causes bleeding into or around the brain. Hemorrhagic stroke is closely linked to chronic hypertension. Arteriovenous malformation (AVM) is another congenital defect that can result in stroke. Due to hemorrhage and subsequent hematoma, there is increased intracranial pressures with injury to brain tissues and restriction of distal blood flow, leading to ischemia of the brain tissue in that part of the brain supplied by such distal arterial branches. Sometimes, due to a very large intracranial pressure, the brain substances are pushed to the opposite hemisphere, called midline shift/mass effect (which may produce neurological impairments on the other side of the body, which was not expected to be affected due to the primary pathology). Hemorrhagic strokes result from the following types of occurrences:
  a. **Intracerebral hemorrhage (ICH)** is caused by rupture of a cerebral vessel with subsequent bleeding into the brain.
  b. **Primary cerebral hemorrhage** (nontraumatic spontaneous hemorrhage) typically occurs in small blood vessels weakened by atherosclerosis producing an **aneurysm**.
  c. **Subarachnoid hemorrhage (SAH)** occurs from bleeding into the subarachnoid space typically from a saccular or berry aneurysm affecting primarily large blood vessels. Congenital defects that produce weakness in the blood vessel wall are major contributing factors to the formation of an aneurysm.

B. **Classification of stroke depending upon the vascular territories affected.**
- *Anterior cerebral artery stroke (syndrome):* The ACA, which is a branch of the internal carotid artery, supplies the medial aspect of the cerebral hemisphere (frontoparietal lobes), basal ganglia, anterior fornix, and anterior four-fifths of corpus callosum. Stroke involving this artery produces contralateral hemiparesis and sensory loss with greater involvement of the lower extremity (LE) than the upper extremity, causing paresis of opposite foot and leg and to the lesser extent the arm. Patient may also have mental impairments (perseveration, confusion, and amnesia), sensory impairment primarily in the lower extremity, urinary incontinence, aphasia, agraphia, apraxia, etc.
- *Middle cerebral artery stroke (syndrome):* The MCA is the most common site of occlusion in stroke. The MCA supplies the entire lateral aspect of the cerebral hemisphere (frontal, parietal, and temporal lobes) as well as the subcortical structures such as posterior limb of internal capsule, corona radiata, outer part of globus pallidus, most of the caudate nucleus and putamen. The most common characteristics of MCA syndrome are contralateral spastic hemiparesis and sensory loss of the face, upper extremity, and lower extremity, with the face and upper extremity more involved than the lower extremity. Lesions of the parieto-occipital cortex of the dominant hemisphere typically produce aphasia. Lesions of the right parietal lobe of the nondominant hemisphere typically produce perceptual deficits such as unilateral neglect, anosognosia, apraxia, and spatial disorganization. Homonymous hemianopia (a visual-field defect) is also a common finding of this type of stroke.
- *Posterior cerebral artery stroke (syndrome):* The PCAs arise from the basilar arteries and supply the occipital lobes, medial and inferior temporal lobes, as well as the upper brainstem, midbrain, posterior diencephalon. Occlusion distal to the posterior communicating artery typically results in minimal deficits owing to the collateral blood supply from the posterior communicating artery. Occlusion of thalamic branches may produce hemianesthesia (contralateral sensory loss) or central poststroke (thalamic) pain. Occipital infarction produces homonymous hemianopia, visual agnosia, prosopagnosia (inability to identify familiar faces), or, if bilateral, cortical blindness. Temporal lobe ischemia results in amnesia (memory loss). Involvement of subthalamic branches may involve the subthalamic nucleus or its pallidal connections, producing a wide variety of deficits. Contralateral hemiplegia occurs with involvement of the cerebral peduncle.
- *Internal carotid artery syndrome:* The ICA supplies blood to MCA and ACA. Occlusion of the ICA usually causes massive stroke involving middle cerebral artery territories, as the ACA manages to get blood flow through the collateral vessels from the circle of Willis. Significant edema is common in ICA stroke, with possible brain herniation, coma, and death (mass effect).
- *Vertebrobasilar artery syndrome:* The vertebral arteries that arise from the subclavian arteries, merge at the inferior border of pons to form the basilar artery. The basilar artery gives rise to the two posterior cerebral arteries. The vertebral arteries supply the cerebellum (via posterior inferior cerebellar arteries) and the medulla (via the medullary arteries). The basilar artery supplies the pons (via pontine arteries), the internal ear (via labyrinthine arteries), and the cerebellum (via the anterior inferior and superior cerebellar arteries). Pathology involving the vertebrobasilar system produces ipsilateral as well as contralateral features. Various clinical syndromes mentioned below are the manifestations of occlusion of the vertebrobasilar system.

- » Median medullary syndrome: Ipsilateral to lesion: Paralysis with atrophy of half of the tongue with deviation to the paralyzed side on protrusion. Contralateral to lesion: Weakness of upper and lower extremities with tactile and proprioceptive sensory loss.
- » Lateral medullary (Wallenberg's) syndrome: Ipsilateral to lesion: Decreased pain and temperature sensation in face. Vertigo, nystagmus, Horner's syndrome (miosis, ptosis, and decreased sweating), dysphagia and dysphonia may be the manifestations. Contralateral to the lesion: Impairment of pain and temperature sensation over half of the body including face (sometimes).
- » Complete basilar artery syndrome (locked-in syndrome): Tetraplegia (quadriplegia), bilateral cranial nerve palsy with sparing of upward gaze, loss of consciousness (sometimes) are the common presentations. Perception and cognition is usually spared. In 1995, the American Congress of Rehabilitation Medicine defined Locked-in syndrome (LIS) as a syndrome characterized by preserved awareness, relatively intact cognitive functions, and by the ability to communicate while being paralyzed and voiceless. This syndrome is defined by five criteria:
    1. Sustained eye opening
    2. Aphonia or severe hypophonia
    3. Quadriplegia/quadriparesis
    4. Preserved cognitive abilities
    5. A primary mode of communication, that uses vertical or lateral eye movements or blinking of the upper eyelid.
- » Weber syndrome: Weber's syndrome is a form of stroke characterized by the presence of an oculomotor nerve palsy and contralateral hemiparesis or hemiplegia. This lesion is usually unilateral and affects several structures in the midbrain. It is caused by midbrain infarction as a result of occlusion of the paramedian branches of the PCA or of basilar bifurcation perforating arteries. Contralateral hemiparesis and typical upper motor neuron findings are the features. It is contralateral because lesion to the coticospinal tract occurs before the decussation in the medulla. Ipsilateral oculomotor nerve palsy with a drooping eyelid and fixed wide pupil pointed down and out are their presentations. This leads to diplopia.
- *Lacunar stroke:* Strokes involving the deep penetrating arteries in the cerebral white matter is called lacunar stroke. They are strongly associated with hypertensive hemorrhage and diabetic microvascular disease. It could be pure motor stroke (due to involvement of posterior limb of the internal capsule, pons, and pyramid of medulla), or pure sensory stroke (due to involvement of ventrolateral thalamus or thalamocortical projections.
- *Silent stroke:* A silent stroke is a stroke that does not have any outward symptoms, and the patients are typically unaware that they have suffered a stroke. Despite not causing identifiable symptoms, a silent stroke still causes damage to the brain, and places the patient at increased risk for both transient ischemic attack and major stroke in the future. Conversely, those who have suffered a major stroke are also at risk of having silent strokes.

Risk Factors/Etiology

Risk factors for stroke are classified into:
a. Modifiable risk factors (Obesity, cigarette smoking, physical inactivity, and diet). However, oral contraceptive pills, that contain estrogen and progesterone, can also be considered as a modifiable risk factor for stroke.
b. Unmodifiable risk factors (Age, sex, family history, race-African American) that result in following events leading to stroke.
   - Hypertension (Blood pressure 140/90 mm Hg or higher)
   - *Heart disease:* Rheumatic heart disease, endocarditis, coronary artery bypass grafting, valvular heart disease, atrial fibrillation, etc., carry an increased risk of stroke.
   - Diabetes mellitus.
   - Peripheral vascular disease (Atherosclerosis, arteriosclerosis, deep vein thrombosis). Elevated total blood cholesterol (hypercholesterolemia) with value of 240 mg/dL or greater, and elevated low-density lipoprotein (bad cholesterol) with borderline high levels of 130-159 mg/dL, high levels of 160-189 mg/dL, and very high levels of 190 mg/dL or greater. Low levels of high-density lipoprotein (good cholesterol) defined as below 40 mg/dL in adult males and below 50 mg/dL in adult females, also increases the risk of stroke. Fasting triglyceride level of greater than 150 mg/dL in adults is considered elevated and a risk factor for heart disease and stroke.
   - Patients with marked elevations of hematocrit (Packed cell volume) are also at an increased risk of ischemic stroke owing to a generalized reduction of cerebral blood flow.
   - End-stage renal disease and chronic kidney disease also increase the risk of stroke.
   - Sleep apnea is an independent risk factor for stroke, doubling the risk of stroke or death.
   - Women with early menopause (before 42 years of age) and late menopause carry the risk of ischemic stroke. Hormone therapy with estrogen and progesterone also increases the risk of ischemic stroke.
   - Pregnancy, childbirth (amniotic fluid embolism) and early postpartum also increase the risk of stroke.
   - *Overage:* As our age increases, the risk of stroke also increases due either to hypertension or reduction of patency of the arteries because of arteriosclerosis or atherosclerosis.

Changes in lifestyle can greatly reduce the risk of stroke. Controlling blood pressure, taking proper diet, reducing weight, quitting smoking, and increasing physical activity, as well as effective disease management can reduce the incidence of stroke.

Pathophysiology of Stroke

Ischemia that results from vascular occlusion, as in ischemic stroke or from the hematoma as occurs in hemorrhagic stroke leads to cerebral infarction due to nonavailability of oxygen and glucose to brain tissues. The frank blood that accumulates in the brain due to hemorrhage acts as a toxic agent, leading to triggering of brain inflammation and subsequently produces ischemia as a result of compression of capillaries due to mass of accumulated hematoma as well as pressure exerted by inflammatory edema. Collapse of the energy-producing processes and disintegration of cell membrane results in altered cellular metabolism and function. Complete occlusion to brain substance causes severe damage with a zone of infarction. The area surrounding this zone consists of cells that are alive but metabolically less active, termed ischemic penumbra. Within minutes, neurons within the ischemic core tissue die, but majority of neurons in the surrounding penumbra survive for a slight longer time. Without timely reperfusion, cells in the penumbra die ceasing neuronal activities causing expansion of the infarct. The ischemic cascade that results from progressive cellular damage, lead to release of excess neurotransmitters (glutamate and aspartate) causing disturbance of energy metabolism and anoxic depolarization. This results in an inability of brain cells to produce energy, particularly adenosine triphosphate (ATP). This is followed by excess influx of calcium ions and pump failure of the neuronal membrane. Excess calcium reacts with intracellular phospholipids to form free radicals. Calcium influx also stimulates the release of nitric oxide and cytokines. Both mechanisms further damage brain cells.

Following the onset of stroke, cerebral edema begins within a few minutes and reaches its peak by about 4 days; however, it mostly disappears by 2–3 weeks. The resulting cerebral edema causes a raised intracranial pressure and may cause contralateral/caudal shift of brain structure. Due to raised intracranial pressure, level of consciousness is altered (stupor/coma), pulse pressure is widened, heart rate is increased and respiration also becomes irregular. There also occurs vomiting, unreacting pupils, and papilledema.

Clinical Features of Stroke

Stroke symptoms typically start suddenly, over seconds to minutes, and in most cases do not progress further except in hemorrhagic stroke. The peak disability develops suddenly in hemorrhagic and embolic stroke, but it develops gradually in other types of ischemic strokes except embolic type. The symptoms depend on the area of the brain affected.

Paralysis is one of the most common disability resulting from stroke. The paralysis is usually on the side of the body opposite the side of the brain damaged by stroke, and may affect the face, an arm, a leg, or the entire side of the body. This one-sided paralysis is called hemiplegia, if it involves complete inability to move or hemiparesis, if it is less than total weakness. Stroke patients with hemiparesis or hemiplegia may have difficulty with everyday activities such as walking or grasping objects. Some stroke patients have problems with swallowing, called dysphagia, due to damage to the part of the brain that controls the muscles for swallowing.

Damage to a lower part of the brain, the cerebellum, can affect the body's ability to coordinate movement—a disability called ataxia—leading to problems with body posture, walking, and balance.

The more extensive the area of brain affected, the more functions that are likely to be lost. Some forms of stroke can cause additional symptoms. For example, in intracranial hemorrhage, the affected area may compress other structures. Most forms of stroke are not associated with headache, apart from subarachnoid hemorrhage and cerebral venous thrombosis, and occasionally ICH.

Early Recognition of Stroke

Early warning signs of stroke as per the American Heart and National Stroke Association include:
- Sudden numbness or weakness of the face, arm, or leg, especially on one side of the body.
- Sudden confusion, trouble speaking or understanding.
- Sudden trouble seeing in one or both eyes.
- Sudden severe headache with no known cause.
- Sudden trouble walking, dizziness, loss of balance or co-ordination.

Different findings are able to predict the presence or absence of stroke to different degrees. Sudden-onset of face weakness, arm drift (i.e., if a person, when asked to raise both arms, involuntarily lets one arm drift downward), and abnormal speech are the findings most likely to lead to the correct identification of a case of stroke. The significance of recognizing early warning signs rests with prompt initiation of emergency care under the rule that "time is brain".

Altered level of consciousness (coma, decreased arousal level) may occur with extensive brain damage. The Glasgow coma scale that examines the three areas of function such as eye opening (spontaneously-4, to speech-3, to pain-2, no response-1), best motor response (obeys command-6, moves to localize pain-5, flex to withdrarw from pain-4, abnormal flexion-3, abnormal extension-2, no response-1), and verbal response (oriented to time, person and place-5, confused-4, inappropriate words-3, incomprehensible sounds-2, no response-1) is the gold standard method for documenting level of consciousness. Total GCS scores range from a low of 3 to a high of 15. A total score of 8 or less is indicative of severe brain injury and coma, a score between 9 and 12 is indicative of moderate brain injury, and a score from 13 to 15 is indicative of mild brain injury.

The therapist should document levels of consciousness using terminologies such as:
- **Normal**
- **Lethargy:** Lethargy refers to altered consciousness in which a person's level of arousal is diminished. The lethargic patient appears drowsy but when questioned can open the eyes and respond briefly.
- **Obtunded:** Obtunded state refers to diminished arousal and awareness. The obtunded patient is difficult to arouse from sleeping and once aroused, appears confused.

- **Stupor:** It refers to a state of altered mental status and responsiveness to one's environment. The patient can be aroused only with vigorous or unpleasant stimuli.
- **Coma:** The unconscious patient is said to be in a coma, if he/she cannot be aroused. The eyes remain closed and there are no sleep–wake cycles. The patient does not respond to repeated painful stimuli and may be ventilator-dependent.

A patient with intracranial bleed and mass effect may progress from normal level of consciousness to lethargy, to obtund to stupor and coma. However, the reverse pattern of progression is an indication that the patient is improving. Some patients after onset of stroke recover from coma and remain in the vegetative state, which is a minimally conscious state characterized by return of irregular sleep-wake cycles and normalization of vegetative functions such as respiration, digestion, and control of blood pressure. Sometimes patients with severe brain injury recover from coma, but remain in persistent vegetative state for 1 year or more. While recovering from coma, some patients show motor behavior as per "inverted-U-principle", that means at appropriate level of arousal, the motor performance is optimal, but at very low or very high levels of arousal, the motor performance deteriorates.

If the area of the brain affected contains one or more of the three central nervous system pathways, such as the spinothalamic tract, the corticospinal tract, and the dorsal column (medial lemniscus), the patient may present with the following symptoms:
- Initial flaccidity that includes absence of muscle tone on the affected side and loss of ability to swallow and incontinent bladder and bowel. The patient may be applied with a nasogastric tube and urinary catheter (**Fig. 19.1**).
- Subsequently spasticity with hyperreflexia, obligatory synergies, reappearance of certain primitive reflexes, and associated reactions develop. The person may recover following Brunnstrom stages/Bobath stages of recovery.

Synergy patterns, which are abnormal in such patients, are stereotyped, primitive mass movement patterns associated with spasticity, which is triggered either voluntarily or reflexly. These abnormal synergies patterns could be either flexor or extensor types, which make the movements purposeless in such patients. Spastic patterns seen in the patients have components from the abnormal flexor and extensor synergies.

Abnormal Limb Synergies

- The pathological synergy patterns seen in the upper limbs are described in **Tables 19.1 and 19.2**.
- The pathological synergy patterns seen in the lower limbs are described in **Tables 19.3 and 19.4**.

Table 19.1: Pathological flexor synergy pattern in the upper limb (Fig. 19.2).

Body segment	Attitude
Scapula	Elevation and retraction
Shoulder	Flexion, abduction, and lateral rotation
Elbow	Flexion
Forearm	Supination
Wrist and fingers and thumb	Flexion

Table 19.2: Pathological extensor synergy pattern in the upper limb.

Body segment	Attitude
Scapula	Protraction and depression
Shoulder	Adduction, extension, and internal rotation
Elbow	Extension
Forearm	Pronation
Wrist and fingers and thumb	Flexion

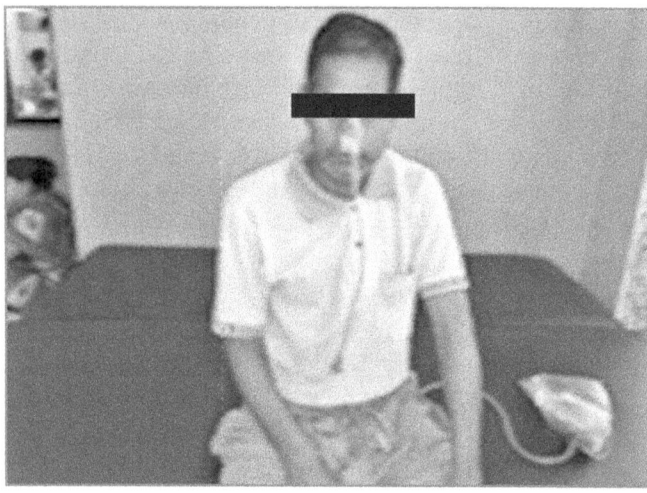

Fig. 19.1: Stroke patient with the nasogastric tube and indwelling catheter.

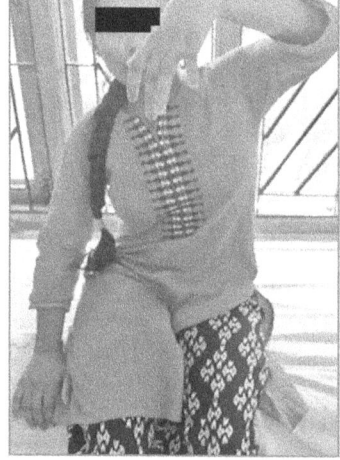

Fig. 19.2: Presentation of abnormal flexor synergy pattern in upper limb.

Chapter 19: Stroke/Cerebrovascular Accident

Table 19.3: Pathological flexor synergy pattern in the lower limb.

Body segment	Attitude
Hip	Flexion, abduction, lateral rotation
Knee	Flexion
Ankle	Dorsiflexion
Foot	Inversion
Toes	Extension

Table 19.4: Pathological extensor synergy pattern in the lower limb.

Body segment	Attitude
Pelvis	Retraction
Hip	Extension, adduction, and medial rotation
Knee	Extension
Ankle	Plantar flexion
Foot	Inversion
Toes	Flexion

Spastic Pattern

- The spastic patterns seen in the upper and lower limbs are described in **Tables 19.5 and 19.6**.

Table 19.5: Spastic pattern in upper limb (Fig. 19.3).

Body segment	Attitude
Scapula	Depression and retraction
Shoulder	Flexion, adduction, and internal rotation
Elbow	Flexion
Forearm	Pronation
Wrist	Flexion
Fingers and thumb	Flexion with adduction of thumb

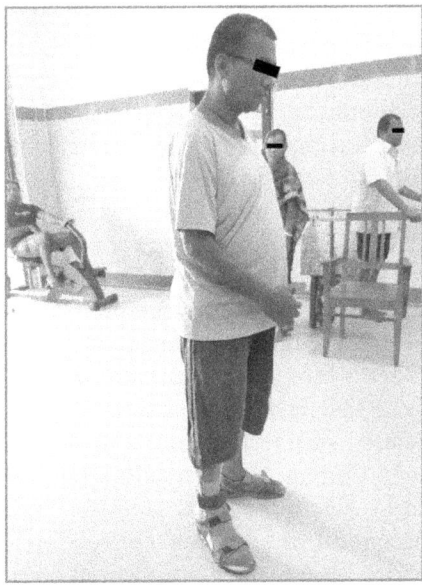

Fig. 19.3: Spastic pattern of the upper limb.

Table 19.6: Spastic patterns in the lower limb (Fig. 19.4).

Body segment	Attitude
Pelvis	Retraction
Hip	Extension, adduction, internal rotation (Though spasticity is found in the hip internal rotators, hip remains externally rotated due to pelvic retraction)
Knee	Extension
Ankle	Plantar flexion
Foot	Inversion
Toes	Flexion

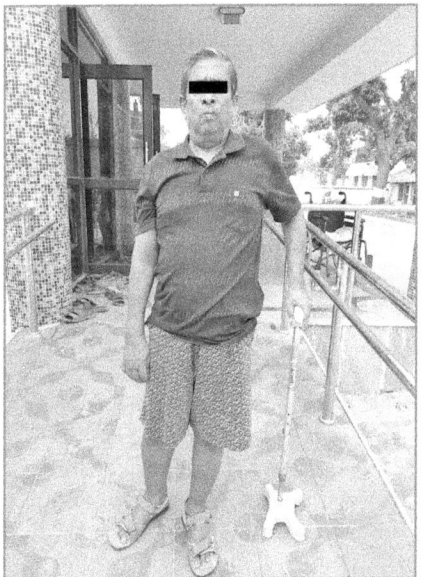

Fig. 19.4: Spastic pattern in the lower limb (right).

Release of Primitive Reflexes

Due to brain lesion, the primitive reflexes that are produced by the lower level of CNS (which were integrated during infancy/early childhood) are released from the inhibitory influences of the higher centers and may reappear again. The common reflexes that are seen in the hemiplegics are:

- **Symmetric Tonic Neck Reflex (STNR):** Flexion of the neck results in flexion of the arms and extension of the legs; extension of the neck results in extension of the arms and flexion of the legs.
- **Asymmetric Tonic Neck Reflex (ATNR):** Head rotation to the left causes extension of left arm and leg and flexion of right arm and leg; head rotation to the right causes extension of right arm and leg and flexion of left arm and leg.
- **Tonic Labyrinthine Reflex (TLR):** Prone-lying position facilitates flexion; the supine position facilitates extension. The reflex can also be thought of as inhibition of extensor tone in the prone position.
- **Tonic Lumbar Reflex:** This is initiated by a change in the position of the upper trunk with respect to the pelvis.

Rotation of the trunk to the right results in flexion of the right upper extremity and extension of the right lower extremity; rotation of the trunk to the left results in extension of the right upper extremity and flexion of the right lower extremity.
- ❖ **Tonic Thumb Reflex:** When the affected upper extremity is elevated above the horizontal with forearm supination, thumb extension is facilitated (pronation is facilitatory to finger extension).

Associated Reactions

These are the abnormal reactions, which usually manifest as an attenuation of the hemiplegics attitude in response to movement either on the same side or occurring in any other parts of the body. A mutual dependency occurs between body parts, that is when one lower limb goes into flexion, the upper limb on same side also moves into flexion.

The common reactions include:
- ❖ **Souques' Phenomenon:** Elevation of the affected arm above the horizontal evokes an extension and abduction response of the fingers.
- ❖ **Raimiste's Phenomenon:** Strenuous movement on one limb produces similar movements on the opposite side. Resistance applied to abduction or adduction of the non-affected lower extremity evokes a similar reaction in the affected lower extremity.
- ❖ **Homolateral Limb Synkinesis:** It has been noted that a dependency exists between the synergies of the involved upper and lower extremities. Thus, flexion of the involved upper extremity will elicit flexion of the involved lower extremity and vice versa **(Fig. 19.5)**.

Motor Programming Deficits

The left (dominant hemisphere) has a primary role in sequencing of movement. The individuals with left CVA

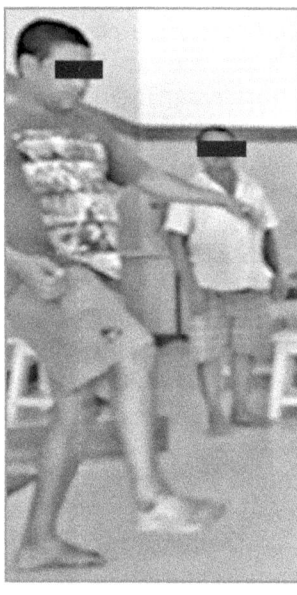

Fig. 19.5: Right-sided homolateral synkinesis, i.e., flexion of knee to clear the ground increases flexion of elbow on the same (right) side.

(i.e., Right hemiplegia) with frontal and posterior parietal lesions may present with deficits in motor planning (Apraxia). Apraxia could be either **Ideomotor** (Movement is not possible on command, but occurs automatically or **Ideational** (Movement is not possible either automatically or on command).

Perceptual Dysfunction

Perceptual dysfunctions include:
- ❖ **Body scheme disorders such as asomatognosia:** Inability to perceive the relationships of the body parts with respect to each other and the relationship of the body parts with respect to the environment).
- ❖ **Anosognosia:** A deficit of self-awareness/the person is unaware of its existence/an inability to acknowledge the reality of the physical impairments resulting from stroke.
- ❖ **Unilateral neglect:** Lack of awareness of the affected side, most commonly the nondominant left side. Unilateral neglect limits movement and use of the more involved extremities. The patient typically does not react to sensory stimuli such as visual, auditory, or somatosensory, presented on the more involved side.
- ❖ **Spatial relations disorder:** Difficulty in perceiving the relationship between self and two or more objects in the environment such as impairments in figure-ground discrimination, topographical disorientation, etc.
- ❖ **Agnosia:** Inability to recognize incoming information (despite intact sensory capacities) which includes visual object agnosia, auditory agnosia, or tactile agnosia (astereognosis),
- ❖ Prosopagnosia—inability to identify familiar faces.

The perceptual dysfunctions are very common in lesions involving the right parietal lobe (left hemiplegics).

Cognitive Dysfunctions

Stroke survivors may have dramatically shortened attention spans or may experience deficits in short-term memory. Individuals also may lose their ability to make plans, comprehend meaning, learn new tasks, or engage in other complex mental activities.

Cognitive dysfunction may be present with lesions involving the cortex and includes impairments in alertness, attention, orientation, memory, or executive functions. Memory disorders (long-term memory is usually preserved, but short-term memory is impaired), Confabulation (Memory gaps are filled with inappropriate words or fabricated stories), Perseveration (continued repetition of words, are not related to the current contexts). Altered attention results from lesions in the prefrontal cortex and reticular formation. Short-term memory loss is associated with lesions of the limbic system, limbic association cortex (orbitofrontal areas), or temporal lobes. Long-term memory loss is associated with lesions of the hippocampus of the limbic system. Confabulation results from lesions in the prefrontal cortex, whereas Perseveration results from lesions in the premotor and/or prefrontal cortex.

Patients with lesions of the prefrontal cortex typically demonstrate impairments in executive function (planning purposeful movements) including lack of abstract thinking, impaired organization and sequencing, decreased insight, impaired planning ability, and impaired judgment. They are unable to realistically appraise their environment and the people and events in it. They also demonstrate difficulty in self-monitoring and self-correcting behaviors, thereby posing safety risks. Delirium (also known as acute confusional state) is characterized by a clouding of consciousness or dulling of cognitive processes and impaired alertness is found in some patients in the acute stage.

Emotional Disturbances

Many people who survive a stroke feel fear, anxiety, frustration, anger, sadness, and a sense of grief for their physical and mental losses. These feelings are a natural response to the psychological trauma of stroke. Some patients with stroke may demonstrate pseudobulbar affect, also known as emotional lability or emotional dysregulation syndrome, which is characterized by emotional outbursts of uncontrolled or exaggerated laughing or crying that are inconsistent with mood. This altered emotional state is the result of lesions of the brain affecting the frontal lobe, hypothalamus, and limbic system. Depression which is considered as one feature of stroke is characterized by persistent feelings of sadness accompanied by feelings of hopelessness, worthlessness, and/ or helplessness. Patients with lesions of the left hemisphere may experience more frequent and more severe depression than patients with right hemisphere or brainstem strokes.

Pusher's Syndrome

Ipsilateral pushing (Pusher's syndrome) is an unusual motor behavior, characterized by the patient's strong lateral lean toward the hemiplegic side. This poses a difficulty to manage the patient in the flaccid stage/early-recovery stage, as buckling of the knee occurs on leaning to affected side, threatening the posture and balance.

Dysphagia

Some patients have difficulty in swallowing, particularly in acute stage. A few others who suffer from brainstem stroke also have difficulty in swallowing, resulting in drooling of saliva.

Aphasia/Dysphasia/Dysarthria

At least one-fourth of all stroke survivors experience language impairments, involving the ability to speak, write, and understand spoken and written language. A stroke-induced injury to any of the brain's language-control centers can severely impair verbal communication. The dominant centers for language are in the left side of the brain for right-handed individuals and many left-handers as well.

Patients of stroke, who have brain lesion in the dominant hemisphere (left side of brain), may show complete loss of speech (aphasia) or partial loss of speech called dysphasia. The aphasia could be motor (Broca's aphasia-non fluent aphasia) or sensory (Wernick's aphasia-fluent aphasia).

Damage to a language center located on the dominant side of the brain, known as Broca's area, causes expressive aphasia. People with this type of aphasia have difficulty conveying their thoughts through words or writing. They lose the ability to speak the words they are thinking and to put words together in coherent, grammatically correct sentences. Damage to a language center located in a rear portion of the brain, called Wernicke's area, results in receptive aphasia. Sometimes there is coexistence of both motor and sensory type aphasias, called global aphasia. Patients may also show articulate speech disorder called dysarthria, as a result of incoordinated movement of lips, jaw, and tongue.

Bladder and Bowel Involvement

The loss of urinary continence is fairly common immediately after a stroke and often results from a combination of sensory and motor deficits. Stroke survivors may lose the ability to sense the need to urinate or the ability to control bladder muscles. Some may lack enough mobility to reach the toilet in time. Loss of bowel control or constipation also may occur. Permanent incontinence after a stroke is uncommon, but even a temporary loss of bowel or bladder control can be emotionally difficult for stroke survivors. Disturbances of bladder function are common during the acute phase, when the patient remains in the state of shock. Urinary incontinence can result from bladder hyperreflexia or hyporeflexia, disturbances of sphincter control, and/or sensory loss. Patients with ACA stroke usually suffer from urinary incontinence. Persistent incontinence is associated with a poor long-term prognosis for functional recovery. Disturbances of bowel function can include incontinence and diarrhoea or constipation and impaction.

Sexual Dysfunction

This could be due to mood disorder, physical impairments, and the fear of rise of blood pressure.

Muscle Weakness

The muscles in the affected extremities and lower part of face become weak, due to flaccidity in the acute stage, and subsequent spasticity. The spastic muscles remain weak as they contract in the inner range, and the antagonistic muscles to spastic groups suffer weakness due to prolonged stretch induced by a pull of the spastic muscles. The trunk muscles remain weak in the acute stage, but subsequently they retain power as they have bilateral innervations like the upper part of the face. Secondary weakness of trunk may result from inactivity and deformity of lateral trunk bending to the affected side.

Sensory Impairment

Stroke patients may lose the ability to feel touch, pain, temperature, or position. Sensory deficits also may hinder the ability to recognize objects that patients are holding and can even be severe enough to cause loss of recognition of one's own limb. Some stroke patients experience pain, numbness, or odd sensations of tingling or prickling in paralyzed or weakened limbs—a symptom known as paresthesia. Superficial (pain, touch, and temperature), Deep (kinesthesia—ability to perceive the joint in motion, proprioception—ability to perceive joint position at rest, vibration sensation), and cortical sensation (Two-point discrimination—the minimum distance where two points are perceived as one, stereognosis—ability to recognize objects by touch, barognosis—ability to perceive light and heavy, graphesthesia—ability to recognize drawings made on skin) are expected to be impaired depending upon the site of lesion.

Tightness/Contracture/Deformity

Due to improper positioning and inadequate exercises in the acute (flaccid) stage, and pull of the muscles in the spastic stage, and abnormal synergistic and spastic patterns, the patients develop joint stiffness (commonly in shoulder and hand), Deformities (Equinovarus foot, knee flexion/genu recurvatum deformity, scoliosis, wrist flexion deformity, etc.).

Abnormal Gait

Stroke patients show abnormal walking pattern both in stance and swing phases of gait, as well as very high-energy-consuming gait, which could be due to muscle weakness, abnormal synergies, and fear of fall. The common stance phase anomalies include lack of 30 degree hip flexion, neutral knee extension and plantigrade ankle at heel strike, lack of controlled knee flexion of about 0–15 degree at foot flat to midstance, lack of neutral hip extension with excessive lateral horizontal shift of pelvis with excessive downward tilt of pelvis on the opposite side at mid stance, lack of hip extension, knee flexion, and ankle plantar flexion at push off.

The common swing phase anomalies include excessive forward rotation of pelvis with lack of adequate hip and knee flexion and ankle dorsiflexion to clear the ground.

Pain

Stroke survivors frequently have a variety of chronic pain syndromes resulting from stroke-induced damage to the nervous system (neuropathic pain). In some stroke patients, pathways for sensation in the brain are damaged, causing the transmission of false signals that result in the sensation of pain in a limb or side of the body that has the sensory deficit. The most common of these pain syndromes is called "thalamic pain syndrome" (caused by a stroke to the thalamus, which processes sensory information from the body to the brain), which can be difficult to treat even with medications. Complex regional pain syndrome, also called reflex sympathetic dystrophy is a painful disorder that may complicate in some patients. Shoulder impingement/shoulder subluxation and adhesive capsulitis of shoulder is also the cause of pain. Deformity of joints also leads to the secondary arthritic changes precipitating pain in joints.

Shoulder Subluxation and Pain

Patients with hemiplegia develop shoulder pain in both the stages, i.e., (1) Flaccid and (2) Spastic.
1. In Flaccid stage, proprioceptive impairment, lack muscular tone and strength in the rotator cuff muscles and the muscles that produce force couples in shoulder stabilizing the humeral head in the glenoid, such as middle deltoid and supraspinatus muscle force couple is the cause of shoulder subluxation and pain. At this stage, the stability of shoulder depends mostly on ligaments and capsules and bony contour of glenoid and humeral head. The normal orientation of glenoid fossa, which is upward, outward, and forward, keeping the superior capsule taut and stabilizing the humeral head, mechanically is lost, causing shoulder subluxation. In the absence of supporting musculature, any abduction and forward flexion of shoulder in the presence of shoulder depression, reduces shoulder stability causing subluxation. The subluxation is initially very mild, which may not be very painful. Subsequently by the traction exerted while handling the patient, and gravitational forces acting upon the flaccid limb in upright posture, increase shoulder subluxation causing pain **(Fig. 19.6)** The normal scapulohumeral rhythm is lost in such patients, which may result in shoulder impingement, due to glenohumeral friction and compression stresses, occurring between the humeral head and superior soft tissues, during flexion and abduction movements.
2. In spastic stage, abnormal muscle tone causing scapular depression, retraction and downward rotation, also results in shoulder subluxation and pain. Impingement of soft tissues in the suprahumeral space may also occur in this stage, due to poor scapular position.

Besides the above, poor handling and positioning the affected upper limb also produce micro trauma to soft tissues around shoulder, which may also lead to adhesive capsulitis (frozen shoulder) causing pain and movement limitations. Reflex sympathetic dystrophy (shoulder hand syndrome) is also another factor for painful shoulder.

Recovery of Stroke

The recovery process involved includes:
a. **Early recovery (local process):**
   – Resolution of poststroke edema.
   – Reperfusion of ischemic penumbra.

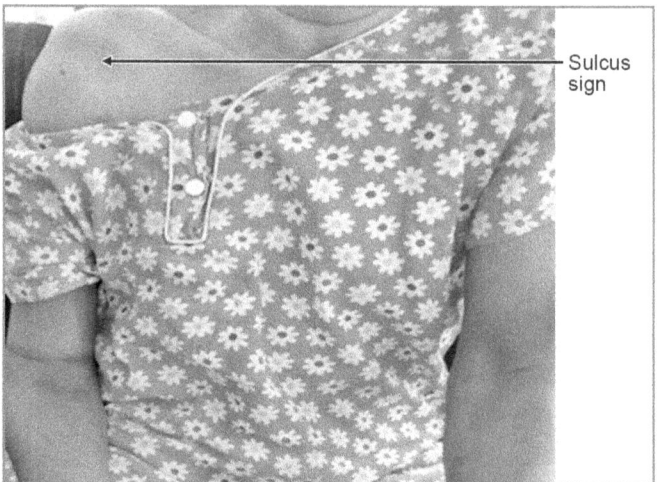

Fig. 19.6: Shoulder subluxation in flaccid stage showing sulcus sign.

- Resorption of local toxins.
- Recovery of partially damaged ischemic neurons.
b. **Late recovery (Neuroplasticity):** Ability of the nervous system to modify structural and functional organization. The process involves:
   - Collateral sprouting of new synaptic connections.
   - Unmasking of previously latent functional pathways.
   - Reversibility from diaschisis (Diaschisis has been defined as a loss of function within a region distant to the site of the lesion and results from deafferentation of neurons as a result of axon damage caused by stroke. This results in reduced metabolic activity in the regions affected by the loss of neuronal input).
   - Denervation supersensitivity (Denervation hypersensitivity is the sharp increase of sensitivity of postsynaptic membranes to a chemical transmitter after denervation. It is a compensatory change).

Brunnstrom's Stages of Recovery

a. **Recovery of stroke patient proceeds through six stages as per Brunnstrom:**
   1. *Stage-1:* Flaccid and no movement.
   2. *Stage-2:* Spasticity begins and basic limb synergies may be seen as associated reaction.
   3. *Stage-3:* Limb synergies are produced voluntarily.
   4. *Stage-4:* Some movement combinations not belonging to synergy may appear, spasticity starts declining.
   5. *Stage-5:* More difficult movement combinations are learned.
   6. *Stage-6:* Spasticity disappears, isolated movement possible.
b. **Brunnstrom's stages of recovery of hand function in stroke:**
   - *Stage 1:* Flaccidity
   - *Stage 2:* Little or no active finger flexion
   - *Stage 3:* Mass Grasp, use of hook grasp but no release, no voluntarily finger extension, reflex extension of the digits occurs.
   - *Stage 4:* Lateral prehension, release by thumb movement, semivoluntary finger extension present in small range.
   - *Stage 5:* Palmar prehension, possible cylindrical and spherical grasp, awkwardly performed and with limited functional use; voluntary mass extension of the digits in variable range.
   - *Stage 6:* All prehension types under control; skills improving; full range voluntary extension of digits; individual finger movements present, and less accurate than opposite side.
c. **Recovery of stroke patients as per Bobath occurs in three stages:**
   1. Flaccid.
   2. Spastic.
   3. Stage of spontaneous recovery.

Assessment of Stroke Patients

The components of assessment are:
A. **Demographic data:** Name, age, sex, address, etc.
B. **Complaint:** Complaint of patient from most priority to less priority.
C. **History:** History of present illness, past history, family history, personal history, socioeconomic history, and treatment history.
D. **Observation:** Observation of patient, as he/she enters the assessment clinic, observation of posture from standing to lying.
E. **Examination:**
   - *Higher function testing:* Speech, hearing, vision, memory, orientation, attention span, etc.
   - *Cranial nerve testing:* Mostly, 2nd, 7th, 9th, 10th, and 12th cranial nerves need to be tested.
   - *Sensory examination:* Superficial (pain, touch, and temperature), Deep (proprioception and kinesthesia, vibration), Cortical (Stereognosis, barognosis, and graphesthesia, tactile localization, and tactile discrimination, two point discrimination).
   - *Motor examination:*
     » Tone: Tone grading scale: 0: Flaccid, 1+: Hypotonic, 2+: Normal, 3+: Mild to moderate hypertonia, 4+: Severe hypertonia.
     » Spasticity: Graded using scales such as: Modified-Modified Ashworth Scale: 0-No increase in muscle tone, 1-Slight increase in muscle tone, manifested by catch followed by release, or minimum resistance at the end of the passive ROM, when the muscle is elongated, 2-Considerable increase in muscle tone, throughout the range of motion, but passive movement is possible, 3-Significantly increased muscle tone, making passive movement difficult, 4-Very high muscle tone, making the limb rigid.
     » Reflexes/Reaction: Superficial reflex (plantar response), deep tendon reflexes, primitive reflexes, protective reactions, and associated reactions. Deep tendon reflexes are graded using the DTR grading scale: 0: Absent, 1+: Diminished (Slight response), 2+: Normal, 3+: Mild hyperreflexia (Brisk reflex), 4+: Moderate to severe hyperreflexia with clonus (very brisk reflex/exaggerated reflex response).
     » Coordination: For upper limb, finger to nose test, and for lower limb heel to shin test is commonly performed.
     » Involuntary movements (if any).
     » Postural control and balance: Static posture of the patient in lying, sitting and standing need to be analyzed and documented. During quiet sitting and standing the degree and direction of sway should be determined and documented.

Balance is the condition in which all the forces acting on the body are balanced such that the center of mass (COM) is within the stability limits. The overall goals of the postural control system, stability and function, are achieved through integrated CNS systems of control. Reactive postural control (response to external forces acting on the body, e.g., perturbations) as well as proactive postural control/anticipatory postural control (anticipation of internally

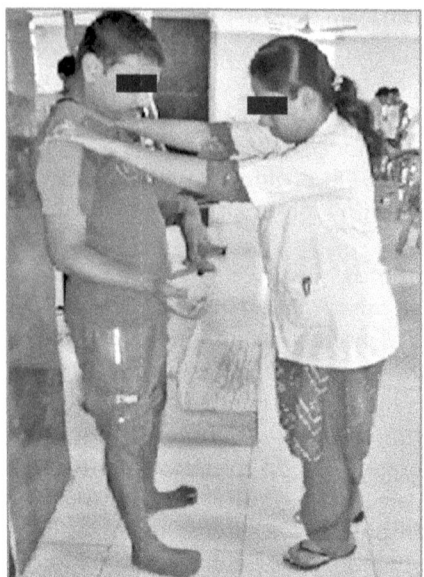

Fig. 19.7: Assessment of ankle strategy.

generated destabilizing forces imposed on the body's own movements are usually impaired which need to be tested.

In standing the ability to recruit fixed-support strategies (movement strategies used to control the COM over a fixed BOS) such as Ankle strategy (shifting the COM forward and backward by moving the body as relatively a fixed pendulum about the ankle joint) **(Fig. 19.7)** and hip strategy (shifting the COM by flexing or extending at the hips) as well as the ability to recruit change-in-support strategy (movements of lower or upper limbs to make a new contact with the support surface) such as the stepping strategy (realigning the BOS under the COM by using rapid steps or hops in the direction of the displacing force) to be assessed and documented.

The Berg Balance Scale (BBS) developed by Berg et al., the Functional Reach (FR) Test developed by Duncan et al., the Timed Get Up and Go (GUG) Test developed by Mathias et al., and the Performance-oriented Mobility Assessment (POMA) developed by Tinetti et al., are tools used to asses balance quantitatively. The functional balance grading system that grades balance from: Poor: (Static—patient requires handhold support and moderate to maximal assistance to maintain position, Dynamic—patient is unable to accept challenge or move without loss of balance), Fair: (Static—patient is able to maintain balance with hand held support, may require occasional minimal assistance, Dynamic—patient accepts minimal challenge, and is able to maintain balance while turning the head/trunk), Good: (Static—patient is able to maintain balance without hand hold support with limited postural sway, Dynamic—patient accepts moderate challenge, and is able to maintain balance, while picking objects off the floor), Normal: (Static—patient is able to maintain steady balance without hand hold support, Dynamic—patient accepts maximal challenge and can shift weight easily within full range in all directions).

❖ **Range of Motion**
  – Tightness/Contracture/Deformity.

– **Muscle power:** If movements performed against gravity/resistance do not increase the muscle tone, MRC grading should be performed to assess muscle power. However, if the tone is altered on doing movements for MRC grading, the voluntary motor control (VMC) grading, using STREAM scoring system/some conventional grading system is used.
– *The STREAM scale:* Stroke Rehabilitation Assessment of Movements is a clinical measure of voluntary movements and basic mobility in stroke patients. It assesses the voluntary movements of upper limb, lower limb as well as basic mobility such as rolling, bridging, sit to stand, standing, stepping, walking, and stair climbing. The scores in the scale indicate, whether the movements produced by the patient are done fully or partially, and whether they are done normally fully controlled by the individual or there are abnormal components (synergies), which are not under control of the individual.

For limbs, voluntary movements produced are scored using a 3-point scale: 0-Unable to perform, 1-partial performance of movements abnormally/ normally and full performance of movements abnormally, having three components, such as 1.a- Able to perform part of the movement with marked deviation from normal pattern, 1.b- Able to perform part of the movement in a normal pattern, 1.c-Able to perform the movement fully, with marked deviation from normal pattern. 2- Full performance of movement normally.

The basic mobility are scored using a 4-point scale such as 0-Unable to perform the test movement through appreciable range, 1.a-Able to perform the activity partially with or without an aid with deviation from normal pattern, 1.b- Able to perform part of the activity, with or without an aid, normally, 1.c- Able to perform the test activity fully with or without an aid with marked deviation from normal pattern, 2- Able to perform the activity normally with an aid, 3-Able to perform the activity normally without an aid. The maximum STREAM score is 70, with each limb subscore worth 20 points and functional mobility subscore worth 30 points. As application of STREAM is time consuming, a simple objective grading method discussed here may be followed to grade voluntary motor control as per the school of thought of the Institution.

Voluntary motor control grading for assessing movement (in synergy pattern):
» Grade 0: No contraction present.
» Grade 1: Flickering contraction/movement initiation.
» Grade 2: Half range of motion in synergy/abnormal pattern.
» Grade 3: Full range of motion in synergy/abnormal pattern.
» Grade 4: Initial half range of motion, performed in isolation, and the remaining half performed in synergy/abnormal pattern
» Grade 5: Full range of motion produced in isolation, but goes into pattern when resistance is applied.

» Grade 6: Full range of motion against resistance, produced in isolation.
- Bladder bowel control.
- **Functional evaluation:** Evaluation of ADL skills, mobility skills on bed and out of bed as well as instrumental ADL such as writing, typing skills, etc., should be tested.
- **Gait:** Observational analysis of stance and swing phase activities, gait laboratory assessment and assessment of energy consumption during walking should be assessed and documented as per availability of infrastructure.

Goal Setting

For stroke patients duration of short-term goal (such as rolling on bed over sound side) is 1 month, and duration of long-term goal (such as hand function skill improvement)/walking independently, etc., is usually 6 months. The goal that is realistic and achievable during this period is set.

Management

When an acute stroke is suspected by history and physical examination, the goal of early assessment is to determine the cause. Treatment varies according to the underlying cause of the stroke, such as: thromboembolic (ischemic), or hemorrhagic. Good nursing care is fundamental in maintaining skin care, feeding, hydration, positioning, and monitoring vital signs, such as temperature, pulse, and blood pressure.

Medical and Surgical Management in Acute Stage

For ischemic stroke

Definitive therapy is aimed at removing the blockage by breaking the clot down (thrombolysis), or by removing it mechanically (thrombectomy). The philosophical premise underlying the importance of rapid stroke intervention was crystallized as "Time is Brain" in the early 1990s. Years later, that same idea that rapid cerebral blood flow restoration results in fewer brain cells dying, has been proved and quantified.

For hemorrhagic stroke

People with ICH require neurosurgical evaluation to detect and treat the cause of the bleeding, although many may not need surgery. Anticoagulants and antithrombotics, key in treating ischemic stroke, can make bleeding worse. People are monitored for changes in the level of consciousness, and their blood pressure, blood sugar, and oxygenation are kept at optimum levels.

Large territory strokes can cause significant edema of the brain with secondary brain injury in surrounding tissue. This phenomenon is mainly encountered in strokes of the middle cerebral artery territory, and is also called "malignant cerebral infarction" because it carries a poor prognosis. Relief of the pressure may be attempted with medication, but some require hemicraniectomy, the temporary surgical removal of the skull on one side of the head (the removed part of the cranium is sometimes preserved in the peritoneal cavity of abdomen or may be preserved in bone bank for reimplantation later on). This decreases the risk of death, although some more people survive with disability, who would otherwise have died.

Stroke unit

Ideally, people who have a stroke are admitted to a "stroke unit", an Intensive Care Unit (ICU), or a ward or dedicated area in hospital staffed by nurses and therapists with experience in stroke treatment. It has been shown that people admitted to a stroke unit have a higher chance of surviving than those admitted elsewhere in hospital, even if they are being cared for by doctors without experience in stroke.

Physiotherapy to stroke patients in ICU/ Acute care set up

The Physiotherapist has to maintain co-ordination with the ICU Medical officer, ICU Nurse, while delivering services to the stroke sufferers in the ICU. The duties of the physiotherapist in ICU include:

1. Monitoring the vital parameters such as pulse rate, blood pressure, respiratory rate, oxygen saturation level etc.
2. Checking the catheters and drainage tubes for blockage (if any)
3. Regular turning of the patient from supine to side-lyings if permitted by the treating neurologist/neurosurgeon. If the same is not permissible, and the patient has been placed on a tilt bed, the therapist needs to monitor that the bed is

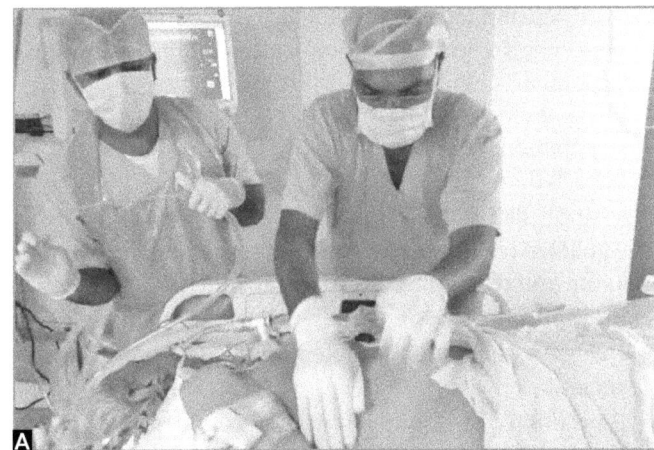

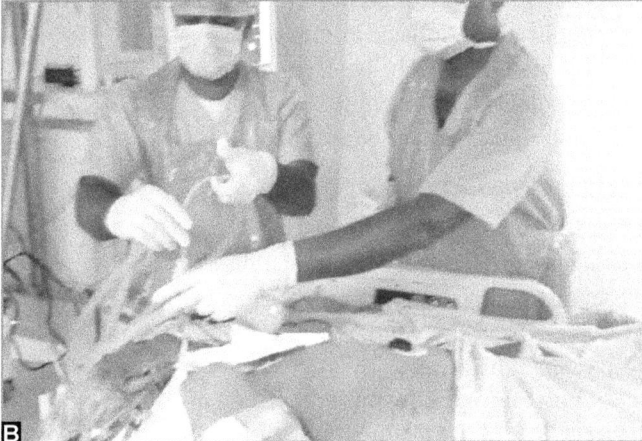

Figs. 19.8A and B: (A) Chest percussion applied by physiotherapist in ICU; (B) Suction application by nurse and physiotherapist.

tilting at regular intervals to cause pressure relief and no complication arises from the tilting of the bed.
4. Positioning the patients limbs in the anti-synergistic/anti-spastic postures.
5. Regular relaxed passive movements are given by the therapist to promote venous return, prevent development of joint stiffness, and maintain soft tissue flexibility.
6. Assisted breathing (if the patient is not ventilator dependent) exercises are given at periodic intervals.
7. Chest percussion/vibration are given by the therapist (if not contraindicated) **(Fig. 19.8A)**.
8. Drainage of secretions are made through huffing and coughing, if the patient can produce such reflexes, either spontaneously or when stimulated. If patient can not throw out secretions, voluntarily/reflexly, the physiotherapist and the ICU nurse should work together to apply suction for draining secretion from the airways **(Fig. 19.8B)**.

Medical/Surgical Management in the Recovery Stage

As the patient recovers, abnormal synergies and spastic patterns dominate the patient's movements. Antispastic drugs may be prescribed by the physician to control the spasticity. Sometimes, patients report to the rehabilitation team late, with contracture and deformities, which need surgical lengthening.

Besides the medical and surgical management, therapeutic and orthotic managements should start from the very acute stage, once the patient is medically stable. Therapeutic management includes:
- Physiotherapy.
- Occupational therapy.
- Speech therapy.
- Orthotic management.

The goals of treatment in the acute stage when the patient is stable and treated in the hospital bed:
- Prevent ignorance or unawareness of the hemiplegic side.
- Decrease the tendency to develop strong synergy in later stages.
- Prevention of any joint restriction or stiffness.
- Prevention of deconditioning complications such as: chest complications, muscle atrophy, etc.
- Promote early weight-bearing.
- Psychological counseling.
- Family and caregiver education.

Physiotherapy Treatment

Physiotherapy treatment involves: (A) Acute care management. (B) Stroke rehabilitation.
A. **Acute management:** This starts either in the ICU (discussed above), or in the ward, depending on the stability of the patient. It involves:
  - **Positioning of the patient**: In the early stages, emphasis is given for arrangements of patient's room, so that every article/person are presented at the hemiplegic side and the affected side faces the door, with an aim

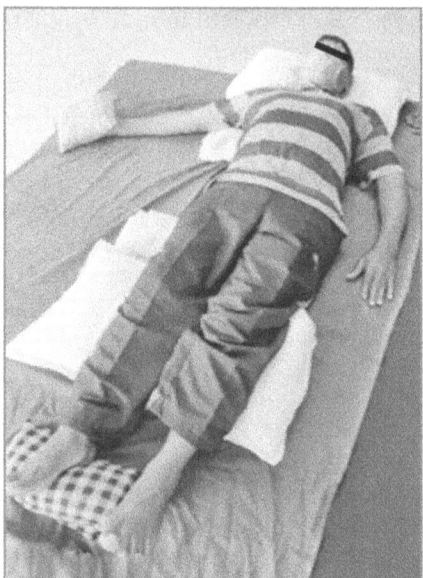

Fig. 19.9: Positioning in supine lying.

of prevention of sensory deprivation and stimulation of awareness of hemiplegic side.

Positioning of the patient in an appropriate way is essential to control the intensity of development of spasticity and to help faster improvement in the later stages. While positioning, supine postures are much discouraged and lying on the sides is preferred. Shoulder joint should be supported throughout the flaccid stage initially through a triangular sling, followed by some dynamic shoulder support that supports the shoulder freeing the elbow and hand to perform function. Once the patient develops spasticity, a hand splint and elbow gaiter should be considered for the upper limb, which should be used consistently, when the patient is not doing exercise/activities. As the patient tolerates upright posture, a knee immobilizer (if the knee buckles on

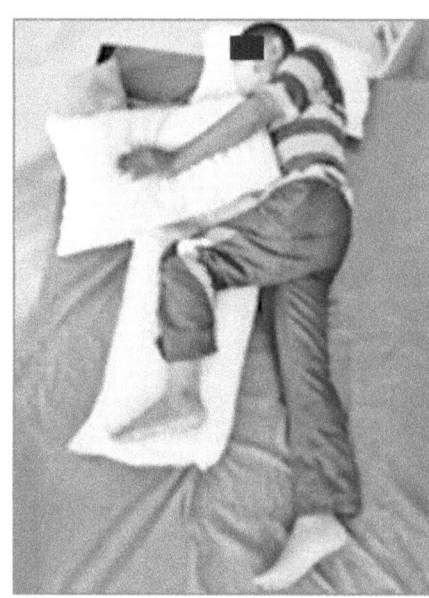

Fig. 19.10: Side lying on the affected side.

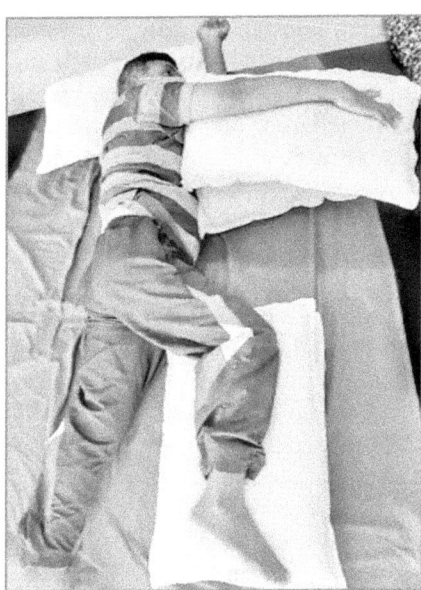

Fig. 19.11: Side lying on the sound side.

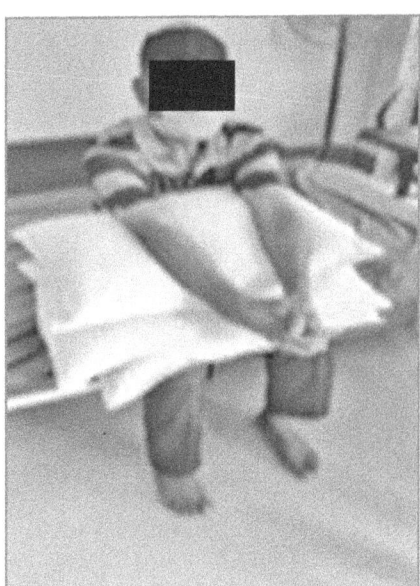

Fig. 19.12: Positioning in sitting.

weight bearing) and a toe pick-up splint (hinged AFO) may be considered.
- **Positioning on bed (supine lying) (Fig. 19.9):** A pillow should be placed under head to minimize the effect of tonic labyrinthine reflex which has an impact on increasing extensor tone. Support should be given under the scapula and pelvis to prevent retraction. Pillow should be positioned along the lateral aspect of thigh to prevent lateral rotation of hip. For upper limb, the shoulder should be in abduction and lateral rotation, elbow should be in extension, forearm should be in supination and wrist and fingers in extension and thumb in abduction. For lower limb, the hip should be in neutral position, with knee in extension and ankle in plantigrade position without any deformation of foot. Use of a polypropylene ankle-foot orthosis (L type splint) as a resting splint should be made carefully, as pressure on the ball of toes may increase tone, as the area is a zone of hypersensitivity. In the absence of L-type splint, a sand bag can be used to keep the ankle plantigrade.
- **Positioning on bed (In side lying over affected side) (Fig. 19.10):** The affected shoulder is kept in flexion with elbow in extension and forearm in supination and wrist and fingers in neutral extension and thumb in abduction. The affected lower limb is maintained with hip in slight extension, knee in slight flexion, and ankle plantigrade. The sound upper and lower limbs are supported on pillow for comfort.
- **Positioning on bed (In side lying over sound side) (Fig. 19.11):** The affected upper limb should be supported on pillow with scapula in protraction, shoulder in flexion, elbow in extension, wrist and finger in neutral extension, and thumb in abduction. The affected lower limb is positioned over pillow with hip and knee in partial flexion and ankle in plantigrade position.

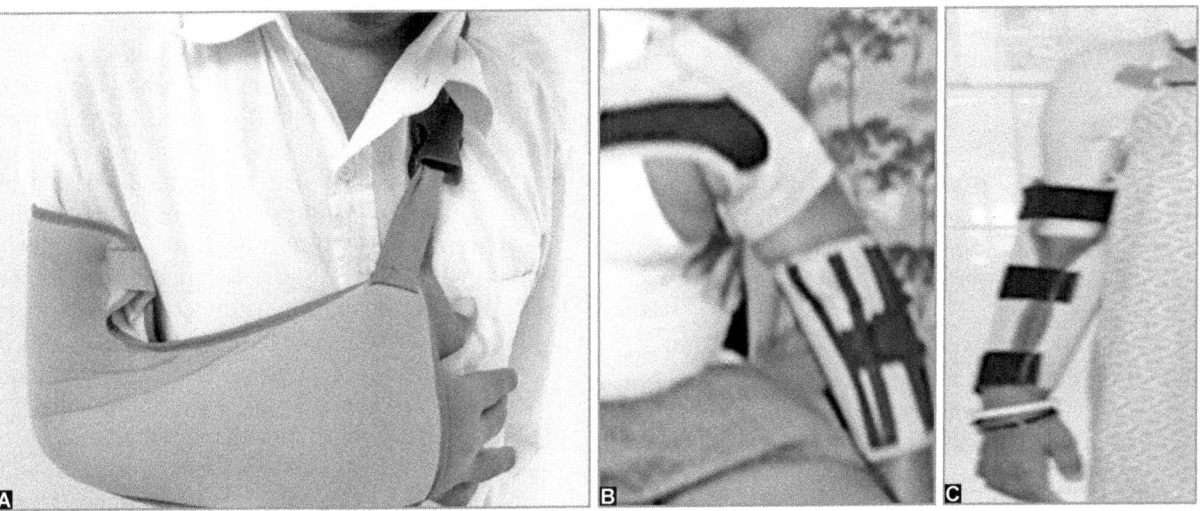

Figs. 19.13A to C: (A) The triangular sling; (B) Neoprene shoulder support; (C) Polypropylene shoulder support.

Section 3: Physiotherapy for Neurological Conditions

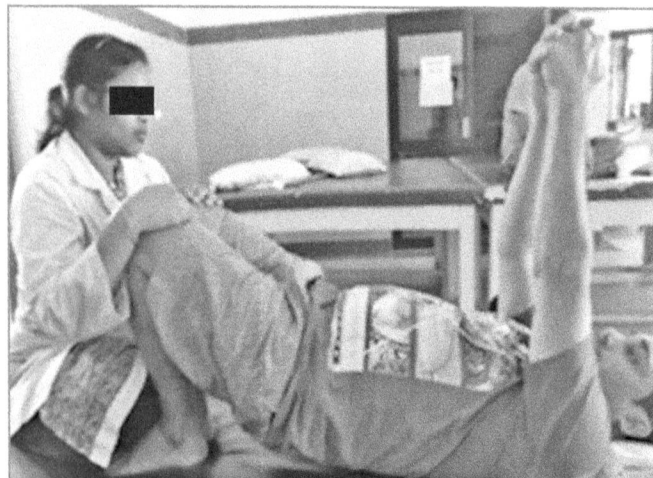

Fig. 19.14: Pelvic bridging exercise.

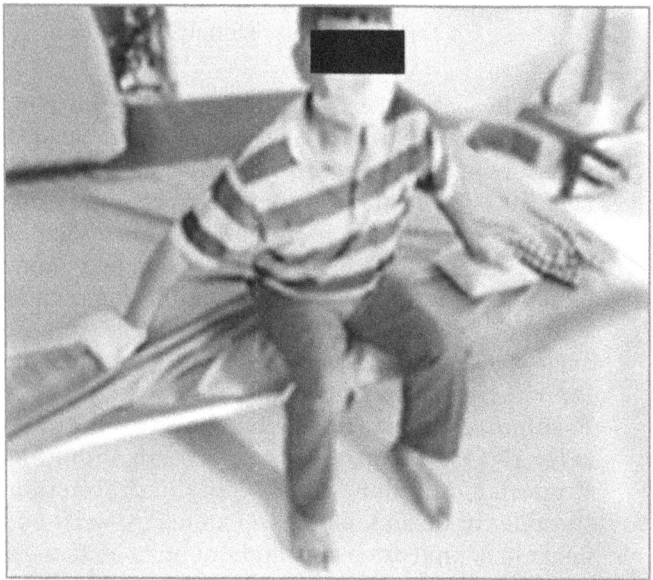

Fig. 19.15: Weight-bearing through affected (right) upper and lower limbs.

- **Positioning in sitting (Fig. 19.12):** The patient is made to sit on a bed, with a pad of towel under the affected buttock. Both the feet are made to touch the floor and the clasped hands rest on the pillows placed on the lap.
- **Shoulder support:** During the early stage, when the muscles are flaccid, the shoulder joint should be supported by a triangular sling **(Fig. 19.13A)**. As the tone returns, a dynamic shoulder brace made of neoprene material **(Fig. 19.13B)** or polypropylene **(Fig. 19.13C)** may be considered.

Conventional exercises in the acute stage: Traditional stroke rehabilitation integrates a variety of treatment strategies, with varying degrees of evidence-based support. Often, treatment incorporates repetitive exercise, used to facilitate motor learning, and build muscle strength. In the acute phase, treatment may integrate passive ROM, in order to maintain the integrity of physical structures in anticipation of subsequent neurological recovery. As recovery occurs, therapeutic exercise typically advances to active-assistive movements, in which a clinician uses physical cues and graded support to aid completion of simple movements. The strategies used in the acute stage are:

- Daily ROM exercises.
- Active assisted/ free exercises.
- Pelvic bridging exercises **(Fig. 19.14)**.
- Bed mobility and mat exercises.
- Sitting development and weight bearing through affected upper and lower limb **(Fig. 19.15)**.
- Chest physiotherapy.
- Oropharyngeal retraining.
- Bladder/bowel retraining.

B. **Stroke rehabilitation:** As the acute symptoms subside and the patient is found medically stable, he/she is subjected to stroke rehabilitation.

The goals of rehabilitation are to help survivors become as independent as possible and to attain the best possible quality of life. Even though rehabilitation does not "cure" the effects of stroke in that it does not reverse brain damage, rehabilitation can substantially help people achieve the best possible long-term outcome.

Rehabilitation helps stroke survivors relearn skills that are lost when part of the brain is damaged. For example, these skills can include coordinating leg movements in order to walk or carrying out the steps involved in any complex activity. Rehabilitation also teaches survivors new ways of performing tasks to compensate for any residual disabilities. Individuals may need to learn how to bathe and dress using the affected hand, or how to communicate, when verbal communication is not possible.

Rehabilitative therapy begins in the acute-care hospital after the person's overall condition has been stabilized, often within 24-48 hours after the stroke. The first steps involve promoting independent movement because many individuals are paralyzed or seriously weakened. Patients are prompted to change positions frequently while lying in bed and to engage in exercises to maintain joint mobility and facilitate/ strengthen their stroke-impaired limbs. Depending on many factors—including the extent of the initial injury—patients may progress from sitting up and being moved between the bed and a chair to standing, bearing their own weight, and walking, with or without assistance. Rehabilitation nurses and therapists help patients who are able to perform progressively more complex and demanding tasks, such as bathing, dressing, and using a toilet, and they encourage patients to begin using their stroke-impaired limbs while engaging in those tasks. Beginning to reacquire the ability to carry out these basic activities of daily living represents the first stage in a stroke survivor's return to independence.

For some stroke survivors, rehabilitation will be an ongoing process to maintain and refine skills and could

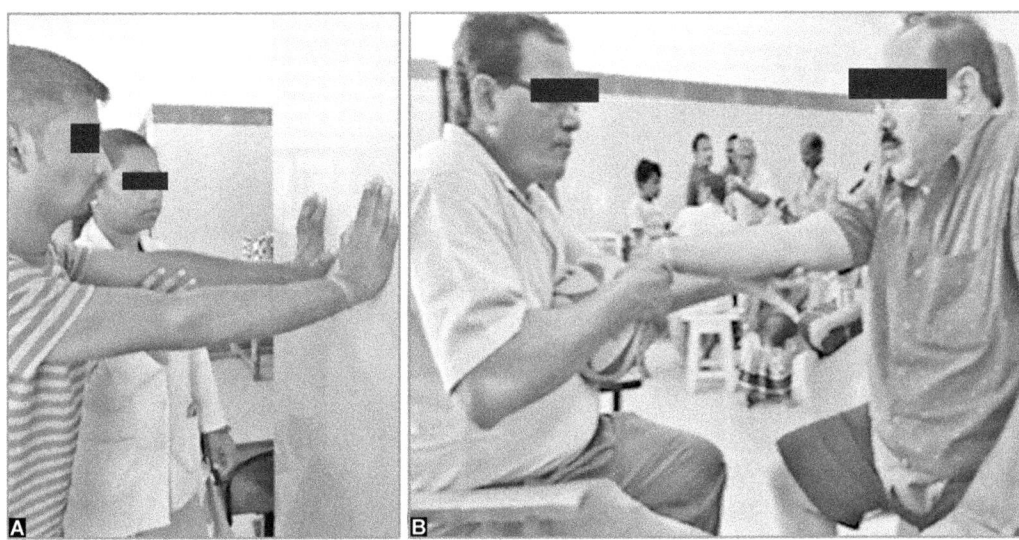

Figs. 19.16A and B: (A) Functional stretching; (B) Passive stretching.

involve working with specialists for months or years after the stroke.

Poststroke rehabilitation involves physicians; rehabilitation nurses; physiotherapist, occupational therapist, recreational therapist, speech-language pathologist, orthotist, vocational therapist; and mental health professionals.

Physiotherapy for stroke survivors in the recovery/rehabilitation phase:

Physiotherapists help stroke survivors regain the use of stroke-impaired limbs, teach compensatory strategies to reduce the effect of remaining deficits, and establish ongoing exercise programs to help people retain their newly learned skills. Affected people tend to avoid using impaired limbs, a behavior called learned nonuse. However, the repetitive use of impaired limbs encourages brain's neuroplasticity (reorganization capacity).

Strategies used by physiotherapists to encourage the use of impaired limbs include selective sensory stimulation such as tapping or stroking, active and passive ROM exercises, and temporary restraint of healthy limbs while practicing motor tasks (constraint-induced movement therapy).

In general, physiotherapy emphasizes practicing isolated movements, repeatedly changing from one kind of movement to another, and rehearsing complex movements that require a great deal of coordination and balance, such as walking up or down stairs or moving safely between obstacles. People too weak to bear their own weight can still practice repetitive movements during hydrotherapy (in which water provides sensory stimulation as well as weight support) or while being partially supported by a harness (body weight supported standing/ walking). A recent trend in physiotherapy emphasizes the effectiveness of engaging in goal-directed activities, such as playing games, to promote coordination. Physiotherapists frequently employ selective sensory stimulation to encourage use of impaired limbs and to help survivors with neglect regain awareness of stimuli on the neglected side of the body. Common therapeutic methods employed are:

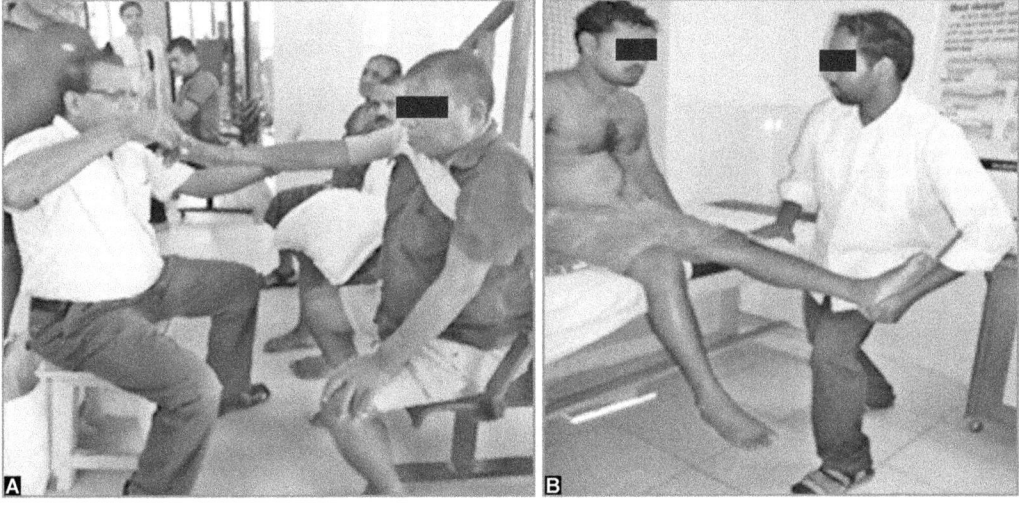

Figs. 19.17A and B: (A) Facilitation of muscles of upper limb; (B) Facilitation of knee extensors.

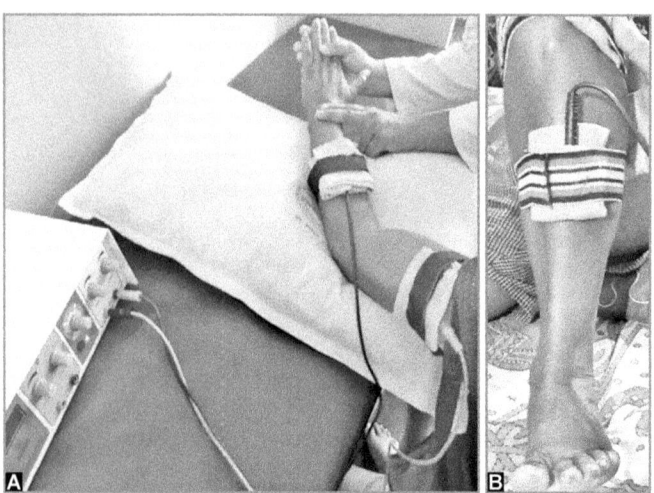

Figs. 19.18A and B: (A) Faradic stimulation to facilitate wrist extensors; (B) Faradic stimulation to facilitate ankle dorsiflexors.

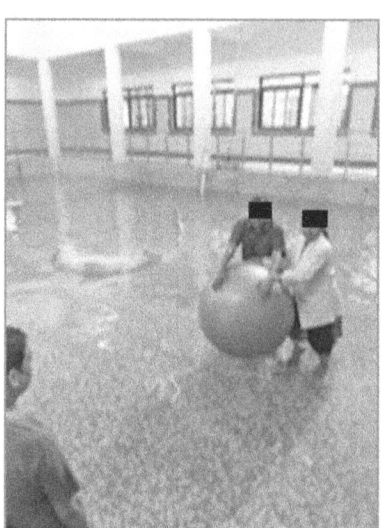

Fig. 19.19: Hydrotherapy to promote standing with shoulder flexor facilitation.

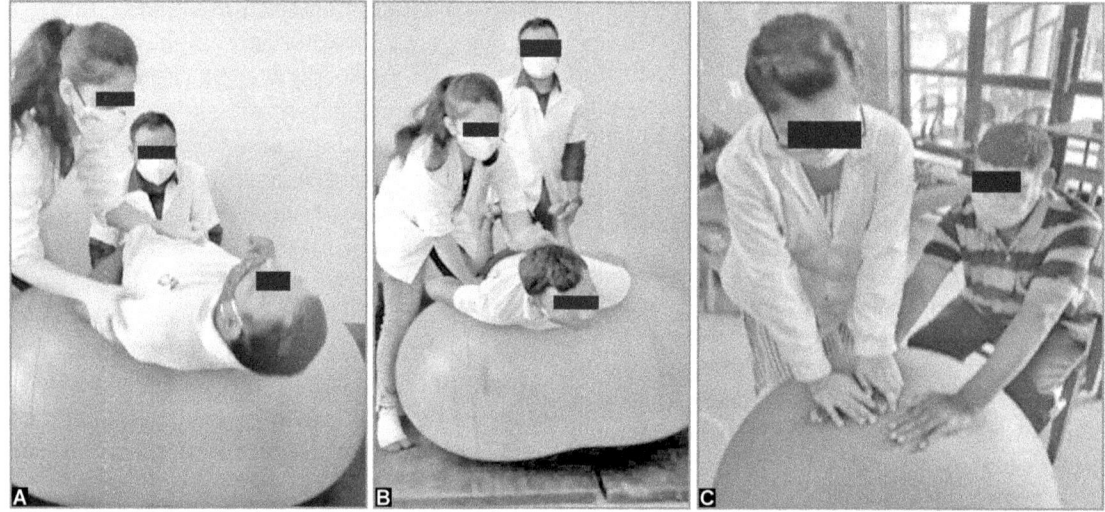

Figs. 19.20A to C: (A) Facilitation of abdominals; (B) Facilitation of back extensors; (C) Facilitation of upper limb muscles.

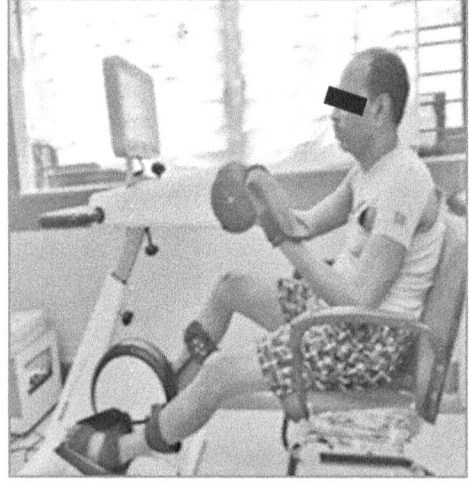

Fig. 19.21: Upper limb/lower limb ergometry exercises.

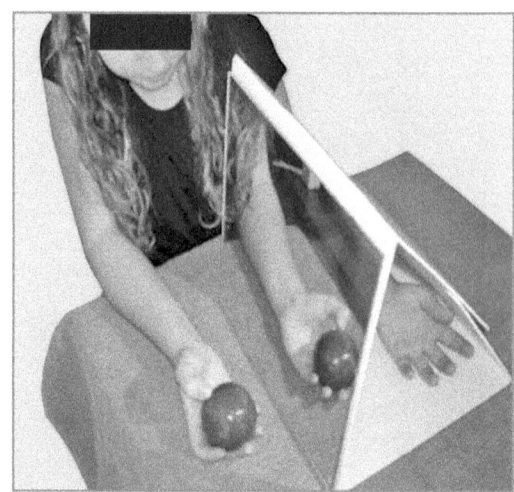

Fig. 19.22: Mirror therapy.

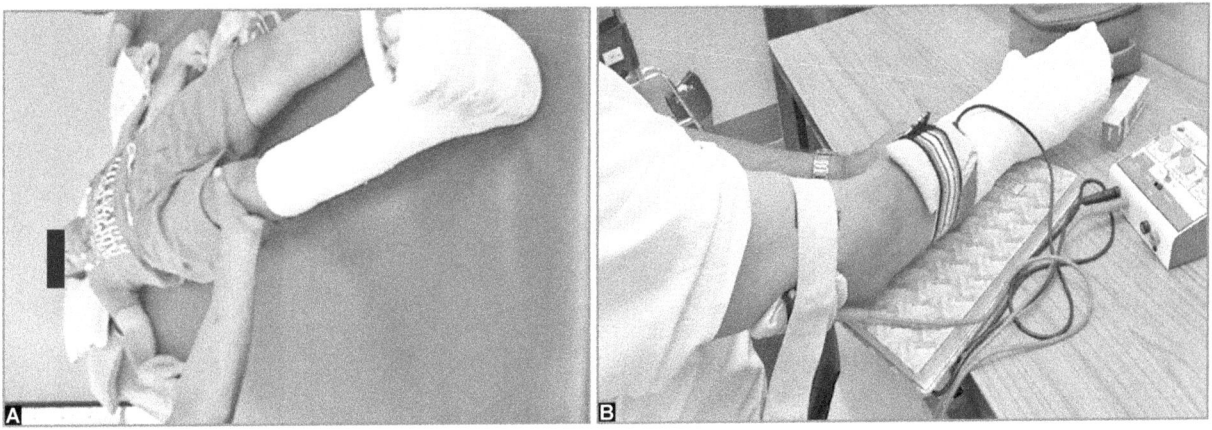

Figs. 19.23A and B: (A) POP casting to reduce tone and tightness of ankle plantar flexors; (B) POP casting for hand (**Note:** The wrist extensors are facilitated through electrical stimulation with the cast applied, preventing disuse).

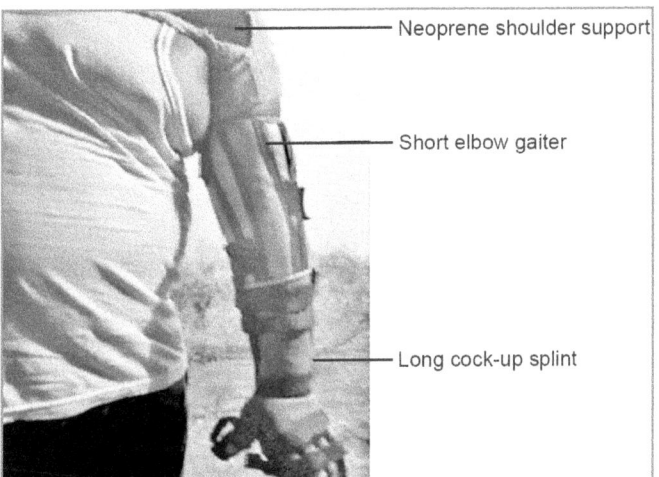

Fig. 19.24: Use of orthotic devices in the upper limb while walking for normal alignment of upper limb.

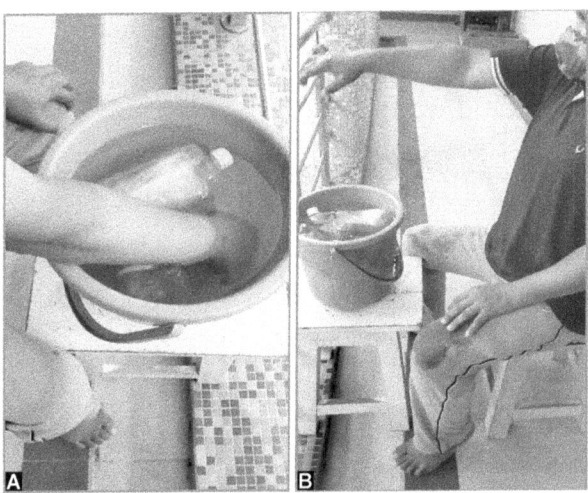

Figs. 19.25A and B: (A) Cold immersion to reduce spasticity of hand; (B) Immediate active movement facilitation after the immersion.

1. **Conventional exercises:** Exercises for stroke patients in recovery/ rehabilitation phase are designed to achieve the following:
    a. Maintain and improve soft tissue flexibility, joint ROM, muscle strength and as normal a posture of body as possible. Strategies used by physiotherapists to achieve the same include:
      » Positioning as done during the acute stage should continue throughout the phases of rehabilitation.
      » Relaxed passive movements.
      » Passive/functional stretching (**Figs. 19.16A and B**)
      » Active exercises to strengthen/facilitate muscles (**Figs. 19.17A and B**), electrical stimulation using Faradic type currents (**Figs. 19.18A and B**), hydrotherapy (**Fig. 19.19**), Swiss ball exercises (**Figs. 19.20A to C**), static cycle/bi-cycle ergometry exercises (**Fig. 19.21**), mirror therapy (**Fig.19.22**), mat exercises, etc., are used to strengthen/facilitate muscles.
    b. Reduce spasticity and inhibit abnormal reactions: Strategies applied include:

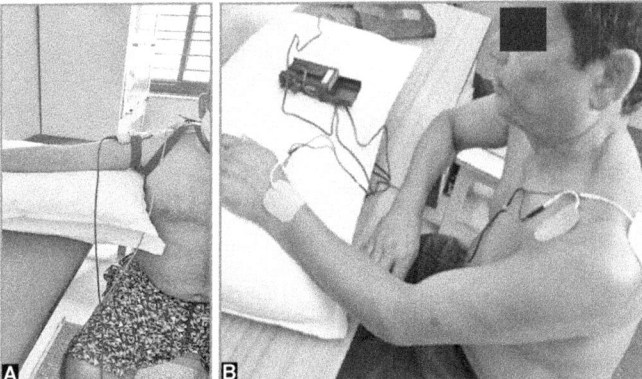

Figs. 19.26A and B: (A) Faradic stimulation to deltoid supraspinatus force couple; (B) TENS for shoulder hand syndrome.

   » Positioning/maintaining antispastic alignments with or without positional devices (sand bags, splints/ orthosis). This should be consistently performed, when the patient is not doing exercises/functional

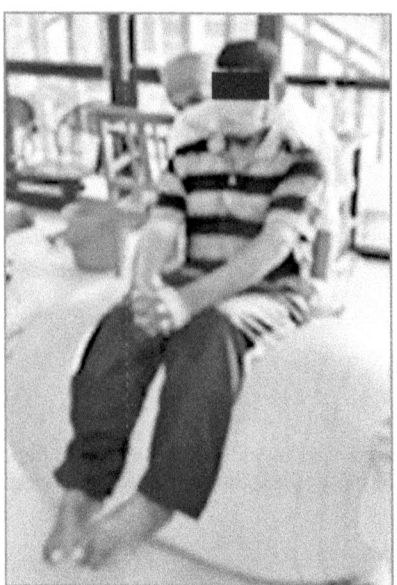

Fig. 19.27: Balancing on Swiss ball.

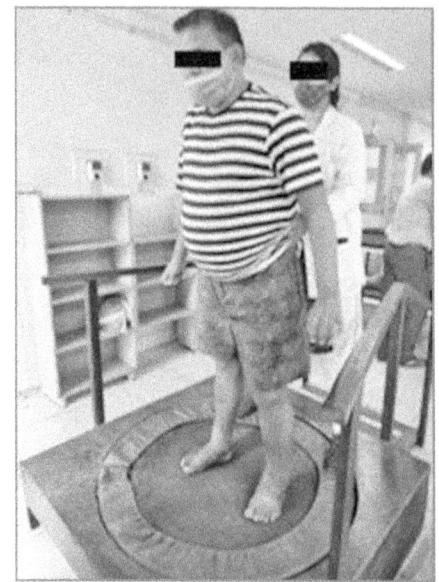

Fig. 19.28: Balancing on trampoline.

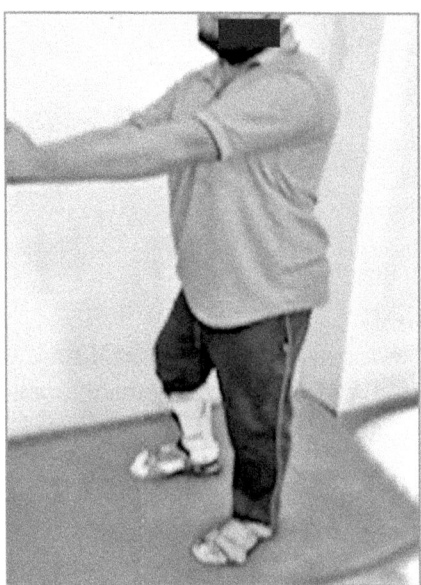

Fig. 19.29: Balancing on wobble board.

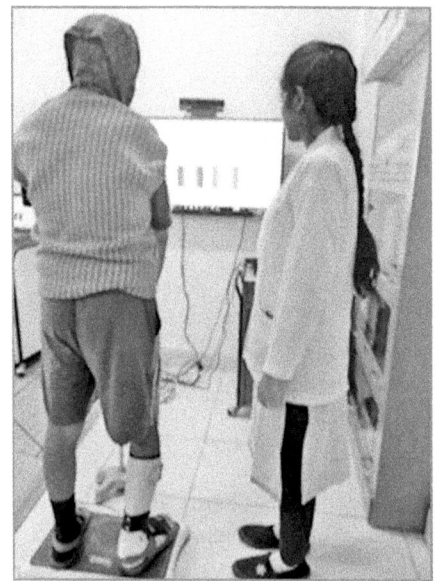

Fig. 19.30: Virtual therapy for balancing.

activities. Antispastic POP casts (**Figs. 19.23A and B**), and tone reducing splints (**Fig. 19.24**) may be requested as an adjunct as required.
- » Sustained stretching of spastic muscles.
- » Use of orthosis/ splints/ POP casts (**Figs. 19.23A and B and 19.24**).
- » Cryotherapy: Cold immersion (**Figs. 19.25A and B**), Ice massage.
- » Active movements.
- » Electrical stimulation to antagonistic muscle groups.
- » Biofeedback.
- » Weight shifting exercises.

c. Reduce shoulder pain and prevent/correct shoulder subluxation as well manage complications such as

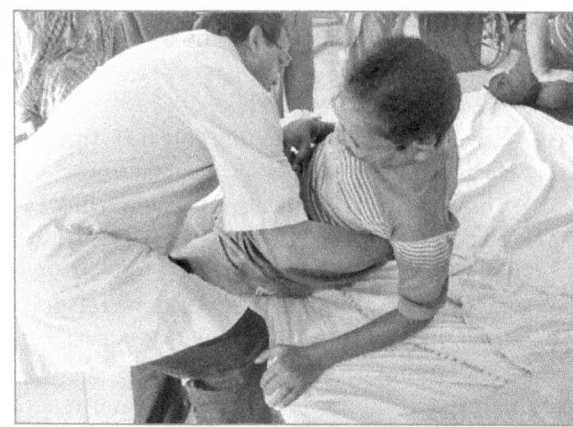

Fig. 19.31: Bed mobility exercises.

shoulder hand syndrome (RSD). Strategies applied include:
- » Use of shoulder orthosis.
- » Shoulder care, i.e., not to pull the patient, holding the affected arm.
- » Strengthening muscles of force couples of shoulder.
- » Faradic type current stimulation and TENS **(Figs. 19.26A and B)**
- » Contrast bath.

d. Improve posture and balance: Strategies applied include:
- » Postural re-education, development of balance strategies in sitting, standing (ankle/hip and stepping strategies), Swiss ball exercises **(Fig. 19.27)**, Trampoline exercises **(Fig. 19.28)**, Wobble board exercises **(Fig. 19.29)**, Virtual rehabilitation **(Fig. 19.30)**, etc.

e. Improve function and gait: Strategies applied include:
- » Mat exercises to improve bed mobility **(Fig. 19.31).**

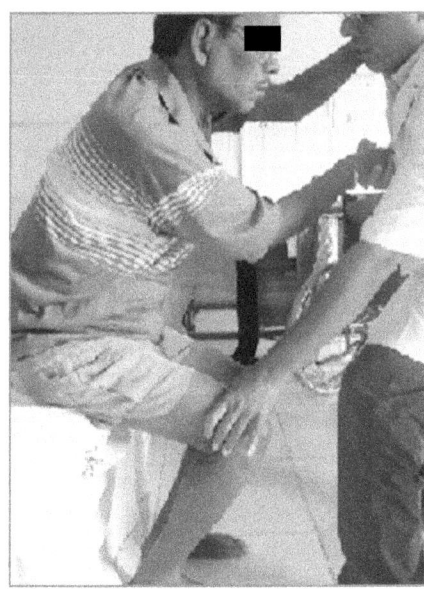

Fig. 19.32: Teaching transitions from sitting to standing.

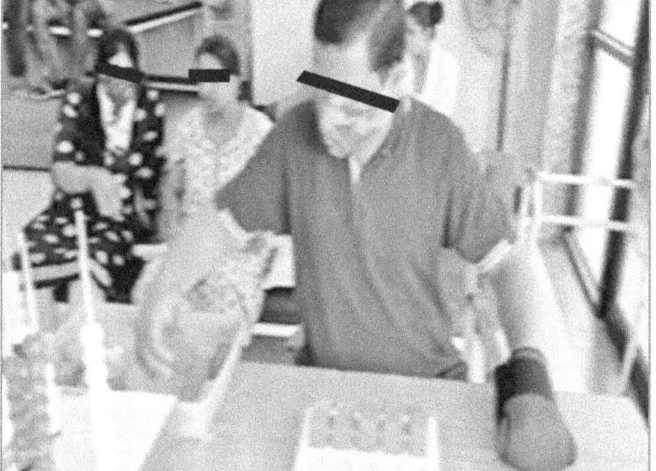

Fig. 19.33: CIMT to improve function with the affected right hand.

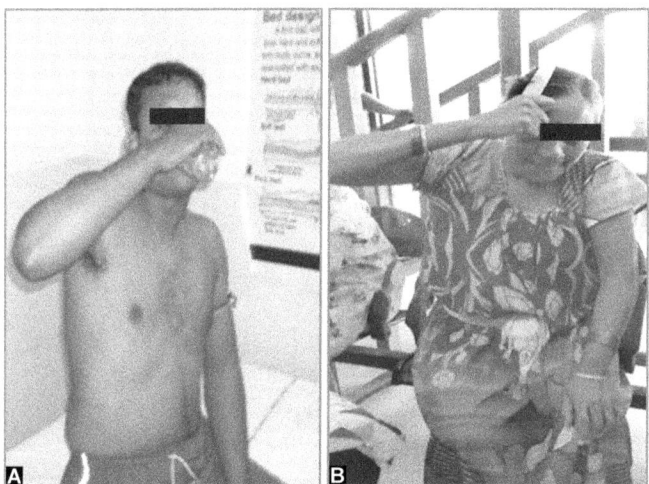

Figs. 19.34A and B: (A) Drinking water with affected hand; (B) Combing hair with affected hand.

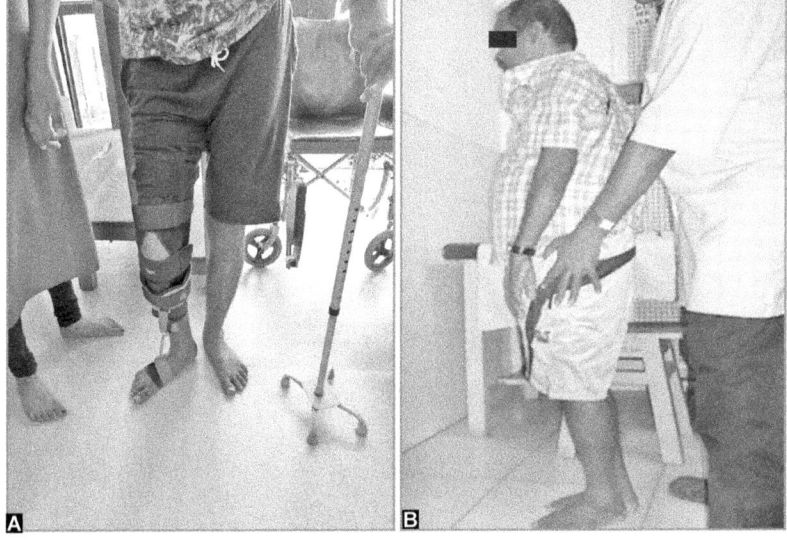

Figs. 19.35A and B: (A) Walking on leveled surfaces with knee immobilizer and toe pick up splint; (B) Gait training in progress.

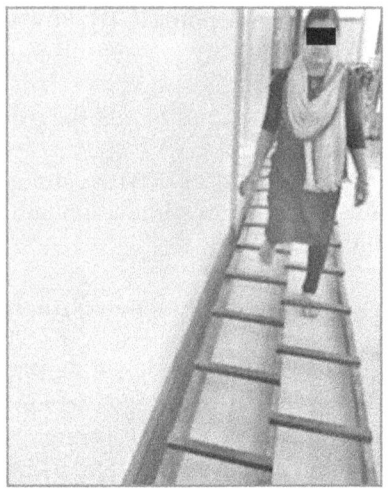

Fig. 19.36: Gait training on gait ladder.

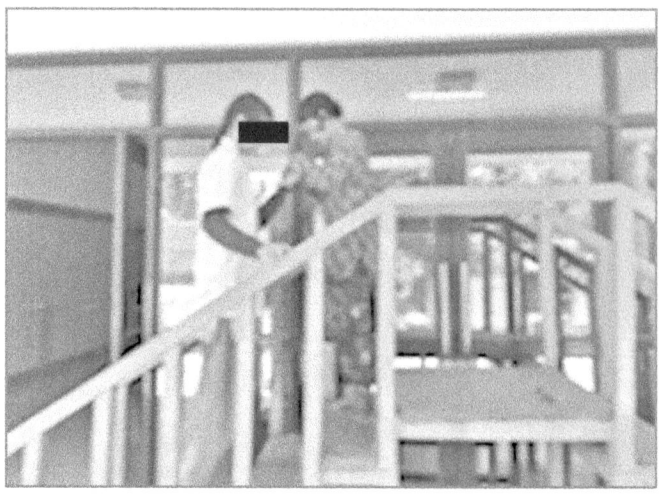

Fig. 19.37: Gait training on staircase.

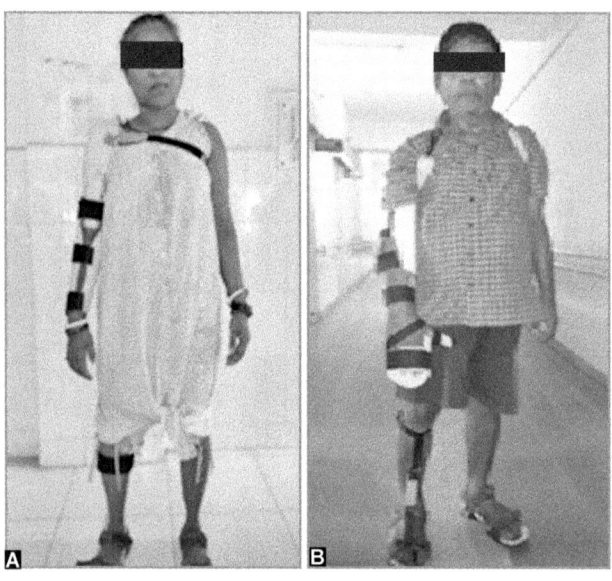

Figs. 19.38A and B: (A) Gait training with dorsiflexion-assist AFO; (B) Gait training with toe pick-up splint.

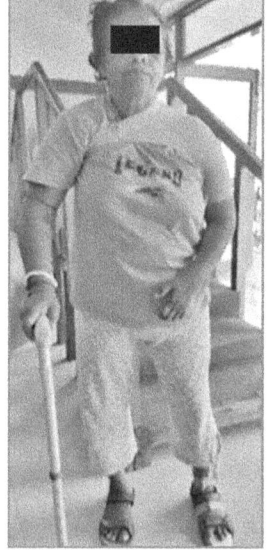

Fig. 19.39: Gait training with tripod stick.

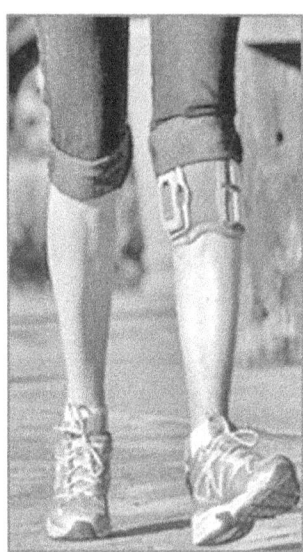

Fig. 19.40: Gait training with FES (Walk-aid system).

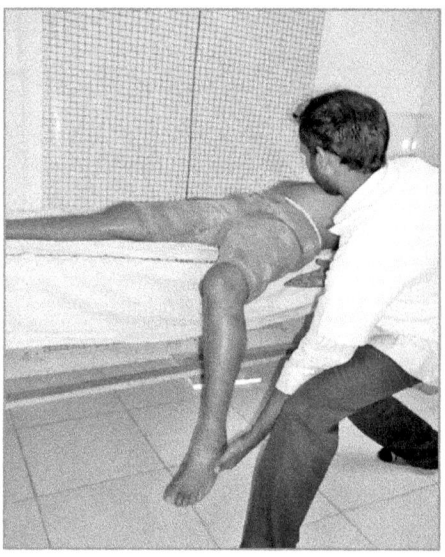

Fig. 19.41: Facilitation of hip extensors in supine lying.

Chapter 19: Stroke/Cerebrovascular Accident

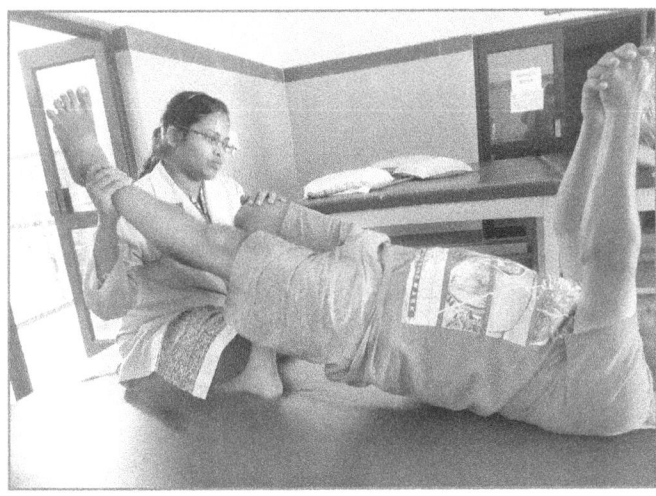

Fig. 19.42: Unilateral bridging exercise.

» Teaching transitions such as sitting to standing **(Fig. 19.32)**.
» Enhancing use of the affected limb through constrained-induced movement therapy (CIMT) **(Fig. 19.33)**.
» Self-care training **(Figs. 19.34A and B)**.
» Gait training: Body weight supported treadmill walking, walking on leveled surfaces **(Figs. 19.35A and B)**/gait ladder **(Fig. 19.36)**/staircase **(Fig. 19.37)**. As required, gait training should be given with orthosis, such as a Toe pick up splint/Dorsiflexion assist AFO **(Figs. 19.38A and B)**. Though use of walking aids such as sticks/tripod/tetrapod are discouraged, selection of such assistive devices may be done carefully to avoid learned nonuse (not taking load on the affected side) **(Fig. 19.39)**. Homolateral synkinesis, i.e., flexion of affected elbow, when the patient tries to flex the hip and knee to clear the ground in swing phase should be controlled by using an elbow splint (elbow gaiter). If the ankle goes into plantar flexion impairing knee flexion during swing phase (as knee extension and ankle plantar flexion are associated as components of abnormal extensor synergy), a toe pick-up splint/dorsiflexion-assist AFO/Functional electrical stimulation (FES) system) **(Fig. 19.40)**, should be considered for effective ground clearance during swing phase.

Exercises/activities are performed in different positions, such as (a) Lying, (b) Sitting, (c) Kneeling, (d) Standing, etc., which are briefly demonstrated below:
a. Exercise in lying **(Figs. 19.41 and 19.42)**.
b. Exercises in sitting **(Figs. 19.43A to C)**.
c. Exercises in kneeling/half kneeling **(Figs. 19.44A to C)**:
d. Exercises in standing **(Figs. 19.45A to E)**:

Fitness Training

Besides the exercises as per need of the individual patient, breathing exercises, low-intensity aerobic exercises on multigym **(Fig. 19.46)**, low-intensity sports **(Fig. 19.47)**, static cycle exercises, etc., may be considered to improve fitness of the patient.

2. **Specific treatment approaches:**
   a. **Neurodevelopmental/Neurophysiological approaches:**
   Various neurodevelopmental/neurophysiological approaches are used by therapists for the rehabilitation of the hemiplegic patient in the rehabilitation unit/physiotherapy departments. The approaches can be applied in isolation, or in combination (eclectic approach).
   The commonly used approaches are:
   » NDT by Bobaths.
   » Synergistic Movement Patterns by Brunnstrom.

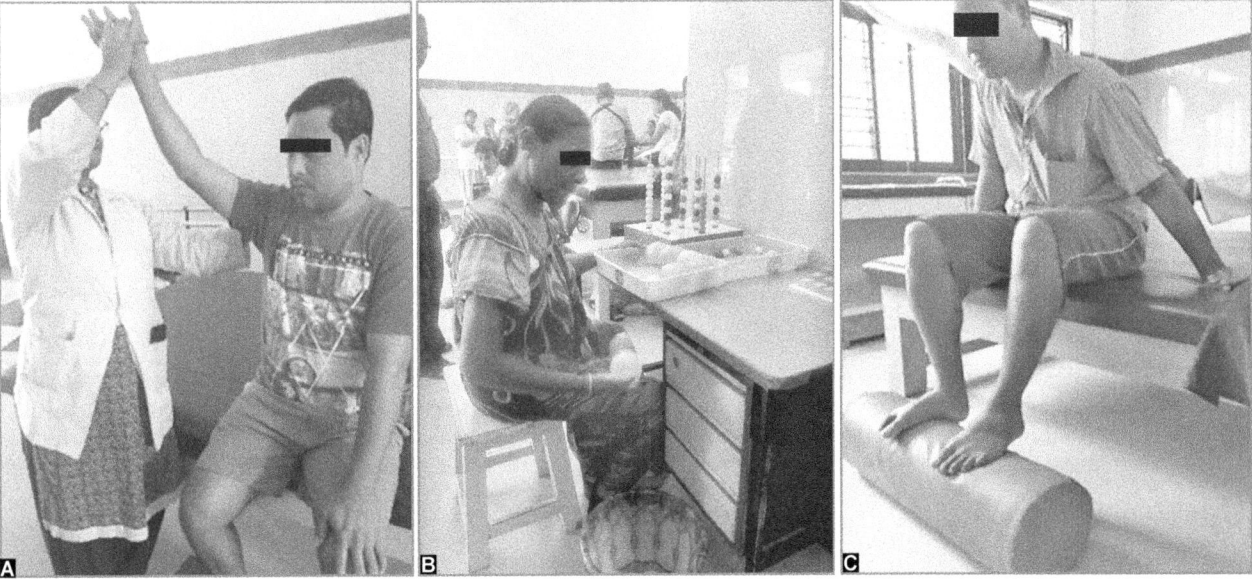

Figs. 19.43A to C: (A) Antispastic pattern of upper limb; (B) Functional use of upper limb; (C) Facilitation of knee flexion through bolster.

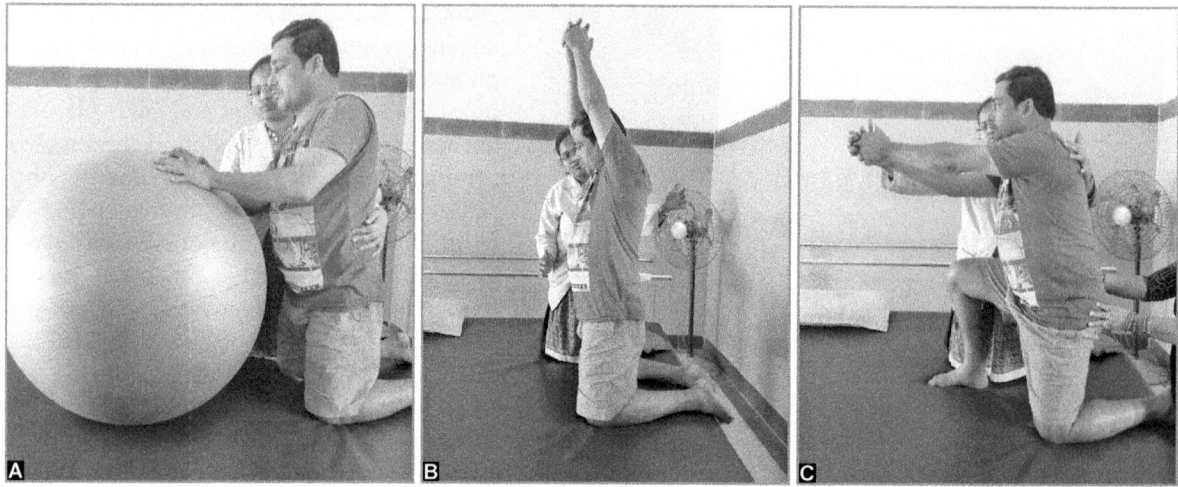

Figs. 19.44A to C: (A) Kneel standing balance training using Swiss ball; (B) Kneel standing with upper limb exercises; (C) Half kneeling with trunk rotation.

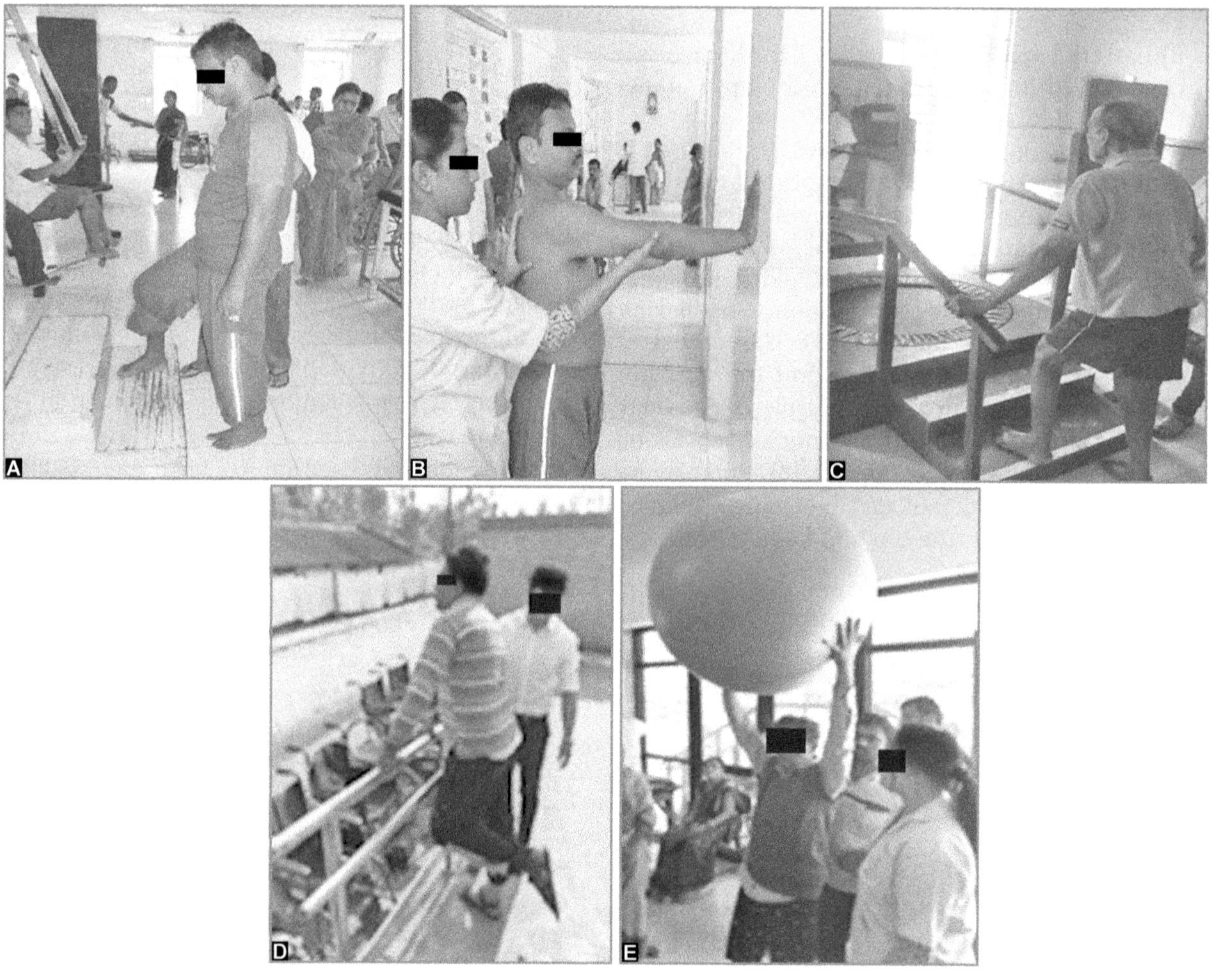

Figs. 19.45A to E: (A) Standing on sound side and stepping up and down with the affected limb to promote hip and knee flexion and vice-versa to promote weight bearing on the affected lower limb; (B) Standing wall push to elongate spastic muscles of upper limb and learn protective strategy; (C) Improvement of hip and knee flexion on affected side through small steps and postural mirror biofeedback; (D) Single leg stance on affected side to promote weight-bearing; (E) Lowering/raising Swiss ball to improve standing balance and upper limb function.

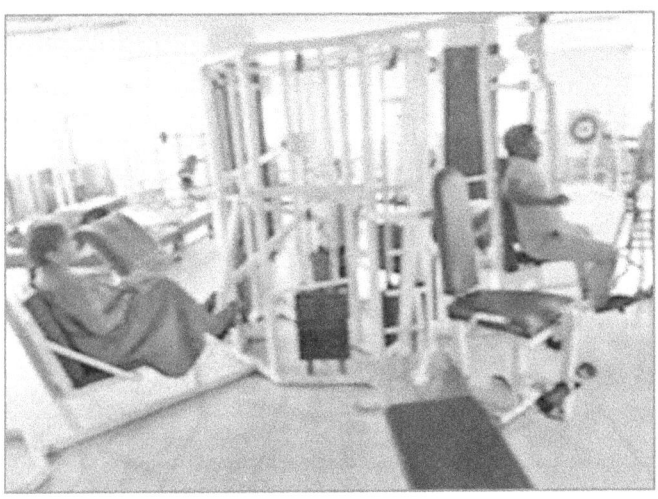

Fig. 19.46: Exercise on multigym.

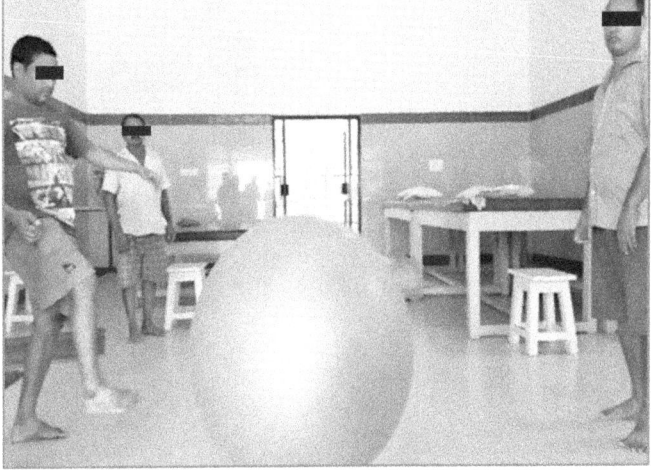

Fig. 19.47: Playing.

- Motor Relearning Program by Janet Carr and Roberta Shephards.
- Conductive Education by Andrews Peto.
- Treatment Technique by Johnstone.
- Sensory Stimulation for Activation and Inhibition by Margarett Roods.
- Proprioceptive Neuromuscular Facilitation by Dr Herman Kabat, Margarett Knotts and Dorothy Voss.
- Sensory Integration Therapy by A Jean Iyers.

The treatment approaches are briefly described as under:

1. **Neurodevelopmental Therapy (NDT):** The Bobath concept is defined as a problem-solving approach to the assessment and treatment of individuals with lesions of the CNS such as stroke. It is based on the dynamic system model of motor control and utilizes the Selectionist model of intervention.

The techniques of inhibition, such as reflex inhibitory positions (**Figs. 19.9 to 19.12**), slow sustained stretching (**Fig. 19.16B**), etc., are utilized to inhibit abnormal tone, abnormal movement synergies/spasticity. Techniques of facilitation such as reflex inhibitory patterns (**Figs. 19.48A and B**), weight bearing/ weight shifting (**Fig. 19.15**), etc., are applied to promote functional movements. Key point stimulation is combined with techniques of inhibition and facilitation to inhibit abnormal pattern and promote normal posture and functional movement pattern (**Figs. 19.49A and B**). As the patient learns normal movement pattern through repeated practice (motor learning strategies), gradually task is added to movement (**Figs. 19.50A and B**). After he/she is able to perform the task, gradually assistance is withdrawn (fading of control), so that, the activities are performed independently (**Fig. 19.51**). The family members should be advised to provide the patient opportunities and guidance to perform functional activities at home.

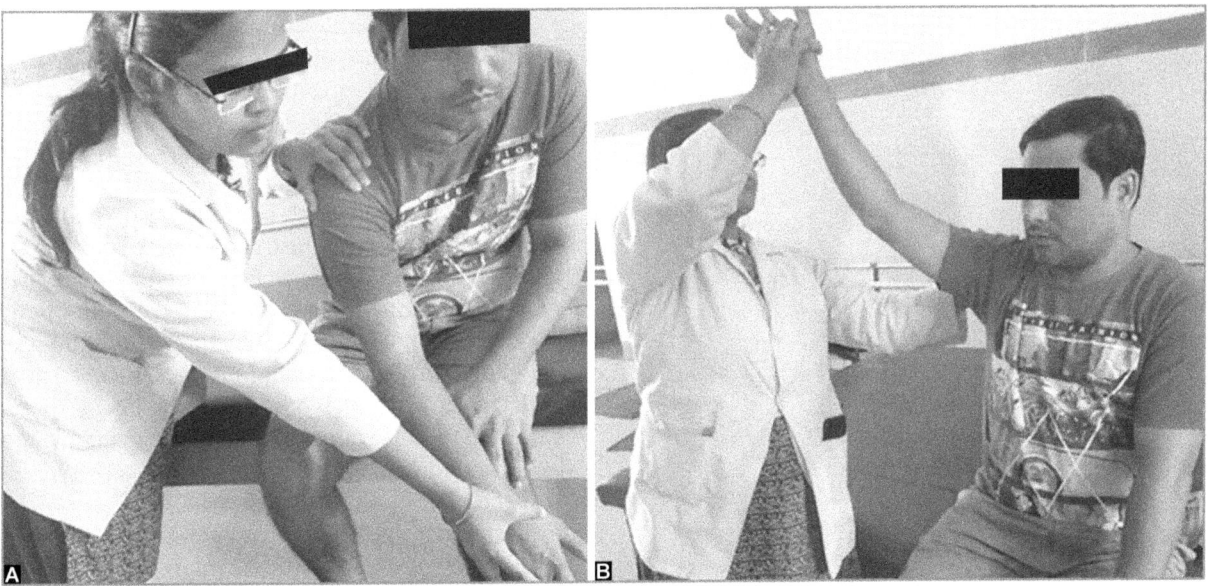

Figs. 19.48A and B: (A) Reflex inhibitory pattern with proximal and distal key point stimulation, to facilitate forward and downward movements; (B) Reflex inhibitory pattern with proximal and distal key point stimulation, to facilitate upward and sideway movements.

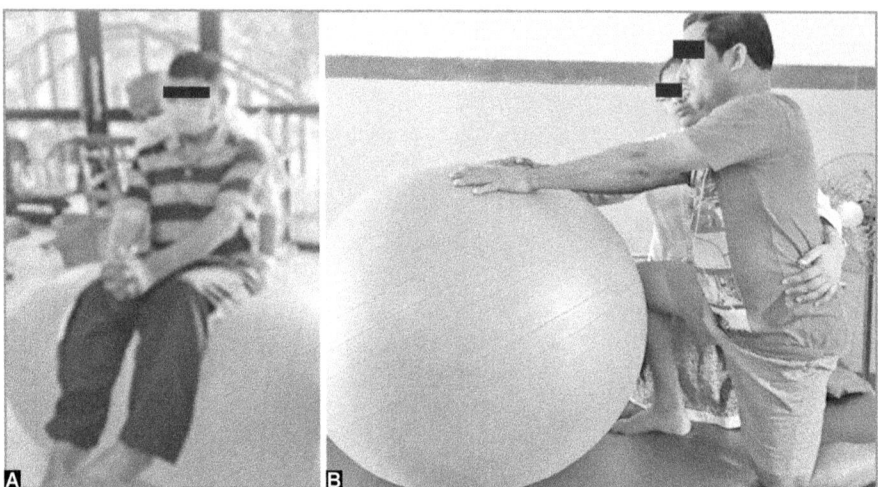

Figs. 19.49A and B: (A) Facilitation of sitting through key point (pelvis) stimulation on Swiss ball; (B) Facilitation of uprighting and inhibition of extensor tone in the right lower limb and flexor tone in the right upper limb, through proximal (pelvis) key point stimulation using the Swiss ball.

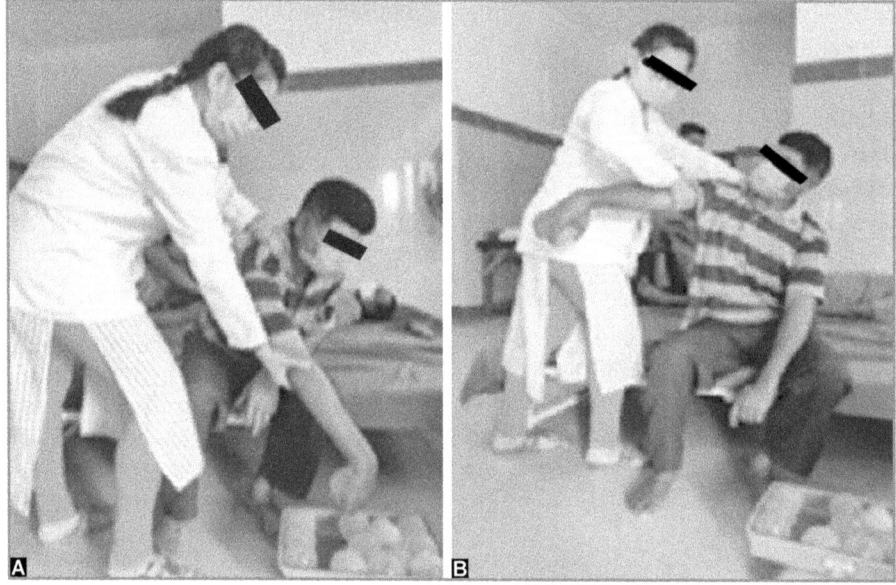

Figs. 19.50A and B: Reflex inhibitory pattern with key point stimulation for manipulation of functional task.

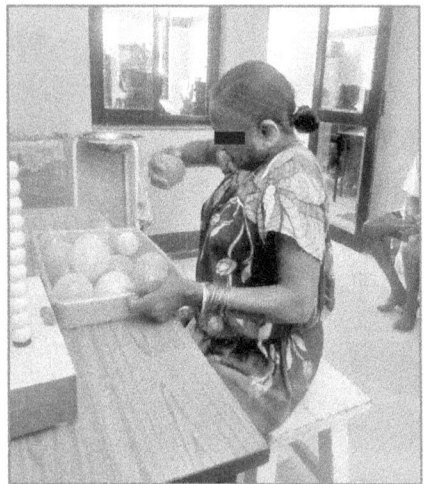

Fig. 19.51: Independent performance of the task.

2. **Motor Relearning Program:** This approach given by Janet Carr and Roberta Shepherd focuses on training of functional tasks, through ongoing observational analysis of motor performance, use of feedback, and discouraging compensatory movements. Emphasis of MRP is on practice of specific real-life activities, the training of cognitive control over muscles and movement components of the activities and conscious elimination of unnecessary muscle activity. The program is based on the following three factors essential for relearning of motor control following stroke:
   – Elimination of unnecessary muscle activity.
   – Feedback.
   – Practice.
   All the seven areas of function are emphasized in the training program, such as:
   – Upper limb function.

- Orofacial function.
- Sitting up from supine.
- Sitting.
- Standing up and sitting down.
- Standing.
- Walking

The steps of the technique involve:

Step-1: Analysis of function **(Fig. 19.52)** to find the missing components of movements through:
- Observation.
- Comparison.
- Analysis.

Step-2: Practice of missing components **(Fig. 19.53)** through:
- Explanation + instruction.
- Practice (with verbal feedback and manual guidance)

Step-3: Practice of activity (whole task) **(Fig. 19.54)**
- Explanation + instruction.
- Practice (with verbal feedback and manual guidance)
- Progression: Increase complexity, add variety, decrease feedback + guidance.

Step-4: Transference of learning through:
- Opportunity for practice.
- Consistency of practice.
- Involvement of relatives and staff.
- Positive reinforcement.
- Stimulating environment.

3. **The Brunnstrom Approach:** This treatment approach was developed by the Swedish physical therapist Signe Brunnstrom. It emphasizes the use of the synergistic patterns of movement for accomplishing function which develops during recovery from hemiplegia. This approach encourages development of flexor and extensor synergies during early recovery, with the intention that synergic activation of muscles will, with training, result in transition into voluntary activation of movements.

The approach is based on use of motor patterns available to patient at any time in the recovery process (i.e., use what you have). Use of synergies/primitive reflex patterns and abnormal movement patterns are made before

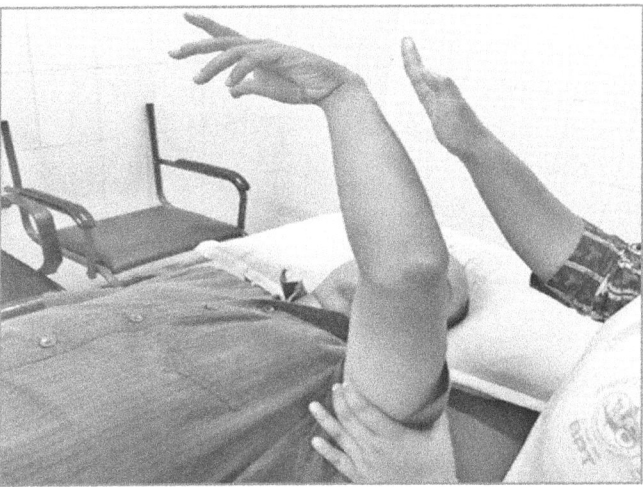

Fig. 19.53: Practice of shoulder flexion/elbow extension.

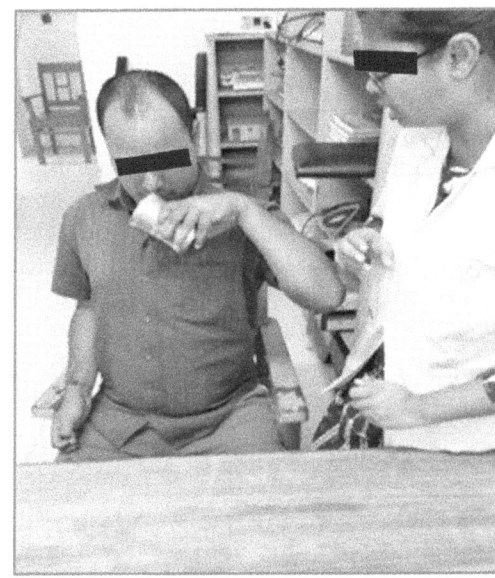

Fig. 19.54: Practice of the task of taking water to mouth with guidance from the physiotherapist.

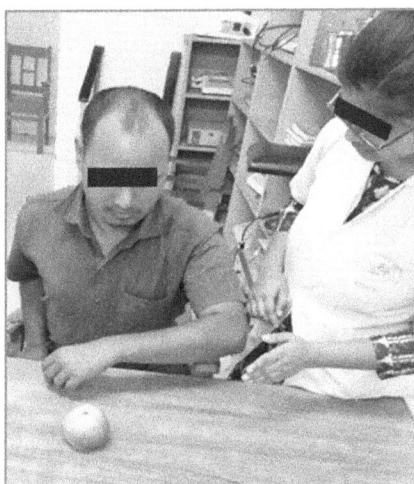

Fig. 19.52: Analysis of reaching/grasping/releasing.

development of voluntary movements **(Fig. 19.55)**. Prognosis may be rapid or slow and could cease at any time.

4. **Conductive Education:** Conductive education is an educational system that has been specifically developed for children and adults who have motor disorders of neurological origin. Like cerebral palsy, it can also be used for stroke patients with hemiplegia. It is a group therapy, which motivates other patients to initiate/produce movements by observing movements produced by the co-performer **(Figs. 19.56A and B)**.

5. **Proprioceptive Neuromuscular Facilitation (PNF):** This is a concept of treatment. Its underlying philosophy is that all human beings, including those with disabilities, have untapped existing potential (Kabat, 1950). PNF uses the body's proprioceptive system to facilitate or inhibit muscle contraction. One of the pioneers in the use of PNF, Dorothy Voss, defined it as a method of promoting or hastening the

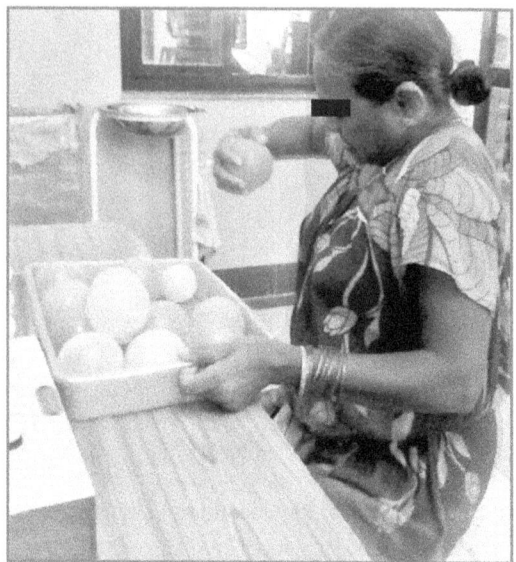

Fig. 19.55: Use of flexor synergy for performing functional tasks, which can be utilized for taking food to mouth.

response of the neuromuscular mechanism through the stimulation of proprioceptors.

Proprioceptive neuromuscular facilitation is one of the major therapeutic approaches aimed at improving the important features necessary for the functional ambulation of hemiplegic patients, such as muscular tone, strength, and flexibility.

The approach encompasses mass movement patterns that are spiral and diagonal in nature and resemble movements seen in functional activities **(Figs. 19.57 and 19.58)**.

6. **Sensory integration therapy:** This technique of treatment was devised by A Jean Iyers, a trained Occupational therapist. Sensory integration is the ability to take in information through the senses of touch, movement, smell, taste, vision, and hearing, and to combine the resulting perceptions with prior information, memories, and knowledge-already stored in the brain, in order to derive coherent meaning from processing the stimuli. Stroke patients with impairment of sensory integration, fails to maintain posture and balance besides loss of other functions such as stereognosis, co-ordinated movements, etc. This therapy when applied to such patients is of great benefit to them like cerebral palsy. The following figures **(Figs. 19.59A and B)** demonstrate a few treatment strategies.

7. **Rood's Approach:** Margaret Rood, a Physiotherapist and Occupational Therapist gave this approach, which focuses on eliciting motor response through various afferent stimuli.

There are four components:
1. Normalization of tone: Through sensory stimulation; necessary for correct motor response.
2. Sensorimotor control is developmentally based:
   a. Therapy must start at developmental level of the patient.
   b. Use is made of facilitation and inhibition techniques to normalize muscle tone and movements.
   c. Treatment starts at head and works downward.
   d. Treatment is directed from proximal to distal.
   e. Stimulate flexors then extensors then adductors then abductors.
3. Movement is purposeful:
   a. Patient focused on end goal (pick up glass) vs. movement.
   b. Patient gains control over movement that has been elicited reflexively (through natural movement)
4. Repetition:
   a. Necessary for learning
   b. Activities provide purpose and repetition (reaching for cones, standing up)

Techniques used:

a. Facilitatory technique:
   » To normalize the muscle tone from a flaccid state: Icing, fast brushing, tapping, stroking, and quick stretch.

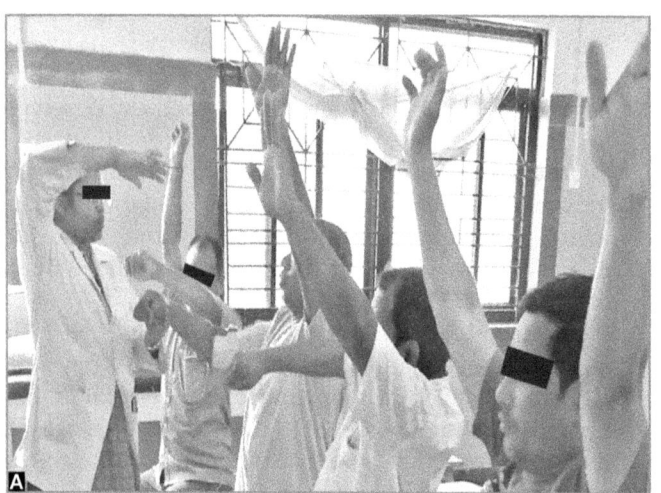
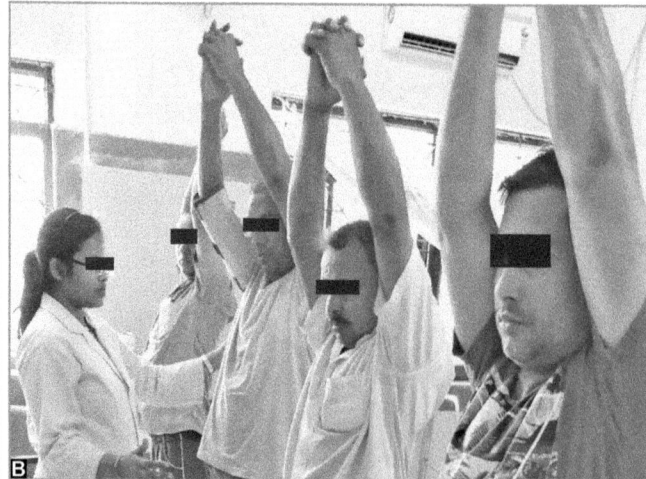

Figs. 19.56A and B: The conductive education program in progress.

Chapter 19: Stroke/Cerebrovascular Accident

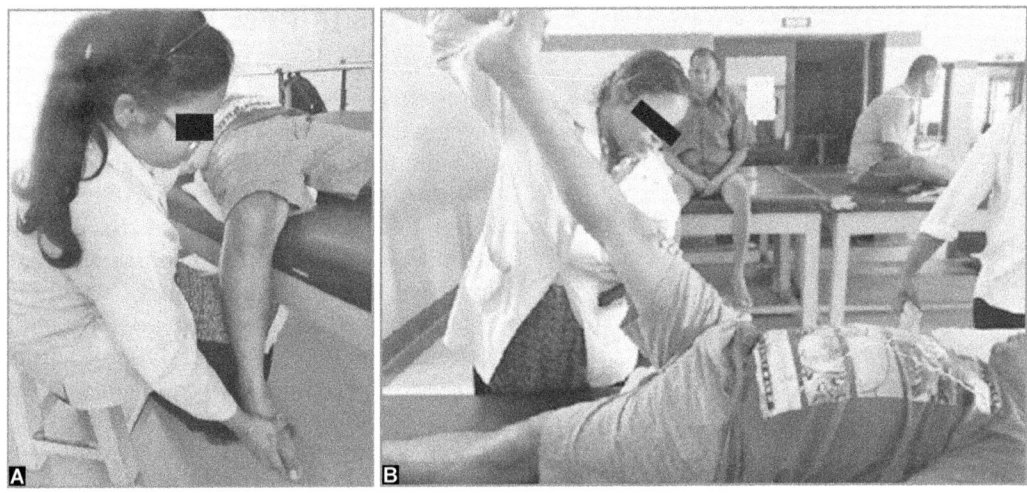

Figs. 19.57A and B: (A) D1 Extension with knee flexion; (B) D1 Flexion with knee extension.

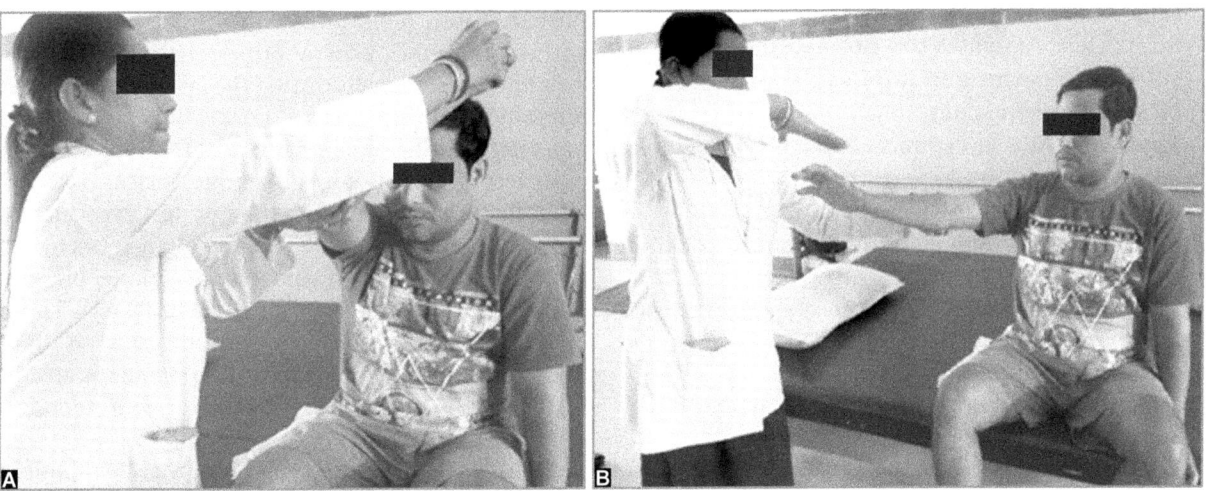

Figs. 19.58A and B: (A) D1 flexion with elbow flexion; (B) D1-extension with elbow extension.

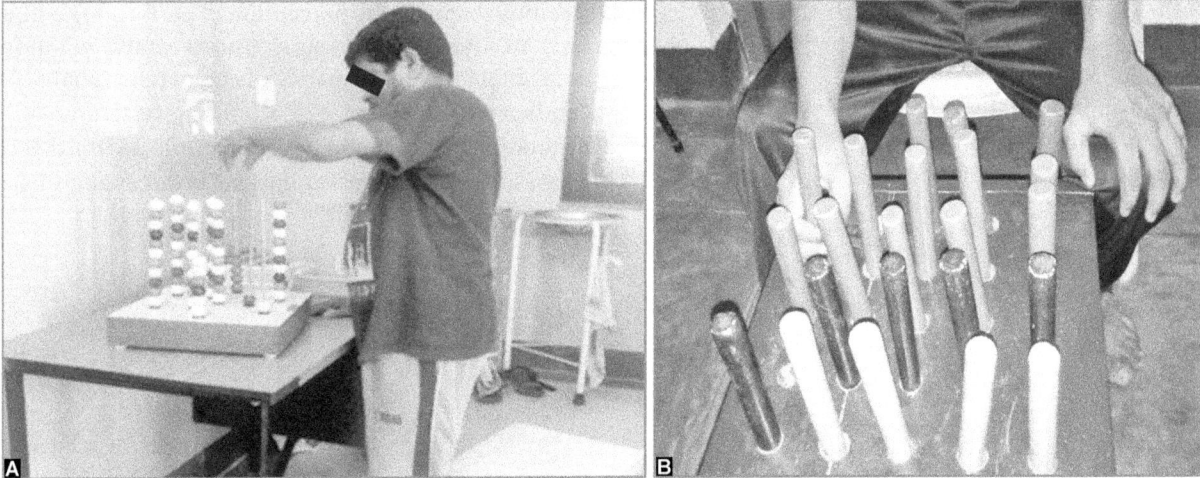

Figs. 19.59A and B: Sensory integration therapy.

Controlled sensory input for facilitation:
- Light moving touch (3 to 5 strokes with 30 seconds between stimuli).
- Fast brushing (by battery-operated brush).
- Quick icing (Good for hypotonic muscles, as it elicits reflex response or withdrawal).

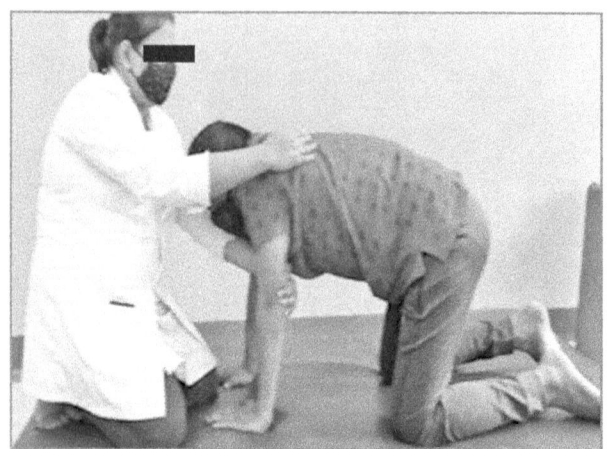

Fig. 19.60: Application of joint compression in prone kneeling.

» Heavy joint compression (side lying, prone kneeling **(Fig. 19.60)**, prone on elbow).
» Stretching: Activates the proprioceptors in the selected muscles and implies the principles of reciprocal innervations.
» Resistance (Muscle contracts through application of resistance).
» Tapping (Over muscle belly).
» Vestibular: Movement through planes: rocking, rolling, spinning, swinging.
» Vibration: Use of vibrator over muscle belly to activate contraction.

b. **Inhibitory technique:**
» To normalize the muscle tone from hypertonic or spastic state.
» Deep pressure, slow rolling **(Figs. 19.61A and B)**, and slow rocking.
» Neutral warmth: Wrapping the patient in blanket for 15–20 minutes, which helps in reducing muscle tone.
» Gentle shaking/rocking (slow/rhythmical).

Slow rolling: Side-lying, rolling upper body and lower body segmentally.

8. **Johnstone Approach:** This approach follows developmental sequences, focusing on proximal stability. It makes use of orally inflated pressure splints.

Orthotics and Assistive Devices

As we know the stroke patient movements are dominated by abnormal movement synergies, and associated reactions, to develop the schema of normal posture and movements, it is essential that the patient should always maintain a normal posture of the body segments, and should move as normally as possible. Further, it is also realized that neuroplasticity is promoted by repeated use of the affected body parts for function, and initially function without assistive and orthotic devices are usually not possible. The Author strongly recommends for the use of dynamic functional orthotic devices to enhance function and static orthotic devices should only be recommended as positional devices.

Some of the orthotic devices used for stroke patients are shown in the **Figures 19.62A to K**.

Robotic Rehabilitation

Research into rehabilitation robotics has grown rapidly and the number of therapeutic rehabilitation robots has expanded dramatically during the last two decades. Robotic rehabilitation therapy can deliver high-dosage and high-intensity training, making it useful for patients with motor disorders caused by stroke. Robotic devices used for motor rehabilitation include end-effector and exoskeleton types. Both end-effector and the exoskeleton devices have proven to be effective complements to conventional physiotherapy in patients with subacute stroke **(Fig.19.63)**. The present evidence supports the use of robot-assisted therapy for improving motor function in stroke patients as an additional therapeutic intervention in combination with the conventional rehabilitation therapies.

There are several strategies employed by robotic systems to retrain movement after stroke. Workstation devices can either use simple games to encourage and guide movements, or integrate simulations of real-life tasks such as cooking or cleaning to create the perception of performing a functional task. An alternative strategy is to use wearable robotic devices to facilitate the performance of actual functional tasks. This can be conceived either as a training system to encourage restoration of motor abilities after removal of the device, or as an assistive device to assist the user on an ongoing basis. This

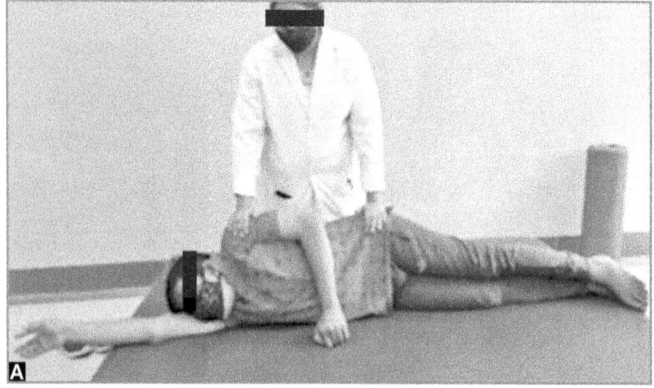
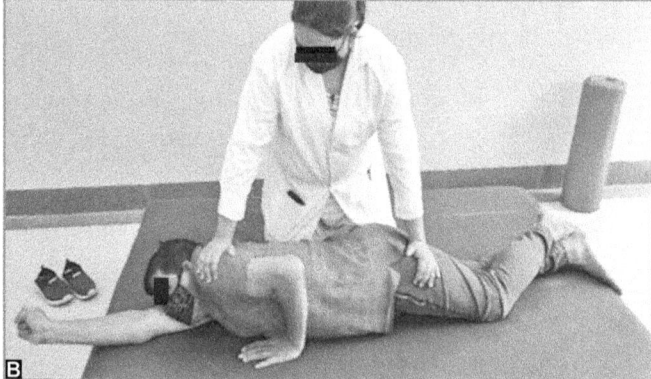

Figs. 19.61A and B: Rolling as a technique of inhibition.

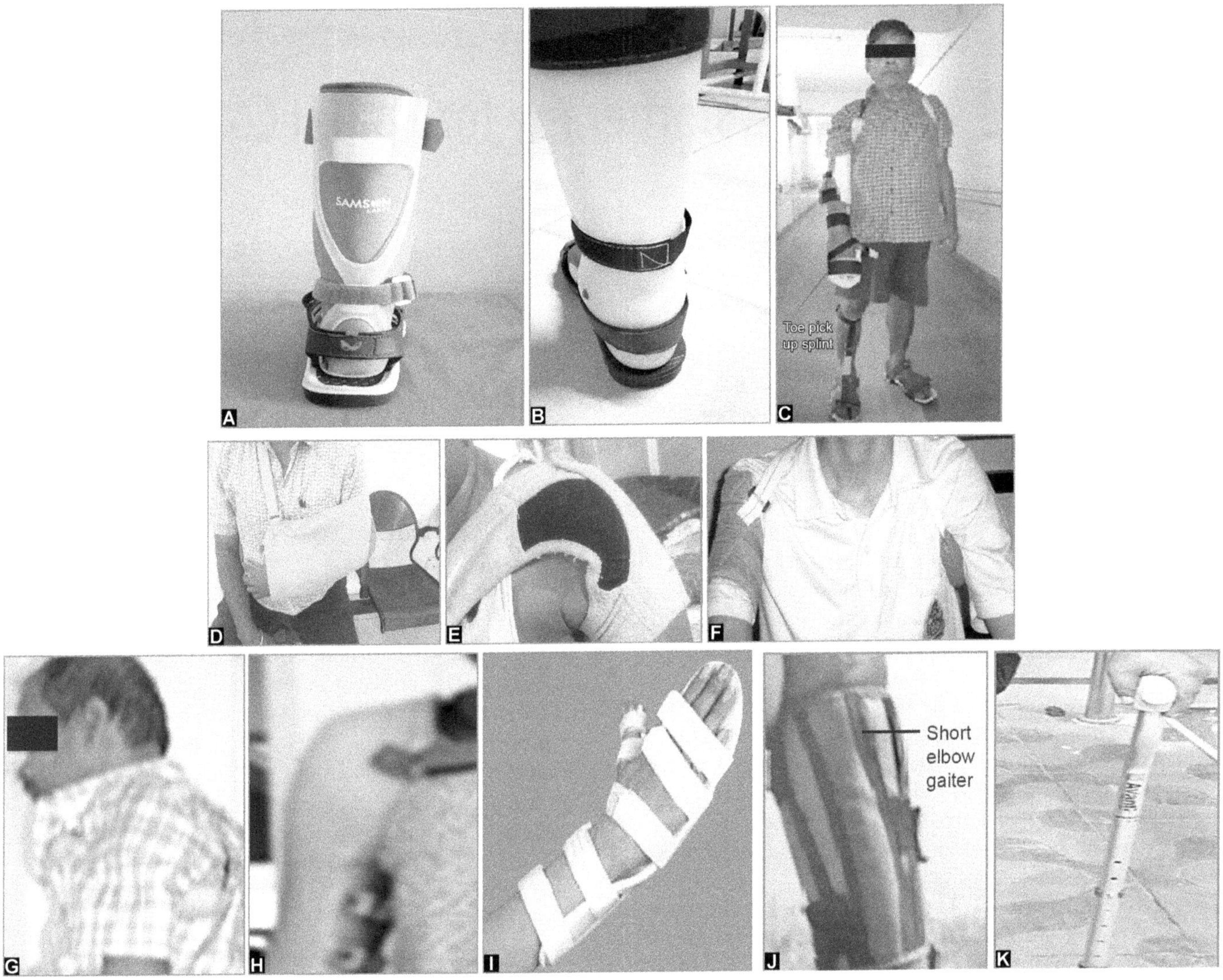

Figs. 19.62A to K: (A) Leaf spring AFO; (B) Dorsiflexion assist AFO; (C) Toe pick up splint; (D) Triangular sling; (E) Neoprene shoulder support; (F) Humeral cuff; (G) Axillary pad; (H) Polypropylene shoulder orthosis; (I) Long cock up splint; (J) Elbow gaiter; (K) Tetrapod stick.

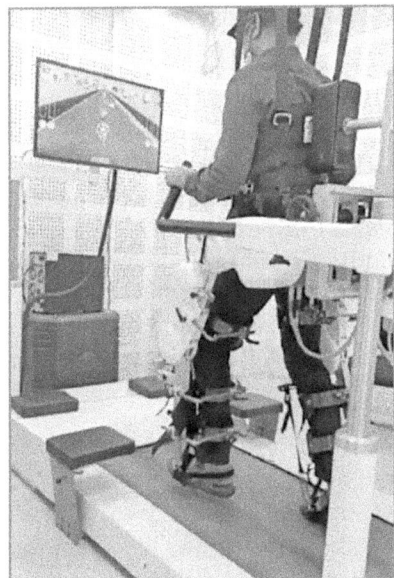

Fig. 19.63: Stroke patient exercising with exo-skeletal type of robotic device.

latter approach is sometimes termed a powered orthosis, or else a neuroprosthesis.

Stem Cell Therapy

Clinical trial for stem cell therapy for stroke patients has not yet yielded satisfactory result. There is evidence that combined with clot busting and mechanical thrombectomy, this therapy enhances recovery. Stem cells injected into distant arteries or veins travel to the site of a stroke in the brain to fuel the repair process. The optimal time for introducing stem cells seems to be between 36 and 72 hours after the stroke.

Physiotherapy for Spinal Cord Injury

INTRODUCTION

In the industrial world, the incidence of spinal cord injury (SCI) is increasing day by day, affecting the individual, the family, society, and the country to a great extent due to the high cost of the disability associated with the disorder. The quality of life of most of the patients becomes miserable due to decreased mobility, loss of job, dependency for self-care, bladder, bowel, and sexual dysfunction.

A spinal cord injury is damage to spinal cord that causes temporary or permanent loss of motor, sensory, and autonomic function in the parts of the body served by the spinal cord below the level of injury. Injury can occur at any level of the spinal cord and can be complete injury, with total loss of sensory and motor function, or incomplete, where some nervous signals are able to travel past the injured area of the cord, with retention of some motor and sensory function below the site of lesion.

Rehabilitation of the spinal cord injured is an important element toward achieving a fulfilling and active life after SCI. A good team work of different professionals, combined with support from Government and Nongovernment Organizations make the living of the affected individuals comfortable.

Spinal cord injury is divided into two categories depending on the etiology:
1. Traumatic SCI, caused by road traffic accidents, industrial trauma, domestic trauma, fall from heights, gunshot injury, sports injury, etc.
2. Nontraumatic SCI, caused by thrombosis, embolism, tumors, infections, etc.

About 50% of spinal cord injuries occur in cervical spine, while nearly 15% injuries occur each in thoracic spine, thoracolumbar spine, and lumbar spines.

The injury is typically divided into two broad functional categories such as:
1. **Tetraplegia (Quadriplegia)/Quadriparesis:** It refers to complete paralysis/incomplete involvement of all four extremities and trunk, including the respiratory muscles, and results from lesions of cervical cord.
2. **Paraplegia/paraparesis:** It refers to complete paralysis/incomplete involvement of all or part of the trunk and both lower extremities, resulting from lesions of thoracic or lumbar spinal cord and cauda equina.

Anatomy of Spinal Cord

There are 31 pairs of spinal nerves such as:
- 8 Cervical.
- 12 Thoracic.
- 5 Lumbar.
- 5 Sacral.
- 1 Coccygeal.

The nerve roots for C1–C7 exit above the corresponding vertebrae. The C8 root exits below the C7 vertebra. The remaining nerve roots exit in a downward direction and do not exit at the corresponding vertebral level. During fetal development, the spinal cord fills the entire length of the vertebral canal and the spinal nerves run in a horizontal direction. As the vertebral column elongates and the person grows, the spinal cord, which does not elongate at the same rate, is drawn upward ending at the lower border of L1.

In adults the spinal cord ends in conus medullaris at L1 vertebral level. The nerve roots assume an increasingly oblique and downward direction, and runs in an almost vertical direction in the lumbar area giving the appearance of a horse's tail (Cauda equina). Because of this the vertebral injury does not correspond with the spinal cord segmental level injury.

The relationship between vertebral levels and corresponding spinal segments are given in **Table 20.1**.
The spinal tracts include **(Fig. 20.1)**:
- **Descending tracts (Motor):** Anterior corticospinal tract, lateral corticospinal tract.
- **Ascending tracts (Sensory):** Spinothalamic tract, spinocerebellar tract, the dorsal column tracts.

The descending spinal tracts and their functions are described in **Table 20.2**.
The ascending spinal tracts and their function are described in **Table 20.3**.

Determination of Level of Lesion

The determination of level of lesion after SCI is important, as the extent of neurological involvement and planning of management is decided from the level of lesion. The extent of loss of motor and sensory function after injury has a large impact on medical and rehabilitation management of the individual.

Table 20.1: Relation between spinal segment and vertebrae.

Regions of spinal column	Spinal segments	Vertebral level	General rule
Upper cervical	C2	C2	Same level
Lower cervical	C6	C5	Add: 1 to the vertebral level to get the corresponding spinal segment.
Upper thoracic	T5	T3	Add: 2 to the vertebral level to get the corresponding spinal segment.
Lower thoracic	T10	T7	Add: 3 to the vertebral level to get the corresponding spinal segment.
Lumbar	L1–L5	T10–T11	The lumbar segments are located 3–5 vertebrae above the corresponding lumbar vertebrae.
Sacral and coccygeal	S1–S5 C X 1	T12–L1	The sacral and coccygeal segments are located, 6–10 vertebrae above the corresponding sacral and coccyx vertebrae.

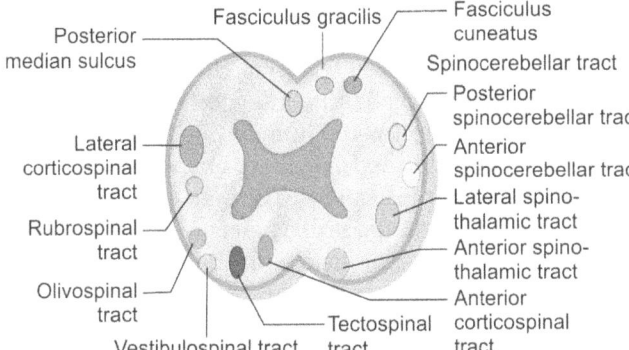

Fig. 20.1: The tracts in the spinal cord.

Table 20.2: The descending spinal tracts and their function.

Tract	Function
Lateral corticospinal tract	Voluntary movements
Anterior corticospinal tract	Voluntary movement of axial muscles
Medial vestibulospinal tract	Positioning of head and neck
Lateral and medial vestibulospinal tracts	Posture and balance
Lateral and medial reticulospinal tract	Posture, balance and automatic gait-related movements
Rubrospinal tract	Movement of limbs

Table 20.3: The ascending spinal tracts and their function.

Tract	Function
Spinothalamic tract (Lateral)	Pain and temperature
Spinothalamic tract (Anterior)	Light touch and pressure
Posterior column pathways	Deep touch and pressure Discriminative touch Proprioception Vibration
Dorsal and ventral spinocerebellar tract	Conveys unconscious proprioception maintaining posture and coordination.

The neurological level is defined as the most caudal level of the spinal cord with normal motor and sensory function on both sides of the body. The motor level is referred to as the most caudal segment of the spinal cord with normal motor function in the key muscles bilaterally. Sensory level is defined as the most caudal segment of the spinal cord having intact sensation to light touch and pin prick over the key dermatomes bilaterally (score-2).

For myotome, that are not clinically testable, i.e., C1–C4, T2–L1, S2–S5, the motor level is considered same as the sensory level.

Classification of Spinal Cord Injury

Clinicians all over the world classify SCI using a method developed by the International Standards for Neurological Classification of Spinal Cord Injury (ISNCSCI).

The ISNCSCI is based on three scores:
1. **American Spinal Injury Association (ASIA) motor score, which grades muscle strength and movement:** Key muscle strength grading **(Fig. 20.6)**.
2. **The ASIA sensory score, which grades light touch and pinprick feeling:** Key sensory point grading **(Fig. 20.6)**.
3. The ASIA Impairment Scale grade, which determines whether the injury is complete or incomplete.

❖ **Key muscle strength grading:** Grading of the key muscles (Elbow flexors: C5, wrist extensors: C6, elbow extensors: C7, finger flexors: C8, finger adductors: T1, hip flexors: L2, knee extensors: L3, ankle dorsiflexor: L4, great toe extensor: L5, ankle plantar flexor: S1) are done using the MRC grading system starting from: 0—No contraction, 1—Flickering of muscle contraction. 2—Full range of movement with gravity elimination. 3—Full range of movement against gravity without resistance, 4—Full range of movement against gravity with minimum resistance, 5—Full range of movement against gravity with maximum resistance.

❖ **Key sensory point grading**: Scoring of sensation for light touch and pin prick is based on a 3-point ordinal scale, having scores: 0—Absent, 1—Impaired, 2—Normal. Those areas could not be tested should be mentioned "NT". The total sensory score is 112 for light touch (28 points left + 28 points right = 56 × 2 = 112) and 112 (28 points left + 28 points right = 56 × 2 = 112) for pinprick.

❖ **The ASIA Impairment Scale** assigns the SCI a grade based on its severity. Grades range from A to E, with A being the most severe injury and E being the least severe. The ASIA grades include:

- *Grade A:* Complete sensory or motor function loss below the level of injury.
- *Grade B:* Sensation is preserved below the level of injury, but motor function is lost.
- *Grade C:* Motor function below the level of injury is preserved, with more than half of the key muscles receiving a less than 3 grade on the ASIA motor score.
- *Grade D:* Motor function below the level of injury is preserved, with more than half of the main muscles receiving at least a 3 or greater grade on the ASIA motor score.
- *Grade E:* Normal sensation and motor function.

Complete, Incomplete Injury, and Zone of Partial Preservation

- **Complete injury:** Clinically an injury is said to be complete, if there is no sensory or motor function in the lowest sacral segments (S4-S5), which are determined from absence of perianal sensation and loss of ability to contract the external anal sphincter voluntarily.
- **Incomplete injury:** An injury is said to be incomplete, if some motor and/or sensory functions are preserved below the neurological level, including sensory and/or motor function at S4-S5. The anal sphincter is innervated by the S4-S5 cord and represents the end of the spinal cord. The anal sphincter is a critical part of the SCI examination. If the person has any voluntary anal contraction, regardless of any other finding, that person is by definition a motor incomplete injury. With incomplete SCI, some function and feeling remain below the injury level. Typically, one side of the body may have more function or feeling than the other side. There are different types, or syndromes, of incomplete SCI described below, that include central cord syndrome, Brown-Séquard syndrome, anterior cord syndrome, and posterior cord syndrome.
- **Zone of partial preservation:** Zone of partial preservation (ZPP) is said to exist, if some sensory and/or motor function exists below the neurological level, without sensory and/or motor function in areas supplied by S4-S5. The areas of intact motor and/or sensory function below the neurological level are termed as ZPP.

Sacral sparing

The presence of any sacral sparing indicates an incomplete SCI. Sacral sparing can be sparing of sensory, motor, or reflex function, which can be evaluated through tests of great toe flexor activity, rectal motor function, and perianal sensation.

Clinical Syndromes Associated with Spinal Cord Injury

Central Cord Syndrome

Central cord syndrome **(Fig. 20.2)** is the most common incomplete SCI syndrome, occurring in 15–25% of traumatic SCIs. This is common in elderly patients with a history of cervical spondylosis and spinal stenosis who suffer an SCI from a traumatic fall. This usually results from hyperextension injury to cervical spinal cord. The central aspect of the spinal cord is affected with hemorrhage and edema. The upper extremities are more severely affected (due to more central location of cervical tracts) by neurological involvement than the lower extremities (as the lumbar and sacral tracts are more peripherally located). Sensory impairments are less severe than motor impairments. The patients usually retain normal bladder, bowel, and sexual function. Patients typically recover the ability to ambulate with some degree of distal upper extremity weakness.

Brown-Sequard Syndrome

Brown-Sequard syndrome results from injury to one half of the spinal cord (hemisection) **(Fig. 20.3)**, mostly due to penetrating wounds such as gun-shot wounds. The patient presents with asymmetrical features, such as: Ipsilateral to lesion, there is muscle paralysis due to damage to the lateral corticospinal tract, and loss of light touch, proprioception, and vibratory sensation due to damage to the dorsal column, and contralateral to the lesion, damage to the spinothalamic tract results in loss of pain and temperature sensation. Patients with this syndrome gain good function with rehabilitation therapies.

Anterior Cord Syndrome

Anterior cord syndrome results from flexion injury to cervical spinal cord from fracture/dislocation/disc prolapse, resulting in damage to the anterior portion of the spinal cord **(Fig. 20.4)**. It is characterized by loss of

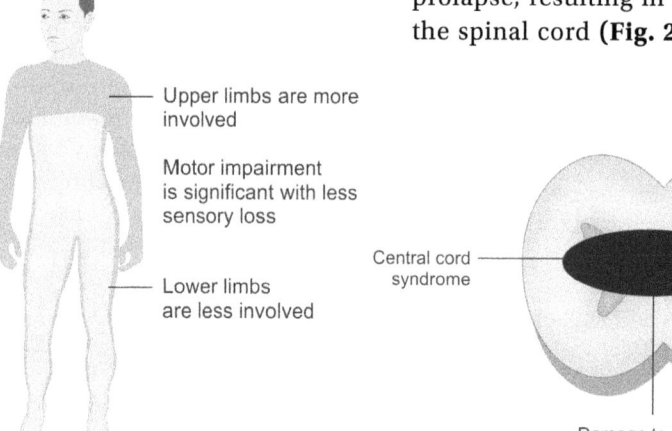

Fig. 20.2: Central cord syndrome.

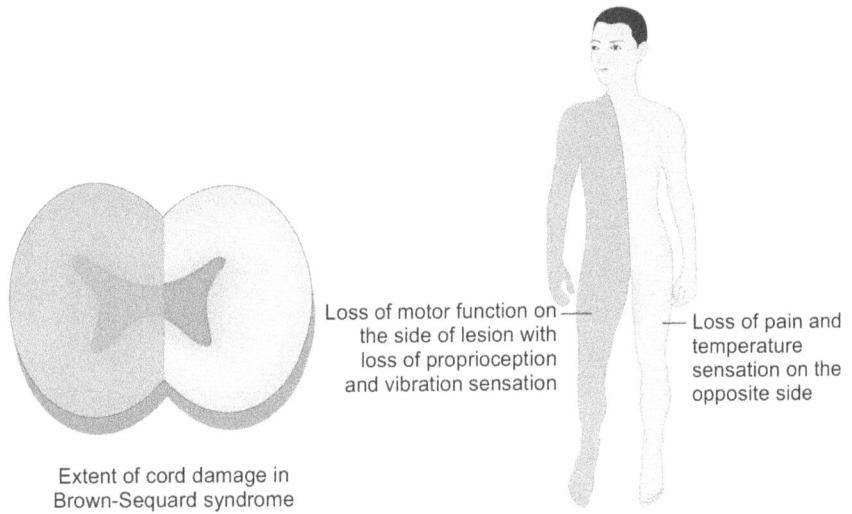

Fig. 20.3: Brown-Sequard syndrome.

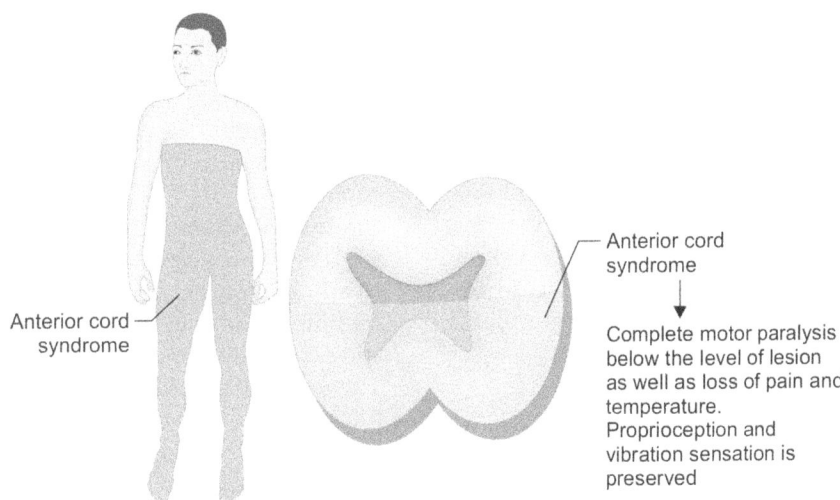

Fig. 20.4: The anterior cord syndrome.

motor function (due to damage to the corticospinal tract), and loss of pain and temperature sensation (spinothalamic tract damage), below the site of lesion. Proprioception, light touch, and vibratory senses are usually preserved, as they are mediated by the posterior column. Individuals with this syndrome require longer hospitalization compared to other syndromes.

Posterior Cord Syndrome

Posterior cord syndrome is the least frequent syndrome affecting the dorsal column of the spinal cord. Injury to the posterior column **(Fig. 20.5)** results in the loss of fine touch, proprioception, kinesthesia, and vibration with intact motor function below the level of lesion.

Cauda Equina Syndrome

In this syndrome, the lesion occurs to the spinal cord below the conus medullaris, where collection of long nerve roots, called cauda equina exists. This lesion is frequently anatomically incomplete, owing to the greater number of nerve roots involved and the comparatively, the large surface area they encompass.

Individuals with cauda equina injury exhibit variable paralysis of muscles of lower limb, saddle anesthesia, areflexic bladder, and bowel. Cauda equina lesions are lower motor neuron (LMN) injuries, behaving like peripheral nerve injuries and have the same potential for recovery like peripheral nerve injuries. The rate of regeneration gradually slows and usually stops after 1 year.

Clinical Features of Spinal Cord Injury

Stage of Spinal Shock

Following SCI, there is a period of spinal shock, which usually develops between 24 and 72 hours after the injury. Spinal shock is manifested by absence of bulbocavernosus reflex, hypotension, bradycardia, and complete loss of motor function, sensation, and reflexes. Bulbocavernosus reflexes are tested by compressing the glans penis in males or by applying pressure to the clitoris in females and observing contraction of

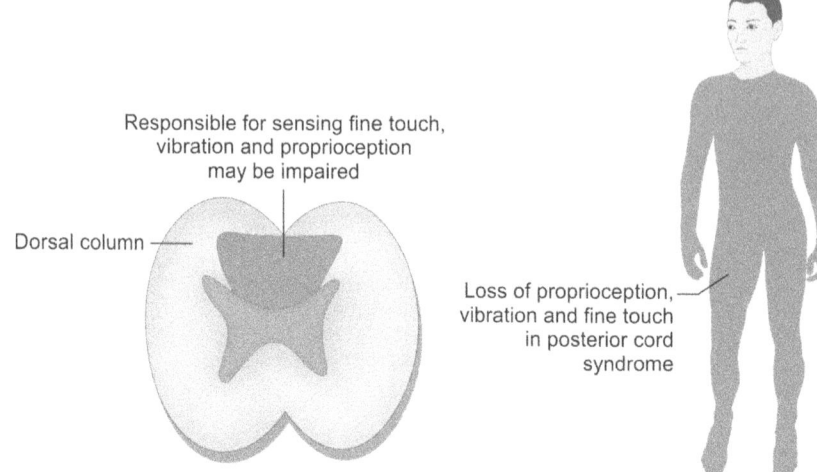

Fig. 20.5: The posterior cord syndrome.

the anal sphincter. This is an oligosynaptic reflex that is used to assess the integrity of sacral sensory and motor fibers, as well as the sacral spinal cord segments, S2-S4.

Spinal shock evolves over time. The initial period of total areflexia lasts approximately 24 hours. This is followed by a gradual return of reflexes 1-3 days after injury, a period of increasing hyperreflexia lasting for 1-4 weeks, and final hyperreflexia, spasticity, clonus (ankle/patellar) developing 1-6 months after injury. The mechanism of spinal shock involves sudden loss of conduction in the spinal cord as a result of migration of potassium ions from the intracellular to the extracellular spaces.

Motor Features

For lesions above the conus medullaris, spastic hypertonia causing paraplegia/quadriplegia typically emerges below the level of lesion after spinal shock subsided. Spastic hypertonia increases gradually during the first 6 months of injury reaching the peak at about 1 year after injury. Patients with cauda equina lesion develop flaccid paraplegia/paraparesis, and those with conus medullaris lesion develop paraplegia/paraparesis having both upper and lower motor features in the lower limbs. Those having lesion above the conus medullaris develop spastic paraplegia/hemiplegia/quadriplegia, depending on the site of lesion.

Lesions above the conus medullaris results into two types of manifestations such as:

- **Paraplegia in extension:** This results from incomplete injury to spinal cord, where only pyramidal tracts are involved. The lower limbs take an extension attitude. This type of paraplegia carries a better prognosis as compared to paraplegia in flexion.
- **Paraplegia in flexion:** This results from complete injury to the spinal cord, where both pyramidal and extrapyramidal tracts are involved. The lower limbs take an attitude of flexion. This type of paraplegia carries a poor prognosis.

Paraplegia can be graded into four types depending on the severity of the lesion, which are described below:

- **Grade I-Negligible:** The patient is unaware of neurological deficits. Clinicians detect ankle/patellar clonus and extensor plantar response, while examining a patient for neck or back problems.
- **Grade II-Mild:** The patient is aware of deficits and has signs of spasticity. He/she manages to walk with/without support.
- **Grade III-Moderate:** The patient is usually nonambulatory, with severe weakness and paraplegia in extension.
- **Grade IV-Severe:** The patient is unable to walk with paraplegia in flexion with complete sensory loss and sphincter disturbances.

The motor features are variable, which is as per the part of the spinal cord involved. The motor (physical features) depending upon the sites of injury are briefly discussed below.

Cervical cord injuries:

- **High-cervical cord injury (C1–C4):**
  - Paralysis/paresis of upper limbs, trunk, and lower limbs resulting in tetraplegia/quadriplegia.
  - Patient may not be able to breathe on his or her own, cough, or control bowel or bladder movements.
  - Ability to speak is sometimes impaired or reduced.
  - Requires complete assistance with activities of daily living, such as eating, dressing, bathing, and getting in or out of bed.
  - May be able to use powered wheelchairs with special controls to move around inside home on their own.
- **Low-cervical cord injury (C5-T1):**
  - *C5:* Likely to have some or total paralysis of wrists, hands, trunk, and legs. Needs assistance with most activities of daily living, but once in a power wheelchair, can move from one place to another independently.
  - *C6:* Paralysis of hands, trunk, and legs. Wrist extension is not possible. Can speak and use diaphragm, but breathing will be weakened. Can move in and out of wheelchair and bed with assistive equipment and can propel a modified manual wheel chair indoor and manages to move outside using the powered wheel chair.

- *C7:* Paralysis/paresis of elbow extensors and some finger extensors, though movement of shoulder and bending of elbow is possible. Paralysis/paresis of trunk and lower limbs are present. Can do most activities of daily living by themselves with adaptive devices, such as a modified spoon, pen, comb, etc. He/she may need assistance with more difficult tasks. Can propel a modified wheel chair on plain surface for short distance. Manages to move outdoor using the powered wheel chair.
- *C8:* Paralysis/paresis affects hand movements as well as paralysis/paresis of muscles of trunk and lower limbs. Patient may try to grasp objects using tenodesis grasp (described later). In a tenodesis grasp, extension of wrist produces shortening of the finger flexors, due to passive insufficiency of the long flexors of hand, resulting grasping movement of hand. The patients can do most activities of daily living by themselves, but may need assistance with more difficult tasks. He/she can propel a manual wheel chair indoor, and can move outdoor using powered mobility.

Thoracic cord injury:
- **T1–T5:**
  - Upper limb function is usually normal. Paraplegia affecting the trunk and lower limbs is the sequel.
  - Patient can use a manual wheelchair.
  - Can stand in a standing frame/parapodium, while some walk (physiological walking) using braces such as HKAFO, with trunk support and walker/crutches.
- **T6–T12 injuries:**
  - Paraplegia affecting the trunk (back extensor and abdominals), and lower limbs depending on the level of injury.
  - Can manage a manual wheelchair.
  - Most of the patients are able to walk with braces [Knee-Ankle-Foot Orthoses (KAFOs/HKAFO/Scot craig orthosis/RGO) and walker/crutches, though the walking is usually physiological.

Lumbar and sacral nerve injuries

Results in LMN type of paralysis/paresis (Cauda equina injury) involving the muscles of the lower limbs, as well LMN type of dysfunction of bladder and bowel. Most patients can manage to walk with KAFOs/AFOs and crutches.

Sensory Features/Pain in SCI

Depending upon the involvement of sensory tracts, the patient may have variable sensory loss (touch/pain/temperature/proprioception/kinesthesia), which may range from complete sensory loss to hypoesthesia.

Nonpainful sensory phenomena or "phantom" sensations are common after SCI. However, the physiological mechanism responsible for these sensations is poorly understood. These postural illusions seem to be due to functional changes in CNS that may occur immediately after SCI. These sensations may be related to strong sensory memory "imprint", that has been established before injury.

A large number of patients with SCI present with diffuse, on-going dysesthesias below the level of lesion, which are burning in quality and usually functionally limiting. The central pain syndrome includes spontaneous, continuous and intermittent pain as well as evoked pain (pain is evoked by non-noxious stimulation of skin-allodynia). The exact mechanism of such pain in SCI patients is not yet understood fully.

Respiratory Function Impairments

Impairments of respiratory function in patients with SCI result from paralysis of muscles of inspiration and expiration, rib fractures, pneumothorax/hemothorax. Paralysis of diaphragm that results from high cervical cord injury, results in paradoxical breathing, where the abdominal wall retracts during inspiration and protrudes during expiration. Alteration in the chest wall, lung and abdominal compliance, in tetraplegic/tetraparesis patients result in increased work of breathing, causing respiratory muscle fatigue.

Autonomic Dysreflexia

A pathological autonomic reflex, which may be life-threatening, typically occurs in patients with lesion to spinal cord above T6. It is triggered by either noxious or non-noxious stimuli, resulting in sympathetic stimulation and hyperactivity. The most common causes include bladder or bowel over distention, from urinary retention and fecal impaction, respectively. Cutaneous or visceral stimulation, below the level of the injury, initiates afferent impulses to the intermediolateral grey columns of the spinal cord, that elicit abnormal reflex sympathetic nervous system activity from T6 to L2. The sympathetic response is exaggerated, due to lack of compensatory descending parasympathetic stimulation and intrinsic post-traumatic hypersensitivity. This leads to diffuse vasoconstriction in the lower 2/3rds of the body, and a significant rise in blood pressure, despite maximum parasympathetic vasodilatory efforts above the level of injury. The symptoms of autonomic dysreflexia include hypertension, bradycardia, headache, profuse sweating, increase spasticity, restlessness, vasoconstriction, constricted pupils, nasal congestion, piloerection, and blurred vision. The uncontrolled hypertension, may result in mild symptoms, such as sweating above the lesion level with goose bumps, blurred vision or headache. The severe hypertension, that results, may also lead to life-threatening complications, including seizure, intracranial bleed, or retinal detachment. There occurs piloerection, pale and cool skin, etc., below the level of the lesion. Sometimes it may also be asymptomatic. If untreated, it can cause seizures, retinal hemorrhage, pulmonary edema, renal insufficiency, myocardial infarction, cerebral hemorrhage and ultimately death. Though the resting systolic blood pressure in SCI patients is less than normal, during episodes of autonomic dysreflexia, systolic blood pressure may rise to 250–300 mm Hg, and diastolic blood pressure may rise to 200–220 mm Hg.

Bladder Dysfunction

Spinal cord injury alters the complex reflexive and voluntary control of micturition. The spinal control for micturition, that originates from the sacral segments S2, S3, S4, is affected in lesions above the conus medullaris and sacral segments resulting in spastic/automatic/hyperreflexive/UMN bladder. A hyper reflexive bladder contracts and reflexively empties urine in response to a certain filling pressure. However, there is lack of coordination between detrusor and sphincter (detrusor sphincter dyssynergia) resulting in hesitancy, whereas lesion of the sacral segments or conus medullaris result in an autonomous/flaccid/areflexic/LMN bladder. A flaccid detrusor muscle that results from flaccid bladder leads to storage of excessive urine, causing overflow incontinence.

Bowel Dysfunction

Dysfunction of bowel is a major concern after SCI, affecting the social activities and quality of life of patients significantly. After spinal shock subsided, two types of neurogenic bowel conditions develop, depending on the level of injuries. In lesions above S2 there is a spastic or reflex bowel, as the parasympathetic and internal sphincter connections from S2-S4 are intact. Reflex defecation occurs when the rectum is filled with stool. In cauda equina lesion, where S2-S4 segments are affected, a flaccid/areflexic bowel develops, where reflex emptying of bowel does not occur, causing impaction of feces, as well as incontinence due to flaccidity of external sphincter.

Sexual Dysfunction

Spinal cord injury not only affects the physiological ability to have intercourse, but also affects the psychological aspect of sexuality, significantly affecting the quality of living.

In males erectile capacity is greater in UMN lesions than LMN lesions and greater in incomplete lesions as compared to complete lesions. Two types of erections, i.e., reflexogenic and psychogenic are significantly affected in sufferers of SCI. Reflexogenic erections occur in response to external physical contact for which intact reflex arc mediated through S2-S4 are required. Psychogenic erection mediated from cerebral cortex in response to the desire through thoracolumbar or sacral cord centers are also significantly affected in the SCI patients resulting in sexual dysfunction. There is also a higher incidence for ejaculation in LMN and incomplete lesions as compared to UMN and complete lesions.

In females, with UMN lesions, the reflex arc is intact, hence sexual arousal will likely take place through reflexogenic stimulation, but psychogenic response may be lost. However, with LMN lesions, psychogenic response may be preserved, but reflex response will be lost. In women, fertility is not affected severely as like that of men with SCI. Though the menstrual cycle is interrupted for 4–5 months following injury, subsequently the monthly cycles return, and the potential for conception exists.

Spinal Cord Injury Pain

Pain which develops in approximately in 2/3rd of patients with SCI, is broadly classified as nociceptive (pain arising from the nociceptors in musculoskeletal structures with preserved sensation which result from overuse of arms and back as occurs in prolonged wheelchair propulsion), or neuropathic (pain arising from damage to somatosensory nervous system). Nociceptive pain usually responds to medical management, whereas neuropathic pain is difficult to treat, which significantly affects the quality of life of the patient.

Other Features

Besides the major manifestations in SCI, pressure ulcers, impaired temperature control, postural hypotension, heterotopic ossifications, contractures/deformities are other manifestations found in such patients.

Assessment of Spinal Cord Injury

The clinicians use the ICF model for the assessment and management of the patients with SCI. Besides motor/sensory assessment, contextual factors such as environmental and personal issues need to be assessed to make the rehabilitation process successful.

Assessment of a patient with SCI depends upon the stage when the therapists are involved for management of such patients. In the acute stage, just after trauma, assessment focuses on finding the level of consciousness, higher functions, vital signs, site of injury, nature of injury, level of lesion, completeness (if any) of the lesion. The levels of the lesion are decided from intact motor and sensory function in the particular spinal cord segment, below which, the motor and sensory function are impaired. The ASIA system of assessment is used to establish whether the lesion is complete/incomplete **(Fig. 20.6)**.

Once the patient becomes stable with or without surgery to stabilize the fracture/dislocation (if any), the following assessment protocol are followed for the rehabilitation of the patient.

Subjective Assessment/Examination

It includes demographic data and histories such as:
- **History of present condition/illness:**
  - *Date of SCI:*
  - *Cause of SCI:* Traumatic/nontraumatic.
  - *Progression of the condition:* Whether there is any change in signs and symptoms since the causation of SCI indicated from change of grade as per ASIA impairment scale.
  - *Result of specific investigations:* The clinician should review the results of specific investigations both radiological/serological, which helps him in planning and progressing management.
- **Pastmedical history:**
  - Presence of any comorbidities such as diabetes, hypertension, cardiac disease, etc., which has some impact on management.
  - *Previous neurological disorders:* History of any previous neurological disorders, which have some impact on function.
  - Use of any special equipment, such as walking aids, seating devices, etc., before onset of injury.
  - Any past surgery conducted.
- **Medical history:**
  - Whether the condition was managed conservatively or surgically.

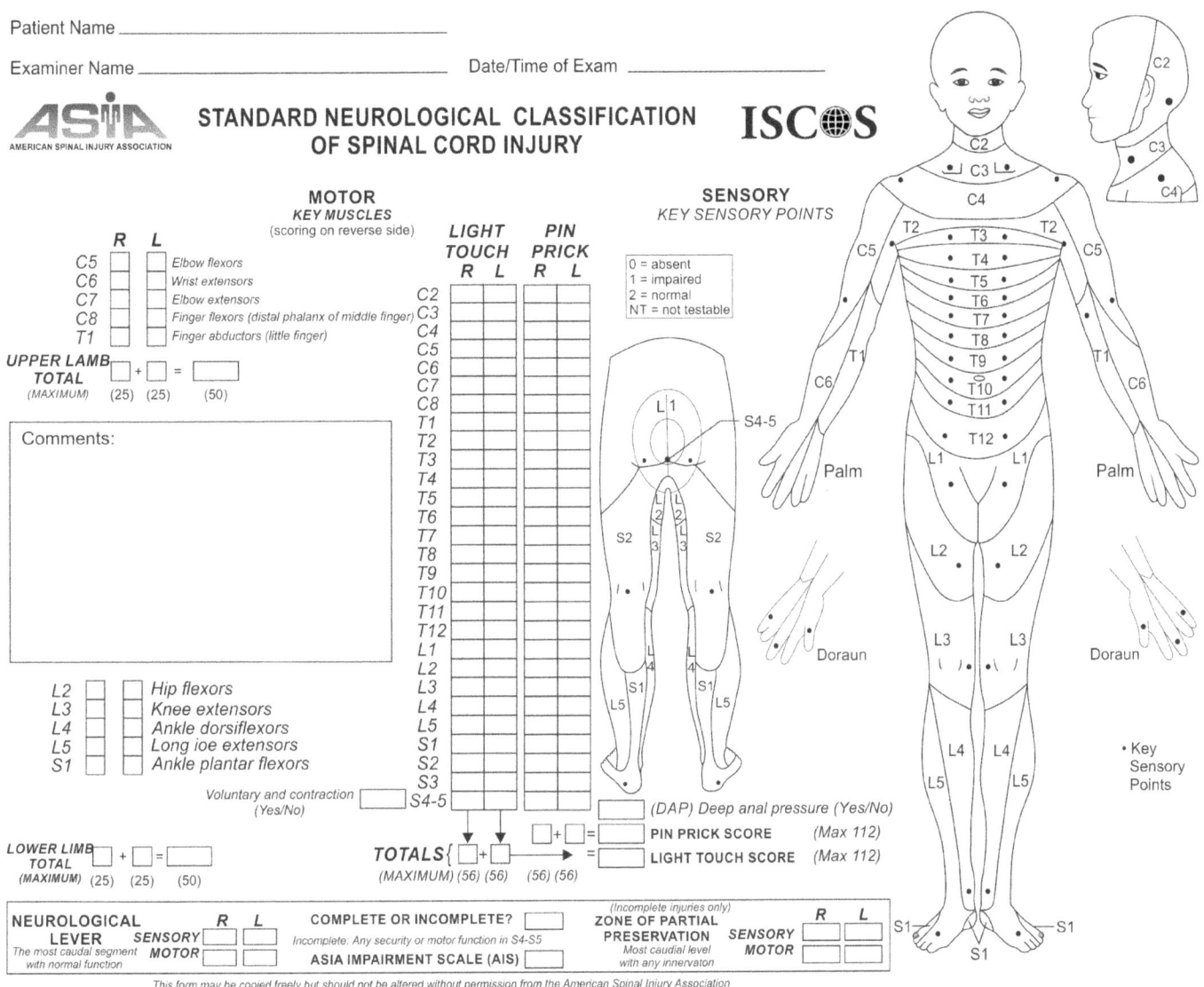

Fig. 20.6: The ASIA system of assessment of spinal cord injury.

- *Previous therapy given:* Whether any physiotherapy, occupational therapy, and orthotics were provided to the client previously.
❖ **Socioeconomic history:** Understanding the patient's social situation and social support systems help the clinicians effectively plan the patient's rehabilitation, hence social data need to be collected for each patient, which include:
  - *Social situation:* Data about the individual's background, e.g., occupation, family, hobbies/recreation.
  - *Social support structures:* It involves finding out of the social supports the individual has from family, friends, colleagues, and dependents.
  - *Accommodation:* The information regarding the living place such as: urban/rural, nature of house such as single or multistoreyed building, access such as stairs with railings, ramps, lifts, etc., need to be collected.
  - Financial status of the family/person.

❖ **Personal/occupational history:** This includes, marital status, hobbies, addiction(if any), educational background, occupation, etc.
❖ **Patient's expectations:** The expectations of the patient in terms of physical achievements need to be explored, which will be taken into consideration for setting goals by the clinician after completing objective assessment.

Objective Assessment/Examination

The functional consequences of an individual with SCI largely depends on an accurate objective assessment, that describe the individual's neurological functions (mostly motor and sensory functions) enabling prediction of future functional achievements from the current impairment status. The key impairments that lead to activity limitations and participation limitations are given emphasis in objective assessment. The components of objective assessment are:

- **Higher functions assessment:** Such as speech, hearing, vision, cognition, and perception in case of associated head injuries.
- **Sensory assessment:** Tactile-light touch and pressure, proprioception, pain, and temperature, all are expected to be affected in SCI; hence, these modalities of sensation need to be assessed. The sensation is assessed using the sensory assessment of the International Standards for Neurological Classifications of SCI to grade the degree of injury (complete/incomplete) and to find the level of injury. Emphasis is given on testing light touch using either cotton, or camel hair brush, as well as pain (finding the ability to perceive pin prick using an alpin). While testing sensation over the trunk, the sensory key points located over the dermatomes aligned along the midclavicular line are tested and while stroking the skin with cotton/brush, the direction followed is outward to inward and maximum length of area stroked should not exceed 1 cm. The same principles are also followed for testing light touch sensation over the sensory key points of the limbs.
- **Motor assessment:** Assessment of muscle nutrition, i.e., atrophy/hypertrophy (if any) is done through observation and limb-girth measurement. Assessment of muscle tone that includes presence of hypotonicity/hypertonicity (spasticity) is done using tone-grading scale having grades from 0 (Flaccid) to 4+ (Moderate to severe hypertonia). Assessment of spasticity is done using Modified-modified Ashworth scale or the Tardieu scale.

Assessment of reflexes:
- **Deep tendon reflexes are graded using the reflex grading scale with a score:** 0 (Absent) to 4+ (Hyperreflexia with clonus).
- **Superficial reflexes that are graded include:**
  - *Babinski's sign:* It refers to dorsiflexion of great toe with or without fanning of other toes and withdrawal of the leg on plantar stimulation of foot. A positive sign indicates pyramidal tract lesion.
  - *Hoffmann's reflex:* Hoffmann's reflex, named for Johann Hoffmann, involves tapping the nail or flicking the terminal phalanx of the middle or ring finger, which produces a positive response in the form of flexion of terminal phalanx of thumb. A positive response is indicative of corticospinal tract lesion.
  - *Abdominal reflex:* Roots involved T7–T12: The procedure involves the patient lying in relaxed supine position with abdomen undressed. The clinician applies stroking over the four quadrants of abdomen from lateral to medial. Response obtained normally is contraction of abdominals and drawing of the umbilicus toward the stimulation side. These reflexes are either reduced or absent in UMN lesions, above their segmental level in spinal cord. They may indicate segmental level of thoracic spinal cord lesion from their absence.

Assessment of muscle strength:
Assessment of muscle strength assists the physiotherapist in establishing the level of lesion as well as in clinical reasoning to decide strengthening programs for rehabilitation of the client. Muscle strength can be assessed by various methods described below such as manual, mechanical, and functional.
- **Manual muscle testing:** The MRC grading is used to assess the power of the key muscles to grade the degree of injury, i.e., complete/incomplete. The muscle power of the trunk and neck and other muscles of the limb are also graded to plan strengthening exercises.
- Repetition maximum testing is defined as the weight that can be lifted through an entire range of motion a set number of times. Most commonly one repetition maximum (1 RM) or ten repetition maximum (10 RM) are used.
- Hand-held myometry, small devices that measure isometric strength of hand muscles may be performed.
- Isokinetic dynamometry that measures torque during dynamic contractions at constant angular velocity may be performed.
- **Joint range of motion assessment:** Measurement of joint range of motion is done through goniometry. There are three primary elements related to joint range of motion such as:
  - Passive range of motion is typically practiced on a joint that is inactive.
  - Active-assistive range of motion is movement completed with some manual assistance from the physiotherapist.
  - Active ranges of motion are movements performed solely by the patient.
- **Assessment of balance:** Balance, especially sitting balance, is essential for individuals with SCI, as many individuals are wheelchair bound. Balance is required in order to remain in upright posture and prevent a fall from occurring, while the upper limbs are used either to propel a wheel chair or to hold a pair of crutches.

Balance control is determined by the ability to perform:
- *Static balance:* Ability to maintain upright posture.
- *Dynamic balance:*
  » Proactive balance: Ability to maintain balance during voluntary movements.
  » Reactive balance: Ability to regain balance after a balance is lost.

The sitting balance score (SBS) that grades balance from a score of 1 (poor)-Unable to maintain a static position, 2 (fair)-Able to maintain static position without difficulty, 3 (good)-Able to maintain a static position without difficulty, but requiring assistance for righting when perturbed, 4 (normal)-Able to perform test without any physical assistance, may be used to grade and document sitting balance.

The motor assessment scale (MAS), item-3: balanced sitting, that grades balance from a score of 1 (sits with support), 2 (sits unsupported for 10 seconds), 3 (sits unsupported with weight well forward and evenly distributed), 4 (sits unsupported, turns head and trunk to look behind), 5 (sits unsupported, reaches forward to touch the floor and returns to the starting position), 6 (sits on stool, unsupported, reaches sideways to touch the floor), can also be used to grade and document sitting balance.

The functional reach test can be modified from standing to sitting to grade sitting balance.
- **Respiratory function assessment:** Respiratory function needs to be assessed with a comprehensive respiratory examination, paying particular attention to other associated thorax injuries. The components of respiratory examination include:
  - Observation of respiratory rate and pattern
  - Type of ventilation.
  - Effectiveness of cough.
  - Chest auscultation.
  - Spirometry to find vital capacity and FEV1.
- **Assessment of cardiovascular fitness:**
  Assessment of cardiovascular fitness is important for prescription and monitoring exercise programs for patients with SCI. Cardiovascular fitness can be assessed using the following methods:
  - *Peak oxygen consumption test (test for VO2 max):* Measures expired gas while undergoing exercise that is gradually increased to maximal intensity. This is considered a gold standard method for measuring cardiovascular fitness in individuals with SCI.
  - *Submaximal arm tests (Cooper's test):* This test does not require an individual to exercise to exhaustion. It is a method of estimating VO2 max or cardiovascular fitness, where the intensity or workload is increased at a steady rate up to 85% of maximum heart rate. Portable gas analysis, heart rate, and perceived exertion using Borg scale are used to quantify the response to exercise.
  - *Field tests:* Tests like 6-minute walk test, where distance covered in a set time of 6 minutes also help in finding the level of fitness.
- **Assessment of pain:** Patients with SCI present with variable types of pain both in onset, pattern, and intensity affecting the patients exercise and activity and quality of life, which can be assessed by detailed subjective and objective assessment.
- Assessment of bladder/bowel functions for the ability/inability to void voluntarily.
- **Assessment of sexual function:** International standards for assessment of autonomic function after SCI (ISAFSCI) document the impact of SCI on sexual responses including psychogenic and reflex arousal (erection or lubrication), orgasm, ejaculation, and sensation of menstruation. Responses are described, based upon a 0–2 scale, with: 0-absent, 1-altered, 2-normal response.
- **Assessment/grading of pressure ulcer:** Intact skin surrounding the ulcer should be assessed for redness, warmth, hardness (induration), swelling, or any sign of infection. There are various stages of pressure ulcer **(Figs. 20.7A to D)** such as:
  - *Stage 1:* Erythema of the skin.
  - *Stage 2:* Erythema with the loss of partial thickness of the skin, including epidermis and part of the superficial dermis.
  - *Stage 3:* Full-thickness ulcer that might involve the subcutaneous fat.

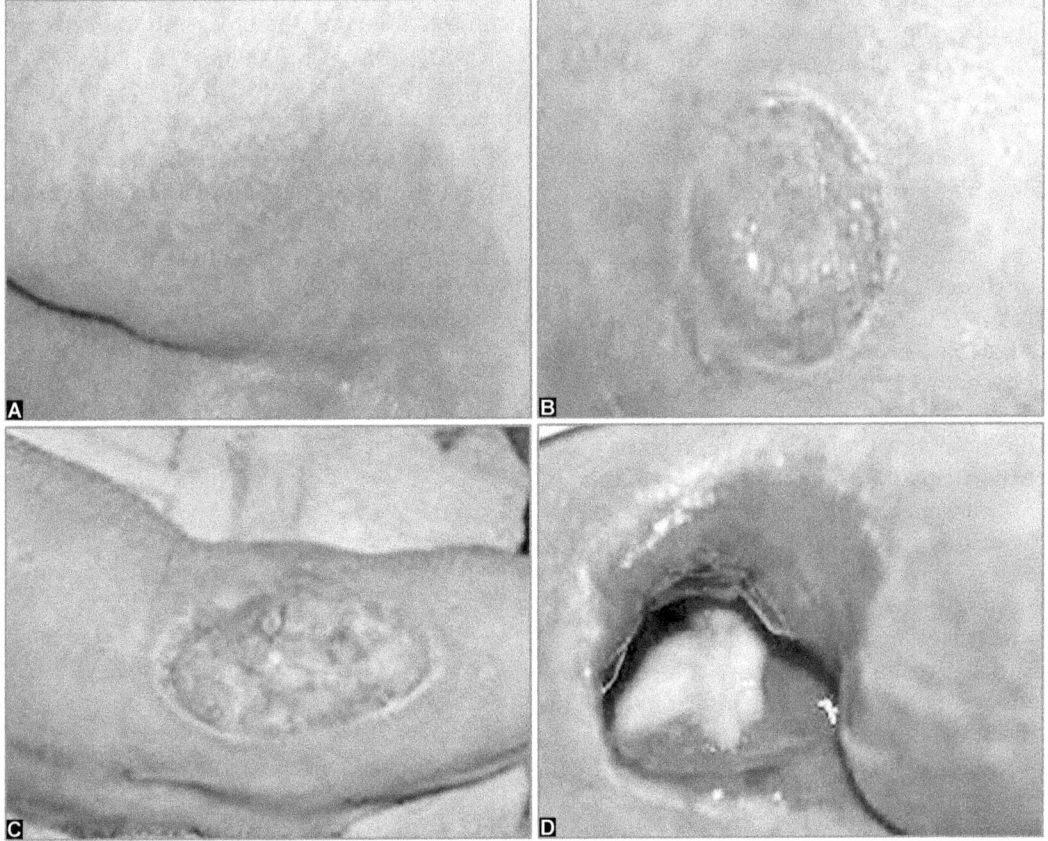

Figs. 20.7A to D: (A) Stage-1; (B) Stage-2; (C) Stage-3; (D) Stage-4 pressure ulcers.

– *Stage 4:* Full-thickness ulcer with the involvement of the muscle or bone.

For stage 3/4 ulcers, the length × width = area of the ulcer and depth and volume (area × depth) should be measured. For stage 1/2 ulcers the length × width = area of the ulcer should be measured and documented. Various methods for calculation of area and volume of the ulcer are available, such as: measuring the length (maximum), width (maximum), depth (maximum) using a sterile millimeter scale and multiplying the length into width to get the area, and multiplying the area into depth to get the volume. Tracing the margin of the ulcer using a sterile transparent sheet and calculating the area from a graph paper is also described as a method of measurement of area of the ulcer. The volume of ulcer is also calculated by filling the ulcer with the measured amount of saline.

Besides measurement of size of the ulcer, the presence of slough, oozing, granulation, etc., should also be documented.

- **Assessment of activity/function:** Impairment in an individual with SCI leads to significant activity/functional limitations. As with assessment of impairments, different standardized assessment scales are available for activity assessment in patients with SCI and the most commonly used assessment scale specific to SCI are the Spinal Cord Independence Measure (SCIM) and The Walking Index for Spinal Cord Injury (WISCI). Commonly assessed activity limitation domains in SCI include:
  - *General mobility that includes bed mobility and transfers:* The outcome measures that could be used include Functional Independence Measure (FIM), Spinal Cord Independence Measure, Quadriplegic Index of Function, and the Clinical Outcomes Variable Scale.
  - *Wheelchair mobility:* Outcome measures that assess wheelchair mobility are the Wheelchair Skills Test, the Wheelchair Circuit, and the Quebec User Evaluation of Satisfaction with Assistive Technology.
  - *Gait:* Outcome measures that assess gait are the 10 meter Walk Test, 6 Minute Walk Test, Walking Index for SCI and the SCI Functional Ambulation Inventory.
  - *Upper limb activity and hand function:* Outcome measures that assess upper limb and hand function are the Sollerman Hand Function Test, Jebsen Hand Function Test, Common Object Test, Tetraplegia Hand Activity Questionnaire, Grasp and Release Test.
- **Assessment of participation:** Understanding the individual's involvement in various activities such as family, society/community, education, work, leisure, etc., before SCI, helps the clinician assess the degree of participation limitation, and designing strategy to overcome such limitations.
- **Environmental Assessment:** Environmental factors are external factors which include the physical, social and attitudinal environment in which the individual will be living after discharged from the rehabilitation center. A thorough assessment of the living environment is required to find out the barriers, so that appropriate environmental modification could be done for an enhanced quality of living.
- **Vocational assessment:** Toward the terminal stage of rehabilitation therapy, a thorough vocational assessment needs to be done for the patient in coordination with the Vocational counselor and/or Occupational therapist for vocational rehabilitation of the client.

Imaging Studies

Imaging studies are helpful in the early stage to identify the site and extent of lesion, for planning of management. Plain X-rays have largely been superseded by computed tomography (CT) and magnetic resonance imaging (MRI). Heterotopic ossification, a common complication in SCI, can easily be identified with the X-rays **(Fig. 20.8)**. Early total body CT is crucial in excluding other life-threatening injuries in traumatic, patients with a cord injury to exclude occult hemorrhage as usual physiological response to shock is impaired. Therefore, neurogenic shock may mask other injuries such as ruptured spleen/fractured pelvis, etc., and the patient may also be unable to describe pain below the level of injury. Spinal reformatting of CT images will aid immediate assessment of vertebral column, assist in spinal clearance, and give some information on cord integrity. Early MRI has a role in investigating cord integrity and guiding early surgery (e.g., epidural hematoma identification).

Management of Spinal Cord Injury

Management of traumatic SCI starts from the phase of transfer from the accident site, ending with vocational rehabilitation and community participation phase. Early immobilization and treatment are the most important factors in achieving recovery from SCI. Aggressive rehabilitation and assistive devices helps people with severe spinal cord injuries to interact in society and remain productive.

The components of management are:
- **Transfer from accident site to hospital:** One important step in treatment of an SCI is immobilization. This often occurs at the time of injury prior to being transported to the hospital. Up to six members (four members for transferring the patient from the site of injury to spine

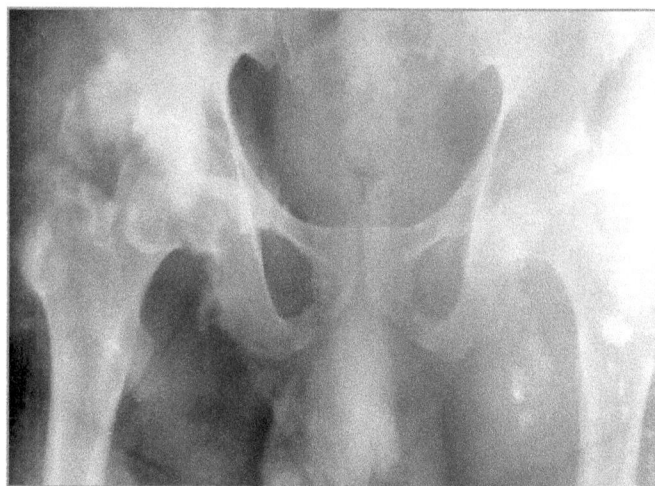

Fig. 20.8: Heterotopic ossification in the hip joints in an SCI patient.

board/stretcher and two members for transferring the patient on spine board/stretcher to ambulance/nearby hospital), may be required to work together in order to undertake routine turning and transfer procedures and they must have supreme confidence in their ability to work as a team. The log roll method **(Figs. 20.9A to E)** can be used for transfer of the patient from the site of injury to the hospital. All moving and handling must be coordinated by a nominated team leader and undertaken with a quiet confidence in the team's ability. The team leader for any maneuver will always be identified as the person in the position closest to the patient's head from where the patient's alignment throughout the maneuver can be monitored. The team leader is also responsible for checking and recording the patient's sensory and motor function in all four limbs at the beginning and end of a maneuver. Where applicable, manual support of the head and neck should be maintained during any flat surface transfers as an additional safeguard—even if a cervical collar is in situ. If cervical traction is in place, the traction cord should be shortened to maintain the pull of the traction weights during transportation.

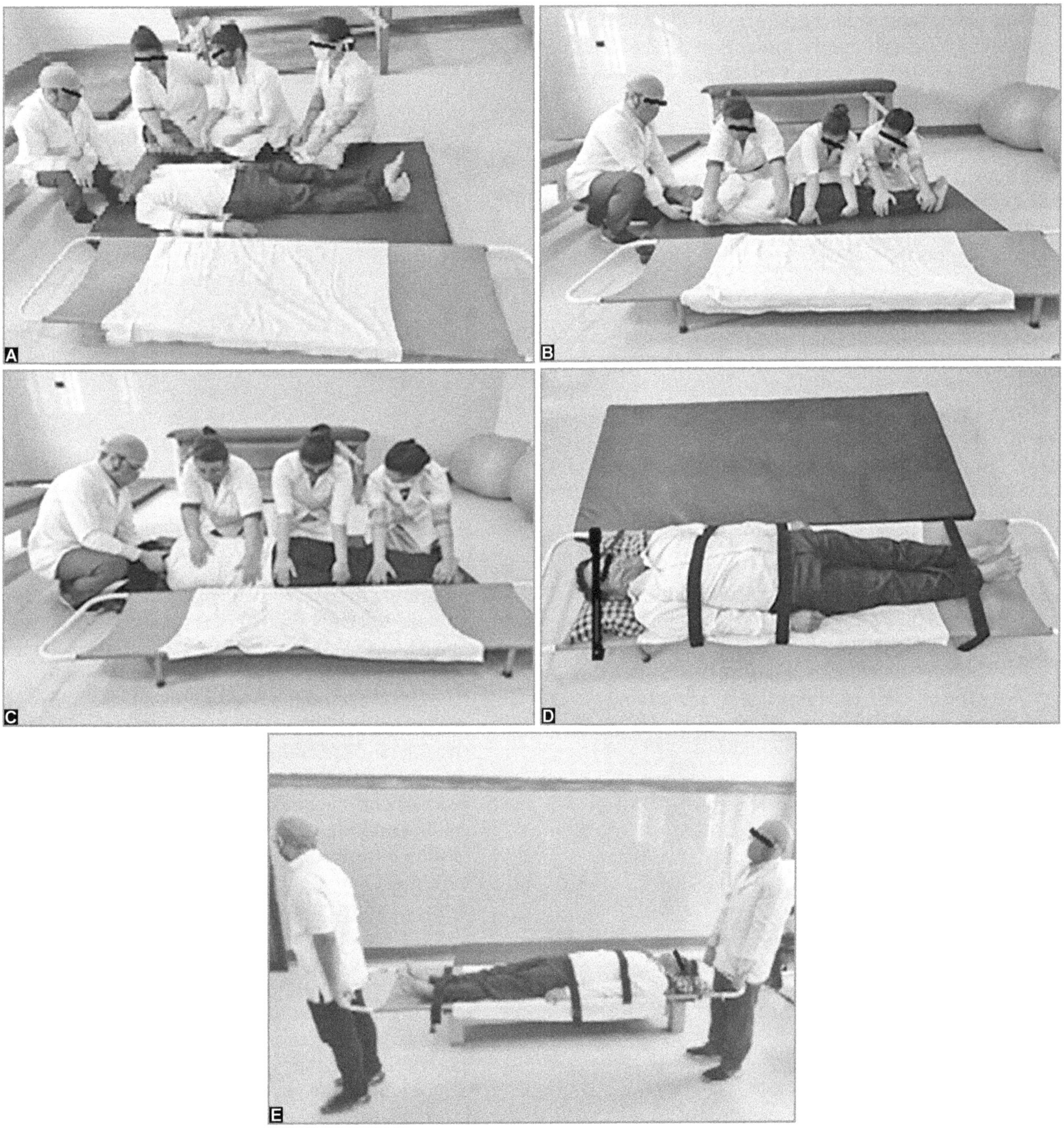

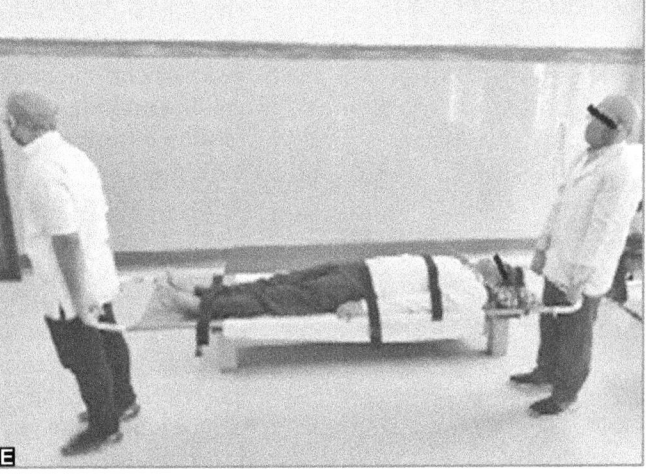

Figs. 20.9A to E: The log roll method of patient transfer.

The risk of secondary complications in patients with traumatic SCI is increased for those who do not obtain acute care in a specialized SCI unit within 24 hours from the time of injury. Parent et al. have systematically reviewed the impact of specialized spinal cord injury unit (SCIU) care on traumatic SCI complications and mortality, concluding that it reduced lengths of stay, mortality risk, and the number and severity of complications. Specific immobilization methods used are cervical collars, head immobilizer, and spinal board **(Fig. 20.10)**.

❖ **Early hospitalization phase:** The best chance for recovery of function following SCI is through prompt treatment. Early surgical decompression and stabilization leads to better recovery. Aggressive physiotherapy and rehabilitation after surgery also maximizes recovery. The majority of recovery occurs within the first 6 months after injury. Any remaining loss of function present after 12 months is much more likely to become permanent.

In this phase, pressure area care through turning every 1-2 hourly, maintaining spinal precautions is essential. Specialized beds and suitable mattresses (Air mattress, water mattress: **Figs. 20.11A and B**) may be selected depending on the patient's condition and stability of fracture.

Monitoring of oxygen saturation through arterial blood gas analysis, pulse oximetry, vital capacity measurement should be done. In case of respiratory distress, resulting in poor or deteriorating vital capacity, tracheotomy, and intubation may be considered. Early catheterization is essential not only to act as a marker of renal perfusion, but also to avoid overdistension of bladder, that may precipitate bradycardia. Various neuroprotection strategies are followed in this stage, which are described below:

- *Vasopressor support:* Early vasopressor support has been advocated to ensure adequate spinal cord perfusion pressure and reduce secondary cord injury.
- *Therapeutic hypothermia:* While early investigations have evaluated the beneficial effects of more profound levels of local hypothermia (less than 30°C) treatment following SCI, recent studies have concentrated on the

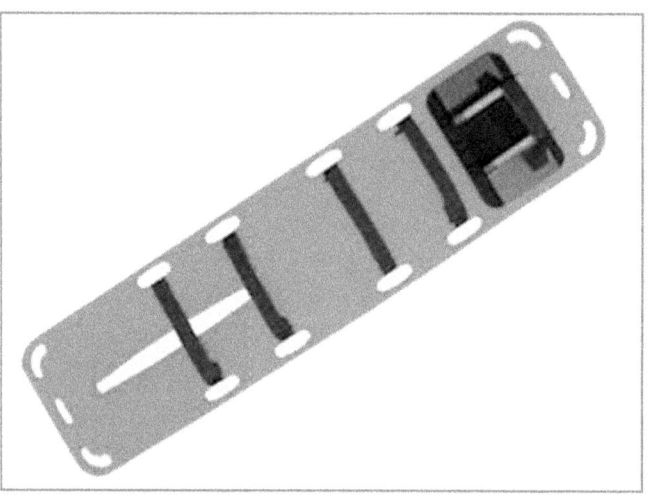

Fig. 20.10: The spine board.

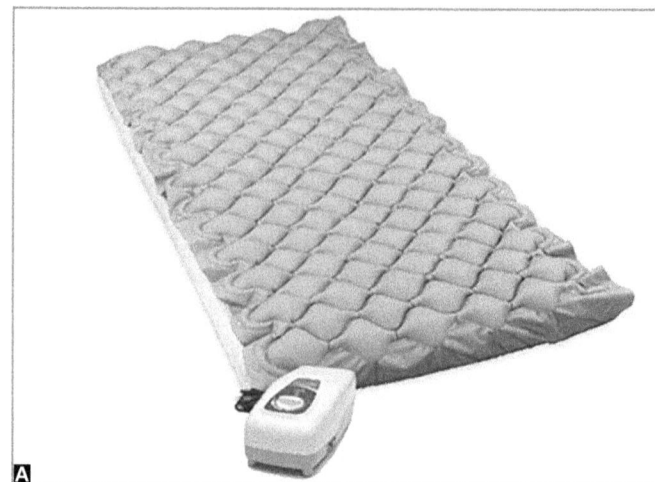

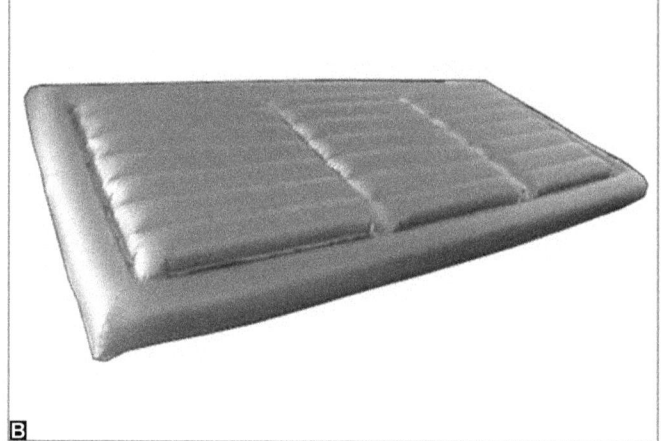

Figs. 20.11A and B: (A) Air mattress; (B) Water mattress.

benefits of mild hypothermia (33°C) in protecting and promoting functional recovery in established animal models. Recently the effects of modest hypothermia (30-32°C) in severely injured SCI patients have been tested and found to be both safe and achievable.

In general two methods of induced hypothermia are used currently such as surface cooling and endovascular cooling. Surface cooling methods include convective air blankets, water mattresses, alcohol bathing, cooling jackets, and ice packing. The advantage of surface cooling over endovascular cooling are that, it does not require advanced equipment or expertise in catheter placement and avoids the risks associated with central venous catheter placement.

- *Use of steroids:* After SCI is diagnosed, the physician might start a high dose of steroids. This could help decrease the amount of damage to the spinal cord by reducing inflammation and swelling.
- *Traction to cervical spine:* The patient suspected to have a cervical spine injury may be placed in traction or a halo device around the head to try to stabilize the spine and prevent further damage **(Fig. 20.12)**.
- *Surgery:* There are two major goals of surgery, such as:

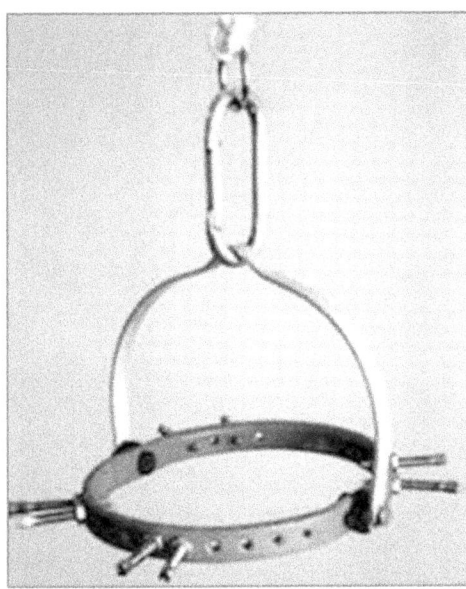

Fig. 20.12: The halo device.

» The first goal is to relieve any pressure on the spinal cord. This could involve removing portions of the vertebrae that have broken and are compressing the spinal cord.
» The second major goal of surgery for SCI is to stabilize the spine. If the vertebrae are weakened from fracture, tumor, or infection, they may not be capable of supporting the normal weight from the body and protecting the spinal cord. A combination of metal screws, rods and plates may be necessary **(Fig. 20.13)** to help hold the vertebrae together and stabilize them until the bones heal.

Besides neuroprotection strategies, the following strategies of management should be followed in the early hospitalization period.

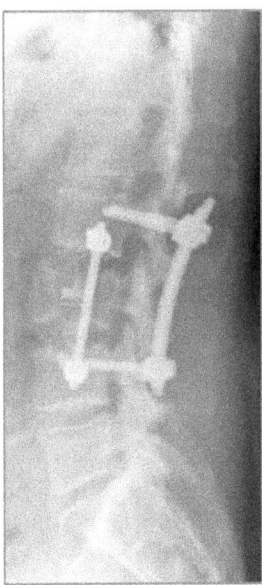

Fig. 20.13: Spinal stabilization by metallic implant.

- ❖ **Thromboprophylaxis:** Deep vein thrombosis and subsequent pulmonary embolism that result from immobility and increased thrombogenicity secondary to trauma, need to be prevented through anticoagulant therapy (usually restricted in the first 48–72 hours, because of risk of bleeding around the cord), limb elevation, regular passive movements, intermittent calf compression and application of compression stockings, etc. Sometimes inferior vena cava filter is also considered to prevent pulmonary embolism.
- ❖ **Pressure sore prevention:** Pressure sores are devastating for cord injured patients leading to prolonged immobilization or severe sepsis. These usually develop in the first few days after hospital admission, which result from immobility, poor perfusion of skin, hypoxia, and nursing the patient on hard beds. Appropriate mattresses, regular turning, good skin care measures, earlier spinal stabilization all help in prevention of pressure ulcer.
- ❖ **Orthotics consideration:** To provide support to the unstable segments, particularly to cervical spine, orthotic devices such as a Philadelphia collar **(Fig. 20.14A)**, Halo device to support cervical spine in case of fractures **(Fig. 20.12)**, Sterno-Occipitoal Mandibular Immobilization (SOMI) brace **(Fig. 20.14B)**, Minerva jacket **(Fig. 20.14C)**, etc., that provide good stability to cervical spine promoting faster rehabilitation is the consideration. The cervical orthoses are usually considered in the early stage, when the patient is confined to bed. However, for thoracolumbar spine a Taylor's brace/Knight spinal brace **(Figs. 20.15A and B)** can be considered when the patient is made upright.

Physiotherapy in early hospitalization phase/Acute phase: In this phase, intervention focuses on:

a. **Respiratory care:** Respiratory care depends on the level of injury and the patient's breathing ability. Patients with injury above C5, may require mechanical ventilation using intermittent positive pressure ventilation (IPPV). Ventilatory support can be provided through tracheotomy or through noninvasive positive pressure ventilation. In thoracic and lumbar spine injuries, assisted/deep diaphragmatic breathing combined with costal breathing exercises are performed to ventilate all parts of the lungs. In patients with high cervical injury with paralysis of diaphragm, glossopharyngeal breathing is given, once the ventilatory support is withdrawn.

The position of the patient for breathing exercises and secretion removal depends on the level of injury. Those with cervical and upper thoracic injury with abdominal weakness/paralysis are benefited when breathing exercises and secretion removal are performed in supine lying, as compared to sitting. In sitting, lack of abdominal musculature support results in falling of the abdominal contents forward pulling on the central tendon of the diaphragm, affecting movement of the diaphragm, when it contracts during inspiration resulting inefficient breathing pattern, as well coughing. Therefore, patients

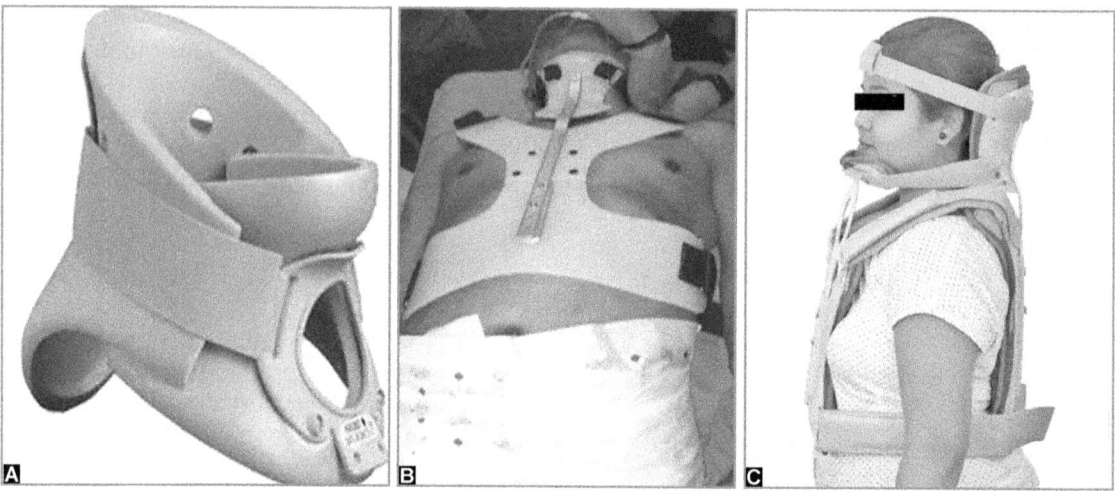

Figs. 20.14A to C: (A) The Philadelphia cervical collar; (B) SOMI brace; (C) The Minerva jacket.

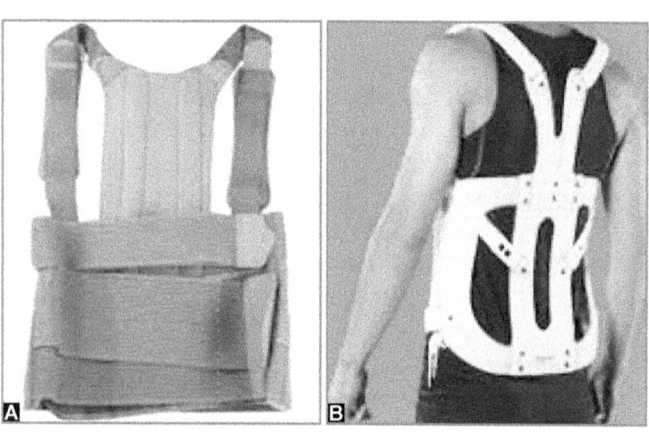

Figs. 20.15A and B: (A) Taylor's brace; (B) Knight spinal brace.

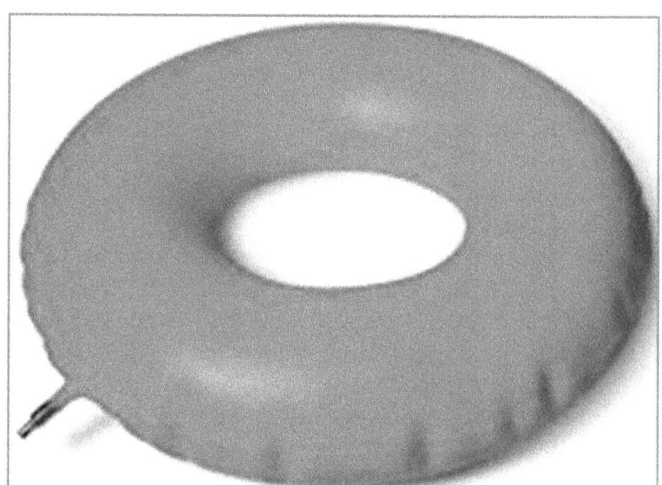

Fig. 20.16: Donut pillow for pressure ulcer.

with abdominal paralysis/weakness, should be given chest therapy in supine lying, instead of sitting.

Air shift maneuvers to inflate a lung/part of the lung, in case of reduced expansion to prevent consolidation/collapse. Abdominal support using abdominal binder can be used in case of abdominal paralysis affecting huffing/cuffing for clearance of secretions. Gentle chest clapping, assisted coughing, huffing techniques are performed to remove secretions.

b. **Skin care to prevent development of pressure ulcer:** The procedures involve:
   - Periodic turning (every 2 hourly) on bed.
   - Regular inspection of skin over pressure-sensitive areas.
   - Use of moisturizing lotions/powders.
   - Use of pressure-relieving pillows (donut pillows) **(Fig. 20.16)**, mattresses (air mattress/water mattress).
   - Periodic exercises (passive/active), as the movements result in increased blood flow and avoid constant load on skin/pressure-sensitive areas.

c. **Maintenance joint range of motion:** The procedures involve:
   - Regular passive movements (Overhead movement of shoulder, i.e., movement of shoulder beyond 90 degrees of abduction/flexion for cervical spine injuries and flexion of hips beyond 70 degrees with the knee straight and 90 degrees with knees flexed, for lumbar spine injuries are to be avoided in the first 3–4 weeks to prevent acceleration of injury.
   - *Joint positioning:* The joints should be positioned by sandbags/pillows/splints to prevent deformity, say for example, a sand bag may be placed under the sole of foot or a well-padded polypropylene AFO may be applied to the foot, to prevent TA tightness and subsequent equinus deformity.

d. **Prevention of indirect impairments and secondary complications:** Heterotopic ossification, contracture/deformities, etc., should be prevented from developing to the extent possible. It is understood that secondary complications like heterotopic ossifications, which is most commonly found in the hip joints are accelerated, if crude maneuvers such as massage, vigorous passive stretching are applied to patients with SCI. Appropriate joint protection strategies, medications may help in prevention of such complications. Regular passive/active movements, positioning of joints may help in prevention of soft tissue contractures, deformities in joints as well as deep vein thrombosis.

e. **Gradual orientation to vertical position**: As early as possible, the patients should be made to sit following joint protection measures such as use of a spinal brace to avoid orthostatic hypotension and to improve function:
   – Measures to promote emptying of bladder and bowel: The therapist should coordinate with the medical and nursing team regarding the procedures to be undertaken for emptying the bladder, such as applying pressure to lower abdomen to avoid accumulation of residual urine. Assisting the patient to make pelvic bridging is also emphasized for insertion of bedpan for emptying the bowel.

Physiotherapy intervention in the active phase (Rehabilitation phase):

The emphasis of treatment in this phase is to maximize functional independence, train bladder and bowel strategies, train strategies for skin care, sexual, and psychosocial management, etc. All the procedures followed in the acute stage are continued in this stage in addition to the followings:

- Training patient to examine own skin using mirror and to try relieve pressure through rolling, pelvic bridging (**Figs. 20.17A to D**), sitting push-ups (**Fig. 20.18**) on bed and wheel chair.
- Relaxed passive movements, gentle stretching of tight structures, active assisted (**Fig. 20.19**)/free/resisted exercises to recovering and normal muscles as appropriate.
- Tilt table standing: Starting from an angle of 30 degrees from horizontal and gradually increasing to 90 degrees as the patient tolerates. This helps in prevention of tightness and contractures in the lower limbs in addition to facilitation of bone mineralization due to gradual weight bearing. It helps in prevention of orthostatic hypotension (**Fig. 20.20**).
- Mat exercises/activities that include:
  – Rolling (**Fig. 20.21**)
  – Prone on elbow positioning.
  – Sitting with or without support.
  – Prone kneeling.
  – Transfers (Transferring from bed to chair and vice versa).
  – Medicine ball exercises.
  – Sitting push-ups.

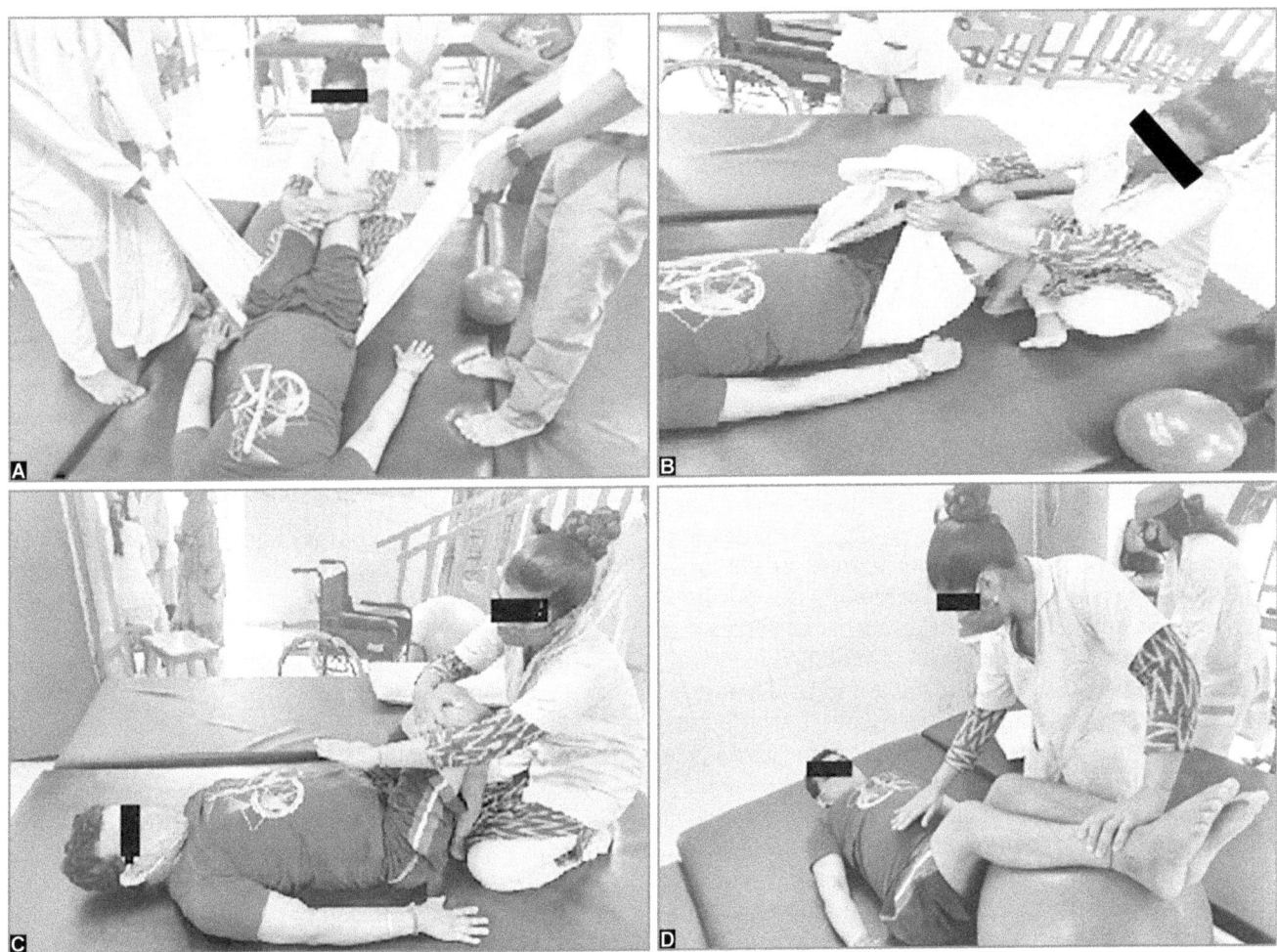

Figs. 20.17A to D: (A and B) Bridging with assistance; (C) Bridging unassisted; (D) Bridging using Swiss ball.

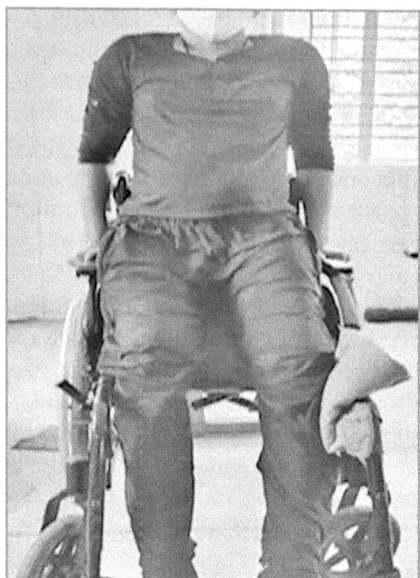

Fig. 20.18: Sitting push-ups on wheel chair to relieve pressure from the buttocks, when sitting for a prolonged period on wheel chair.

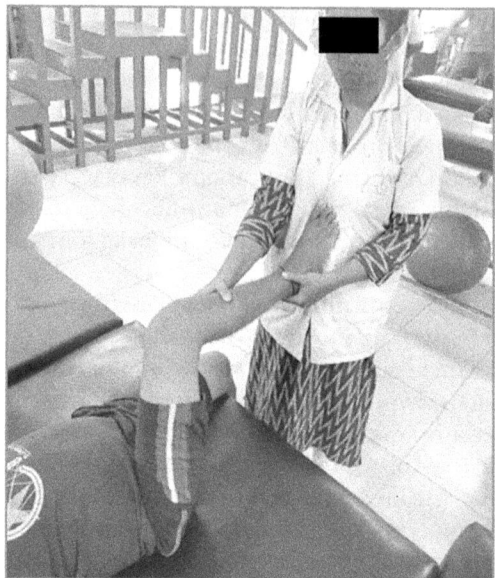

Fig. 20.19: Active assisted exercise for lower limbs.

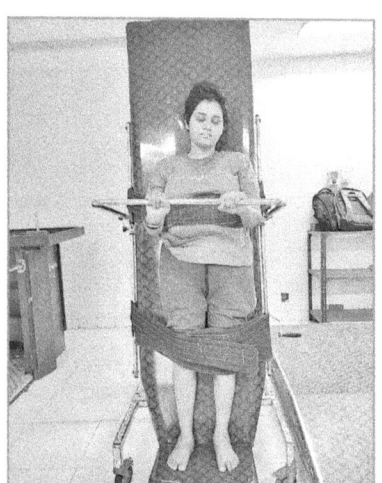

Fig. 20.20: Tilt table standing for a paraplegic/quadriplegic patient.

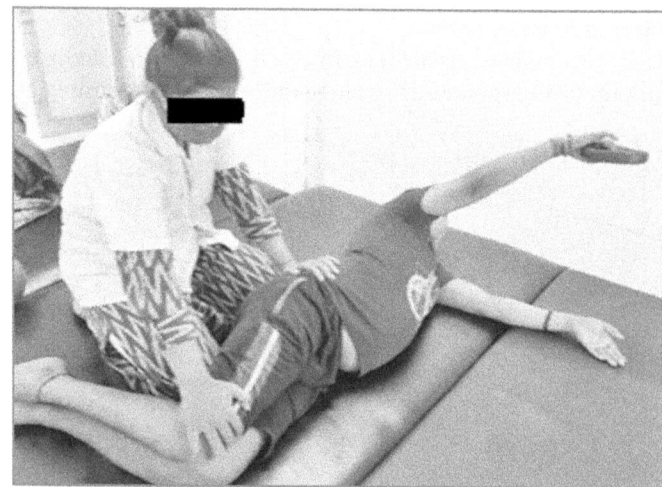

Fig. 20.21: Rolling on mat (Assistance is given by therapist in addition to mechanical assistance obtained by holding a weight in the hand.

- Balancing exercises in sitting **(Figs. 20.22A to D)**.
- **Spasticity management:** Spinal spasticity results from the removal or destruction of supraspinal control, leading to increased excitability of motor neurons, resulting in spasticity. The patient should be carefully assessed about the beneficial role of spasticity (if any). It has been seen that a grade-1 spasticity as per Modified-modified Ashworth scale helps the patient stabilize joints and hold a posture and move. If high-grade spasticity persists affecting posture and movements, the following strategies need to be followed to reduce spasticity and improve function. Treatment for spasticity usually involves a combination of physiotherapy, orthosis and medical/surgical management.
  - *Exercise:* Stretching, positioning and exercises/activities that may help maintain range of motion and prevent shortening or tightening of the muscles, help reducing spasticity.
  - Antispastic splints/casts.
  - Oral medications.
  - Botulinum toxin (Botox) injections applied into the spastic muscles help to reduce spasticity for a period of 3–6 months, during which time, the therapists try to train and achieve function. Phenol or alcohol injections into the peripheral nerve supplying the spastic muscles may reduce spasticity.
  - *Intrathecal baclofen therapy:* This method of treatment provides medicines administered directly into the fluid surrounding the spinal cord 24 hours a day that reduce hypertonicity. This is done by inserting a pump into the abdomen (intrathecal baclofen pump).
  - *Neurosurgery and orthopedic surgery procedures:* Surgical procedures to destroy (ablate) motor nerves corresponding to sensory spinal roots may stop the spasticity.

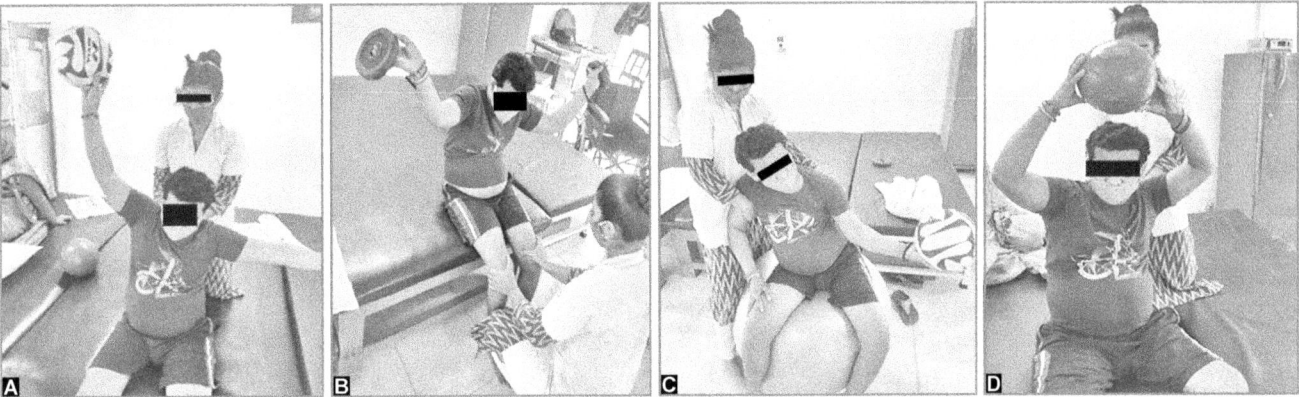

Figs. 20.22A to D: Sitting balance developments: (A) High guard holding a light ball; (B) High guard holding weights in both hands; (C) Balancing on Swiss ball; (D) Balancing with medicine ball.

- **Pressure sore management:** Frequent turning, making use of air/water mattress, early mobility, regular exercises, etc., help in prevention of pressure sore. If a pressure sore has developed, infrared radiation (least used nowadays due to the dry heating effect), pulsed ultrasound to the margin of the ulcer, low-intensity LASER **(Fig. 20.23)**, UVR, HVPGC, kneading to the margin of the ulcer, gentle ice massage to the margin of ulcer may be considered as per the available evidences. Surgical intervention in the form of skin grafting/skin flaps application is usually required for a stage-3/stage-4, ulcer that does not heal with conservative management.
- **Bladder training:** Successful bladder training is an interdisciplinary function involving Urologists, Physiotherapists, and Occupational therapists. The objective of bladder training after SCI is to maintain the patient's bladder at the appropriate volumes for optimum overall health. Methods of bladder retraining are supplemented by monitoring fluid intake to prevent urinary tract infections and control urine volume and concentration, developing scheduled times for urination and using body positions to facilitate voiding.

Management of flaccid/autonomous bladder: Initially, when the patient is in spinal shock and confined to bed, an indwelling catheter is applied to void urine. As the patient recovers and gets the ability to sit with or without support and has good upper limb functions, bladder training in the form of clamping the catheter and periodic voiding through suprapubic stimulation after clamp removal (helpful in flaccid/areflexic bladder), Crede's maneuver, intermittent catheterization **(Figs. 20.24A to D)** may be considered. Exercises to strengthen the sphincters are also emphasized.

Crede's maneuver: This maneuver is considered for patients who have autonomous bladder (flaccid/areflexic bladder) due to a LMN (cauda equina injury), where the voiding reflex is impaired, causing distention of bladder. In this maneuver manual pressure is applied to the lower abdomen either by the patient (if possible) or the caregiver, to assist in emptying of bladder.

Management of spastic/automatic bladder: It comprises fluid intake advice and bladder training, supplemented by antimuscarinic drugs if necessary. Bladder training is one of the primary treatments for spastic bladder. It involves teaching the bladder to be able to hold urine for a longer period of time. This helps to lower the number of times the patient needs to use the bathroom in a day. The components of training of the spastic bladder are:

1. Keeping a bathroom schedule with the intention of urinating at regular intervals throughout the day
2. Slowly increasing the length of those intervals by 5, 10, 15, or 20 minute periods.
3. Avoiding going to the bathroom without a strong urge to urinate
4. Trying to wait a few moments before urinating, despite any strong urge to urinate.

If urodynamic results reveal more and more accumulation of residual urine, the same should be drained through periodic intermittent catheterization.

Every patient after SCI should be subjected to urodynamic assessment preferably 3–4 months after SCI, as by this time

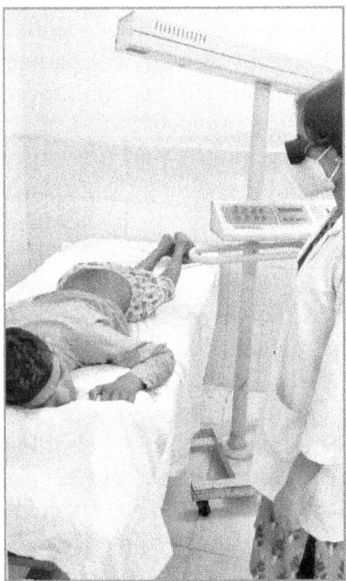

Fig. 20.23: Pressure sore treatment using LASER.

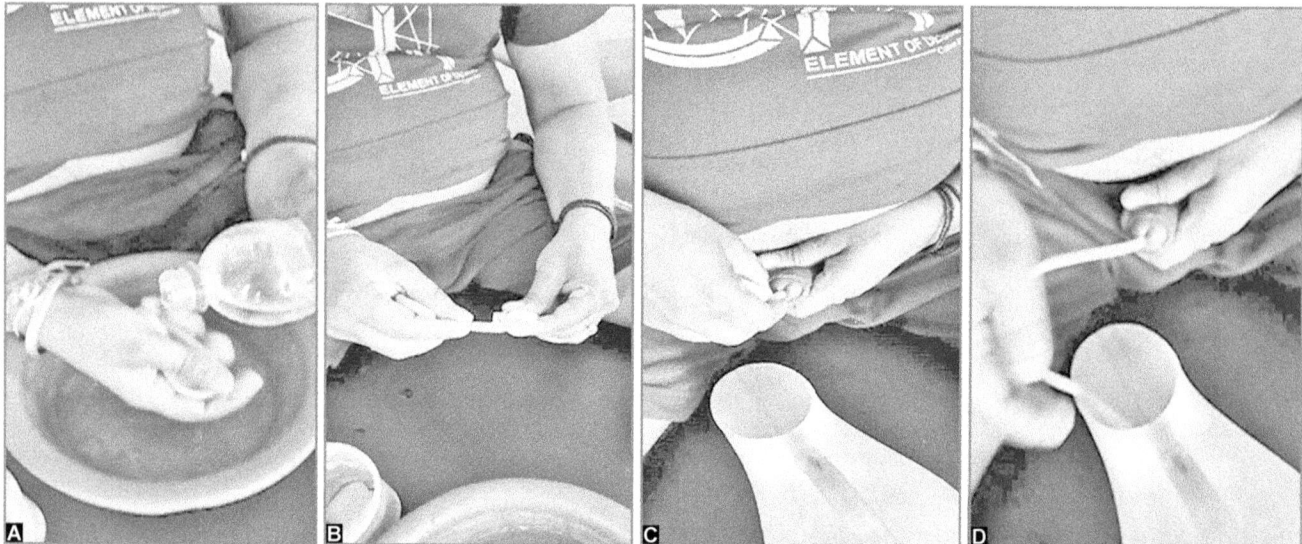

Figs. 20.24A to D: Paraplegic patient performing self-intermittent catheterization: (A) Cleaning the catheter; (B) Applying xylocaine gel; (C) Inserting the catheter into urethra; (D) Evacuating urine.

the patient is expected to have recovered from spinal shock, and detrusor contraction is present. Periodically, the patient should also be subjected to urodynamic studies to monitor the amount of residual urine, so that complications like hydronephrosis could be prevented.

- **Bowel management:** Patients of SCI develop constipation resulting in precipitation of increased muscle tone and autonomic dysreflexia, as well as bowel incontinence resulting in voiding without knowledge any where such as on bed, in workplace, etc.

  An interdisciplinary bowel management program managed by dietician, physician, physiotherapist, nurse, patient, and care givers provide bowel training to the patient. The program consists of:
  - Advice on drinking liquids such as water, juice, and milk and avoiding drinking liquids with caffeine as caffeine can cause constipation and diarrhea.
  - Advice on eating a variety of healthy foods, high in fiber such as vegetables, whole-grain breads and cereals, and beans. Fiber may help decrease constipation by adding bulk to the bowel movements.
  - Exercises and activities that assist bowel movements, such as changing position on bed, moving from lying to sitting/standing with or without assistance, performing passive/active movements need to be performed regularly.
  - Eating or drinking 15–30 minutes before bowel evacuation is tried.
  - Adopting a sitting posture (if possible), to assist bowel contents to move down through the colon.
  - *Massaging lower abdomen:* Massaging the lower abdomen in a circular, clockwise motion from right to left increases bowel mobility. The patient/caregiver is advised to place the palm of the hand on the lower right part of the abdomen pressing inward moving up to the ribs. Maintaining the pressure, the hand is moved to left side and pressure is applied in a downward direction in the left abdomen. The maneuver is repeated 10 times with an interval of 30 seconds between each maneuver.
  - *Digital stimulation:* If bowel evacuation is not performed satisfactorily with the above maneuvers causing impaction of feces, digital stimulation by the patient (if he/she has good sitting balance) or the caregiver may be performed to evacuate the bowel.

    The procedure of digital stimulation involves: Washing the hands followed by putting the gloves and lubricating one of the fingers. The lubricated finger is inserted 2–3 inches inside the rectum, pointing toward the belly button, moving in a circular manner for about 20 seconds. The procedure is repeated every 5–10 minutes, until bowel movement is felt. Any feces impacted in the rectum can also be scooped out by the fingers.
  - *Inserting suppository or enema:* If in spite of all efforts, satisfactory voiding of bowel is not possible, suppository/enema should be applied to empty the bowel. This can be done by the patient, if he/she has good sitting balance, or else the procedure should be performed by the caregiver.

- **Management of sexuality and infertility:** The physical condition after SCI may change aspects of sexual function and affect the patient's physical, mental and social-well being related to sexual health
  - *Treatment for sexual dysfunction:* Men and women who have/had spinal cord injuries may face difficulty in resuming sexual activities, needing intervention to resolve the issue. To overcome the physical dysfunction, treatment should be tailored to resume sexual activity in men and women. The following points should be considered regarding sexuality and fertility in SCI patients.
  - *Psychological therapy:* The patients should be counseled for development of self-confidence in establishing and maintaining intimate relationships after SCI, in the same manner, he/she was doing before the injury.

- Men, who have difficulties with sexual function, may be treated by medications, assistive devices or implants.
- Women with SCI usually can become pregnant and deliver normally.
- Fertility counseling and sexuality education should be provided to the patient and his/her partner by the treatment team.

❖ **Pain management:** Besides pharmacological management (which is helpful for nociceptive pain arising from musculoskeletal structures), nonpharmacological management of pain that includes cognitive behavioral pain therapy, activity pacing, relaxation techniques, desensitization (making the patient continuously exposed to pain episodes), functional activities/exercises, breathing exercises, sustained stretching, hydrotherapy, TENS, wheel chair modifications, ergonomic advice are helpful for controlling both nociceptive and neuropathic pain in individuals with SCI.
❖ Training of wheel chair skills, i.e., wheel chair transfers, such as sliding board transfer **(Fig. 20.25)**, pivot transfer **(Figs. 20.26A to D)**, and wheel chair propulsions.
Patients with cervical injury, who cannot propel a manual wheel chair, a power wheel chair **(Fig. 20.27)** is recommended.
❖ Standing in parallel bar/holding fixed support with above knee wooden slab/below knee wooden slab/polypropylene KAFOs/AFOs/parapodium **(Figs. 20.28A to D)**. A parapodium is considered for very high thoracic lesions, with no trunk control.
❖ Body weight-supported standing/walking **(Fig. 20.29)**.
❖ Standing balance and gait training with crutches (Axillary crutches/elbow crutches) and orthosis **(Fig. 20.30)**. Patients with complete thoracic level injury usually manage to stand with support of orthosis and walking aids and walk for a short distance on level surfaces. However, such walking is considered physiological and cannot be considered walking for function, as it is very much energy-consuming and carries a risk of fall when the patient desires to sit at need. However, those with cauda equina lesion, manage to walk in community with bilateral AFOs and crutches. Even though community walking is not possible

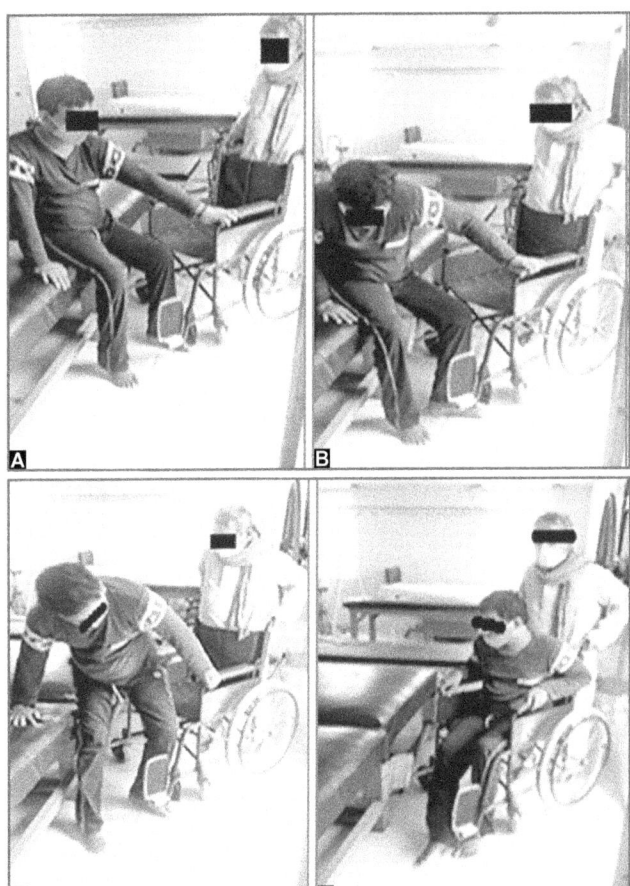

Figs. 20.26A to D: Various stages of sitting pivot transfer: (A) Aligning the wheel chair at an angle of 30–45 degrees to bed and reaching for the arm of wheel chair; (B) Pushing the bed and wheel chair arm; (C) Pushing the body up and pivoting towards wheel chair; (D) Sitting on wheel chair.

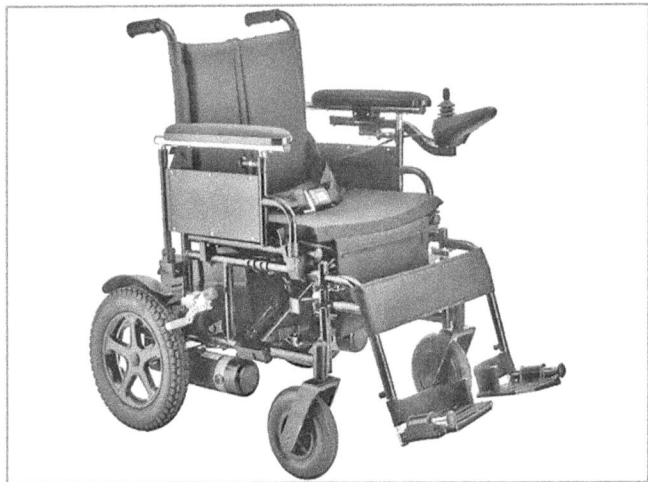

Fig. 20.27: The power wheel chair.

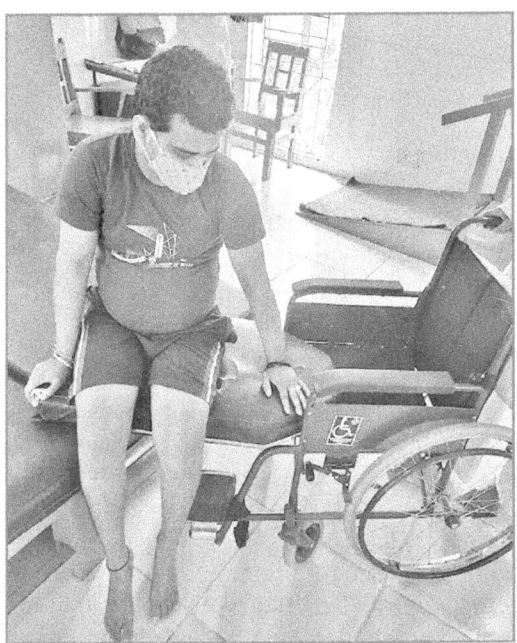

Fig. 20.25: Sliding board wheel chair transfer.

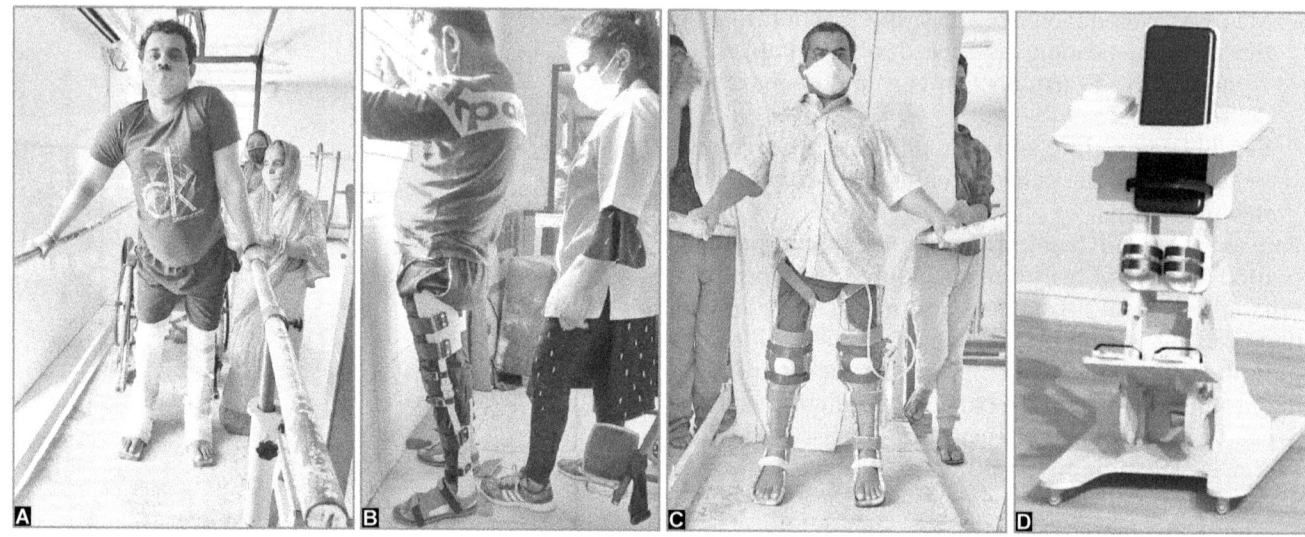

Figs. 20.28A to D: (A) Paraplegic patient standing in parallel bar with bilateral AK wooden slabs; (B) Standing, holding on window railings with bilateral KAFOs; (C) Standing and walking in parallel bar with bilateral KAFOs; (D) Standing on a parapodium and moving indoor.

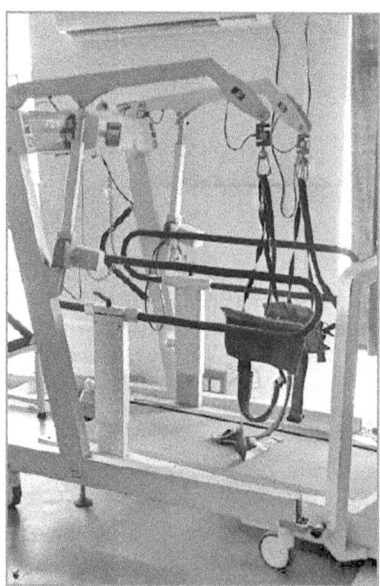

Fig. 20.29: Body weight-supported walking device with treadmill.

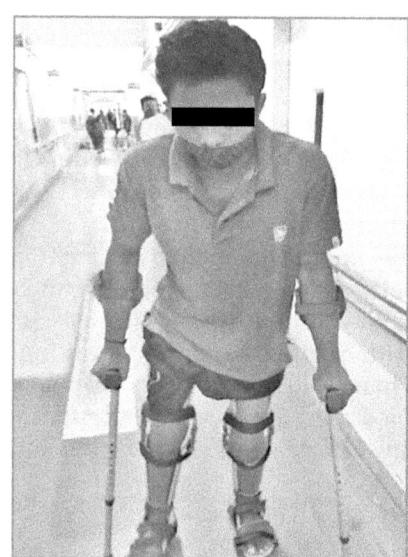

Fig. 20.30: Paraplegic patient walking with bilateral KAFOs and a pair of elbow crutches.

in most of the SCI patients, walking in the form of exercises should be performed several times a day to maintain physical and mental health of the patient. The patient should be trained on donning and doffing techniques of orthosis and transitions (sitting on chair to standing and vice versa).

The crutch gaits used for patients of SCI are of the following types:
- *Swing to gait:* This gait is commonly used for patients of SCI, who have bilateral lower extremity involvement. This gait involves forward movements of both crutches simultaneously, shifting weight to the hands and swinging the lower extremities to the crutches, not crossing the crutch line.
- *Swing through gait:* In this gait which is also used for patients with SCI, the crutches are moved forward together, weight is shifted onto the hands and the lower extremities are swung beyond the crutches. This gait is a progression from swing to gait.
- *4-point crutch gait:* This gait pattern is used when there is lack of coordination, poor balance and muscle weakness in both lower extremities (for paraparetic patients). In this gait pattern one crutch is advanced and then the opposite leg is advanced. For example, the left crutch is moved forward, then the right leg, followed by the right crutch and then the left leg.
- *2-point crutch gait:* This gait pattern is similar to the four-point gait. However, it is less stable as only two points of floor contact are maintained and the use of such gait requires better balance. This pattern more closely simulates normal gait, i.e., opposite lower extremity and upper extremity move together. That means left lower

extremity and right upper extremity moves as one point, and right lower extremity and left upper extremity move as another point, making the two-point gait pattern.

❖ **Functional electrical stimulation to promote hand function for self-care/ankle dorsiflexion for efficient gait:** Functional electrical stimulation (FES), also called as neuroprosthesis, can be used instead of a hand splint or ankle foot orthosis (AFO) to improve function. It stimulates the muscles causing muscular contractions and producing joint movements, helping the patient during walking to clear the ground and extending the wrist to make a grasp for use of hand. The pads acting as electrodes are either attached to the skin or surgically implanted.

❖ **Orthotic considerations for ambulation:** The orthotic recommendation varies according to the level of lesion. The patient with a cauda equina lesion is usually benefited by an AFO. However, patients with complete thoracic lesions may require KAFOs **(Figs. 20.31A to E)**, such as conventional KAFO, HKAFO/HKAFO with trunk support, Scott-Craig KAFO, reciprocal gait orthosis (RGO), HKAFO with trunk support is considered (for very thigh thoracic paraplegia with instability of trunk).

Scott-Craig orthosis, is also known as the double-bar hip stabilizing orthosis: This orthosis is most commonly prescribed bilaterally for patients with complete paraplegia with level of injury at or above L1 to T7. The reciprocal gait orthosis (RGO) is usually recommended for patients with thoracic level SCI. An RGO **(Fig. 20.31D)** can enable patients with lower body weakness or paralysis to stand upright unassisted and walk with the help of crutches/walker. This orthosis consists of bilateral KAFOs and a trunk section. The KAFO section immobilizes the knees and ankles to allow the patient to balance the body in a standing position, while the RGO/trunk section allows the hip motion and pelvic rotation, imitating a functional walking gait.

❖ **Management of tetraplegic hand to improve function:**
  – *The tenodesis action and use of tenodesis splint:* Though most patients with cervical spine injury have enhanced longevity due to advanced medical/surgical and rehabilitative measures, hand function restoration has always remained a challenge, which significantly affect the quality of life of the patient. Although the tenodesis mechanism **(Figs. 20.32A and B)** is widely used by therapists to improve hand function, sometimes the passive insufficiency of long flexors resulting in shortening of the flexor tendons at the interphalangeal joints to grasp objects is inadequate to generate the required force for the grasp. When tenodesis action is trained to improve hand function, weight-bearing exercises with hands open should not be performed, as the same will result in over-stretching of the long flexors, which is not desired. A tenodesis splint **(Fig. 20.33)**, that promotes grasping of objects in C6-C7 tetraplegic patients, who have no finger flexion, but have the ability to extend the wrist is recommended for such patients. The splint is strapped onto the user's forearm, hand and fingers.
  – *Surgical reconstruction of the tetraplegic hand:* Various hand surgery procedures are carried out for patients with SCI with tetraplegia to improve function and overall rehabilitation of the patient. Erik Moberg is recognized as the Father of upper extremity tendon transfers in patients with SCI.

Various tendon transfer procedures are undertaken to restore elbow extension, wrist extension, forearm rotation, and hand grasp and release. Elbow extension is restored by transferring the posterior and all or part of the middle deltoid to triceps brachii, though current evidence suggests transfer of biceps brachii to triceps gives superior results.

Wrist extension provides tenodesis grasp, in the absence voluntary finger flexion, and when wrist extension is not possible, transfer of brachioradialis to extensor carpi radialis brevis restores passive prehension enhancing accomplishing the ADLs. Tendon transfers are also performed to restore active finger and thumb flexion for pinch, grasp, and hand opening. Tendon transfers for thumb and finger extension, make release of objects possible.

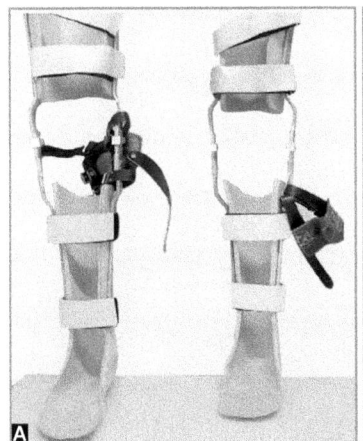 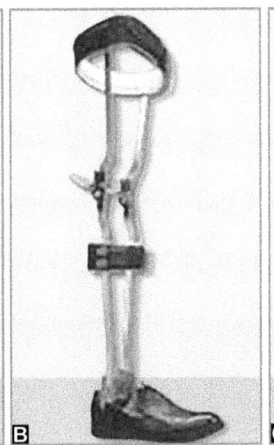 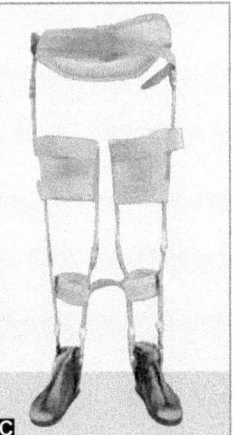 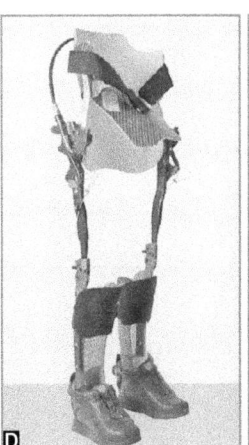 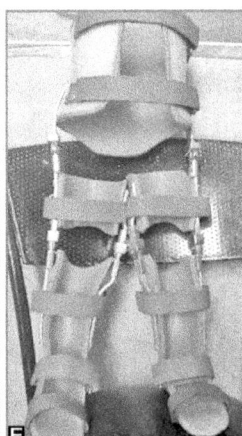

Figs. 20.31A to E: (A) Conventional KAFO; (B) Scott-Craig orthosis; (C) HKAFO (D) Reciprocal gait orthosis (RGO); (E) HKAFO with trunk support.

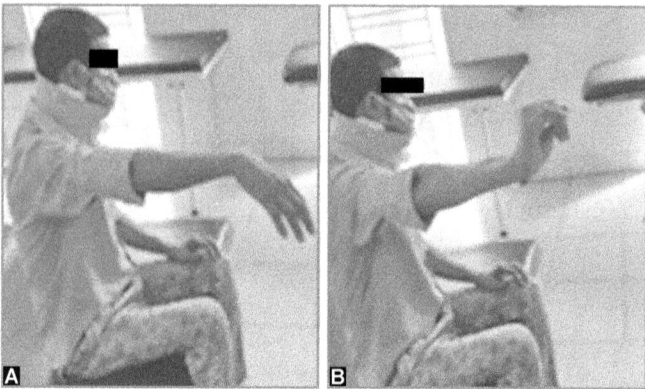

Figs. 20.32A and B: (A) Tetraplegic hand; (B) Grasping with tenodesis action.

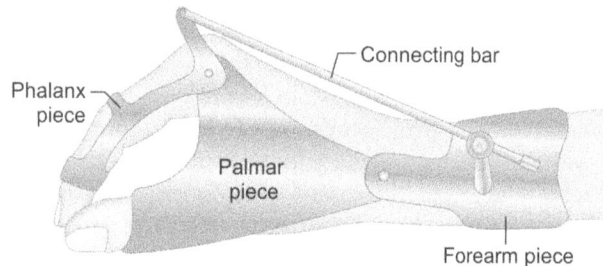

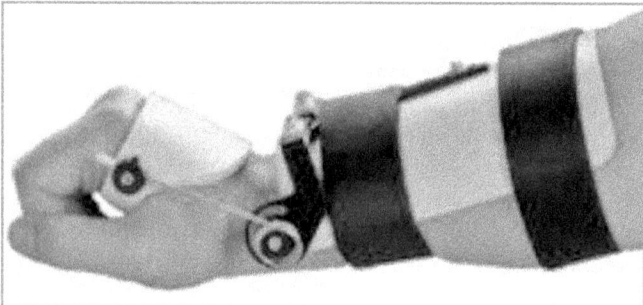

Fig. 20.33: The tenodesis splint.

Restoration of active grasp and release eliminates the need for adaptive equipment for eating, brushing teeth, catheterizing, and other ADLs.

- **Use of adaptive devices to improve hand function:** Tetraplegic patients who have impairments in using hands for function need variable adaptive equipment starting from a mouth piece to operate the key board (mostly C5 lesion) **(Fig. 20.34A)**, or an adapted spoon to take food to mouth (mostly C8 lesion) **(Figs. 20.34B and C)**. The Physiotherapist should coordinate with the Occupational therapist for designing appropriate adaptive devices and training on the use of such devices to achieve function.
- **Fitness training:** Aerobic exercises such as hydrotherapy (if no pressure sore, incontinence of bladder and bowel) **(Fig. 20.35)**, Static cycle exercises (lower limb and upper limb ergometry) **(Fig. 20.36)**, indoor and outdoor sports such as wheel chair basket ball, wheel chair race, etc., need to be organized to improve fitness.

Vocational Rehabilitation Programs

Vocational rehabilitation programs can help individuals with disabilities such as SCI to obtain employment. Through these programs, a wide range of services are available to help people identify their career interests and skills; acquire the relevant education or training; find and apply for jobs; and get work accommodations. Designing effective vocational programs for persons with SCI is essential for improving return to work and integration to family and community. Support, training and job placement help the patient achieve effective vocational rehabilitation. Every effort should be made to overcome physical, financial and attitudinal barriers, so that the patient is placed in a productive and financially yielding vocation.

In India, the 1% reservation out of the total of 4% available to persons with disabilities (as per the PWD act-2016, can

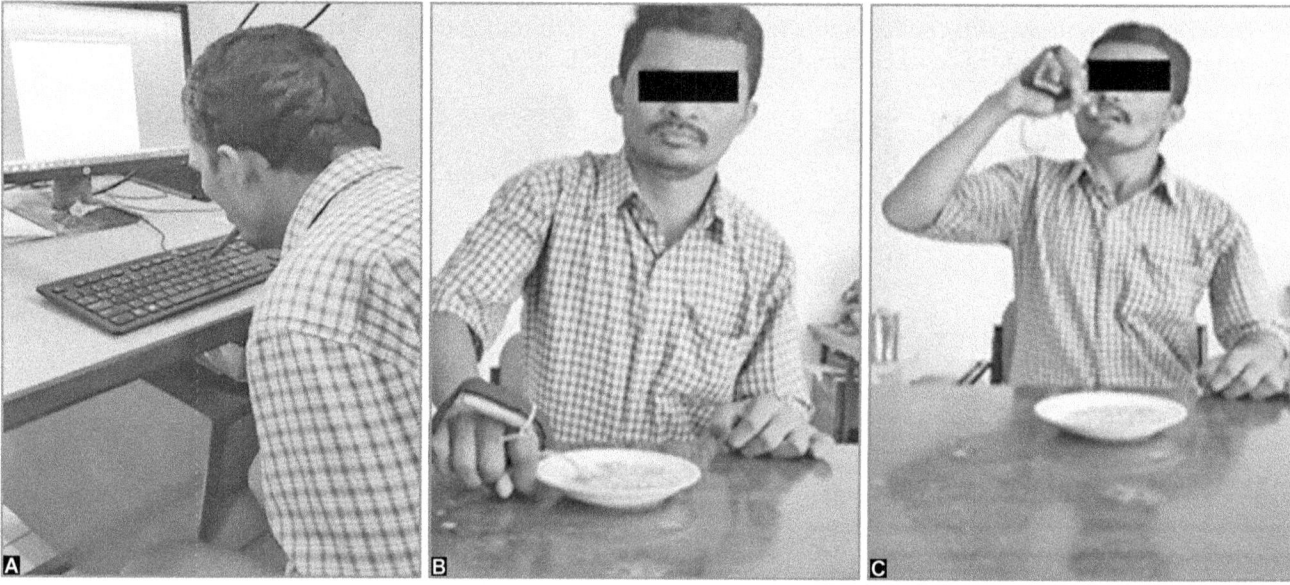

Figs. 20.34A to C: (A) Operating keyboards with a stick in mouth; (B and C) Using adapted spoon to take food to mouth.

Chapter 20: Physiotherapy for Spinal Cord Injury

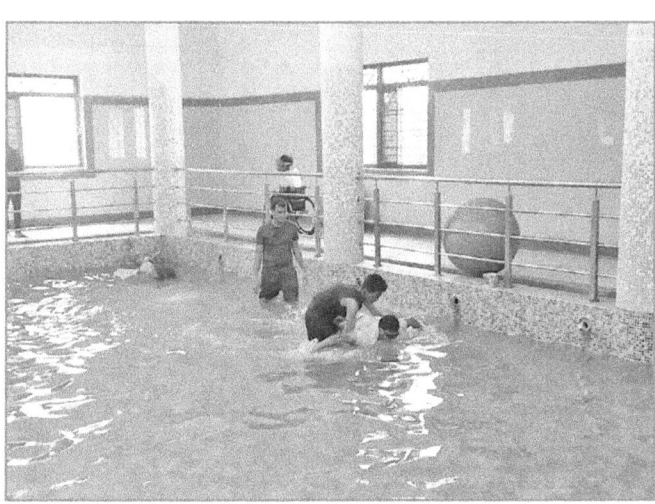

Fig. 20.35: Paraparetic patient exercising in hydrotherapy pool.

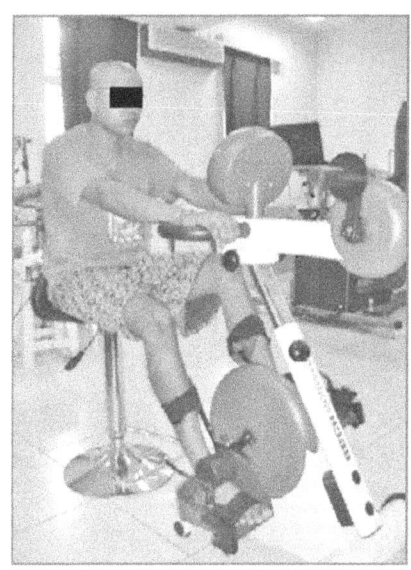

Fig. 20.36: Lower limb ergometry exercise.

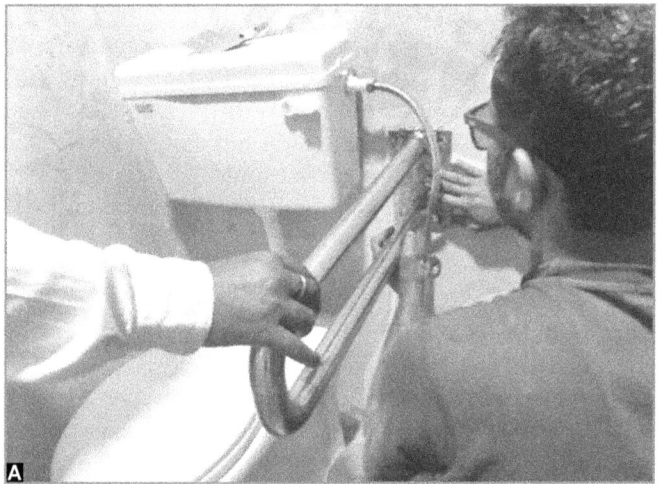
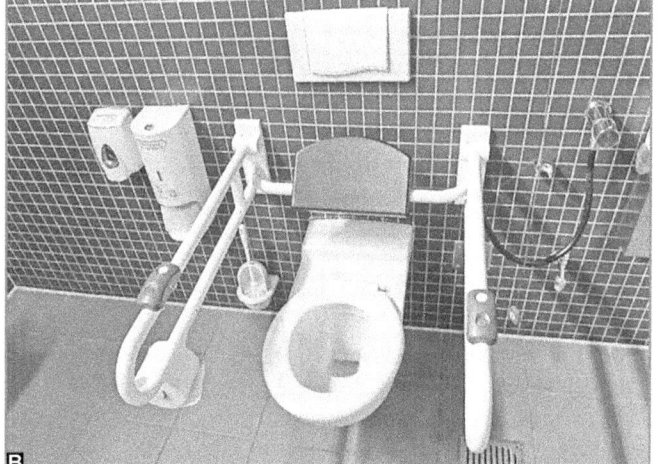

Figs. 20.37A and B: (A) Modification of the toilet is being done for a wheel chair user; (B) Modified, barrier-free toilet.

be availed by the SCI patients, particularly paraplegics, depending on his/her age, educational qualification and percentage of disabilities. Those having requisite qualification, can also avail loan from National Handicapped Finance Development Corporation for establishing their own business establishment.

Planning for Discharge

The most important component of management of SCI patients is discharge planning. Before the patient is sent home, it is the responsibility of the rehabilitation team to visit the patient's home, to assess, whether the home environment is barrier-free or any modification is required to have free access of the patient with crutches/wheel chairs, etc., to toilet, rooms for a comfortable living. If any modification is needed, the same are done **(Figs. 20.37A and B)** with the advice of the team.

Parkinson's Disease

INTRODUCTION

Parkinson's disease is a chronic progressive disorder of the extrapyramidal system of the central nervous system that leads to shaking (coarse tremors), stiffness (rigidity), slowness of movement (bradykinesia) impairment of balance, coordination, difficulty in walking and impairment of cognitive and executive function.

The term Parkinsonism is a generic term used to describe a group of disorders with primary disturbance in the dopamine systems of the basal ganglia, which could be attributed to genetic or environmental causes.

Parkinson's disease or idiopathic parkinsonism is the most common parkinsonian disorder, affecting almost 78% of patients with Parkinsonism. This disorder also called as paralysis agitans or shaking palsy, was first described by James Parkinson in 1817. The disease was categorized into following types:
- Postural instability and gait disturbed.
- Tremor predominant (tremor as the main feature).

The term parkinsonism-plus syndrome refers to those conditions, that resemble Parkinson's disease in some respects, but the symptoms are caused by other neurodegenerative disorders.

EPIDEMIOLOGY AND ETIOLOGY

The disease affects both men and women; however, men are affected more than women. More than 2% of people older than 65 years of age have Parkinson's disease.

One important risk factor for Parkinson's disease is age. Though, most people first develop the disease at about 60 years, about 5-10% of sufferers have early onset disease, which develops before the age of 50 years. Early onset forms of Parkinson's disease are sometimes inherited and linked to specific gene mutations. Although some cases of Parkinson's appear to be hereditary, and a few can be traced to specific genetic mutations, in most cases the disease occurs randomly and does not seem to run in families.

The exact cause of Parkinson's disease is not known (i.e., idiopathic), though researchers now believe that Parkinson's disease results from a combination of genetic factors and environmental factors such as exposure to toxins. However, secondary parkinsonism results from a number of different identifiable causes, including viruses, toxins, drugs, tumors, etc.

PATHOPHYSIOLOGY

Parkinson's disease develops, when the nerve cells or neurons in dopamine producing cells of substantia nigra of basal ganglia, that controls movement become impaired and/or die. The dopamine is produced in the cells in pars compacta of substantia nigra. When the neurons die or become impaired, they produce less dopamine, a neurotransmitter, resulting in movement problems. About 70-80% of loss of neurons in substantia nigra occurs before symptoms develop. Loss of dopamine activating neurons and the production of Lewy bodies within the pigmented substantia nigra neurons are the hallmarks of idiopathic parkinsonism.

The direct pathway facilitates basal ganglia output to thalamus and motor area (**Fig. 21.1**). The underactive direct pathway is responsible for bradykinesia. The indirect pathway (**Fig. 21.2**) disinhibits substantia nigra and in turn inhibits thalamus and motor areas. Loss of dopamine results in an overactive indirect pathway that is thought to underlie akinesia and rigidity. The basal ganglion that plays an important role in planning and programming movements by selecting and inhibiting movement strategies are affected leading to the impairments.

People with Parkinson's disease also lose the nerve endings that produce norepinephrine, the main chemical messenger of the sympathetic nervous system, which controls many

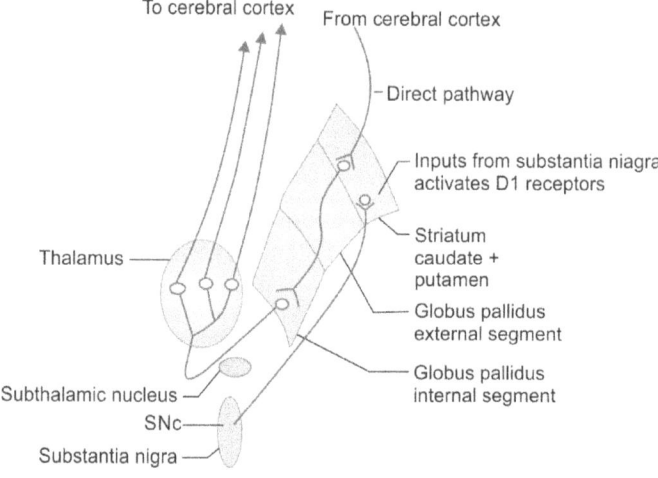

Fig. 21.1: The basal ganglia circuit-direct pathway. (SNc: substantia nigra pars compacta)

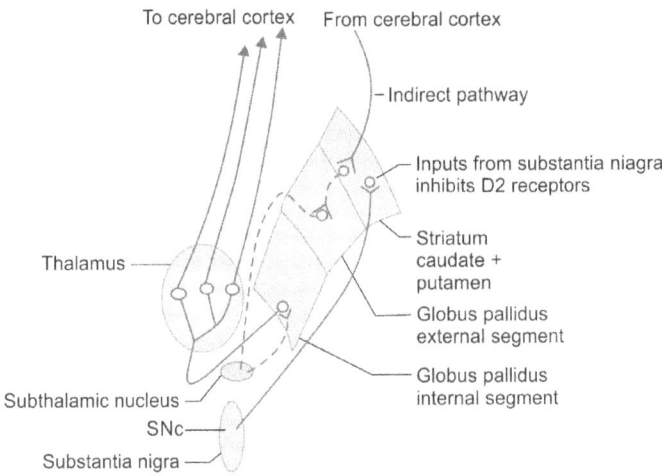

Fig. 21.2: The basal ganglia circuit: Indirect pathways. (SNc: substantia nigra pars compacta)

automatic functions of the body, such as heart rate and blood pressure. The loss of norepinephrine might help explain some of the non-movement features of Parkinson's, such as fatigue, irregular blood pressure, decreased movement of food through the digestive tract, and sudden drop in blood pressure when a person stands up from a sitting or lying-down position.

CLINICAL FEATURES

Parkinson's symptoms usually begin gradually and get worse over time (**Fig. 21.3**). As the disease progresses, people may have difficulty walking and talking. They may also have mental and behavioral changes, urinary problems, constipation, sleep problems, swallowing, chewing and speech problems, depression, memory difficulties, and fatigue.

Symptoms often begin on one side of the body or even in one limb on one side of the body. As the disease progresses, it eventually affects both sides. However, the symptoms may still be more severe on one side than on the other.

The four main features of the disease are:

1. **Tremor:** Tremor is the initial symptom of patients in about 70% of cases. Resting tremor, which is involuntary oscillation of body parts occurring at a rate of 4–6 Hz. It is peel-rolling type in hands and affects legs, jaw, and head also.

2. **Rigidity:** Both cogwheel (resistance at intervals) and lead pipe (resistance throughout) rigidity may be found. It affects shoulder and neck first and later on face and extremities are affected.
3. **Bradykinesia:** Slowness of movements—movements are reduced in speed, range and amplitude. Moments of freezing may occur and is characterized by sudden block or break of movement.
4. **Postural instability:** Narrow base of support, depression, dynamic destabilizing activities lead to postural instability. Weakness of trunk extensors as compared to flexors, leads to stooped posture (Camptocormia—also known as bent spine syndrome) characterized by an abnormal flexion of the trunk, appearing in standing position, increasing while walking, and ablating in supine lying position). Impairment of balance and coordination leads to fall affecting the quality of life significantly.

Masked face (face lacking normal expression), lack of normal limb movements while walking, akinesia (difficulty in initiating movement), Slow shuffle gait (that includes a tendency to lean forward, small quick steps as if hurrying forward, and reduced swinging of the arms), distorted hand writing (micrographia) are the common presentations.

Freezing episodes with periods of off (full inactivity) followed by periods of on (alertness/physically active), poverty of movement, akathisia (a movement disorder that causes an urge to move, which one fails to control), contracture and deformities, kyphotic posture, frequent falls, dysphagia, dysarthria, dementia, bradyphrenia (slowness of thoughts), sailorrhea (excessive drooling of saliva), seborrhea (red, itchy rash on the skin), mutism, low blood pressure, impaired respiratory function, constipation, excessive sweating, and abnormal hot and cold sensations may be present. Sleep disturbances, decreased ability to smell, mental fatigue, motor planning deficits affecting performance of complex movements may be present.

Poor gait, dementia, depression, postural hypotension, involuntary movements increase the risk of fall. The fear of fall increases the levels of immobility and dependency, deteriorating the quality of life of the patient.

Gait: Festinating/freezing gait—festinating gait (from Latin festinare-to hurry) is the type of gait exhibited by patients suffering from Parkinson's disease. It is characterized by stucking in one place when initiating a step or turning with increased risk of falling. The patient walks with a reduced stride length/stride width and reduced speed of walking (**Figs. 21.4A and B**). Cadence is normal, but may reduce in late stages. Double limb support is increased with deficient hip, knee flexion and ankle dorsiflexion and shuffling steps present. There is insufficient heel strike with loading on fore foot. There is reduced trunk rotation and arm swing with difficulty in turning and walking with diverted attention.

STAGES OF PARKINSON'S DISEASE

Hoehn and Yahr classification regarding stages of Parkinson's disease is given in **Table 21.1**.

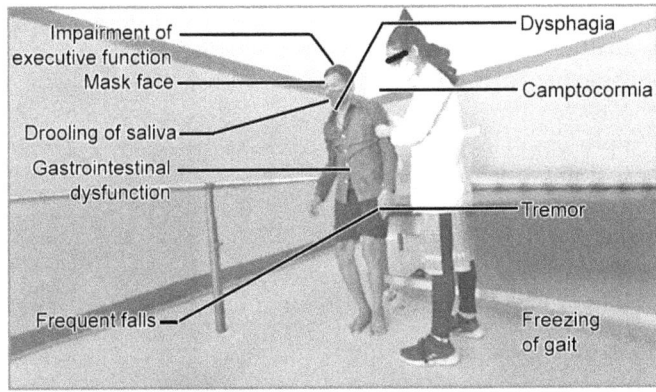

Fig. 21.3: Features of Parkinson's disease.

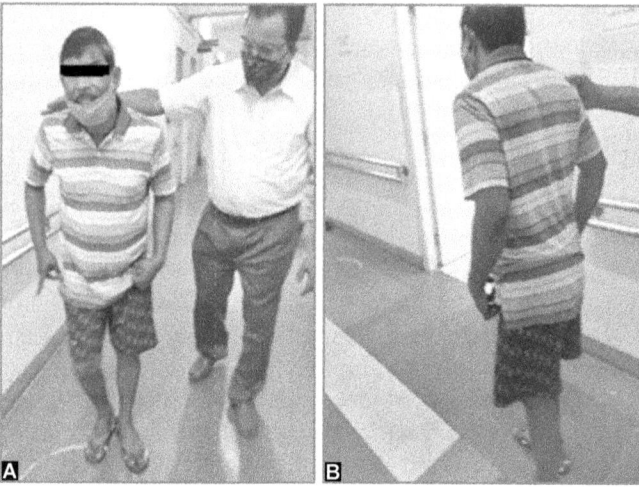

Figs. 21.4A and B: Festinating gait in Parkinson's disease: (A) Anterior view; (B) Posterior view.

Table 21.1: Stages of Parkinson's disease.

Stages	Characters of disability
I	Minimal or absent, unilateral if present
II	Minimal bilateral or midline involvement, balance is not impaired
III	Impaired righting reflexes. Unsteadiness when turning and rising from chair. Some activities are restricted, but patients can live independently and continue some form of employment
IV	All symptoms present and severe, standing and walking possible only with assistance
V	Confined to bed or wheel chair

DIAGNOSIS OF PARKINSON'S DISEASE

A number of disorders can cause symptoms similar to those of Parkinson's disease. People with Parkinson's-like symptoms that result from other causes are sometimes said to have parkinsonism. While these disorders initially may be misdiagnosed as Parkinson's disease, certain medical tests, as well as response to drug treatment, may help to distinguish them from Parkinson's disease. Since many other diseases have similar features but require different treatments, it is important to make an exact diagnosis as soon as possible.

There are currently no blood or laboratory tests to diagnose nongenetic cases of Parkinson's disease. Diagnosis is based on a person's medical history and a neurological examination. Improvement after initiating medication is another important hallmark of Parkinson's disease.

TREATMENT

Although there is no cure for Parkinson's disease, medicines, surgical treatment, and other therapies can relieve symptoms, considerably and improve the person's quality of life. The most common treatment includes drug therapy combined with rehabilitation therapies such as physiotherapy, occupational therapy and other therapies. Surgery is considered, when no improvement occurs with conservative management.

Drug Therapy

The main drug therapy for Parkinson's is levodopa, also called L-dopa. Nerve cells use levodopa to make dopamine to replenish the brain's reduced supply. Usually, people take levodopa along with another medication called carbidopa. Carbidopa prevents or reduces some of the side effects of levodopa therapy—such as nausea, vomiting, low blood pressure, and restlessness—and reduces the amount of levodopa needed to improve symptoms.

Physiotherapy

The physiotherapist performs a comprehensive assessment of the patient, before intervention and derives a problem list and establishes the plan of care. The components of assessment include:

- Complain and history.
- **Examination of higher functions:** Speech/hearing/vision.
- Mini mental state examination (MMSE) or Folstein test is a 30-point questionnaire that is used for measurement of cognitive impairment, mostly to screen for dementia.
- Depression inventory.
- **Sensory examination:** For presence of paresthesia, if any.
- Motor examination:
  - *Tone/rigidity:* Rigidity can be graded by using Webster's rigidity grading scale, such as: 0—nondetectable rigidity, 1—Detectable rigidity in the muscles of neck and shoulder. One or both arms show mild resting rigidity. 2—Moderate rigidity in the neck and shoulders. Resting rigidity is present. 3—Severe rigidity is present in the neck and shoulder. Resting rigidity cannot be relieved by medicines.
- Range of motion.
- Manual muscle test/voluntary motor control (VMC) grading.
- Tightness/contracture/deformity.
- **Posture/balance:**
  - Dynamic posturography.
  - Functional reach test.
  - Timed get-up and go test.
- **Endurance test:** 6-minutes walk test/10 minutes walk test.
- **Functional evaluation:** Functional independence measure (FIM).
- Gait.

Problem list: The problems associated with the patient are:
- Poor posture and balance.
- Reduced joint ROM.
- Weakness of muscles.
- Muscle stiffness/rigidity.
- Episodes of freezing.
- Inability/difficulty in turning.
- Fatigue.
- Pain.
- Abnormal gait.
- Impaired aerobic capacity/endurance.

Goals of Physiotherapy

- Induce relaxation.
- Improve joint range of motion and mobility.

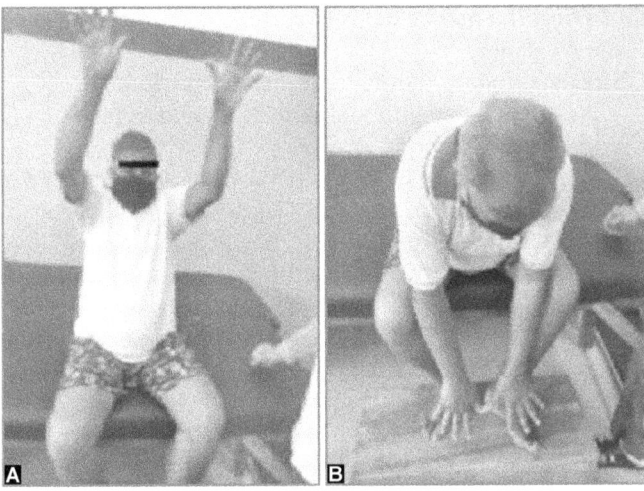

Figs. 21.5A and B: Breathing combined with upper limb movements: (A) Inspiration with arm elevation; (B) Expiration with lowering of arms.

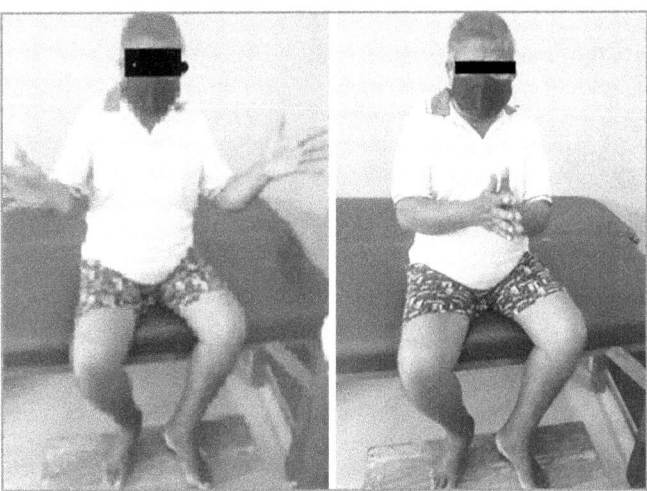

Fig. 21.6: Clapping to overcome freezing/bradykinesia and tremor.

- Improve posture and balance.
- Strengthen weak muscles.
- Improve turning skill.
- Reduce pain.
- Reduce fatigue.
- Improve gait.
- Improve aerobic capacity/endurance.

Physiotherapy Intervention

Relaxation exercises

Deep breathing exercises, such as breathing in with arms elevated, breathing out with arms lowering **(Figs. 21.5A and B)**. Relaxed passive exercises, gentile rocking on Swiss ball, slow rhythmic rotational movements of extremities and trunk, rhythmic initiation technique of PNF where movement progresses from passive to active assisted to active to low load active resisted exercises helps to overcome rigidity and induce relaxation. Activities such as clapping with both hands, playing musical instruments with hands help in inducing relaxation.

Flexibility Exercises

Passive stretching exercises, hold-relax, contract-relax, ROM exercises.

Strategies to overcome bradykinesia/akinesia

High-velocity exercises and activities combined with rhythmic excitatory command help in overcoming bradykinesia. Rhythmic initiation technique of PNF, helps in movement initiation, there by overcomes akinesia. Kicking and throwing a ball, clapping **(Fig. 21.6)**, playing musical instruments such as tabla, are also found to improve the quality and quantity of movement.

Strategies to reduce tremor

Weight bearing/weight shifting over the hands **(Figs. 21.7A and B)**, clapping, playing musical instruments, use of a light weight cuff **(Fig. 21.7C)** tied to forearm, while doing functional activities help in minimizing tremor.

Strengthening exercises

Strength training is most effective during the "on" phase, i.e., 45 minutes to 1 hour after taking medications. Isokinetic exercises are effective as compared to isometric exercises in developing strength and endurance in such individuals. Functional training such as kicking balls **(Figs. 21.8A to C)** and hydrotherapy, static cycle exercises are effective to build up strength and endurance of muscles.

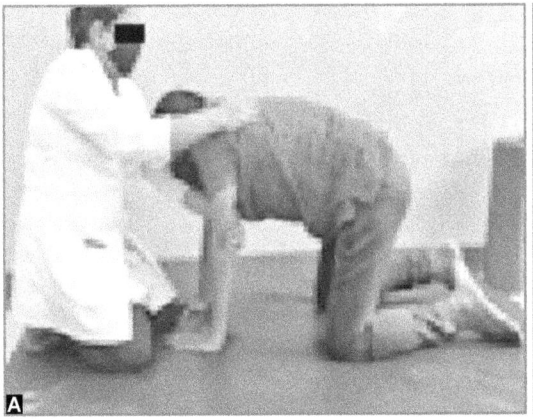 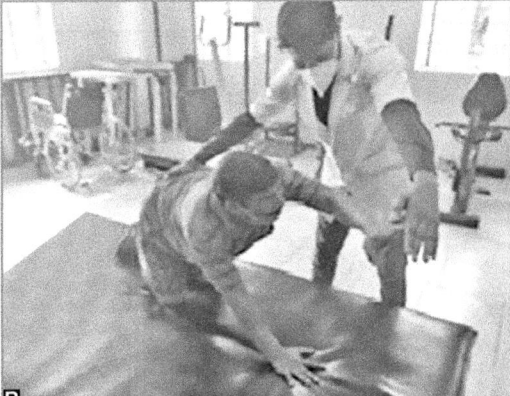 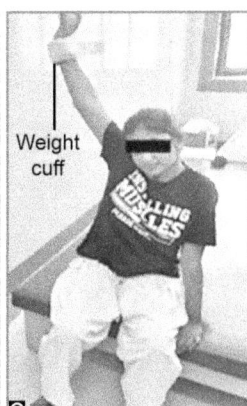

Figs. 21.7A to C: (A) Weight-bearing/weight shifting exercise; (B) Weight-bearing with reaching/weight shifting; (C) Grasping and releasing objects with a weight cuff tied to lower forearm.

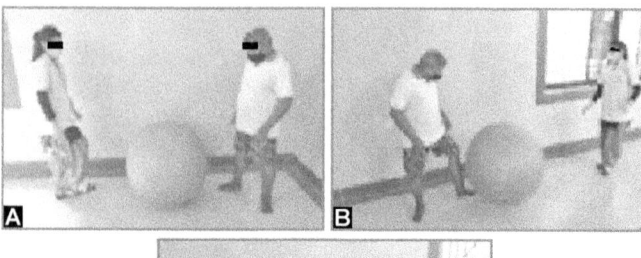

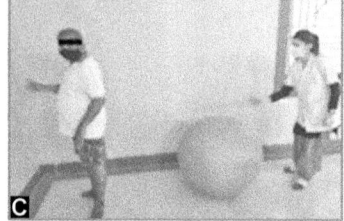

Figs. 21.8A to C: (A) Kicking a ball forward; (B) Kicking a ball sideways; (C) Kicking a ball backward.

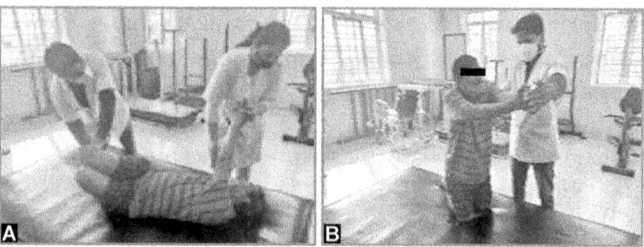

Figs. 21.9A and B: Axial rotation: (A) Lying; (B) Kneel standing.

Strategies to improve posture

- Stretching of tight pectorals (corner stretch), hip flexor stretching, hamstrings stretching, TA stretching.
- Strengthening of neck, trunk and hip extensors on Swiss ball.
- Strengthening of quadriceps femoris muscle.
- Postural biofeedback training using mirror.
- **PNF:** Rhythmic stabilization.
- **Balance training:** Emphasis should be on development of both static and dynamic balance. Standing/sitting in front of a postural mirror, helps to correct posture and develop static balance.
- Strategies to improve dynamic balance include:
  - Practice of dynamic stability tasks such as reaching in different directions.
  - Axial rotation of head and trunk (**Figs. 21.9A and B**).
- Balance exercises on Swiss ball (**Fig. 21.10A**), wobble board (**Fig. 21.10B**), trampoline (**Fig. 21.10C**).
- Catching and throwing a ball from different directions (**Fig. 21.11**).
- Lifting a Swiss ball in standing and turning the ball from left to right (**Fig. 21.12**).
- Stepping/marching on plain surface (**Fig. 21.13**)/over steps.
- Kitchen sink exercises (**Figs. 21.14A to C**) to improve balance. Patient stands facing the kitchen sink, with the feet a comfortable distance apart, feet pointing straight forward. He/she holds onto the edge of the sink as needed for balance, and performs the exercises. Such exercises include:
  - Sink squat.
  - Movement transitions such as sitting to standing, half-kneeling to standing.
  - Standing exercises such as standing heel raises, standing toe offs, partial squat, etc.
  - Single limb stance, and side kicking, and backward kicking a ball, and marching in one place.
- **Functional training:**
  - Bed mobility exercises such as rolling on bed, supine to sitting, quadruped weight shifting are helpful.
  - Sitting on bed/chair and performing peg board activities.
  - Pelvic bridging exercises (**Fig. 21.15**).
  - Pelvic clock exercises on Swiss ball.
  - Sit to stand and stand to sit activities.
  - Training of self-care skills.
  - Training to get up after fall.
  - Facial exercises.
- **Locomotor/gait training:**
  - Mental rehearsing the walking pattern before walking.

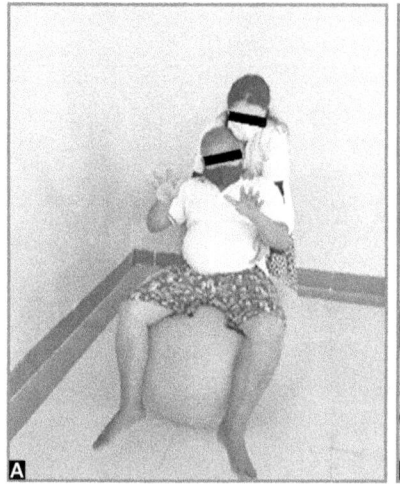
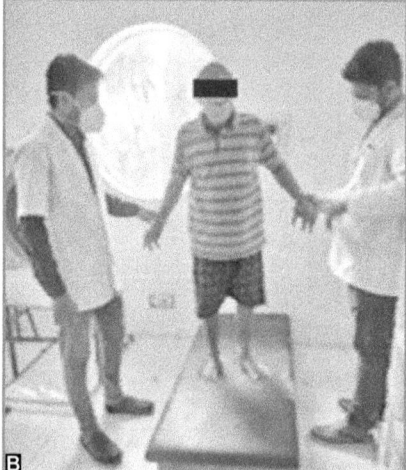
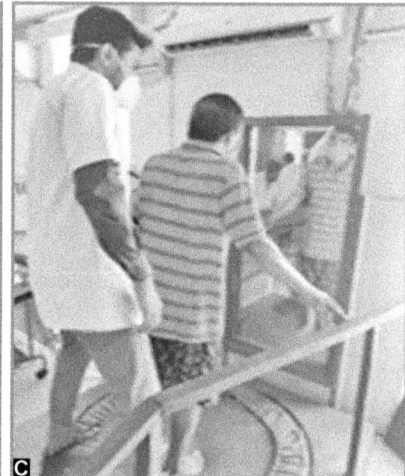

Figs. 21.10A to C: (A) Sitting balance development on Swiss ball; (B) Standing balance development on wobble board; (C) Standing balance development on trampoline.

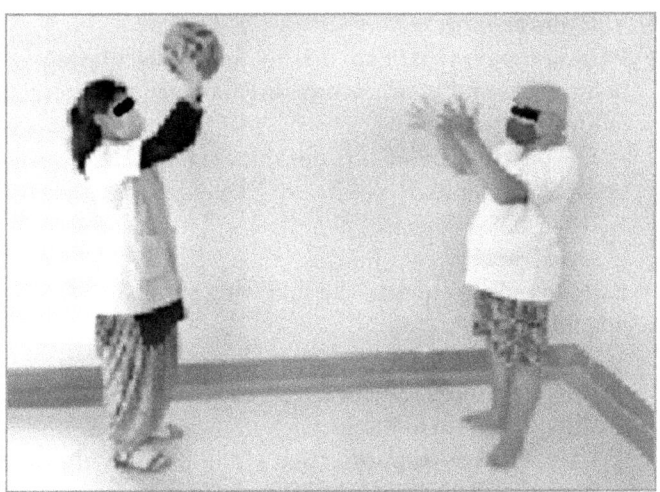

Fig. 21.11: Catching and throwing ball to improve standing balance and upper limb function.

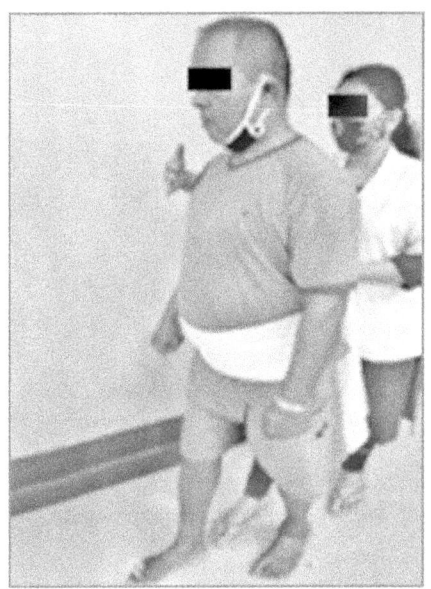

Fig. 21.13: Stepping/marching on plain surface.

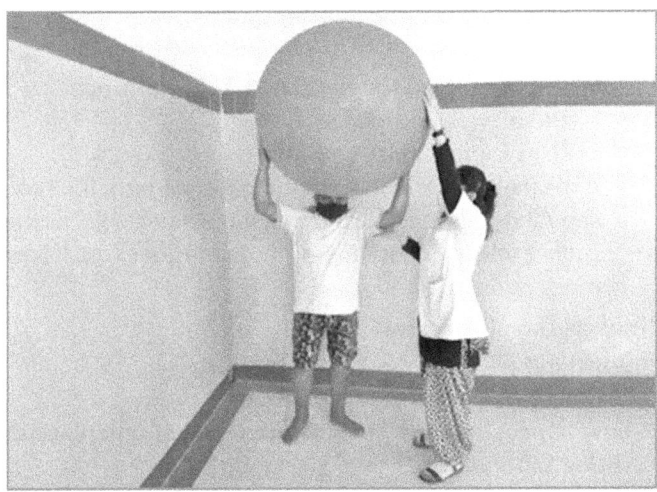

Fig. 21.12: Development of standing balance (static/dynamic).

- Walking on gait mat/foot prints on floor/gait ladder **(Fig. 21.16)** to increase step and stride length/stride width.
- Gait training using declarative learning strategies with increased velocity.
- Enhancing arm swings through the use of two sticks, one end each of the sticks held by the patient and other end held by therapist **(Fig. 21.17)**.
- Turning and changing direction while walking through sudden opening of an umbrella in front of the patient.
- Postural mirror biofeedback training.
- PNF activity of braiding (side stepping/alternate cross stepping).
- Walking into side stepping, walking backwards, fast walking, and walking on incline surfaces.
- Step climbing and descending.
- Gait training with walker/tripod stick/walking stick.

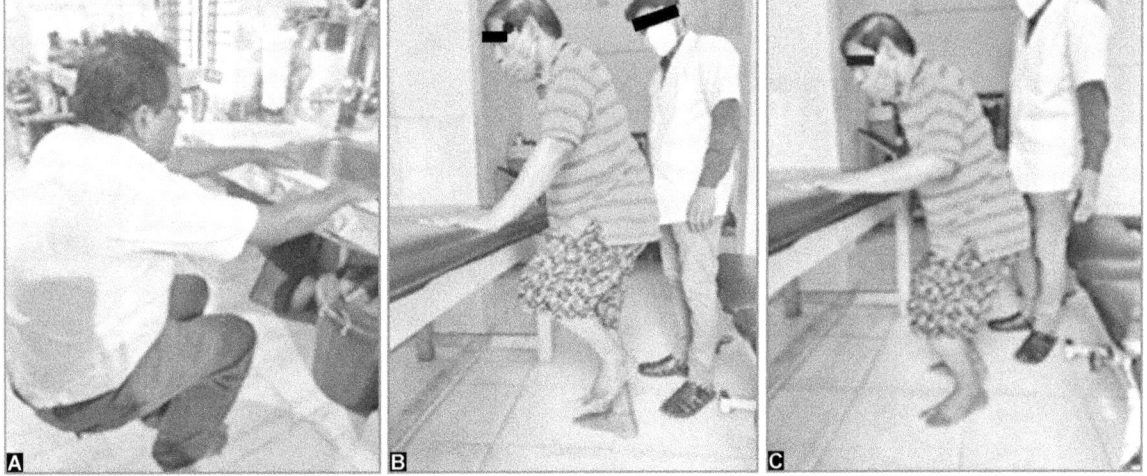

Figs. 21.14A to C: Kitchen sink exercises: (A) Sink squat; (B) Single limb stance; (C) Standing heel raises.

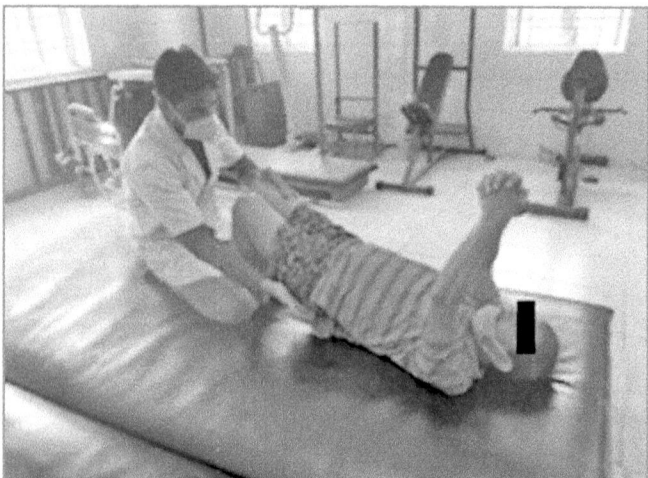

Fig. 21.15: Pelvic bridging exercise.

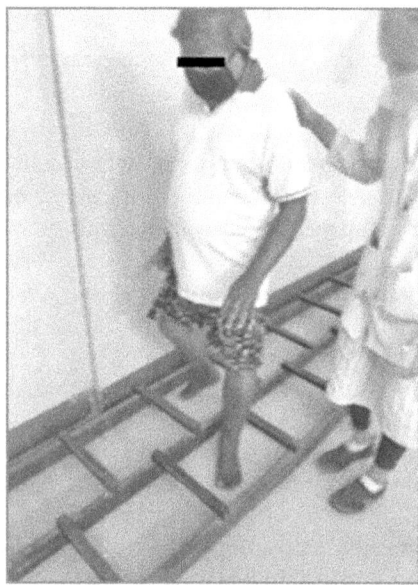

Fig. 21.16: Walking on gait ladder.

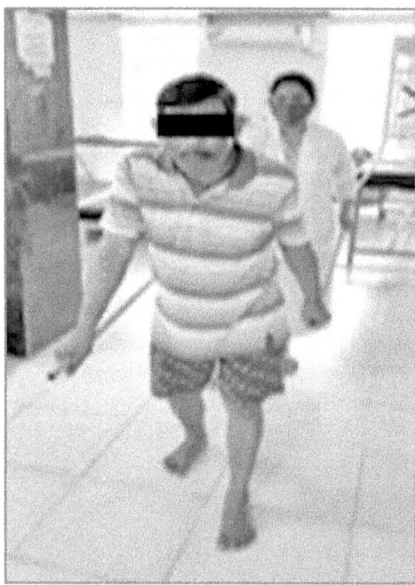

Fig. 21.17: Gait training using two sticks.

- ❖ **Cardiopulmonary/fitness training:**
  - Deep breathing exercises.
  - Upper and lower extremity ergometry.
  - Hydrotherapy.
- ❖ **Pain management:** Pain arising from musculoskeletal deformities and poor posture are managed through the following strategies:
  - Use of orthotics, such as ASH brace **(Fig. 21.18)**.
  - Moist hot packs.
  - IFT/TENS.
  - Hydrotherapy.
- ❖ **Fatigue management:** The following strategies may be helpful:
  - Activity pacing/energy conservation techniques.
  - Deep breathing exercises.
  - Circuit interval training.
  - Use of adaptive/supportive equipment to improve posture and function: An occupational therapist designs the appropriate adaptive devices and trains the patient for its use. The spinal brace should be custom made for the patient, fabricated by the orthotist. Such devices include:
    » Use of raised toilet sheets and bars for support in toilet.
    » Use of adapted spoon **(Fig. 21.19)**/comb/pen.
    » Use of walking aids.
    » Use of spinal brace (ASH brace).
  - If the patient walks in a shuffling gait pattern, the shoe should have a leather or hard composition sole, as the rubber sole does not slide easily on the floor, which may result into a fall.

Group and home exercises
This include:
- ❖ Clapping/playing musical instruments.
- ❖ Low impact aerobics such as marching in one place in sitting and standing.

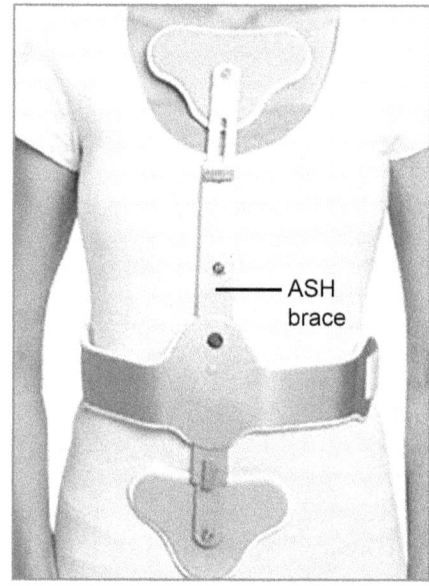

Fig. 21.18: The ASH brace.

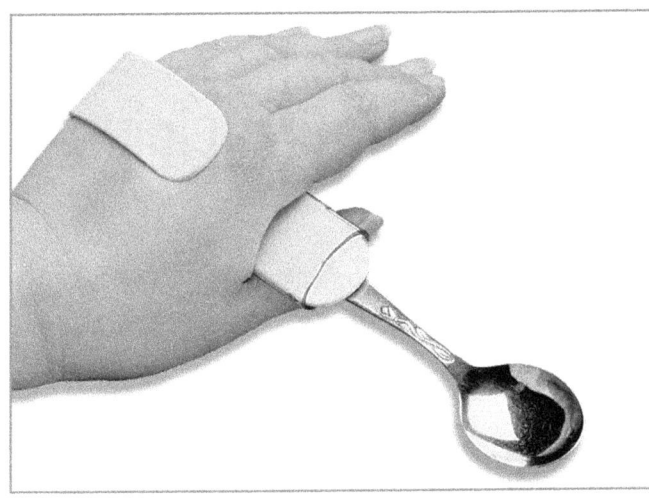

Fig. 21.19: The adapted spoon.

* Singing.
* Dancing in tune with music.

Surgical Intervention

If, no response in improvement of symptoms takes place with medical and therapeutic management, surgery is the next choice of management in selected cases. Surgical procedures undertaken include ablative surgery, such as:

* **Pallidotomy:** A neurosurgical procedure, where a tiny electrical probe is placed in the globus pallidus (one of the basal nuclei of the brain), which is then heated to 80°C for 60 seconds, to destroy a small area of brain cells.
* **Thalamotomy:** This is a surgical procedure used to treat tremor. It involves destroying a tiny area in a part of the brain called the thalamus.

Deep Brain Stimulation

Deep brain stimulation (DBS) is a surgical procedure in which surgically implanted electrodes are inserted into part of the brain and connects them to a small electrical device implanted in the chest. The device and electrodes painlessly stimulate the brain in a way that helps stop many of the movement-related symptoms of Parkinson's, such as tremor, slowness of movement, and rigidity.

Neural transplantation: This surgery involves replacement of dopaminergic neurons in patients with Parkinson's disease.

Traumatic Brain Injury

INTRODUCTION

Traumatic brain injury (TBI) is defined as an insult to the brain from an external force that leads to temporary or permanent impairment of physical, cognitive, or psychosocial function. It is a form of acquired brain injury, which may be open (penetrating) or closed (nonpenetrating) and can be categorized as mild, moderate, or severe, depending on the clinical presentation.

It is a disruption of normal function of brain, due to a blow, bump, or jolt to the head, or penetration into the brain by a bullet or fractured piece of skull, causing injury to the brain tissue, resulting in motor, sensory, and higher function (cognitive, perceptual, speech, hearing, and vision) impairments and persistent vegetative state to death in few cases.

Etiology

The most common cause of TBI is road traffic accidents (RTA). The other causes include fall from height, domestic and community violence resulting in fall/hit on head, bullet injury/blast injury (defence war, robbery, by violent mobs), fall in bathroom, direct contact sports, etc. Violent shaking of a baby (Shaken baby syndrome) can also cause TBI in infants.

Risk factors for the disorder include:
- Children of age group of 1–4 years.
- Young adults between the age of 15 and 24 years.
- Old men/women over the age of 60 years.
- Males as compared to females, due to more involvement in outside works.

Types of Traumatic Brain Injury

The injury to the brain could be:
- **Mild TBI**: In this the brain tissue is affected temporarily, and good prognosis can be expected from such injury. The injury is mostly of concussion.

  Concussion: A concussion is a type of injury that affects brain function temporarily. The features include headaches and problems with concentration, memory, balance, and coordination.
- **Moderate to severe TBI**: It results in bruising, tearing, bleeding and physical damage to brain tissues. The damage to brain tissues could be of the following types:
  - *Contusion:* A *contusion* is an *injury* that causes bleeding and tissue damage. It is a bruise of the brain tissue, resulting in an *injured* capillary or blood vessel leaking blood into the surrounding area. *It is* a type of *hematoma*, which refers to any collection of blood outside of a blood vessel **(Fig. 22.1)**.
  - *Laceration:* Cerebral lacerations are tears in brain tissue, caused by a foreign object or pushed-in bone fragment from a skull fracture. Motor vehicle crashes and blows to the head are common causes of bruises and tears of brain tissue. Symptoms of moderate to severe head injury may develop.

Mechanism of Traumatic Brain Injury

There are various mechanisms producing TBI that result in physiologic or structural brain damage. The mechanisms include:

Blunt, Nonpenetrating TBI

Blunt, nonpenetrating TBI results from a direct impact to the head or from head acceleration or deceleration without impact. Brain injury from this mechanism has two phases. The first phase occurs as a direct result of the initiating traumatic event that results in death immediately before emergency medical care is initiated. Direct impact of the brain against the bony cranial vault and shearing of the neurovascular structures result in neuronal damage. Further, during

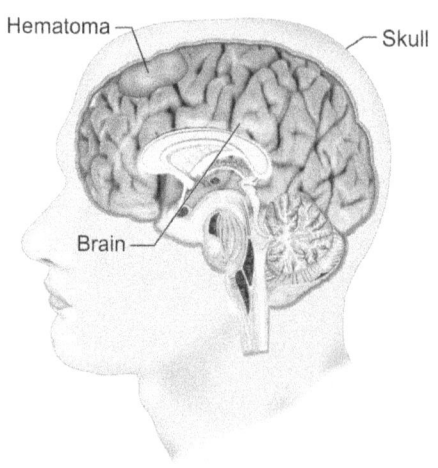

Fig. 22.1: Contusion of brain, producing hematoma.

acceleration/deceleration, movement of the brain in the fluid filled compartment inside the skull, result in striking the brain tissues against the inner aspect of the skull both anteriorly and posteriorly, resulting in **coup-contrecoup injury**.

The second phase that begins after the primary/first phase, involves a cascade of several neuropathologic processes continuing for weeks to months after the initial injury. There occurs a progression of axonal injury, with shifts in ionic flux leading to axonal swelling, a loss of axonal transport, and altered neurotransmission. Mitochondrial failure results in an energy crisis for the neuron, leading to a loss of neuronal function and apoptosis (programmed cell death). This secondary phase might also involve necrosis and neuronal demyelination.

Penetrating TBI

A penetrating TBI occurs when physical, external forces affect the brain and an object enters the brain tissue. Missile injuries such as gunshot wounds are either penetrating (where the object/bullet enters and lodges inside the cranial cavity) or perforating types (where the object/bullet, traverses the cranial cavity and leaves through an exit wound).

Blast-induced TBI

Blast-induced type of injury most commonly occurs in military personnel. The neurologic injury results both from a direct shock wave effect and an indirect transfer of the shock wave through blood vessels and cerebrospinal fluid (CSF) to the brain. Exposure to blast overpressure initiates a cascade of cellular pathologic processes in the brain, including damage to the microvasculature and blood-brain-barrier integrity, followed by increased permeability. The breakdown of the microvessels can result in brain edema and an increase in intracranial pressure (ICP), accompanied by the activation of secondary brain injury by impairing cerebral perfusion and oxygenation.

Recovery of Function after TBI

Recovery of function following brain injury occurs through two processes:
1. **Spontaneous recovery:** Repair of central nervous system (CNS), early after brain injury, including regression of diaschisis (sudden change of function in a portion of brain, connected to a distant, but damaged brain area).
2. **Function-induced recovery:** The process is based on promotion of neuroplasticity in response to activity practice and environmental stimulation. The principle of experience dependent neuroplasticity are:
    - *Use it or lose it:* Not using the body for function causes deterioration.
    - *Use it and improve it:* Using body for function results in improvement.
    - *Specificity:* Neuroplastic changes are determined by specific types of task performed.
    - *Time matters:* Different time of training is related to different neuroplastic changes. Task practice during recovery phase causes increased neuroplasticity.
    - *Repetition:* Sufficient repetitions of task practice are required to intensify neuroplasticity.
    - *Intensity/progressive practice of task:* Tasks performed in progressive and complex manner leads to greater neuroplasticity.
    - *Silence matters:* Tasks with a proper meaning induces better neuroplasticity.
    - *Age:* Neuroplasticity is better in young people compared to older.
    - *Neuroplasticity induces transference:* Neuroplastic changes following practice of one task might help in performing tasks of similar in nature.

Diagnostic Tests in TBI

Imaging Tests

- **Computerized tomography (CT) scan:** This test is usually the first performed test in an emergency room for a suspected TBI. A CT scan can quickly visualize fractures and reveals evidence of bleeding in the brain, blood clots (hematomas), bruised brain tissue (contusions), and brain tissue swelling.
- **Magnetic resonance imaging (MRI):** An MRI uses powerful radiowaves and magnets to create a detailed view of the brain. This test may be used after the patient's condition stabilizes, or if symptoms don't improve soon after the injury.
- **Intracranial pressure monitor:** A probe is inserted through the skull to monitor intracranial pressure.

Clinical Features

Traumatic brain injury produces a wide-range of physical and psychological effects on the affected individual. Some signs or symptoms may appear immediately after the traumatic event, while others may appear days or weeks later. The features of TBI depend on the severity of the condition, i.e., mild or moderate to severe.
- **Features of mild TBI:** Headache, nausea, vomiting, dizziness, loss of consciousness for few seconds to minutes, memory deficits, sleep disturbances, blurring of vision, impairment of smell and taste, etc.
- **Features of moderate to severe TBI:** Prolonged or permanent changes in person's state of consciousness that include:
    - *Coma:* The person in this state of unconsciousness, is unaware of the environment. This results from wide spread damage to all parts of the brain. The person may recover from the state of coma in a few days/weeks or may enter into vegetative state.
    - *Vegetative state:* Widespread damage to the brain can result in a vegetative state. The person may be unaware of surroundings; he or she may open eyes, make sounds, respond to reflexes, or move. The person may remain in the vegetative state, permanently or may progress to a minimally conscious state.
    - *Minimally conscious state:* It is a condition of severely altered consciousness, with persistence of some

awareness of one's environment. It is sometimes a transition between coma/vegetative state and state of recovery.
- *Brain death:* In this there is no measurable activity in the brain/brainstem. This condition is usually irreversible and patient survives with life support systems. Removal of breathing devices results in cessation of breathing and heart failure.

Besides, changes in consciousness level discussed above, patients with moderate to severe head injury also exhibit the followings:
- Headache and vomiting.
- Seizure disorders.
- Vertigo.
- Hydrocephalus.
- Cognitive perceptual dysfunction.
- Mood disorders (excessive anxiety/depression).
- Speech loss (aphasia)/impairment (dysphasia/dysarthria).
- Impairment of emotion and executive functions.
- Cranial nerve dysfunctions leading to loss/impairment of smell, taste, vision, hearing and swallowing functions.
- Sensory impairment.
- Motor impairment leading to spasticity (though initially, the patient is flaccid, soon after, he/she develops spasticity. A recent study concludes that "Signs of spasticity can often be noted within the first 4 weeks after brain injury and is more common in the upper than lower extremity), and so also for rigidity, dystonia, ballismus, chorea, ataxia presenting with severe weakness of muscles of face, neck, trunk, and limbs depending upon the part of brain affected". Two types of postures are exhibited by the patient, such as:
  1. Decorticate posture (pathology is in the cortex, the neck and legs remain in extension, hips medially rotated and feet plantar flexed with upper limbs in flexor pattern) **(Fig. 22.2)**.
  2. Decerebrate posture (pathology is in the brainstem or cerebellum; abnormal breathing pattern, extension pattern in upper and lower limbs) **(Fig. 22.3)**.

The patient may present with quadriplegia/quadriparesis, monoplegia/monoparesis, and hemiplegia/hemiparesis with severe impairment of gross motor/fine motor functions.
- Bladder/bowel/sexual dysfunction.
- Impairment in family and social participation.

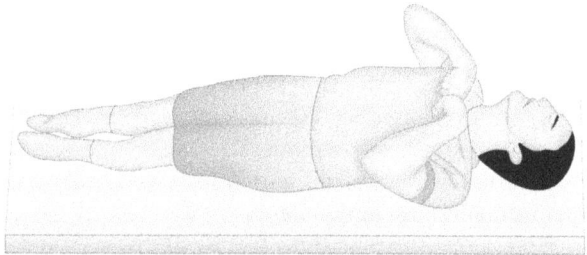

Fig. 22.2: Decorticate posture.

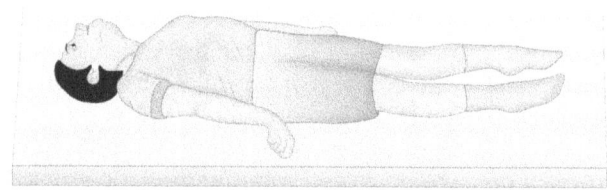

Fig. 22.3: Decerebrate posture.

Assessment of a Patient with Traumatic Brain Injury

The assessment includes:
a. **Immediate assessment after trauma:** Once a patient is brought to the hospital/trauma care center, the clinical team should assess the followings:
   - Status of the airways (to find whether the airway is intact or blocked by the tongue falling backward, broken teeth, etc.).
   - *Breathing:* Whether the patient is able to breath air efficiently or has breathing difficulties (may be due to associated rib fractures) or there is cessation of respiration, necessitating intubation and ventilator application.
   - *Circulation:* Heart rate, peripheral pulsation should be assessed to know the functioning of cardiovascular system.
   - *Level of consciousness:* The Glasgow Coma Scale (GCS) is a clinical scale used to reliably measure the person's level of consciousness after a brain injury. A person's level of consciousness is graded based on his/her ability to open the eye, speak and move the body. The GCS score ranges from 3 (completely unresponsive) to 15 (fully responsive). In clinical situations, where it is not possible to test for the various items such as, eye opening in case of blindness, verbal response in case of intubation motor response in case of muscle paralysis, it should be mentioned: NT = Not tested.
   - *Bladder function:* As the patient very often remains in cerebral shock, the ability to void urine may be affected, necessitating application of indwelling catheter. Hence, it is essential to assess bladder function shortly after head injury.

b. **Assessment during recovery and rehabilitation phase:** The assessment by the physiotherapist in this stage commences when the patient is medically stable. It includes:
   - Demographic data.
   - Subjective examination.
   - Observation of posture (including decorticate/decerebrate postures, if any), mobility and breathing status.
   - Examination of interacting systems of the body such as:
     » Level of consciousness.
     » Higher function examination: Speech, hearing, vision, memory, perception, cognition, executive function, etc.
     » Examination of cranial nerves.
     » Sensory system examination.

- Motor system examination, that includes:
  - Tone.
  - Spasticity/rigidity/dystonia/ataxia.
  - Reflexes: Superficial/deep/primitive reflexes.
  - Muscle power (MRC-grading system)/voluntary motor control (VMC): When spasticity grade is >1, as per Modified/modified-Ashworth scale, and movements alter the muscle tone, VMC, grading should be performed in place of manual muscle testing. Though different experts have described different VMC grading systems, the following system of grading, which is done in line with the Stroke Rehabilitation Assessment of Movement (STREAM) scale described for stroke patients seems reasonable for VMC grading in patients with UMN lesions including TBI. Six grades of voluntary motor control are:
    - Grade 0: No contraction
    - Grade 1: Flicker of contraction present or initiation of movement
    - Grade 2: Half range of motion in synergy or abnormal pattern
    - Grade 3: Full range of motion in synergy or abnormal pattern
    - Grade 4: Initial half range is performed in isolation and the latter half in pattern
    - Grade 5: Full range of motion in isolation but goes into pattern when resistance is offered
    - Grade 6: Full range of motion in isolation against resistance.
  - Tightness/contracture/deformity.
  - Coordination.
  - Involuntary movements.
  - Balance.
  - Exercise tolerance/endurance.
  - Bladder/bowel/sexual function.
  - Respiratory system examination.
  - Functional ability.
  - Need of assistive/mobility devices.
  - Gait.

After a thorough assessment, the clinician/therapist prepares a problem list and sets goal for the patient.

Goal Settings

The patients with TBI have impairment in multiple systems affecting their family and community participation, and overall quality of life. Once the patient is medically stable, and attends rehabilitation clinic, specific, measurable, achievable, realistic, timely (SMART) goal should be set by the rehabilitation team having short-term and long-term components in the same line as done with stroke patients.

Management of Traumatic Brain Injury

Management of TBI is based on the severity of injury, i.e., whether the injury is mild or moderate/severe, are briefly discussed:

- **Mild injury:** The patient needs rest, medications to control headache and vomiting (if any) and regular health status monitoring. The treatment team should decide, when the patient should return to work involving physical and cognitive stress.
- **Moderate to severe injury:** The patients with moderate to severe brain injury, need immediate care for oxygenation, blood supply, maintenance of blood pressure and prevention of further injuries to head and neck. The major facets of management are:
  - Medical management consists of antiseizure medicines (as most patients with TBI get seizure within 1 week following head injury), diuretics (are given intravenously to reduce raised ICP in the brain) and other drugs to reduce complications as needed.
  - *Surgery:* Emergency surgery may be indicated to prevent further damage to brain tissue. It includes:
    - Surgery to remove hematoma that has developed due to bleeding in or outside the brain, causing raised ICP.
    - Surgery to control bleeding.
    - Surgery to repair skull fractures.
    - Surgery to reduce ICP by creating a window in the skull that provides room for the brain tissue, which is compressed/displaced due to raised ICP.
  - *Rehabilitation:* Once the patient is medically stable, rehabilitation of the patient is very important, which aims at achieving as much functional independence as possible and enabling return to family/community and providing a qualitative living to the clients. The facets of rehabilitation are:
    - Medical management for spasticity/dystonia and epilepsy (if any).
    - Physiotherapy: Physiotherapy to TBI patients starts in the very early stage when the patient is in ICU/trauma care unit, and continues throughout recovery/rehabilitation phases. Physiotherapy in the early stage focuses on:
      - Chest care: Through secretion removal techniques and breathing exercises.
      - Joint positioning through pillows, positional braces, sand bags, etc. To prevent development of peripheral limb edema and subsequent deep vein thrombosis (DVT), as well as to prevent development of tightness/contracture and deformity that interferes with the patient's rehabilitation.
      - Regular passive movements: Relaxed passive movements to the limbs are to be given regularly to maintain circulation, maintain joint range of motion and prevent DVT.
      - Regular turning from supine to side lying through use of special beds or manually, if permitted by the neurosurgeon.
      - Active assisted/free exercises and up-righting (sitting) as per the patient's health status.

Physiotherapy During Recovery/Rehabilitation Phase

During this phase physiotherapy focuses on:
- Restorative interventions for reactivation of penumbra and diaschisis and restoring premorbid movements—promotion of neuroplasticity.
- Compensatory strategies to accomplish function through use of unaffected body parts/assistive and adaptive technologies.
- Preventing interventions to reduce complications and minimize barriers for activity and participation limitations. The physiotherapy interventions provided are:
  - *Therapeutic exercises:* It includes relaxed passive exercises, passive stretching, and range of motion (ROM) exercises, and active exercises/motor control training **(Figs. 22.4A and B)**, developmental therapies [Neurodevelopmental treatment (NDT)/Rood's approach/proprioceptive neuromuscular facilitation (PNF) technique/sensory integration therapy, etc.] to normalize tone and improve posture and mobility **(Figs. 22.5 and 22.6)**, functional re-education with or without adaptive devices and weight cuff to minimize involuntary movements (if any) in the upper limbs **(Figs. 22.7A to C)**, biofeedback to enhance posture and movements, balance training **(Fig. 22.9)**, resistance training, mobility and transfer skill training, standing tolerance development and gait training with or without orthosis and walking aids/modified (weighted walker, if ataxia dominates) **(Figs. 22.8A and B)**. Ataxia and dyskinesia, if present, should be managed by weight-

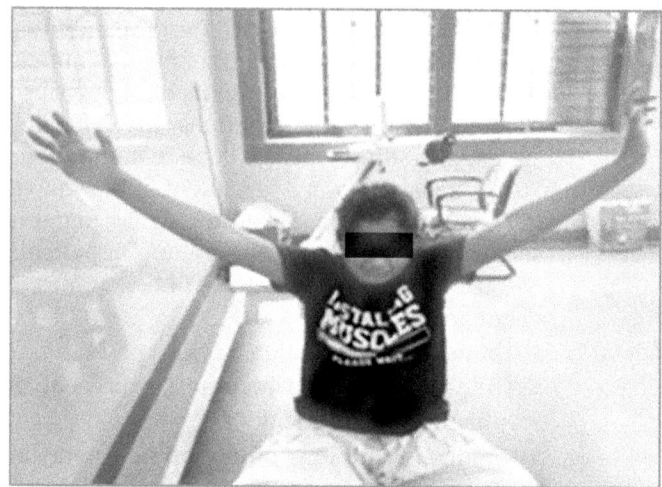

Fig. 22.5: Proprioceptive neuromuscular facilitation: Upper limb pattern in sitting.

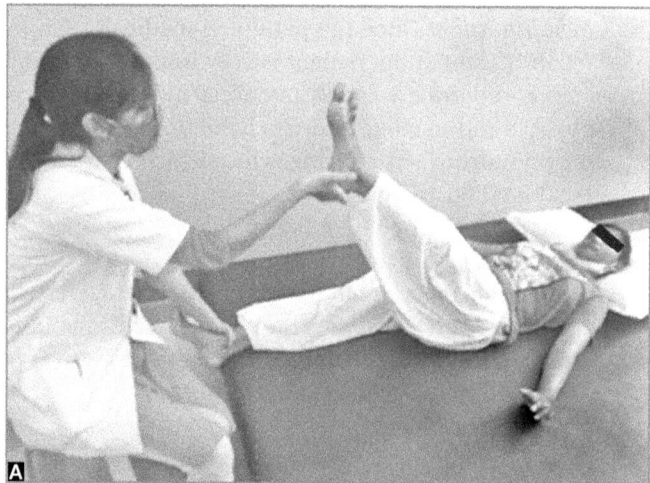

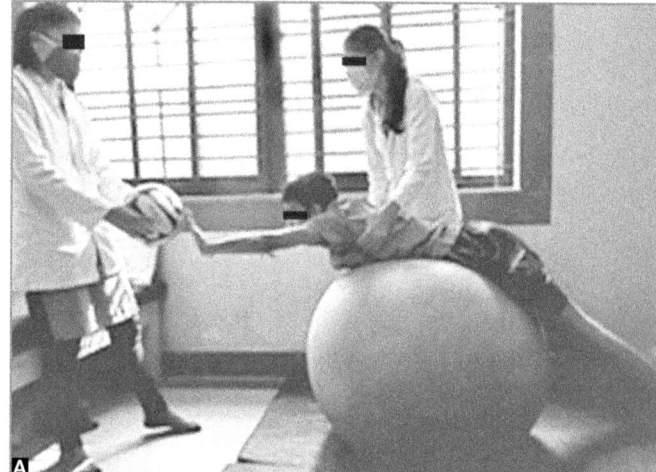

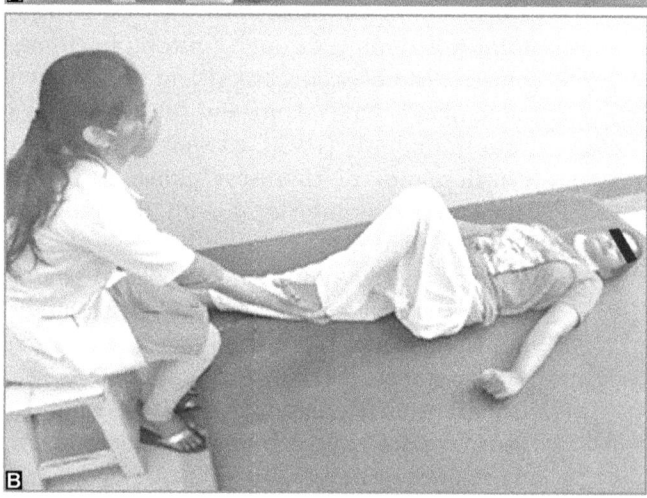

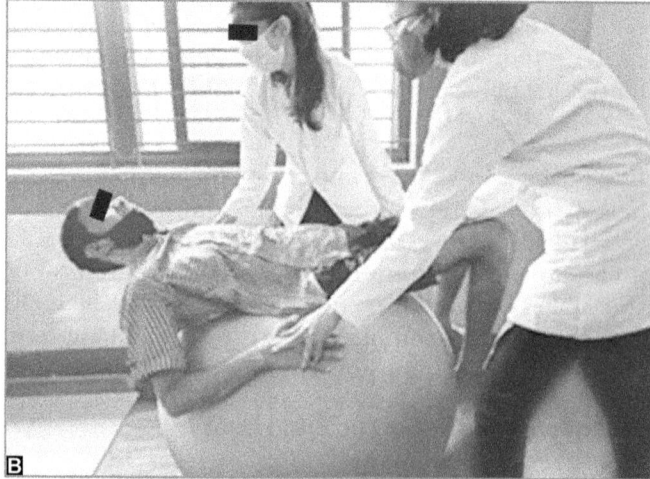

Figs. 22.4A and B: Motor control training for reciprocal motion of lower limbs used during walking.

Figs. 22.6A and B: Neurodevelopmental treatment: Trunk facilitation on Swiss ball—(A) Extension; (B) Flexion.

Chapter 22: Traumatic Brain Injury

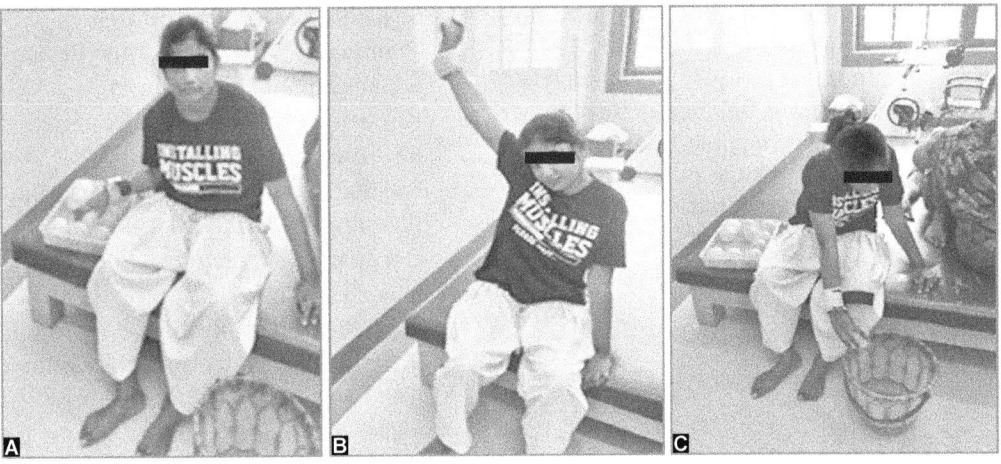

Figs. 22.7A to C: Functional re-education training using weight cuff in hand to reduce tremor.

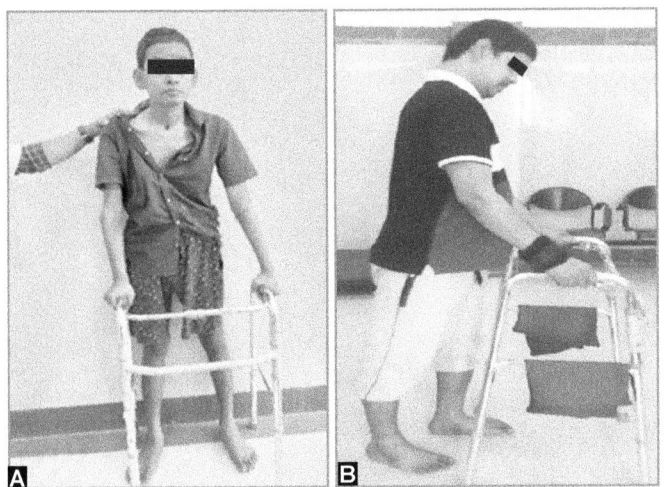

Figs. 22.8A and B: (A) Standing and initiating stepping with walker; (B) Gait training with modified/weighted walker.

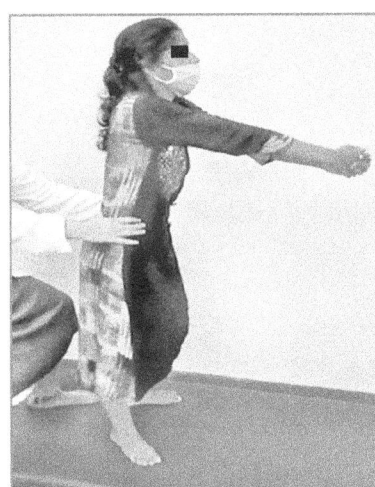

Fig. 22.9: Balance training on wobble board.

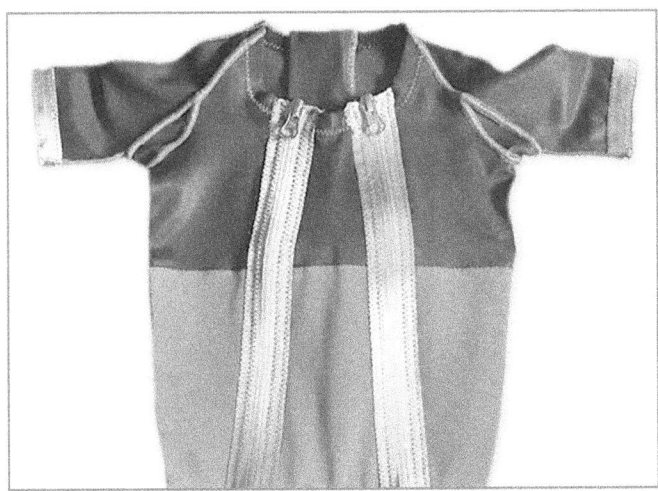

Fig. 22.10: Lycra weight jacket.

bearing exercises, rhythmic stabilization exercises, and by the use of weight cuffs and weight jackets (lycra weight jacket) **(Fig. 22.10)**.
- Body weight supported by standing may be used initially to develop standing tolerance, if standing, holding on to support is not possible.
- Static cycle exercises (bicycle ergometry for upper and lower limbs), hydrotherapy, etc., may be used to facilitate movement and train fitness.
- *Chest physiotherapy:* Air way clearance techniques—it consists of chest clapping, vibrations, and postural drainage with huffing and coughing/suctioning. Breathing exercises in the form of diaphragmatic breathing, costal breathing, air shift maneuver, etc., are performed and taught to improve vital capacity and fitness.
- Use of physical agents like ice/heat, electrical stimulation, etc., are used to reduce hypertonia, and facilitate movements.

- Functional electrical stimulation (FES) may be considered to improve function.
- Strategies to prevent and treat pressure ulcers, such as regular turning, pressure relief techniques such as sitting push ups, using pressure relieving mattresses/pillows, using modalities like high voltage pulsed galvanic current (HVPGC), LASER, ultrasound, iontophoresis, etc., to cause healing of pressure sores.
- Recommendation for appropriate orthotics/adaptive devices and walking/mobility aids.
- Wheel chair training/gait training.
- Bladder/bowel training.
- Sexuality and fertility counseling.
- Training on the use of adaptive devices in collaboration with occupational therapists.
- Recommending modification of home/work environment.
- Facilitating family and community integration.
- Planning for discharge.
- Occupational therapy.
- Speech therapy.
- Psychological counseling.
- Vocational guidance and job placement.

Physiotherapy in Multiple Sclerosis

INTRODUCTION

Multiple sclerosis is a chronic complex neurodegenerative disease of the central nervous system (CNS), widely believed to be autoimmune in nature, characterized by chronic inflammation, demyelination, gliosis and neuronal loss in brain, spinal cord, and optic nerves, affecting function of multiple systems of the body producing muscle spasticity, and weakness, sensory loss, visual disturbances, speech impairments with impairment of cognitive/perceptual function, gastrointestinal disturbances, impairment of bladder, bowel, and sexual function.

The disease may be relapsing-remitting or progressive in nature and the lesions in the CNS occur at different times and in different locations of CNS, due to which, the lesions are sometimes said to be disseminated in time and space.

EPIDEMIOLOGY

In India, no large scale studies are available regarding the incidence and prevalence of multiple sclerosis. In an earlier study by Singhal et al., the prevalence of this disease in India was estimated to be approximately 1.33 per 100,000 populations. The disease prevails across the globe, with the number of female sufferers 2–3 times more than their male counterparts. The common age groups affected are individuals between the ages of 20 and 40 years and the disease rarely affect children and adults over the age of 50 years.

ETIOLOGY

The exact cause of the disease is unknown, and the most accepted theory regarding etiology is autoimmune pathology, preferentially destroying the CNS, and sparing the peripheral nervous system. The demyelination of the CNS causes the symptoms.

There are various factors believed to be involved in the causation of the disease, such as:

- **Immunologic factor:** The body's own immune cells attack the CNS, destroying the myelin sheaths and there by impairing nerve conduction. The T cells (one type of white blood cells in the immune system, becomes sensitized to proteins in the CNS, producing inflammation and damage of the myelin sheath. Once in the CNS, these T cells, not only damage myelin, but also secret chemicals that damage nerve fibers (axons).
- **Environmental factors:** Multiple sclerosis appears to be more prevalent in areas, farther from the equator, in a colder climate. People who live closure to the equator are exposed to greater amount of sunlight round the year. As a result, they tend to have higher levels of naturally produced vitamin D, which is thought to have a beneficial impact on immune function, and may help protect against autoimmune diseases like multiple sclerosis.
- **Genetic factors:** Though, the disease is not considered to be hereditary, the risk of getting the disease increases in a person, who has a first degree family member with the disease.
- **Infectious factor:** There is a possibility, that viruses and other infectious agents may trigger the onset of multiple sclerosis.
- **Gut microbiome factor:** It is hypothesized that, gastrointestinal microbiota might play an important role in the pathogenesis of multiple sclerosis. Recent evidence suggests that, gut microbiota is one of the key environmental factors for the causation of autoimmune diseases like multiple sclerosis.

PATHOPHYSIOLOGY

The disease greatly impacts the CNS, when the body's own immune cells attack the myelin, which exposes the nerve and creates a disconnection between the brain and rest of the body (**Figs. 23.1A and B**). The pathophysiologies involved are

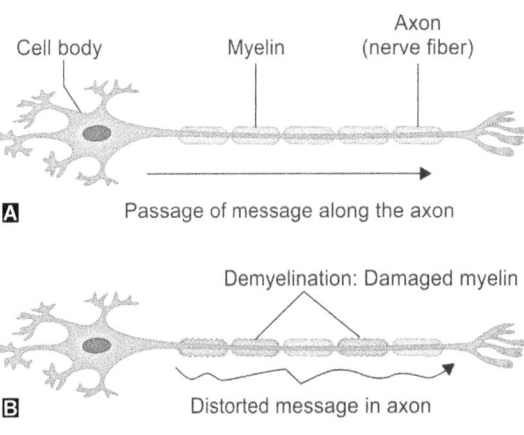

Figs. 23.1A and B: (A) Normal nerve; (B) Demyelination in multiple sclerosis.

inflammatory lesions resulting in neuronal demyelination, axonal damage, and subsequent neurological dysfunctions following the formation of multiple plaques in the gray and white matter of brain and spinal cord. The disease is dominated by diffuse gray and white matter atrophy and is characterized by low grade inflammation.

CLINICAL FEATURES

The onset of symptoms is usually sudden and occurs rapidly over a period of minutes or hours, except in very rare cases, where the onset is insidious, taking several weeks to months for the symptoms to develop.

The symptoms of the disease include:
- **Musculoskeletal impairments:** Tingling numbness and weakness of the muscles occur early as the demyelination starts. Subsequently, as the disease progresses, spasticity, ataxia, in-coordination, impaired balance, and abnormal gait develop.
- **Sensory impairment:** It may start with tingling numbness (paresthesia) in the limbs, trunk, and extremities, however, complete loss of any single sensation (anesthesia) is rare. Focal sensory deficits with loss of joint position and vibration senses in the lower limbs are commonly found.
- **Visual disturbances:** Vision disturbances are a common first symptom in multiple sclerosis that comes on suddenly in one or both eyes. Visual disturbances, such as blurred or double vision, pain in the eyes, impaired ocular movements may be seen.
- Fatigue, dizziness, vertigo, and sometimes seizures are also present.
- **Pain:** Headache, chronic neuropathic pain, paroxysmal limb pain, may be present.
- Cognitive symptoms, such as short-term memory deficits, diminished attention/ concentration and executive function, may be present.
- Affective symptoms such as confusion, depression, anxiety, and personality changes may be present.
- **Respiratory dysfunction:** The decreased function of the respiratory muscles due to nerve damage can create speech as well as breathing difficulties, which worsen as the disease progresses.
- Speech and swallowing impairment such as dysarthria, dysphonia, and dysphagia may be present.
- **Bladder/bowel symptoms:** Spastic (automatic) or flaccid (autonomous) bladder with incontinence of urine and feces, constipation/diarrhea may be present, due to involvement of the nerves connecting bladder, rectum, and sphincters.
- **Sexual symptoms:** Impotence, decreased libido, decreased ability to achieve orgasm, may be present due to involvement of the nerves to the sexual organs as well as spasticity of muscles limiting movements, impairment of mood, etc.
- Integumentary system may be affected causing skin breakdown and pressure ulcers.

The clinical features of multiple sclerosis are determined by the exact neuroanatomical location of the plaque and differ from person to person. The onset of the neurological manifestations may be sudden, or the disease may present with a relapsing remitting manner, which is characterized by short attack to CNS producing symptoms, followed by a complete or partial return to normal functioning. Secondary progressive multiple sclerosis is a subgroup of this disease that begins as a relapsing-remitting course, accompanied by a steady decline in function. Primary-progressive multiple sclerosis is the progression of the disease, where a steady decline in function is experienced by the patient from the onset of the disease. Progressive-relapsing multiple sclerosis, is progression of the disease causing a decline of function with additional characteristics of acute attacks. The symptoms get aggravated with an increase in body temperature, as many patients have sensitivity to heat. This adverse reaction to heat is known as Uhthoff's symptom/phenomenon. This transient increase in symptoms following a raise in core temperature is termed as pseudoexacerbation, which occurs due to transient increased blockade of nerve conduction in demyelinated fibers.

DIAGNOSIS

Diagnosis of the disease is done by the neurologist from the history, clinical features, and performing diagnostic tests.

Diagnostic Tests in Multiple Sclerosis

- **MRI:** Shows plaques in the white matter of brain and spinal cord.
- **Lumbar puncture:** The cerebrospinal fluid (CSF) is tested for an abnormal amount of white blood cells, proteins, and other abnormalities that are secondary to multiple sclerosis.
- **Evoke potential studies:** It measures electrical signals in the nerves sent from the brain in response to a stimulus This test helps detect whether there is a lesion to a nerve, in the optic nerve, brainstem and spinal cord even though a person may not be presenting with any neurological signs of nerve damage.
- Blood tests to rule out other infective and inflammatory lesions of the nervous system.

MANAGEMENT

- **Medical management:** Immunosuppressants and anti-inflammatory drugs to reduce brain swelling. Plasmapheresis, disease modifying drugs, etc., are used by the medical team to prevent progression of the disease. Drugs to reduce symptoms such as pain, spasticity, etc., may be prescribed by the physician as per need.
- **Physiotherapy:** Physiotherapy plays an essential role in the management of multiple sclerosis, as it helps the patient remain functional and fit in the family and community. The aims of physiotherapy are:
  – To normalize muscle tone and re-educate and maintain voluntary control.
  – To prevent abnormal movements.
  – To maintain and re-educate posture.

- To stimulate all sensory and perceptual experiences.
- To improve activities of daily living (ADLs)/instrumental activities of daily living (IADL) by incorporating treatment techniques into living requirements.
- To provide bladder and bowel training.

PHYSIOTHERAPY ASSESSMENT

Before therapy is instituted, the physiotherapist makes a detailed assessment of the patient focusing on posture and movements, functional abilities, and limitations, presence of early fatigue and pain that limit function, degree of spasticity present, tightness/contracture/deformity, gait abnormalities, etc.

Physiotherapy Treatment Strategies

* **Exercise therapy:**
  - Exercise therapy in the form of relaxed passive exercises, passive stretching exercises, breathing exercises, active assisted/free exercises that, does not increase the body temperature significantly, low and moderate intensity resistance training **(Fig. 23.2)**, aerobic/endurance training, weight-bearing/weight-shifting exercises, balancing, and coordination exercises **(Figs. 23.3A to C)**, etc., are recommended to normalize muscle tone, improve posture, balance, and function.
  - Special techniques of treatment such as neurodevelopmental treatment (NDT), propioceptive neuromuscular facilitation (PNF) are applied to improve posture and movements.
  - Aquatic exercise/hydrotherapy with water maintained at normal temperature is beneficial for inducing relaxation, improving strength and endurance.
  - *Aerobic exercises:* Aerobic exercise training with low to moderate intensity can result in the improvement of aerobic fitness and reduction of fatigue in patients with multiple sclerosis affected with mild or moderate disability. Circuit training/circuit interval training, such as leg press on multigym, followed by rest for few minutes and then elbow curl, followed by rest for few minutes, and then arm raise is an example of circuit interval training **(Figs. 23.4A to C)**, which helps in increasing fitness and avoids fatigue.
* **Hippo therapy:** This therapy in the form of horse back riding is helpful for improving posture, balance in ambulatory patients with multiple sclerosis.
* **Motor imagery:** Motor imagery with rhythmic auditory stimulation is beneficial in improving motor control and gait in patients with multiple sclerosis.
* **Cognitive behavioral therapy (CBT):** It is a type of psychotherapeutic treatment that helps people with multiple sclerosis learns how to identify and change destructive or disturbing thought patterns that have a negative influence on behavior and emotions. It focuses on changing the automatic negative thoughts that can contribute to and worsen emotional difficulties, depression, and anxiety. Through CBT, these thoughts are identified, challenged, and replaced with more objective, realistic

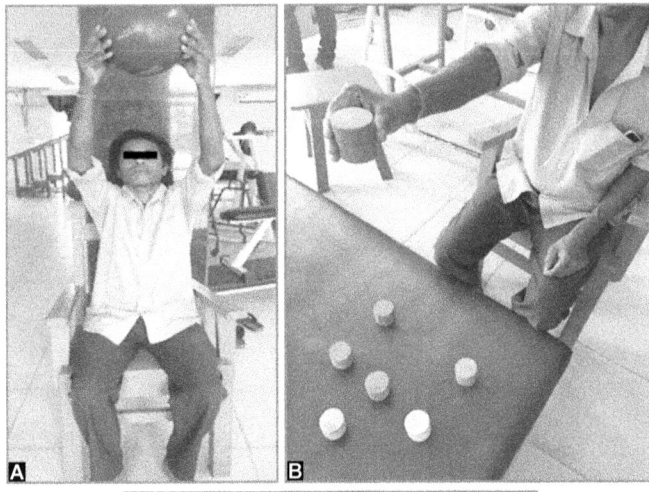
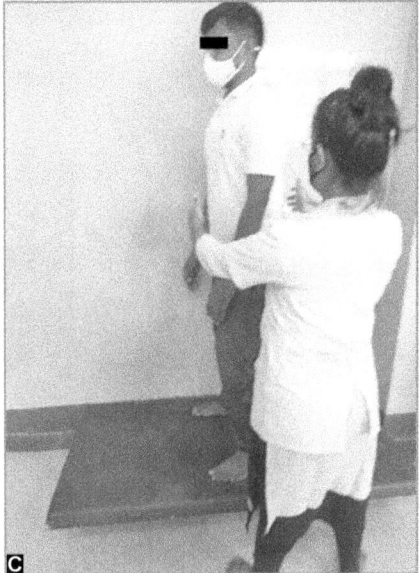

Figs. 23.3A to C: (A) Static sitting balance development using medicine ball; (B) Eye hand coordination exercises; (C) Dynamic balance exercise in standing on wobble board.

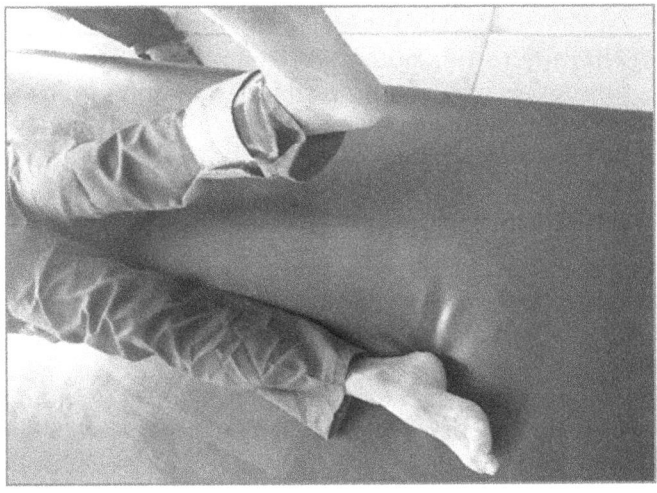

Fig. 23.2: Low intensity resistance training with weight cuff.

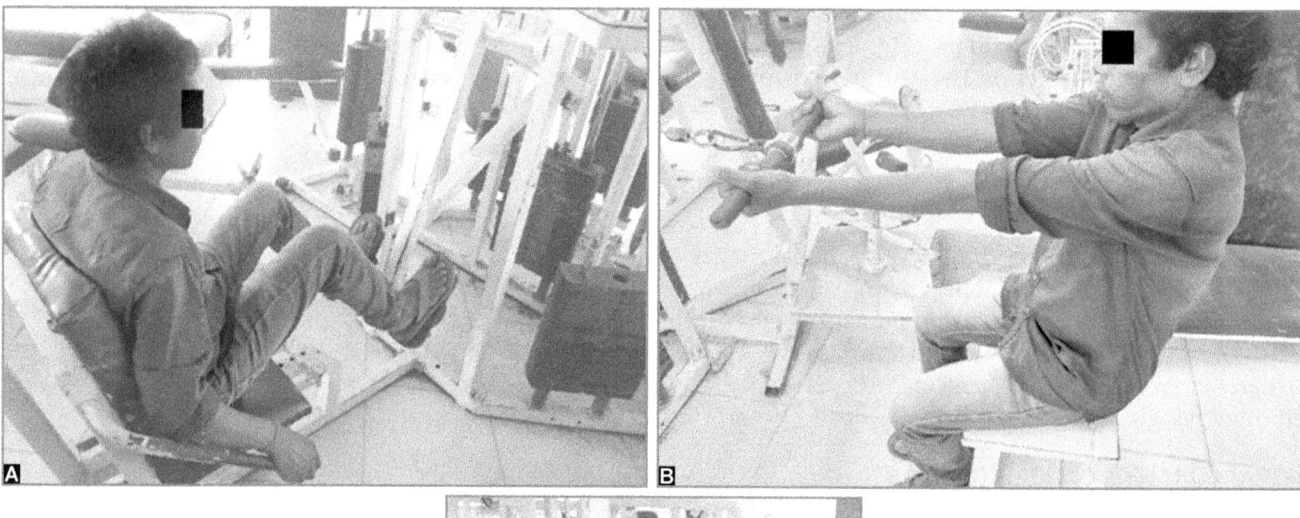
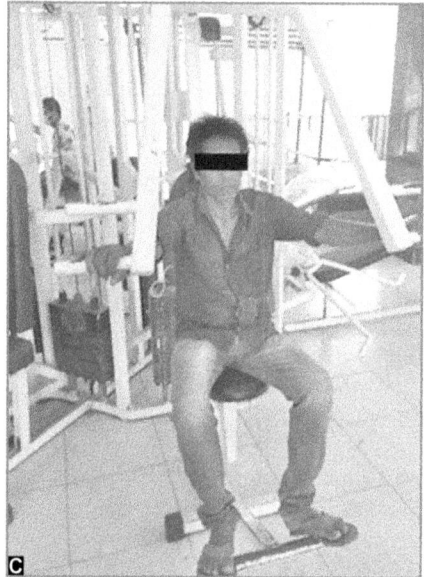

Figs. 23.4A to C: Circuit interval training. (A) Leg press; (B) Elbow curl; (C) Arm raise.

thought. It is focused on using a wide range of strategies to help people with multiple sclerosis overcome these thoughts and achieve an enhanced quality of life. Such strategies may include journaling, role-playing, relaxation techniques, and mental distractions.

- **Therapy to reduce pain:** Pulsed ultrasound therapy, Low intensity LASER therapy, hydrotherapy with normal temperature of water, interferential therapy (IFT), transcutaneous electrical nerve stimulation (TENS), etc., may be selected to reduce pain from the disease or from secondary musculoskeletal complications. However, heat producing modalities should be avoided.
- **Therapy for spasticity reduction:** Sustained stretching, cryotherapy, hydrotherapy, relaxed passive exercises, etc., are applied to reduce spasticity.
- **Therapy for sensory deficits:** Tapping and verbal cues during exercise and resistance training can help improve proprioception losses. Education regarding posture and movements in home and work environments due to reduced vision (as a result of blurred/double vision) is provided to the patient. Pressure relieving techniques on bed/chair/wheel chair are taught to prevent pressure sore formation, which is precipitated due to sensory deficits.
- **Therapy to improve mobility and function:** The physiotherapist should recommend for appropriate orthotics, walking aids and adaptive devices to improve mobility and function.

PROGNOSIS

Multiple sclerosis itself is rarely fatal, but complications may arise from severe type of the disease, in the form of chest or bladder infections, or swallowing difficulties. The average life expectancy for people with the disease is around 5–10 years lower than average. The treatment team should focus on maintenance of muscular and cardiorespiratory endurance.

Physiotherapy for Muscular Dystrophies, Motor Neuron Disease and Spinal Muscular Atrophies

A. MUSCULAR DYSTROPHY

INTRODUCTION

Muscular dystrophy was first described in the 1830s by Charles Bell. The word "dystrophy" is from the Greek word "dys", meaning "difficult" and "troph" meaning "nourish".

Muscular dystrophy is a group of muscle diseases that results in progressive weakness of skeletal muscles of the body, leading to minimal disabilities to fatal consequences in sufferers. These conditions are generally inherited, and different muscular dystrophies follow various inheritance patterns. The muscular dystrophy group contains thirty different genetic disorders and the most common types include:

i. Duchenne Muscular Dystrophy/Pseudohypertrophic Muscular Dystrophy (PHMD)

Duchenne muscular dystrophy (DMD) is the most common childhood form of muscular dystrophy. This condition represents about half of all cases of muscular dystrophy and affects 1 in 5,000 males at birth. Males are affected more than females, who are the carriers. This is a rare progressive disease, which eventually affects all voluntary muscles and involves the heart and breathing muscles in later stages.

Etiopathology

The disorder is X-linked recessive. About two-thirds of cases are inherited from a person's mother, while one-third of cases are due to a new mutation. Mutation of the dystrophin gene at locus Xp21, located on the short arm of the X chromosome leads to deficiency of muscle protein dystrophin. Deficiency of dystrophin impairs function of fast muscle fibers, and these muscle fibers degenerate first, followed by degeneration of other muscle fibers, degeneration proceeds until the entire muscle is replaced by fatty and fibrous tissue.

Dystrophin is responsible for connecting the cytoskeleton of each muscle fiber to the underlying basal lamina (extracellular matrix), through a protein complex containing many subunits. The absence of dystrophin permits excess calcium to penetrate the sarcolemma (the cell membrane). Alterations in calcium and signaling pathways cause water to enter into the mitochondria, which then burst. In skeletal muscle dystrophy, mitochondrial dysfunction gives rise to an amplification of stress-induced cytosolic calcium signals and an amplification of stress-induced reactive-oxygen species production. In a complex cascading process, that involves several pathways and is not clearly understood, increased oxidative stress within the cell damages the sarcolemma and eventually results in the death of the cell. Muscle fibers undergo necrosis and are ultimately replaced with adipose and connective tissue.

Clinical Features

Though the affected child shows delayed motor development, the signs are more marked when the child attends school by 4–5 years of age. The boy demonstrates awkward manner of walking, stepping, running, and gets frequent fall while walking/running. The proximal muscles are affected first, especially those of the hips, pelvic area, thighs, and calves. It eventually progresses to the shoulders and neck, followed by arms, respiratory muscles, and other areas (**Fig. 24.1**).

To compensate for weakness of quadriceps, the affected child walk on toes, resulting in shortening of tendoachilles. To compensate for weakness of hip extensors affected children stand and walk with increased lumbar lordosis (**Fig. 24.2A**). There is also waddling gait due to weakness of hip abductors (**Fig. 24.2B**). Anterior pelvic tilt, chest deformities,

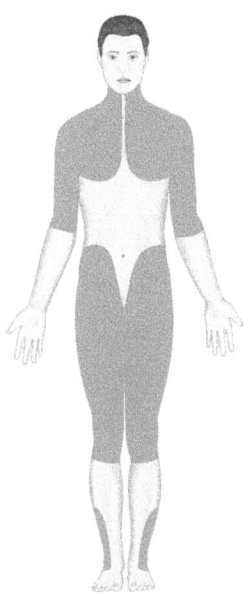

Fig. 24.1: Muscles affected in Duchenne and Becker muscular dystrophy.

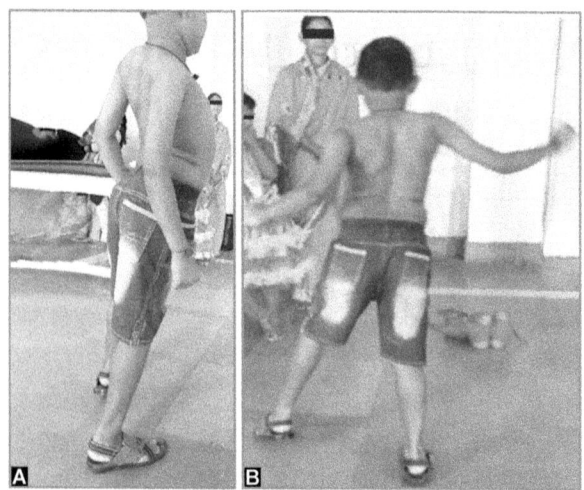

Figs. 24.2A and B: (A) Anterior pelvic tilt with increased lumbar lordosis; (B) Waddling gait.

scoliosis, etc., are also seen. Another characteristic sign is pseudohypertrophy (enlarging) of the muscles of the tongue, calf, buttocks, and shoulders (around age 4 or 5 years). The muscle tissue is eventually replaced by fat and connective tissue, hence the term pseudohypertrophy **(Fig. 24.3)**. The affected child demonstrates significant difficulties while standing from sitting/lying exhibiting positive Gower's sign **(Figs. 24.4A and B)**.

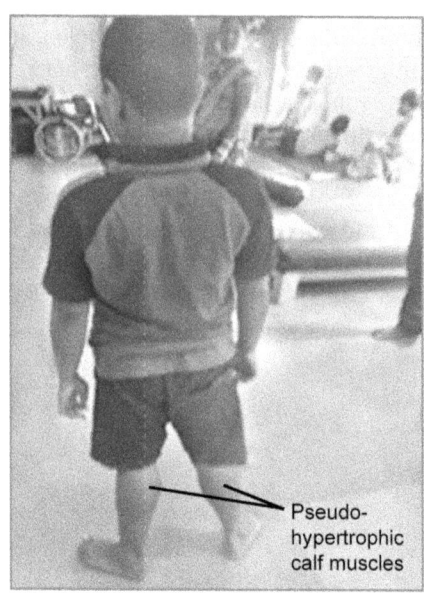

Fig. 24.3: Pseudohypertrophy of calf muscles.

Some children become wheel chair bound by 9–10 years. The approximate rates of progression of the disease are:
Ambulatory stage → Up to 7 years of age.
Wheel chair bound → By the age of 12 years.
Bed bound → 19–20 years.

The disease is staged as under:
Stage I → Ambulatory.
Stage II → Ambulates, but climbs stairs with support.
Stage III → Can stand from sitting.
Stage IV → Needs to be lifted for standing, but can walk when made to stand.
Stage V → Wheel chair bound, but independent in wheel chair activities.
Stage VI → Wheel chair bound, and dependent for wheel chair activities.
Stage VII → Confined to bed, but independent in most of self-care activities.
Stage VIII → Confined to bed and dependent for all ADL activities.

Diagnosis

Diagnosis is made from:
- Clinical features.
- **Blood test:** Serum creatinine phosphokinase (CPK-3) level is highly raised due to leaking of this enzyme into blood stream as a result of muscle damage. The CPK normal range for a male is between 39 and 308 U/L, while in females the CPK normal range is between 26 and 192 U/L.
- **EMG:** Increased interference pattern with low amplitude spikes. The **Figures 24.5A and B** shows EMG features of normal and myopathic muscles.
- **DNA test:** DNA testing and analysis identifies the specific type of mutation and confirms the diagnosis in most cases.
- **Muscle biopsy:** A small sample of muscle tissue is extracted using a biopsy needle. The key tests performed on the biopsy sample for DMD are immunohistochemistry, immunocytochemistry, and immunoblotting for dystrophin, and should be interpreted by an experienced neuromuscular pathologist.
- **Prenatal tests:** A prenatal test can be considered when the mother is a known or suspected carrier. These tests can tell whether the unborn child has one of the most

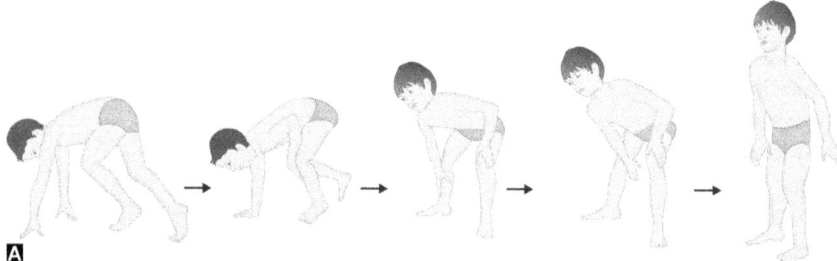
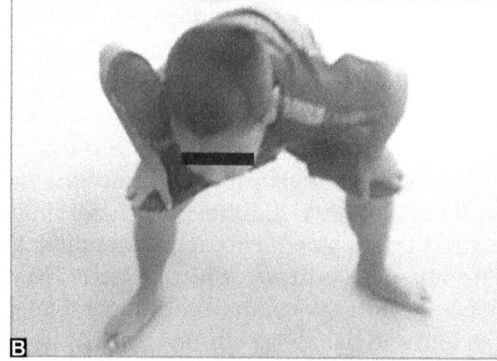

Figs. 24.4A and B: (A) Demonstrates stages of positive Gower's sign; (B) A child using Gower's maneuver to stand up from sitting.

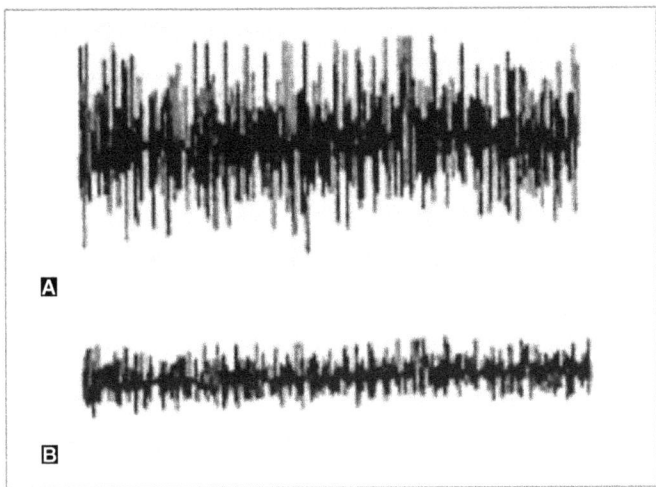

Figs. 24.5A and B: EMG features of normal and myopathic muscles: (A) Normal muscle; (B) Myopathic muscle.

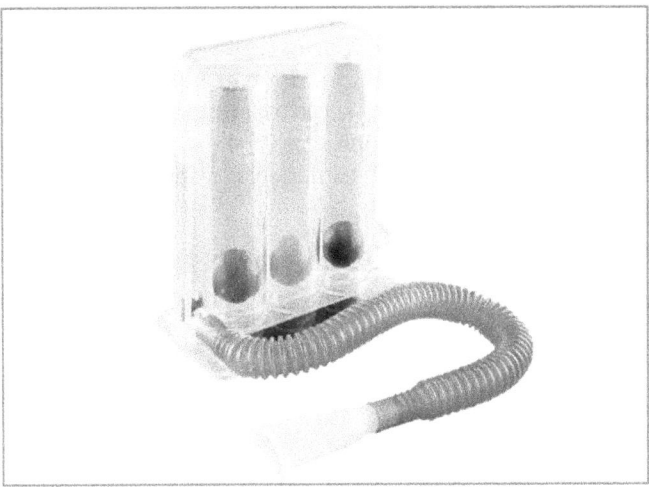

Fig. 24.6: The incentive spirometer.

common mutations. Amniocentesis can be done after 15 weeks, fetal blood sampling can be done around 18 weeks. Another option in the case of unclear genetic test results is fetal muscle biopsy.

Management

Treatment is generally aimed at controlling the onset of symptoms to maximize the quality of life. It consists of:
- **Medical management:** Corticosteroids lead to short-term improvements in muscle strength and function up to 2 years and also has been reported to help prolong walking.
- **Physiotherapy:** Physiotherapy is helpful to maintain muscle strength and endurance, flexibility, cardio respiratory fitness, and function. It also helps in preventing tightness, contracture deformities and improves the quality of life.

Physiotherapists are concerned with enabling patients to reach their maximum physical potential. The aims of physiotherapy are:
- Prevent/minimize the development of contractures and deformity through a program of exercises, positional devices, such as appropriate chairs, positional braces such as L-type splint for the ankle, spinal braces to prevent progression of scoliosis, etc.
- Maintain muscle strength and endurance.
- Periodic monitoring of respiratory functions and maintain/improve the same through breathing exercises and secretion removal techniques.
- Counseling the parents with assistance from clinical psychologist and pediatrician.
- Advice on measures to improve the quality of life of the patient.

Physiotherapy Techniques

- Deep breathing exercises that include incentive spirometry **(Fig. 24.6)**, breathing games such as blowing pieces of paper are used to increase vital capacity. As respiratory muscle weakness progresses, a sleep apnea device might help to improve oxygen delivery at night.
- Postural drainage to remove secretions (if any).
- Gentile passive stretching exercises and passive ROM exercises to maintain and improve joint range of motion.
- Active assisted/free exercises.
- Circuit training/circuit interval training.
- Low-load high-repetition endurance exercises without producing fatigue.
- Low impact aerobics such as hydrotherapy, static cycle exercises, low impact sports, etc.
- Functional training for self-care with or without adaptive devices.
- Gait/mobility training with or without elbow crutches/walking frames, walking sticks, wheel chairs.

Orthotic management

Lightweight functional orthoses and positional devises such as L-type polypropylene AFOs, lightweight spinal braces can be considered.

Surgery

Orthopedic surgery such as tendoachilles lengthening is strictly contraindicated for ambulatory children, as once, the deformity at ankle is corrected and heel touched the ground, the knee may buckle (due to line of gravity falling posterior to knee joint, causing a flexion moment), and patient may fail to walk. Surgery for spinal deformities may be considered, if breathing restrictions due to the deformity occurs. Patients who need ventilator support, tracheostomy may be considered, if required. Cardiac function may be improved with a pacemaker.

ii. Becker's Muscular Dystrophy

Becker muscular dystrophy (BMD) is a less severe variant of DMD and is caused by the production of a truncated, but partially functional form of dystrophin. It is an X-linked recessive inherited disorder characterized by slowly progressing muscle weakness of the legs and pelvis, with loss of muscle mass (atrophy). Muscle weakness also occurs in the arms, neck, and other areas, but not as noticeably severe as in the lower half of the body. Though, calf muscles initially enlarge during the age of 5–15 years (as an attempt by the body to compensate for loss of muscle strength), subsequently, the enlarged muscle tissue is replaced by fat and connective tissue producing pseudohypertrophy. Survival is usually into old age and affects only boys (with extremely rare exceptions).

Management

Same as that described under DMD. However, as the sufferers have a longer life span as compared to DMD, they are evaluated for light vocational activities and appropriate vocational training and placement should be done.

iii. Facioscapulohumeral Muscular Dystrophy/ Landouzy-Dejerine Disease

Facioscapulohumeral muscular dystrophy (FSHD) is an inherited and progressive muscle disorder. Initially, it affects the muscles of the face (most commonly orbicularis oculi/oris as well as the zygomaticus major), shoulders, and upper arms with progressive weakness affecting the leg (commonly the tibialis anterior muscle) and trunk (mostly abdominals) muscles also **(Fig. 24.7)**.

Symptoms usually develop in early adulthood (late teens); affected individuals become severely disabled. The pattern of inheritance is autosomal dominant, though a number of spontaneous mutations occur. It occurs both in males and females. Life expectancy may be normal as the cardiac muscles are not involved. The clinical features **(Fig. 24.8)** include:
- Severe weakness of facial and shoulder girdle muscles.
- Weakness of extraocular muscles with inability to close the eye during sleep.
- Winging of scapula with loss of deltoid contour.
- Wasting and weakness of arm muscles such as biceps and triceps.
- Weakness of anterior tibial and peroneal muscles causing foot drop.

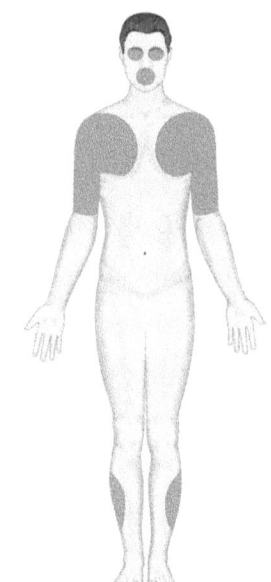

Fig. 24.7: Muscles affected in facioscapulohumeral type of muscular dystrophy.

- Weakness of muscles of chest and upper back.
- **Poly hill sign:** A positive Poly hill sign that shows multiple projections in the upper part of the scapula **(Fig. 24.9)**, due to atrophy of upper trapezius, displacement of acromioclavicular joint, atrophy of proximal deltoid with normal bulk of distal deltoid.
- **Beevor's sign:** A positive Beevor's sign that result in upward movement of the umbilicus, when the patient tries to raise the head and trunk in supine position.
- Weakness of muscles of thigh and pelvis may develop.
- Camel back gait with protrusion of buttock, associated with foot drop.

Management

Physiotherapy consists of:
- Relaxed passive exercises/joint ROM exercises.

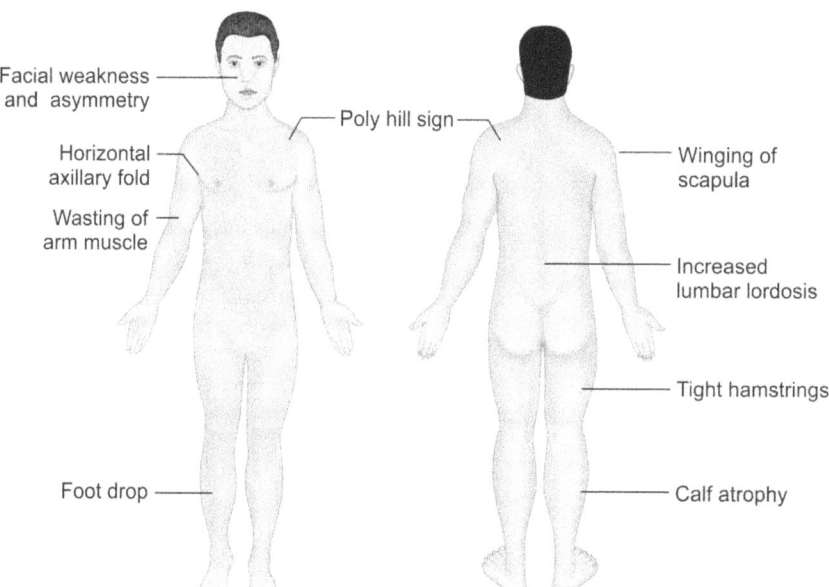

Fig. 24.8: Features of facioscapulohumeral type of muscular dystrophy.

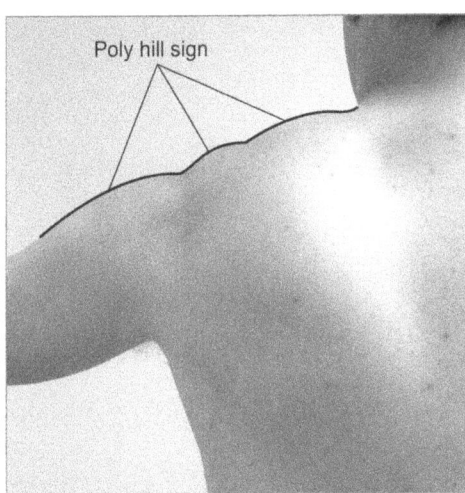

Fig. 24.9: Poly hill sign in facioscapulohumeral type of muscular dystrophy.

- Gentile stretching of tight muscles (if any).
- Deep breathing exercises.
- Low-load endurance exercises.
- Orthotic recommendation for deformities such as foot drop.
- Recommendation for walking aids and gait training.
- Counseling.

Besides, physiotherapy, occupational therapy and orthotic management, vocational evaluation, training and placement should be provided to the patients to increase the quality of living.

iv. Myotonic Muscular Dystrophy

Myotonic muscular dystrophy is the most common form of muscular dystrophy that begins in adulthood. Myotonic muscular dystrophy is an autosomal dominant condition that presents with myotonia (delayed relaxation of muscles), as well as progressive muscle wasting and weakness. The patients complain of inability to relax the muscles after use, say for example, while moving the door, may have difficulty in releasing the grip at the door knob/ door handle. The patients may have a slurred speech or temporary locking of the jaws. This condition varies in severity and manifestations and affects many body systems in addition to skeletal muscles, including the heart, endocrine organs, and eyes. Myotonic dystrophy type-I, is the most common adult form of muscular dystrophy, whereas myotonic dystrophy type-II is the rarer form from this variety, which shows mild symptoms as compared to type-I.

The muscle weakness in type-I occurs mostly in muscles farthest from the center of the body (distal muscles), such as the muscles of the lower legs, hands, neck and face. Muscle weakness in type-II, occurs in muscles closer to the center of the body (proximal muscles), such as muscles of the neck, shoulders, elbows, and hips.

Management

It consists of physiotherapy, occupational therapy, orthotic management, vocational training, and placement. Physiotherapy consists of:

- Relaxed passive exercises.
- Breathing exercises.
- Low intensity strength and endurance training.
- Balancing exercises.
- Gait training with/or without orthosis and walking aids.
- Functional training.

Congenital Muscular Dystrophy

Congenital muscular dystrophy is a general term for a group of genetic muscle diseases that occur at birth (congenital) or early during infancy. The disease is generally characterized by hypotonia, which is sometimes referred to as "floppy baby"; progressive muscle weakness and atrophy, abnormally fixed joints that occur when thickening and shortening of tissue such as muscle fibers cause deformity and restrict the movement of an affected area (contractures); spinal rigidity, and delays in reaching motor milestones such as sitting or standing unassisted. Feeding difficulties and breathing (respiratory) complications can develop in some cases, which may result in a shorter life span of the child. Muscle weakness may improve, remain stable or worsen. Some forms of the disease may be associated with structural brain defects and, intellectual disability. The severity, specific symptoms, and progression of these diseases vary greatly.

This disease is caused by defects in proteins thought to have some relationship to the dystrophin-glycoprotein complex and to the connections between muscle cells and their surrounding cellular structure. Some forms of congenital muscular dystrophy show severe brain malformations, such as lissencephaly (smooth brain, where, whole or part of the surface of the brain appears smooth) and hydrocephalus.

Management

It includes physiotherapy, occupational therapy, orthotics, and appropriate wheel chair to improve mobility, function, and the quality of life of the patient. Physiotherapy focuses on chest care, i.e., secretion removal and breathing exercises, passive ROM exercises, low intensity aerobic exercises, postural control training, play and recreational therapy, functional training, etc.

v. Distal Muscular Dystrophy

Distal muscular dystrophy (distal myopathy) is a general term for a group of rare progressive genetic disorders characterized by wasting (atrophy) and weakness of the voluntary distal muscles. Distal muscular dystrophies' occur at about 20–60 years, and the symptoms include weakness and wasting of muscles of the hands, forearms, and lower legs. The progress of the disease occurs slowly and is not life-threatening. Miyoshi myopathy, one of the distal muscular dystrophies, causes initial weakness in the calf muscles, and is caused by defects in the same gene responsible for one form of limb-girdle muscular dystrophy. Welander distal myopathy, occur in individuals greater than 40 years of age, where the intrinsic muscles of the hands and feet as well as the long finger/toe extensors are predominantly affected.

The severity, specific symptoms, and progression of the distal myopathies vary greatly, even among members of the same family. Slowly progressive weakness and degeneration of the voluntary distal muscles characterizes these disorders. In some cases, additional muscles including various proximal muscles may become involved.

Management

No cure exists for the distal myopathies. Treatment is aimed at the specific symptoms present in each individual. Specific treatment options may include physiotherapy, occupational therapy to improve muscle strength, endurance, and function. Appropriate orthotic devices and walking aids should be provided to the clients to improve mobility and function. Vocational evaluation, training and placement help the patients achieve a better quality of life. Genetic counseling may be of benefit for affected individuals and their families.

vi. Limb Girdle Muscular Dystrophy

Limb girdle muscular dystrophy (LGMD) represents a group of progressive hereditary myopathies that mainly affects muscles of hip and shoulder girdles. LGMD affects both boys and girls. It rarely appears before middle and late childhood or the disease appearance may be deferred until early adult life. Many forms of this disease have been identified, showing different patterns of inheritance (autosomal recessive vs. autosomal dominant). In an autosomal recessive pattern of inheritance, an individual receives two copies of the defective gene, one from each parent. The recessive variants are more frequent than the dominant forms, and usually have childhood or teenaged onset. The dominant LGMDs usually show adult onset. Some of the recessive forms have been associated with defects in proteins that make up the dystrophin-glycoprotein complex. Though a person normally leads a normal life with some assistance, in some extreme cases, death from LGMD occurs due to cardiopulmonary complications. The clinical features include:

- Onset with involvement of pelvic girdle or shoulder girdle muscles **(Fig. 24.10)**.
- Involvement of muscles may be asymmetrical.
- Disease progression is usually slow, and proximal muscle weakness may be followed by weakness of distal muscles.
- Development of lordotic posture.
- Weakness of neck flexors and extensors.
- Calf muscle hypertrophy and TA contracture is seen in few cases.

Management

Like other myopathic conditions, the management consists of physiotherapy, occupational therapy, orthotic management, vocational evaluation, training and placement. Physiotherapy consists of:

- Relaxed passive exercises and passive stretching.
- Deep breathing exercises.
- Low-intensity strengthening and endurance exercises: Though, there are some studies available, highlighting the effectiveness of exercises for limb girdle muscular

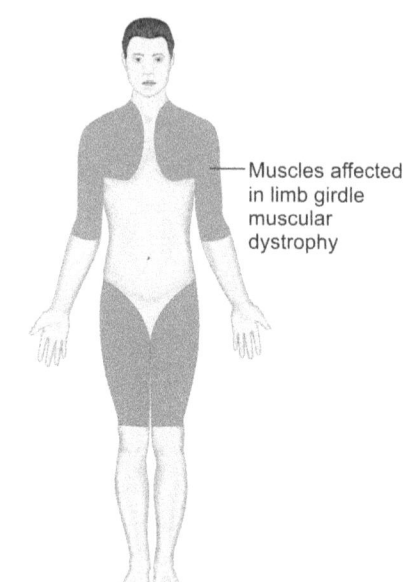

Fig. 24.10: Muscles affected in limb girdle muscular dystrophy.

dystrophy, few studies also reveal that intense muscle contracting exercises, may damage the muscle permanently. Hence, exercises that produce vigorous muscle contraction should be avoided.
- Hydrotherapy.
- Mobility and functional activity training with orthotic and assistive devices.

vii. Emery-Dreifuss Muscular Dystrophy

Emery-Dreifuss muscular dystrophy is a condition that mainly affects muscles used for movement, such as skeletal muscles and also affects the cardiac muscle; it is named after Alan Eglin H Emery and Fritz E Dreifuss.

Three types of Emery-Dreifuss muscular dystrophy are identified from their pattern of inheritance: X-linked, autosomal dominant, and autosomal recessive. X-linked types generally have cardiac involvement, whereas autosomal dominant types have both involvement of skeletal muscles and heart. Autosomal recessive variants demonstrate cardiac issues such as arrhythmias.

The age of onset, severity, and progression of the disease varies greatly from case to case, even among individuals of the same family. Some affected individuals may experience childhood onset with rapid disease progression and severe complications; others may experience adult onset and a slowly progressive course.

Signs and symptoms include:
- Symmetric weakness of biceps and triceps with sparing of deltoids
- Face, thigh, and hand weakness is uncommon and occurs later in the disease.
- Toe walking
- Cardiomyopathy (which may lead to heart failure)
- Atrioventricular block.
- Atrial paralysis.
- Fainting due to effect on heart

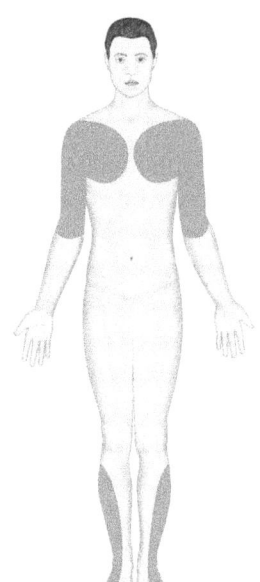

Fig. 24.11: Muscles affected I Emery-Dreifuss muscular dystrophy.

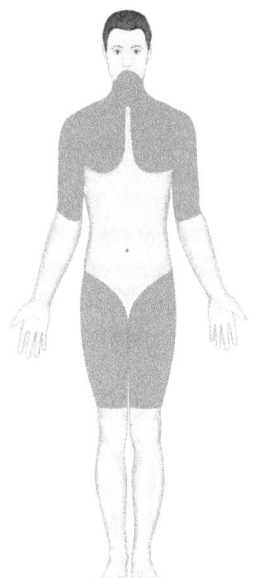

Fig. 24.12: Muscles affected in oculopharyngeal muscular dystrophy.

- The disease is characterized by a triad of: (a) Joint contractures that begin in early childhood; (b) Slowly progressive muscle weakness and wasting, initially in a humero-peroneal distribution, that later extends to the scapular and pelvic girdle muscles; (c) Cardiac involvement.
- Early contractures of Achilles tendon, elbow flexors and posteri or cervical muscles may be seen.
- Progressive atrophy of muscles of humeroperoneal distribution (i.e., proximal muscles of upper limbs and distal muscles of lower limbs may be seen) **(Fig. 24.11)**. Late into the disease, proximal limb girdle musculature becomes weak as well.
- Cardiac conduction defects may be seen.

Management

Physiotherapy, occupational therapy, and orthotic management are provided to the patient to minimize disability and lead a better quality of life. The components of physiotherapy are:
- Passive and active stretching exercises.
- Low intensity strengthening and endurance exercises.
- Deep breathing exercises/assisted coughing/respiratory muscle training.
- Training mobility and function through the use of orthotic and mobility devices, such as crutches, sticks, wheel chairs, etc.

viii. Oculopharyngeal Muscular Dystrophy

Oculopharyngeal muscular dystrophy is a rare genetic muscle disorder with onset during adulthood most often between 40 and 60 years of age. It is characterized by slowly progressive muscle disease affecting the muscles of the upper eyelids, face, and the throat, followed by weakness of muscles of pelvic and shoulder girdle **(Fig. 24.12)**. It can be autosomal dominant (most common), or autosomal recessive type of disease.

Management

Currently no cure or specific treatment exists to eliminate the symptoms or stop the disease progression. As involvement of throat muscles lead to dysphagia, the patients suffer from severe malnutrition, needing a balanced diet as per the advice of the dietician. Physiotherapy in the form of breathing exercise, active assisted/free exercise, endurance training, mobility and functional training with the help of mobility and adaptive devices are helpful. Speech therapy is provided by the speech therapist as needed.

B. MOTOR NEURON DISEASE

Motor neuron disease refers (MND) to a heterogeneous group of rare neurodegenerative conditions, characterized by degeneration of lower motor neurons (those that have cell bodies in the cranial nerve nuclei or in the anterior horn of the spinal cord and synapse directly on the muscles) and/or upper motor neuron (those that have cell bodies in the brain and synapse on the lower motor neuron).

Epidemiology and Etiology

The disease affects both children and adults. The disease can appear at any age, but symptoms usually appear after the age of 40 years. In adults, men are more commonly affected than women.

Most cases of MND are sporadic and their causes are usually not known. It is thought that, environmental, toxic, viral, and genetic factors are associated for causation of this disease. About 10% cases of MND are thought to have a hereditary cause and remaining 90% are sporadic.

Types

i. Amyotrophic lateral sclerosis (ALS)

This is also called as Lou Gehrig's disease. It affects both upper and lower motor neurons (neurons in the brain and spinal cord), resulting in severe weakness of muscles of arms, legs, mouth, and respiratory system. The disease has both lower motor neuron and upper motor neuron features.

- Lower motor neuron features: Atrophy of muscles **(Fig. 24.13)** fasciculation, muscle weakness, muscle cramps, difficulty in chewing, swallowing, and difficulty in moving face and tongue.
- Upper motor neuron features: It includes clumsiness, muscle stiffness (spasticity), hyperreflexia, extensor plantar response, muscle weakness, slowness of movement, and emotional lability.
- The main features of ALS are muscle weakness, which is mild at first, but gradually become worse. The first symptoms commonly develop in the hands and arms or in the feet and legs. Less commonly, the first symptoms are in the muscles around the face and throat (bulbar muscles). In ALS, the patient may have asymmetric distal weakness without sensory loss and/or symmetrical focal midline proximal weakness involving neck, trunk, and bulbar muscles.

Initially, the patient may have reduced grip strength, wasting of muscles of hands, dragging of feet while walking, early fatigue, slurring of speech, swallowing difficulties, muscle cramps, fasciculation, jerky movements in arms, or leg at rest.

Subsequently, the patient may have impairment of walking, impairment in doing functional tasks, difficulty in drinking, eating, and swallowing. He/she may develop breathing difficulties on exertion.

- Sensation is usually retained with retained control of bladder, bowel, and sexual function. Emotional lability may be present in some case.
- The survival time from onset of symptoms is 2–5 years.

Diagnosis: Clinical features and laboratory investigations help in diagnosing this disease. The tests performed are EMG/NCV **(Figs. 24.14A and B)**, transcranial magnetic stimulation, and MRI of brain.

Management of ALS: There is no cure for MND. Treatment may slow progression and maximize the individual's independence and comfort.

- **Medical management:** Riluzole is a medicine prescribed by neurologist for this disease.
- **Stem cells therapy:** This may be beneficial in this disease.
- **Supportive therapies:** That include:
  - *Physiotherapy:* Aims of physiotherapy:
    » To maintain joint ROM and prevent development of tightness/contracture/deformities.
    » To improve oro-motor function and improve respiratory function.
    » Maintain muscle endurance as much as possible.
    » Maintain mobility with or without walking aids/mobility devices.
    » Maintain the ability to perform self-care tasks and improve the quality of life as much as possible.
  - Methods of physiotherapy are relaxed passive exercises, active assisted/free exercises, low impact aerobic exercises such as swimming, static cycle exercises, circuit training/circuit interval training, etc. Chest care measures that include deep breathing exercises, breathing exercises using incentive spirometer,

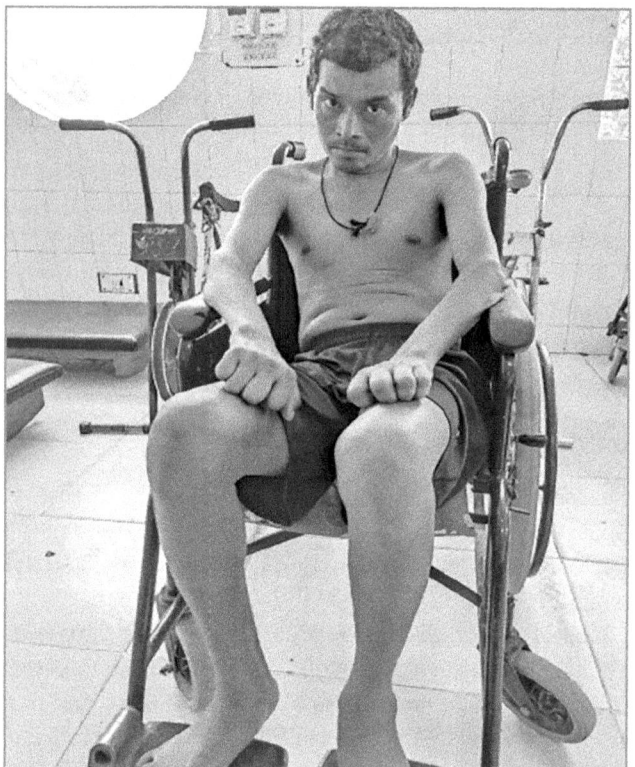

Fig. 24.13: Muscle wasting in MND.

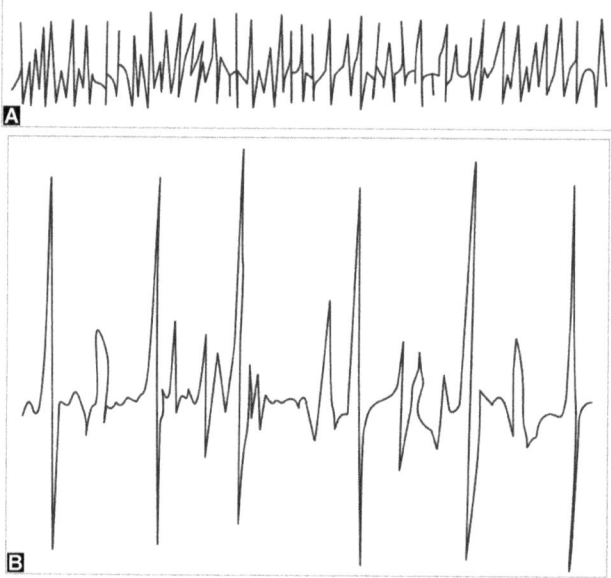

Figs. 24.14A and B: (A) Normal EMG on volition; (B) EMG picture in MND on volition.

breathing games and secretion removal techniques if required. Functional training/gait training with adaptive and assistive devices. Wheel-chair training (using manual/motorized wheel chairs) in later stages is given to maintain function and mobility.
- Occupational therapy and speech therapy are included to maintain function including communication.
- **Orthotic management:** Lightweight supportive devices such as polypropylene AFO or a hand splint may be used to improve mobility and function.

ii. Progressive bulbar palsy (PBP)
It affects brain stem. The condition causes frequent choking spells, difficulty in swallowing, speaking, eating, etc. It may be associated with ALS also. The survival time from start of symptoms is 6 months to 3 years.

Treatment: Supportive treatment to improve the quality of life is the focus. Physiotherapy focuses on: Relaxed passive exercises, active assisted/free exercises, breathing exercises, etc.

iii. Progressive muscular atrophy (PMA)
This is a rare condition affecting the lower motor neurons in the spinal cord. It causes slow but progressive muscle wasting especially in the arms, legs, and mouth **(Fig. 24.15)**. The survival time from start of symptoms is 2-4 years.

Treatment: Physiotherapy and other supportive treatments are given as discussed under ALS above.

iv. Primary lateral sclerosis (PLS)
It affects the neurons in the brain. It is a rare form of MND that progresses very slowly than ALS. Though it is not fatal, it affects the person's quality of living. It has a variant, called juvenile primary lateral sclerosis, which affects children. The survival time from start of symptoms is 8-10 years.

Treatment: Physiotherapy and other supportive treatments are given as discussed under ALS above.

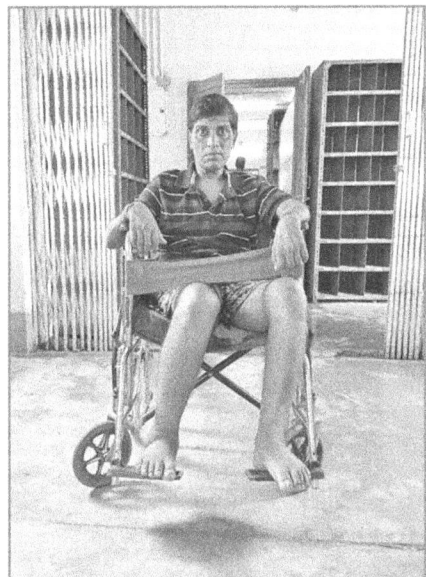

Fig. 24.15: Muscle wasting in progressive muscular atrophy.

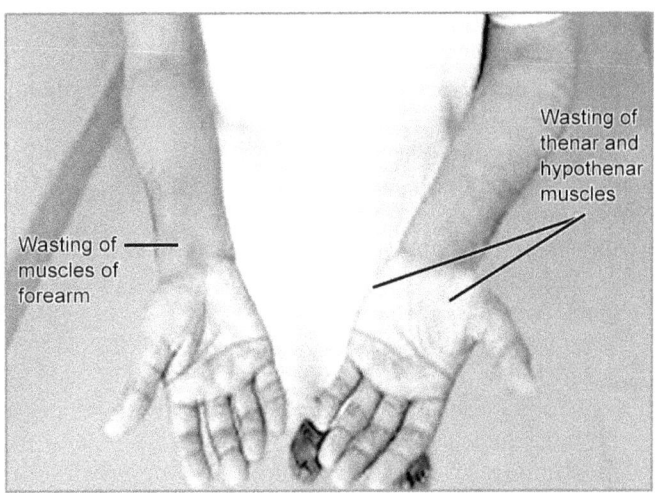

Fig. 24.16: Muscle wasting in distal upper extremities in Hirayama disease.

v. Monomelic amyotrophy
Monomelic amyotrophy (MMA) also known as Hirayama disease is a rare disease that cause muscle weakness in the upper extremities. It affects the lower motor neurons. There is muscle weakness and atrophy in the distal upper extremities **(Fig. 24.16)** during adolescence, followed by spontaneous halting in progression, and stabilization of symptoms. The onset is insidious in nature.

Treatment: Physiotherapy focuses on maintenance of muscle strength and endurance, maintenance and improvement of lungs function and improvement of function and quality of life.

C. SPINAL MUSCULAR ATROPHY

Spinal muscular atrophy (SMA) is a group of genetic neuromuscular disorders, that result in loss of motor neurons in the spinal cord and brain stem leading to progressive muscle wasting, weakness and twitching. It affects the arm, leg, and respiratory muscles initially and leads to progressive disability with problems of swallowing, deformities in spine, such as scoliosis and limb deformities. It is a leading genetic cause of death in infants.

Epidemiology/Etiology

It is a common childhood disability affecting more than 10 lakh cases per year in India. It affects approximately 1 in 8,000–10,000 babies in the world. It is an autosomal recessive disorder, caused by mutation in the survival motor neuron 1 gene *SMN1*.

Clinical Features

The features of this disease depends upon the type of SMA (discussed below), and stage of the disease. The common features include:
- Muscle weakness, atrophy, hypotonicity, tendency to flop when made to sit.
- The child has difficulty in controlling head and is not able stand and walk.

- Areflexia in the extremities, i.e., absent or markedly decreased deep tendon reflexes (e.g., Knee-jerk)
- Delayed development of motor milestones, resembling, and confusing with atonic cerebral palsy.
- Respiratory muscle weakness, that leads to dyspnea, difficulty in coughing, and clearing secretions.
- Adaptation of a frog leg position in sitting,
- Bell-shaped torso in severe type of disease due to use of abdominal muscles for respiration.
- Spinal deformity (Scoliosis).
- Difficulty in sucking, swallowing, feeding with fasciculations in the tongue.
- Faster deterioration of symptoms due to nonavailability of pharmacological treatment.
- If left untreated, majority of children diagnosed as SMA-type-0, I do not reach the age of 4 years.
- In SMA-type-II, the disease shows a slower progression, though the life expectancy is less than the normal population.
- SMA-type-III has normal or near normal life expectancy, whereas SMA-type-IV, is adult onset in nature and causes mobility impairment without affecting life expectancy.

Types of Spinal Muscular Atrophy

Spinal muscular atrophy (SMA) manifests over a wide range of severity, affecting infants to adults. The commonly used classification as per the National Institute of Neurological disorders and stroke is as follows:

- **SMA-type-I:** This is also called Werdnig–Hoffmann disease. It is a serious condition that usually appears before the age of 6 months. The child may be born with breathing problems, and other symptoms include muscle weakness, hypotonicity (floppy baby syndrome) **(Fig. 24.17)**, muscle twitching, etc. These children never sit unsupported and have severe respiratory complications. Pneumonia-induced respiratory failure is the most frequent cause of death. If untreated, these children usually do not survive beyond 2 years of age.

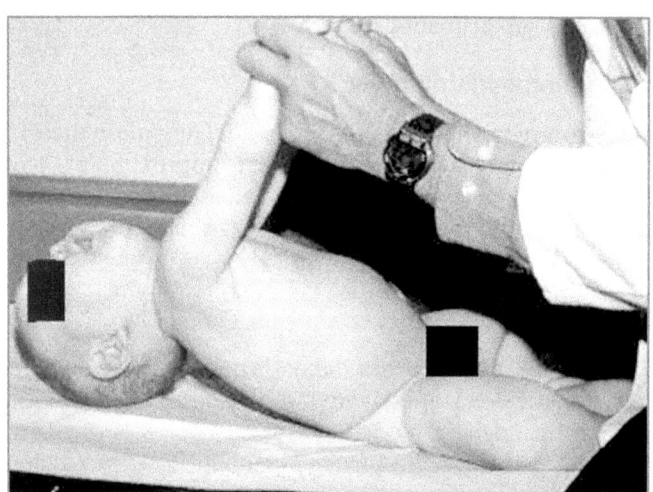

Fig. 24.17: SMA-type-I, showing significant floppiness.

- **SMA-type-II:** Also called as Dubowitz disease. Symptoms of SMA-type-II usually appear at the age of 6–12 months. The infant can sit without support, when placed, but they will never be able to stand or walk. In some cases, without treatment, the individual may lose their ability to sit.

  Life expectancy depends on whether breathing problems are present. Most people with SMA-type-II, survive into adolescence or young adulthood.
- **SMA-type-III:** Also called as Kugelberg-Welander disease. It appears after the age of 18 months. The child may exhibit mild muscle weakness, difficulty in walking and frequent respiratory infections. The individual may have scoliosis or contractures, a shortening of the muscles or tendons, which can prevent the joints from moving freely. Most of the sufferers are able to walk, but they may have an unusual gait and experience difficulty running, climbing steps, or rising from a chair. There may also be a slight tremor of the fingers. Complications include a higher risk of respiratory infections. With appropriate treatment, the individuals may have normal life expectancy.
- **SMA-type-IV:** The adult onset form, sometimes called as late onset SMA-type-III, usually manifests after the third decade of life with gradual weakness of leg muscles and frequently requiring walking aids. The life expectancy of such individuals is not affected.

Besides, the above four types of SMA, another variant called SMA-type-0, which develops during prenatal period, is sometimes described. The affected infants, usually survive for a few weeks after birth, even with intensive respiratory support.

Diagnosis

Spinal muscular atrophy is sometimes difficult to diagnose, as the features resemble other conditions, such as muscular dystrophies, flaccid cerebral palsy, etc. The condition is diagnosed from the clinical features and developmental history (revealing delayed motor development). Very occasionally other tests such as EMG and muscle biopsy, serum CPK examination may be needed to differentiate the disease from other similar conditions and to confirm the diagnosis.

Treatment of Spinal Muscular Atrophy

Though, there is no curative treatment for this disease, physiotherapy, occupational therapy, and orthotic devices help to improve mobility and function enhancing the quality of life of the patients.

Physiotherapy for SMA

It includes:
- **Physiotherapy assessment:** It consists of health and developmental history, examination of posture and movements, muscle power grading, respiratory system examination, functional activity level, participation with family and friends, and quality of life.

- **Physiotherapy intervention:**
  - *Therapeutic exercises:* The physiotherapist designs therapeutic exercises for the children with SMA, to keep them active and mobile, so that their quality of life is maintained and enhanced. The exercises recommended include:
    » Deep breathing exercises and breathing games, such as blowing balloon, blowing paper pieces, and incentive spirometry.
    » Progressive resisted strength training for SMA-Type-II, III, IV. Studies performed by Lewelt et al., in 2015, to find the effect of progressive resistance strength training in children with SMA-type-II, III, reveal improvement of strength and motor function with progressive resistance strength training.
    » Static cycle exercise: Studies performed to find the benefit of bicycle ergometry exercises on type-III SMA patients, reveal 12 weeks of exercise training, is associated with an improvement of maximum oxygen uptake (VO_2 max), though fatigue was precipitated.
    » Low intensity circuit training/circuit interval training.
    » Hydrotherapy:
  - Secretion removal techniques with teaching of huffing and coughing.
  - Functional education with or without spinal brace and assistive devices.
  - Mobility/gait training with or without mobility devices (manual/power wheel chair, elbow crutches, polypropylene orthotic devices). Orthotic care is an important aspect of treatment SMA in order to deal with the clinical problems caused by muscle weakness, i.e., scoliosis or other spinal deformities. Spinal braces, KAFOs, AFOs, cock up splints, etc., should be recommended as per the patient's requirement.

Physiotherapy for Peripheral Nerve Injuries

INTRODUCTION

Peripheral nerves are structures that suffer injuries like those seen in other tissues, resulting in significant motor and sensory disabilities. It is estimated that, the incidence of traumatic peripheral nerve lesions is as high as 500,000 cases per year in some countries, where 2.8% of the patients become permanently disabled due to prolonged nerve regeneration time.

The causes of peripheral nerve injuries include cuts, firearm lesions (gun shot injuries), thermal injuries, prolonged or acute compressions, mechanical traction, infections, and toxins. There are also different injury mechanisms such as laceration, avulsion, section, stretching, compression, and crushing. The injuries can damage the tissue integrity, causing important dysfunctions in the innervated structures of the damaged nerve, with consequent changes in the nerve pathway and axonal transport.

Structure of a Nerve

The nerve has an outer covering, which forms a sheath around the nerve, called epineurium. The nerve fibers which consist of neurons are organized into bundles known as fascicles, with each fascicle surrounded by the perineurium. Between individual nerve fibers, there is an inner layer of endoneurium (**Fig. 25.1**). The structure of a neuron is shown in **Figure 25.2**.

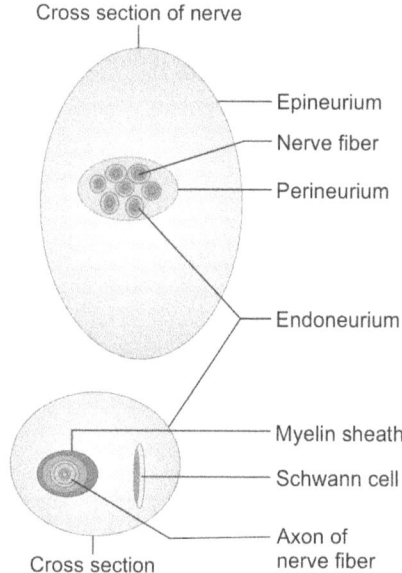

Fig. 25.1: Cross section of nerve and nerve fiber.

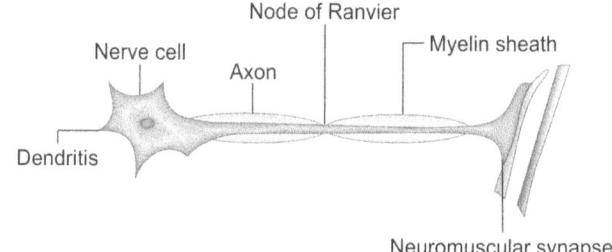

Fig. 25.2: Structure of a neuron.

Classification of Nerve Injuries

* **Seddon's classifications:** As per Seddon's classification, nerve injuries are classified into three types, such as (**Fig. 25.3**):
  1. *Neuropraxia:* Temporary paralysis of a nerve caused by lack of blood flow or compression/stretching of the affected nerve with no loss of structural continuity.
  2. *Axonotmesis:* In this type injury caused by violent stretch of a nerve, results in intact of the neural tube, but the axons are disrupted. The nerves are likely to recover spontaneously.
  3. *Neurotmesis:* This type of injuries that result mostly from cut injuries involve severing of the neural tube and axon, i.e., complete disruption of nerve occurs. Spontaneous recoveries are not possible without surgical repair.

* **Sunderland's classification:** There are five grades of nerve injury as per Sunderland's classification, such as:
  – *Grade I:* Same as Seddon's neuropraxia, i.e., temporary paralysis of a nerve caused by lack of blood flow or compression/stretching of the affected nerve with no loss of structural continuity. There is disruption of myelin.
  – *Grade II:* Same as Seddon's axonotmesis, i.e., there is intact of the neural tube, but the axons are disrupted. There is disruption of myelin and axon.

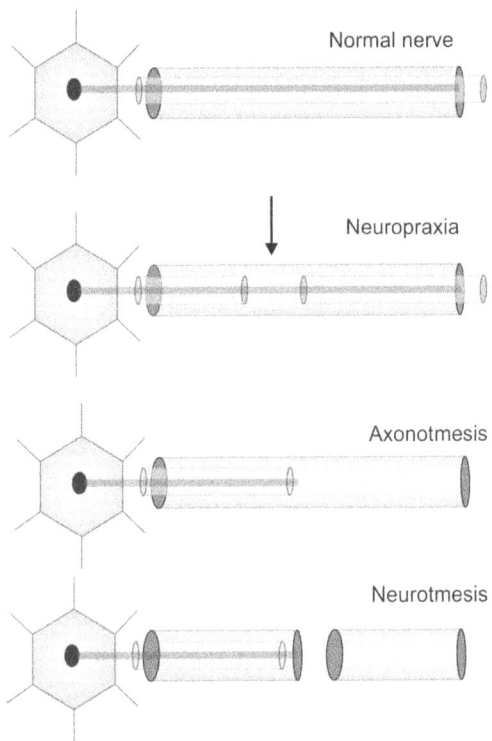

Fig. 25.3: Shows nerve injury types as per Seddon's classification.

- *Grade III:* Neurotmesis with preservation of perineurium. There is disruption of myelin, axon, endoneurial tube and its contents.
- *Grade IV:* Neurotmesis with preservation of the epineurium. There is disruption of myelin, axon, endoneurial tube, and perineurium.
- *Grade V:* Complete transection of the nerve trunk.

Neuronal Degeneration and Regeneration

Any part of the neuron detached from its nucleus (anterior horn cells for spinal nerves and nuclei in the brain stem for the cranial nerves) degenerates and is destroyed by phagocytosis. Wallerian degeneration, takes place, where the nerve degenerates distal to the site of injury and up to the first node of Ranvier proximal to the site of injury except Seddon's neuropraxia and Sunderland's grade-I injuries. Though the time required for degeneration varies between sensory and motor fibers, Wallerian degeneration of motor nerves is completed by 2 weeks, after which regeneration may start. Advancing Tinel sign and motor march phenomenon are the signs of regeneration. Regeneration occurs at the rate of 1 mm per day or about 25 mm a month.

BRACHIAL PLEXUS INJURY

The brachial plexus **(Fig. 25.4)** is the network of nerves that sends signals from the spinal cord to the upper limbs. A brachial plexus injury occurs when these nerves are stretched, compressed, or in the most serious cases, ripped apart or torn away from the spinal cord.

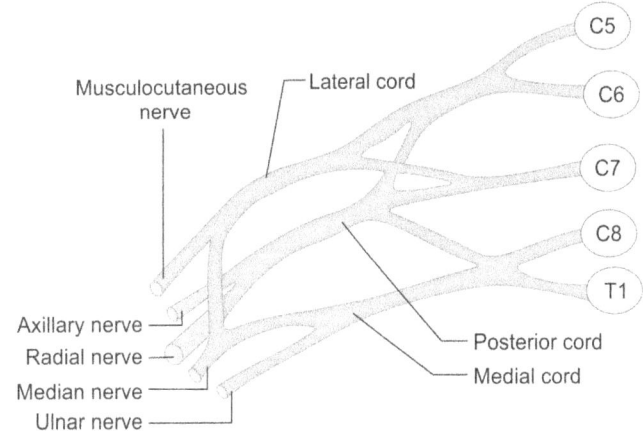

Fig. 25.4: The brachial plexus.

Causes of Brachial Plexus Injuries

The most severe brachial plexus injuries usually result from automobile or motorcycle accidents, which results in paralysis and deformities in the upper limbs and loss of function. Damage to the upper trunk occurs when the shoulder is forced down, while the neck is stretched in the opposite direction, causing abnormal separation of the head from the shoulders. Injury to the lower trunk occurs in events, where the arm is forcibly moved towards the head. The events that lead to such injuries are:

- **Contact sports:** Such as football playing, where brachial plexus is stretched beyond its limits during collision with other players.
- **Birth trauma:** High birth weight breech presentation or prolonged labor may lead to brachial plexus injury in infants.
- **Trauma:** Several types of trauma such as motor vehicle accidents, heavy falls with stretching of the neck, bullet injuries, and industrial trauma can result in brachial plexus injuries.
- **Assault with sharp objects.**
- **Tumors and cancer treatments:** Tumors such as that developing in the upper lobe of the lungs can grow in or along the brachial plexus, or put pressure on the brachial plexus or spread to the nerves, causing injury to the brachial plexus.
- **Iatrogenic:** Surgeries in the posterior triangle of neck, radiotherapy to neck and chest.

Classification of Brachial Plexus Injury

Brachial plexus injuries can be classified in different ways such as:
- **As per site of lesion:**
    - Root level injury
    - Trunk level injury
    - Cord level injury
    - Nerve level injury
    - Often a mixture of all
- **As per severity of lesion:**
    - *Preganglionic (supraclavicular) lesion:* Caused either by trauma or birth injury. The characteristic feature is

presence of Horner's syndrome (decreased size of pupils, drooping of eye lid, and decreased sweating on the affected side of face) and the ability to elevate scapula. Tinel's sign may be localized to supra scapular region only (strong Tinel sign without distal transmission). This carries a poor prognosis. Horner's syndrome is characterized by:
» A persistently small pupil (miosis)
» A notable difference in pupil size between the two eyes (anisocoria)
» Little or delayed opening (dilation) of the affected pupil in dim light
» Drooping of the upper eyelid (ptosis)
» Slight elevation of the lower lid, sometimes called upside-down ptosis
» Sunken appearance to the eye
» Little or no sweating (anhydrosis) either on the entire side of the face or an isolated patch of skin on the affected side
- *Postganglionic lesion:* This carries somewhat better prognosis as compared to preganglionic lesion. There is no Horner's syndrome and Tinel's sign (tapping 2–3 cms above the clavicle at the Erb's point, produces tingling sensation distally) is elicitable in the later stages.
❖ **As per part of plexus affected:**
- *Upper plexus:* C5, C6 with or without C7
- *Lower plexus:* C8T1
- *Global:* C5, C6, C7, C8, T1
❖ **Relation to clavicle:**
- Supraclavicular
- Retroclavicular
- Infraclavicular

Pathophysiology of Brachial Plexus Injury

The trauma from motor vehicle accidents involve traction on the plexus caused by an abnormal neck, shoulder angle while the person is being thrown from the vehicle after the impact. If the shoulder is in adduction at the time of injury, then the upper plexus is affected involving the C5, C6 with or without C7. If the shoulder is in abduction the stress is directed to the lower plexus, i.e., C8T1 roots. If the transfer of momentum is massive due to the high combined velocity of the two vehicles involved, then all roots can be damaged resulting in a flail upper limb.

Pathophysiology of Pre and Postganglionic lesion

Lesions proximal to the dorsal root ganglion (DRG) on the sensory side and at the level of the rootlets from the anterior horn cells (AHC) on the motor side are preganglionic and those distal to these structures, i.e., in the mixed spinal nerve emerging out of the foramina of the cervical spine are postganglionic **(Fig. 25.5)**. Preganglionic lesions essentially signal a permanent loss of that root and the axons within it. Postganglionic lesions are amenable to repair from the root stump since they represent axons distal to the cell body, which can regenerate.

The following pathomechanics are involved in brachial plexus injury:
❖ **Avulsion:** The nerve is torn away from its attachment from the spinal cord leading to the most severe type of

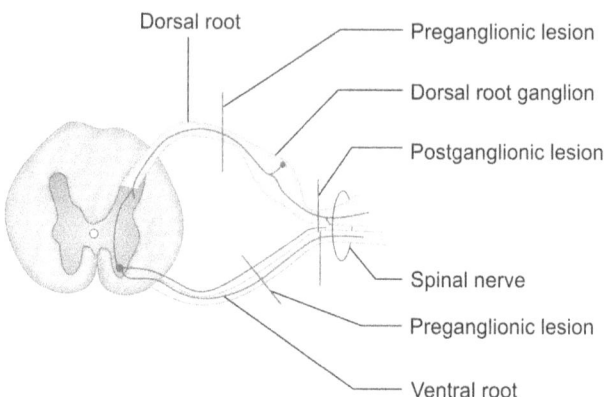

Fig. 25.5: Shows pre and postganglionic brachial plexus lesions.

preganglionic lesion, resulting in complete paralysis of muscles supplied and Horner's syndrome.
❖ **Rupture:** The nerve may be torn at trunk, cord or branch level, causing weakness/paralysis of muscles supplied by the same nerve.
❖ **Neuroma:** Scar tissue developed around the injured site puts pressure on the injured nerve resulting in development of neuroma (nerve bundle), hence preventing the nerve to send signal to the supplied muscles.
❖ **Neuropraxia:** The nerve gets stretched not torn or avulsed, causing loss of function.

Signs and Symptoms

❖ **Motor symptoms:** Pattern of muscle paralysis/weakness in the upper extremity depends on the /roots branches of the nerve that is affected. There is atrophy and weakness/paralysis of muscles. Summary of root wise motor function is shown in the **Table 25.1**.
❖ Decreased/loss of sensation in the involved upper extremity depending upon the branch/nerve root affected. It is represented in the **Table 25.2**.
❖ **Pain:** Pain from the most severe types of brachial plexus injuries has been described as a debilitating, severe crushing sensation or a constant burning. It results from damage of nerves and may be chronic.
❖ **Joint stiffness/deformity:** This results from lack of mobility and muscular imbalances.
❖ **Disability:** People who get severe type of complete brachial plexus injuries particularly with all preganglionic lesions and some postganglionic lesions sometimes lose function in the affected upper extremity and are permanently disabled.

Table 25.1: Nerve roots affected and functions lost.

Root value	Gross functions involved
C5, C6	Shoulder abduction and elbow flexion
C6, C7	Elbow extension and wrist extension
C8, T1	Hand function
C5–T1	Flail upper limb

Table 25.2: Nerve roots and area of skin affected.

Root value	Area of skin affected
C5	Skin over the upper arm (deltoid region)
C6	Thumb and index finger
C7	Middle finger
C8	Ulnar two fingers
T1	Medial forearm
T2	Inner aspect of arm

Diagnosis

Diagnosis of brachial plexus injury is done from history, clinical examinations, and diagnostic tests. The tests performed are:
- X-ray of shoulder and cervical spine.
- EMG/NCV.
- MRI.
- CT/CT myelography.
- S-D curves/Faradic–IDC tests.

Management of Brachial Plexus Injury

Brachial plexus injuries are managed through nonsurgical methods/conservative method in most of the cases. However, if nonsurgical methods fail to improve, or there is a rupture at trunk, cord or branch level surgery in the form of neurosurgery/orthopedic surgery, may be performed followed by rehabilitation therapies such as physiotherapy/occupational therapy/orthotic management.

The aim of conservative treatment is to maintain the range of motion of the extremity, to maintain muscle properties and prevent muscle fibrosis, to strengthen the remaining functional muscles, to protect the denervated dermatomes, manage pain and manage complications such as paralytic edema.

Chronic edema may appear as a result of hypokinesia, loss of vascular tone due to sympathetic denervation, and any other soft tissue injury. Limb elevation, splinting and application of tensile bandaging help in decreasing edema. Appropriate physiotherapy in the form of passive/active exercises, electrical stimulation should be provided, otherwise stiffness may be the final outcome, especially in the hand.

Management of anesthesia-denervated dermatomes is the same as with diabetic neuropathy, with the patients avoiding extreme temperatures. The methods of management could be: Nonsurgical methods such as—
- Physiotherapy.
- Occupational therapy.
- Orthotic management.

Physiotherapy

Immediately after brachial plexus injury the shoulder should be supported by using a triangular splint/aeroplane splint (Figs. 25.6A and B). Therapeutic interventions consist of:
- Relaxed passive exercises/joint range of motion exercises.
- Interrupted galvanic stimulation to paralyzed muscles using labile technique, preferably after 2 weeks of injury.

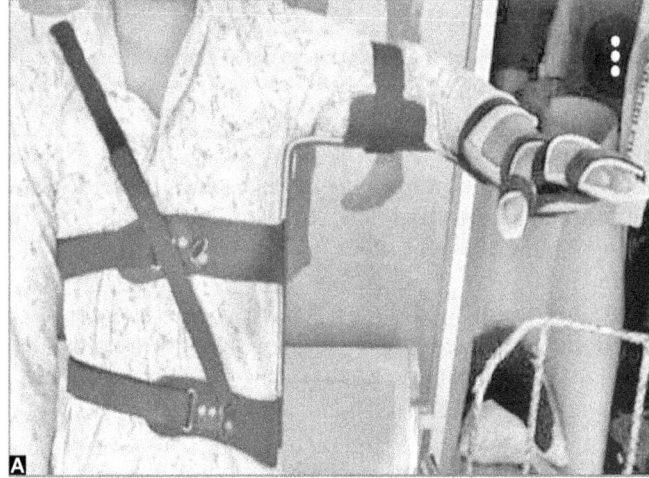
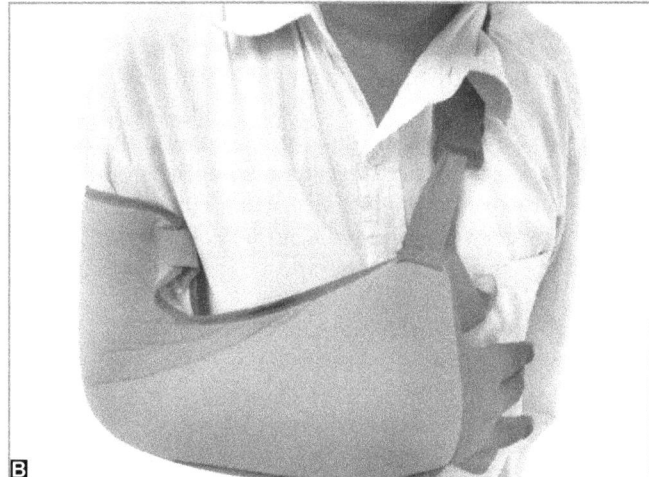

Figs. 25.6A and B: (A) Airplane splint; (B) Triangular sling.

- Surged faradic current to innervated muscles after performing simple tests such as S-D curves/Faradic-IDC tests.
- Active assisted/free/resisted exercises.
- PNF-Irradiation techniques to facilitate weaker muscles by over flow of impulse from the stronger intact/recovered muscles.
- Sensory education and skin care measures such as advice on avoiding exposure to fire.
- **Pain control:** Pain from the most severe types of brachial plexus injuries has been described as a debilitating, severe crushing sensation or a constant burning. This pain can be managed by application of TENS, patient counseling and medical management. If conservative methods can't control the pain, surgical procedure to interrupt the pain signals coming from the damaged part of the spinal cord may be considered.
- **Edema control:** Limb elevation/contrast bath (after testing temperature sensitivity), tensile bandaging, effleurage massage, passive/active exercises, etc., may be considered to treat edema.

Besides physiotherapy and shoulder supports, occupational therapy and hand splints are considered in the nonsurgical management (Figs. 25.7A and B).

Robotic Rehabilitation of Brachial Plexus Injury

Studies on robotic rehabilitation training with a newly developed upper limb single-joint hybrid assistive limb (HAL-SJ) for elbow flexor reconstruction (intercostobrachial anastomosis, i.e., intercostals nerve crossing to musculoskeletal nerve) after brachial plexus injury, where biofeedback techniques are applied with the robot, reveal significant improvement of power of biceps brachii even from a MRC grade of 1.

Assistive/adaptive devices: Assistive devices such as a functional arm brace **(Fig. 25.8A)** and adaptive devices such as adapted spoon **(Fig. 25.8B)**, may be used to improve function using the affected hand.

Surgical Management of Brachial Plexus Injuries

Neurosurgery

A physiotherapist treating a patient of brachial plexus injury should be knowledgeous about various surgical procedures performed, as through periodic assessment of the patient, while therapy is continued, the physiotherapist communicates with the Surgeon about selection of a particular patient either for neurosurgery or orthopedic surgery. A physiotherapist also provides preoperative therapy before surgery and takes measures to protect the repaired nerve/tendon after surgery is performed and provides postoperative physiotherapy till the patient is physically rehabilitated (functional).

Surgery to repair brachial plexus nerves should generally occur within 6 months after the injury. Surgeries that occur later than 6 months have lower success rates. Microsurgical nerve repair may be undertaken as early as 3 months after injury. Primary nerve repair is typically completed by approximately 6 months following injury.

The time frame for surgical repair is an important consideration for recovery from injury. If the muscles are not connected to nerves within 18 months of injury, it may not be possible to achieve muscle contraction subsequently, as gross structural changes take place in the muscles there after. For avulsion and rupture injuries, there is no potential for full recovery, unless surgical intervention is done in a timely manner. However, for pre-ganglionic lesions, direct repair at the injured site, may not produce significant recovery of function. For neuropraxic injuries, spontaneous recovery is significantly possible, where as for neuromas, recovery may occur with surgery.

Preoperative physiotherapy

It consists of maintenance and improvement of joint range of motion, prevention/correction of deformities, maintenance

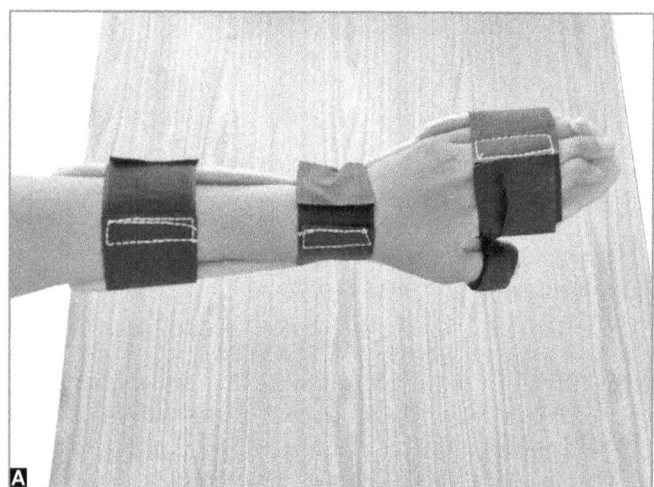

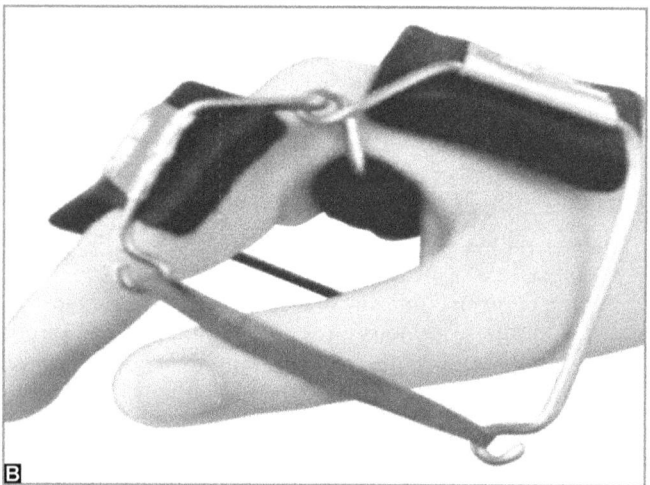

Figs. 25.7A and B: (A) Pancake splint; (B) Knuckle bender splint.

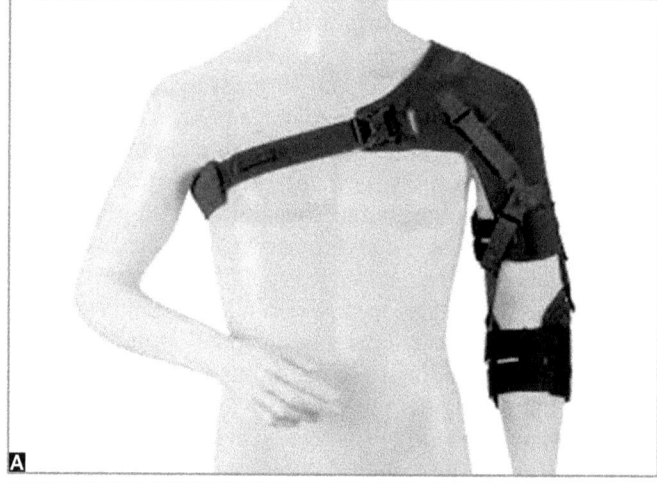

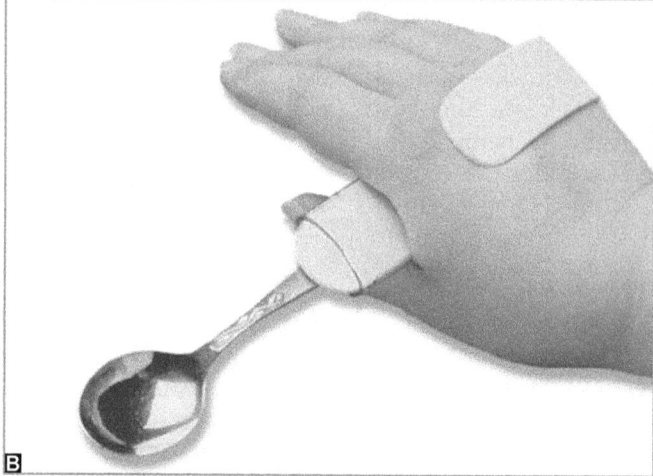

Figs. 25.8A and B: (A) The functional arm brace; (B) Adapted spoon.

of muscle properties (prevent fibrosis of muscles, as even after surgery, the recovery may take several months, and, if muscle properties are not maintained both preoperatively, as well as postoperatively, it may not be possible to get muscle contraction after nerve recovery occurred). Preoperative physiotherapy also focuses on improvement of lung function and counsels the patient for the surgery.

The surgical procedures

Adult traumatic brachial plexus injuries can have devastating effects on upper extremity function. Although neurolysis, nerve repair, and nerve grafting, neuroma excision, etc., have been used to treat injuries to the plexus, nerve transfer makes use of an undamaged nerve to supply motor input over a relatively short distance to reinnervated a denervated muscle. The procedures used include:

a. **Neurolysis:** Removal of connective scar tissue surrounding the nerve. This procedure consists of freeing up the nerve from scar tissue.
b. Neuroma excision and nerve repair.
c. **Nerve grafting:** In this procedure, the damaged part of the brachial plexus is removed and replaced with sections of nerves taken from other parts of your body. This provides a bridge for new nerve growth over the time.
d. **Neurotization/nerve transfer:** This is used generally in those cases where there is an avulsion. Donor nerves are used for the repair. The parts of the roots still attached to the spinal cord can be used as donors for avulsed nerves. When the nerve root has been torn from the spinal cord, surgeons often take a less important nerve that is still working and connect it to a nerve that is more important but not working. This provides a bypass for new nerve growth. The followings are some of the important nerves considered for transfer in brachial plexus injury.
   – *Spinal accessory nerve transfer:* The spinal accessory nerve is a pure motor nerve, which innervates the sternocleidomastoid and trapezius muscles. It is essential to protect branches to the upper and middle trapezius to preserve function when this nerve is used as a donor. Proximity of the spinal accessory nerve to the suprascapular nerve allows direct micro approximation without graft. Although transfers to the more distal musculocutaneous nerve and axillary nerves have been described, both require use of an interposition nerve graft.
   – *Intercostal nerve transfer (intercostobrachial anastomosis):* The intercostal nerves are a mixed motor and sensory nerve with a finite number of available axons, necessitating transfer of multiple nerves to any particular recipient nerve. Transfer of intercostal nerves (2nd to 4th intercostal nerves) for elbow (Intercostobrachial anastomosis) or shoulder reinnervation is usually reserved for use when other available donor nerves are unavailable or injured. The author has successfully worked with an orthopedic surgeon, on a patient, subjected to intercosto brachial anastomosis, and could achieve an elbow flexor grade of 3 as per MRC grading postoperatively with use of elbow orthosis to prevent stretching of the nerve, active assisted/ free exercises, electrical stimulation, etc. Subsequently the patient was advised to continue home exercise program and to make use of the hand for light functional activities.
   – *Triceps nerve branch to axillary nerve:* Functional restoration of shoulder abduction can be achieved by transferring a nerve branch of the long head, lateral head, or medial head of the triceps muscle to the distal deltoid motor branch of the damaged axillary nerve.
   – *Ulnar nerve to musculocutaneous nerve (Oberlin transfer):* Christophe Oberlin described transfer of one or more ulnar nerve fascicles to the motor branch (es) of the biceps muscle. This is performed to restore elbow flexion in patients who have an irreparable upper trunk injury or avulsion, and an intact lower trunk.
   – *Double fascicular transfer for elbow flexion:* In this, transfer of motor fascicles from both the ulnar and median nerves to the biceps and brachialis branches of the musculocutaneous nerve are done respectively.
   – *Medial pectoral nerve transfer for elbow flexion:* The proximity of the medial pectoral nerve to musculocutaneous recipient provides an advantage for early recovery (which may take 6-8 months).

Orthopedic Surgery

❖ **Tendon transfer:** Tendon transfers are useful in restoring upper extremity function after brachial plexus injury. An absolute indication for tendon transfer is upper or lower brachial plexus traumatic injury with only partial paralysis. Before tendon transfer intensive preoperative physiotherapy is required to mobilize stiff joint, correct deformities (if any) and to achieve a grade of 4 as per MRC grading for the muscle to be transferred. It must be kept in mind by the team of clinicians that transferring a tendon over stiff joints is usually useless, hence intensive physiotherapy (with surgical intervention if required) should be undertaken before tendon transfer surgery. Postoperatively, tendon re-education exercises and splinting to be done accordingly.
   – *Tendon transfer techniques for shoulder:*
     » Trapezius to deltoid transfer as described by Elhassan et al. in 2000 to restore abduction of the shoulder.
     » Latissimus dorsi transfer as described by L'Episcopo, to improve shoulder external rotation.
     » Anterior transfer of the posterior part of the deltoid muscle to restore nonfunctional anterior segment.
   – *Tendon transfer techniques for elbow:* Restoration of elbow flexion is of great importance for a good clinical and functional outcome. Depending on the level of injury and the degree of reinnervation there are different types of surgical procedure. The surgical goal is to restore good muscle strength through a range of elbow

motion (30–130 degrees). The most commonly used procedures are as follows:
- » Transfer of the common origin of the forearm flexor muscles to a proximal section as described by Steindler.
- » Transfer of latissimus dorsi muscle to the tendon of the biceps brachii provides great muscle strength, but this muscle is often denervated.
- » Transfer of pectoralis major brachial branch tendon to biceps brachii to achieve elbow flexion (Clark technique).
- *Tendon transfer techniques for hand:*
  - » Intrinsic balance (claw hand correction): Transfer of flexor digitorum superficialis.
  - » Thumb opposition: Transfer of extensor indicis, FDS, abductor digiti minimi.
  - » Thumb flexion: Transfer of pronator teres, FDS, brachioradialis.
  - » Thumb extension: Transfer of palmaris longus, brachioradialis, and extensor indices.
  - » Finger flexion: Transfer of brachioradialis, ECRL.
  - » Finger extension: Transfer of brachioradialis, flexor carpi radialis, flexor carpi ulnaris, and extensor indices.
  - » Wrist extension: Transfer of brachioradialis, pronator teres.

Arthrodesis: In complete traumatic brachial plexus injuries involving the upper trunk, arthrodesis resulting in shoulder stabilization at an angle of 20 degrees of abduction, 30 degrees flexion, and 30–40 degrees of internal rotation **(Fig. 25.9)** allows the patient to be independent in his daily life. When planning shoulder arthrodesis certain parameters should be taken into consideration. First, good scapulothoracic functionality is of great importance. Second, the motion, mobility of the peripheral hand is important as shoulder arthrodesis has no clinical effect on a paralytic hand whatsoever.

OBSTETRICS BRACHIAL PLEXUS INJURIES

Erb's Palsy

Erb's palsy also called as Erb-Duchenne palsy is one of the obstetrics brachial plexus injury that results from injury to

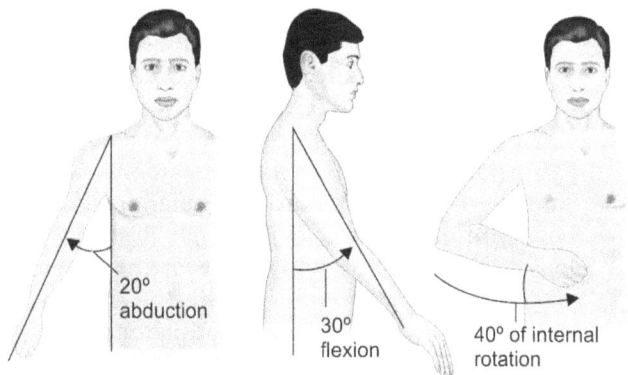

Fig. 25.9: Positions of arthrodesis of shoulder in BPI.

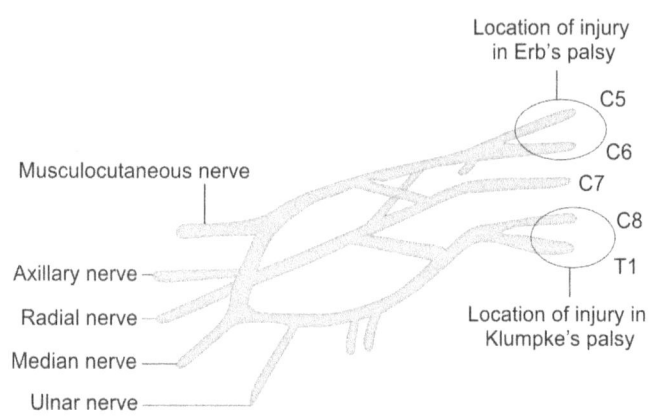

Fig. 25.10: Location of injury in Erb's palsy/Klumpke's palsy.

the upper brachial plexus at birth. The injury can stretch, rupture or avulse the roots of the plexus that form the upper trunk **(Fig. 25.10)**.

Etiopathology

The most common cause of Erb's palsy is excessive lateral traction or stretching of the baby's head and neck in opposite directions during delivery such as Forceps or Breech delivery, where the baby's head may be deviated from the axial plane. This may cause the brachial plexus to be stretched and ruptured.

Clinical Features

There is paralysis of muscles of baby's shoulder, arm, and forearm with minimal involvement of muscles of wrist. The baby develops an attitude of shoulder extension, adduction and medial rotation, elbow extension, forearm pronation and wrist slight flexion due to paralysis/weakness of muscles supplied by C5, C6 such as the deltoids, shoulder lateral rotators (supraspinatus, infraspinatus, and teres minor) elbow flexor (biceps brachii), fore arm supinator and partial involvement of wrist extensors. The affected upper limb assumes the police man's tip hand/Waiter's tip hand position **(Figs. 25.11A and B)**. The baby develops the attitude of upper limb, similar to the attitude of upper limb made by the traffic police at the traffic post to make vehicles stop, those are coming from behind. The baby may also exhibit sensory loss in the lateral aspects of arm and forearm both in the front and back.

Diagnosis of Erb's Palsy

Diagnosis of Erb's palsy is made through:
- ❖ History of birth.
- ❖ Physical examination.
- ❖ Special diagnostic tests such as MRI, NCV.

Management

Recoveries in most cases occur spontaneously between 4 months to 2 years, though a majority of children show spontaneous recovery by 9 months. Physiotherapy, occupational therapy, orthoses/splints, etc., are used to promote recovery and achieve function when recovery progresses. However, if movement at shoulder, i.e. deltoid contraction does not recover by 3 months and electrophysiological tests do not show signs of recovery,

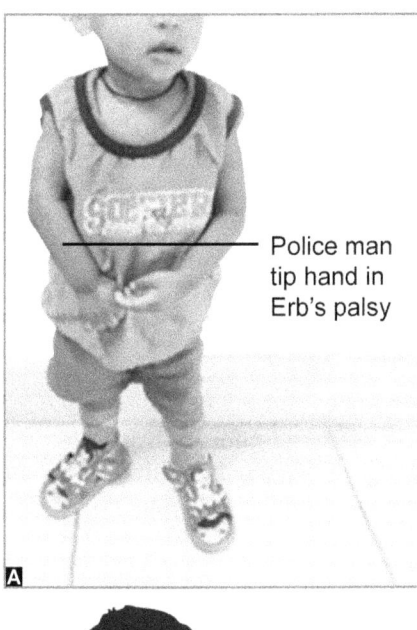

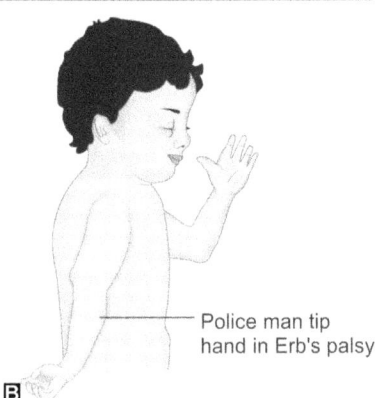

Figs. 25.11A and B: Deformed attitude of upper limb in Erb's palsy: The police man's tip hand.

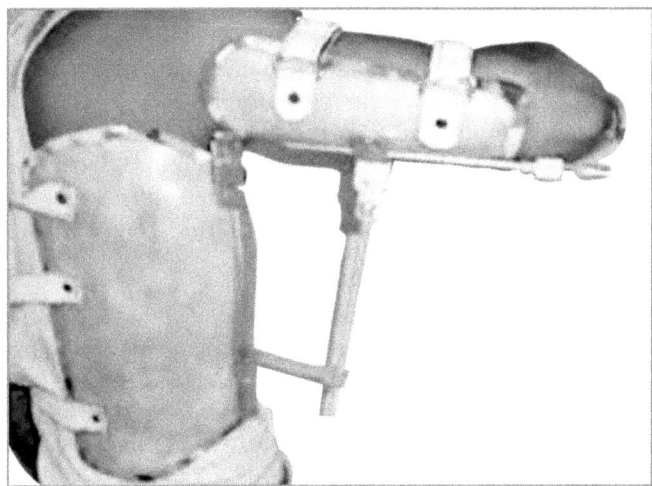

Fig. 25.12: Aeroplane splint applied to a child with Erb's palsy.

surgery is to be considered. The conservative management consists of:

- ❖ **Physiotherapy:** It includes :
  - Positioning the affected upper limb in shoulder abduction and external rotation, elbow flexion and forearm supination and wrist in few degrees of extension, through positioning on bed and by use of airplane splint **(Fig. 25.12)**.
  - Passive ROM exercises to maintain ROM.
  - Gentle stretching of the tight muscles to prevent development of tightness/contracture and deformities.
  - Interrupted galvanic current stimulation to paralyzed muscles, preferably through finger stimulation. In finger stimulation, the indifferent electrode is placed over the infant's thigh and the stimulating electrode is strapped over the therapist's forearm. The therapist places his/her finger tip (preferably index finger) over the muscle belly for denervated muscles using galvanic type of currents/motor point for innervated muscles using faradic type of currents.
  - Surged faradic type current stimulation is used for recovering/innervating muscles.
  - Active assisted/free/resisted exercises.
  - Constraint induced movement therapy (CIMT).
  - Kinesio taping.
  - Sensory education.
  - Play therapy.
  - *Virtual reality:* Virtual reality (VR) refers to a computer-generated simulation in which a person can interact within an artificial three-dimensional environment using electronic devices, such as special goggles with a screen or gloves fitted with sensors.
  - Functional education.
  - A systematic review suggests constraint-induced movement therapy, kinesio taping. Electrotherapy, virtual reality, and use of splints or orthotics have positive outcomes for the affected upper limb functionality in obstetric brachial palsy from birth to 10 years.
- ❖ **Surgical management:** Surgery is only considered when conservative treatment fails and/or there is no sign of recovery of shoulder muscles by 3 months. Surgery involves nerve transplants or tendon transfer of functioning muscles. Nerve transplants are usually performed on babies under the age of 9 months since the fast development of younger babies increases the effectiveness of the procedure, and are not usually carried out on patients older than this age. Release of subscapularis muscle and transfer of latissimus dorsi muscle to achieve shoulder abduction is also helpful.

Prognosis: Many children show a near complete recovery, but for those unfortunate not to recover fully, it is important to focus on helping a child to adapt to tasks and work on different strategies to complete activities in their daily life. The prognosis is dependent on the severity of injury, timing of treatment and associated injuries such as fractures. Mild cases of Erb's palsy may resolve significantly in 3–6 months with conservative treatment. The condition resolves almost completely in 70–80% of children in the first year of life with prompt treatment. Majority of children recover if treatment begins within first 4 weeks of birth.

Klumpke's Palsy

Klumpke's palsy is one obstetric brachial plexus injury, which is named after Augusta Dejerine-Klumpke.

This is the injury to the lower trunk of the brachial plexus that result from a difficult child birth. Usually the 8th cervical (C8) and 1st thoracic (T1) roots are injured either before or after they have joined to form the lower trunk **(Fig. 25.10)**.

Etiopathology

The condition is usually caused by undue abduction of the arm that usually occurs in breech presentations. This injury can cause a stretching, tearing (avulsion and rupture), or scarring (neuroma) of the brachial plexus nerves. Most infants with Klumpke paralysis have the more mild form of injury (neuropraxia) and often recover within 6 months.

Clinical Features

There is paralysis/weakness of the intrinsic muscles of hand (T1), or ulnar flexors of wrist and fingers (C8), causing claw hand deformity **(Fig. 25.13)**. There is also supination of forearm and wrist extension with loss of sensation along the medial aspects of the arm, forearm and hand along the C8, T1 dermatome. Horner's syndrome may be present. Features of good shoulder and bad hand are present.

Diagnosis of Klumpke's Palsy

Diagnosis of Klumpke's palsy is made through:
- History of birth.
- Physical examination.
- Special tests such as MRI, NCV.

Management of Klumpke's Palsy

The affected arm may be immobilized across the body for 7–10 days. Following which physiotherapy and orthotic management is considered.

Physiotherapy focuses on:
- Maintenance of joint range of motion and prevention of deformities.
- Maintenance of muscle properties and improve muscle strength.
- Recommendation for use of appropriate splint.
- Educate functional use of the hand.

Physiotherapy Methods
- Joint range of motion exercises.
- Passive stretching exercises.
- Active assisted/free exercises.
- Interrupted galvanic/surged faradic current stimulation using therapist's finger as stimulating electrode, depending upon denervation/innervations.
- Make use of a light weight, well-padded polypropylene/Orfit made hand splint **(Fig. 25.14)**.
- Play therapy.
- Virtual reality.

Surgery

Surgery (nerve grafts/neuroma excision), as well as tendon transfer (at the age of 3 years or more) may be considered, if there is an avulsion/rupture and spontaneous recovery is not possible.

Bell's Palsy

Bell's palsy is a lower motor neuron type of facial palsy, affecting the whole of the face on the affected side. The condition is named after Scottish anatomist Charles Bell, who was the first to describe the condition.

Causes of Bell's Palsy

Bell's palsy occurs when the seventh cranial nerve becomes swollen or compressed, resulting in facial weakness or paralysis. The exact cause of this damage is unknown, but many medical researchers believe it's most likely triggered by a viral infection. Exposure to cold, such as travelling in a bus/car sitting near the windows in winter, is found as a causative factor in many individuals.

The viruses/bacteria that have been linked to the development of Bell's palsy include:
- Herpes simplex, which causes cold sores and genital herpes
- HIV, which damages the immune system
- Sarcoidosis, which causes organ inflammation
- Herpes zoster virus, which causes chickenpox and shingles
- Epstein-Barr virus, which causes mononucleosis
- Lyme disease, which is a bacterial infection caused by infected ticks.

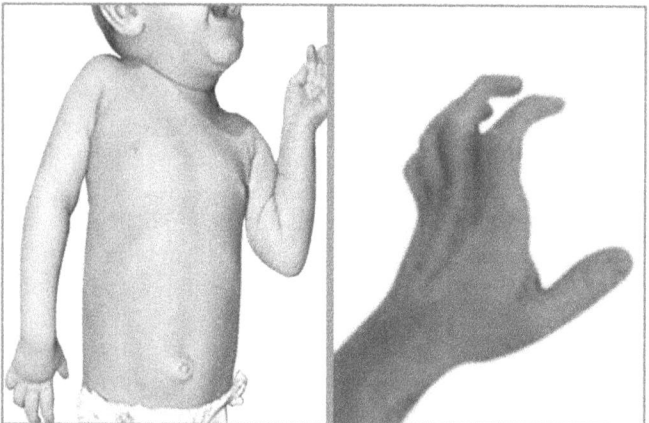

Fig. 25.13: Claw hand deformity in Klumpke's palsy.

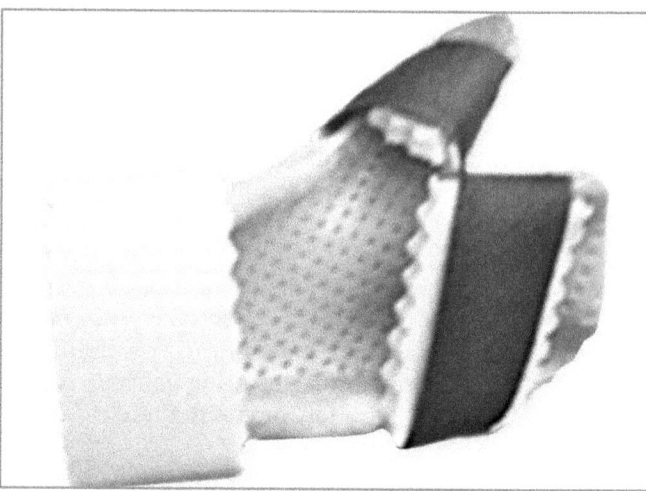

Fig. 25.14: Hand splint for Klumpke's palsy.

Epidemiology

Bell's palsy most commonly occurs between the ages of 10 and 40 years. The reason is not clear, but most cases are probably due to a viral infection/exposure to cold. Most people make a full recovery within 2–3 months. Anyone can get Bell's palsy, and it affects both men and women equally.

Clinical Features

The symptoms of Bell's palsy may develop 1–2 weeks after someone has a cold exposure/suffering from cold, ear infection, or eye infection. They usually appear abruptly, and the sufferer may notice them when he/she wakes up in the morning or try to eat or drink.

The condition is marked by a dropping of angle of mouth **(Fig. 25.15A)** and the inability to open or close the eyes on the affected side **(Fig. 25.15B)**. In rare cases, Bell's palsy may affect both sides of the face. The patient may also have other features, such as:

- Facial weakness affecting the whole of the face on the affected side.
- Drooling of saliva.
- Difficulty in eating and drinking. Food collecting in the inner wall of cheek.
- Inability to make facial expressions, such as smiling or frowning.
- Muscle twitches in the Face
- Dry eye and mouth.
- Crocodile tears: "Crocodile tears syndrome", also known as Bogorad syndrome, is the shedding of *tears* while eating or drinking in patients recovering from Bell's palsy.
- Headache
- Sensitivity to sound
- Irritation of the eye on the involved side.

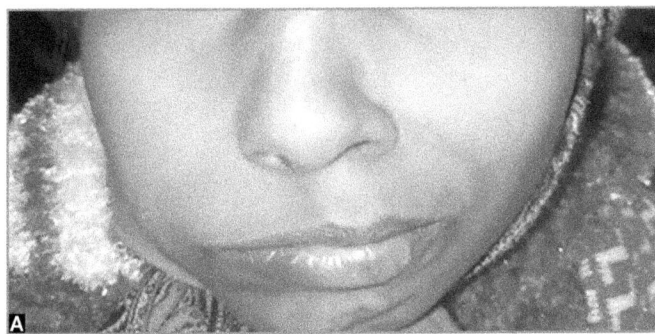

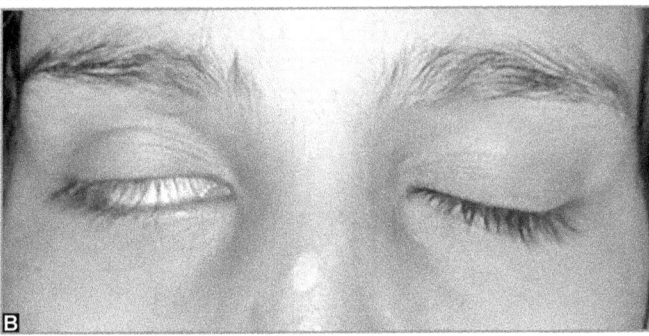

Figs. 25.15A and B: (A) Drooping of angle of mouth; (B) Inability to close the eyes.

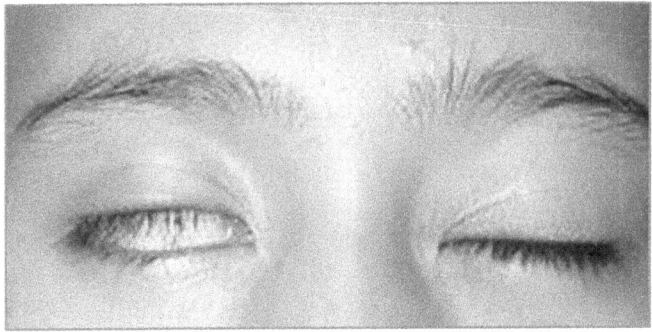

Fig. 25.16: Positive Bell's sign: The eye ball rolling upward, as the patient tries to close the eyes.

- Positive Bell's sign **(Fig. 25.16)**: When the patient tries to close the eye, the eye balls roll upwards.

Diagnosis of Bell's Palsy

Diagnosis is made from history of onset, clinical features, and laboratory tests such as blood test to find the presence of virus/bacteria. Sometimes CT scan/MRI of head is recommended to establish diagnosis in the absence of definite history.

Treatment/Management

- **Medical management:**
  - Corticosteroid drugs, which reduce inflammation are prescribed by the physician.
  - Antiviral or antibacterial medication, which may be prescribed by the physician, if a virus or bacteria caused Bell's palsy
  - NSAIDs
  - Antibiotic drops for eye.
- **Physiotherapy:** Physiotherapy for Bell's palsy consists of:
  - Use of a S-hook splint to prevent stretching of the paralyzed/weak muscles **(Fig. 25.17)**.
  - *Facial massage:* Gentle finger kneading and effleurage.
  - *Interrupted galvanic stimulation:* Even though the injury is neuropraxic in nature and the muscles are innervated, faradic type current stimulation is not applied to facial muscles, as it causes secondary muscle tightness/contracture. Hence, interrupted galvanic current stimulation to facial muscles are applied.
  - Application of moist heat/pulsed shortwave diathermy (PSWD) to the affected side of face, over the stylomastoid foramen, avoiding the eyes.

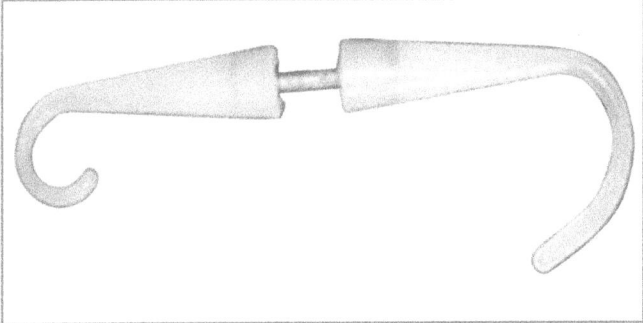

Fig. 25.17: The S-hook splint.

Section 3: Physiotherapy for Neurological Conditions

- *Facial exercises:* Facial exercises help strengthen the facial muscles and should be done 4–5 times a day in front of a mirror. Facial exercises for Bell's palsy involve doing basic actions with the different muscle groups throughout face. The facial workouts involve, sitting relaxed in front of a mirror and performing the followings:
  » Gently raising the eye brows with assistance using own fingers (if required) **(Fig. 25.18A)**.
  » Pulling the eye brows together and frowning **(Fig. 25.18B)**.
  » Wrinkling of the nose **(Fig. 25.18C)**.
  » Breathing in deeply and flaring the nostrils and breathing out, slowly bulging the cheeks **(Fig. 25.18D)**.
  » Moving the corners of the mouth outward **(Fig. 25.18E)**.
  » Pulling one side of the mouth up, then the other, to form a smile **(Fig. 25.18F)**.
  » Bringing the lips together and forward (making purse lip) **(Fig. 25.18G)**.
  » Keep the head still, and look down. Place one index finger gently over one eyelid to hold it closed **(Fig. 25.18H)**.
  » Exercise to promote closure of eye and prevent tightness of upper eye lid **(Fig. 25.18I)**.
  » Gently try pressing the eyelids together using the hands **(Fig. 25.18J)**.

Factors to be considered while doing facial exercises:
- Facial exercises can be performed at home, 4–5 times a day.
- Repetitions and frequency of exercises should be modified according to improvement status.
- Exercises should be done in short sessions, but the frequency of exercises can be increased.

Precautions to be followed by the patient:
The main concern is to ensure the eye is protected and is kept moistened. At night-time, it is probably best to use a soft, surgical, eye pad, taped to ensure the eye remains closed during sleep. Protection from dust and dirt can be achieved by wearing suitable glasses. The patient should avoid exposure to cold.

Prognosis of Bell's palsy
In most people the function of the nerve gradually returns to normal. Symptoms usually start to improve after about 2–3 weeks, and resolve within 2 months. In some cases, it can take up to 12 months to recover fully.

In some cases, symptoms do not completely go. Some weakness may remain as residual weakness, which may not be markedly noticeable. It is uncommon to have no improvement at all; however, some people are left with some degree of permanent facial weakness, resulting in deviation of angle of mouth or inability to close the eye fully (requiring tarsorrhaphy).

ULNAR NERVE INJURY

The ulnar nerve (C8, T1), gives motor supplies to the flexor carpi ulnaris, flexor digitorum profundus (medial part) in the forearm.

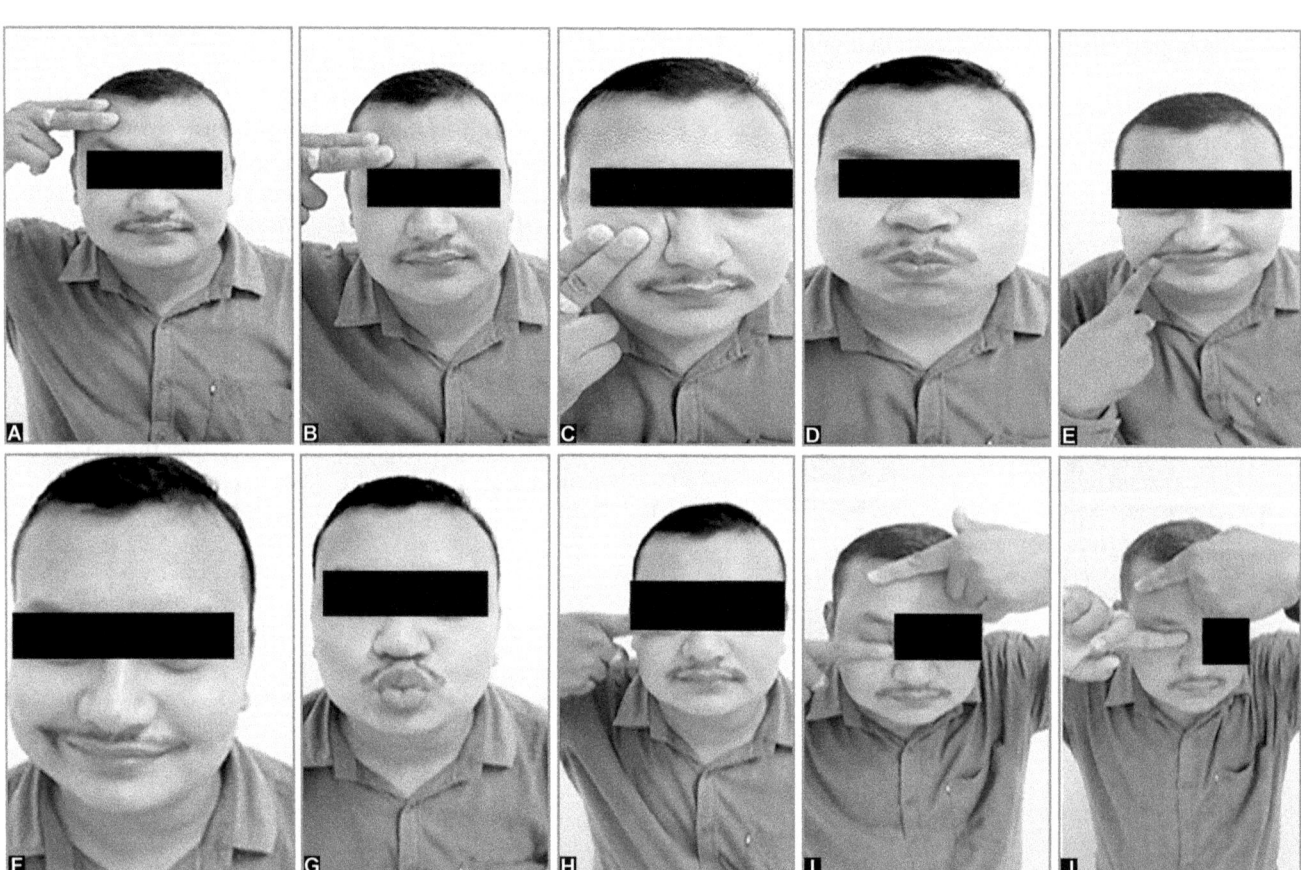

Figs. 25.18A to J: Facial exercises.

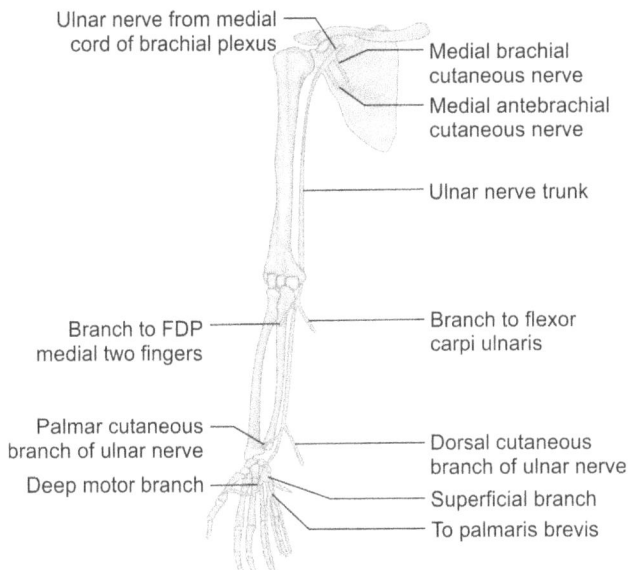

Fig. 25.19: Shows the course of ulnar nerve and the muscles it supplies.

It also supplies the muscles of hypothenar eminence, medial two lumbricals, and all the interossei muscles as well as adductor pollicis in the hand **(Fig. 25.19)**. The nerve also gives sensory supply to the medial aspect of hand (both volar and dorsal).

Causes of Ulnar Nerve Injury

The nerve may be damaged by chemical, mechanical (trauma/entrapment in various tunnels, such as cubital tunnel at elbow, Guyon's tunnel at wrist), neoplastic, iatrogenic, and infective (Hansen's disease) factors at various levels such as:
- ❖ **Axilla:** Crutch pressure, aneurysm of axillary vessels, trauma are the causes.
- ❖ **Arm:** Trauma (fracture shaft of humerus), bullet injuries.
- ❖ **Elbow:** Fracture of medial condyle of humerus, chronic stretching of the nerve as occurs in tardy ulnar palsy, cubitus valgus deformity, cubital tunnel syndrome (CBTS).
  - *Cubital tunnel syndrome:* It is an irritation or injury of the ulnar nerve in the cubital tunnel at the elbow. It is a progressive entrapment neuropathy of the ulnar nerve at the medial aspect of the elbow. The cubital tunnel extends from the medial epicondyle of the humerus to the olecranon process of the ulna. The roof of the cubital tunnel is formed by the cubital tunnel retinaculum, which is about 4 mm between the medial epicondyle and the olecranon. The floor of the tunnel consists of the elbow joint capsule and the posterior band of the medial collateral ligament of the elbow. The nerve runs superficial to the ulnar collateral ligament (UCL) and deep to the aponeurotic attachment of the flexor carpi ulnaris (FCU), which is also known as Osborne's ligament. Once the ulnar nerve reaches the proximal border of Osborne's ligament, it is located in the cubital tunnel. This is also termed as ulnar nerve entrapment and is the second most common compression neuropathy in the upper extremity after carpal tunnel syndrome.

It represents a source of considerable discomfort and disability for the patient and may, in extreme, cases lead to a loss of function of the hand.
- ❖ **Forearm:** Fracture both bones of forearm. Glass cut injury at lower forearm (very common).
- ❖ **Wrist:** Fracture of hook of hamate. Compression at Guyon's canal/ulnar tunnel (a semi-rigid longitudinal canal at wrist that allows passage of ulnar nerve and ulnar artery into hand).
- ❖ **Hand:** Burn injuries, blunt injury to hand.

Clinical Features

The features of ulnar nerve injury depend upon the site of injury, and are described briefly as under:
- ❖ **High ulnar nerve injury:** When injury occurs at the region of the elbow, entire function of ulnar nerve is lost. Cubital tunnel syndrome (CBTS) that affects the ulnar nerve at the elbow manifests in three grades such as:
  - *Grade I:* Mild symptoms including:
    » Intermittent paresthesia
    » Minor hypoesthesia of the dorsal and palmar surfaces of the fifth and medial aspect of fourth digits
    » No motor changes
  - *Grade II:* Moderate and persistent symptoms including:
    » Paresthesia
    » Hypoesthesia of the dorsal and palmar surfaces of the fifth and medial aspect of fourth digits and medial aspects of hand **(Fig. 25.20)**
    » Mild weakness of ulnar innervated muscles.
    » Early signs of atrophy of muscles.
  - *Grade III:* Severe symptoms including:
    » Paresthesia
    » Obvious loss of sensation of the dorsal and palmar surfaces of the fifth and medial aspect of fourth digits and medial aspects of hand.
    » Significant functional and motor impairment.
    » Muscle atrophy of the intrinsic of hand.
    » Possible digital clawing of fourth and fifth digits (sign of benediction) **(Fig. 25.21)**.
- ❖ **Low ulnar nerve injury:** When injury occurs below the elbow (commonly occurring at the junction of middle and lower third of the forearm), functions of flexor digitorum profundus and flexor carpi ulnaris are spared, but there is

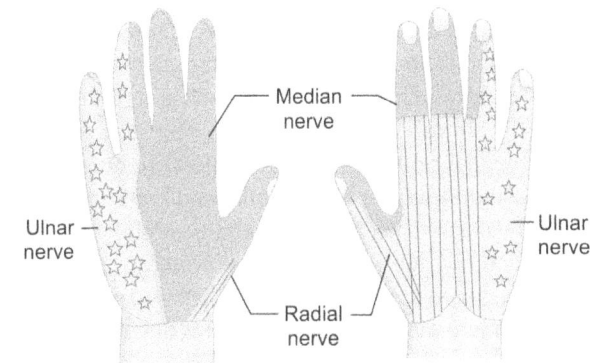

Fig. 25.20: Sensory innervation of hand.

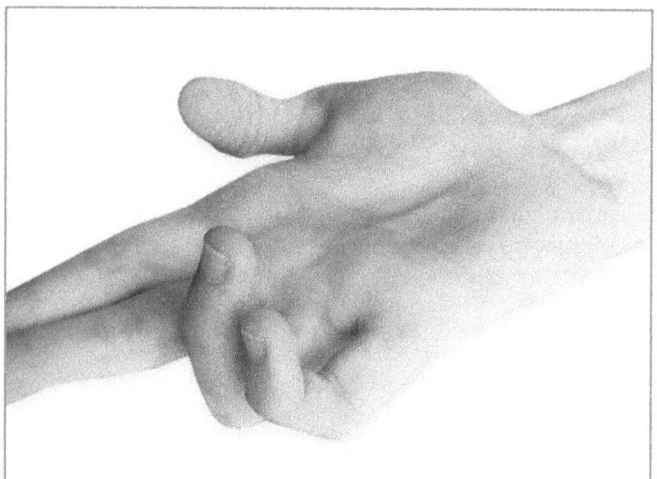

Fig. 25.21: Atrophy of intrinsic muscles with ulnar claw hand deformity.

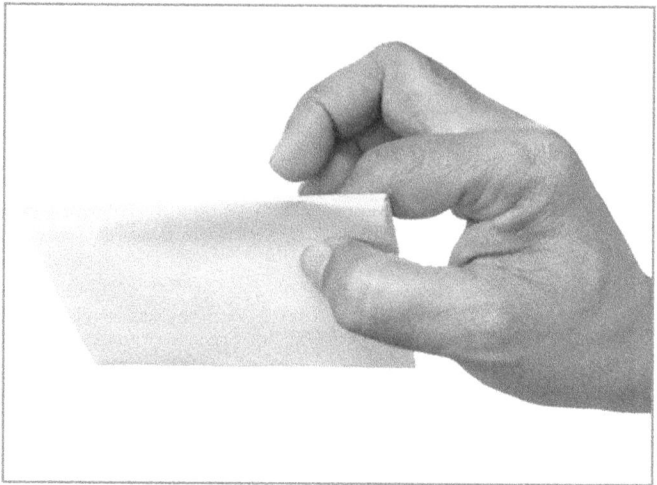

Fig. 25.22: Test showing positive Froment's sign.

paralysis/paresis of hypothenar muscles, interossei, medial two lumbricals and sensory loss over the medial aspects of hand (both dorsally and volarly). The patient may also show a positive Wartenberg's sign (Wartenberg's Sign refers to the slightly greater abduction of the fifth digit, due to paralysis of the adducting palmar interosseous muscle and unopposed action of the radial innervated extensor muscles such as ext. digiti minimi, extensor digitorum communis).

If the injury to nerve occurs proximal to Guyon's canal (a semi-rigid longitudinal canal in the wrist, that allows passage of ulnar artery/ulnar nerve into hand), flexor digitorum profundus (medial part), flexor carpi ulnaris and sensation over the dorsal aspect of hand supplied by ulnar nerve will be spared, but sensation over volar aspect in the medial side will be lost.

Diagnostic Procedure

Diagnosis of ulnar nerve injury/entrapment is done through history, physical examination, and electrodiagnostic studies and imaging. Besides the loss/impairment of motor and sensory function, a positive Tinel sign (which usually progresses distally as the nerve grows) is also helpful in making diagnosis. A positive Tinel's sign is the reproduction of tingling and numbness in the ulnar nerve distribution on the involved side, when the nerve is tapped with tip of fingers from distal to proximal along the course of the nerve. Froment's sign (The patient is asked to make a strong pinch between the thumb and index finger and grip a flat object such as a piece of paper between the thumb and index finger. The examiner then attempts to pull the object out of the subject's hands. If there is weakness of the adductor pollicis innervated by the ulnar nerve, the patient will fail to keep IP joint relatively straight; instead, the flexor pollicis muscle which is innervated by the median nerve is substituted for the adductor pollicis and will cause the IP joint to go into a hyperflexed position) **(Fig. 25.22)**, which tests the integrity of adductor pollicis muscle is also helpful in diagnosis.

The card test **(Fig. 25.23)** (Where a patient fails to hold a card placed between the fingers, due to weakness of palmar interossei that adducts the fingers), may also be positive suggesting ulnar nerve injury.

The Egawa's sign test **(Fig. 25.24)**, which is done to find weakness of dorsal interossei of middle finger supplied by ulnar nerve: The test involves moving the middle finger actively sideways with the palm flat on the table. Weakness/difficulty in moving the middle finger sideways is a positive Egawa test.

Electrophysiological studies: Nerve conduction velocity (NCV) measurement (NCV of ulnar nerve <50m/s, at the elbow is suggestive of CBTS), S-D curve plotting, Faradic-IDC tests etc., are helpful in making diagnosis.

Imaging studies: High resolution neuro-ultrasonography (helps to know the size and position of ulnar nerve at elbow), magnetic resonance neurography (to know the structural changes of the ulnar nerve and its environment), X-ray of cervical spine/elbow/wrist may be recommended as indicated to establish diagnosis.

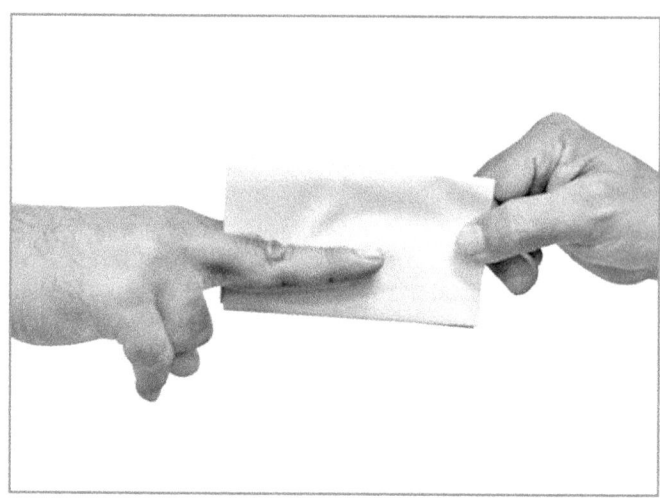

Fig. 25.23: The card test.

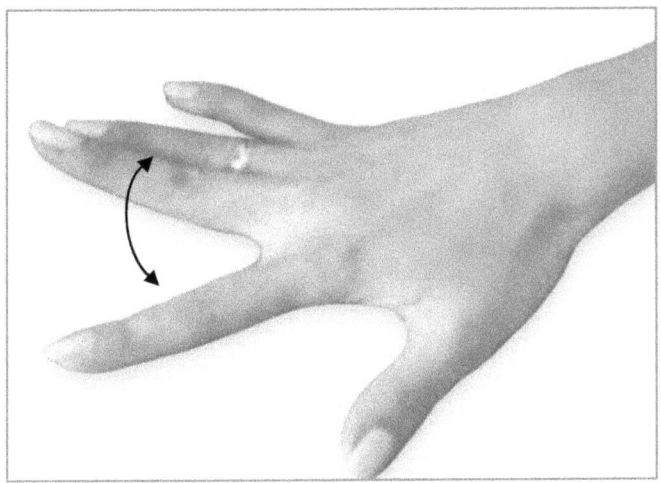

Fig. 25.24: Demonstrates Egawa test to find ulnar nerve injury.

Management of Ulnar Nerve Injury

It consists of medical/surgical management, physiotherapy, orthotic management, and occupational therapy.

- **Medical/surgical management:** In closed injuries, medical management in the form of NSAIDs/steroids are prescribed by the physician in combination with rest and splint.

  In acute open ulnar nerve injury, immediate exploration and primary neurorrhaphy is recommended as long as the repair can be achieved under minimal tension. For contaminated wounds, for which immediate repair would be imprudent, a delayed repair can be performed ideally in less than 72 hours, but up to 7 days without detriment to outcome. Delays in repair increase the likelihood for nerve grafting. Full recovery from ulnar nerve injuries may take as long as 5 years. Tendon transfer should be considered as a second-line treatment when motor loss is deemed permanent after nerve repair.

  For compressive injuries like CBTS, anterior transposition of ulnar nerve may be considered, if conservative treatment fails to improve symptoms.

- **Physiotherapy:** In case of compressive injuries such as CBTS, or Guyon's tunnel syndrome, an impairment-based approach is used to address deficits in strength and range of motion, pain and loss of function. For compression of the ulnar nerve at elbow, an elbow brace that prevents elbow flexion beyond 45 degrees with a hand splint that keeps the wrist slightly flexed and MCP joints flexed, IP joints extended and thumb adducted may be worn during night hours during the course of the treatment **(Fig. 25.25A)**. For injuries occurring around the wrist, a hand splint, that keeps the wrist slightly flexed, MCP joints flexed, IP joints extended and thumb adducted may be worn in the similar manner as described for injuries occurring around the elbow. If the patient has developed an ulnar claw hand deformity, a hand splint (knuckle bender splint) **(Fig. 25.25B)**, may be advised.

- **Electrotherapy:** Ice therapy to reduce pain and inflammation during the first 72 hours of onset, Ultrasound therapy, high power laser therapy, iontophoresis

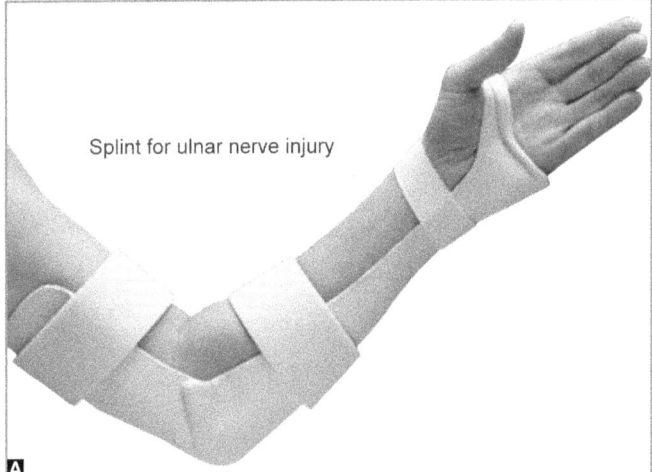
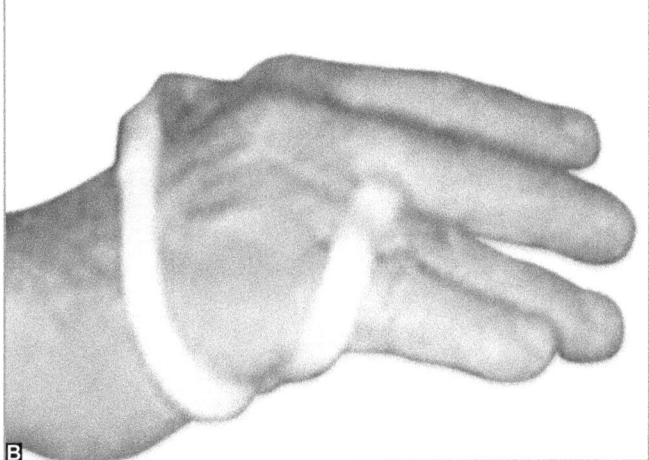

Figs. 25.25A and B: (A) Resting splint for high ulnar nerve injury; (B) Knuckle bender splint for ulnar clawing.

for sclerolytic effect, etc., may be used at the site of compression to mobilize tight tissues and to reduce pain. Interrupted galvanic current (if muscles are denervated)/surged faradic current (if muscles are innervated) stimulation may be considered to maintain/increase muscle properties/muscle power. TENS may be used to reduce pain.

Massage: Friction massage as tolerated, kneading, etc., may be applied at the site of compression to relieve the nerve off pressure.

Exercises: Nerve gliding exercises for ulnar nerve **(Figs. 25.26A to E)**, active assisted/free exercises are given to mobilize the nerve and strengthen muscles. For ulnar nerve gliding exercises, each position shown below is held for 5 seconds and the series (1–5) are repeated 3–5 times in a session.

Home exercises: Exercises such as finger parting and closing with or without resistance offered by elastic bands **(Fig. 25.27A)**, grasping a book/register between fingers and thumb **(Fig. 25.27B)**, grasping a sheet of paper between the fingers, stretching of fingers, grasping and releasing exercises, functional re-education, sensory education while doing functional activities are emphasized.

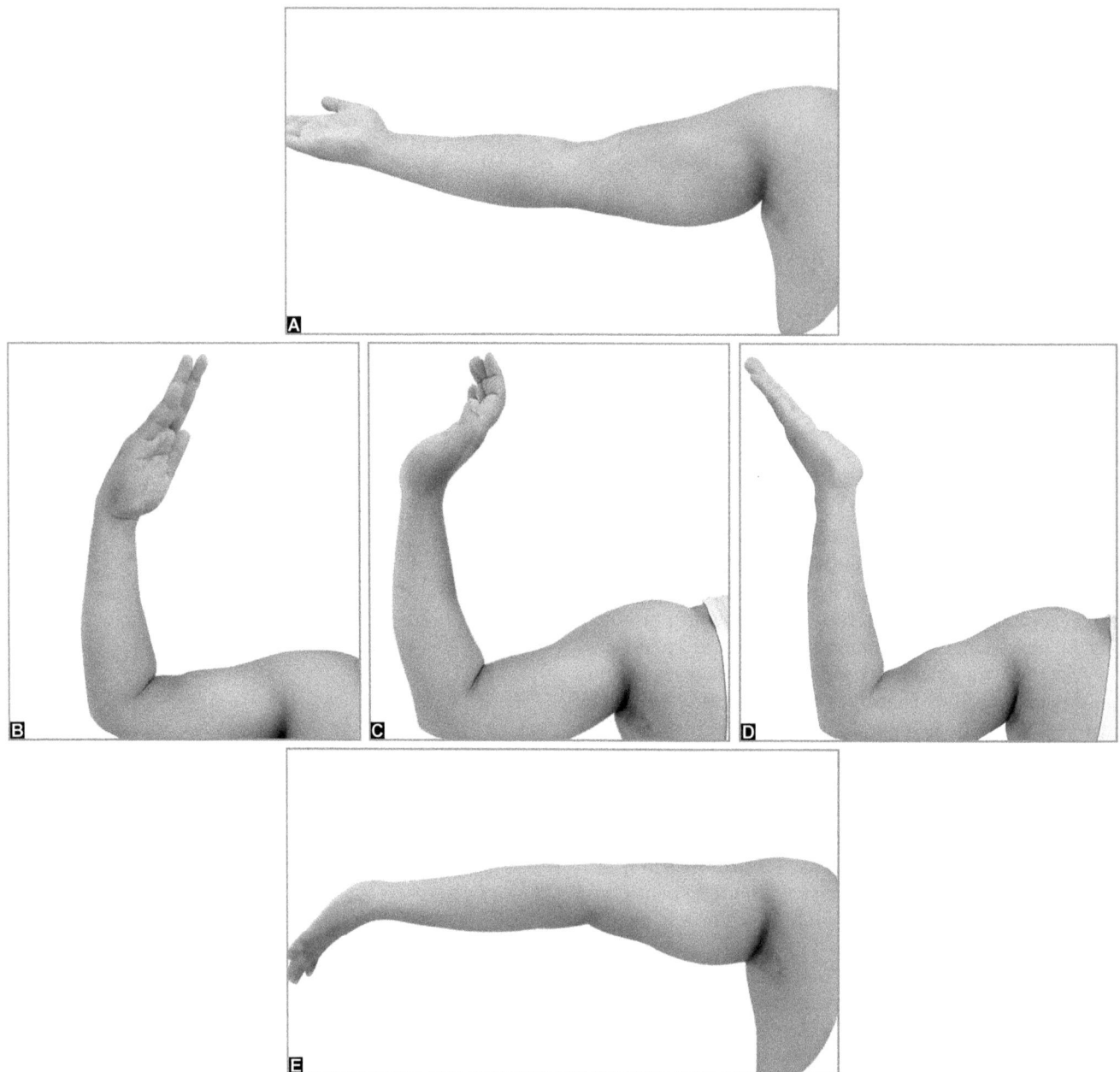

Figs. 25.26A to E: Nerve gliding exercises for ulnar nerve. (A) Begin with arm out, palm facing up; (B) Bend the elbow towards you, with palm side facing you; (C) Rotate the palm outward and bend wrist backwards; (D) Twist the wrist, so that palm faces up; (E) Stretch the arm out with wrist bending backward, fingers bent toward the floor.

Postoperative Rehabilitation

If surgery (ulnar nerve transposition/repair) is performed, the following rehabilitation protocol may be followed:

- **Phase I:** Immediate postoperative phase (week: 0–1).
  - *Goal:* Allow soft tissue healing, decrease pain and inflammation, retard muscle atrophy.
  - *Intervention given:* Posterior splint at 90 degree elbow flexion and wrist in neutral or slight flexion is applied (a sling may be applied for comfort). The splint is used for 7–10 days. Compression dressing is applied at the site of surgery.
  - *Exercises:* Passive ROM exercises for wrist, gripping and releasing for fingers, isometric exercises for shoulder without producing shoulder external rotation.

- **Phase II:** Intermediate phase (weeks: 3–7).
  - *Goal:* To restore full pain free range of motion, improve strength, power, endurance of muscles of upper limb, increase function.

  Intervention given:
  - *Weeks 3–5:* Progress elbow range of motion exercises with emphasis on full elbow extension. Initiate flexibility and strengthening exercises for the elbow (flexion/extension), forearm (supination/pronation), and wrist (flexion/extension). Electrical stimulation after performing Faradic-IDC tests can be applied to denervated/innervating muscles. Shoulder muscle strengthening exercises are to be performed.

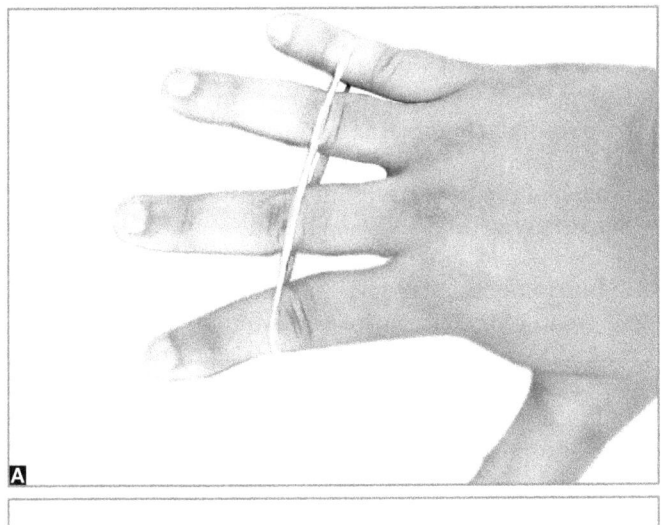

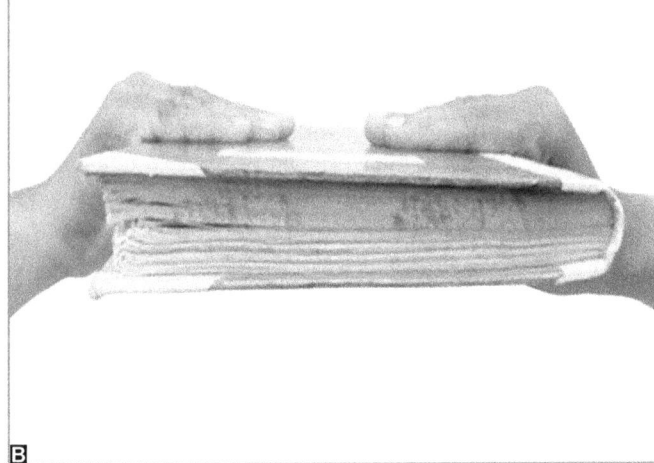

Figs. 25.27A and B: (A) Strengthening the interossei using elastic bands; (B) Exercise to strengthen lumbricals.

- *Weeks 6-7:* All exercises listed above for weeks 3-5 are to be performed with addition of light sports and functional activities.
- **Phase III:** Advanced strengthening program (week 8-12)
  - *Goal:* To improve strength/power/endurance.
  - *Intervention given:* Initiate sporting/functional activities. Initiate eccentric exercise program for the muscles supplied by ulnar nerve, initiate plyometric drills, continue strengthening and flexibility exercises for shoulder and elbow. Initiate interval training/throwing program for throwing athletes.
- **Phase IV:** Return to activity (Weeks 14-32): Gradual return to activity and competitive program.
  - Splints as required may be considered.
  - *Occupational therapy:* Occupational therapy is applied to enhance function.

MEDIAN NERVE INJURY

Median nerve injury is a mixed nerve (containing both sensory and motor fibers). The root value of this nerve that runs in the medial plane of forearm is: C5, 6, 7, 8, and T1. The nerve arises in the axilla from the combination of branches from the lateral and medial cord of the brachial plexus. The nerve runs down the arm, where it passes on the medial side of the arm between the biceps brachii and brachialis muscles. At the elbow joint, the nerve lies medial to brachial artery and the relationship at elbow from lateral to medial is Biceps tendon→Brachial artery→Median nerve.

At the cubital fossa, the median nerve gives branches to four muscles, such as pronator teres, palmaris longus, flexor digitorum sublimis, and flexor carpi radialis. The anterior interosseous branch of the nerve gives branches to three muscles, such as pronator quadratus, lateral half of flexor digitorum profundus, and flexor pollicis longus **(Fig. 25.28)**.

The nerve enters the forearm between the two heads of pronator teres. At about 5 cm above the wrist, it lies on the lateral side of flexor digitorum sublimis and becomes superficial just above the wrist. It gives the palmar cutaneous branch about 3 cm above the wrist, which supplies sensory innervation to the lateral part of volar aspect of the palm. It passes under the transverse carpal ligament of carpal tunnel to supply muscles of thenar eminence (such as: abductor pollicis brevis, opponens pollicis, and flexor pollicis brevis), 1st and 2nd lumbricals. The palmar digital branches supplies cutaneous innervation to lateral 3 and ½ digits and their nail beds.

The anterior interosseous nerve, which is one branch of the median nerve, only accounts for the movement of the fingers of the hand and does not have any sensory supply. The anterior interosseus nerve syndrome is purely a motor neuropathy. Individuals suffering from this syndrome have impaired movements of fingers and thumb.

The median nerve can be torn partially or fully or compressed at the elbow or wrist. The common compression injuries of median nerve are:
- Pronator teres syndrome (where the median nerve is compressed between the two heads of pronator teres).
- Carpal tunnel syndrome (where the nerve is compressed inside the carpal tunnel).

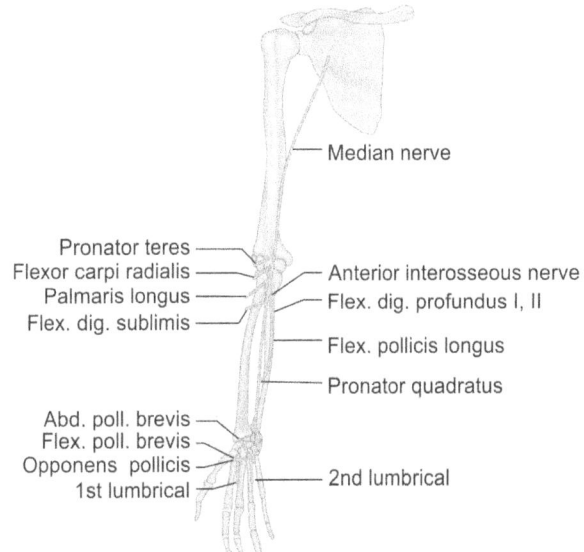

Fig. 25.28: The median nerve and muscles supplied by it.

Injuries to the nerve producing disruption of continuity/conduction could be of two types such as:

a. **High median nerve injury:** The injury to the nerve occurs at cervical spine, arm and around the elbow.
   - *Causes:* Cervical spondylosis/PIVD, elbow dislocation, supracondylar fracture of humerus, gunshot injury, stab injury, fracture both bones of forearm.
   - *Features:* Paralysis of all muscles supplied by median nerve in the forearm, such as: flexor pollicis longus, flexor carpi radialis and radial portion of flexor digitorum profundus, pronator teres, flexor digitorum superficialis, pronator quadratus and palmaris longus and hand such as: muscles of the thenar eminence i.e., abductor pollicis brevis, superficial portion of flexor pollicis brevis, opponens pollicis and lumbricals 1 and 2. Sensory impairment/anesthesia over the median nerve distribution in the hand.

b. **Low median nerve injury:** Injury to the nerve occurs at or below the distal third of the forearm and wrist.
   - *Causes:* Fracture both bones in the distal 1/3rd, Colle's fracture, Carpal tunnel syndrome.
   - *Features:* Sparing of muscles of forearm such as pronator teres, flexor carpi radialis etc. Paralysis/paresis and wasting of muscles of the thenar eminence such as abductor pollicis brevis, superficial portion of flexor pollicis brevis, opponens pollicis and lumbricals 1&2. Sensory impairment/loss over the median nerve distribution in the hand may be present.

Besides high and low median nerve injuries, where the nerve is torn partially/completely, the nerve may also be affected by compression at different sites resulting in two common clinical syndromes such as:

a. **Carpal tunnel syndrome:** It is caused by compression of the median nerve as it passes under the carpal tunnel. Tests such as nerve conduction velocity tests, Phalen's test, reverse Phalen's test, Tinel's sign, etc., are performed to confirm the diagnosis. Another typical feature found in the patients is shaking movements of the hand, as if shaking a thermometer, done to relieve symptoms.

b. **Pronator teres syndrome:** Also known as pronator syndrome is the compression of the median nerve between the two heads of the pronator teres muscle. The pronator teres test, where, the patient is asked to pronate the forearm against the clinician's resistance and to extend the elbow simultaneously, if produces pain, indicates the syndrome as the cause of patient's pain. A positive Tinel sign over the area around the heads of pronator teres, and an enlarged pronator teres muscle confirms the diagnosis. A key difference of this syndrome from carpal tunnel syndrome is absence of pain while sleeping.

Diagnosis of Median Nerve Injury

An early, accurate diagnosis of the nerve injury is essential to plan treatment, which could be conservative or surgical and to determine the prognosis.

Assessment of Median Nerve Injury

- **Muscle strength/power examination:** Manual muscle testing for median nerve innervated muscles, e.g., flexor carpi radialis in forearm, abductor pollicis brevis in the hand. The prehension and pinch muscle strength are evaluated using the Jamar and Pinch Gauge dynamometer.
- **Sensory charting:** Sensory charting for the skin supplied by the median nerve in the hand using Semmes-Weinstein monofilaments should be done and documented.
- **Checking for deformities:** Ape thumb deformity (**Fig. 25.29A**), claw hand involving lateral two fingers, pointing index deformity (**Fig. 25.29B**), (caused by injury to median nerve in the mid forearm, causing paralysis of flexor digitorum superficialis muscle), if any should be found and examined for their flexibility.
- **Performing clinical tests such as:**
   - *Pen test for abductor pollicis brevis:* Hand placed flat on the table. The clinician holding a pen above the patient's palm, asks him/her to touch the pen with the thumb (**Fig. 25.30**). Inability to touch the pen with the thumb indicates positive test suggesting injury to median nerve.
   - *Benedict sign:* The hand of benediction also known as Benedict's sign or preacher's hand occurs as a result of

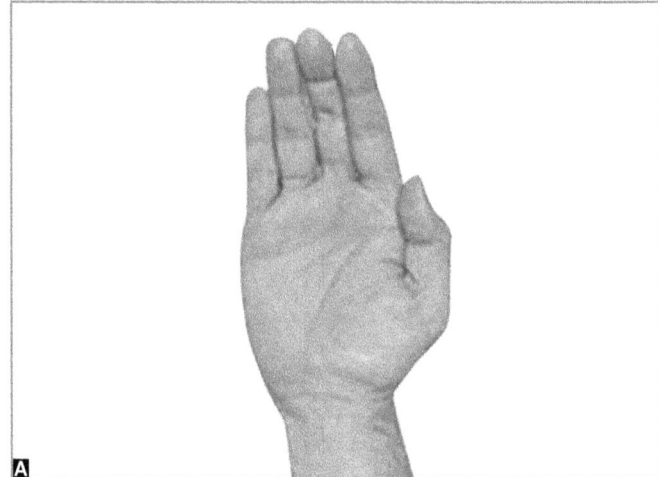

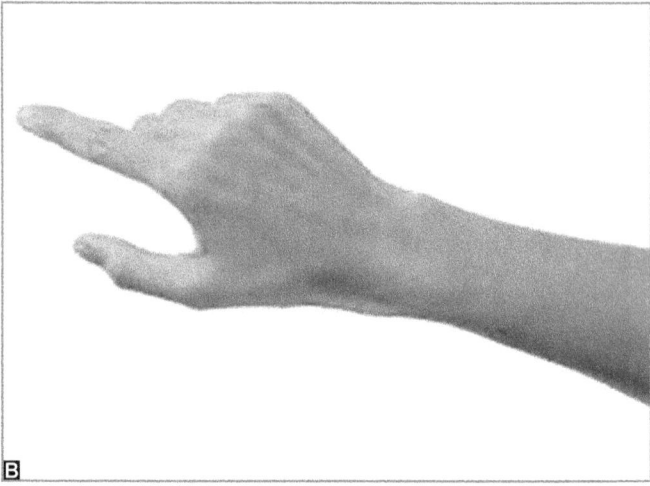

Figs. 25.29A and B: (A) Ape thumb deformity; (B) Pointing index deformity.

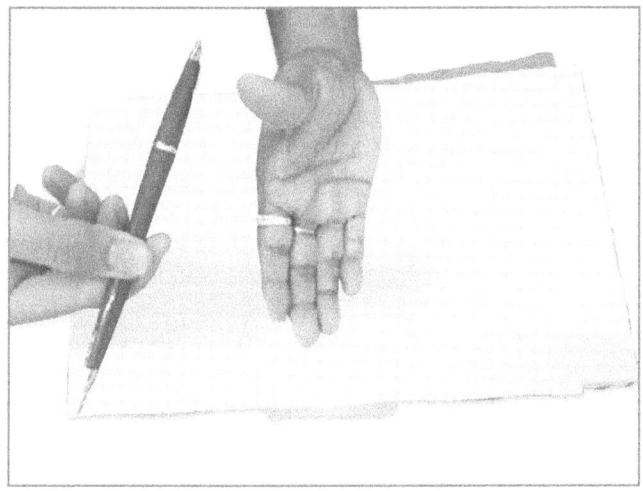

Fig. 25.30: The pen test.

injury to the median nerve at the upper forearm or elbow **(Fig. 25.31)**. The patient, when asked to clasp his hand, the index, middle, and thumb fail to flex due to paralysis of FDS, FDP (index and middle) and FPL. Sometimes, the patient is able to flex middle finger, because of the connection between the FDP tendons of middle, ring and little fingers (due to sharing of a common muscle belly), which is called the quadrigia phenomena, resulting in a pointing index deformity.
- *Pointing index sign/deformity:* The patient is asked to clasp his hand on the affected side. When there is a median nerve injury, the index remains straight due to paralysis of flexor digitorum superficialis and flexor digitorum profundus connecting the index finger.
- *Functional evaluation:* The DASH (disabilities of arm, shoulder and hand) questionnaire can be used to assess function involving the affected hand.

Laboratory Tests for Median Nerve Injury

Electrophysiological studies: Nerve conduction velocity measurement, S-D curve plotting, Faradic-IDC tests, etc., are helpful in making diagnosis. X-ray of cervical spine may be considered as per indication.

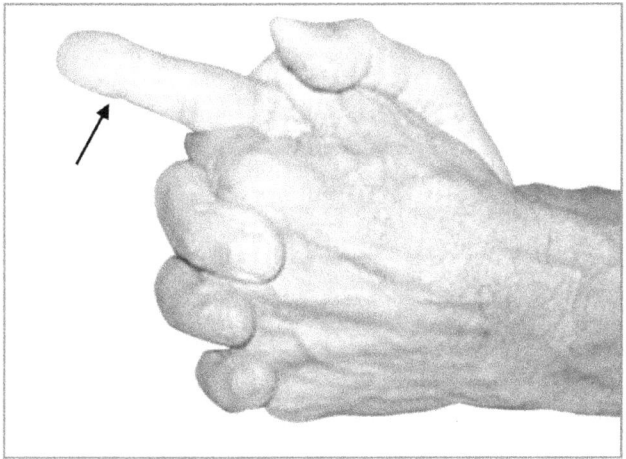

Fig. 25.31: The Benedict sign.

Management of Median Nerve Injury

Depending on the severity of lesion, a conservative or surgical management is considered. A conservative management is basically selected for neuropraxia and axonotmesis as well as compressive injuries, where as for neurotmesis surgical repair of the nerve may be considered. In case of injuries that do not improve with nerve repair tendon transfer surgeries may be considered to improve function. For compressive lesions like carpal tunnel syndrome and pronator teres syndrome, if conservative treatment fails to improve symptoms, decompression surgeries may be considered.

A. Conservative management: It consists of:
- *Use of splints:* Immediately after a median nerve injury, a suitable splint depending upon the site of injury to be applied. For low median nerve injury, a dorsal blocking splint **(Fig. 25.32A)** to prevent stretching of the nerve and lumbricals/short opponens splint **(Fig. 25.32B)**, (to maintain the 1st web space) may be selected, however, for high median nerve injury, a dorsal blocking splint with elbow in 90 degrees flexion, and forearm in neutral position to prevent stretching of the nerve may be selected. The use of the splint prevents over stretching of the injured nerve and the denervated muscles. It also prevents joint stiffness and maximizes functional use of the hand. For compressive injuries like carpal tunnel syndrome, a resting hand **(Fig. 25.32C)** splint may be beneficial.
- Relaxed passive movements to the affected hand are given to maintain and increase the joint range of motion.
- *Electrical stimulation:* There are some evidences that, regeneration of peripheral nerves can be accelerated by low intensity electrical stimulation, which begins to appear by third postoperative week and continues to happen for about 90 days. Initially interrupted galvanic current stimulation is applied after 2 weeks of injury (after completion of Wallerian degeneration) after performing Faradic-IDC tests. If the muscles show signs of innervation the stimulation can be changed to surged faradic current to innervating muscles.
- *Therapeutic modalities:* It is well known now a days that physical agents like electricity, magnetic field and ultrasound may positively influence the outcome of healing process of different tissues like skin, bone, muscles, tendons, and peripheral nerves. The use of therapeutic modalities for peripheral nerve regeneration has been investigated currently. It has been found that, low power laser, ultrasound, and electrical stimulation are beneficial in accelerating regenerative process in order to achieve early functional recovery. Studies on laser therapy using continuous emissions has shown to have a positive outcome for nerve regeneration.

Ultrasound has been studied in the area of enhancing recovery after peripheral nerve injuries by reducing pain and improving function with entrapment neuropathies and facilitating nerve regeneration. There are some evidences regarding beneficial effects of ultrasound on

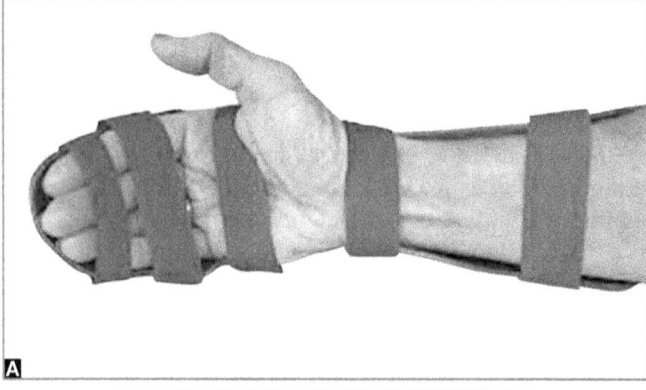

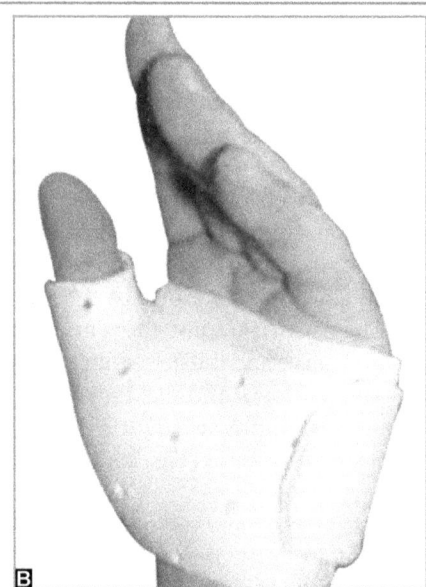

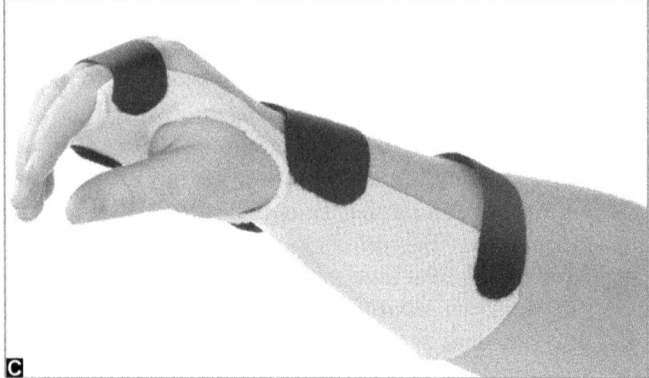

Figs. 25.32A to C: (A) Dorsal blocking splint; (B) Short opponens splint; (C) Resting hand splint.

peripheral nerve regeneration. It has been concluded that, treatment with low intensity therapeutic ultrasound, can improve regeneration of a peripheral nerve with compressive lesion, but a delayed regeneration can result from high intensity applications. Regeneration of the nerve was enhanced with SATA intensity of 0.25 W/cm² and frequency of 2.25 MHz.

- *Active exercises:* Active exercises in the form of active assisted, free and resisted exercises are given to the recovering muscles as per the muscle power detected through manual muscle testing. Keeping in mind the need of tendon transfer, in cases, where conservative treatment fails, and the muscles to be transferred, need isolation and strengthening to have a minimum grade of 4.
- *Sensory re-education:* Regarding the hand sensation recovery, various sensory re-education strategies have been introduced in the rehabilitation process with the aim of enhancing patient's capacity to reinterpret altered sensory stimuli due to injury sustained in the hand. An important aim of sensory re-education is to facilitate sensory integration with the cortex area and to promote an interaction between tactile, visual, auditory stimuli, so that preservation of the hand's cortical map representation is maximized during the early phase following injury.
- *Rehabilitation of the injured hand following nerve injury:* Rehabilitation is based on exercises, use of splints to augment function and promote neuroplasticity. If functional gain using the impaired part is not possible, adaptive devices may be recommend/used to improve function.

Surgical Management

Nerve repair: It involves immediate repair of the nerve, if there is complete disruption of connectivity (neurotmesis as per Seddon's classification). The upper limb is immobilized in a splint/POP slab after repair to prevent further injury.

For repairs on high median nerve injury, as stated above under the conservative management the hand is immobilized in a dorsal blocking splint/POP slab with elbow flexed to 90 degrees and forearm in neutral position in order to prevent further injury to the nerve.

For repairs on low median nerve injury, the wrist is immobilized in a splint/POP slab in flexion.

Postoperative management following median nerve repair: After immobilizations are removed, the patient is expected to have stiffness of elbow and/or wrist depending on whether the elbow and/or wrist are immobilized. Postoperative exercises are directed at gradually recovering elbow and wrist extension and restoration of movements of thumb and fingers. Initial movements given are active-free exercises. Active assisted and passive exercises are introduced gradually to achieve elbow and wrist extension depending upon the patient's progress, following specific precautions not to over stretch the repaired nerve. Therapy is gradually tailored to improve full range of motion in elbow, forearm and wrist and to gain adequate elbow muscle and grip strength.

Pulsed ultrasound/PSWD/LILT and electrical stimulation of denervated/innervated muscles are applied as required to facilitate recovery/regeneration and maintain muscle properties/power respectively.

Any pain developing after surgery due to nerve compression from incisional scar can be managed by ultrasound/iontophoresis/TENS.

Decompression surgeries: For carpal tunnel syndrome and pronator teres syndrome, if the patient is not relieved of symptoms, decompression surgery may be considered.

Tendon Transfers following Median Nerve Injury

Most important factor for loss of function in the hand following low median nerve injury is loss of thumb opposition. Many tendon transfers have been shown to restore opposition of the thumb by providing thumb and finger flexion.

For patients with low median nerve palsy, it has been shown that the flexor digitorum superficialis of long and ring fingers or the wrist extensors best approximate the force and motion, that is required to restore full thumb opposition and strength, hence can be considered as donor muscles for transfer. Appropriate tendon transfer may be considered for correction of partial claw hand deformity involving the index and middle fingers.

For high median nerve palsy, the brachioradialis or extensor carpi radialis longus transfer is more appropriate to restore lost thumb flexion. To restore independent flexion of the index finger, pronator teres (if available), or extensor carpi radialis/ulnaris tendon muscle units transfer can be considered.

Postoperatively, protection of the transferred tendon, tendon re-education (isolation, strengthening, and functional integration) are followed.

RADIAL NERVE INJURY

The radial nerve (**Fig. 25.33**) is the branch of the posterior cord of the brachial plexus and has a root value C5, C6, C7, C8, and T1. The nerve arises in the region of the axilla and exits the axilla inferiorly and supplies branches to the long and lateral head of the triceps brachii. The nerve then descends down the arm traveling in the radial groove, where it supplies branches to the medial head of the triceps brachii and anconeus muscle. In the arm, it also gives branches to brachioradialis and extensor carpi radialis longus muscles.

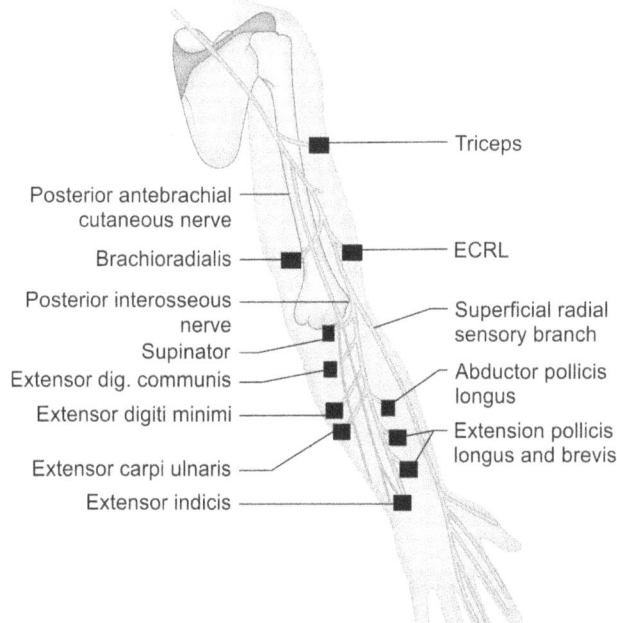

Fig. 25.33: The radial nerve.

To enter the forearm, the nerve travels anterior to the lateral epicondyle of the humerus, through the cubital fossa, and then divides into deep and superficial branches. When the deep branch of the radial nerve penetrates the supinator muscle, it is termed as the posterior interosseous nerve. The two branches of the radial nerve in the forearm are:

1. **Deep branch (motor):** The posterior interosseous nerve; innervates the muscles on the back of the forearm, such as extensor carpi radialis brevis, extensor digitorum, extensor digiti minimi, extensor carpi ulnaris, supinator, abductor pollicis longus, extensor pollicis longus, extensor pollicis brevis, and extensor indicis.
2. **Superficial branch (sensory):** This is a terminal division of the radial nerve, which provides sensory innervation to the dorsal surface of the lateral three and half digits and the associated area in the dorsum of the hand.

Sensory Functions of Radial Nerve

Besides the superficial branch discussed above, there are the following branches of the radial nerve that provide cutaneous innervations to the arm and forearm.

1. **Lower lateral cutaneous nerve of the arm:** It innervates the lateral aspect of the arm, inferior to the insertion of deltoid muscle.
2. **Posterior cutaneous nerve of the arm:** It innervates the posterior surface of the arm.
3. **Posterior cutaneous nerve of the forearm:** It innervates a strip of the skin down the middle of the posterior forearm.

Clinical Significance

The features of radial nerve injury at three different sites of lesion are briefly discussed below:

1. **In the axilla:** The radial nerve can be damaged in the axilla, by a dislocation of shoulder, surgical drainage of an abscess, fracture of proximal humerus, pressure from badly fitting crutches, etc. The following features may be observed in injury at this site.
    - *Motor functions affected:* The triceps brachii and the muscles in the back of forearm are affected. The patient may develop a wrist drop (**Fig. 25.34**) due to the inability to extend the wrist and fingers.
    - *Sensory functions affected:* All the four cutaneous branches of the radial nerve are affected. There might be a loss of sensation over the lateral and posterior aspect of the arm, posterior aspect of the forearm, and dorsolateral aspect of the hand, including the dorsal surface of the lateral three and half digits.
2. **In the radial groove:** The radial nerve is very much prone to be damaged with a fracture of the shaft of the humerus resulting in the following impairments:
    - *Motor functions:* As the branches to long and lateral head of triceps arise proximal to the radial groove, there will be no loss of power in long and lateral head, but the triceps will be weak due to injury of the branch that supplies the medial head of the triceps.

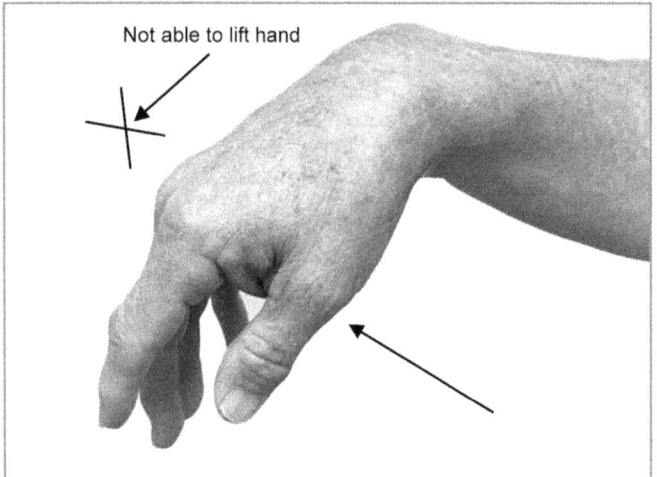

Fig. 25.34: Wrist drop deformity.

The muscles of posterior forearm are affected resulting lack of forearm supination and wrist drop.
- *Sensory functions:* As the cutaneous branches to the arm and forearm have already arisen before the nerve entered the radial groove, only the superficial branch of the radial nerve will be affected, resulting in sensory loss to the dorsal surface of the lateral three and half digits and the associated area on the dorsum of the hand **(Fig. 25.20)**.
3. **In the forearm:** There are two terminal branches of the radial nerve located within the forearm such as:
    - *Superficial branch:* The nerve may be affected by stabbing or lacerated wound in the forearm. There is no motor loss, but sensory loss is found over the lateral 3 and ½ digits and the adjoining area over the dorsum of hand.
    - *Deep branch:* The nerve may be affected by fracture of radial head, or posterior dislocation of radius. Majority of muscles in the posterior forearm are affected. Complete wrist drop is not found, as extensor carpi radialis longus, which is innervated from the branch of radial nerve above the elbow is spared. There is no sensory loss if this deep branch of the radial nerve is affected.

Saturday Night Palsy

Saturday night palsy refers to the compression injury to the radial nerve in the spiral groove of the humerus, caused while sleeping in a position where the arm is constantly placed over a hard surface such as the arm rest/back of a chair. This happens when the person falls asleep, when heavily medicated or under the influence of alcohol. The resultant injury is neuropraxia of radial nerve, which leads to wrist drop and paralysis/paresis of muscles supplied by the radial nerve at and below the radial groove with sensory impairment over the lateral aspects on dorsum of hand.

Posterior interosseous palsy/posterior interosseous nerve syndrome

Posterior interosseous nerve syndrome usually develops spontaneously and is caused by compression injuries to the upper extremity, mostly in the arcade of Frohse (arcade of Frohse is a site of posterior interosseous nerve entrapment, causing progressive paralysis of muscles supplied by the nerve with or without injury). It is the area where the nerve enters the supinator muscle and is the most common place for a compression of the nerve. Posterior interosseous nerve syndrome is characterized by motor deficits in the distribution of the posterior interosseous nerve. While the posterior interosseous nerve does have afferent fibers that transmit pain signals from the wrist, it does not carry any cutaneous sensory information (as it is a motor nerve). It differs from, typical radial nerve palsy by preservation of elbow extension, partial wrist drop, and no impairment of sensation over the lateral aspect of hand and wrist.

Crutch Palsy

Crutch palsy is a form of paralysis, which can occur when the radial nerve or part of the brachial plexus is under constant pressure due to poorly fitting crutch. The muscles supplied by the radial nerve are partially or fully paralyzed, resulting in wrist drop. The injury is neuropraxic in nature, which improves quickly with therapy.

Honeymoon Palsy

Honeymoon palsy results from another individual sleeping on one's arm overnight and compressing the radial nerve as well anterior interosseous nerve. The radial nerve is usually compressed near the elbow. This is referred honeymoon palsy, due to the closer sleeping habits of newlyweds.

Handcuff Neuropathy

It develops from tight fitting hand cuffs compressing the superficial branch of the distal radial nerve resulting sensory impairment over the dorsolateral aspect of the hand. This is also called as cheiralgia paresthetica (compression neuropathy of superficial radial nerve).

Diagnosis of Radial Nerve Palsy

Diagnosis is done based upon:
- History of injury (e.g., trauma, pressure, Saturday night palsy).
- Clinical features.
- **Electrodiagnosis:** NCV, EMG, S-D curve plotting, Faradic-IDC tests.
- **Imaging studies:** X-ray, ultrasound, MRI.

Management of Radial Nerve Injury

It depends on the type of injury the individual has sustained.
- **For compressive injuries:** If the injury is a neuropraxia of the radial nerve, either in the axilla/arm, a triangular shoulder sling **(Fig. 25.35)** is used to support the shoulder, arm and wrist, so that neither the nerve nor the paralyzed muscles will be overstretched and this also allows the nerve to heal.

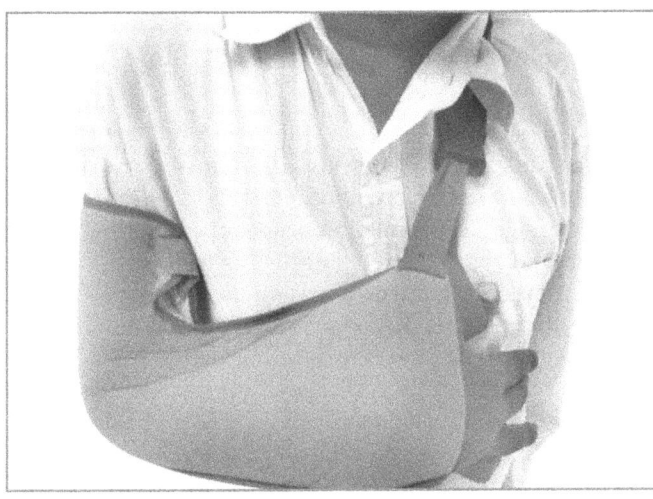

Fig. 25.35: The triangular sling.

NSAIDS are prescribed by the physician/surgeon, to reduce inflammation/swelling at the affected site.

Physiotherapy: Application of ice over the area of compression to relieve swelling, PSWD/pulsed ultrasound/LILT over the area of compression may be helpful. Gentle ROM exercises, electrical stimulation (interrupted galvanic stimulation for denervated muscles, faradic type stimulation for innervating muscles), active assisted/free/resisted exercises to the affected muscles as they recover, sensory re-education, functional integration are helpful.

❖ **For moderate to severe injuries:** In cases of axonotmesis of radian nerve that usually develops from fracture shaft of humerus, or draining an abscess in the axilla, full recovery is expected in majority of cases without surgery. A hand splint (cock-up splint—**Fig. 25.36A**) is applied to prevent wrist drop that stretches the wrist and finger extensors. A volar/dorsal short cock-up splint may be applied, as besides prevention of wrist drop, it allows functional use of the hand. After 2 weeks of injury, once the Wallerian degeneration is completed, electrical stimulation to the paralyzed muscles following Faradic-IDC test is started. PSWD/LILT/pulsed ultrasound may be applied at the site of injury to promote nerve regeneration. Sensory mapping, motor evaluation and Tinel's sign testing should be done periodically to judge the recovery. When there is some recovery of power in the wrist extensors, a dynamic wrist drop splint (**Fig. 25.36B**) may be considered.

❖ For severe injuries like neurotmesis, nerve repair (nerve grafting/nerve transfer) may be performed by the orthopedic surgeon/neurosurgeon/plastic surgeon. The physiotherapy treatment after nerve repair starts after the POP cast is removed. A cock-up splint as indicated is applied and general physiotherapy treatment follows the same as discussed for axonotmesis.

Surgery for Radial Nerve Injury

If nerve reconstruction is not possible, or it fails to improve, the muscle power, tendon transfer is the option. For achieving

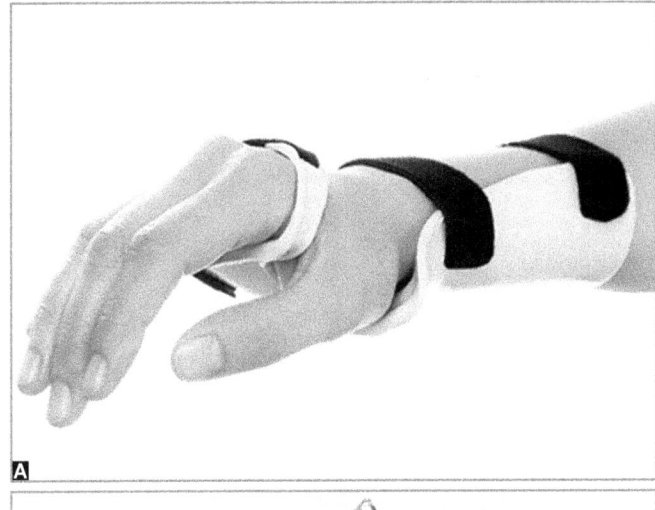

Figs. 25.36A and B: (A) Static volar short cock up splint; (B) Dynamic wrist drop splint.

wrist extension after a high radial nerve palsy, transfer of pronator teres (PT) to ECRB/ECRL is the choice. For achieving thumb extension, the palmaris longus or the flexor digitorum superficialis of ring finger is transferred to EPL. MCP joint extension of fingers can be re-established by transferring FCR (brand procedure)/FCU/FDS (Boyes, procedure) tendon to EDC.

After tendon transfer a POP cast is applied for 4-6 weeks for the tendon to heal, followed by the application of a cock-up splint and tendon re-education exercises.

SCIATIC NERVE INJURY

The sciatic (root values-L4, L5, S1,S2, and S3) nerve is the longest nerve in the human body, which is the continuation of the lumbosacral plexus. It is a thick flat structure approximately 2 cm in width. The nerve emerges from the pelvis through the greater sciatic foramen, inferior to piriformis muscle. The nerve divides into the terminal branches, i.e., posterior tibial nerve and common peroneal nerve usually just below the mid-thigh (**Fig. 25.37**). It

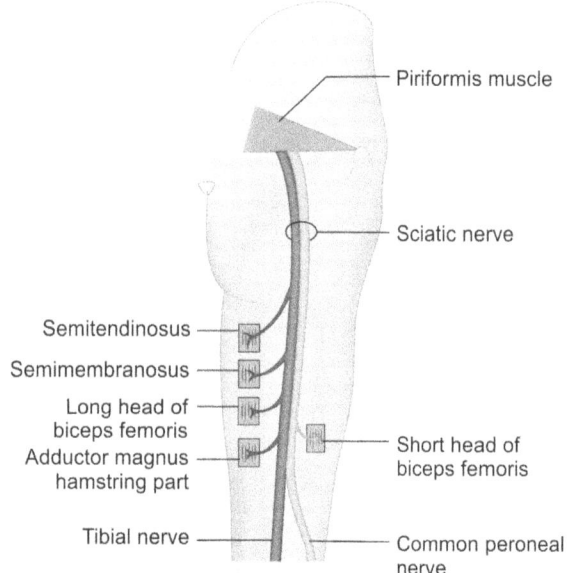

Fig. 25.37: The sciatic nerve and its branches.

supplies muscles on the posterior thigh, i.e. hamstrings, and the hamstring portion of the adductor magnus and all the muscles in the leg and foot. The two terminal branches of the nerve and their motor and sensory functions are discussed below:

- **Tibial nerve (posterior tibial nerve):**
  - *Motor functions:* It innervates the calf muscles (Gastrocnemius and soleus), tibialis posterior and some of the intrinsic muscles of the foot.
  - *Sensory functions:* It supplies the skin of the posterolateral leg, lateral foot, and sole of the foot.
- **Common peroneal nerve:**
  - *Motor functions:* It innervates muscles of the anterior leg (tibialis anterior, extensor dig. longus, ext. hallucis longus), lateral leg (peroneus longus and brevis) and the remaining intrinsic foot muscles.
  - *Sensory functions:* It innervates the skin of the lateral leg and dorsum of the foot **(Fig. 25.38)**.

Causes of Sciatic Nerve Injury

Injury to sciatic nerve occurs due to trauma (pressure, stretch, direct invasion such as puncture due to injections or cut), resulting in significant impairment and functional limitations, hence need proper understanding for its prevention and management. Stretch, compression, ischemia, and direct damage are the chief mechanisms. The lithotomy, frog leg, and sitting positions have been implicated in injury to this nerve perioperatively (hyperflexion of the hip, abduction, and extension of the leg causes stretching). Hyperflexion of the hips may occur if a patient in the lithotomy position slips or is pulled caudad during surgery. Regional anesthetic techniques and hip arthroplasty may cause injury. The causes of injury can be categorized as:

- **Spinal causes:** It includes: PIVD of lumbar spine, lumbar Spondylolisthesis/spondylosis, lumbar canal stenosis, etc.
- **Non-spinal causes:** It includes piriformis syndrome, pregnancy, posterior dislocation of hip, trauma, etc.
- **Iatrogenic causes:** Injection injuries (injection palsy) **(Fig. 25.39)**, hip surgeries such as total hip replacement.

Features of Sciatic Nerve Injury

The features depend upon the level of the lesion/injury, which are briefly described:

- **High level lesion:** Injury to the nerve occurs above the knee joint, resulting in loss of functions in all muscles supplied by the posterior tibial and common peroneal nerves. The common peroneal component is usually more affected, as it is more posterior, lateral, and superficial compared to the tibial component. Paralysis of the hamstring muscles and all the muscles below the knee leading to a weak knee flexion and foot drop **(Fig. 25.40)** are the manifestations. All the sensations below the knee except sensation over the medial aspects of leg and foot are impaired.

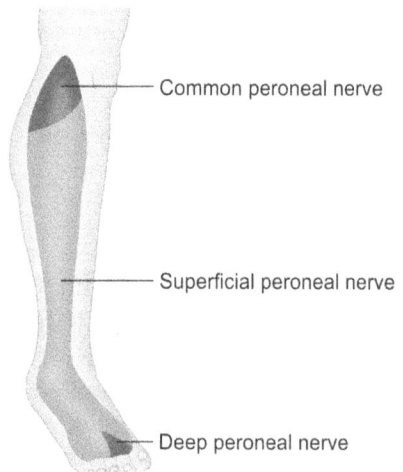

Fig. 25.38: Sensory supply by common peroneal nerve.

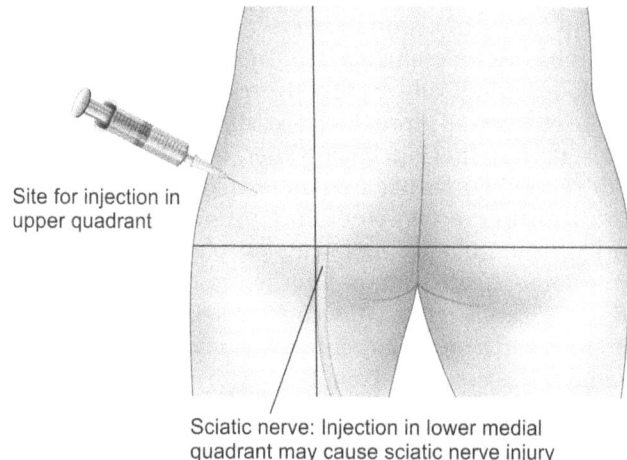

Fig. 25.39: Shows the quadrant to inject for prevention of injection palsy.

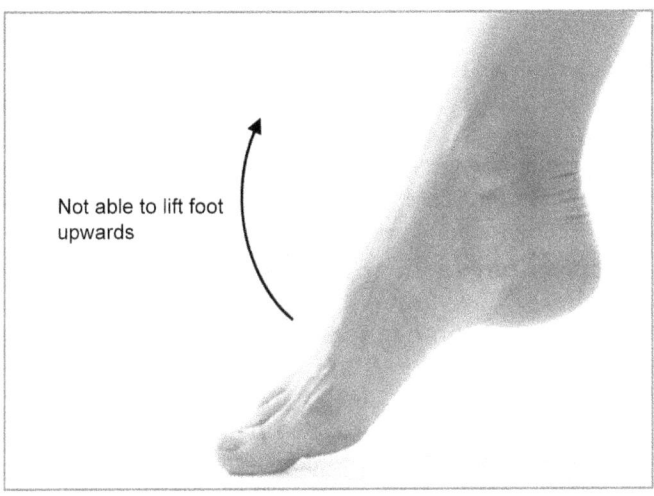

Fig. 25.40: Shows foot drop deformity due to sciatic nerve injury.

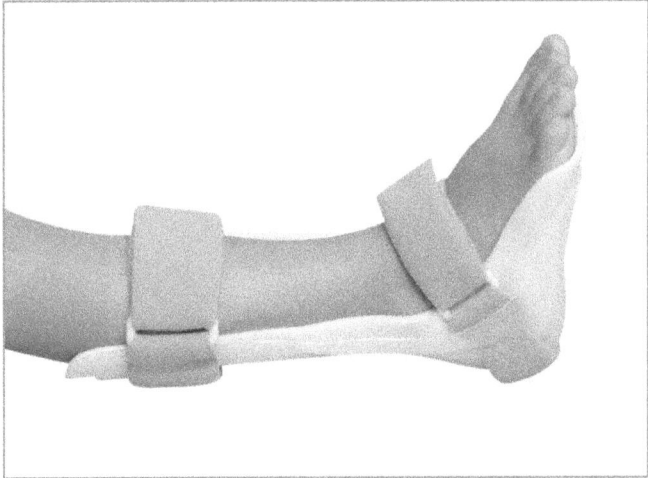

Fig. 25.41: Night splint for foot drop deformity.

- **Low level lesion:** Injury to the nerve occurs below the knee. It could be of the following types:
  - *Type: 1 (Anterior tibial nerve injury):* Muscle paralysis/paresis of tibialis anterior, extensor dig. Longus, extensor hallucis longus and sensory loss/impairment over the 1st web space occurs.
  - *Type: 2 (Superficial peroneal nerve/musculocutaneous nerve injury):* All the muscles supplied by anterior tibial nerve will be spared. There will be paralysis/paresis of peroneus longus and brevis, and sensory loss/impairment over the outer leg and foot.

Diagnosis of Sciatic Nerve Injury

Sciatic neuropathy is diagnosed mostly from clinical features. However, electrodiagnostic studies such as: NCV, EMG, S-D curve plotting, Faradic-IDC tests, etc., are performed to decide the site and nature of lesion and progression of injury. Radio diagnostic tests such as: X-ray, MRI, etc., may be performed to establish spinal, hip and knee pathologies.

Management

- **Medical management:** NSAIDS to reduce inflammation is very often prescribed by the physician/surgeon. Muscle relaxants help to some extent to relieve pain arising due to lumbosacral pathologies. The use of methyl prednisolone via transsacral block/intravenously/orally is sometimes considered by the physician/surgeon to reduce pain and motor/sensory deficits. The pathologies of spine (PIVD), or hip (hip posterior dislocation), etc., are treated either by conservatively or surgically.
- **Physiotherapy:** The aim of physiotherapy is to reduce pain, maintain and increase muscle properties and strength, and to improve function. The methods followed include:
  - *For pain relief:* Use of modalities such as PSWD, pulsed ultrasound, TENS/IFT, laser therapy, etc., may be employed. Gentle massage and stretching of soft tissues (piriformis muscle, if involved) may help.
  - *To promote nerve regeneration:* PSWD, pulsed ultrasound, low intensity laser, etc., may help.
  - *For maintenance of joint ROM and prevention of deformities:* Use of L-type of splint at night **(Fig. 25.41)**, relaxed passive movements, gentile stretching of tendoachilles and mobilization exercises are all helpful.
  - *For maintaining and improving muscle properties and strength:* Electrical stimulation of denervated/innervated muscles, low intensity high repetition exercises for strengthening the recovering muscles are used.
  - To improve gait, gait training with a dorsiflexion assist AFO/toe pick up splint **(Figs. 25.42A and B)** may help.
  - *To manage anesthetic foot:* Sensory re-education/education, use of MCR (microcellular rubber) lined sandals/chappals **(Fig. 25.43)** are helpful.

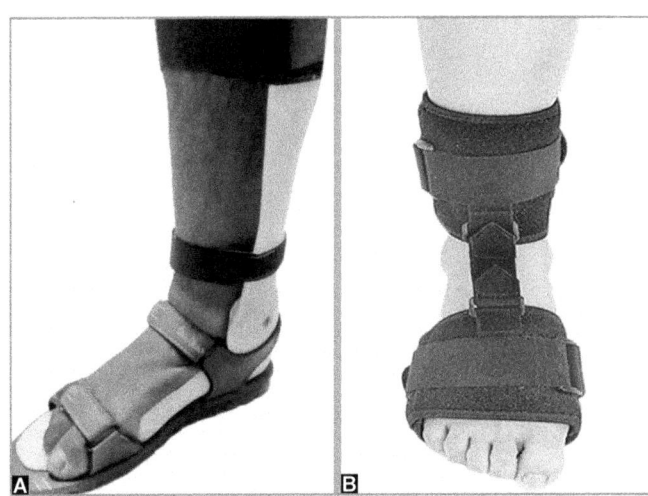

Figs. 25.42A and B: (A) Dorsiflexion assists AFO; (B) Toe pick up splint.

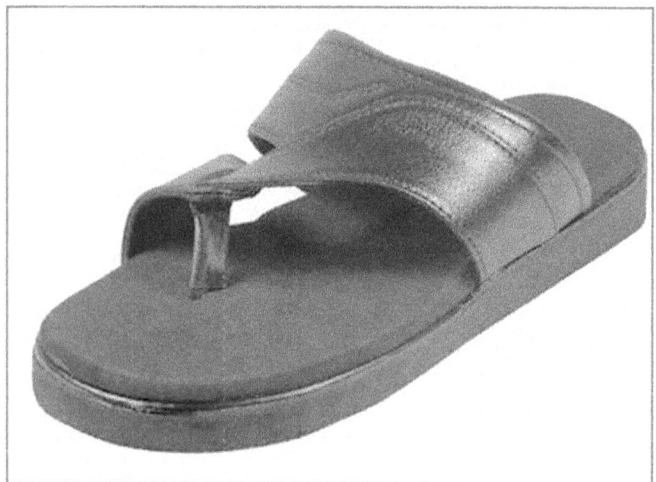

Fig. 25.43: MCR-lined chapel.

Surgery for Sciatic Nerve Injury

Neurosurgery: Clinical evidence reveals that for transection of a nerve, that nerve may be explored and repaired without waiting for electrophysiological confirmation. Delay in recognition and therefore treatment contributed to the poor outcome in many cases. Simple neurolysis is performed in cases of compression by hematoma or stricture by scar tissue.

Orthopedic surgery: In cases where, recovery is not possible with conservative or neurosurgical procedures, tendon transfer is the option. In case of common peroneal nerve injury, tibialis posterior can be transferred for the ankle dorsiflexion. In case of deep peroneal nerve injury, the peroneus brevis can be transferred for ankle dorsiflexion.

Postoperatively, tendon re-education exercises and use of a hinged/dorsiflexion assist AFO is emphasized till the transferred tendon is fully functional.

Physiotherapy in Guillain-Barré Syndrome: Acute Inflammatory Demyelinating Polyneuropathy and Chronic Inflammatory Demyelinating Polyneuropathy

GUILLAIN-BARRÉ SYNDROME

Guillain-Barré syndrome (GBS), also known as Landry's palsy is a self-limited autoimmune, classic lower motor neuron disorder, in which the body's immune system attacks part of the peripheral nervous system presenting as acute generalized weakness. It is called as a syndrome, because it presents a broad group of demyelinating inflammatory polyradiculopathies.

Guillain-Barré syndrome commonly called as acute inflammatory demyelinating polyneuropathy (AIDP), is characterized by ascending motor paralysis/paresis peaking within 4 weeks, diminished or absent muscle stretch reflexes, sensory symptoms with minimal objective sensory loss, electrophysiologic evidence of a demyelinating neuropathy, and CSF albuminocytologic dissociation.

Classification

The disease is classified into following types:
- **Acute inflammatory demyelinating polyneuropathy (AIDP)**: In this type, the immune response damages the myelin coating and interferes with the transmission of nerve signals.
- **Acute motor axonal neuropathy (AMAN)**: AMAN is a variant of GBS. It is characterized by acute paralysis and loss of reflexes without sensory loss. Pathologically, there is motor axonal degeneration with antibody-mediated attacks of motor nerves and nodes of Ranvier.
- **Acute motor sensory axonal neuropathy (AMSAN)**: It is a rare and severe variant of GBS that has a prolonged recovery course.
- **Miller Fisher syndromes**: It is a rare, acquired nerve disease that is considered to be a variant of GBS. It is characterized by abnormal muscle coordination, paralysis of the eye muscles, and absence of the tendon reflexes. Like GBS, symptoms may be preceded by a viral illness.

Causes

The exact cause of GBS is not known. Two-thirds of patients report symptoms of an infection of the respiratory or digestive tract, 6 weeks preceding the onset of symptoms. Rarely, recent surgery or vaccination can trigger GBS. Recently, there have been cases reported following infection with the Zika virus.

The risk factors include:
- Old aged persons (though people of all ages may be affected).
- Males are more affected compared to females.
- Certain infections:
  - Infections by *Campylobacter* (a type of bacteria found in undercooked poultry), *Mycoplasma pneumonia*.
  - Certain viral infections such as influenza virus, *Cytomegalovirus*, Epstein-Barr virus, Zika virus, Hepatitis A, B, C, and E, HIV, etc.
  - Surgeries and trauma.
  - Hodgkin's lymphoma.
  - Rarely vaccinations performed in childhood.

Pathophysiology

The pathophysiology of GBS is complex. It is an autoimmune disease triggered by preceding bacterial or viral infection.

In the AMAN form of GBS, the infecting organisms probably share homologous epitopes (parts of an antigen that is recognized by the immune system) to a component of the peripheral nerves and, therefore, the immune responses cross-react with the nerves causing axonal degeneration. The target molecules in AMAN are likely to be gangliosides GM1, GM1b, GD1a, and GalNAc-GD1a expressed on the motor axolemma.

In the AIDP form, immune system reactions against target epitopes in Schwann cells or myelin result in demyelination. When myelin is destroyed, destruction is accompanied by acute inflammation, which may be present for several days after onset of symptoms. The nerve conduction is interrupted or completely blocked. This demyelination prevents nerves from transmitting signals to and from the brain, causing numbness, weakness, or paralysis.

Even though the Schwann cells that produce myelin in the peripheral nervous system are destroyed, the axons are left intact in all except the most severe cases. After 2-3 weeks of demyelination, the Schwann cells begin to proliferate, inflammation subsides, and remyelination begins.

The progression of demyelination appears different in AMAN type of GBS versus AIDP type. Nadir (the development of peak disability) is the point of greatest severity and patients with AMAN type reach it earlier, as compared to AIDP.

Clinical Features

Guillain-Barré syndrome often begins with tingling and weakness starting in the feet and legs and spreading to the upper body and arms. In about 10% of people with the disorder, symptoms begin in the arms or face. As GBS progresses, muscle weakness can evolve into paralysis.

People with GBS usually experience their most significant weakness within 2 weeks after symptoms begin. Signs and symptoms of GBS may include:

- Prickling, pins, and needles sensations in the fingers, toes, ankles, or wrists
- The patient may present with finger dysesthesias and proximal muscle weakness of the lower extremities. The weakness may progress over hours to days to involve the arms, truncal muscles, cranial nerves, and muscles of respiration. Variants of GBS may present as pure motor dysfunction.
- Though sensory symptoms are minimal in GBS, a 2001 publication in journal of Neurology by Shin J Oh, Chris LaGanke, Gwen C Claussen, reveal sensory variant of GBS.
- Sensory GBS, an acute demyelinating neuropathy that presents clinically with only sensory peripheral nerve involvement. This entity is recognized by the sensory neuronopathy pattern (absent sensory CNAP in the presence of normal motor nerve conduction) in the NCS.
- Unsteady walking or inability to walk or climb stairs
- Difficulty with facial movements, including speaking, chewing, or swallowing
- Double vision or inability to move eyes
- Severe pain that may feel achy, shooting, or cramp-like and may be worse at night
- Difficulty with bladder control or bowel function
- Rapid heart rate
- Low or high blood pressure
- Difficulty breathing: This is a serious and potentially fatal complication that develops due to paralysis or weakness of the muscles that control breathing.
- Complications like deep vein thrombosis (DVT), pressure sore, etc., may arise due to prolonged immobility.
- Relapse: 2-5% of people with GBS experience a relapse.

Diagnosis

Guillain-Barré syndrome can be difficult to diagnose in its earliest stages, as its signs and symptoms are similar to those of other neurological disorders and may vary from person to person. Besides clinical features, the following diagnostic tests may be performed:

- **Spinal tap (lumbar puncture):** During the acute phase of the disease, characteristic findings on cerebrospinal fluid (CSF) analysis include albuminocytologic dissociation, which is an elevation in CSF protein (>0.55 g/L) without an elevation in white blood cells. The increase in CSF protein is thought to reflect the widespread inflammation of the nerve roots.
- **Electromyography:** Earliest findings reveals prolonged distal latencies with decreased amplitude of compound muscle action potential (CMAP) in muscles of upper and lower extremities. The F-wave latency is also prolonged.
- **Nerve conduction velocity:** In the late stage of the disease, slowing of conduction velocities/conduction block may be seen.
- **Sensory nerve action potential (SNAP):** Occasionally, SNAP may be normal in the feet, but abnormal in the arms (sural sparing).

Treatment

There is no definite treatment for GBS, however, timely medical management, ventilator support (if needed), physiotherapy and rehabilitation helps to save life (in those with respiratory muscle paralysis) and minimize disability and improve function. The treatment/management includes:

Medical Management

- **Plasmapheresis:** It is a process in which, the liquid part of the blood or plasma, is separated from the blood cells. Typically, the plasma is replaced with another solution, such as saline or albumin, or the plasma is treated and then returned to the body.
- **Immunoglobulin therapy:** Immunoglobulin containing healthy antibodies from blood donors is given through a vein (intravenously). High doses of immunoglobulin can block the damaging antibodies that may contribute to GBS.
- Medical management for relief of pain, and prevention of blood clot formation.

Physiotherapy

Physiotherapy can be started from the very acute stage, when the patient is hospitalized including admission to ICU and continues through the recovery and postrecovery period. The aims of physiotherapy and intervention strategies in the acute stage are:

- **Prevent DVT and maintain circulation:** Regular passive movements respecting pain, limb elevation, effleurage (if swelling persists), active assisted exercises if muscles contract and inhibition due to pain does not exist help for maintenance of circulation, thereby preventing DVT.
- **Maintain clear airways and promote ventilation:** Postural drainage, assisted breathing for patients who do not require ventilator support, chest vibration, and clapping and suctioning of secretions for those who are on ventilator support helps for maintenance of airways and promotes ventilation.
- **Maintain joint ROM and prevent deformities:** Positioning of extremities, relaxed passive movements, all help in maintaining joint range of motion and to prevent deformities.
- **Prevent development of pressure sore:** Regular turning on bed at 2 hourly intervals, for patients who are completely

paralyzed. If a patient has developed pressure sore, it should be promptly treated by ice cube massage to the periphery of ulcer/UVR/LASER/HVPGC/PSWD, etc.
- **Reduce pain:** Mild warmth, transcutaneous electrical nerve stimulation (TENS) are helpful.
- Provide psychological support to the family members through counseling.

The aims of physiotherapy in the rehabilitation stage: In this phase, the aims of management include the same as described for the acute stage plus the followings:
- **To improve muscle strength:** Strengthening exercises involve use of isometric, dynamic or isokinetic exercises. Active assisted/free/resisted exercise (using theraband/weight cuff) **(Fig. 26.1A)** are applied as per the patient's muscle power. In the presence of long-flexor weakness compromising grasp, tenodesis grasp (wrist extension combined with finger flexion) **(Fig. 26.1B)**, is promoted.

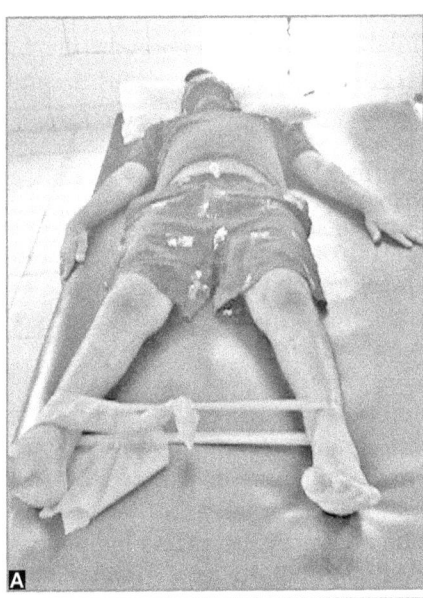

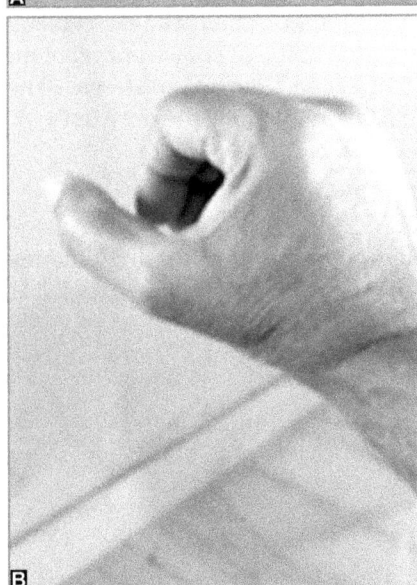

Figs. 26.1A and B: (A) Shows use of theraband to strengthen hip abductors in supine; (B) Tenodesis grasp.

Electrical stimulation after faradic-galvanic tests (galvanic type current stimulation for denervated muscle groups, and faradic type current stimulation for innervated muscle groups may be considered, when using galvanic current stimulation, the labile technique is safe to use, than the stabile technique.
- **To retrain normal movement pattern:** Normal functional movements involving self-care and mobility are made to be performed with assistance.
- **To improve posture:** Postural control training in sitting, standing, are imparted in front of a postural mirror.
- **To improve coordination and balance:** Coordination exercises, balance retraining on Swiss ball, balance board, etc., are performed.
- **To improve proprioception:** Proprioceptive training in the form of weight bearing, placing joints in different positions, holding and moving all help in improving proprioception. However, in the presence of weakness of hand muscles, weight bearing on hands should not be performed, as it stretches the long flexors, further decreasing grip strength.
- **To improve respiratory function:** Chest percussion, vibration, postural drainage, breathing exercises **(Fig. 26.2A)**, incentive spirometry, resistive inspiratory muscle training, etc., are performed to clear the airways and to reduce the work of breathing.
- **To improve aerobic capacity/endurance:** Endurance training given, involves progressively increasing the intensity and duration of functional activities such as walking or stair-climbing/hydrotherapy/static cycle exercises **(Fig. 26.2B)**.
- **To reduce pain:** Moist heat, TENS may be helpful.
- Training functional independence with everyday tasks with or without assistive/adaptive devices.
- **To improve standing balance and locomotion:** For patients who develop the potential for ambulation, standing balance training **(Fig. 26.3A)** gait re-education is done without/with orthosis and walking aids like walker/elbow crutches and walking sticks. **Figure 26.3B** shows the therapist preparing the patient walk with elbow crutches,

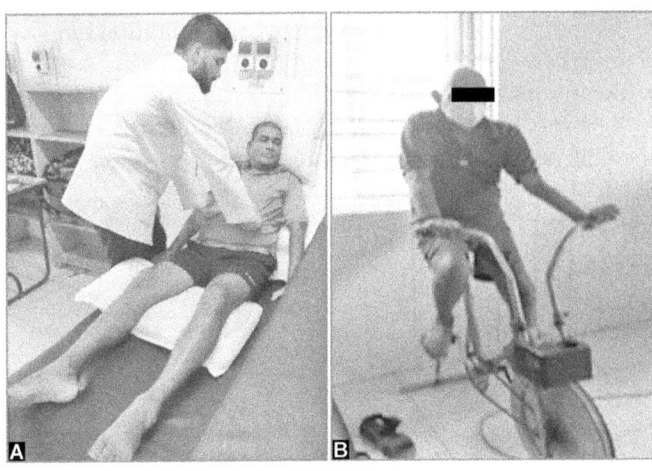

Figs. 26.2A and B: (A) Assisted diaphragmatic breathing exercise; (B) Static cycle exercise.

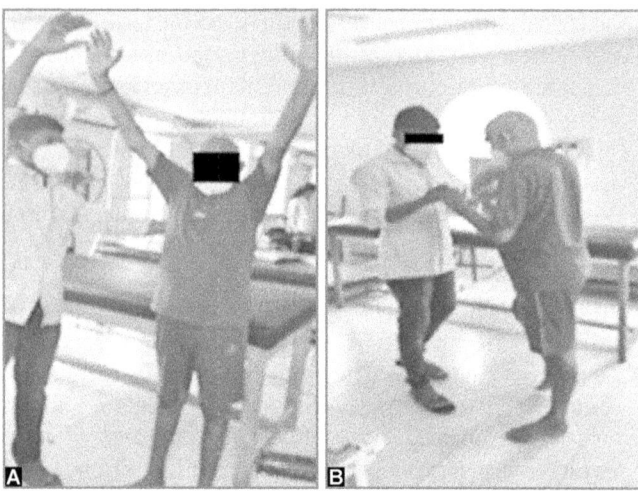

Figs. 26.3A and B: (A) Standing balance training; (B) Gait training.

once, the patient is able to grasp the therapists hands and walk, gait training with elbow crutches should be started.
- **To improve overall function:** Retraining of dressing, washing, bed mobility, transfers, and ambulation activities comprise a big part of the rehabilitation process. Balance and proprioception retraining in all these functional activities should also be included, while motor control can be achieved by doing proprioceptive neuromuscular facilitation (PNF) techniques.

Orthotic Management

Patients of GBS very often have a residual foot drop/wrist drop deformities. Cock up splints for wrist drop and ankle foot orthosis (AFO) for foot drop may be considered. Those who have poor grasp due to long flexor weakness, are benefited by a tenodesis splint.

Prognosis and Recovery

About 90% of patients with GBS recover maximally, 5% are left with disabilities and 5% die of respiratory complications. Although some people can take months and even years to recover, most people with GBS experience the following general timeline:
- After the first signs and symptoms, the condition tends to progressively worsen for about 2 weeks
- Symptoms reach a plateau within 4 weeks
- Recovery begins, usually lasts for 6–12 months, though for some people it could take as long as 3 years.

CHRONIC INFLAMMATORY DEMYELINATING POLYNEUROPATHY

Chronic inflammatory demyelinating polyneuropathy (CIDP) is the most common autoimmune polyneuropathy in adults.

Etiology

The exact cause of this disease is still not known. Autoimmune factors are regarded as the cause to produce demyelination.

Pathophysiology

The pathologic features in CIDP described by Dyck were "onion bulb" formations, perivascular inflammatory infiltrates, and segmental demyelination in teased fibers. These have led to two assumptions: (1) that CIDP is a primarily demyelinating disorder, and (2) that inflammation or autoimmunity is a key feature of the pathogenesis. Humoral immune factors have been presumed to be involved given the response of most patients to corticosteroids, intravenous immunoglobulins (IVIg), or plasma exchange.

Clinical Features

The key features are:
- Weakness (both proximal and distal extremities and trunk, with less involvement of bulbar muscles).
- Subacute to chronic onset of symptoms (greater than 8 weeks).
- Areflexia.
- Electrodiagnostic features of conduction block and asymmetric conduction velocity.
- Features of cytoalbuminologic association (elevated CSF protein without a pleocytosis).

Chronic inflammatory demyelinating polyneuropathy is distinguished from AIDP, the most common form of GBS, by time course and steroid responsiveness. Unlike AIDP, CIDP typically has a more indolent course and all of the published criteria for CIDP recognize time to greatest weakness of longer than 8 weeks to differentiate CIDP from AIDP (which reaches nadir in 4 weeks or less).

Management

Chronic inflammatory demyelinating polyneuropathy is managed in the same lines as discussed under AIDP (GBS).

Physiotherapy in Ataxias (Ataxic Disorders)

INTRODUCTION

Ataxia is the term for a group of neurological diseases (diseases related to the nervous system) that affect movement and coordination. People with ataxia often have trouble with balance, coordination, swallowing, and speech. Ataxia usually develops as a result of damage to a part of the brain that coordinates movement (cerebellum).

Causes of Ataxia

Causes of ataxia, depends upon its type. Persistent ataxia usually results from damage to the part of the brain (cerebellum) that controls muscle coordination. The conditions that can cause ataxia are:
- Trauma.
- Intoxication due to drug and alcohol.
- Vitamin deficiencies such as, Vitamin E deficiency which may cause ataxia and dysarthria.
- Stroke, tumor, cerebral palsy, brain degeneration, multiple sclerosis, cancers, infections.
- Inherited defective genes.
- Idiopathic causes.

Clinical Features of Ataxia

The clinical features of ataxia depend on its types. However, the features common to ataxia are as follows:
- Poor limb coordination, such as dysmetria (undershooting/over shooting), dysdiadochokinesia (inability to perform rapid alternating movements, such as supination and pronation of forearm).
- Dysarthria (slurred and slow speech).
- Tremors (coarse tremors/fine tremors/head shaking-titubation).
- Difficulty in balancing.
- **Nystagmus:** Involuntary back-and-forth eye movements.
- **Loss of joint position sensation:** Impairment of kinesthesia and proprioception are commonly seen in sensory ataxia.
- Muscle weakness (asthenia), flaccidity.
- Difficulty in swallowing.
- Unsteady gait.

Types of Ataxia

There are different types of ataxia occurring as per the causes, such as:
- Cerebellar ataxia.
- Sensory ataxia.
- Vestibular ataxia.
- Frontal ataxia.
- Mixed ataxia.
- Ataxia telangiectasia.
- Episodic ataxia.
- Friedreich's ataxia.
- Spinocerebellar ataxia.

Cerebellar Ataxia

Cerebellar ataxia develops due to lesions to the cerebellum, and/or the afferent and efferent connections of the cerebellum, responsible for perception, coordination, and motor control. Cerebellar ataxia can be observed in diseases such as spinocerebellar ataxia and hereditary ataxias such as Friedreich's ataxia, chronic alcoholism, paraneoplastic cerebellar degeneration, pontocerebellar angle tumors, and multiple sclerosis.

The extent of symptoms depends on parts of the cerebellum which are damaged, and whether lesions occur on one side (unilateral) or both sides (bilateral).
- If the vestibulocerebellum is affected, the patient's balance and eye movement control will be affected. The patient will typically stand with feet wide apart in order to gain better balance and avoid swaying backward and forward.
- If the spinocerebellum is affected, the patient will have an unusual gait with unequal steps, sideways steps, and stuttering starts and stops. The spinocerebellum regulates body and limb movements.
- If the cerebrocerebellum is affected, the patient will have problems with voluntary, planned movements. The head, eyes, limbs, and torso may tremble as voluntary movements are carried out. Speech may be slurred.
- If the cerebellar vermis is affected, titubation occurs.

The features typical of cerebellar ataxia are:
- Hypotonic muscles.
- Deep tendon reflexes are usually maintained, but become pendular type.

- ❖ Wide-based stance with staggering gait.
- ❖ Impaired coordination and balance.
- ❖ Romberg sign may be positive/negative.
- ❖ Positive finger to nose and heal to shin test.
- ❖ **Asthenia**: Generalized muscle weakness.
- ❖ Tremor/titubation (shaking movement of the head and upper trunk). The tremor could be: kinetic tremor (oscillation that occur during movements), intention tremor (increase of tremor toward the end of movement) and postural tremor (tremor that occur when the limb is held in a static position).
- ❖ Difficulty in accurately estimating how much time has passed (dyschronometria/distorted time perception).
- ❖ Incoordination/dysmetria (overshooting/undershooting).
- ❖ **Dyssynergia:** In coordination between agonists and antagonists to carry out a purposeful movement.
- ❖ Nystagmus.
- ❖ Dysarthria.
- ❖ **Disdiadochokinesia**: Inability to perform rapid alternating movements, such as rapid supination/pronation.
- ❖ **Dysmetria**: Inability to judge distance.

Sensory Ataxia

Sensory ataxia affects patients with significant proprioceptive loss. Characteristically, the patient looks down and walks as if throwing his feet, which tend to slap on the ground. Sensory ataxia is distinguished from cerebellar ataxia by the presence of near-normal coordination when the movement is visually observed by the patient, but marked worsening of coordination when the eyes are shut, indicating a positive Romberg's sign.

Causes of sensory ataxia

Sensory ataxia can be a manifestation of sensory large fiber peripheral neuropathies and conditions causing dysfunction of the dorsal columns of the spinal cord, causing loss of proprioception due to a variety of disorders, infectious (e.g., tertiary syphilis), autoimmune, metabolic, toxic, vascular, and hereditary diseases.

Clinical features

- ❖ A patient with sensory ataxia typically has an unsteady stamping gait.
- ❖ The patient has difficulty in walking in dark/poorly lit environments, as there is no proprioception, and visual stimuli used by the patient to maintain balance is not available in dark places.
- ❖ Romberg's sign is usually positive, i.e., when the patient is made to stand with eyes closed, there is excessive body sway, with a tendency to fall.
- ❖ The patient may find it difficult to perform smoothly coordinated voluntary movements/actions using limbs, trunk, pharynx, larynx, and eyes.
- ❖ Finger to nose test/heel to shin test, may be positive/negative.

Vestibular Ataxia

The term vestibular ataxia is used to indicate ataxia due to dysfunction of the vestibular system (made up of the inner ear and the semicircular canals that contain the semicircular fluid, which senses the position of head in space, helping in balance and spatial orientations), which in acute and unilateral cases is associated with prominent vertigo, nausea, and vomiting and loss of balance and spatial orientation. In slow-onset chronic bilateral cases, the patient may only experience unsteadiness.

Causes of vestibular ataxia

Middle or inner ear infection. Geriatric vestibular ataxia is a disease in which the precise cause may never be identified. Hypothyroidism and tumors in the ear or skull are also the causes.

Clinical features

The features of vestibular ataxia are:
- ❖ Problems in maintaining standing and sitting.
- ❖ Vertigo.
- ❖ Staggering gait.
- ❖ Difficulty in walking in a straight line.
- ❖ Nausea and vomiting.

Frontal Ataxia

Frontal ataxia (also known as gait apraxia) is observed when tumors, abscesses, cerebrovascular accidents, and normal pressure hydrocephalus affect the frontal area of the brain.

Causes

As stated, above, this ataxia is caused by tumors, brain abscesses, CVA, normal pressure hydrocephalus, etc.

Clinical features

It has the following features:
- ❖ Difficulty in standing erect, as the trunk is upright, but head leans forward.
- ❖ The legs get crossed in standing.
- ❖ Association of frontal dementia, incontinence of urine, perseveration along with ataxia.
- ❖ Slow shuffling gait maintaining a wide base. There is excess swing of arms.
- ❖ Difficulty in turning with frequent falls.
- ❖ Romberg test may be positive/negative.

Mixed Ataxia

Mixed ataxia refers to the type of ataxia when symptoms of two or more types of ataxia are observed together, such as occurrence of sensory and cerebellar ataxia symptoms.

Ataxia Telangiectasia

Ataxia telangiectasia (AT) is also known as Louis–Bar syndrome. This is an inherited condition typically developing in babies or young children.

Clinical features

- ❖ Appearance of enlarged (dilated) blood vessels known as telangiectasias in the eyes and on the skin of the face.
- ❖ Increasing difficulty in walking, coordinating movements, looking from side to side.
- ❖ Difficulty in speaking.

Episodic Ataxia

With episodic ataxia, people have recurring troubles with movement and balance. These episodes can happen multiple times per day or just one or two times in a year. It can develop at any age.

Causes

The causes include stress, medications, alcohol, illness, and physical exertion.

Features

The features are difficulty in moving, balancing, nausea, vomiting, dizziness, and headache.

Friedreich's Ataxia

Friedreich's ataxia is named after Nikolaus Friedreich, a German physician. It is a rare inherited disease, that causes progressive nervous system damage and movement problems. It is the most common type of genetic ataxia, typically developing in children and adolescents between the ages of 5 and 15 years, with worsening muscle coordination. In rare cases the disease may also start in the adulthood.

The disease primarily affects the brain, spinal cord, peripheral nerves, heart, and pancreas.

Clinical features

- The early feature that appears is difficulty in walking with poor balance.
- Slowness of movements with dysarthria.
- Gradually worsening ataxia is found in limbs and trunk.
- As muscle weakness progresses, most affected individuals develop increased muscle tone (spasticity).
- The deep tendon reflexes are gradually lost.
- Difficulty in swallowing also results from impaired coordination of muscles of tongue and throat.
- Sensory loss in the arms and legs is often a presentation in few sufferers.
- Loss of vision and hearing may also occur.
- Palpitations in heart and shortness of breath are also seen.

Prognosis

The symptoms of Friedreich's ataxia get gradually worse over time. The sufferers have a shorter life expectancy as compared to normal. Most of the sufferers live up to their 30s, though a few also live up to their 60s, or beyond.

Spinocerebellar Ataxia

These are a group of hereditary ataxias, characterized by degenerative changes in the cerebellum and its tracts in brain, brainstem, and spinal cord, but the peripheral nervous system is less commonly affected. Involvement of upper motor neuron, leads to spasticity and hyper-reflexia, where involvement of the peripheral nervous system, leads to motor and sensory features. Symptoms of spinocerebellar ataxia can develop at any age. It often progresses more slowly than other types of ataxia.

Clinical features

- Problems with coordination and balance.
- Gait incoordination.
- Spasticity/hypotonicity.
- Hyper-reflexia/hyporeflexia.
- Muscle weakness with sensory loss.
- Dysarthria.
- Poor eye hand coordination.
- Nystagmus.
- Difficulty in information processing.

Assessment of Ataxia

It consists of:
- Examination of muscle tone for spasticity/hypotonicity.
- Muscle power examination.
- Sensory testing, mostly focusing on proprioception (joint position sense at rest) and kinesthesia (joint position sense on motion).
- Romberg test/Sharpened Romberg test.
- **Examination of coordination:** Finger to nose test, heel to shin test **(Figs. 27.1A and B)**.
- Examination of posture.
- Measurement of balance, using balance scales such as Berg balance scale, functional reach test, etc.
- Examination of function and gait.

Diagnosis of Ataxia

Diagnosis of the ataxias is made from:
- Complain of patient, clinical features, and assessment findings.
- MRI/CT scan.
- Genetic tests/blood tests/urine tests.

Management of Ataxia

The goal of ataxia treatment is to improve the quality of life and requires an individualized approach. Symptomatic medical management, nutritional advice, physiotherapy, occupational therapy, speech and language therapy, form the main components of management.

Physiotherapy in Ataxia

Physiotherapy focuses on:
- Improvement of muscle strength and overall endurance.
- Improvement of posture.
- Improvement of coordination.
- Improvement of balance.
- Improvement of gait.
- Improvement of function and quality of life.

Physiotherapy intervention strategies:
- Active-free exercises/low-intensity resisted exercise without inducing fatigue.

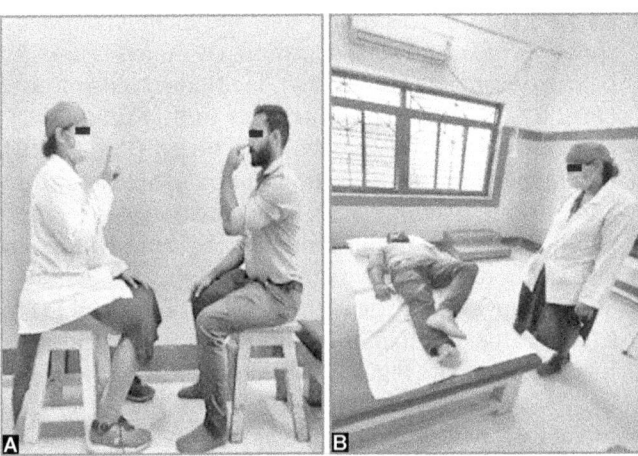

Figs. 27.1A and B: (A) Finger to nose test; (B) Heel to shin test.

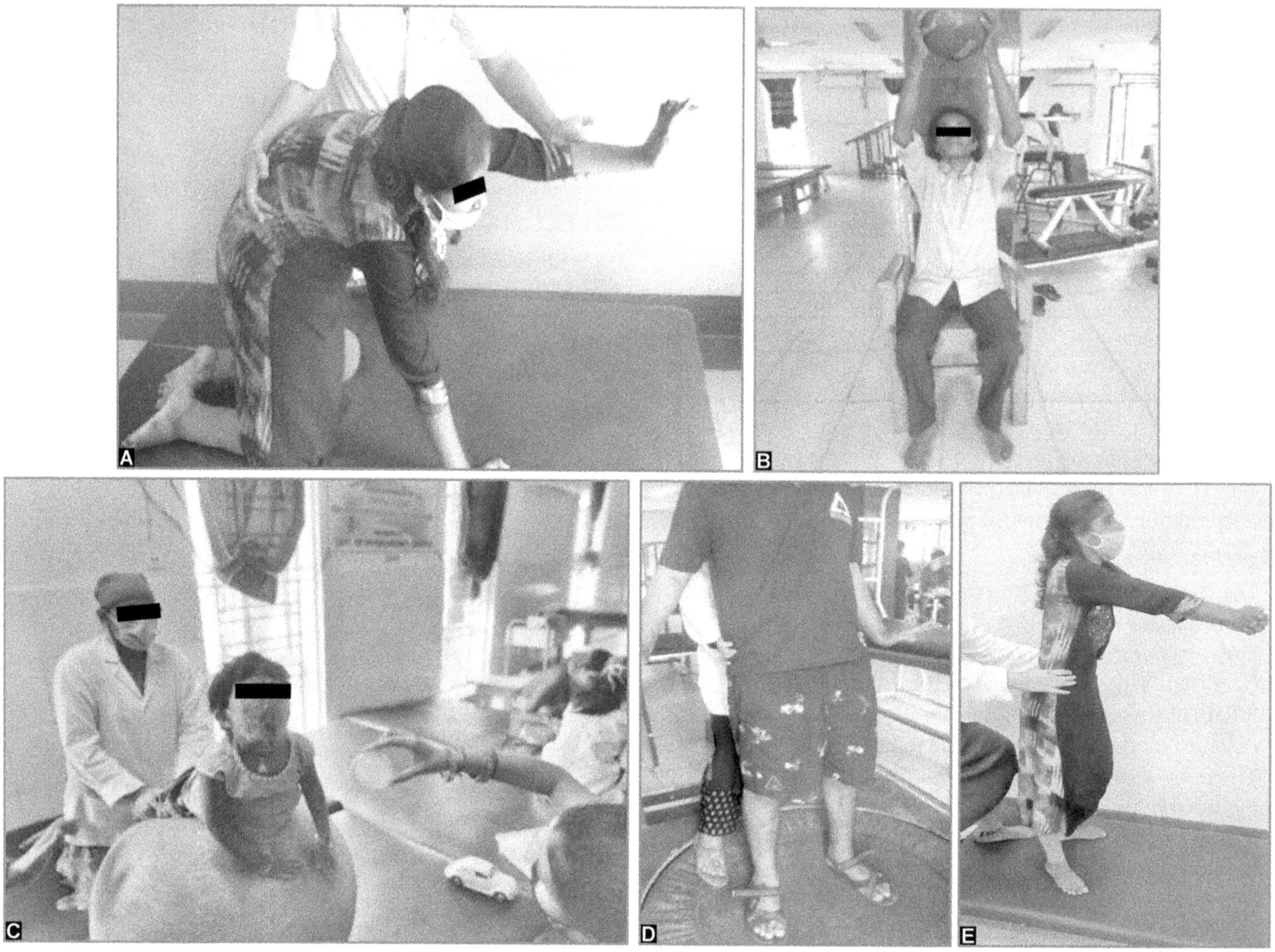

Figs. 27.2A to E: (A) Weight bearing exercise to improve proprioception; (B) Medicine ball exercise; (C) Exercise on Swiss ball; (D) Exercise on trampoline; (E) Exercise on balance board/wobble board.

- Deep breathing exercise/incentive spirometry.
- **Proprioceptive training:** The aim is to increase proprioceptive input by mechanically stimulating the joint surfaces, muscles and tendons, and decreasing postural instability by improving body awareness.

  Proprioceptive neuromuscular facilitation (PNF), rhythmic stabilization, slow reversal techniques, resistive exercises, use of Johnstone pressure splints, gait exercises on different surfaces (hard, soft, and inclined surfaces) with eyes open and closed, plyometric exercises, weight-bearing exercise **(Fig. 27.2A)**, medicine ball exercises **(Fig. 27.2B)**, exercise on Swiss ball **(Fig. 27.2C)**/trampoline **(Fig. 27.2D)**/balance board **(Fig. 27.2E)**, etc., help in improving proprioception to hold a posture, and perform activities with balance. Strategies to apply vibration to the muscle/tendon using a tuning fork are also methods to improve proprioception.
- Suit therapy using vests with pockets to add weight **(Fig. 27.3A)** can be used to improve proprioception, posture/balance and gait **(Fig. 27.3B)**. Methods, which develop body awareness, such as the Feldenkrais (the Feldenkrais method is a type of exercise therapy, claimed to reorganize connections between the brain and the body and so improve body movement and psychological state) and Alexander techniques, yoga, and body awareness exercises, can be included in the program.
- Frenkel's exercises for sensory ataxia **(Figs. 27.4A and B)**.

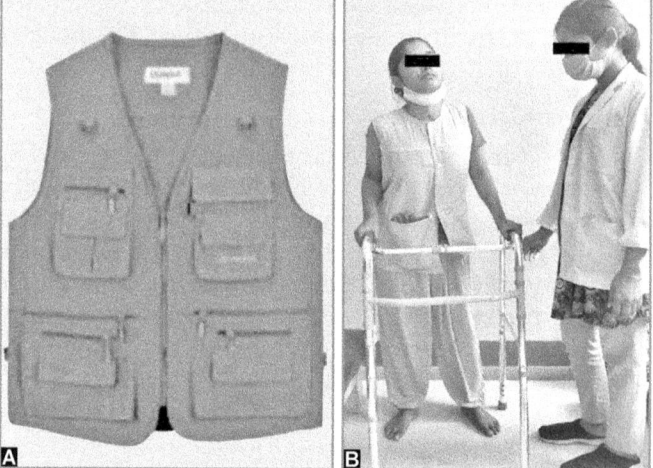

Figs. 27.3A and B: (A) Vests with weight pockets to improve proprioception; (B) Gait training using vest with weight pockets.

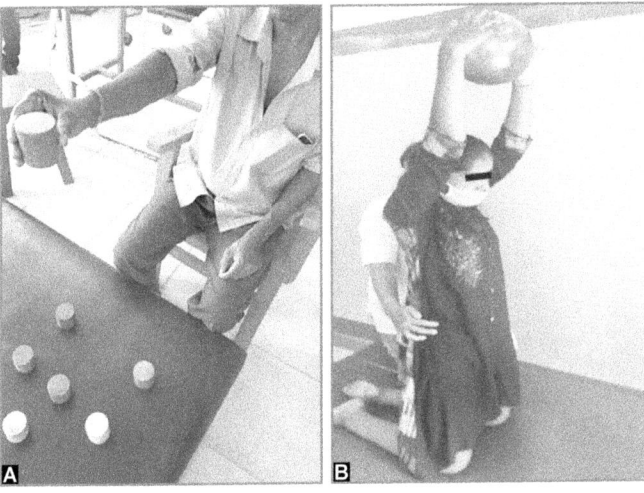

Figs. 27.4A and B: Frenkel's exercises for upper limbs.

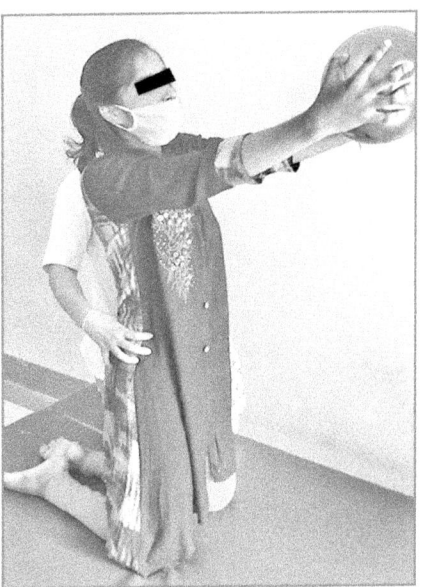

Fig. 27.5: Turning body repeatedly from left to right—habituation exercise.

- Rhythmic stabilization technique of PNF to improve posture of trunk and extremities. Combination of isotonics also helps in controlling ataxia of extremities.
- Habituation exercises for vestibular ataxia. A vestibular exercise program consists of repetitive, progressively more difficult, eye, head, and body movements, such as turning the body from left to right in sitting, standing, kneel standing holding a ball, etc., **(Fig. 27.5)** designed to encourage movement and facilitate sensory substitution.
- **Coordination dynamic therapy (CDT):** It was developed by Giselher Schalow, which "improves the self-organization of the neuronal networks of the CNS for functional repair by exercising extremely exact coordinated arm and leg movements on a special device (GIGER MD—Modern therapeutic device for repair of the CNS) and, in turn, result in the coordinated firing of the many billions of neurons of the human CNS".
- Balance training on Swiss ball/wobble board/trampoline.
- Gait training using weight jacket/weight cuffs attached to extremities **(Fig. 27.6A)**, weighted walkers **(Fig. 27.6B and C)**.

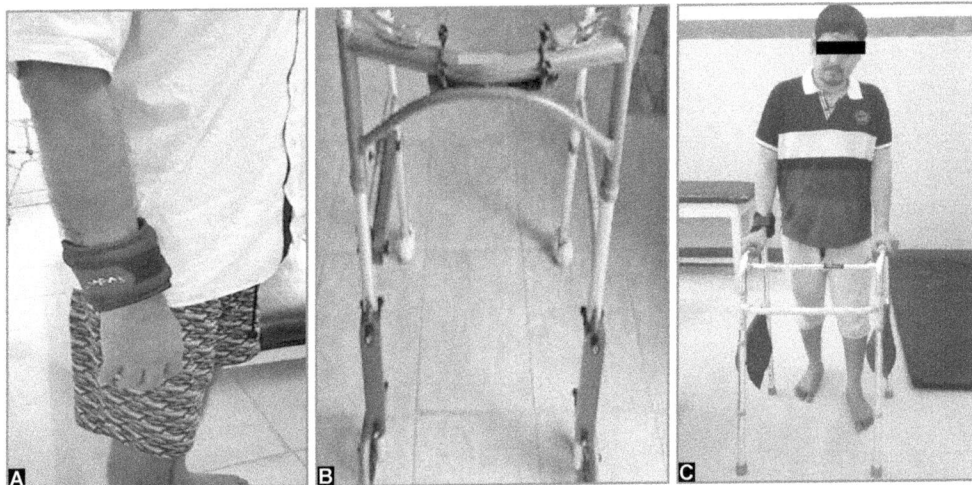

Figs. 27.6A to C: (A) Weight cuff in hand to control ataxia; (B) Weighed walker rollator; (C) Patient walking with weighted walking frame.

SECTION 4

Physiotherapy in Obstetrics and Gynecology

Section Outline

Chapter 28: Physiotherapy in Obstetrics
Chapter 29: Physiotherapy in Gynecological Diseases

Physiotherapy in Obstetrics

INTRODUCTION

Gestation is an important time in woman's life. Preparation of the woman, who wants to be a mother, should begin long before pregnancy, as well as during pregnancy to eliminate complications of pregnancy as well to prepare the pregnant mother to have a safe and uncomplicated labor. Physiotherapy is also given to the mother during childbirth (normal vaginal delivery) to have a safe, painless labor. Postnatal exercises are very important to the mother whether child birth was a normal vaginal delivery or through a cesarean section delivery to eliminate complications of pregnancy and child birth. A pregnant mother goes through the three phases concerning pregnancy and childbirth such as prenatal phase (conception to onset of labor), perinatal phase (the child birth period to 1 week following birth), postnatal phase (the period following child birth, i.e., from 1 week following child-birth upto 2 years). Physiotherapy in all the three phases of pregnancy and child birth is required to avoid complications of pregnancy, and to have a safe child birth as well to live better quality of living during postpartum period. Appropriate exercises are prescribed and taught to the pregnant woman by the physiotherapists to have safe pregnancy, uncomplicated child birth and to minimize and treat the musculoskeletal complications after child birth.

PREGNANCY, ITS COMPLICATIONS, AND MANAGEMENT

Normal pregnancy lasts between 38 and 40 weeks or 280 days. During this period, the musculoskeletal system of the pregnant woman undergoes significant changes, which are partly due to abnormal postural changes, and partly due to hormonal changes leading to laxity of soft tissues and joints. Postural changes because of the displacement of the center of gravity, as the pregnant woman stoops forward due to protrusion of abdomen, result in an anterior pelvic tilt, and movement of the upper body backward as a compensatory strategy leads to a lordotic posture **(Fig. 28.1)**. Both the postural and hormonal changes result in musculoskeletal complications such as low back pain, joint pain, tendinitis, fasciitis, and compression syndromes (e.g., Carpal tunnel syndrome). Prenatal physiotherapy helps to minimize these complications and prepares the woman for a safe child birth.

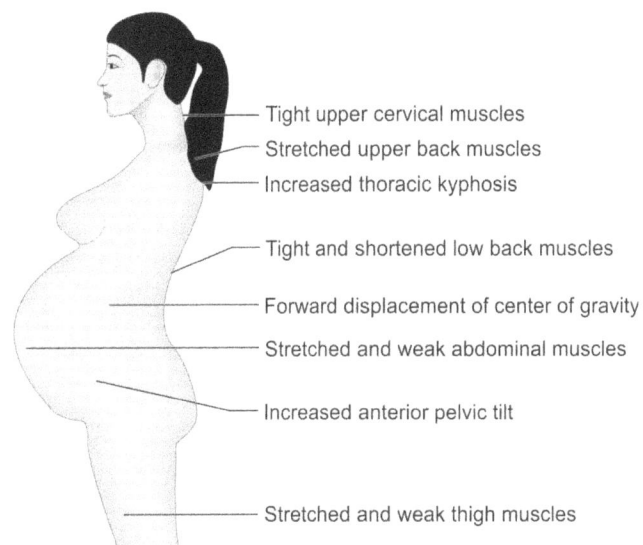

Fig. 28.1: Changes in different structures that lead to abnormal posture during pregnancy.

Common musculoskeletal complications of pregnancy and their management are briefly discussed here:

- ❖ **Diastasis recti abdominis muscle:** The rectus abdominis muscles of both sides separate abnormally (gap between both sides >25 mm) **(Fig. 28.2)**, which may occur during pregnancy as well as during expulsive stage of labor.

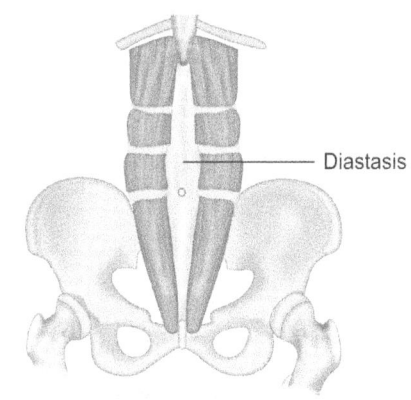

Fig. 28.2: Diastasis recti abdominis during pregnancy.

Management
- Abdominal strengthening exercises **(Fig. 28.3)**
- Posterior pelvic tilt exercises **(Figs. 28.4A and B)**
- Use of abdominal binder **(Fig. 28.5)**

❖ **Low back pain and pelvic pain:** Low back pain could be due to both postural changes and sacroiliac joint dysfunction. The pain is usually located to posterior pelvis and may radiate to back of thigh and leg.

Management of low back pain:
– Relative rest
– Moist hot pack to low back with gentle massage to paraspinal muscles to reduce pain and spasm in side lying.
– If facet joint dysfunction is noted, gentle mobilization to the same may be performed in side lying.
– Transcutaneous electrical nerve stimulation (TENS) may be considered in very acute nonremitting pain considering current evidences on its use.

❖ **Varicose veins:**
Management of varicose veins: Varicosities are caused by increased venous distensibility due to inadequate venous return (venous stasis). It is aggravated during pregnancy due to increased uterine weight.
Management:

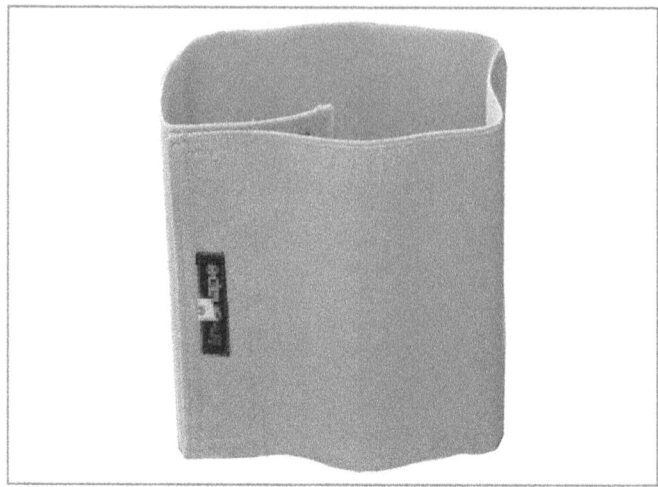

Fig. 28.5: Abdominal binder.

– Limb elevation
– Use of elastic support stockings **(Fig. 28.6)**
– Active exercises to lower limbs

❖ **Pelvic floor dysfunction:** Management of pelvic floor dysfunction:
The process of labor in vaginal delivery can produce significant trauma to the muscles of pelvic floor. Subsequently, after child birth, it may lead to:
– Prolapse of uterus/rectum
– Incontinence
– Pain

Pelvic floor rehabilitation (Kegel's exercises—discussed later) is performed during pregnancy, which also continues postpartum.

❖ **Joint laxity:** Due to hormonal changes during pregnancy, the joints become lax, increasing the chance of injury.
Management: Nonweight bearing and less stressful exercises such as swimming/hydrotherapy, static cycle exercises, etc., are advised during the period of pregnancy in the presence of joint laxity.

❖ **Osteitis pubis and diastasis of symphysis pubis:** The width of symphysis pubis increases during pregnancy, producing

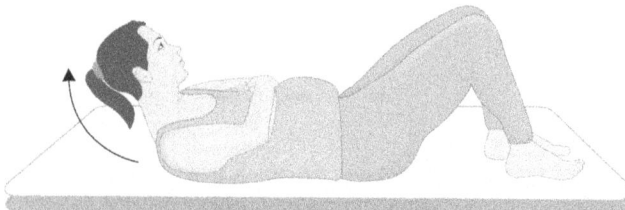

Fig. 28.3: Abdominal strengthening exercise.

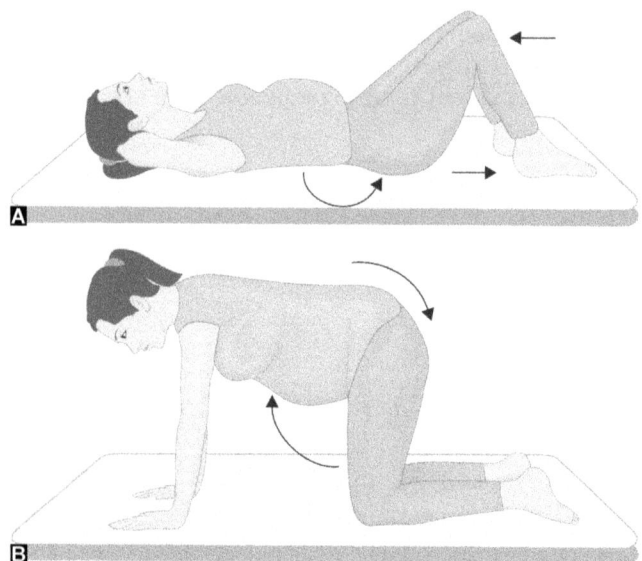

Figs. 28.4A and B: Posterior pelvic tilt exercises. (A) Combined with hip and knee flexion; (B) Quadruped position.

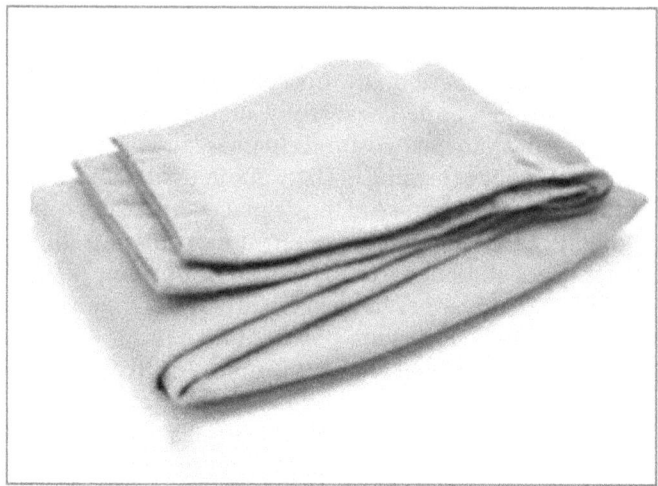

Fig. 28.6: Elastic support stockings for varicose vein.

transient pain that may radiate to the medial aspect of thigh. Movement dysfunctions such as difficulty in turning on bed, walking, squatting, and abducting hips may result.
Management: If the pain is acute, bed rest with hips in flexion and adduction is advised.
Ice pack to the painful area, 2–3 times a day is advised and the pregnant lady is provided with a walking stick if she has difficulty in walking.

- **Muscle cramps:** Cramps in calf muscles, feet, and thigh may occur during pregnancy, due to calcium deficiency, ischemia and nerve root pressure, fluid retention, etc.
  Management:
  - Gentle stretching exercises
  - Active exercises
  - Massage: Deep kneading
  - Referral to physician for nutritional supplements
- **Upper back pain:** This could be due to changes in posture combined with tendinitis of muscles connecting the thorax with scapula.
  Management:
  - Moist hot packs
  - Upper back extension in sitting
  - Shoulder shrugs in sitting
  - Massage to musculotendinous structures
  - Posture correction
- **Osteoporosis**: This results from calcium deficiency.
  Management:
  - Referral to a physician for nutritional advice
  - Active exercises
- **Coccydynia:** It results from a change of posture during late stages of pregnancy.
  Management:
  - Sitz bath
  - Coccydynia pillow **(Fig. 28.7)**
- **Nerve compressions:** Nerve compressions such as carpal tunnel syndrome, thoracic outlet syndrome, etc., are very common during pregnancy and after child birth.
  Management:
  - Posture correction, nerve gliding exercises and TENS (for thoracic outlet syndrome)
  - Pulsed ultrasound, flexor retinaculum stretching, carpal mobilization exercises, tendon gliding exercises (for carpal tunnel syndrome)

Besides the specific complications during pregnancy and their management, physiotherapy in obstetrics is provided through the following three stages such as:

Prenatal Physiotherapy

Physiotherapy is of great importance in the prenatal period not only to reduce discomfort, but also to prepare the woman for labor, particularly if she opts for vaginal delivery. The physiotherapist must place emphasis on directing and training pregnant women to ensure that their newly assumed posture does not overstress any body segment, since the outcome of this could be fatigue, microtrauma and pain. Kinesiotherapeutic exercises that are performed at this period help strengthening the muscles that help during normal labor. Stretching exercises, relaxation exercises, pelvic floor proprioceptive exercises, breathing exercises, and postural re-education are performed to help the woman to reduce the discomfort and to have a safe child birth. This helps in promoting relief of pain during the period of contractions that occur during labor and reduces labor time.

Bavaresco et al., sought to show the work of physiotherapy within obstetrics, not only working on analgesia, but also for stimulation of ambulation, breathing, active exercises that help relaxation at the time of delivery, and provide the necessary strength to the pregnant woman at the time of baby's expulsion. TENS, with the electrodes placed on the paravertebral and sacral region, may be used for relief of pain during pregnancy, though many controversies exist in this regard, and current evidences on use of TENS during pregnancy should be considered, while using this modality. However, as per the study done by Mazzali and Goncalvez, TENS can be used as a method of pain relief during labor.

According to Bim et al., physiotherapist has an important role to play with pregnant women who have weakness of pelvic floor muscles, as these muscles participate actively during the expulsive phase of child birth. Kegel's exercises are the best known techniques for the strengthening of these muscle groups.

Principles of exercises during pregnancy

- All women should remain physically active during pregnancy, except where contraindications for exercises exist.
- Pregnant women should accumulate a minimum of 150 minutes of moderate-intensity physical activity in each week, to achieve health benefits and to reduce the risks for complications during pregnancy.
- The pregnant woman should remain active daily. The physical activities should be accumulated over 3 days per week.
- A combination of aerobics, resistance training, breathing exercises and stretching should be encouraged.
- Pelvic floor muscle training should be performed daily to assist in labor as well as to prevent urinary incontinence.

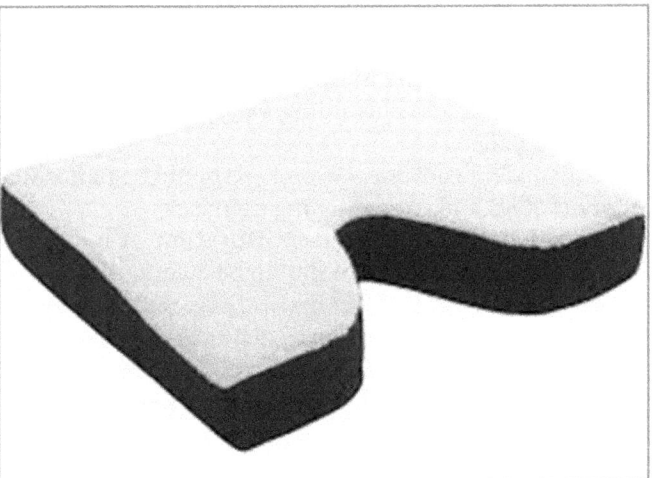

Fig. 28.7: Coccydynia pillow.

Contraindications to exercises during pregnancy:
- **Absolute contraindications:** Even though certain pregnant women have absolute contraindications to exercise, they should continue with their usual daily activities and should avoid moderate to vigorous activities. The absolute contraindications are:
  – Placenta previa (placenta previa occurs, when a baby's placenta partially or totally covers the mother's cervix, resulting in bleeding throughout the pregnancy).
  – Ruptured membrane.
  – Unexplained vaginal bleeding.
  – Preeclampsia.
  – Incompetent cervix.
  – Intrauterine growth retardations.
  – Higher order multiple pregnancy (twins/triplets).
  – Uncontrolled high BP, diabetes, thyroid disease.
  – Serious disorders such as cardiovascular and respiratory illness.
- **Relative contraindications:** When relatively contraindicated, the pregnant woman should perform exercises/activities as per the advice of the healthcare provider/physiotherapist. The relative contraindications include:
  – Gestational hypertension
  – History of spontaneous preterm birth
  – Anemia with symptoms
  – Malnutrition
  – Eating disorder/nausea and vomiting
  – Any significant medical illness

Prenatal exercise safety:
While doing exercises, certain safety precautions should be explained to the pregnant woman, so that, if any complications to exercise arise, the same could be prevented/minimized. These include:
- Avoiding exercises in excessive heat and humidity.
- Avoiding exercises that involve physical contact such as playing hockey.
- Avoiding scuba diving.
- Avoiding physical activities at high altitude, if they live in lower land.
- Maintaining adequate nutrition and hydration.
- Stopping exercises if any adverse reaction such as persistent dyspnea, severe chest pain, vaginal bleeding, decreased fetal movement, dizziness/faintness, etc., develop.

Benefits of prenatal exercises:
- **Exercise improves cardiorespiratory fitness:** Pregnancy is accompanied by many cardiac and respiratory changes beginning during the 5th week of gestation and lasting up to 1 year after child birth. Cardiac output and blood volume as well as tidal volume and oxygen consumption (VO_2) all increase to supply nutritional and oxygen requirement of the fetus. Exercising during pregnancy maintains these cardiorespiratory parameters.
- **Exercise improves psychological well-being:** Pregnancy produces many emotional changes, resulting in alterations of mood and prenatal depression. By regular exercises, the fitness is maintained, which induces relaxation, and enhances better coping with emotional and physiological stresses of pregnancy.
- **Exercise prevents and improves low back pain:** The postural and emotional changes such as increased lumbar lordosis, result in low back pain in pregnant women. A general whole body exercise program and lumbar stabilization exercises help to reduce low back pain.
- **Exercises help for uncomplicated labor:** Pregnant women, who maintain regular exercise routine, may experience less labor pain and have shorter labor time.
- **Exercise prevents urinary incontinence:** Exercises, particularly those done to strengthen muscles of pelvic floor, help in preventing urinary incontinence after child birth.
- **Exercises help to prevent diastasis recti abdominis:** Diastasis recti is a separation between the right and left side of rectus abdominis muscle (**Fig. 28.2**) that develops in pregnant women above the age of 35 years or those who have multiple pregnancies. It is thought that regular exercises during pregnancy can minimize this complication.

Frequency, intensity, time and types of exercise recommendations for exercise during pregnancy:
As per the American College of Obstetricians and Gynecologists, in the absence of contraindications, a pregnant woman should be encouraged to perform regular moderate intensity physical activities and exercises. Moderate intensity physical activity is defined as an activity with an energy requirement of 3-5 metabolic equivalents (METs).

Recommendations and guidelines for exercises during pregnancy are:
- Physical examination should be done before engaging the woman in performing exercises.
- Frequency: For aerobic exercises, 3 or more days in a week, however, for resisted exercises 2-3 nonconsecutive days in a week.
- Intensity: Moderate-intensity exercises for aerobic activities (Energy requirement of 2-3 METs and a rate of perceived exertion score of 12-13 on the 6-20 Borg scale). Resistance activities/exercises should be performed to the point of moderate fatigue (8-10 reps or 12-15 reps). Beginning of exercises should be with low weights and multiple repetitions. In general, low resistance high-repetition exercises avoiding valsalva maneuvers are recommended.
- Warm up and cool down exercises should be performed for aerobics and strengthening exercises.
- Time/duration of exercises: Duration of moderate intensity aerobic exercise should be 30 minutes.
- Type of exercises: Exercises that use large muscle groups in a continuous rhythmic manner such as aerobic exercises in the form of walking, running, dancing, jogging, swimming, cycling, rowing, skating, skipping, etc., are beneficial.
- Exercises in supine position after the first trimester should be avoided.

Unsafe exercises during pregnancy:
- Bilateral straight leg raising

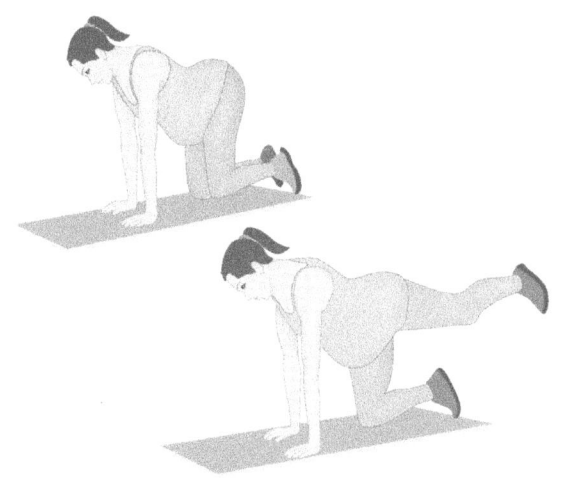

Fig. 28.8: Fire hydrant exercises.

- **Fire hydrant exercises:** It is a glute exercise, done in quadruped, to build up gluteus maximis, medius and deep core muscles, as well as spinal stabilizers. Quadruped hip extension is an example of fire hydrant exercise **(Fig. 28.8)**.
- Unilateral weight-bearing exercises

The prenatal exercises are:
- **Deep breathing exercises**
- **Kegel's exercises:** Kegel's exercises were initially devised and described by Arnold Kegel a renowned gynecologist from the University of South California, in the year 1948. These exercises strengthen the pelvic floor muscles, which support the uterus, bladder, small intestine, and rectum. These exercises prevent or control urinary incontinence and other pelvic floor dysfunctions after child birth. The procedure involves:
  - **Finding the right muscles:** To identify the pelvic floor muscles, the woman is asked to stop urination in midstream. Once she has identified the pelvic floor muscles she can do the exercises in any position, e.g., Crook lying, crook lying with pelvic bridging, semi-Fowler position with legs resting on Swiss ball, sitting on Swiss ball, mini squat position, etc. **(Figs. 28.9A to E)**, although she might find it easiest to do them lying down at first.
  - **Perfecting the technique:** To do Kegel's exercises, she is asked to imagine as if she is sitting on a marble and try to tighten the pelvic muscles as if lifting the marble upward. She is asked to tighten the pelvic floor muscles for five seconds (counting: 1—one thousand, 2—one thousand, 3—one thousand, 4—one thousand, 5—one thousand), followed by relaxation of the muscles. 10-15 repetitions of exercises, three times each day are performed.
  - **Maintaining the focus:** For best results, she is asked to focus on tightening only the pelvic floor muscles, and not to contract the muscles of the abdomen, thighs or buttocks. She should avoid holding the breath, and should breathe freely during the exercises.

Frequency of exercises: She should aim to perform the exercise for at least three times in a day, each session consisting of 1 set of exercises with 10-15 repetitions.

Benefits of Kegel's exercises:

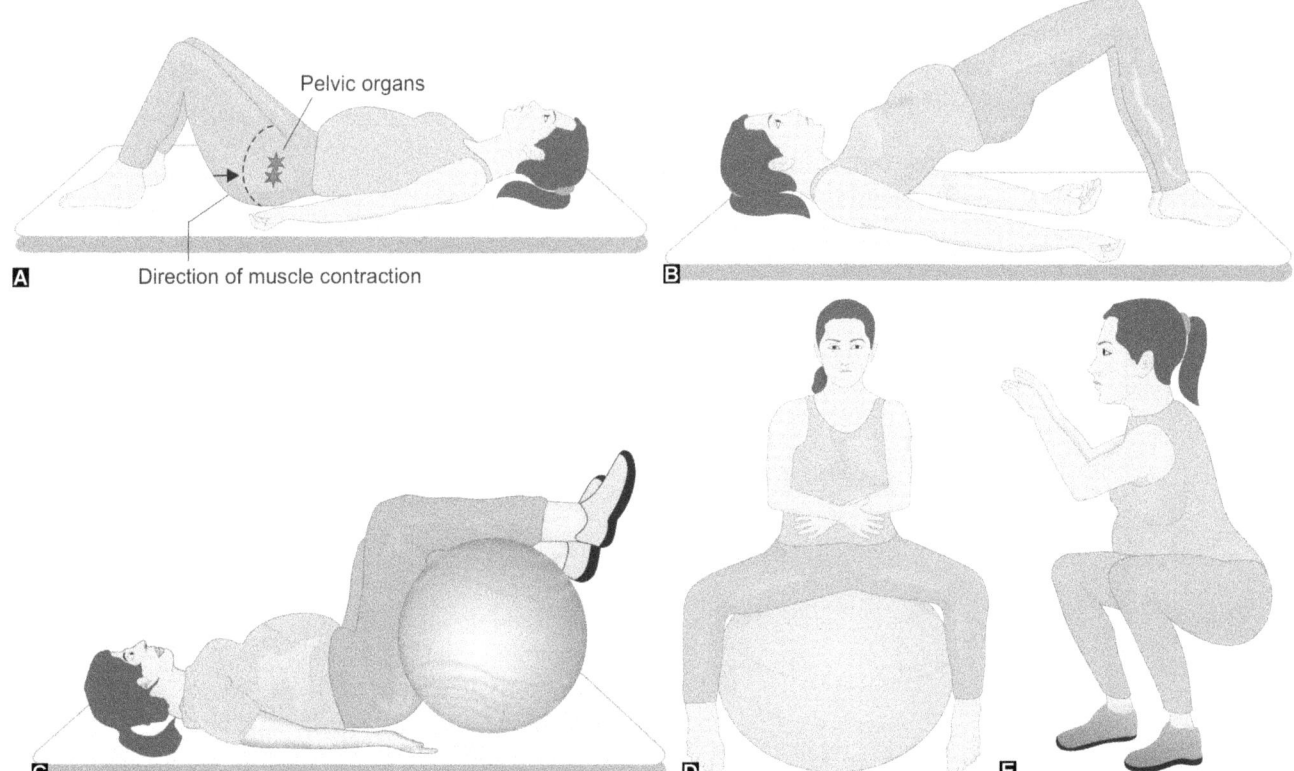

Figs. 28.9A to E: Kegel's exercises. (A) Crook lying; (B) Crook lying with pelvic bridging; (C) Semi-Fowler position with legs resting on Swiss ball; (D) Sitting on Swiss ball; (E) Mini squat position.

- Strengthens muscles of pelvic floor, thereby improving bowel incontinence and urine leakage issues
- Increases blood flow to pelvic region
- Restores vaginal muscle tone and improves vaginal health
- Promotes recovery from physical stress of child birth

❖ **Wall slide squats:** The woman is advised to stand against the wall with feet slightly apart and slowly slide down to semi-squat position, hold the position for 3–5 seconds and then slide up. She should then relax and repeat the same for 5–10 times. This exercise strengthens the muscles of pelvic floor, buttock, and lower limbs and improves endurance for a safer child birth **(Fig. 28.10)**.

❖ **Walking lunge:** From the walk standing position, the woman is asked to go forward and down, slowly and come to the starting position again. The maneuver should be repeated by performing lunge with the opposite leg. A few repetitions of the exercise as tolerated should be performed daily, which improves strength, endurance, and flexibility for a safer child birth **(Fig. 28.11)**.

❖ **Knee extension in sitting:** The woman is asked to extend the knee one after the other in sitting on a chair. The exercise should be repeated as tolerated and performed to improve fitness **(Fig. 28.12)**.

❖ **Neck rotation in sitting:** This exercise helps in improving flexibility of cervical spine, which may be affected due to postural changes during pregnancy **(Fig. 28.13)**.

❖ **Stepping exercises:** This exercise helps in improving aerobic endurance of the woman, helping for a safe, uncomplicated child birth **(Fig. 28.14)**.

❖ **Hip abduction in side lying:** This exercise helps in enhancing flexibility of the perineum, and improves strength and endurance **(Fig. 28.15)**.

❖ **Groin stretch in tailor sitting:** This exercise improves the flexibility of perineum and prepares the woman for a safer child birth **(Fig. 28.16)**.

❖ **Standing wall press:** This exercise helps in stretching the tight pectorals, corrects posture, and strengthens the

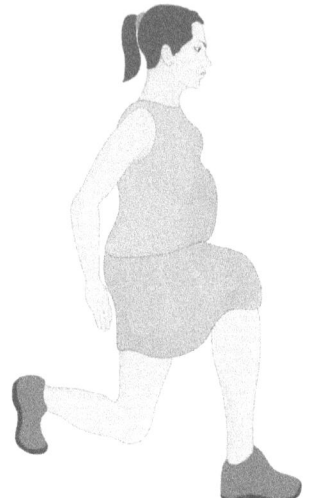

Fig. 28.11: Walking lunge exercise.

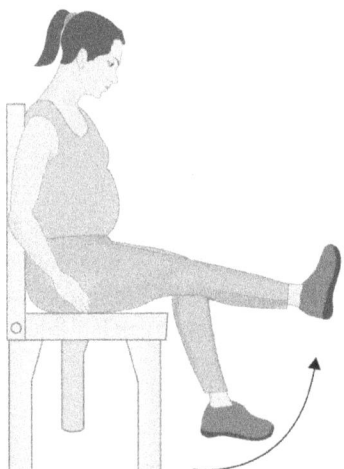

Fig. 28.12: Knee extension in sitting.

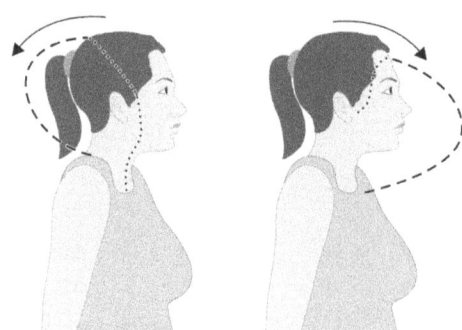

Fig. 28.13: Neck rotation exercise.

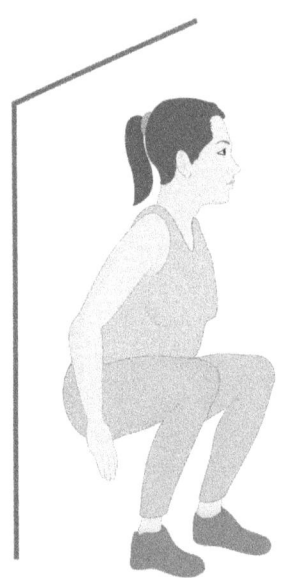

Fig. 28.10: Wall slide squatting exercise.

muscles of upper body for a comfortable pregnancy and safer child birth **(Fig. 28.17)**.

❖ **Chest muscle exercises:** These exercises combined with breathing help in strengthening chest muscles, which results in improved air intake, in the presence of weakness of diaphragm that results during late stage of pregnancy **(Figs. 28.18A and B)**.

Chapter 28: Physiotherapy in Obstetrics 485

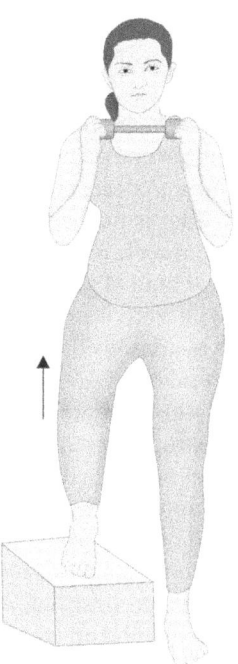

Fig. 28.14: Side stepping exercise in standing.

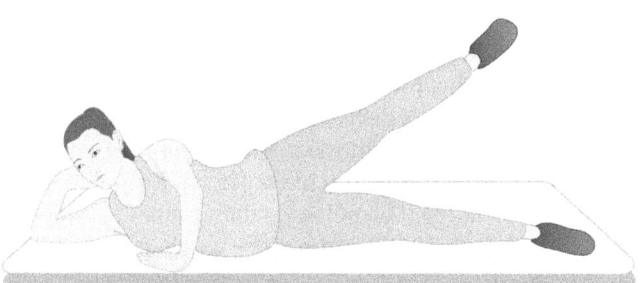

Fig. 28.15: Hip abduction exercise in side lying.

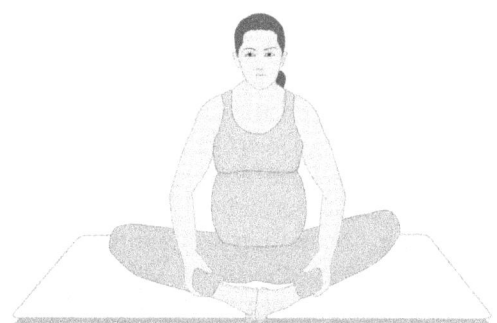

Fig. 28.16: Groin stretch in tailor sitting.

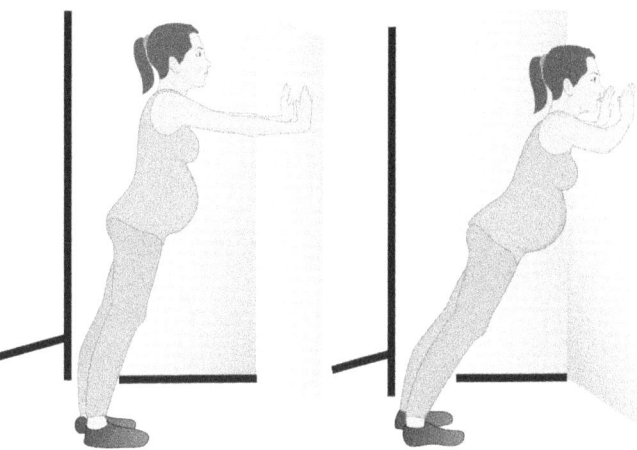

Fig. 28.17: Standing wall press.

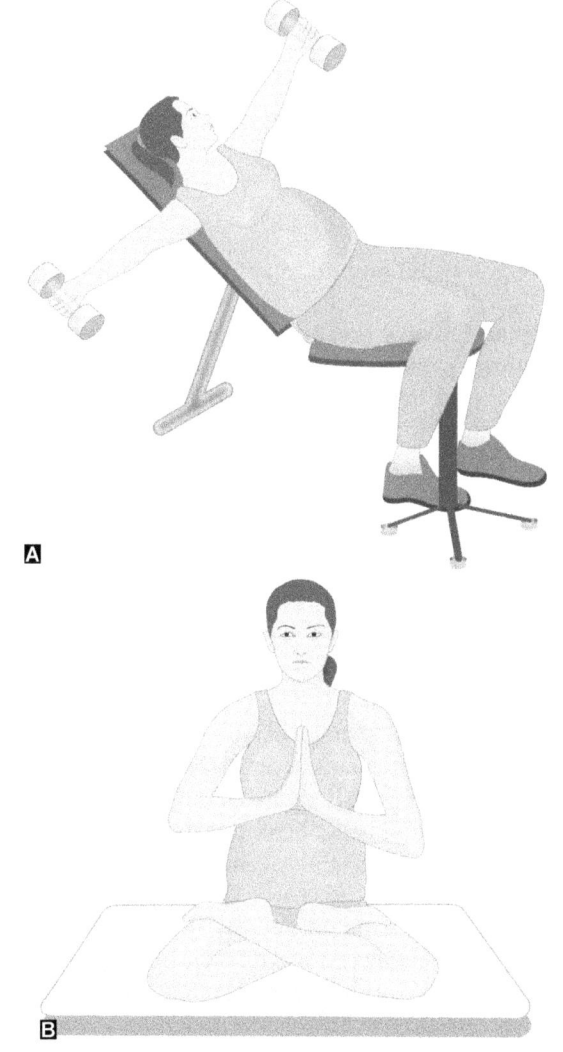

Figs. 28.18A and B: Chest muscle exercise. (A) With dumbbells held in hand; (B) With hands clasped and pressing each other.

❖ **Theraband exercise:** This exercise improves breathing, strength and endurance of chest and upper limb muscles, which helps for a safer child birth **(Fig. 28.19).**

Perinatal Physiotherapy (Physiotherapy during Childbirth)

When the time of delivery arrives, many physiological changes occur in the body of the pregnant woman. The most significant changes are the dilatation of the cervix, contractions generated by secretion of hormones, distention of uterine fibers and birth canal.

There are different types of childbirth, such as:

A. **Vaginal delivery:** In this method, the pregnant woman can exercise her choices regarding: Normal child birth,

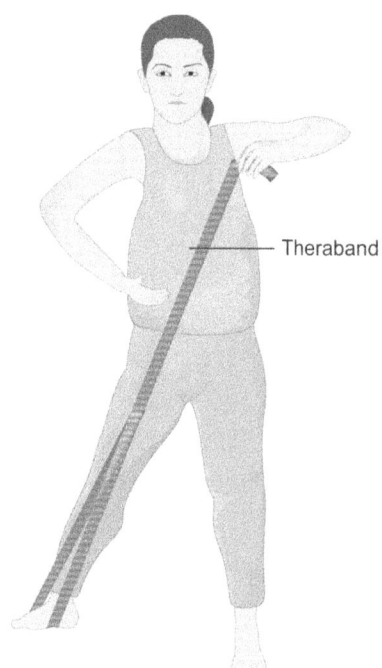

Fig. 28.19: Theraband exercise in standing.

delivery in water and delivery in the squatting position, etc.
B. **Surgical delivery (cesarean section delivery):** This is sometimes performed as per the choice of the pregnant woman, and other times, there is no option (where normal child birth may be at risk), only child birth to occur using this method.

Labor/child birth/vaginal delivery and physiotherapy during and after child birth: Labor/child birth is the process of expulsion of the baby out of the uterus through the birth canal. Labor typically occurs between the 37th and 42nd week of gestation, and can be classified into three stages:

Stages of labor:

- ❖ **First stage:** The first stage of labor begins with the onset of regular rhythmic contraction of uterus and culminates when the cervix is fully dilated to about 10 cm. The first stage of labor can further be divided into three phases: the latent phase, the active phase and the transitional phase, discussed here.
  - *Latent phase:* This phase lasts approximately for 6–8 hours, producing cervical dilatation of about 3–4 cm.
  - *Active phase:* In this phase cervical dilatation occurs more rapidly, reaching a total dilatation of about 7 cm.
  - *Transitional phase:* In this phase, cervical dilatation slows down and cervix reaches full dilatation of 10 cm.
- ❖ **Second stage:** The second stage of labor begins when the cervix is fully dilated and ends when the baby is born. The second stage can be divided into two phases such as: *latent phase and active phase* (discussed later). The average duration of second stage of labor is 50 minutes for primigravida mothers and 20 minutes for multigravida mothers.
  - *Latent phase:* During this phase the mother feels no urge to push. The baby's head continues to descend down by uterine contractions. As the baby is descending down, it changes its position frequently to navigate the curvature of the birth canal. Several pelvic tissues are displaced, as the baby continues to descend through the birth canal such as: the bladder is pushed up into the abdominal cavity, flattening of rectum and thinning of levator ani muscles and stretching of perineum.
  - *Active phase:* The active phase of stage two begins once the baby's head is visible at the vaginal orifice. In this phase, the fetal head exerts increased pressure on the rectum and pelvic floor, resulting in initiation of Ferguson reflex, which provides the mother the urge to push. The mother can adopt different birthing positions to increase diameter of the birth canal, so that the baby's head could be accommodated. During pushing, women should be encouraged to avoid prolonged breath holding, and excessive pushing, as, this can interfere with placental perfusion and compromises the fetus.

  During the second stage, between each contraction and push the uterus relaxes and the baby recedes. At a certain point of time crowning of the baby's head occurs and the head of the baby will be visible. Once the head exits, the shoulders and body will follow it, and the baby is born.
- ❖ **Third stage:** The third stage of labor, which lasts from 5 to 30 minutes, involves delivery of the placenta and control of bleeding to prevent hemorrhage. Placement of the baby onto the breast can also help to achieve placental separation and assist with control of bleeding via the release of oxytocin.

Physiotherapy during time of child birth (Perinatal period): The female physiotherapist may be deployed in the labor room to assist the Obstetrician in inducing as pain free a labor as possible. The therapeutic interventions in this period include:

1. **Positioning of the mother:** The position a woman adopts during labor varies depending on which stage of birth they are in. Birthing positions can be divided into two different categories: (a) Vertical/upright positions; and (b) Horizontal or recumbent/semirecumbent positions.
   a. The vertical positions include:
      » Squatting: The mother is supported by a partner/midwife.
      » Kneeling: The mother kneels with the trunk upright and hands resting on a cushion.
      » Sitting: The mother sits on a bed/chair with trunk inclined forward at an angle of 45 degrees.
   b. Horizontal/Recumbent/Semirecumbent positions:
      » Supine lying: The mother is either lying on her back or lying on the back with the trunk slightly raised (less than 45 degrees from horizontal).
      » Lithotomy position: The mother is lying flat on her back, with the hips flexed and abducted and the knees flexed, and the legs are placed into stirrups **(Fig. 28.20)**.
      » Lateral position: The mother is lying on her side, with the upper leg close to the chest.

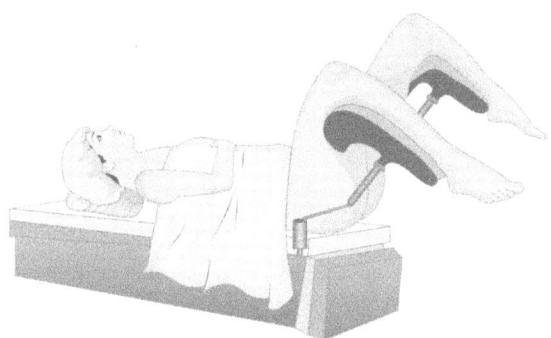

Fig. 28.20: Lithotomy position.

2. **Application of TENS:** This modality provides a non-pharmacological method for relief of pain, and is beneficial during the first stage of labor. However, the mother should not have any contraindications to TENS such as having a cardiac pacemaker. During labor, electrodes are typically positioned over the areas of the skin, that overlie the thoracic (T10), lumbar (L1), and sacral nerve endings (S2-S4) **(Fig. 28.21)**. The mother may also operate the unit herself to control the frequency and intensity of the impulses during labor.

3. **Massage therapy:** This therapy may be used to relax the tense muscles, producing pain relief during labor. Massage can be given by the female physiotherapist/midwife or the woman's partner. Deep tissue massage/trigger point massage/neuromuscular massage, etc., may be given as per the indications. Massage to the lumbosacral region may be performed to reduce back pain associated with labor. Gentle effleurage over abdominal region, may be used to produce stress relief, whereas stroking massage may help in releasing oxytocin. Though massage therapy is said to be beneficial during labor, strong evidence on its efficacy is still lacking. A Cochrane review, published by Smith and colleagues (2018), found low quality evidence regarding the analgesic effects of massage therapy during the first/second/third stages of labor. Perineal massage provides a method to gently stretch the pelvic floor in preparation for birth of the baby. A Cochrane review written by Aasheim and colleagues (2017), states that there is moderate quality evidence in favor of perineal massage to reduce the incidence of third and fourth degree perineal tears, while performed during the second stage of labor. Perineal massage also helps to retain intactness of the perineum following labor.

4. **Heat/cold therapy:** Warm compressions are used during labor to reduce perineal pain, through increase of blood flow, relaxation of muscles and interruption of pain transmission. A study done by Dahlen and colleagues (2009), reported significant pain relief with hot compression in the second stage of labor in a group of women, as compared to the other group who got only the standard care. However, a review done by Smith and colleagues (2018), shows low-quality evidence regarding benefits of warm compression in the first stage of labor. In third stage of labor, heat enhances the mother's comfort, releases endorphin, and oxytocin and assists in delivery of placenta. Ganji and colleagues (2013) examined the effects of simultaneous application of heat and cold on management of labor pain, and reported that local warming with intermittent cold packs to the low back, lower abdomen, and perineum, could reduce labor pain in the first and second stages of labor. As regards the benefits of cold pack, the works of Waters and Raislers report reduction of labor pain, when ice massage is applied to the large intestine meridian.

5. **Acupuncture/acupressure:** We know acupuncture is the technique of inserting needles to different parts of the body, whereas acupressure is the application of pressure to different parts of the body using thumb and fingers. Though many studies highlight the role of acupuncture and acupressure in reducing labor pain, a recent systemic review conducted by Smith and colleagues (2017), found no evidence of acupuncture and acupressure in inducing labor. However, Smith and colleagues (2020) stated that acupuncture may increase the woman's satisfaction with relief of labor pain and may reduce labor pain.

6. **Relaxation techniques:** Relaxation techniques during labor, help the woman to cope with the labor pain, by slowing down breathing, lowering blood pressure and providing the sense of wellbeing. The techniques include: progressive relaxation, breathing exercises and guided imagery (imagining a pleasant relaxing experience).

7. **Breathing techniques:** Several studies have reported that breathing exercises in combination with other techniques (i.e., massage, relaxation techniques) are effective in reducing the perception of pain by women during labor. Breathing techniques can interrupt the transmission of pain from the uterus to the brain, by decreasing sympathetic activity and providing emotional regulation. The techniques include soft sleep breaths performed in between contractions, blissful belly breaths performed during contractions for pain relief, cleansing calming breaths to be used following contractions during the transition period of labor, and gentle birth breaths to be used during the second stage of labor to encourage descent of the baby. Other breathing exercises described in the literature include deep diaphragmatic breathing, slowed inhalation (5 sec in duration) during

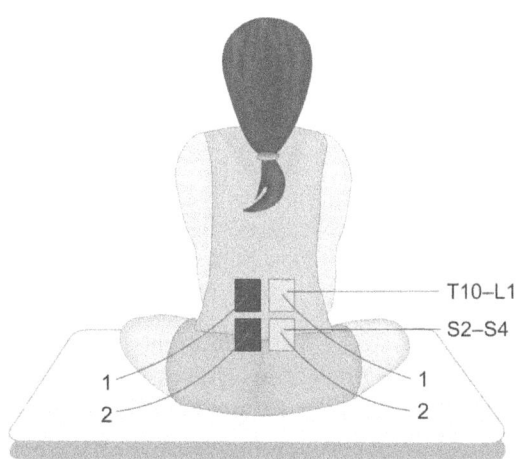

Fig. 28.21: Placement of TENS electrodes during labor.

the first stage of labor, shallow breathing during the active phases of labor, pursed-lip breathing during contractions and the "pant-blow" technique during, pushing in the second stage of labor.

Postnatal Physiotherapy

After normal childbirth, physiotherapy is provided to the woman with the following objectives:
- To improve posture and reduce weight.
- To reduce back pain and prevent development of spondylolisthesis.
- To strengthen the abdominals (to correct diastasis recti).
- To strengthen muscles of pelvic floor, to overcome pelvic floor dysfunctions and subsequent complications.
- To treat complications such as tendinitis, varicose veins, compression neuropathies, etc.

Posture correction, use of modalities, such as moist hot packs, TENS, etc., for back pain and postnatal exercises are considered during the postnatal period. Immediately after child birth, the following three steps may be followed:

1. **Rest:** After childbirth, the pregnant woman should be advised to lie flat on the back for at least 30 minutes twice daily, to provide rest to muscles of pelvic floor and the abdominals.
2. **Ice:** Within the first 72 hours following vaginal delivery, ice/cold pack should be applied to the perineum to reduce pain and swelling and to promote recovery.
3. **Exercises:** Exercises to strengthen the muscles of the pelvic floor can be started as early as possible, after an uncomplicated labor.

Postnatal exercises:

The postnatal exercises can be started as soon as the woman feels that she is comfortable to perform physical activities. After a normal vaginal delivery, exercises can be started a week after delivery. But, if cesarean section delivery was performed, simple exercises are started a week after delivery, but abdominal exercises can be started after 8 weeks (cesarean section delivery and postoperative exercises are discussed separately).

All prenatal exercises performed by the woman can also be performed safely during the postpartum period. The exercises after a normal vaginal delivery are performed gradually through three phases:

1. **Phase I:** It includes diaphragmatic breathing exercises, Kegel's exercises **(Fig. 28.9)** posterior pelvic tilt exercises **(Fig. 28.4)**, upper back stretching, and strengthening exercises **(Figs. 28.22A to C)**, posture correction.
2. **Phase II:** All the exercises of phase-I, plus pelvic swing (bridging) exercises and bilateral straight leg raise exercises **(Figs. 28.23A and B)**.
3. **Phase III:** All the exercises performed during phase-I, II plus straight and diagonal curl ups for abdominal strengthening, provided if the patient does not have diastases recti (or a muscle separation > 2 finger width). The following exercises are performed gradually to return the woman back to function.

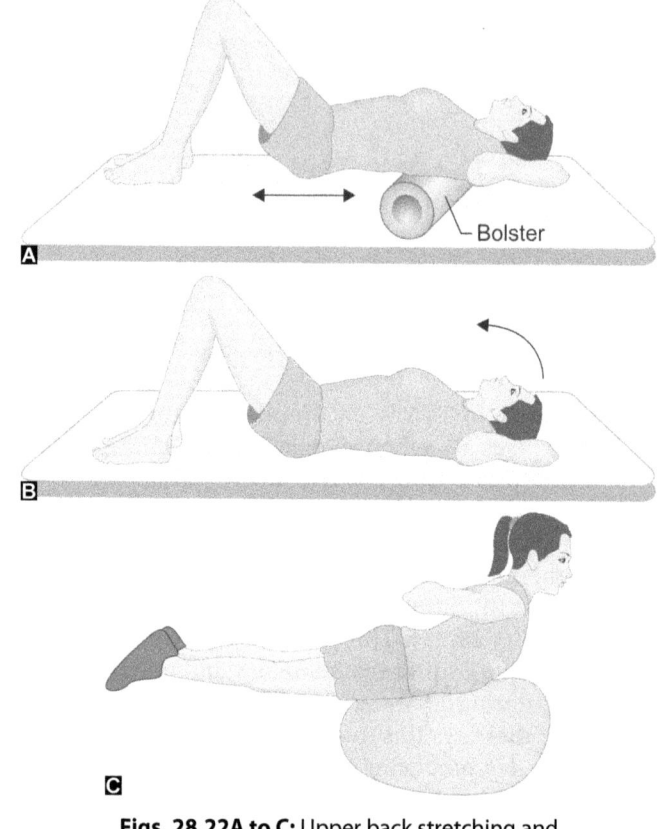

Figs. 28.22A to C: Upper back stretching and strengthening exercises.

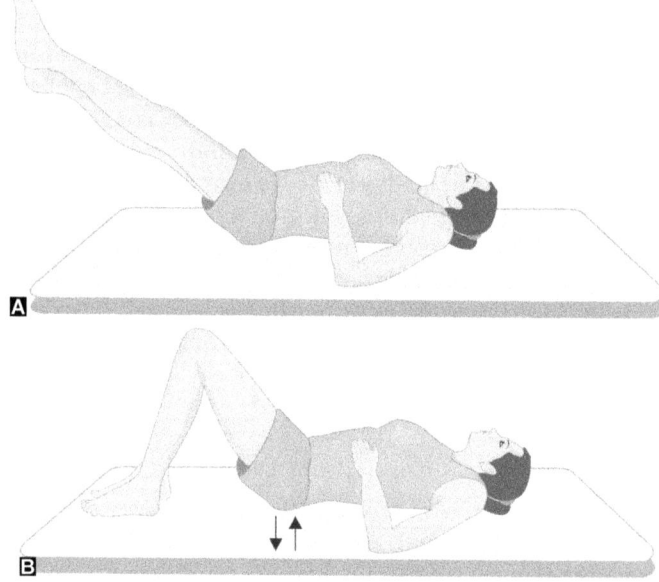

Figs. 28.23A and B: (A) Bilateral straight leg raise exercise; (B) Pelvic swing (bridging) exercise.

Pelvic floor exercise (Kegel's exercise-1): This exercise helps to build the strength and endurance of the muscles of the pelvic floor. The procedure involves:

The woman is either in sitting, lying or standing. She is advised to tighten the muscles around the anus (back passage) and vagina (front passage), as if trying to stop flow of urine or flatus. The contraction should be held as long as possible preferably for 10 seconds, followed by relaxation for 4 seconds. The contraction and relaxation should be performed for 10 times in a session and 3 sessions in a day should be performed in combination with pelvic floor exercise-2.

Pelvic floor exercise (Kegel's exercise-2): This exercise prepares the pelvic floor muscles to respond quickly to sudden stresses such as coughing, laughing correcting stress incontinence.

The following procedures are followed: The woman is either in sitting, lying or standing. She is advised to tighten the pelvic floor and hold the contraction for 1 second, before releasing the muscle. The contraction followed by relaxation is repeated for 10 times in a session and 3 sessions in a day should be performed along with exercise-1. **Figure 28.24** shows one pelvic floor muscle strengthening exercise.

Besides the pelvic floor strengthening exercises, other exercises performed are:

Knee rolls: The patient is asked to lie on back, with both the knees bent to 90 degrees and feet flat on bed. Keeping the knees together, she is asked to rotate both the knees toward right, followed by left. 3-5 rotations are made on each side **(Fig. 28.25)**.

Pelvic tilt exercise: In standing/sitting/lying, quadruped, the patient is asked to pull the lower abdominal muscles in and squeeze the buttock and gently flatten the small of the back. The muscle contractions are held for 10 seconds, while breathing normally. The muscles are then relaxed and 10 repetitions of the exercise 3 times a day is advised **(Fig. 28.26)**.

Besides the above, the followings are usually performed for gradual return to function **(Figs. 28.27A to F)**.

❖ Brisk walking
❖ Swimming
❖ Aqua aerobics
❖ Pilates **(Fig. 28.27A to F)**
❖ Yoga
❖ Low impact aerobics (Calisthenics exercises): Calisthenics is a form of strength training consisting of a variety of movements that exercise large muscle groups, such as standing, grasping, and pushing, catching and throwing a ball, kicking a ball, squat reaching, squat tap down, etc. These exercises are often performed rhythmically and with minimal equipment.
❖ Light weight resistance training **(Figs. 28.28A and B)**
❖ Static cycling exercises.

Besides the above, modalities such as TENS/IFT, etc., may be considered for relief of back pain. Lumbosacral belt/abdominal binder, etc., may be recommended if required. Other complications such as tendinitis, nerve compression syndromes, flat feet, etc., should be managed appropriately.

Physiotherapy after cesarean section delivery:
A cesarean section is a procedure in which the delivery of a baby is performed through an incision in the abdominal wall and uterus rather than through the pelvis and vagina.

Types of incision: Two types of incisions are used in cesarean section procedure such as:

❖ Lower segmental (Transverse incision): This incision is also known as "Pfannenstiel or bikini line incision", and is given over the lower segment of the uterus. This incision is made in the lower segment of the uterus, which heals faster and successfully than the incision in the upper segment of the uterus **(Fig. 28.29A)**.
❖ Upper segment/vertical/classical incision: This incision is given over the fundus and body of the uterus. The healing of the incisional wound is poorer as compared to lower segmental incision **(Fig. 28.29B)**.

The transverse incision is preferred over vertical incision as the wound heals faster in transverse incision with less bleeding and there is a chance of normal child birth in subsequent pregnancies. However, the condition of the mother and the fetus determines which type of incision will be used. The surgery is performed most commonly under spinal anesthesia, however, in some individuals, general anesthesia may be applicable. The optimum interval between uterine incisions and delivery of the baby should be less than 90 seconds.

Postoperative physiotherapy after cesarean section delivery

Like the postpartum management given to mothers who deliver normally, postoperative physiotherapy is also imparted to mothers who deliver through cesarean section, which is

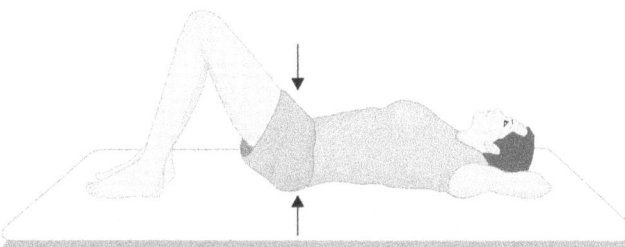

Fig. 28.24: Pelvic floor muscle strengthening exercise.

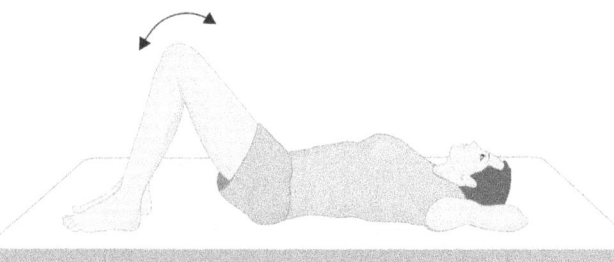

Fig. 28.25: Knee rolling.

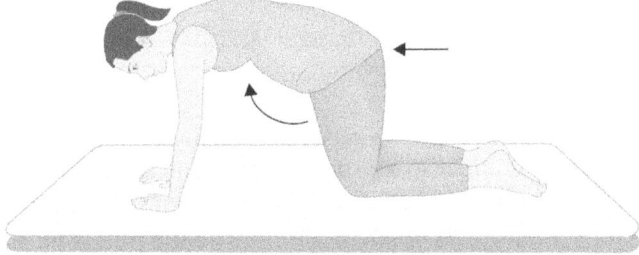

Fig. 28.26: Pelvic tilt exercise.

Section 4: Physiotherapy in Obstetrics and Gynecology

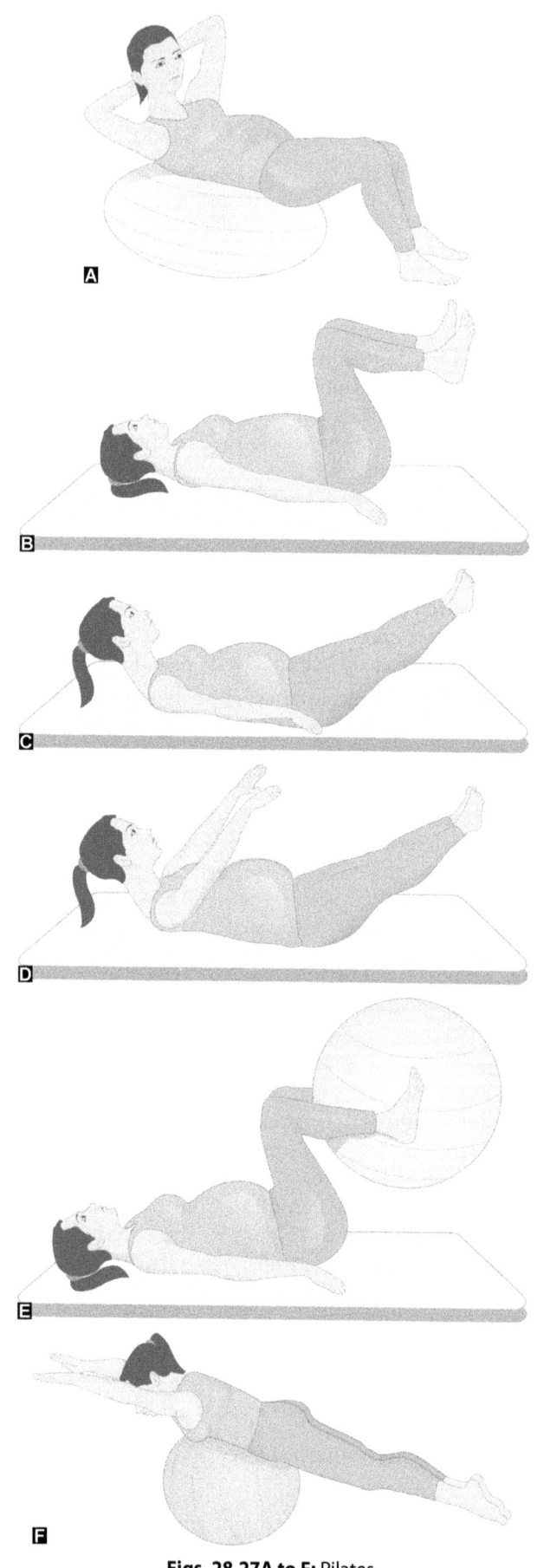

Figs. 28.27A to F: Pilates.

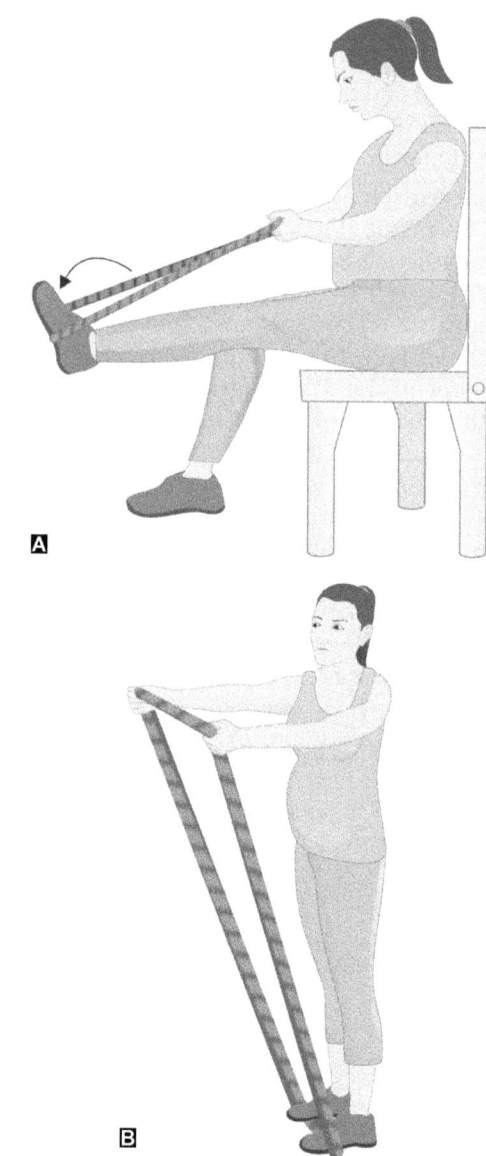

Figs. 28.28A and B: Light weight resistance training.

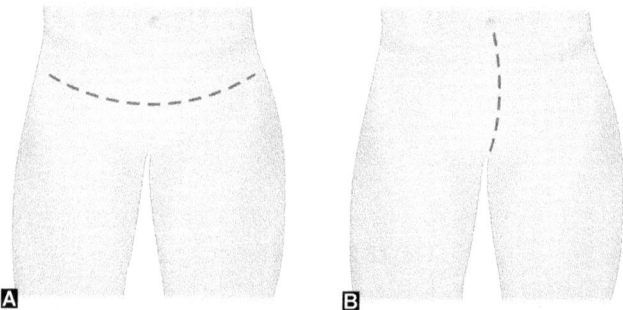

Figs. 28.29A and B: Types of incision: (A) Transverse incision; and (B) Vertical incision.

one major abdominal surgery. The patient may suffer from pulmonary complications, nonhealing of incisional wound, incisional wound pain and adhesions, sagging of abdomen due to weak abdominals, gastrointestinal complications, vascular complications, etc., which need intervention from a physiotherapist. Postoperative physiotherapy for these complications is discussed here.

a. **Management of incisional wound/incisional pain and incisional scar/adhesions:** The incisional wound, that is having poor healing, can be managed by using modalities such as low-intensity laser (LILT)/PSWD/IR/iontophoresis, etc., as applicable. If the woman is having incisional pain TENS with electrodes placed on either side of incision is applied at a frequency of 120 Hz, pulsed width 60 μs, intensity evoking strong tingling sensation and treatment duration 30 minutes. For tight incisional scar, abdominal myofascial release and deep scar mobilization may be beneficial.

b. **Management of pulmonary complications:** Immediately following surgery, gentle breathing exercises, huffing techniques to clear airways, protecting the incisional wound is advised. Gradually, after the incisional wound is healed, deep breathing exercises, thoracic expansion exercises, huffing and coughing techniques using abdominal support are performed to prevent pulmonary complications.

c. **Management of gastrointestinal complications:** Postoperative ileus (POI) where there is prolonged absence of bowel function, is a common gastrointestinal complication experienced following cesarean section surgeries. Postoperative ileus occurs when there is blockage of the intestines and is associated with failure of peristalsis (or the involuntary contractions of the digestive tract). Symptoms of POI include accumulation of gastrointestinal secretions and gas, distension of the abdomen, constipation, vomiting, and nausea. Acupressure, acupuncture, connective tissue massage are helpful for the management of this condition. Connective tissue massage is a type of reflex therapy that involves applying a shear force to the different fascial interfaces of the skin to stimulate autonomic nerve endings. Karakaya and colleagues (2012) reported benefits of connective tissue massage (CTM) in conjunction with posterior pelvic tilt exercises in the early return of intestinal function during post-cesarean section period.

d. **Management of vascular complications:** It is seen that the incidence of thromboembolism is five times higher in pregnant women as compared to normal population, the risk increases by 20 times during postpartum period. Pulmonary edema and edema in the lower limbs are also found in the woman during pregnancy. Passive

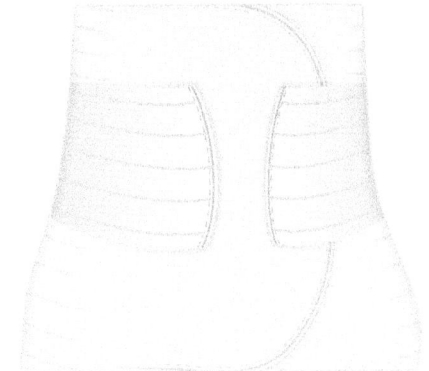

Fig. 28.30: Abdominal binder.

and active range of motion exercises, in combination with breathing exercises help in preventing these complications. Karakaya and colleagues (2012) stated that lower extremity exercise in combination with breathing exercises help to improve blood circulation, allow for early ambulation and reduce the side effects experienced from the anesthesia postoperatively.

e. **Retraining of function:** Following cesarean section delivery, lower limb exercises performed in combination with breathing exercises help to improve mobility, preventing complications and reducing the period of hospitalization, thereby enhances function. Studies reveal that early mobilization, sometimes between 6 and 24 hours postoperatively, helps to improve pulmonary function, reduces the risk of embolism, and decreases the length of hospital stay. Kinesio taping over the abdominals is also considered beneficial in combination with exercises to strengthen the abdominals and early return to function. A study by Gursen and colleagues (2016) looked at the effects of Kinesio taping (KT) combined with exercise and found that Kinesio taping application over rectus abdominis muscle, as well as the oblique muscles of the abdomen performed two times weekly for 4 weeks, led to significant improvement of abdominal strength and reduced pain. Use of an abdominal support **(Fig. 28.30)** postoperatively also helps in early return of function. Ghana and colleagues (2017) found that the use of abdominal binders can reduce postoperative pain and symptoms of distress following cesarean section delivery. The patient should be encouraged to perform light functional activities as tolerated with use of abdominal binder, which should be gradually progressed.

Physiotherapy in Gynecological Diseases

PHYSIOTHERAPY AFTER RADICAL MASTECTOMY

Breast cancer is the most common malignant lesion found in women. The management of breast cancer is in constant evolution. Fortunately, survival rates continue to improve, likely due to improved individualized treatment as well as earlier detection.

The increase in the number of breast cancer survivors necessitates improved care and interventions to improve the overall quality of life for women who have survived breast cancer.

Clinical Presentation of Breast Cancer

- Breast cancer may be asymptomatic and undetectable in its earlier stages.
- The hallmark signs and symptoms of a ductal carcinoma are a lump in the breast and breast tenderness (not usually painful).
- The hallmark signs and symptoms of a lobular carcinoma do not involve a lump. Therefore, a lobular carcinoma may be harder to detect.
- There is often a change in breast texture.
- Axillary lymph node enlargement or breathlessness (features of metastasis) occurs in advanced stage of the disease.

Management of Breast Cancer

The complete management of breast cancer is not described here and is not under the scope of this book. However, certain information relevant to physiotherapists is discussed here.

Physiotherapists have an important role in the rehabilitation process during and after a diagnosis of breast cancer, as well as in the care of survivors, particularly, after breast cancer surgery. An interprofessional teamwork is required to achieve the best possible outcomes. This team includes oncologic and plastic surgeons, medical oncologist, radiation oncologist, pathologist, physiotherapist, radiologist, nurses, and multiple other individuals to discuss about each patient and formulate a treatment plan.

Surgeries for Breast Cancer

There are two main types of surgery performed to remove breast cancer:

1. **Breast-conserving surgery (also called a lumpectomy, quadrantectomy, partial mastectomy, or segmental mastectomy):** In this surgery only the part of the breast containing the cancer is removed. The goal is to remove the cancer as well as some surrounding normal tissue. How much breast tissue is removed depends on where and how big the tumor is, as well as other factors.
2. **Mastectomy:** It is a surgery in which the entire breast is removed, including all of the breast tissue and sometimes other nearby tissues. There are several different types of mastectomies. Some women may also get a double mastectomy, in which both breasts are removed. When breast tissue is removed along with the adjoining lymph nodes, it is called modified radical mastectomy, whereas procedures involving removal of breast tissue, adjoining lymph nodes and underlying muscles of chest, are called radical mastectomy.

Radical Mastectomy

Radical mastectomy is a surgical procedure involving the removal of breast, underlying chest muscles (both pectoralis major and minor), as well as the adjoining axillary lymph nodes as a treatment of cancer of breast **(Fig. 29.1)**.

Modified radical mastectomy: It is a procedure that involves removal of the entire breast, including the skin, breast tissue, areola, and nipple along with most of the axillary lymph nodes. However, most of the chest muscles are left intact.

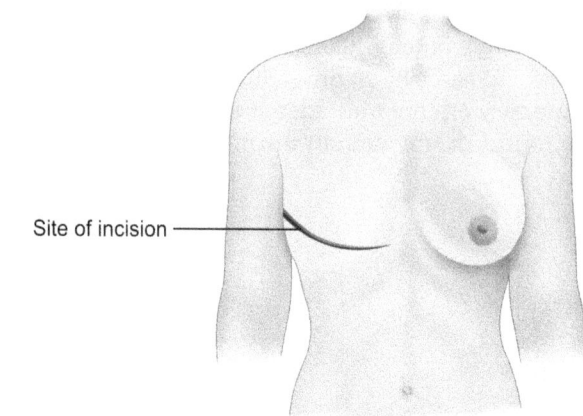

Fig. 29.1: The incision site for mastectomy/radical mastectomy.

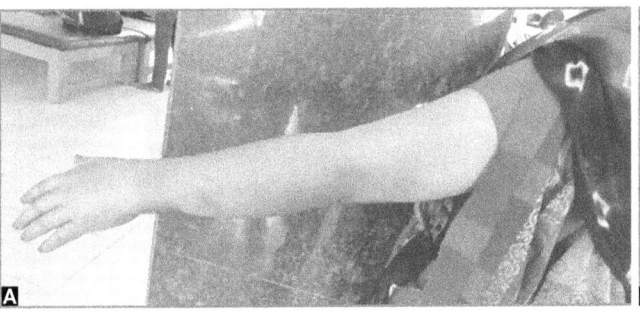 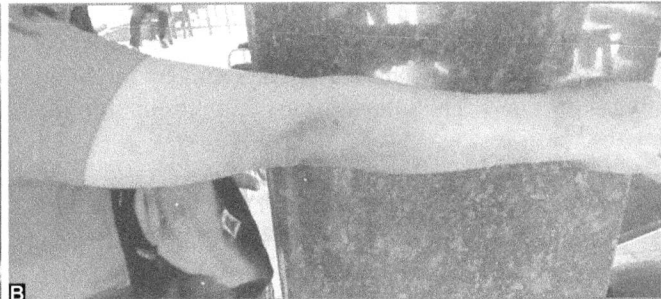

Figs. 29.2A and B: (A) Lymphedema of left upper limb following radical mastectomy; (B) Normal right upper limb.

There are two types of modified radical mastectomy such as:
1. **Patey's operation (Patey modified radical mastectomy):** In this type, the pectoralis major muscle is maintained, but the pectoralis minor muscle removed.
2. **Auchincloss modified radical mastectomy:** In this type, both the pectoralis major and pectoralis minor are maintained.

Complications after radical mastectomy
- **Swelling over the affected side upper limb (lymphedema):** As the lymphatic return from the upper limb is significantly compromised due to removal of the lymph nodes, causing closure of the lymphatic channels that drain fluid from the upper limb to the neck and trunk, swelling develops in the affected side upper limb **(Figs. 29.2A and B).**
- **Stiffness of shoulder:** Frozen shoulder causing pain and stiffness of shoulder is a common complication after modified radical mastectomy/radical mastectomy, which develops due to tight scar that is formed at the site of incision.
- **Nerve sensitivity/numbness at the surgical site:** Numbness and/or nerve sensitivity may develop at the surgical site causing pain and discomfort.
- **Axillary web syndrome or cording:** This complication develops due to dissection of axillary lymph nodes. Cording presents as a moderate to painful tightening, which appears as "cords" emanating from the armpit and extending down the arm. Cording significantly restricts range of motion and arm function, and is also a cause of frozen shoulder in such patients.
- **Chest tightness:** Due to the incisional scar, the patient is likely to develop stiffness of the chest, leading to difficulty in breathing and discomfort.
- **Spinal deformity:** Scoliosis with concavity on the operated side and kyphosis is found in majority of patients after surgery.
- **Psychological issues:** Psychological issues causing depression, and decreased quality of living is found in most sufferers.

Physiotherapy after radical mastectomy
The aims of physiotherapy after radical mastectomy include:
- Reduction of edema of affected side upper limb
- Reduction of chest tightness
- Improves ventilation
- Improves range of motion of shoulder on the affected side
- Increases strength of muscles on the affected side upper limb
- Reduction of pain (if any)
- Improvement of posture by correcting deformities
- Improvement of functional mobility
- Improvement of sensation at the surgical site
- Improvement of quality of life

Physiotherapy early intervention strategies after radical mastectomy

Early rehabilitation is implemented to promote functional movement to restore the patient's previous level of activity. Exercises to maintain shoulder range of motion and arm mobility may be started as early as 24 hours after surgery. The following guidelines may be observed in the early postoperative days:
- Passive shoulder movements are implemented on the first or second-day postoperatively (preferably within first week).
- Active exercises to shoulder and upper limb are started after second week.
- Mobilizations are performed using joint rotations to tolerance but abduction and flexion of shoulder are limited to 40°.
- At day 4, postoperatively, flexion and abduction are gradually increased to 45°, this can be increased furthermore by 10–15° per day depending on the patient's pain tolerance.
- The mobilization techniques are performed by holding the patients arm in 45° flexion or abduction until the drains are removed.
- Secondary lymphedema is very common after the surgery, affecting the patients' quality of life to great extent and the same is managed through complete decongestive therapy (complete decongestive therapy, also called complex decongestive therapy, is an intensive program to reduce secondary lymphedema after breast cancer surgery, that combines many different treatment approaches such as crepe bandaging/compression garments, manual lymphatic drainage, exercises and self-care).

Physiotherapy treatment strategies during the rehabilitation phase after radical mastectomy

Various exercises and interventions are applied during the phase of rehabilitation, to reduce the complications associated with the disease and after surgery. Various exercises are designed by the therapists to restore range of motion, muscle strength and improve circulation (reduce edema). As rehabilitation progresses, these exercises may be modified to meet new goals. The interventions applied include the following:

- Positioning of the affected upper limb, with the hand elevated above the chest level, to prevent fluid accumulation.
- Relaxed passive exercises to the affected upper limb.
- **Active exercises:** Active exercises are advised to improve and maintain tissue extensibility, joint range of motion, venous and lymphatic return and for facilitation of normal movement pattern to improve the muscle strength and endurance. Gradually progressive resisted exercises with the resistance offered by therabands/weight cuffs are applied to the affected upper limb.
- Myofascial release techniques are applied at the surgical site after the wound has healed for enhancing the extensibility of the tight scar/soft tissues.
- Joint mobilization exercises are applied for mobilization of stiff shoulder.
- Neurodynamic techniques are applied to reduce pain in the upper limb.
- Breathing exercises (both diaphragmatic and costal) are advised to improve chest expansion/ventilation, as well as for promotion of venous and lymphatic return.
- Massage (effleurage) are applied to drain fluid from the affected upper limb and to reduce edema.
- Faradism under pressure to the affected side upper limb is applied to reduce edema. Once the edema is reduced, maintenance of circulation in the affected side (upper limb) is obtained through application of crepe bandage/elastic stockings.
- Pain (if any) should be controlled by the use of transcutaneous electrical nerve stimulation (TENS).
- Aerobic exercises such as brisk walking, running, static cycle exercises can be advised to improve cardiorespiratory as well as muscular endurance.
- Functional re-education, using the affected upper limb should be promoted, as possible and tolerated.
- Referral of the patient to the prosthetist should be made for the silicone breast prosthesis.
- Counseling of the patient should be made to use the prosthesis for a better body image, to do regular exercises and functional activities as tolerated to live a better quality of life.

PHYSIOTHERAPY AFTER HYSTERECTOMY

Hysterectomy is an operation for removal of the uterus, and sometimes other reproductive organs such as the ovaries, cervix and the fallopian tubes. The surgery is performed either through general anesthesia (for open abdominal incisions) or through spinal anesthesia (laparoscopic procedures).

There are different types of hysterectomies such as:
- **Total abdominal hysterectomy:** Removal of the uterus and the cervix through an abdominal incision.
- **Subtotal hysterectomy:** In this procedure, only the uterus is removed.
- **Laparoscopic hysterectomy:** In this, the uterus is removed through the vagina, and only small incisions are made in the abdomen to insert the camera and probe.
- **Vaginal hysterectomy:** Removal of uterus and/or cervix by giving an incision in the upper part of vagina.
- **Radical or Wertheim's hysterectomy:** It is done in malignant lesions, where the uterus, cervix, fallopian tubes, and parts of the vagina are removed.

Indications for Hysterectomy

- Uterine fibroids, which are painful
- Prolapsed uterus
- Malignancy

Physiotherapy Prior to a Hysterectomy (Preoperative Physiotherapy)

It includes:
- Upper limb strengthening exercises.
- Pelvic floor muscle strengthening exercises (**Figs. 29.3A and B**)
- Exercises for rectus abdominis (sometimes cut in transverse incisions, and mostly separated) and aponeuroses of oblique and transverse muscles called rectus sheath, that surrounds the rectus abdominis muscle which is cut in open abdominal procedures (**Figs. 29.4A and B**).
- Cardiorespiratory exercises such as breathing exercises, static cycle exercise, walking, hydrotherapy, etc.
- Lower limb strengthening exercises.

Incision for total and subtotal hysterectomy: The incision given could be transverse or vertical type (**Figs. 29.5A and B**). A vertical incision, which starts in the middle of the abdomen and extends from just below the navel to just above the pubic bone. This incision is preferred, as it gives better access to the pelvis. A horizontal transverse bikini-line incision, lies about

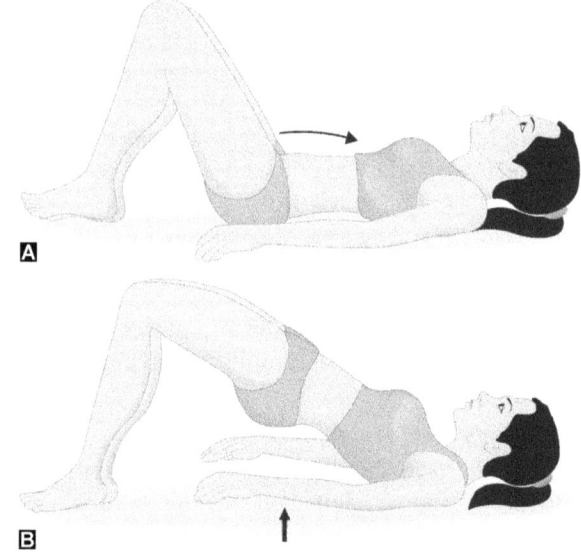

Figs. 29.3A and B: Pelvic floor strengthening exercise: (A) Pelvic floor squeeze and lift; (B) Pelvic bridging exercise.

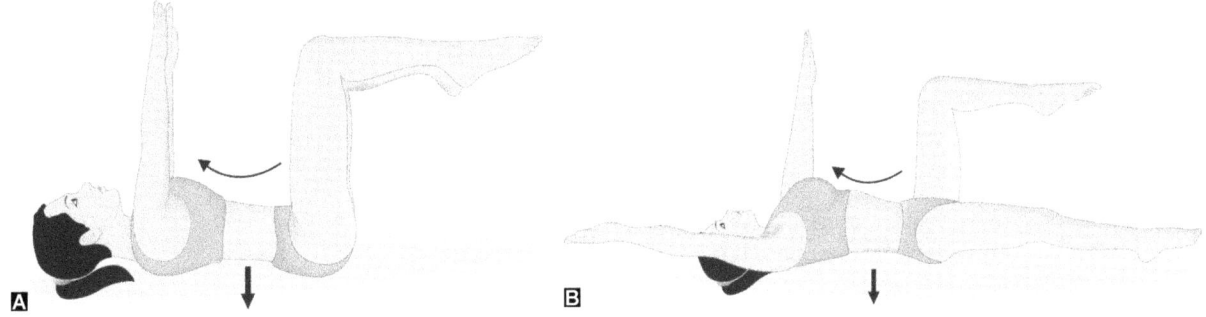

Figs. 29.4A and B: Transverse abdominis strengthening exercises.

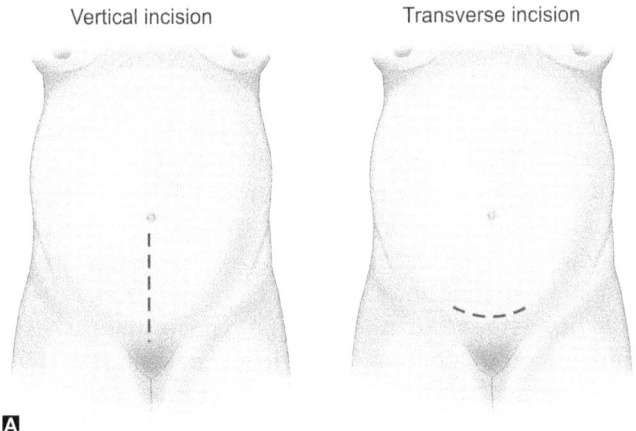

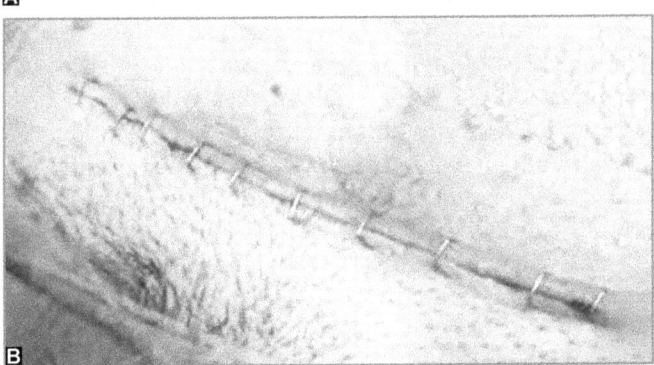

Figs. 29.5A and B: (A) Types of incision—vertical and transverse type; (B) Transverse incision for hysterectomy.

an inch above the pubic bone. This incision produces a thin scar, as it follows the natural lines of skin.

Recovery from a hysterectomy is often quite long and physiotherapy is a very effective way to help gradual return to full fitness as soon as possible.

Physiotherapy Following a Hysterectomy (Postoperative Physiotherapy)

Following surgery, the patient may remain in hospital for 5–7 days, depending on the type of hysterectomy. During this period she is advised to do active ankle and foot exercises, gentile breathing exercises and walk around the bed. Secretions accumulating (if any) in the lungs, should be removed through huffing/coughing, with protection of the incision using a sterile pad/pillow. After discharge from the hospital, week-wise physiotherapy is provided as discussed here, which can be performed as a home exercise program/outpatient basis.

Week 1 (Post-discharge)

- Passive range of motion exercises
- Breathing exercise protecting the incision. Pain after surgery may make breathing difficult. The patient should be advised to take 4–5 deep breaths slowly every hour.
- Lower limb elevation and strengthening exercises
- Scar management after the stiches are removed.
- Pelvic floor strengthening (Kegel's exercises) exercises should be performed to prevent sagging of pelvic organs down. The patient is advised to squeeze the buttock, as if trying to stop flow of urine or flatus. A minimum of 10 long squeezes and 50 quick squeezes should be done every day **(Fig. 29.3)**.
- Transverse abdominis muscle strengthening exercise, should be performed by pulling the belly button up and inwards (slowly during the 1st week, gradually increasing the intensity of exercise, in subsequent weeks) holding for 10 seconds followed by relaxing the muscle. A minimum of 10 contractions should be done daily protecting the incisional sutures **(Fig. 29.4)**. Gradually exercises for rectus abdominis and internal oblique should be added and progressed.
- Pain control at the site of incision by using modalities such as TENS, where electrodes are placed on either side of the incision, the frequency and intensity are controlled to have a strong tingling sensation, without producing contraction of abdominals.

Week 2–6 (Post-discharge)

By this time the patients' symptoms are reduced significantly and the patient is able to return to normal daily routine gradually. Physiotherapy during this period includes:

- Passive range of motion exercises to continue.
- Breathing exercises to continue.
- Strengthening exercises to lower and upper limbs and abdominals (transverse abdominis/rectus abdominis and internal oblique/external oblique).
- Pelvic floor strengthening exercises.
- Functional activities with pacing.

Week 7 onwards (Post-discharge)

The exercises performed during weeks 2–6 are continued in this period. By this time the patient gradually returns to activities, and is able to perform lifting of light load, even though she is advised not to lift heavy load for up to 6 months.

PHYSIOTHERAPY IN PELVIC INFLAMMATORY DISEASE

Pelvic inflammatory disease (PID) is an inflammatory condition of the female reproductive organs (uterus, ovary and fallopian tubes) mostly caused by infection. It primarily affects the upper genital tract in females.

Causes of Pelvic Inflammatory Disease

The disease is caused mostly by bacterial infection, and in most cases the infection spreads through sexual activities. Untreated gonorrhea and chlamydia cause about 90% of PID cases. Other causes include:
- Abortion
- Childbirth
- Pelvic procedures
- Insertion of an intrauterine device (IUD), either copper or hormonal

Pathophysiology

Bacteria entering the reproductive tract cause PID. These bacteria are passed from the vagina, through the cervix, into the uterus, fallopian tubes and ovaries, and into the pelvis, causing infection of these organs and resulting in inflammation. Normally, when bacteria enter the vagina, the cervix prevents them from spreading deeper to other reproductive organs. But sometimes, the cervix becomes infected from infections such as gonorrhea and chlamydia. When this happens, the cervix is less able to keep bacteria out, causing the pathology.

Clinical Features

Common symptoms of this ailment are pain in the lower abdomen along with fever and/or vomiting. There might also be discharge from vagina and irregular menstruation. It might also be accompanied by a severe diarrhea and dysuria (painful urination).

Management of Pelvic Inflammatory Disease

Since the causative agent in 60-70% of cases is microbial infection (gonococcal and chlamydial infections being more common), the first avenue of treatment employs pharmacological agents such as antibiotics that help to control the spread of infection and eradicate the cause. In many cases, antibiotic treatment is supported with physiotherapy to address the other symptoms associated with the disease.

Physiotherapy for Pelvic Inflammatory Disease

Physiotherapy aids the pharmacological treatment of PID in different capacities at different stages of progression of the disease. The physiotherapy management in various stages of the disease is discussed briefly as under:
1. **Acute stage:** In mild and moderate (acute) cases of PID, physiotherapy is used to relieve the pain and inflammation.

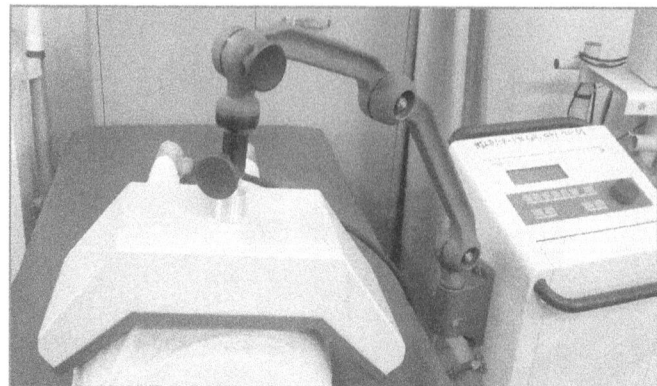

Fig. 29.6: Application of MWD to pelvis.

Pulsed shortwave diathermy (PSWD) using the crossfire technique for a short period (5-10 minutes) three times a week is helpful in this stage. Gradually, the frequency, intensity, and treatment duration of PSWD should be increased to produce mild thermal effect. The heat produced by PSWD, causes increase of circulation, which promotes healing and reduces pain.

2. **Chronic stage:** At the chronic stages of the disease, physiotherapy aims not only to relieve pain and promote healing around the area, but also aims to increase functional movement and treat musculoskeletal dysfunction (if any). Shortwave diathermy thermal dose using crossfire method/ microwave diathermy (MWD) **(Fig. 29.6)** is given for 15-30 minutes, twice a day, three times a week, with an aim to increase circulation and health of pelvic floor muscles and organs, resulting in increase of metabolic activities, helping in loosening of scar tissue and promoting healing.

Transcutaneous electrical nerve stimulation is also applied to the back, if the patient experiences back pain. The patient is also advised to take moist hot packs at home if she feels pain and discomfort.

Pelvic floor muscle rehabilitation is also required in this disease, as these muscles get inhibited during inflammation, because of pain and immobility.

Pelvic Floor Muscle Rehabilitation

Evidence exists regarding pelvic floor muscle dysfunction in women with pelvic disorders. Therefore, pelvic floor rehabilitation is part of the treatment for PID that causes pain and dysfunction. Common treatment interventions for pelvic floor muscles include:
- Kegel's exercises
- Electrical stimulation to pelvic floor muscles
- Electromyography (EMG) biofeedback
- Relaxation exercises

Sometimes, when the extent of damage is more, pharmacology and physiotherapy are not sufficient to treat the disease. Circumstances may call for surgical procedures. However, physiotherapy can help in the recovery of the pelvic muscle action post-surgery.

SECTION

Physiotherapy for Pulmonary and Cardiac Conditions: Pulmonary Rehabilitation and Cardiac Rehabilitation

Section Outline

Chapter 30: Pulmonary Rehabilitation
Chapter 31: Cardiac Rehabilitation

Pulmonary Rehabilitation

INTRODUCTION

Patients suffering from obstructive pulmonary disease such as bronchial asthma, chronic bronchitis, bronchiectasis, emphysema, cystic fibrosis, etc., as well as restrictive pulmonary diseases such as pleurisy, empyema, bronchopneumonia, idiopathic pulmonary fibrosis, etc., have a reduced exercise/activity tolerance, due either to more residual air in the lungs as seen in obstructive pulmonary conditions, or decreased inflation of the lungs as seen in restrictive pulmonary conditions.

Irrespective of the type of pathology, it is clear that chest physiotherapy and pulmonary rehabilitation is of value for all patients in whom respiratory symptoms have resulted in decreased functional capacity resulting in a decreased quality of life.

Besides direct pulmonary pathologies, sufferers of scoliosis, kyphosis, spinal cord injuries, myopathies, motor neuron disease, cardiac disease, etc., also need chest physiotherapy.

INTRODUCTION TO RESPIRATORY SYSTEM

When the respiratory system is mentioned, people generally think of breathing, but breathing is only one of the activities of the respiratory system. The body cells need a continuous supply of oxygen for the metabolic processes that are necessary to maintain life. The respiratory system works with the circulatory system to provide this oxygen and to remove the waste products of metabolism. It also helps to regulate pH of the blood.

Respiration is the sequence of events that result in the exchange of oxygen and carbon dioxide between the atmosphere and the body cells. In every 3–5 seconds, nerve impulses stimulate the breathing process, or ventilation, which moves air through a series of passages into and out of the lungs. After this, there is an exchange of gases between the lungs and the blood. This is called an external respiration. The blood transports the gases to and from the tissue cells. The exchange of gases between the blood and tissue cells is internal respiration. Finally, the cells utilize the oxygen for their specific activities: this is called cellular metabolism, or cellular respiration. Together, these activities constitute respiration.

The respiratory conducting passages/respiratory system are divided into the upper respiratory tract and the lower respiratory tract (**Fig. 30.1**). The upper respiratory tract includes the nose, pharynx, and larynx. The lower respiratory tract consists of the trachea, bronchial tree, and lungs. These tracts open to the outside and are lined with mucous membranes. In some regions, the membrane has hairs that help to filter the air. Other regions may have cilia to propel mucus.

MECHANICS OF VENTILATION/BREATHING

Ventilation or breathing is the movement of air through the conducting passages between the atmosphere and the lungs. The air moves through the passages because of pressure gradients that are produced by contraction of the diaphragm and thoracic muscles. The process of air flowing into the lungs is called inspiration and air flowing out of the lungs is called expiration (described below). In normal breathing that occurs at a rate of 12–16 cycles per minute, the inspiration is an active process brought about by the contraction of diaphragm and external intercostal muscles and expiration is a passive process brought about by the recoil of elastic tissues. However, in forceful expiration, that usually occurs during airways clearance, the abdominals and internal intercostals muscles contract.

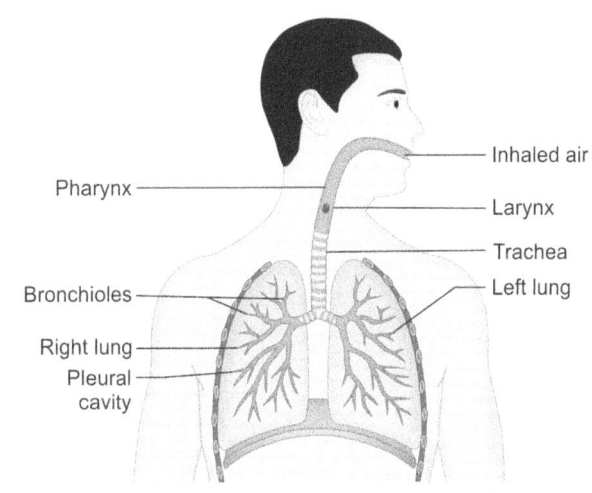

Fig. 30.1: Respiratory system.

Inspiration

Inspiration (inhalation) is the process of taking air into the lungs. It is the active phase of ventilation that results from muscle contraction. During inspiration, the diaphragm, external intercostal muscles, and intercartilaginous portion of the internal intercostals muscles contract, and the thoracic cavity increases in volume. This decreases the intra-alveolar pressure, so that air flows into the lungs. During forceful inspiration/laboured breathing, the accessory muscles also undergo contraction along with diaphragm and external intercostal muscle.

Expiration

Expiration (exhalation) is the process of letting air out of the lungs during the breathing cycle. During expiration, the relaxation of the diaphragm and elastic recoil of tissue decreases the thoracic volume and increases the intra-alveolar pressure. Expiration pushes air out of the lungs. However, during forceful expiration, the abdominals and interosseous portion of internal intercostals muscles contract **(Table 30.1)**.

RESPIRATORY PHYSIOLOGY

When we breathe in, air is inspired through the nose or mouth, through the conducting airways, and reaches the distal respiratory units, which contains the respiratory bronchiole, alveolar ducts, alveolar sacs, and alveoli. At full inspiration, the lungs contain maximum amount of air, called total lung capacity (TLC), which is the combination of so many volumes such as, tidal volume (TV), inspiratory reserve volume (IRV), expiratory reserve volume (ERV), and residual volume **(Fig. 30.2)**.

The lung volumes and capacities and their normal values are discussed below:

Tidal volume (TV): The amount of air inspired or expired, during normal resting ventilation is called tidal volume.

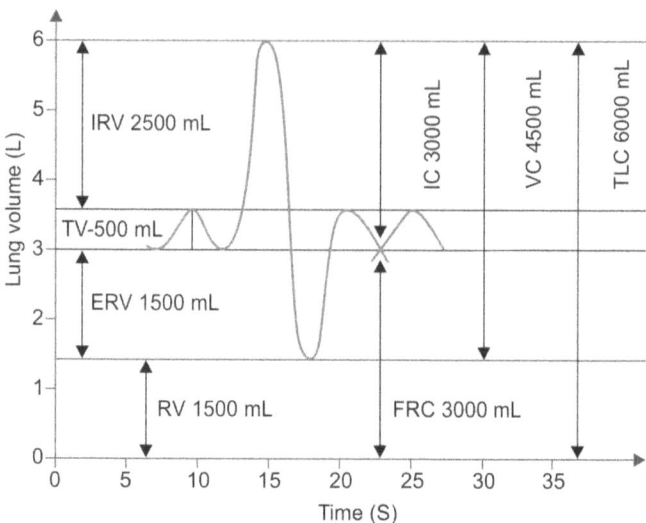

Fig. 30.2: Normal lung capacities and volumes.

Though normal TV is 500 mL, only 350 mL of air takes part in gas exchange and the remaining 150 mL of air remains in the conducting airways and does not take part in gas exchange.

Inspiratory reserve volume (IRV): After tidal inspiration, the amount of air that can be further inspired is called inspiratory reserve volume —2500 mL.

Expiratory reserve volume (ERV): The amount of air that can be expired forcefully after tidal expiration is called expiratory reserve volume—1500 mL.

Residual volume (RV): The amount of air remaining in the lungs after a forceful expiration—1,500 mL.

Inspiratory capacity (IC): It is the amount of air that can be inspired after a tidal expiration. It is the sum of TV and IRV. Its value is 3,000 mL.

Functional residual capacity (FRC): It is the sum of ERV and RV. Its value is 3,000 mL.

Vital capacity (VC): It is the maximum amount of air that can be inspired after a forceful expiration. It is the combination of three lung volumes, i.e., ERV, TV, and IRV. Its value in a healthy adult (male) is 4,500 mL.

Total lung capacity (TLC): It is the total air-holding capacity of lung, which is the sum of RV, ERV, TV, and IRV. Its value is 6,000 mL.

The lung volumes are altered significantly in obstructive and restrictive diseases, which can be understood from **Figure 30.3**.

Lung Compliance

Compliance describes the distensibility of lung tissue. It is defined as the change in lung volume per change in transmural or transpulmonary pressure, expressed symbolically as $\Delta V/\Delta P$. The lung can be compared to a balloon during inspiration, where there exists a tendency to collapse or recoil while inflated. To maintain inflation, the transmural pressure or pressure difference between the intrapulmonary pressure and intrapleural pressure must be

Table 30.1: Muscles of ventilation.	
Muscles of inspiration	**Muscles of forceful expiration**
Primary muscles: Diaphragm, External intercostal muscles, Intercartilaginous portion of the internal intercostals muscles **Accessory muscles:** The sternocleidomastoid, scalenes, serratus anterior, pectoralis major and minor, trapezius, and erector spinae muscles	**Abdominal muscles:** The abdominal muscles include the rectus abdominis, transversus abdominis, and internal and external obliques. These muscles work to raise intra-abdominal pressure when a sudden expulsion of air is required in maneuvers such as huffing and coughing. Pressure generated within the abdominal cavity is transmitted to the thoracic cage to assist in emptying the lungs
	Internal intercostal muscle: The posterior aspect on the internal intercostal muscles is termed as the interosseous portion that depresses the ribs to aid in a forceful expiration

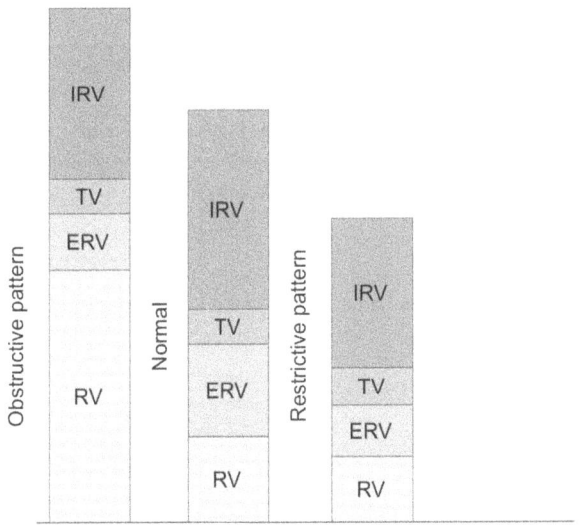

Fig. 30.3: Lung volumes in obstructive and restrictive lung diseases.

maintained. A given transpulmonary pressure, will cause a greater or lesser degree of lung expansion, depending on the distensibility or compliance of the lung. The compliance of the lung is reduced by factors that produce a resistance to distension such as emphysema, pulmonary fibrosis, etc. Also, the compliance is reduced as the lung approaches its TLC, where it becomes relatively stiffer and less distensible. In obstructive and restrictive pulmonary conditions the compliance of the lungs are reduced, affecting exercise tolerance and function, therefore, the need for pulmonary rehabilitation.

Table 30.2 briefly describes the obstructive and restrictive lung diseases.

Physiotherapy Interventions in Pulmonary Conditions

A physiotherapist is actively involved in the management of pulmonary conditions through:
1. Respiratory system assessment.
2. **Application of chest clearance techniques (Postural drainage):** Discussed in pulmonary rehabilitation.
3. **Designing appropriate breathing exercises/breathing strategies/breath control training programs:** Discussed in pulmonary rehabilitation.
4. Pulmonary rehabilitation.

Table 30.2: Obstructive and restrictive lung diseases.	
Obstructive pulmonary diseases	**Restrictive pulmonary diseases**
About the disease: Obstructive lung disease is a category of respiratory disease characterized by airway obstruction. Many obstructive diseases of the lung result from narrowing (obstruction) of the smaller bronchi and larger bronchioles, often because of excessive contraction of the smooth muscle itself. It is generally characterized by inflamed and easily collapsible airways, obstruction to airflow, and problems in exhaling air. At the end of a full exhalation, an abnormally high amount of air may still remain in the lungs (high residual volume)	**About the disease:** • Restrictive lung disease refers to a group of lung diseases that prevent the lungs from fully expanding with air. This restriction makes breathing difficult. Many forms of restrictive lung disease are progressive, getting worse over time. However, some causes of restrictive lung disease can be reversed • Restrictive lung diseases are a category of extrapulmonary, pleural, or parenchymal respiratory diseases that restrict lung expansion resulting in a decreased lung volume, an increased work of breathing, and inadequate ventilation and/or oxygenation. Pulmonary function test demonstrates a decrease in the forced vital capacity
Types a. Chronic obstructive pulmonary disease (COPD), which includes emphysema and chronic bronchitis b. Asthma c. Bronchiectasis ➢ Cystic fibrosis	**Types** • Interstitial lung disease, such as idiopathic pulmonary fibrosis • Sarcoidosis, an autoimmune disease • Obesity, including obesity hypoventilation syndrome • Scoliosis • Neuromuscular disease, such as muscular dystrophy or amyotrophic lateral sclerosis (ALS) • Pneumonia • Pulmonary tuberculosis • Lung cancers • Fibrosis caused by radiation • Infant and acute respiratory distress syndrome • Pleural effusions • Empyema • Myasthenia gravis • Rib damage, especially fractures • Ascites, or abdominal swelling connected with liver scarring or cancer • Diaphragm paralysis • Kyphosis, or hunching of the upper back • Diaphragmatic hernia • Heart failure

Contd...

Contd...

Obstructive pulmonary diseases	Restrictive pulmonary diseases
Signs and symptoms: COPD symptoms often don't appear until significant lung damage has occurred, and they usually worsen over time, particularly if smoking and exposure to allergens continues. For chronic bronchitis, the main symptom is a daily cough and mucus (sputum) production at least three months a year for two consecutive years. Other signs and symptoms of COPD may include: • Shortness of breath (dyspnea), especially during physical activities. • Wheezing/crackles. • Chest tightness • Excess expectorations in the morning. • Chronic cough that may produce mucus (sputum) that may be clear, white, yellow or greenish. • Blueness of the lips, tongue, or finger nail beds (cyanosis) • Frequent respiratory infections. • Lack of energy. • Unintended weight loss (in later stages) • Swelling in ankles, feet or legs. People with COPD are also likely to experience episodes called exacerbations, during which their symptoms become worse than usual day-to-day variation and persist for at least several days.	**Signs and symptoms:** • Shortness of breath (Dyspnea), especially with exertion. • Chronic cough, usually dry, but sometimes accompanied by mucoid sputum. • Weight loss • Chest pain • Wheezing. • Fatigue or extreme exhaustion without a logical reason. • Depression • Anxiety

Respiratory System Assessment

The physiotherapist dealing with patients with cardio-respiratory disorders should make a comprehensive assessment of the patient, not only to plan his/her intervention, but also to refer the patient to the appropriate specialists for different medical and surgical issues and to manage complications (if any). The components of assessment are:

Subjective examination: The subjective examination is an important part of the client experience. It allows the clients to express their symptoms from their viewpoints and help to guide the objective examination and plan a treatment program with the client's needs at the forefront. Each subjective examination should include the following components:

❖ **Biological and demographic data:**
  – Name
  – Age
  – Gender
  – Living situation
❖ **Current symptoms/current health:**
  – *Cough:* Note should be made of the nature of cough such as described below, and when and how it developed. The cough types could be:
    » Dry
    » Hacking
    » Hoarse
    » Congested
    » Barking
    » Wheezy
  – *Dyspnea:* Difficulty in breathing is a common manifestation in the sufferers with pulmonary dysfunction. It manifests by shortness of breath, suffocation, chest tightness.
  – *Chest pain:* The physiotherapist/clinician should be able to differentiate between chest pain of cardiac and noncardiac origin. The location, intensity and duration of chest pain help to determine the cause of the chest pain. Pleuritic chest pain is sharp, stabbing type of pain that increases with breathing and chest wall movements and is confined to one location in the chest.
    Angina pectoris (cardiac chest pain) is a heavy, squeezing, and aching sensation with feeling of pressure or tightness in the substernal area and often radiates to neck and arm.
  – *Deposition of secretions:* Whether the individual presents with crepitus sound in the chest, suggesting accumulation of secretions.
  – *Hemoptysis:* It is the expectoration of blood through the mouth. It is commonly found in chronic bronchitis, bronchiectasis, pulmonary tuberculosis, cystic fibrosis, pneumonia, lung cancer, lung abscesses, etc.
  – *Wheeze:* It is the musical sound produced, when air is passed through the partially obstructed or narrowed airways, which may be audible to outside or through the stethoscope.
  – *Crackles (Rales):* Crackles occur, when the small air sacs in the lungs are filled with fluid. This is a series of short explosive sounds like bubbling, rattling or clicking, most likely occurring during inspiration and may also be found during expiration. It could be fine crackles or coarse crackles, suggesting accumulation of secretion in the lungs.
  – *Stridor:* It is the high-pitched whistling sound produced, when air enters through partially obstructed or narrowed airways. It is often heard during the inspiration.
  – Decreased level of activity and decreased quality of life.

- **History:** It includes:
  - *History of present illness:* It includes the following:
    » Onset: Sudden or gradual
    » Site, intensity, type, aggravating factor, and relieving factor (SITAR)
    » Duration: Frequency or chronology (seasonal or daily variations)
    » Characteristics: Quality or severity
    » Current situation: Improving or deteriorating
    » Effect on activity of daily living (ADL)
    » Previous diagnosis of similar episodes
    » Previous treatment and efficacy
  - *Past medical history:* History of any chest infection/injury in the past such as tuberculosis, bronchitis, asthma, or any other upper/lower respiratory tract infections, and any surgery in the chest conducted therein. Any history of diabetes, high blood pressure, etc., should also be collected.
  - *Family health history:* Review should be made of the family data regarding the upper and lower respiratory tract diseases.
  - *Personal history:* It contains information regarding smoking, sleep disturbances, exercise tolerance, occupation, living home environment, etc.
  - *History of allergies:* The client should be asked about the history of allergies and precipitating and aggravating factors for the current illness such as certain foods, medicines, pollens, smoke, fume, dust, etc.
  - *Psychosocial history:* This includes information regarding living and work environment, hobbies, occupation, nutrition, exercise, and stresses faced in family and workplace.
  - *Dietary history:* As maintaining nutritious diet is important for clients with chronic respiratory disease, due to greater workload for the lungs and increased caloric expenditure, the dietary history should be taken.

Systems review: The systems review is a brief examination of all systems that would affect the ability of the patient to "initiate, sustain, and modify purposeful movement for the performance of actions, tasks, or activities that are important for function". The systems review is a limited examination performed prior to the full examination and used as a screening of all the major systems. The systems review includes the assessment of the following:

- Communication ability, affect, cognition, language, and learning style
- The cardiovascular and pulmonary systems, with an examination of the heart rate, respiratory rate, blood pressure, and presence of edema.
- The musculoskeletal system, with an examination of gross symmetry, gross range of motion, gross strength, height, and weight.
- The neuromuscular system, including an examination of gross movement involving balance, gait, locomotion, transfers, and transition as well as motor control and motor learning.
- The integument system, including examination of pliability (texture), presence of scar formation, skin color, and skin integrity.

The results of the systems review should be documented in the chart.

Physical/Objective examination: It includes:

- **Examination of vital signs such as:**
  - Level of consciousness
  - Temperature
  - Pulse
  - Respiratory rate
  - Blood pressure
  - Oxygen saturation (SpO_2)
- **General appearance:**
  - Body weight.
  - Height.
  - Nails – clubbing (**Fig. 30.4A**).
  - Eyes: Pallor (anemia); Plethora (high hemoglobin); Jaundice.
  - Tongue and mouth: Cyanosis (**Fig. 30.4B**)
  - Jugular venous pressure: Increased in right heart failure, chronic lung disease, dehydrated patient.
  - Peripheral edema: Seen in decreased albumin level, impaired venous or lymphatic function.
  - Pressure sores (in bed-bound patients).

Examination of Pulmonary System

Inspection/Observation

- **General appearance:** The patient's level of arousal, body type, posture, skin tone, and need for external monitoring or support equipment should be observed and documented.
- **Facial expression:** The expression of face and effort to breathe are two characteristics that can be observed easily in a patient who is having dyspnea. This gives important information for the clinical evaluation of the patient.
- **Inspection of the neck:** The activity of the neck musculature during breathing and the appearance of the jugular veins should be a part of the standard patient assessment. The presence of hypertrophy or adaptive shortening of the sternocleidomastoid muscles may indicate a chronic pulmonary condition. The presence of jugular venous distension should be assessed with the patient sitting or recumbent in bed with the head elevated at least 45 degrees. Jugular venous distension is said to be present, if the veins distend above the level of the clavicles (**Fig. 30.5**). It is an indication of increased volume in the venous system and may be an early sign of right-sided heart failure (cor pulmonale).
- **Inspection of the chest:**
  - *Chest symmetry and deformity:* The resting chest should be inspected for its symmetry, deformities such as kyphoscoliosis, pectus excavatum (funnel chest, where the anterior chest wall has a concave appearance) (**Fig. 30.6A**), pectus carinatum (pigeon chest, where the sternum and ribs protrude anteriorly) (**Fig. 30.6B**), barrel chest, where the rib cage remains expanded, due

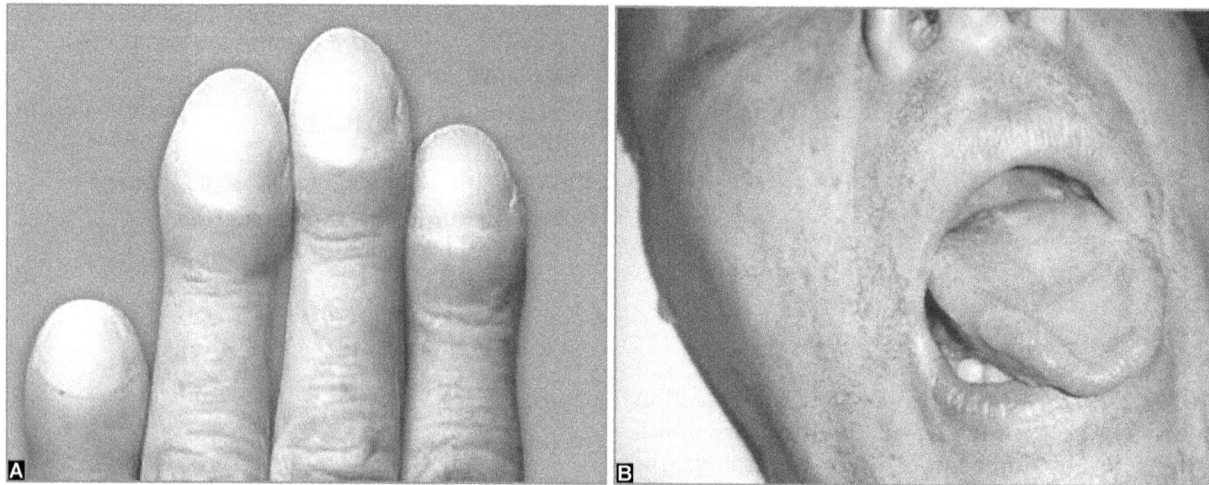

Figs. 30.4A and B: (A) Clubbing of the finger; (B) Cyanosis of tongue.

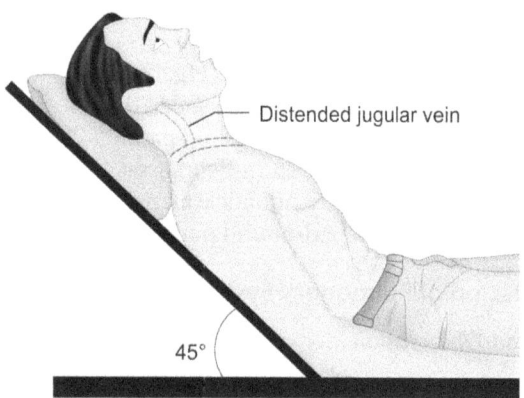

Fig. 30.5: Distension of jugular vein.

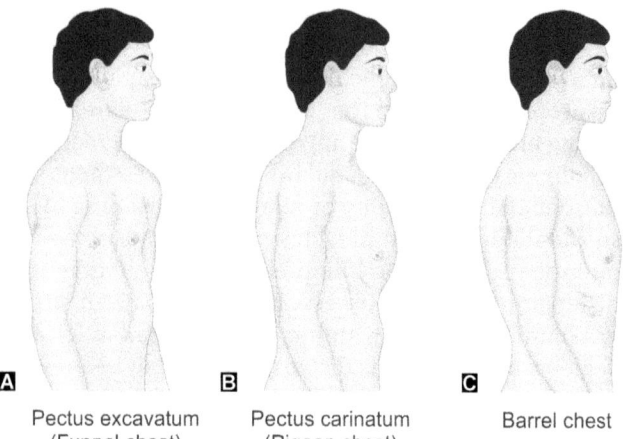

Figs. 30.6A to C: (A) Funnel chest; (B) Pigeon chest; (C) Barrel chest.

to hyperinflation of the lungs, resulting in increased AP diameter of the chest cavity (**Fig. 30.6C**), breathing pattern, breathing rate, inspiratory to expiratory ratios and symmetry of chest wall motion, normalcy of intercostals spaces, rib angles, etc.

Normally, the transverse diameter of the chest is more than the AP diameter (Normal AP diameter is one half of the size of the transverse diameter, measured at shoulder to shoulder). In chronically hyperinflated chest wall, as found in patients with chronic obstructive pulmonary diseases (COPD), the AP diameter increases and may be equal to transverse diameter, resulting in a barrel chest deformity. Normally, rib angles (**Fig. 30.7**) measure less than 90 degrees, and they attach to the vertebrae at approximately 45-degree angles. The intercostal spaces are normally broader posteriorly than anteriorly, but chronic hyperinflation causes the rib angles to increase and the intercostal spaces to become broader anteriorly.

Hoover's sign: Hoover's sign refers to the inspiratory retraction of the lower intercostal spaces that occur with obstructive airway disease. It results from alteration in dynamics of diaphragmatic contraction due to hyperinflation, resulting in traction on the rib margins by the flattened diaphragm. The dome of the diaphragm cannot descend any further during inspiration and diaphragm contraction during inspiration pulls the lower ribs inward (**Fig. 30.8**).

- **Breathing pattern:** Rate of breathing (Typical rate is 12–16 breaths per minute), inspiratory:expiratory ratio [Normal ratio is 1:2, however, in individuals with COPD, particularly with asthmatics, the ratio may be reduced to 1:4 owing to their inability to get rid of air in the lungs], normal pattern

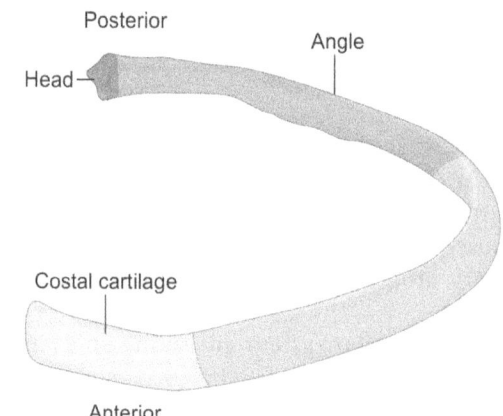

Fig. 30.7: Rib angle.

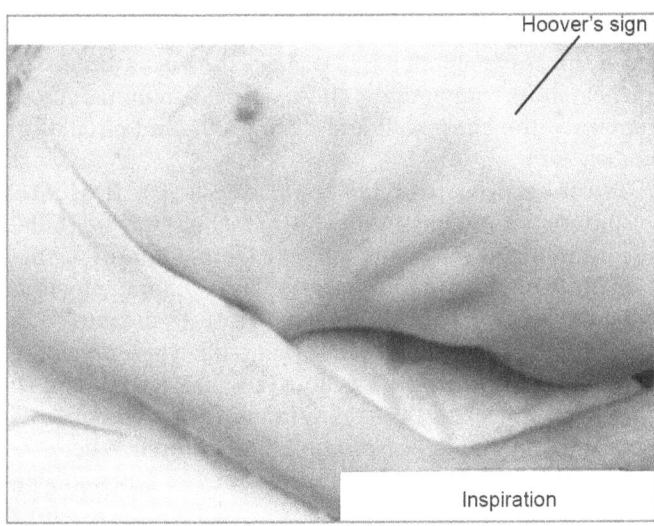

Fig. 30.8: The Hoover's sign.

of breathing is abdominothoracic, however in females, the pattern may be thoracoabdominal.

Presence of abnormal breathing patterns that include:
- *Pursed lip breathing:* The patient uses this breathing to keep the airways open, so that he/she can remove the air that is trapped in the lungs as it occurs in COPD.
- *Kussmaul's respiration:* Characterized by deep rapid breathing pattern performed as an attempt to expel carbon dioxide, which is an acidic compound in the blood.
- *Ataxic breathing:* It is an abnormal breathing pattern characterized by complete irregularity of breathing, with irregular pauses and increasing periods of apnea.
- *Apneustic breathing:* An abnormal breathing pattern characterized by a prolonged inspiratory time with an end inspiratory pause and a shorter expiratory time.
- *Cheyne Stokes respiration:* An abnormal breathing pattern, characterized by progressively deeper and sometimes faster breathing followed by a gradual decrease, that results in a temporary stop of breathing called apnea.
- *Paradoxical breathing:* Where the chest and abdominal wall instead of moving out during inspiration, moves in.

❖ **Observation of phonation and cough**: Evaluation of a patient's speech also is an assessment of shortness of breath at rest. When speech is interrupted for breath, an individual is described as having dyspnea of phonation.

The strength of the patient's cough needs to be assessed, as well as the production of any secretions from the cough (if they are present). Several characteristics of the cough are essential to evaluate, including the effectiveness of the cough (strength, depth, and length of cough). For example, an individual with weak respiratory accessory muscles (e.g., one who has a high spinal cord injury) would have a very weak and therefore ineffective cough. In addition, an individual with bronchospasm may have a very long, drawn out spasmodic cough that is just as ineffective.

The cough should be categorized into acute (< 3 weeks), persistent (> 3 weeks), and chronic (> 8 weeks), depending on the duration of its prevalence. The nature of the cough such as dry cough (irritation), or wet cough (infection) should also be found and documented.

❖ **Inspection of sputum:**
The secretions should be assessed and described with regard to quantity, color, smell, and consistency (Normally, persons may raise 100 mL of mucus—clear to white, per day).
The color of the sputum and their potential causes are given in **Table 30.3**.

❖ **Observation of dyspnea**: The physiotherapist should observe for dyspnea and relate it to the level of function such as:
- Dyspnea at rest or on performing activities such as walking, stair climbing, etc.
- Presence of constant breathlessness.
- Association of paroxysmal nocturnal dyspnea.

Grading of breathlessness (Dyspnea): Dyspnea exhibited by the patients is graded through:

a. **New York Heart Association grading:** This grades dyspnea into: grade 1: No symptoms and limitations in ordinary physical activities, grade 2: Mild symptoms, angina and slight limitation in ordinary activities, grade 3: Marked limitation of activities due to symptoms, even during less than ordinary activities, grade 4: Severe limitations. Experience symptoms even at rest.

b. **Medical Research Council Dyspnea scale:** The MRC dyspnea scale is a questionnaire that consists of five statements about perceived breathlessness: grade 1, "I only get breathless with strenuous exercise"; grade 2, "I get short of breath when hurrying on the level or up a slight hill"; grade 3, "I walk slower than people of the same age on the level because of breathlessness or have to stop for breath when walking at my own pace on the level"; grade

Table 30.3: Color of sputum and the causes.

Color of the sputum	Potential causes
Blood streaked	Inflammation of thorax (larynx, trachea, bronchi), lung cancer
Pink	Blood formed from alveoli and small peripheral bronchi
Copious amounts of blood	Tuberculosis, lung abscess, bronchiectasis, lung infarction, pulmonary embolism
Greenish	Infection
Rust	Pneumonia, tuberculosis
Brownish	Chronic bronchitis, chronic pneumonia
Yellowish green	Bronchiectasis, cystic fibrosis, pneumonia
Whitish grey	Chronic allergic bronchitis
White/ mucoids	Viral infection/asthma
Foamy white	Pulmonary edema
Frothy pink	Severe pulmonary edema
Black specks	Smoke inhalation

4, "I stop for breath after walking 100 yards or after a few minutes on the level"; grade 5, "I am too breathless to leave the house".
  c. **Modified Medical Research Council grading**, which grades dyspnea into: grade 0: No dyspnea except with strenuous exercise, grade 1: Dyspnea when walking up hill or hurrying on level ground, grade 2: Walks slower than most on the level or stops after 15 minutes of walking on the level ground, grade 3: Stops after few minutes of walking on the level ground, grade 4: Dyspnea with minimal activities such as getting dressed.
  d. **American Thoracic Society grading,** which grades dyspnea into: grade 0: No dyspnea on level/uphill, grade 1: Dyspnea at level/uphill, grade 2: Walks slower than persons of same age, grade 3: Stops after 100 yards, grade 4: Breathlessness.
  e. **Modified Borg Dyspnea scale**: The patient is asked about the degree of dyspnea felt at present such as: 0-Nothing, 0.5-Very, very slight, 1-Very slight, 2-Slight, 3-Moderate, 4-Somewhat severe, 5-Severe, 7- Very severe, 9-Very, very severe, 10-Maximal.
- **Information on chest pain:** Chest pain in respiratory patients usually originates from musculoskeletal, pleural, or tracheal inflammation as lung parenchyma and small airways contain no pain fibers. Typical examples of the causes of chest pain include:
  – Pleuritic chest pain
  – Tracheitis
  – Musculoskeletal (chest wall) pain/costochondritis.
  – Angina pectoris
  – Pericarditis
- **Presence of incontinence:** Coughing and huffing increases intra-abdominal pressure, which may precipitate urinary leakage.
- **Other features:** Fever (pyrexia), headache in morning due to nocturnal carbon dioxide retention, peripheral edema (right heart failure), shivering, weight loss, palpitations, vomiting, GI reflux, etc., if present, should be observed.
- **Inspection of the extremities:**
  Observation of the fingers and toes and the calf regions of the legs for swelling/change of color etc., should indicate whether long-term problems with circulation and oxygenation are present or not. Digital clubbing of the fingers and toes indicates chronic tissue hypoxia and is found in many instances of hypoxemia-producing disease. Cyanosis (blueness) of the nail beds may also indicate cardiopulmonary dysfunction.
  For ICU patients: Note should be made of:
  – *Mode of ventilation:* Supplemental oxygen; intermittent positive pressure ventilation
  – *Route of ventilation:* Face mask, nasal cannula, endotracheal tube, tracheostomy
  – *Level of consciousness:* Measured with Glasgow coma scale
  – Central venous pressure (CVP) and pulmonary artery pressure (PAP).

Palpation

The purpose of palpation is to evaluate the mediastinum (for tracheal shift), chest motion, chest wall pain, fremitus, muscle activity of the chest wall and diaphragm, and circulatory status.
- **Trachea position:** Tracheal deviation indicates underlying mediastinum shift. Trachea may be pulled toward in, in collapsed or fibrosed upper lobe or pushed away from, in pneumothorax or large pleural effusion.
- **Chest expansion:** Chest expansion is measured by encircling a measuring tape around the chest at the level of the nipple in males **(Fig. 30.9)** and below the breasts in females and taking the reading from end of deep expiration to the end of deep inspiration. The difference between maximal inspiration and maximal forced expiration gives the value of chest expansion. Normal chest expansion at the level of the nipple is about 2 inches (≥ 5 cm).
- **Chest wall pain or discomfort:** Palpation may also be performed to evaluate chest wall discomfort and should include all areas of the chest wall: anterior, posterior, and lateral regions of the thorax. Patients may often develop musculoskeletal pain from bed rest and inactivity, which are frequently associated with diseases of the cardiopulmonary system. The pain also could arise from a prevalant costochondritis. Musculoskeletal pain must be differentiated from anginal pain, and palpation is an extremely useful tool to distinguish between the two. If chest pain is increased with deep inspiration or if it is increased or reproduced by direct point palpation, it is less likely to be of cardiac origin.
- **Vocal fremitus**: It is the measure of speech vibrations transmitted through the chest wall to the examiner's hands. It is tested by asking the patient to repeatedly say "ggg" or 111 while the examiner's hands are placed flat on both sides of the chest. Vocal fremitus increases in patients, whose lung underneath the chest wall is relatively solid (consolidated). It decreases in patients with pneumothorax or pleural effusion.

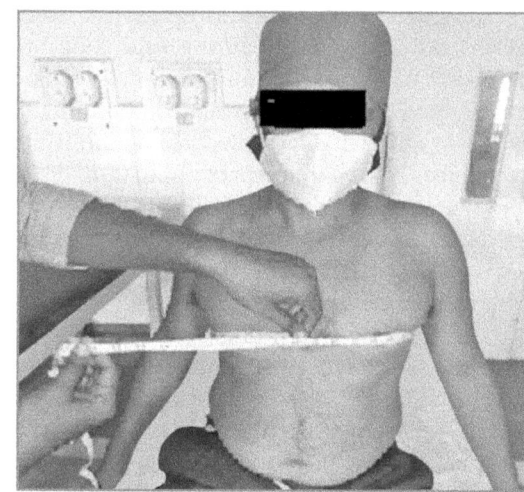

Fig. 30.9: Measurement of chest expansion.

Percussion

It is performed by placing the left hand firmly on the chest wall so that the fingers have good contact with the skin. The middle finger of the left hand is struck over the DIP joint with the middle finger of the right hand of the examiner, at 4-5 cm intervals over the intercostal spaces, moving systematically from superior to inferior and medial to lateral (**Fig. 30.10**).

It may reveal the following:

* **Resonance:** The expected normal sound can usually be heard over all areas of the lungs.
* **Hyperresonance:** Associated with hyperinflation, which may indicate emphysema, pneumothorax, or asthma.
* **Dullness or flatness:** Pneumonia, atelectasis, pleural effusion, pneumothorax, or asthma.
* **Tympany:** This sound is usually associated with percussion over the abdomen.

Auscultation

Auscultation with the stethoscope (**Fig. 30.11**) provides important information to the condition of the lungs and pleura. Auscultation of lung sounds is performed with the diaphragm of the stethoscope preferably in a quiet environment. Auscultation of heart sounds requires both the diaphragm and the bell and, again, a quiet environment.

The lung sounds/breath sounds could be of the following types:

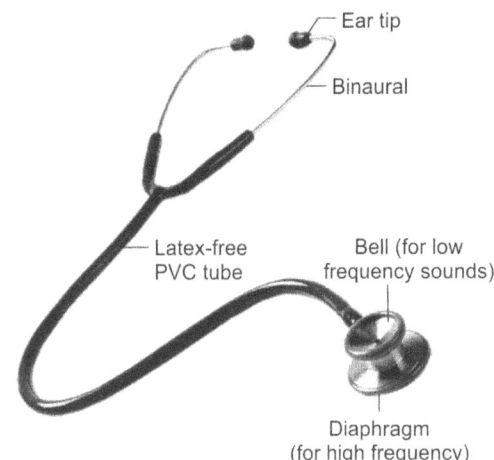

Fig. 30.11: Stethoscope.

* Normal breath sound: Bronchial/Vesicular (**Table 30.4**)
* *Abnormal (adventitious) breath sounds:*
  – *Crackles:* Crackles are also known as alveolar rales and are the sounds heard in a lung field that has fluid in the small airways. The sound crackles created are fine, short, high-pitched, intermittently crackling sounds. The crackles arise from air passing through fluid, pus, or mucus present in the small airways.
  » Rhonchi/wheeze: Rhonchi are coarse, rattling, sounds that resemble snoring. Rhonchi occur when there are secretions or obstruction in the larger airways. These breath sounds are associated with conditions such as: COPD, bronchial asthma, bronchiectasis, pneumonia, chronic bronchitis, or cystic fibrosis.
  Inflammation and narrowing of the airway in any location, from the throat out into the lungs, can result in wheezing. The most common causes of recurrent wheezing are asthma and COPD, which both cause narrowing and spasms (bronchospasms) in the small airways of the lungs.
  » Stridor: Stridor is a loud, high-pitched, musical sound produced by upper respiratory tract obstruction. It is different from wheezing and is louder over the neck than chest wall. It is mainly heard during inspiration.
  » Pleural friction rub: A pleural friction rub is an adventitious breath sound heard on auscultation of

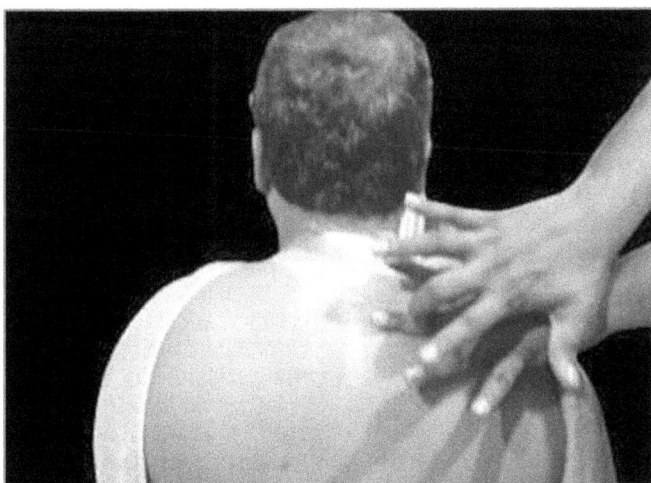

Fig. 30.10: Chest wall percussion.

Table 30.4: The normal breath sounds.					
Type of breath sound	**Pitch**	**Amplitude**	**Duration**	**Quality**	**Normal location**
Bronchial (Tracheal)	High	Loud	Inspiration < Expiration	Harsh/hollow, tubular	Trachea/Larynx
Bronchovesicular	Moderate	Moderate	Inspiration = Expiration	Mixed	Over major bronchi, where fewer alveoli are located.
Vesicular	Low	Soft	Inspiration > Expiration	Rustling, like sound of wind in tree.	Over peripheral lung field, where air flows through smaller airways and alveoli.

the lung. This sound is nonmusical, and described as "grating", "creaky", or "the sound made by walking on fresh snow". Any potential cause of pleural effusion, pleuritis, or serositis can result in a pleural friction rub.
- *Vocal resonance:* Vocal resonance is an assessment of the density of lung tissue, performed by auscultating the chest and asking the patient to speak. Increased vocal resonance suggests increased density, while reduced vocal resonance suggests an increase in the amount of air present. Decrease in resonance is found in emphysema, pneumothorax, pleural thickening, or pleural effusion.
- *Examination of heart sounds:* Auscultation of the chest is usually done by the cardiologist/physician to find the nature of heart sound. However, the knowledge of the heart sound is also required by the physiotherapist, as he/she works as a cardiopulmonary rehabilitation team member and contributes significantly in the rehabilitation process. **Table 30.5** describes the various heart sounds.

Besides the normal and abnormal heart sounds described above, auscultation of heart may also reveal murmurs, which are described below:

Murmurs: Heart murmurs are produced as a result of turbulent flow of blood strong enough to produce audible noise. They are usually heard as a whooshing sound. Most heart problems do not produce any murmur and most valve problems also do not produce

Table 30.5: The heart sounds.

Type of heart sound	Criteria	Clinical implication	Site of auscultation
S1 Normal heart sound associated with heart valve closing.	**Lubb:** Occurs due to mitral and tricuspid valve closure. Indicates start of systole.	The delay of tri-cuspid valve closure, more than normally causes the split S1, which is heard in a right bundle branch block.	Apex of heart: 5th intercostals space on mid-clavicular line on the left side.
S2 Normal heart sound associated with heart valve closing.	**Dubb:** Indicates simultaneous closure of aortic and pulmonary valves. Indicates end of systole and start of diastole.	A widely split S2 can be associated with several different cardiovascular conditions, and the split is sometimes wide and variable whereas, sometimes wide and fixed. The wide and variable split occurs in right bundle branch block, pulmonary stenosis, pulmonary hypertension and ventricular septal defects. The wide and fixed splitting of S2 occurs in atrial septal defect.	Base of heart: 2nd intercostal space on the right side.
S3 The extra heart sound called gallop rhythm, may be found in normal individuals and patients.	This rare sound is called protodiastolic gallop, ventricular gallop, or informally the "Kentucky" gallop (S1 = Ken; S2 = tuck; S3 = y). It occurs at the beginning of diastole after S2 and is lower in pitch than S1 or S2 as it is not of valvular origin.	The third heart sound is benign in youth, some trained athletes, and sometimes in pregnancy but if it re-emerges later in life, it may signal cardiac problems, such as a failing left ventricle as in dilated congestive heart failure (CHF). It is considered as the early sign of congestive heart failure (CHF).	An S3 heart sound is best heard with the bell-side of the stethoscope (used for lower frequency sounds). A left-sided S3 is best heard in the left lateral decubitus position and at the apex of the heart, which is normally located in the 5th left intercostal space at the midclavicular line. A right-sided S3 is best heard at the lower-left sternal border.
S4 The extra heart sound called gallop rhythm, may be found in normal individuals and patients.	S4 when audible in an adult is called a presystolic gallop or atrial gallop. This gallop is produced by the sound of blood being forced into a stiff or hypertrophic ventricle. It sounds like: "ta-lub-dub" or "a-stiff-wall". The combined presence of S3 and S4 is a quadruple gallop, also known as the "Hello-Goodbye" gallop.	It is a sign of a pathologic state, usually a failing or hypertrophic left ventricle, as in systemic hypertension, severe valvular aortic stenosis, pulmonary stenosis and hypertrophic cardiomyopathy.	It is best heard at the cardiac apex with the patient in the left lateral decubitus position and holding his breath.

an audible murmur. Murmurs can be heard in many situations in adults without major congenital heart abnormalities also. Different causes of murmur include:
» Regurgitation through the mitral valve, producing a pansystolic/holosystolic murmur, which is sometimes fairly loud to a practiced ear.
» Stenosis of the aortic valve is typically the next most common heart murmur, producing a systolic ejection murmur.
» Regurgitation through the aortic valve, if marked, is sometimes audible to a practiced ear with a high quality, especially electronically amplified, stethoscope. Generally, this is a very rarely heard murmur, even though aortic valve regurgitation is not so rare.
» Stenosis of the mitral valve, if severe, also rarely produces an audible, low-frequency soft-rumbling murmur, best recognized by a practiced ear using a high quality, especially electronically amplified, stethoscope.

Activity Evaluation

The therapist after examination of the chest should perform an initial evaluation of the patient's responses to exercise. The activity evaluation is an assessment of the patient's responses to the following situations: rest (supine), sitting, standing, some type of activity of daily living (e.g., dressing lower or upper bodies, combing hair, brushing teeth), and ambulation of some distance; in some cases, Exercise tolerance tests are performed to assess the ability to tolerate activity/exercise.

- **Exercise tolerance tests:** Exercise tolerance testing is an integral part of pulmonary rehabilitation (PR) management of patients with cardiopulmonary diseases. Timed walking tests such as 6 minutes walk test can be used to measure exercise capacity before and following rehabilitation. Measuring the distance covered in 6 minutes during a walking test is considered a simple and reproducible way to determine exercise tolerance in patients with chronic lung disease. The 6-minute stepper test (6MST) is a new, well-tolerated, reproducible exercise test, which can be performed without any spatial constraints. Cardiopulmonary exercise testing is useful for determining the causes of exercise limitation and for assessing the maximal exercise capacity of patients with COPD.

Diagnostic Tests

Noninvasive tests: These include:
- **Pulmonary function tests: Spirometry (Fig. 30.12):** This is a simple respiratory test that measures the forced expiratory volume in 1 second (FEV1), the forced vital capacity (FVC), and peak expiratory flow rate (PEFR), which are important measures of ventilatory function.
- **Pulse oximetry:** Pulse oximetry is a noninvasive and painless test that measures the oxygen saturation level, or the oxygen levels in the blood. It can rapidly detect even small changes in how efficiently oxygen is being carried to the extremities furthest from the heart, including the legs and the arms.

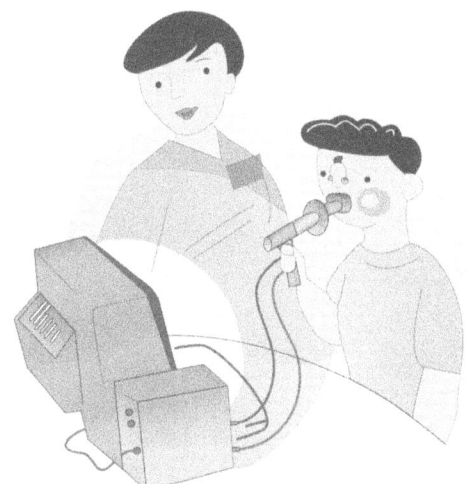

Fig. 30.12: The spirometry.

A beam of light is passed through the tissues. The sensor attached to the fingertip (**Fig. 30.13**), toe, or ear lobe measures the amount of light absorbed by oxygen saturated hemoglobin.

- **Chest X-ray:** Provides information about the chest and helps in establishing the cause of respiratory dysfunction. Chest X-rays are often taken early, if a respiratory disorder is suspected. Chest X-rays also help in establishing diagnosis of pulmonary disorders (**Figs. 30.14A to H**).
- **CT scan/MRI:** Helps in diagnosing peripheral (pleural) or mediastinal disorders.
- **Sputum culture**.
- **ECG:** It records the electrical activity of the heart, which should be interpreted by a physician/cardiologist to establish pathology. The parts of normal ECG are shown in **Figure 30.15**.
- **Arterial blood gas (ABG) analysis:** ABG provides an accurate measure of O_2 uptake and CO_2 removal by the respiratory system as a whole. Typical values are listed below:
  - *Arterial blood pH:* 7.38–7.42.
  - *PaO_2:* The partial pressure of oxygen, also known as PaO_2, is a measurement of oxygen pressure in arterial

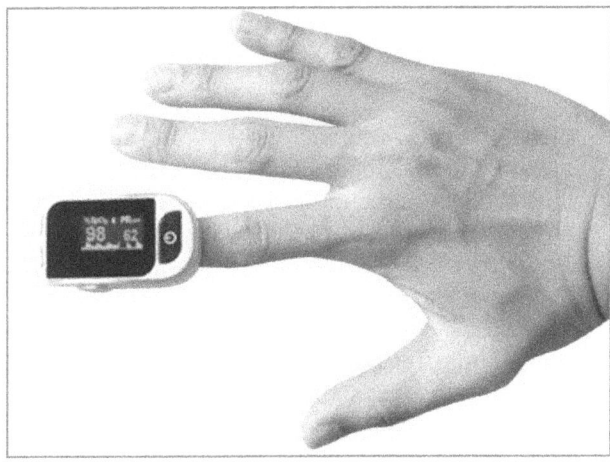

Fig. 30.13: Pulse oximetry.

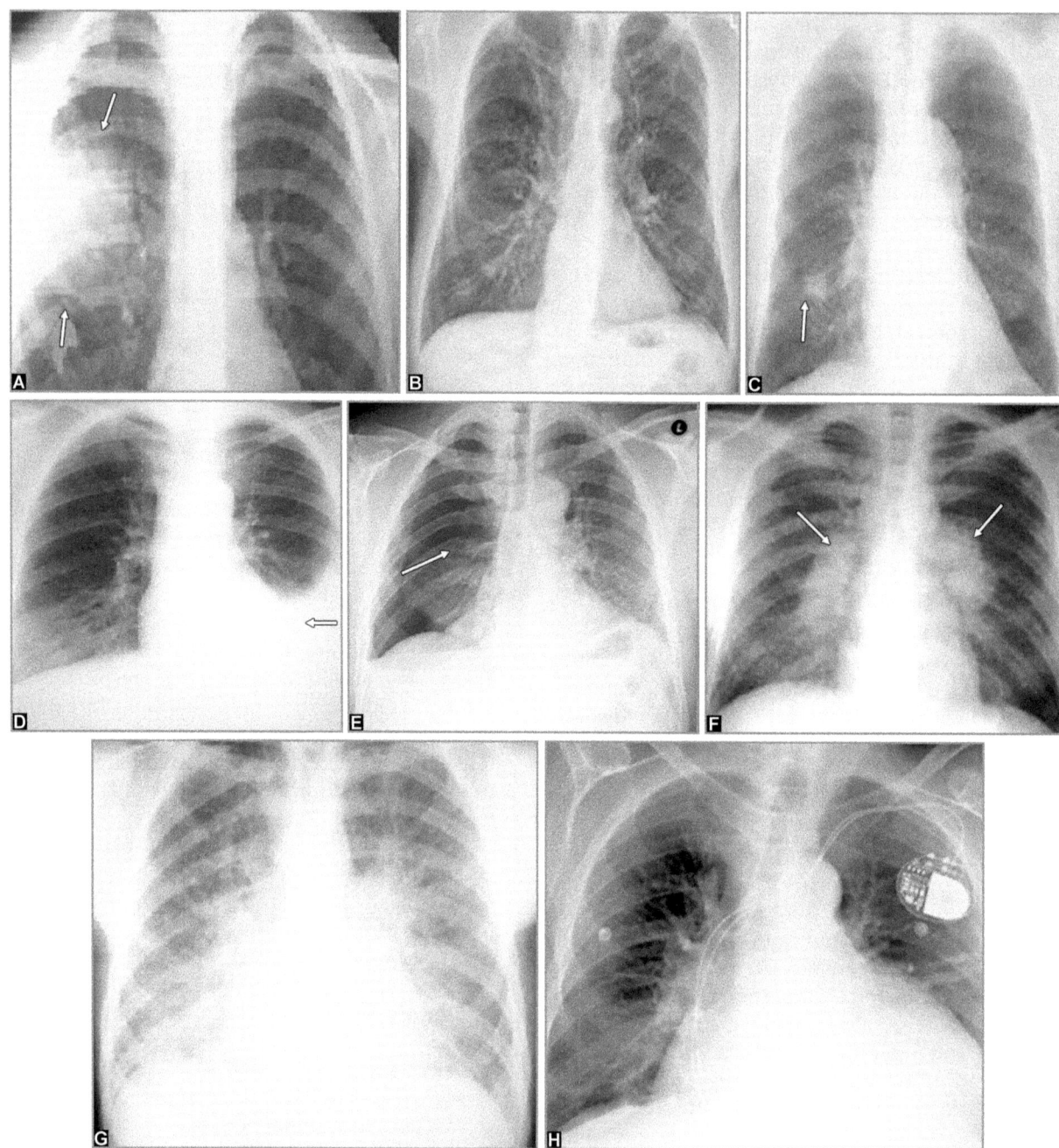

Figs. 30.14A to H: (A) Pneumonia; (B) Emphysema; (C) Lung nodule; (D) Pleural effusion; (E) Rib fracture; (F) Pulmonary tuberculosis; (G) Congestive heart failure; (H) Cardiomegaly.

blood. It reflects how well oxygen is able to move from the lungs to the blood, and it is often altered by severe illnesses. Normal value of PaO_2 is 75-100 millimeters of mercury (mm Hg), or 10.5-13.5 kilopascal (kPa).
- $PaCO_2$: Partial pressure of carbon dioxide ($PaCO_2$): 38-42 mm Hg (5.1-5.6 kPa)
- *Base excess:* A typical reference range for **base excess** is −2 to +2 mEq/L. Comparison of the base excess with the reference range assists in determining whether an acid/base disturbance is caused by a respiratory, metabolic, or mixed metabolic/respiratory problem.

❖ *Invasive test:* It includes:
  - *Bronchoscopy:* It permits visualization of larynx, trachea, and bronchi for therapeutic and diagnostic uses.
  - *Laryngoscopy:* Visual examination of larynx, done to diagnose laryngeal papillomas, nodules, polyps, or cancer.
  - *Biopsy.*
  - *Thoracentesis and pleural fluid analysis:* It involves insertion of a needle into the pleural space for removal of pleural fluid or air.

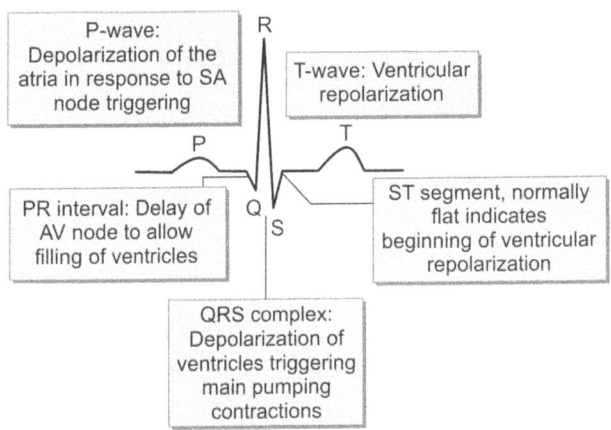

Fig. 30.15: The parts of the ECG graph.

Evaluation

On completion of the full cardiopulmonary examination, including chest examination and activity evaluation, the physical therapist develops a clinical judgment (evaluation) based on the data gathered and formulates a decision regarding interventions to be used. Evaluation includes the development of a diagnosis based on the clinical findings that includes the impact of the findings or problems, otherwise known as functional limitations and disability. This allows the therapist to select from available interventions, a plan of care for the patient that will optimally achieve the expected outcomes in the documented amount of time described in the prognosis associated with the practice pattern.

Objectives of cardiopulmonary physiotherapy interventions: The objectives of cardiopulmonary physiotherapy interventions are:
- To increase air flow to the lungs to maintain lung volumes/ capacities and oxygen saturation.
- To remove secretions from the airways.
- To teach breath control during episodes of dyspnea.
- To increase the strength and endurance of muscles of respiration.
- To increase exercise tolerance/endurance.
- To enhance function.

The interventions provided include:

Breathing exercise: An exercise intended to promote effective and healthy breathing and breath control that helps in improving respiratory function by maintaining lung volumes and capacities and controlling episodes of dyspnea, thereby improving the overall endurance and function. It is an effective tool in pulmonary rehabilitation.

Types of breathing exercises: Breathing exercises performed depend on the conditions for which they are applied. It may be deep breathing (for example in restrictive lung diseases), or controlled relaxed breathing (for example asthma/COPD). Generally breathing exercises are classified into:
- Diaphragmatic breathing exercise:
- Segmental (costal) breathing exercise.
- Ventilatory muscle training.

However, in serious pathological conditions, such as high level cervical spinal cord injuries, severe dyspnea due to asthma, lung collapse/consolidation, etc., the breathing exercises performed are:
- Glossopharyngeal breathing (Upper cervical spinal cord injury)
- Pursed lip breathing (COPD/Asthma).
- Air shift maneuver (Lung collapse/consolidation).

The different types of breathing exercises performed are briefly described as under:

1. **Diaphragmatic breathing exercise:** Diaphragm is the primary muscle for inspiration. Diaphragm controls breathing at an involuntary level. A patient with primary pulmonary disease like COPD can be taught breathing control by optimal use of diaphragm and relaxation of the accessory muscles. This exercise also helps to mobilize secretions in the lungs in postural drainage. This contributes to about 60% of total work of breathing. All breathing exercises start with diaphragmatic breathing, followed by segmental breathing and end with diaphragmatic breathing.

   Procedure: The patient is placed in a relaxed position, where gravity will assist the descent of diaphragm, such as Half flying position with head and trunk elevated by 45 degrees and hips and knees flexed with pillow support (**Fig. 30.16**). Other positions such as supine, sitting, standing may be used as the patient progress during treatment. The therapist places his/her hands over the rectus abdominis, just below the anterior costal margin. The patient is asked to breathe slowly and deeply via nose by keeping the shoulders relaxed and upper chest quiet, allowing the abdomen to rise, followed by slowly letting all the air out using controlled expiration through the mouth. The maneuver is practiced for 3 or 4 times, to avoid hyperventilation. The face of the patient should be turned to sides, to avoid direct exposure to therapist/clinician.

2. **Segmental breathing:** It is performed on a segment of a lung, or a section of the chest wall that needs increased ventilation or movement. Hypoventilation that occurs in certain areas of the lungs, due to chest wall fibrosis, pain after surgery, atelectasis, trauma to chest wall, pneumonia, and post-mastectomy scar can be expanded

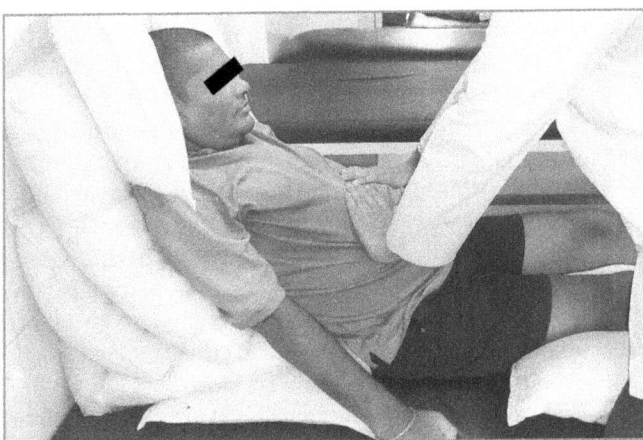

Fig. 30.16: Diaphragmatic breathing exercise.

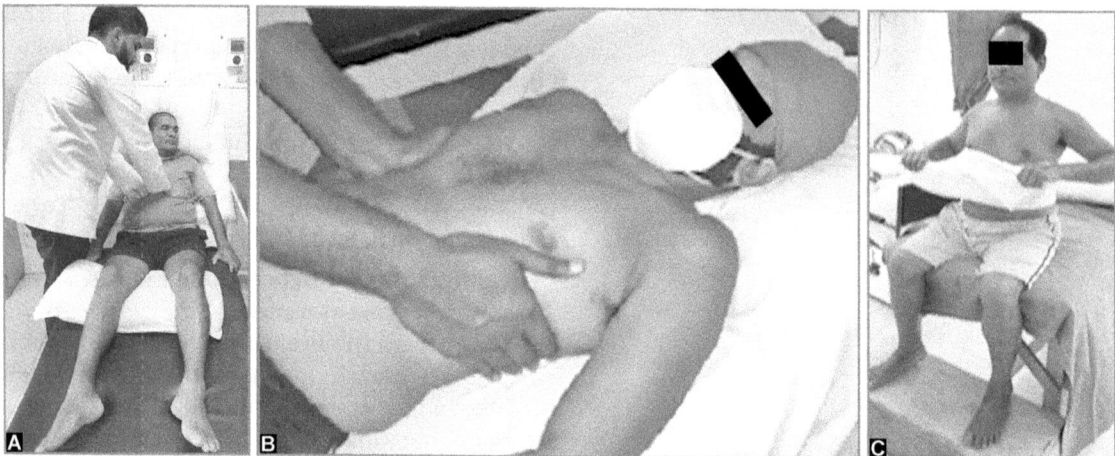

Figs. 30.17A to C: (A) Lateral costal expansion exercise in half-lying; (B) Lateral costal exercise in supine/crook lying; (C) Lateral costal expansion exercise in sitting using a towel.

by this procedure. This exercise when performed, prevents accumulation of pleural fluid and secretions, decreases paradoxical breathing, and panic episodes, and improves chest mobility. The segmental breathing exercises are briefly described below:

a. *Lateral costal expansion/lateral basal expansion exercise:* This exercise may be done unilaterally or bilaterally. The patient may be positioned in half-lying **(Fig. 30.17A)**, sitting or supine/crook lying **(Fig. 30.17B)**. The therapist places the hands along the lateral aspect of the lower ribs and asks the patient to breathe out through the mouth. As the patient breathes out, the therapist applies firm downward pressure into the ribs with the palms of the hands and guides the rib cage to move downward and inward during the phase of expiration. Then the patient is asked to deeply inhale air through the nose, while the therapist applies a quick downward and inward stretch to the chest, to facilitate contraction of external intercostals muscle, guiding the rib cage to move upward and outward. Light manual resistance can be applied to the lower ribs to increase sensory awareness, as the patient breaths in deeply and the chest expands. The procedure is repeated 3–4 times followed by performance of diaphragmatic breathing exercises as described above. The patient may be taught to perform the maneuver independently and to apply resistance with his own hand or towel/belt **(Fig. 30.17C)**.

b. *Posterior basal expansion exercise:* This form of segmental breathing is important for the postsurgical patients who are confined to bed for an extended period of time, as secretion often accumulates over the posterior segments of lower lobes. The patient is either made to remain in half lying **(Fig. 30.18)**/sitting and leaning forward on pillows. The therapist places the hands over the posterior aspect of the lower ribs and follows the same procedure as described for lateral basal expansion exercise described above.

c. *Right middle-lobe or lingular (left) expansion exercise:* Patient is placed in sitting/half-lying. The therapist

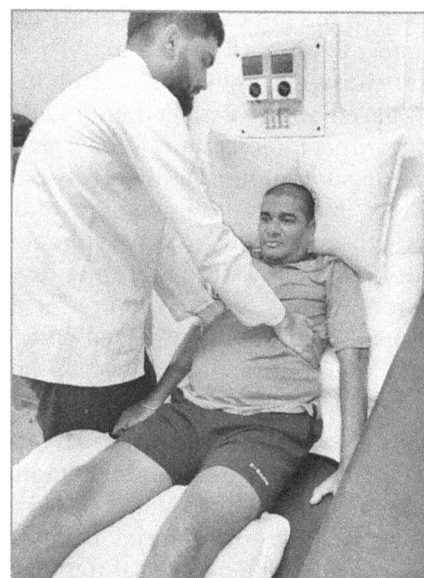

Fig. 30.18: Posterior basal expansion exercise in half-lying.

places the hands on either the right or left side of the patient's chest just below the axilla **(Fig. 30.19)**. The same procedure as above is followed.

d. *Apical expansion exercise:* Patient is placed in half-lying **(Fig. 30.20)**/sitting. The therapist places the hands/hand over the anterior chest below the clavicle(s). The same procedure as above is followed. The patient may also be taught to use his own hand for assisting during expiration and resisting during inspiration.

3. **Active cycle of breathing technique (ACBT):** Active cycle of breathing technique (ACBT) combines different breathing techniques that help clear mucus from the lungs in three phases. It is an independent breathing exercise program consisting of breath control exercise, thoracic expansion exercise, and forced expiratory techniques **(Fig. 30.21)**:

a. *Breath control exercise:* This is the first phase that relaxes the airways. It is the relaxed diaphragmatic breathing,

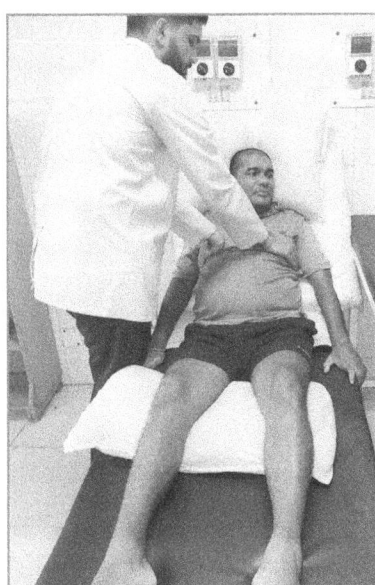

Fig. 30.19: Placement of the hands for right middle and left lingular lobe.

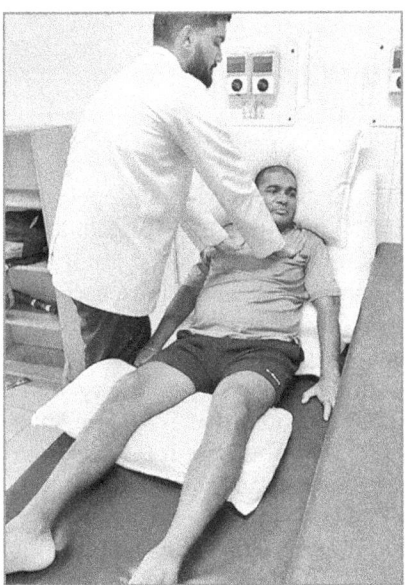

Fig. 30.20: Apical expansion exercise.

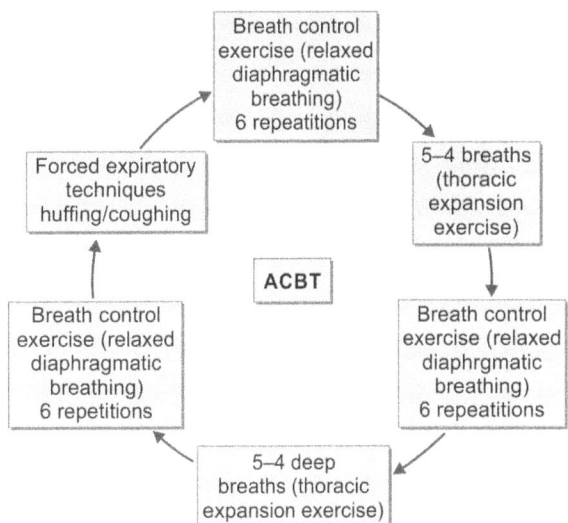

Fig. 30.21: The active cycle of breathing techniques.

where the patient is asked to breathe in through the nose and breathe out through the mouth with very little effort and relaxing the upper chest and shoulders. A good way to do this is to place one hand on the stomach as one breathes. He/she should breathe gently so that the airways are relaxed. By using the pursed lip technique when breathing out a back pressure is created in the airways that stents the airway open longer. The breathing control is repeated for six breaths before moving to thoracic expansion exercises.

b. *Thoracic expansion exercise:* This is the second phase that helps to get air behind the mucus and clear the mucus. The patient is asked to breathe in deeply (Some people use a 3-second breath hold to get more air into smaller airways and behind the mucus) and then breathe out without forcing the air out. This may be done with chest clapping or vibration, followed by another cycle of breathing control.

c. *Forced expiratory technique:* This is the third phase that helps to force the mucus out of the lungs. This is a maneuver used to move secretions, mobilized by deep breathing/thoracic expansion exercises, downstream toward the mouth. A huff is exhaling through an open mouth and throat instead of coughing. Huffing helps to move sputum from the small airways to the larger airways, from where they are removed by coughing, as coughing alone cannot remove sputum from small airways.

4. **Ventilatory muscle training:** The process of improving strength and endurance of muscles of breathing is known as ventilatory muscle training (VMT). This technique usually focuses on primary muscles of inspiration such as diaphragm and intercostal muscles. The procedures involved are:

a. *Diaphragmatic muscle training using weights:* The patient is placed in supine lying/crook lying **(Fig. 30.22)**. Place a small weight (1.30–2.20 kg) over the epigastric region of the abdomen. Tell the patient to breathe out through the mouth followed by deep inspiration through

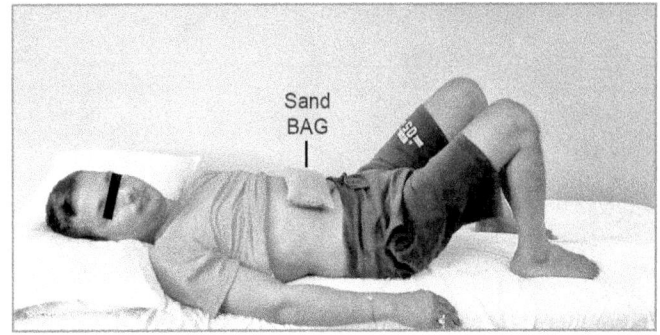

Fig. 30.22: Diaphragmatic muscle training using weight (sand bag).

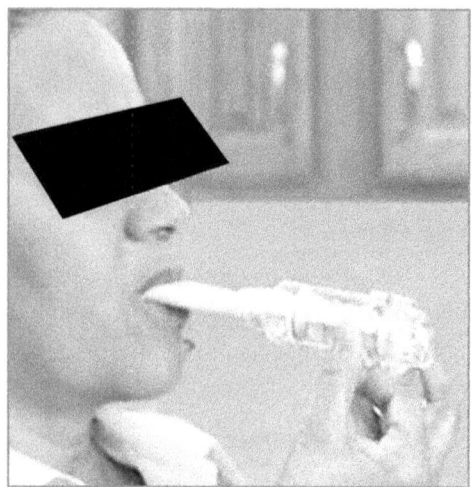

Fig. 30.23: Inspiratory resistance training.

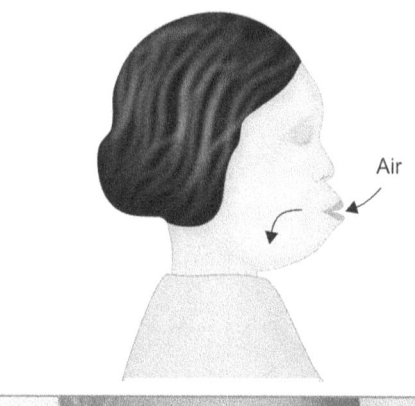

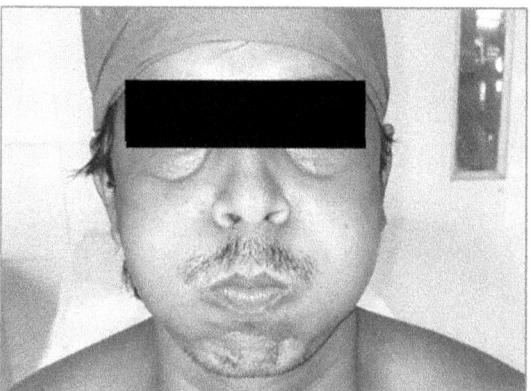

Fig. 30.25: Glossopharyngeal breathing.

the nose, keeping the upper chest quiet. Gradually increase the time, that the patient breaths against the resistance of the weight. Weight can be increased, when the patient can sustain diaphragmatic breathing pattern, without the use of any accessory muscles of inspiration for 15 minutes.

b. *Inspiratory resistance training:* The patient inhales through a hand-held resistive device that he or she places in the mouth **(Fig. 30.23)**. These devices are narrow tubes of varying diameters that provide resistance to airflow during inspiration and improve strength of inspiratory muscles. Gradually, the time is increased to 20–30 minutes.

c. *Incentive spirometry:* This is a form of low-level resistance training, where the patient inhales through a spirometer that provides visual or auditory feedback as he/she breaths deeply, with the mouthpiece placed in the mouth **(Fig. 30.24)**. The patient is placed in a comfortable position. Then, have the patient place mouthpiece of the device in the mouth and maximally inhale through the spirometer and hold the inspiration for few seconds and then exhale air through the mouth by removing the mouth piece.

Glossopharyngeal breathing: Glossopharyngeal breathing (GPB), also called "frog breathing", is a positive pressure breathing technique that uses muscles of the mouth and pharynx to propel small volumes of air ("gulps") into the lungs **(Fig. 30.25)**. It is a means of increasing the patient's inspiratory capacity, when there is severe weakness of muscles of inspiration. It is used primarily for ventilator dependent patients, due to absent or incomplete innervations of the diaphragm because of high cervical cord injury or neuromuscular disorders. The patient takes several gulps of air (6-10 numbers). Then the mouth is closed and the tongue pushes the air back and traps it in the pharynx. The air is then forced into the lungs and the glottis is opened. This increases the depth of the inspiration and the patient's inspiratory and vital capacity.

5. **Pursed-lip breathing exercise:** Pursed lip breathing is a technique that helps people living with asthma or COPD when they experience shortness of breath. Pursed lip breathing helps control shortness of breath, and provides a quick and easy way to slow patient's pace of breathing, making each breath more effective. This is a strategy that involves lightly pursing the lips together during controlled expiration **(Fig. 30.26)**. It helps to improve ventilation and releases trapped air in the lungs.

Have the patient assume a comfortable position. Explain to the patient that expiration must be relaxed and passive and contraction of abdominals must be avoided. Instruct the patient to breathe slowly and deeply through the nose, and then breathe out gently through lightly pursed lips. By providing slight resistance, an increased positive pressure will generate within the airways, which helps to keep open small bronchioles that otherwise collapse. It can be

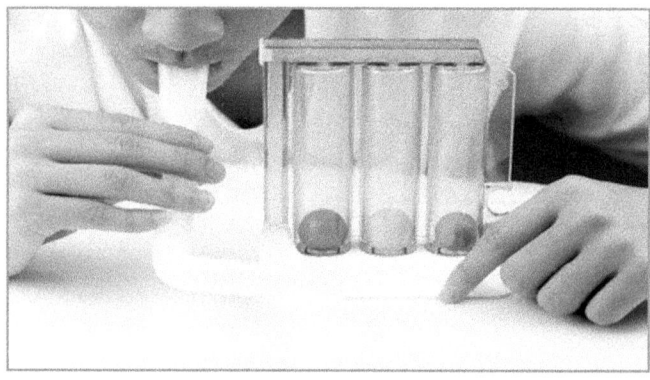

Fig. 30.24: Incentive spirometry.

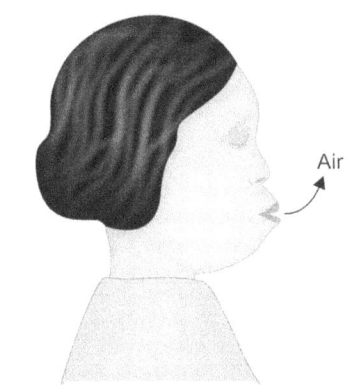
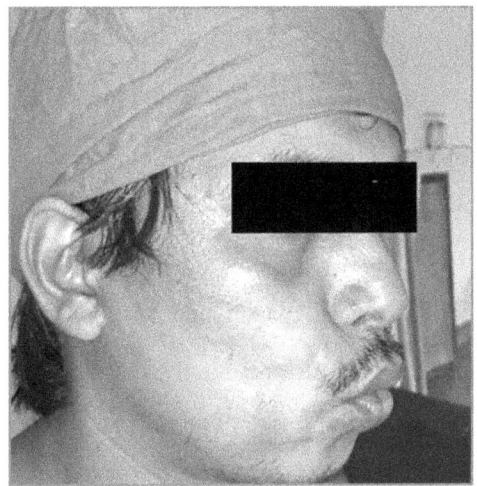

Fig. 30.26: Pursed-lip breathing.

applied as 3–5 minutes "rescue exercise" or an emergency procedure to counteract acute exacerbations or dyspnea in COPD and asthma.

6. **Air shift maneuver:** Any individual with paradoxical breathing or a poorly expanding chest wall (due to intercostals weakness) during inspiration should learn to perform an air shift maneuver. When an individual has a dominant diaphragmatic breathing pattern that results in collapse of the anterior chest wall (as occurs in those with C4-T4 motor complete injuries), the volume of air moving into lungs does not act to expand the chest wall but instead moves in a caudal direction. An air shift is a maneuver in which a person inhales maximally, closes the glottis and relaxes the diaphragm to move the air upward toward the middle and upper lobes of the chest and creates expansion of these regions. This exercise is used to maintain chest mobility or expand the chest from ½ inch to as much as 2 inches.

Position the patient in supine lying. Ask the patient to take deep breath, close the glottis and hold that breath. While holding the breath, therapist asks the patient to suck in the abdomen so that air will move from lower part to upper part of thorax. To learn this technique, the therapist places one hand on the patient's epigastric area, and the other hand on the upper part of the chest, and holds the hands in place. When the patient takes a deep breath, holds it, sucks in the stomach, and moves the air to the upper part of the chest,

the therapist's top hand will rise. The patient is instructed to perform this exercise daily.

Heimlich maneuver/Abdominal thrust: This is an air shift maneuver performed to overcome inability to breathe caused by a blockage in the throat.

BENEFITS OF BREATHING EXERCISE

- **Breathing detoxifies and releases toxins:** The body is designed to release 70% of its toxins through breathing. If the person is not breathing effectively, he is not properly ridding the body of its toxins (CO_2). When one exhales air from the body, he/she releases carbon dioxide that has been passed through from the bloodstream into the lungs.
- **Breathing releases tension, relaxes mind/body and brings clarity:** When a person is stressed, the muscles become tight and breathing becomes shallow. The body does not get adequate amount of oxygen as per need. Slow deep breathing exercises performed in such states of body induces relaxation, brings clarity by diverting attention and providing adequate oxygen to the brain to meet the needs of the body.
- **Breathing relieves emotional problems:** Relaxed deep breathing exercises during negative emotional events and abnormal outbursts of emotion helps to overcome emotional problems.
- **Breathing relieves pain:** During episodes of pain such as labor pain, individuals hold breath. It is found that breathing into the pain helps to ease it.
- **Breathing massages the vital organs:** The movements of the diaphragm during the deep breathing exercise massage the stomach, small intestine, liver, and pancreas. The upper movement of the diaphragm also massages the heart. When air is inhaled, diaphragm descends, and abdomen expands. By this action, massage to vital organs improves circulation in them.
- **Breathing strengthens the immune system:** The oxygen that travels through the bloodstream by attaching to hemoglobin in the red blood cells enriches the body to metabolize nutrients and vitamins, strengthening the immune system.
- **Breathing improves Posture:** Deep breathing techniques over a sustained period of time promotes good posture, thereby helps in correction of spinal deformities such as kyphosis/scoliosis, when combined with spinal exercises and bracing.
- **Breathing improves quality of the blood:** Regular deep breathing exercises remove all the carbon dioxide and increases oxygen in the blood and thus increases the quality of blood.
- **Breathing increases digestion and assimilation of food:** The digestive organs such as the stomach receive more oxygen, and hence operate more efficiently helping in digestion and assimilation of food (into blood).
- **Breathing improves the nervous system:** The brain, spinal cord and nerves receive increased oxygenation and are more nourished. This helps to improve the function of the nervous system.

- **Breathing improves tissue healing:** As breathing helps to provide the required amount of oxygen to the tissues, and helps in tissue metabolism, healing of injured tissues is facilitated more and more. Breathing improves cellular regeneration.
- **Breathing improves the lung function:** As breathing increases lungs function, it can be used to treat obstructive and restrictive pulmonary conditions.
- **Breathing makes the heart stronger:** Breathing exercises reduce the workload on the heart as it leads to more efficient lungs and increases oxygenation of blood. So, the heart doesn't have to work as hard to deliver oxygen to the tissues. Breathing exercises also produce a massaging effect on heart, increasing its efficiency.
- **Proper breathing assists in weight control:** In case of obesity, the extra oxygen burns up the excess fat more efficiently and reduces weight. In case of underweight, the extra oxygen feeds the starving tissues through increase of tissue metabolism.
- **Breathing Boosts Energy levels and improves stamina:** Due to this, breathing exercises are performed as a warm up exercise before resuming vigorous activities/sports.
- **Breathing elevates moods:** Breathing increases pleasure-inducing neurochemicals in the brain to elevate mood and combat physical pain.
- **Breathing improves endurance:** Breathing exercises improve both cardiorespiratory and muscular endurance.

Mechanical Ventilation

When a patient fails to breathe air either spontaneously or through assisted ventilation from an oxygen cylinder, passive ventilation using a mechanical ventilator **(Fig. 30.27)** is considered. A ventilator is a device that supports or takes over the breathing process, pumping air into the lungs. People who stay in intensive care units (ICU) may need the support of a ventilator.

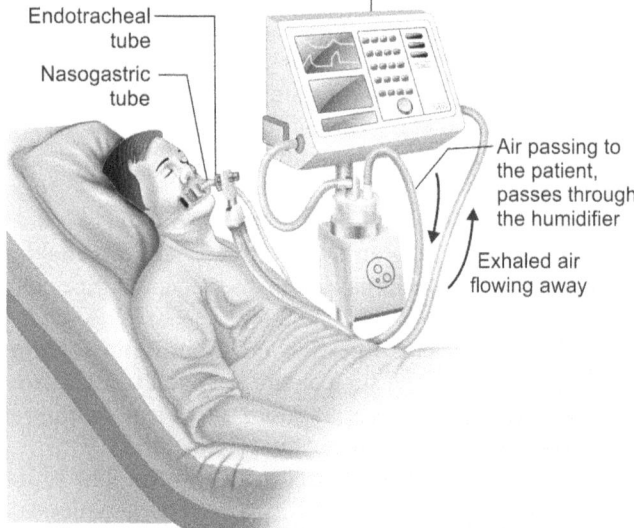

Fig. 30.27: Mechanical ventilation through ventilator.

Ventilators are of different types such as:
- **Face mask ventilator/Noninvasive ventilator:** A face mask ventilator is a noninvasive method of supporting a person's breathing and oxygen levels. It is the use of breathing support administered through a face mask/nasal mask. Air, usually with added oxygen, is given through the mask under positive pressure.
- **Invasive ventilator:** Invasive ventilation is positive pressure delivered to the patient's lungs via an endotracheal tube or a tracheostomy tube.
- **Positive-pressure ventilation:** Positive pressure ventilation is a form of respiratory therapy that involves the delivery of air or a mixture of oxygen combined with other gases by positive pressure into the lungs. It pushes the air into the lungs.
- **Negative pressure ventilator:** It is a type of mechanical ventilator that stimulates an ill person's breathing by periodically applying negative air pressure to their body, to expand and contract the chest cavity.

POSTURAL DRAINAGE

Postural drainage is a means of mobilizing secretions in one or more lung segments to the central airways by placing the patient in various positions so that gravity assists in the drainage process. Postural drainage therapy includes the techniques such as positioning, percussion, vibration, and voluntary huffing and coughing.

Positioning the patient so that the bronchus of the involved lung segment is perpendicular to the ground is the basis of postural drainage.

Aim/Indication of Postural Drainage

- To prevent accumulation of secretions in the lungs in patients confined to bed, as well as postsurgical patients.
- Remove secretion from the lungs in chronic pulmonary disorders.

Contraindications of Postural Drainage

- Hemorrhagic disorders.
- Untreated acute conditions such as congestive heart failure, pleural effusion, pulmonary embolism.
- Cardiovascular instability such as hypertension, myocardial infarction.
- Acute fracture of vertebrae and ribs.
- Recent head injury and craniotomies.

Techniques Applied during Postural Drainage

- **Percussion:** It is a force, rhythmically applied with the therapist's cupped hand **(Fig. 30.28)** to the patient's chest wall, corresponding to the lung segments to be drained. The technique is typically administered for 3–5 minutes over each involved lung segment.
- **Vibration:** It is applied by placing both the hands directly over the chest wall, and gently compressing and rapidly vibrating the chest wall as the patient breathes out. The position of the hand for vibration is shown in **Figure 30.29**.

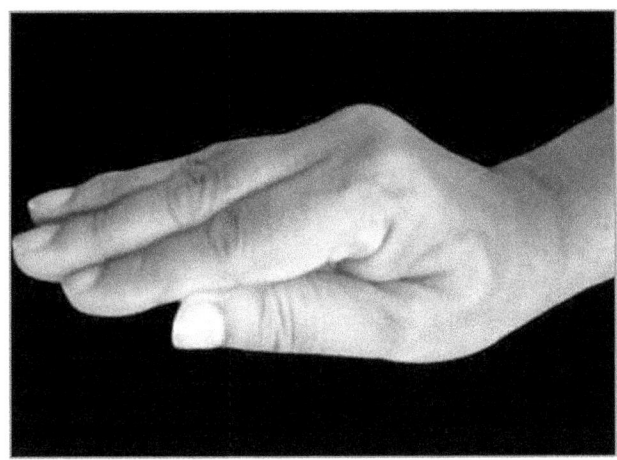

Fig. 30.28: Cupped hands for chest percussion.

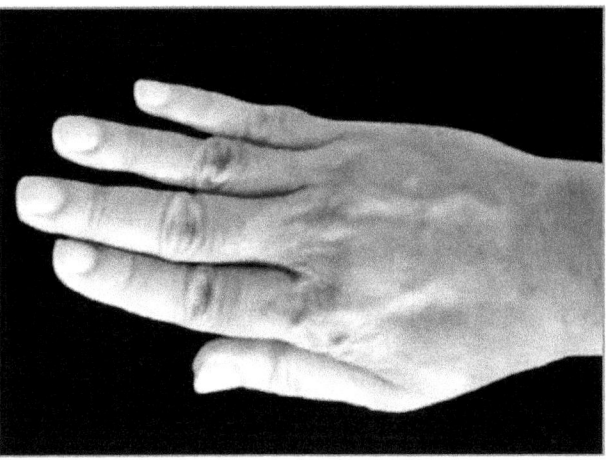

Fig. 30.29: Position of the hand for application of chest vibration.

- **Shaking:** It is applied during exhalation using intermittent bouncing maneuver performed with the wide movement of therapist's hands. Five to seven deep breaths with shaking on exhalation are appropriate to hasten the removal of secretion. Shaking is commonly used following percussion in the appropriate postural drainage position.
- **Airway clearance:** Once the secretions have been mobilized with percussion, vibration and shaking in the postural drainage position, the task of removing the secretions from the airways is undertaken using an airway clearance technique. Coughing is the most common and easiest means of clearing the airway. Coughing involves taking a deep inspiration (glottis closes and vocal cord tightens), followed by explosive expiration (Abdominal contraction, diaphragm elevation, and glottis open). Huffing is an alternative method of airway clearance that is useful for patients with obstructive pulmonary disease. A huff uses many of the same steps of coughing, without creating the high intrathoracic pressures. The patient is asked to take a deep breath and then rapidly contract the abdominal muscles while forcefully saying "Ha, ha, ha". This allows a forced expiration through a stabilized open airway and makes secretion removal more effective. The clinician should have a thorough knowledge of the bronchopulmonary segments (airways) **(Fig. 30.30)**, which will enable for appropriate postural drainage positioning.

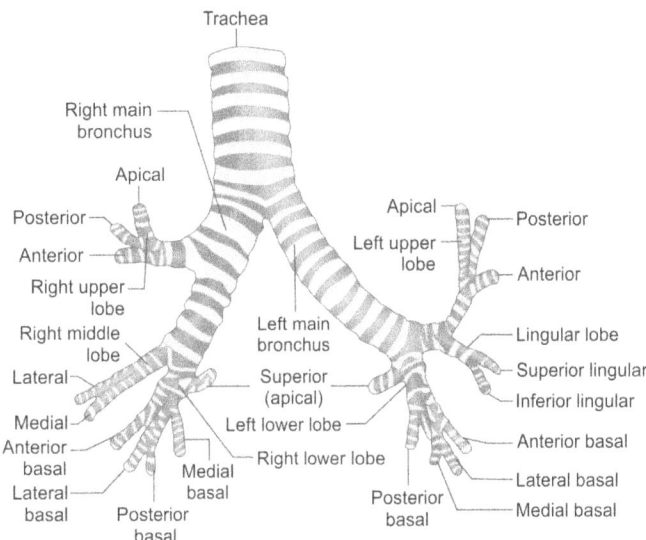

Fig. 30.30: Bronchopulmonary segments.

Nebulization and steam inhalation: Nebulizer is a drug delivery device **(Figs. 30.31A and B)** used to administer medication in the form of a mist inhaled into the lungs. Nebulizers are commonly used for the treatment of asthma, cystic fibrosis, COPD, and other respiratory diseases or disorders. Nebulization therapy helps in liquefying and loosening of the

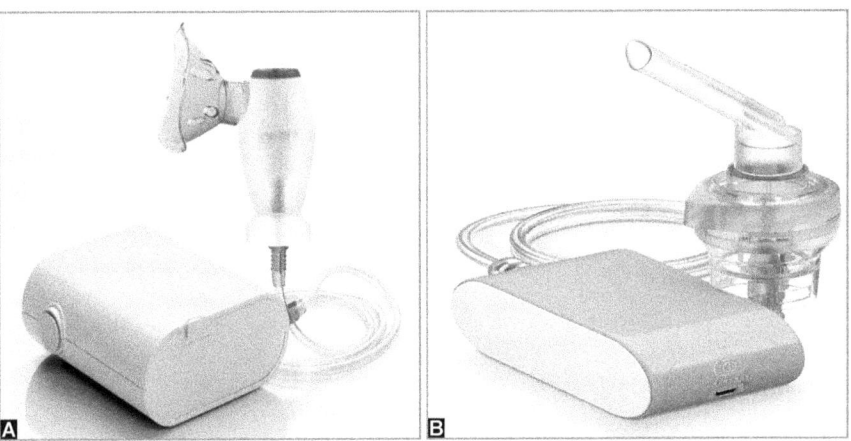

Figs. 30.31A and B: (A) Nebulizer with face mask; (B) Nebulizer with mouth piece.

retained secretions and promotes bronchodilation. Steam inhalation though used by many before postural drainage, there is no strong evidence regarding its efficacy.

Positions and Procedure for Postural Drainage

1. **Upper lobes:**
   – *Apical segments of upper lobe on both sides:* Patient sits comfortably on a bed or chair and leans backward over pillows/ half lying with head resting on pillow/head board **(Fig. 30.32)**. The therapist/ caregiver percusses the chest over the muscular area between the collar bones and upper margin of the scapulae. Subsequently, the patient is asked to take a deep breath and exhale slowly. During the period of exhalation vibration is applied, and the patient is asked to huff/ cough to remove the secretions.
   – *Postural drainage from posterior segments of both upper lobes:* The patient sits comfortably on a chair or over the side of the bed, and leans forward over the pillows **(Fig. 30.33)**. The therapist applies percussion and vibration over the posterior aspects of the scapulae and patient is asked to huff and cough to clear secretions.
   – *Postural drainage from anterior segments of upper lobes:* The patient is flat on the bed with pillows under the knee and head **(Fig. 30.34)**. The therapist/ care giver applies percussion/vibration to the anterior chest between the collar bone and nipple. Secretions are removed through huffing and coughing.

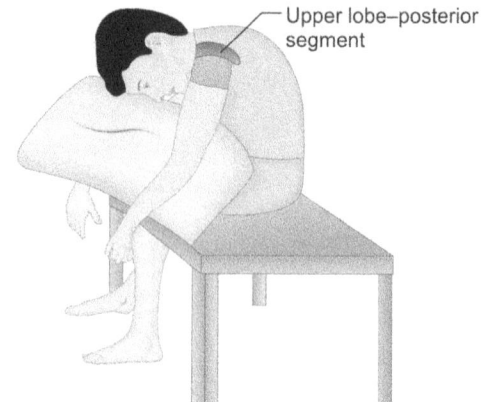

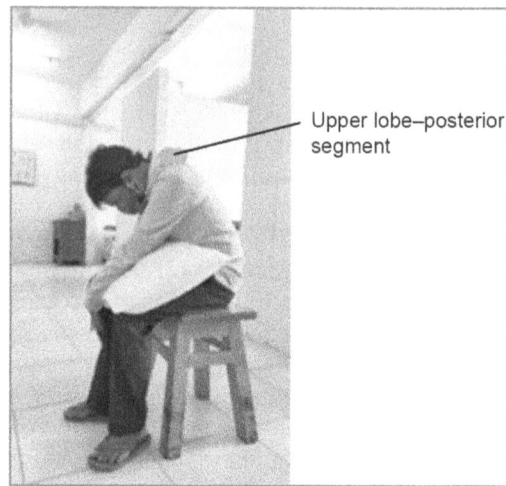

Fig. 30.33: Postural segment from posterior segments of both upper lobes.

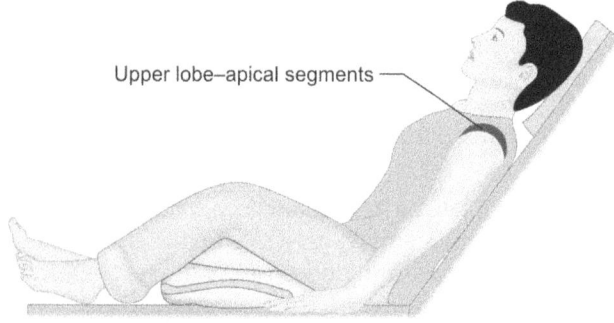

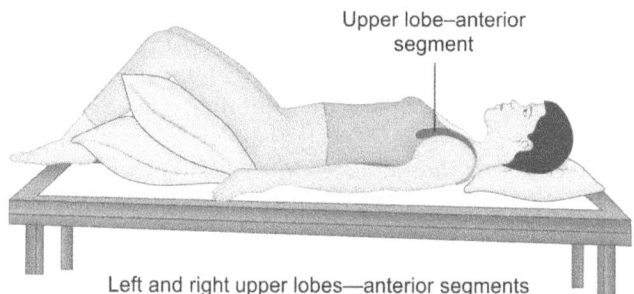

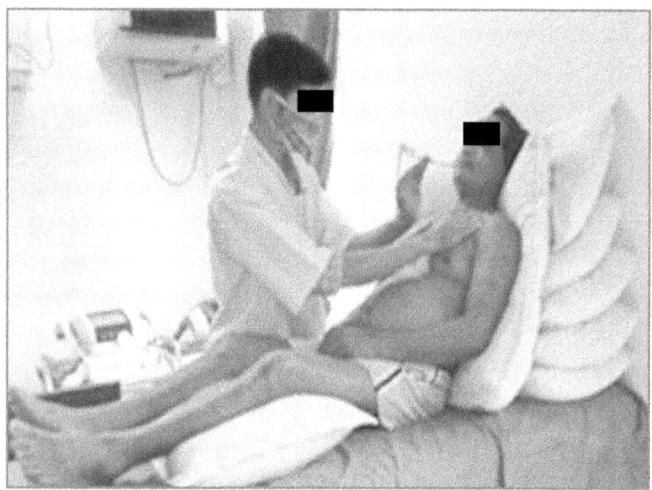

Fig. 30.32: Postural drainage from apical segments of upper lobes.

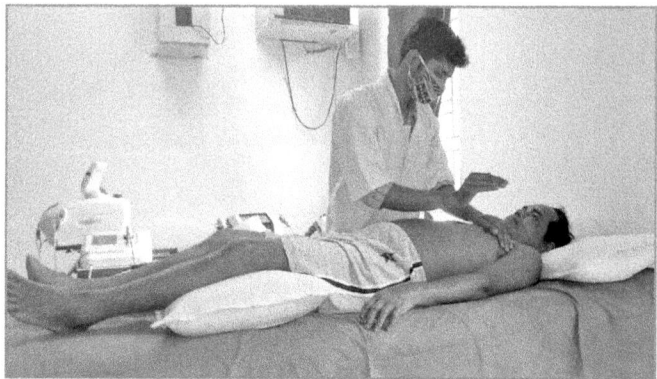

Fig. 30.34: Postural drainage from anterior segments of both upper lobes.

2. **Middle lobes:**
   - *Right middle lobe:* Patient lies on left side lying and turns body backwards by ¼, supported on pillow from shoulder to hip **(Fig. 30.35)**. The knees are flexed. The foot end of the bed is elevated by 16 inches. The therapist applies percussion over the right nipple area. In females, percussion is applied with the cupped hand, with heel of the hand under armpit, and fingers extending forward beneath the breast.
   - *Left lung (Lingular segment):* Patient lies head down on right side. The foot end of the bed is elevated by 16 inches. The body is 1/4 turned backward and supported on pillow from shoulder to hip **(Fig. 30.36)**. The knees should be flexed. The therapist applies percussion over left nipple area with moderately cupped hand. In females, percussion is applied with the cupped hand, with heel of the hand under armpit, and fingers extending forward beneath the breast.
3. **Lower lobes:**
   - *Left and right lower lobes–Anterior basal segments:* Foot of bed or table elevated by 20 inches. The patient lies on side (Right side lying for left anterior basal segment and left side lying for right anterior basal segment), head down and pillow placed behind the back of the body **(Fig. 30.37)**. Therapist applies percussion with slightly cupped hands over the lower ribs.

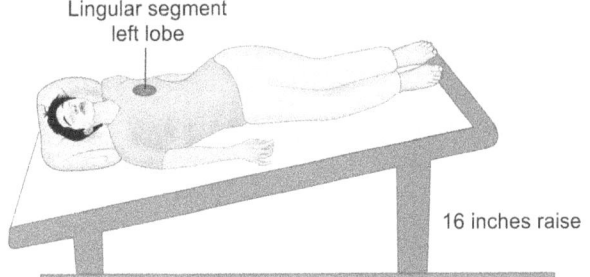

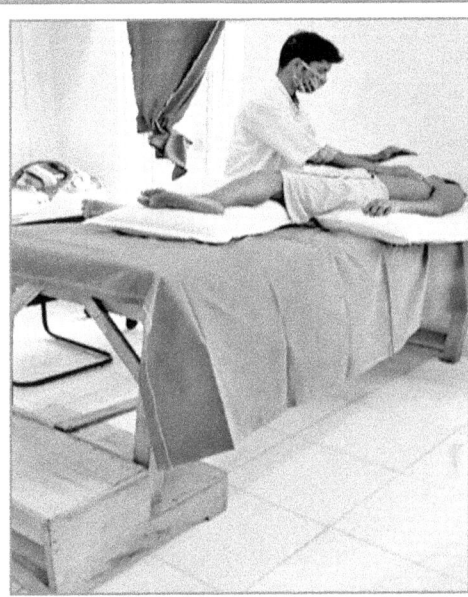

Fig. 30.36: Postural drainage from left lingular lobe.

   - *Left and right lower lobes–Lateral basal segments:* Foot of the bed elevated by 20 inches. Patient lies in prone lying, head down, body rotates ¼ turn upward (turns toward right side for right lateral basal segment, and turns towards left side for left lateral basal segment) **(Fig. 30.38)**. The upper side leg is flexed and supported on pillow. Therapist applies percussion with cupped hands over upper most portions of lower ribs.
   - *Left and right lower lobes–Posterior basal segments:* Foot of the bed elevated by 20 inches. The patient lies in prone position, head down with pillow under hips **(Fig. 30.39)**. Therapist applies percussion with cupped hands over the lower ribs, close to the spine on each side (left and right side).
   - *Left and right lower lobes–Superior segments:* Patient lies on a flat bed in prone position, with two pillows under the hips **(Fig. 30.40)**. Therapist applies percussion with cupped hands over middle of the back, at tip/inferior angle of scapula on either side of the spine.

Airway suctioning: Airway suctioning refers to the collective measures that are used for clearing the airway of a patient, if forced expiratory techniques such as huffing/coughing is either not possible or fails to remove secretions from the airways. It involves suctioning, clearing secretions, and maintaining the patency of the airway. Suctioning can be performed through an endotracheal tube, a tracheostomy tube, the mouth, or the nose. It is done combinedly by the

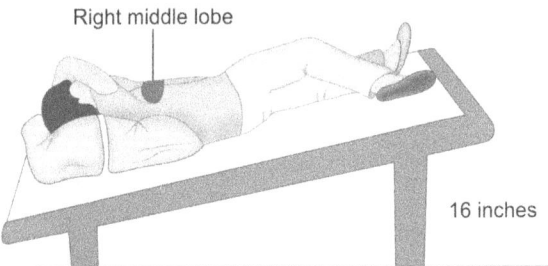

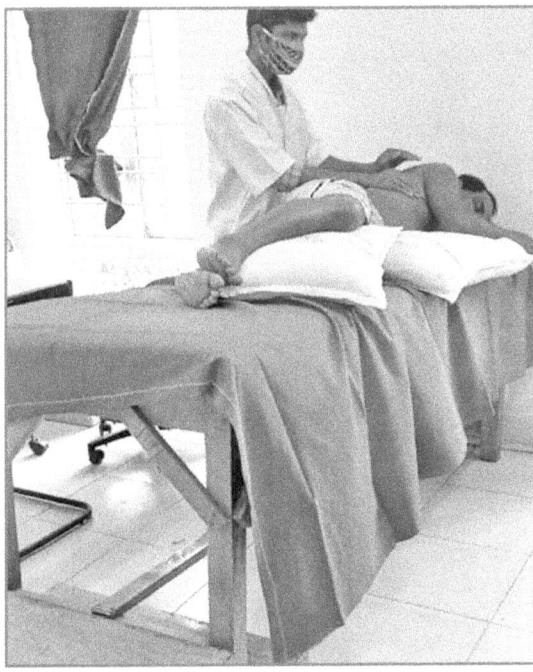

Fig. 30.35: Postural drainage from right middle lobe.

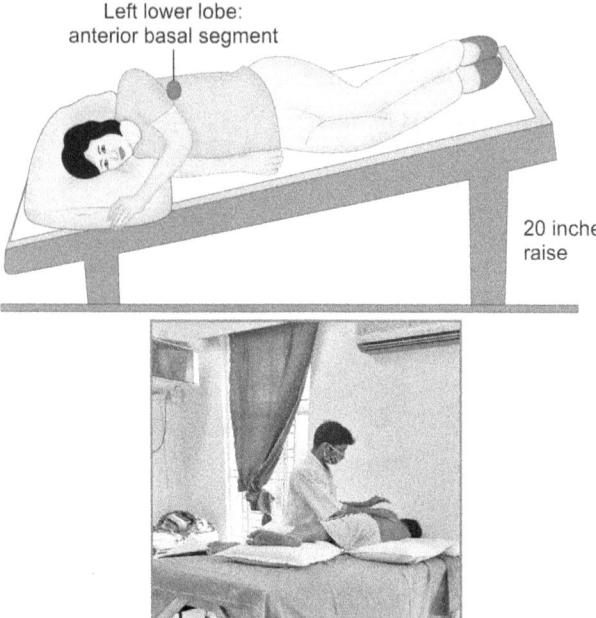

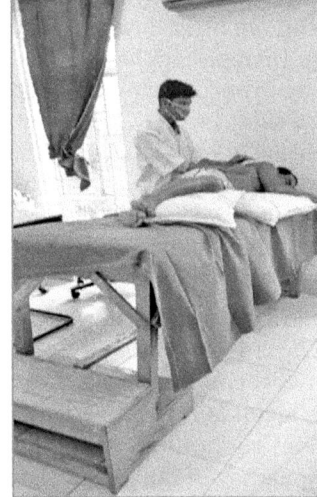

Fig. 30.37: Postural drainage from anterior basal segments of lower lobes (left lower lobe is shown in the figure).

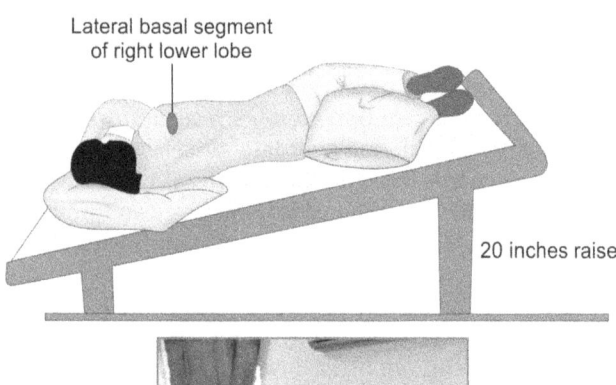

Fig. 30.38: Postural drainage from lateral basal segments of lower lobes (right lower lobe is shown in the figure).

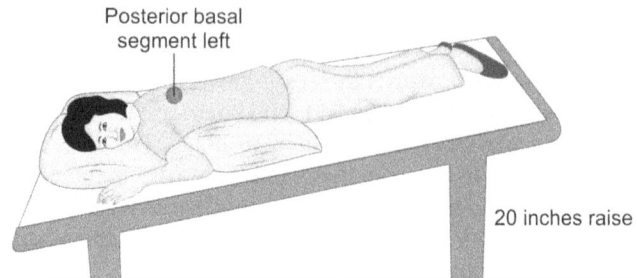

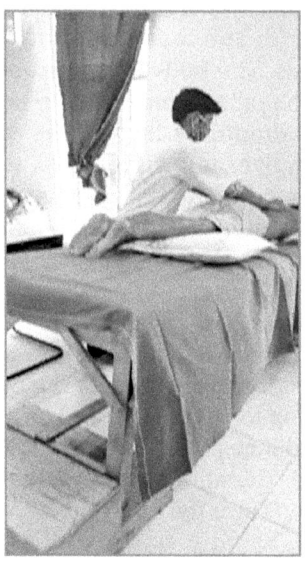

Fig. 30.39: Postural drainage from posterior basal segments of lower lobes (left lower lobe is shown in the figure).

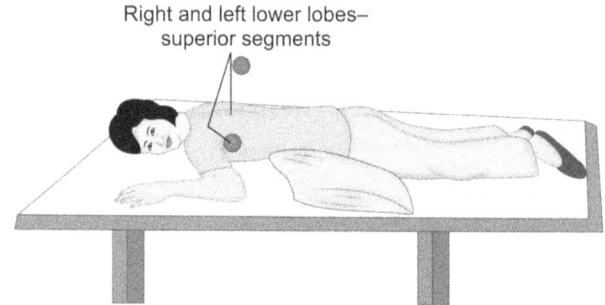

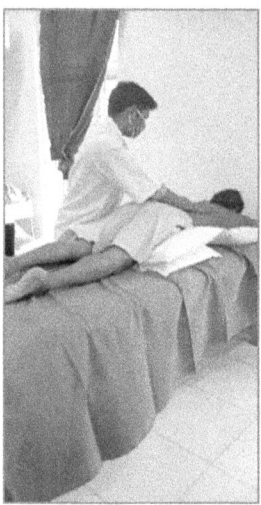

Fig. 30.40: Postural drainage from superior segments of right and left lower lobes.

nurse and physiotherapist. The **Figure 30.41** shows suctioning through the mouth.

Pulmonary Diseases Commonly Requiring Pulmonary Rehabilitation

Pulmonary rehabilitation is a service that is designed for those who experience chronic lung problems which is described in detail later.

Chronic Obstructive Pulmonary Disease (COPD)

Pulmonary rehabilitation should be offered to all patients who consider themselves functionally disabled by COPD with dyspnea grade of 3 ("I walk slower than people of the same age on the level because of breathlessness or have to stop for breath when walking at my own pace on the level") and above as per Medical Research Council grading system for dyspnea.

Chronic obstructive pulmonary disease is a chronic inflammatory lung disease that causes obstructed airflow from the lungs. Symptoms include breathing difficulty, cough, mucus (sputum) production and wheezing. It's typically caused by long-term exposure to irritating gases or particulate matter, most often from cigarette smoke. People with COPD are at increased risk of developing heart disease, lung cancer and a variety of other conditions. These are a group of progressive lung diseases, and the most common types include chronic bronchitis and emphysema.

Chronic bronchitis: It is a type of COPD, characterized by a constant productive cough that produces sputum, lasting for 3 months or more per year for at least 2 years. It also causes shortness of breath, wheezing, low-grade fever and tightness of chest. It is a disease of upper respiratory tract.

Emphysema: It is a chronic respiratory disease, where there is over-inflation of the air sacs (alveoli), causing decrease in lung function and breathlessness. It is a condition in which the alveoli at the end of the smallest air passages (bronchioles) of the lungs are destroyed as a result of damaging exposure to cigarette smoke and other irritating gases and particulate matter.

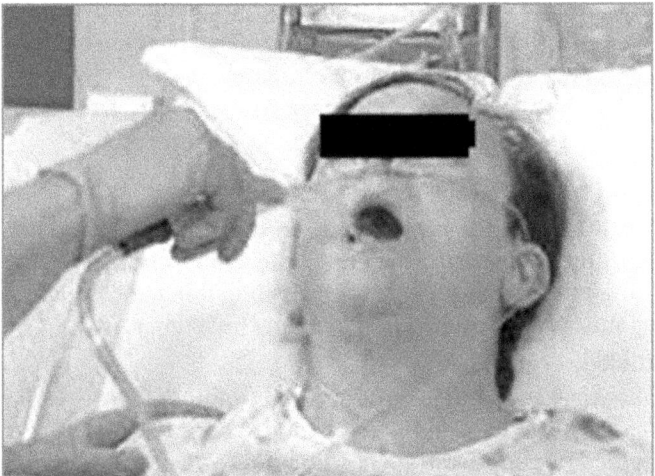

Fig. 30.41: Suctioning of secretion through the mouth.

Although COPD is a progressive disease that gets worse over time, COPD is treatable. With proper management, most people with COPD can achieve good symptom control and quality of life, as well as reduced risk of other associated conditions.

Causes of COPD

- Tobacco smoking.
- Exposures to fumes that occur in cooking.
- **Genetic:** In about 1% of people with COPD, the disease results from a genetic disorder that causes low levels of a protein called alpha-1-antitrypsin (AAt). Alpha-1-antitrypsin is made in the liver and secreted into the bloodstream to help protect the lungs. Alpha-1-antitrypsin deficiency can cause liver disease, lung disease or both.
- Air pollution.
- Exposure to dust.
- **Asthma:** A chronic inflammatory airway disease that may be a factor for developing COPD. The combination of asthma and smoking increases the risk of COPD even more.
- Bacterial infections.

Pathophysiology: Normally air travels from the trachea into the lungs through the bronchi. Inside the lungs, the bronchi divides into the bronchioles, that end in the small air sacs called alveoli. The alveoli have very thin walls lined with capillaries that take part in gaseous exchange.

In **chronic bronchitis,** bronchial tubes become inflamed and narrowed and the lungs produce mucus, which can block the narrowed tubes. The patient develops a chronic cough, trying to clear the airways. Due to production and accumulation of secretions, the bronchial tree and the alveoli, lose the natural elasticity that help in exhaling air and removal of secretions, resulting in over expansion, and accumulation of secretions and trapping of air.

In **emphysema,** there is destruction of the fragile walls and elastic fibers of the alveoli. Small airways collapse when one exhales, impairing airflow out of the lungs.

Clinical features of COPD

- Shortness of breath, especially during physical activities
- Wheezing
- Chest tightness
- A chronic cough that may produce mucus (sputum) that may be clear, white, yellow or greenish
- Frequent respiratory infections
- Lack of energy
- Unintended weight loss (in later stages)
- Swelling in ankles, feet, or legs.
- Periods of remission and exacerbations of symptoms
- Low-grade fever (sometimes).

Diagnosis

COPD is diagnosed from the clinical presentations, history of exposure to lung irritants such cigarette smokes and laboratory tests: The tests include:

- **Lung (pulmonary) function tests:** Spirometry, which reveals reduction of vital capacity and increase of FRC is

performed and the values are documented. Other tests include:
- Measurement of lung volumes using body plethysmography and diffusing capacity (measure of how well oxygen and carbon dioxide are transferred between the lungs and the blood, and can be a useful test in the diagnosis and to monitor treatment of lung diseases).
- 6-minute walk test.
- Pulse oximetry.

- **Chest X-ray:** A chest X-ray **(Figs. 30.42A and B)** is an important diagnostic test to diagnose COPD like bronchitis and emphysema.
- **CT scan:** A CT scan of the lungs can help detect emphysema
- **Arterial blood gas analysis:** This blood test measures how well the lungs are bringing oxygen into the blood and removing carbon dioxide.
- **Laboratory tests:** These tests are performed, when there is a family of COPD, to determine the presence of alpha-1 antitrypsin (AAT) deficiency, which may be the cause of COPD in few patients.

Management

People, with COPD should be advised to avoid exposure to causative agents such as cigarette smokes or polluted work environments. Those with milder symptoms require little therapy and are managed by medical personnel. Patients in the advanced stage of the disease need medical management and pulmonary rehabilitation.

Medical management: Several medicines are used to treat symptoms of COPD, and the most common drugs are:

- **Bronchodilators:** Bronchodilators are medications used to relax the smooth muscles of the airways. They can easily be taken in the form of inhalers, which helps in relieving dyspnea and cough. Depending upon the severity of the disease, the patient may be given a short-acting bronchodilator before activities, or a long-acting bronchodilator, that may be used every day.
- **Inhaled steroids:** Inhalation of corticosteroids help in reducing airways inflammation and prevents exacerbation of the condition.
- **Oral steroids:** This drug may be prescribed by the physician for patients who have moderate to severe acute exacerbations.
- **Phosphodiesterase-4 inhibitors:** This drug decreases airway inflammation and relaxes the airways.
- **Theophylline:** This drug which is less expensive is sometimes prescribed by the physician to prevent episodes of worsening of symptoms.
- **Antibiotics:** As respiratory infections such as acute bronchitis, pneumonia and influenza can aggravate symptoms of COPD, antibiotics may be prescribed by the physician to control such infections.
- **Oxygen therapy:** In case, there is reduction of oxygen saturation in blood, supplemental oxygen can be delivered to lungs through different methods. For patients who are ambulatory and functional, oxygen can be delivered through light weight portable units, which the patient can use while moving also. For patients needing ventilation therapy, oxygen can be delivered in the hospital/home using bilevel positive airway pressure device.
- **Pulmonary rehabilitation program:** This combines education, exercise training, nutritional advice, and counseling. Pulmonary rehabilitation after episodes of worsening COPD, reduces the possibility of re-admission to a hospital, increases the ability to participate in everyday activities and improves the quality of life.
- **Surgery:** This is a treatment option in some sufferers of emphysema, if they do not get benefit with conservative management. Surgeries performed include:
    - *Lung volume reduction surgery:* In this procedure, the surgeon removes small wedges of damaged lung tissue from the upper part of the lungs to create extra spaces, so that the remaining healthier lung tissue can expand. The diaphragm can also function efficiently after the surgery.
    - *Lung transplantation:* This is a treatment option for some sufferers.
    - *Bullectomy:* In emphysema, the destruction of the walls of the air sacs (alveoli), form large airs paces (bullae). These bullae can undergo enlargement causing breathing problems. The bullae may be removed from the lungs to help improve air flow.

Postoperatively, physiotherapy and pulmonary rehabilitation to be started following the precautions and protocols.

Cystic Fibrosis

Cystic fibrosis (CF) is a genetic disorder that affects mostly the lungs, but also the pancreas, liver, kidneys, and intestine. Long-term issues include difficulty breathing and coughing up mucus as a result of frequent lung infections.

Etiology

The disease is inherited through an autosomal recessive manner. It is caused by the presence of mutations in both copies of gene for the CF transmembrane conductance regulator (CFTR) protein. Those with a single working copy are the carriers and are mostly healthy.

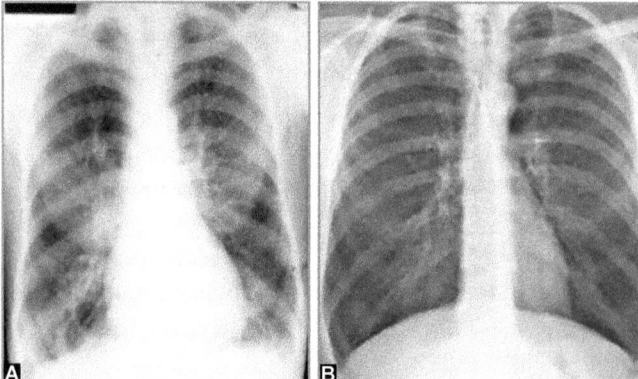

Figs. 30.42A and B: (A) Chest X-ray showing chronic bronchitis; (B) Chest X-ray showing emphysema.

Pathophysiology

Most of the damage in CF is due to blockage of the narrow passages of affected organs with thickened secretions. These blockages lead to remodeling and infection in the lungs, damage to pancreas due to accumulation of digestive enzymes, blockage of intestines by thick feces, etc.

Though several theories exist explaining the defects in protein and cellular function that causes the clinical effects, most current theory suggests that defective ion transport leads to dehydration in the airway epithelia, and thickening mucus. In airway epithelial cells, the cilia exist in between the cell's apical surface and mucus in a layer known as airway surface liquid (ASL). The flow of ions from the cell and into this layer is determined by ion channels such as CFTR. CFTR not only allows chloride ions to be drawn from the cell and into the ASL, but it also regulates another channel that allows sodium ions to leave the ASL and enter the respiratory epithelium. CFTR normally inhibits this channel, but if the CFTR is defective, then sodium flows freely from the ASL and into the cell.

As water follows sodium, the depth of ASL will be depleted of fluid and the cilia will be left in the mucus layer—As cilia cannot effectively move in a thick, viscous environment, mucociliary clearance is deficient and a build-up of mucus occurs, clogging small airways—The accumulation of more viscous, nutrient-rich mucus in the lungs allows bacteria to hide from the body's immune system, causing repeated respiratory infections. The presence of the same CFTR proteins in the pancreatic duct and sweat glands in the skin also cause symptoms in these systems.

Signs and symptoms

Though, the long-term issues include difficulty in breathing and coughing of mucus, the main signs and symptoms are:
* Salty testing skin.
* Poor growth and gain in weight despite normal food intake.
* Frequent chest infections, cough and breathlessness.
* Fatty stool.
* Clubbing of fingers.
* Infertility in males.

Management

Though there is no cure for the disease, recent advances in the treatment of CF lead individuals live a fuller life. The cornerstones of management are:
* Proactive treatment of airway infection, through use of antibiotics.
* Encouragement of good nutrition.
* Encouragement of active lifestyle.

Pulmonary rehabilitation (described below) as a management of CF continues throughout life of the person and is aimed at maximizing organ function and quality of life. Chest physiotherapy that involves chest percussion to loosen the secretions, postural drainage and active cycle of breathing techniques (ACBT) are considered as important components in pulmonary rehabilitation in subjects with CF.

Positive expiratory pressure physiotherapy that consists of providing a back pressure to the airways during expiration, applied by devices that consist of a mask or a mouthpiece in which a resistance is applied only on the expiration phase, helps preventing the early collapse of the small airways during exhalation.

Physical exercise is usually part of outpatient care for people with CF. Aerobic exercise seems to be beneficial for aerobic exercise capacity, lung function, and health-related quality of life.

Those with significantly lower oxygen saturation may be given home-based oxygen therapy.

As the lung condition worsens, mechanical ventilation may be necessary. Bilevel positive airway pressure (BiPAP) ventilators help in preventing low blood oxygen levels during sleep. If the patient's condition worsens, tracheostomy with ventilator support is considered.

Surgery

Some lung infections require surgical removal of the infected part of lung. Lung transplantation may become necessary for individuals with CF as lung function and exercise tolerance decline.

After lung surgeries, pulmonary rehabilitation is provided to improve function and quality of life.

SARCOIDOSIS

Sarcoidosis is a chronic inflammatory systemic disease having unknown cause. The disease involves abnormal collection of inflammatory cells that form lumps known as granulomas.

The disease usually begins in the lungs, skin, or lymph nodes, though it may also affect the eyes, liver, heart, or brain. Localization to the lungs is by far the most common manifestation of sarcoidosis. It can also affect the muscles, bones, and joints, resulting in acute or chronic arthritis. Sarcoidosis patients suffering from acute arthritis often also have bilateral hilar lymphadenopathy (BHL) and erythema nodosum. These three associated syndromes often occur together in Lofgren syndrome. The arthritis symptoms of Lofgren syndrome occur most frequently in the ankles, followed by the knees, wrists, elbows, and metacarpophalangeal joints. Usually, true arthritis is not present, but instead, periarthritis appears as a swelling in the soft tissue around the joints. Enthesitis also occurs in about one-third of patients with acute sarcoid arthritis, mainly affecting the Achilles tendon and heels.

Chronic sarcoid arthritis may involve the ankles, knees, wrists, elbows, and hands often this presents itself in a polyarticular pattern. Dactylitis similar to that seen in psoriatic arthritis that is associated with pain, swelling, overlying skin erythema, and underlying bony changes may also occur.

When it affects the lungs, wheezing, coughing, and shortness of breath or chest pain may be the presentation. The X-ray of lungs shows typical nodularity at the base of the lungs (**Fig. 30.43**).

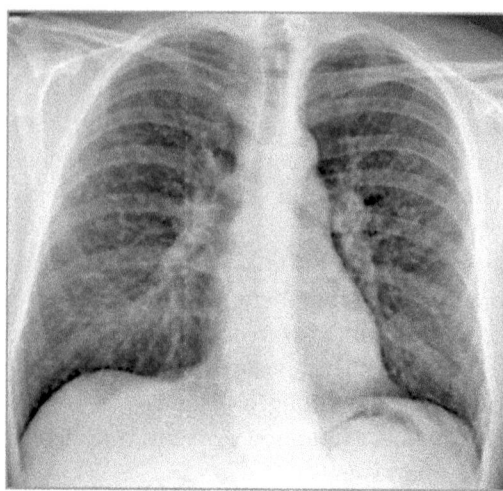

Fig. 30.43: Chest X-ray revealing sarcoidosis.

The four stages of pulmonary involvement are based on radiological stage of the disease, which is helpful in prognosis:
1. **Stage I:** BHL alone.
2. **Stage II:** BHL with pulmonary infiltrates.
3. **Stage III:** Pulmonary infiltrates without BHL.
4. **Stage IV:** Fibrosis

Management

Treatments for sarcoidosis vary greatly depending on the patient. NSAIDs, corticosteroids, antibiotics, immunosuppressant, etc., are prescribed by the physician as per indications.

Physiotherapy and Pulmonary Rehabilitation

Physical therapy, pulmonary rehabilitation, and counseling can help avoid deconditioning and improve social participation, psychological well-being, and activity levels. Key aspects are avoiding exercise intolerance and muscle weakness.

Low- or moderate-intensity exercise training has been shown to improve fatigue, psychological health, and physical functioning in people sarcoidosis without adverse effects. Inspiratory muscle training has also decreased severe fatigue perception in subjects with early stages of sarcoidosis, as well as improving functional and maximal exercise capacity and respiratory muscle strength. The duration, frequency, and physical intensity of exercise need to accommodate impairments such as joint pain, muscle pain, and fatigue.

IDIOPATHIC PULMONARY FIBROSIS

Idiopathic pulmonary fibrosis is a type of chronic scarring lung disease characterized by progressive and irreversible decline in lung function. It is a type of interstitial lung disease.

Cause: The cause of the disease is unknown. However, risk factors include cigarette smoking, certain viral infections and family history of the condition.

Clinical features: Symptoms typically include gradual onset of shortness of breath accompanied with dry cough. Other features include, fatigue, abnormally large and dome-shaped finger and toenails (nail clubbing). The complications of the disease include: pulmonary hypertension, heart failure, pneumonia, and pulmonary embolism.

Management: Pulmonary rehabilitation, oxygen therapy is the treatment of choice. In case of severity of symptoms, lung transplantation may be the option.

Pulmonary rehabilitation may alleviate the overt symptoms of this condition and improve functional status by stabilizing and/or reversing the extrapulmonary features of the disease. Though the number of published studies on the role of pulmonary rehabilitation in idiopathic pulmonary fibrosis is small, but most of these studies have found significant short-term improvements in functional exercise tolerance, quality of life, and dyspnea on exertion in the sufferers. Typical programs of rehabilitation include exercise training, nutritional modulation, occupational therapy, education, and psychosocial counseling.

PULMONARY REHABILITATION

Pulmonary rehabilitation, also known as **respiratory rehabilitation**, is an important part of the management and health maintenance of people with chronic respiratory disease who remain symptomatic or continue to have decreased function despite standard medical treatment.

Definition: It is defined as an evidence-based, interdisciplinary, and comprehensive intervention for patients with chronic respiratory diseases who are symptomatic and often have decreased daily life activities. It refers to a series of services that are administered to patients of respiratory disease and their families, typically to attempt to improve the quality of life for the patient.

It is the use of exercise, education, and behavioral intervention to improve function in daily life and to enhance the quality of life in people with chronic lung disease.

Indications for Pulmonary Rehabilitation

Pulmonary rehabilitation is specific to the individual patient, with the objective of meeting the needs of the patient. The program may benefit patients with lung diseases such as COPD, sarcoidosis, idiopathic pulmonary fibrosis (IPF), and cystic fibrosis, etc. Although the process is focused on the rehabilitation of the patient him/herself, the family is also involved.

It is indicated for patients with chronic respiratory diseases, who have decreased exercise tolerance, exertional dyspnea or fatigue, and/or impairment of activities of daily living. The conditions necessitating pulmonary rehabilitation include:
- COPD that include chronic bronchitis and emphysema.
- Sarcoidosis.
- Pulmonary hypertension
- Lung cancer.
- Pulmonary fibrosis.
- Lung volume reduction surgery.
- Lung transplantation.

Contraindications for Pulmonary Rehabilitation

- Angina pectoris, recent myocardial infarction, severe pulmonary hypertension.
- Congestive heart failure.
- Unstable diabetes.
- Inability to do exercise due to orthopedic diseases or other reasons.
- Psychiatric illness, dementia.
- Severe exercise-induced hypoxemia, not correctable with O_2 supplementation.

Objectives/Goal of Pulmonary Rehabilitation

The goal of pulmonary rehabilitation is to help improve the well-being and quality of life of the patient and their families. It can be summarized as below:

- To reduce symptoms such as dyspnea, cough, etc.
- To improve knowledge on lung condition and promote self-management
- To increase muscle strength and endurance.
- To increase the exercise tolerance.
- To reduce length of hospital stay.
- To help to function better in day-to-day life.
- To help in managing anxiety and depression.
- To improve the quality of life.

Benefits of Pulmonary Rehabilitation

- Reduces periods of hospitalization.
- Reduces COPD symptoms and perceived intensity of breathlessness.
- Improves exercise capacity, physical activity and daily life function.
- Improves emotional health.
- Reduces anxiety and depression.
- Reduces the number of exacerbations in patients who are active and perform exercises.
- Reduces exacerbations post rehabilitation.
- Increases participation in family and social roles.
- Increases health-related quality of life.
- Increases survival.

Settings for Pulmonary Rehabilitation

Pulmonary rehabilitation can be provided in inpatient care set-up, outpatient care set-up as well as in patient's home.

Focus of Pulmonary Rehabilitation

The rehabilitation program focuses on the following impairments/weaknesses in clients with pulmonary diseases:

- Reduction of ventilatory limitation.
- Reduction of gas exchange limitation.
- Minimizing cardiac dysfunction.
- Minimizing skeletal muscle dysfunction.
- Minimizing respiratory muscle dysfunction.

Components of Pulmonary Rehabilitation

The various components of management included in pulmonary rehabilitation are shown in **Figure 30.44**.

- **Medical management**: Medications are used in the process of pulmonary rehabilitation, which include anti-inflammatory agents (inhaled steroids), long-acting bronchodilators, antibiotics, mucolytic agents, oxygen therapy, etc., as prescribed by the physician.
- **Chest secretion clearance techniques**: Airway clearance techniques (postural drainage and ACBT). Airway clearance techniques are defined as manual or mechanical procedures that facilitate mobilization of secretions from the airways. The techniques include postural drainage, percussion, vibration, huffing and coughing techniques, manual hyperinflation, and airway suctioning.

  Active cycle of breathing is also an effective chest clearance technique taught to the patient for clearance of secretion and improvement of ventilation. The ACBT consists of a series of maneuvers (described earlier) performed by the patient to emphasize independence in secretion clearance and thoracic expansion. This forced expiratory technique is as effective as airway clearance techniques performed by a therapist or caregiver.
- **Exercise testing and training:** Exercises are the important components of pulmonary rehabilitation that help the heart and lungs work better. There are various types of exercises performed to improve cardiorespiratory fitness, strength of the skeletal muscles including muscles of ventilation, so that the individual achieves the potential to overcome cardiopulmonary and skeletal muscle dysfunctions and returns to the workplace as early as possible. Although the breathing exercises and exercises to the muscles of ventilation improve lung function, exercises to the skeletal muscles of limb and trunk also produce many physiological adaptations to exercise resulting in improvement of physiological function.

Exercise testing: Testing exercise tolerance is essentially performed by the pulmonary physiotherapist, before subjecting the patient to exercise training. The client's blood oxygen saturation level, lung capacities (Spirometry),

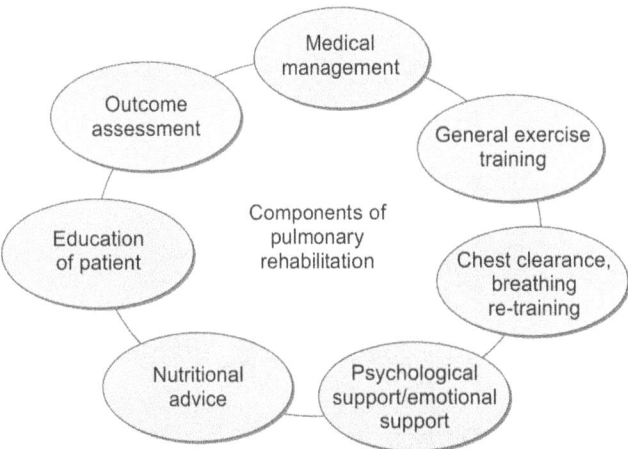

Fig. 30.44: Components of pulmonary rehabilitation.

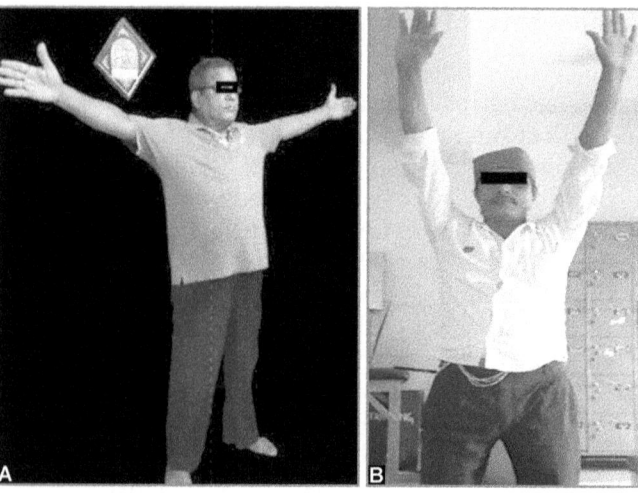

Figs. 30.45A and B: Warm-up exercises during pulmonary rehabilitation.

exercise tolerance, and ability to perform various exercises/activities are to be tested. Various exercise tolerance tests such as the followings may be performed and documented:
- Exercise testing using exercise time.
- Walk tests such as 6-minutes walk test.
- 6-minutes step test.
- Exertion and overall dyspnea using the Modified Borg scale, discussed later.

The exercises recommended to the patients are:
- **Warm-up exercises:** It consists of 5–10 minutes of low intensity warm up exercises as shown in **Figures 30.45A and B**.
- **Lower body exercises:** The exercises that center on leg workouts such as walking around a track or on a treadmill, stair climbing, static cycle exercises, jugging, hopping, etc., which are gradually progressed in intensity and duration are considered beneficial to improve heart and lungs function, hence are an important part of pulmonary rehabilitation. Some of the exercises are shown in **Figures 30.46A and B**.
- **Upper body exercises:** The muscles of the upper body such as muscles of arm, chest, and trunk are important for breathing as well as performance of ADL. Exercises such as bending forward with exhalation and getting vertical with inspiration, theraband exercises, medicine ball exercises, progressive resisted exercises to upper limb, shoulder wheel exercises, etc., are considered in subjects for pulmonary rehabilitation. Some of the exercises are shown in **Figures 30.47A to E**.
- **Breathing training/Breathing exercises:** Diaphragmatic and costal breathing exercises are given to expand all the segments of the lungs. Postural drainage and the ACBT is used to clear secretions from the lungs, and pursed-lip breathing and use of breathing games such as blowing a piece of paper **(Fig. 30.48)**, incentive spirometry, etc., can be used to increase air flow to the lung in COPD.
- **Strength training:** Strengthening or resistance exercises **(Figs. 30.49A and B)** can help in building muscle strength and endurance of muscles including the muscles of respiration.
- **Aerobic exercises:** Aerobic exercises **(Figs. 30.50A and B)** tend to improve the body's ability to use oxygen, by decreasing the heart rate and blood pressure. The exercises include fast walking, running, jogging, dancing, deep breathing combined with movement of upper limb and trunk, etc.
- Stretching exercises to tight soft tissues are given to improve flexibility **(Fig. 30.51)**.
- Pilates can be given to improve breathing and co-ordination **(Figs. 30.52A and B)**.
- **Cool down exercises:** The exercise training should end with 5–10 minutes of low-intensity exercises to smoothly bring the patient's cardiorespiratory function to resting level. **Figures 30.53A and B** demonstrate a cool down exercise.
- **Education about lung disease:** The pulmonary rehabilitation program should offer either one-on-one or

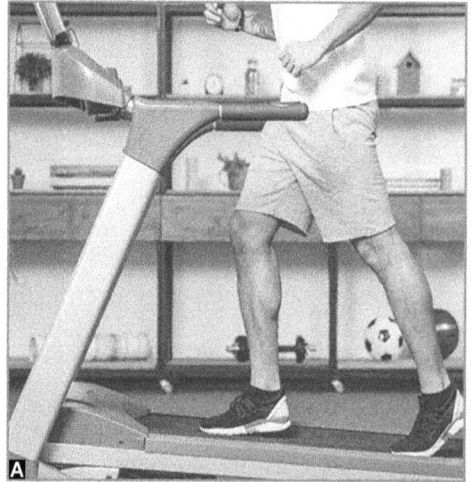
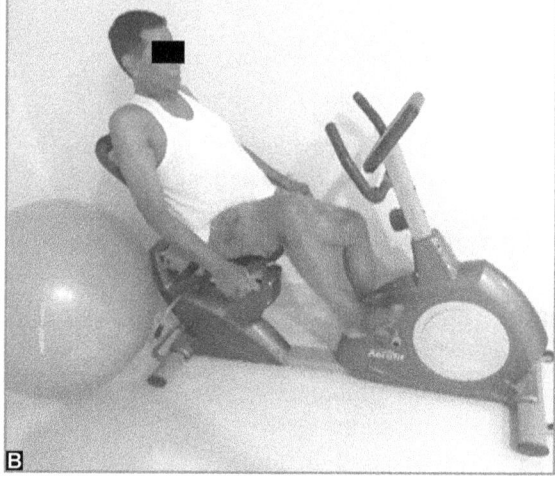

Figs. 30.46A and B: (A) Lower body exercise on treadmill; (B) Static cycle exercise.

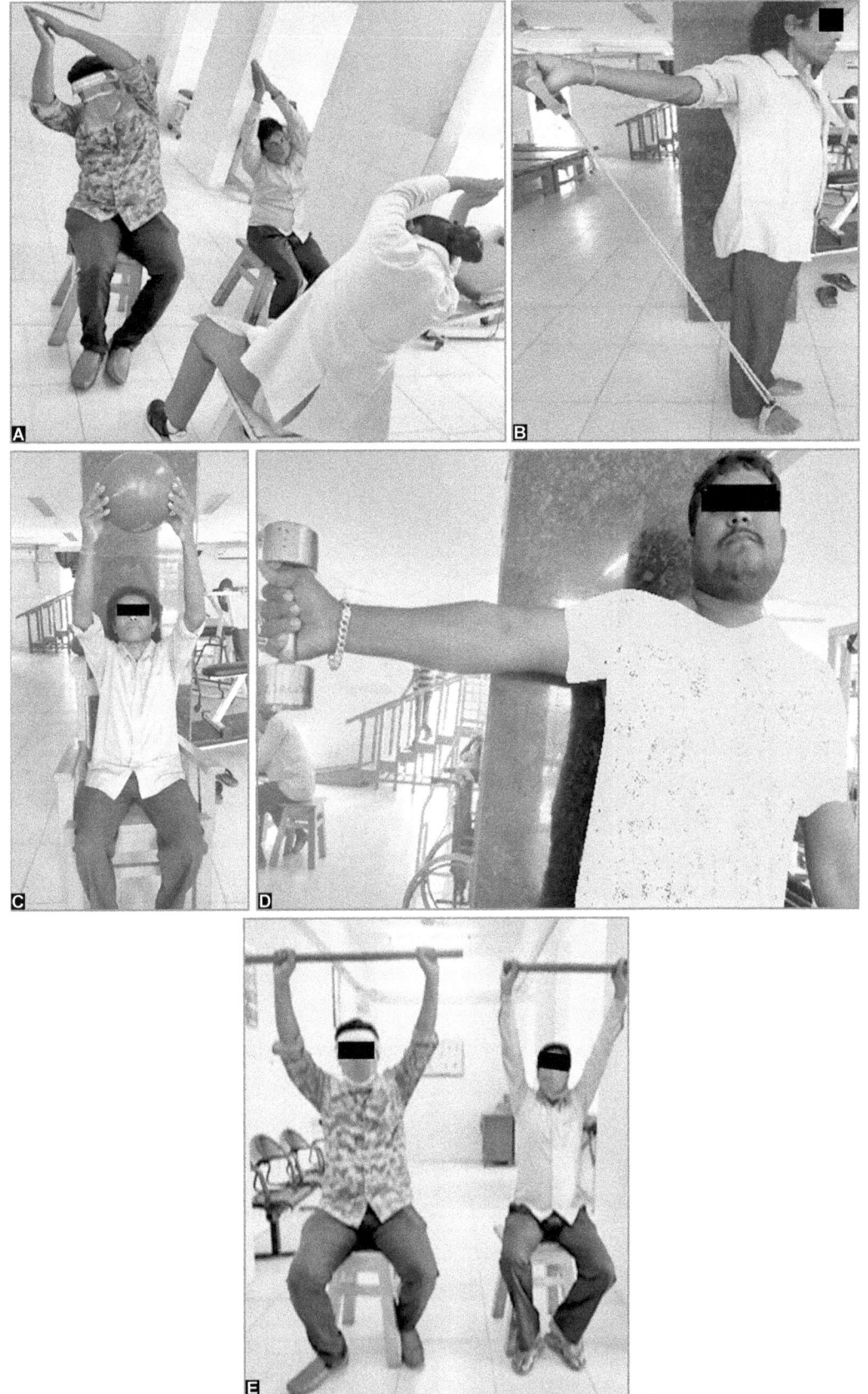

Figs. 30.47A to E: (A) Breathing in combination with upper limb and trunk movements; (B) Theraband exercise; (C) Medicine ball exercise; (D) Resistance training with weight held in hand; (E) Wand exercise for shoulder combined with trunk movement and breathing.

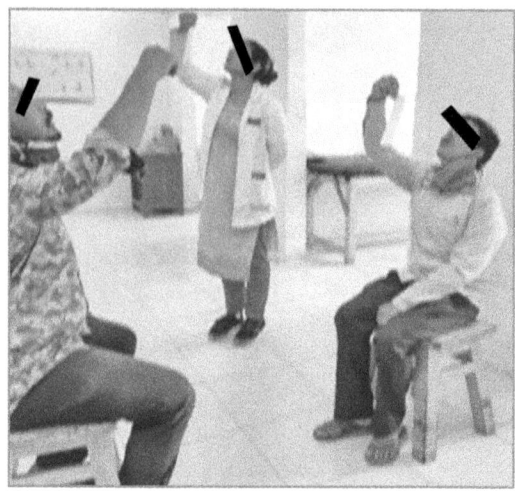

Fig. 30.48: Breathing game.

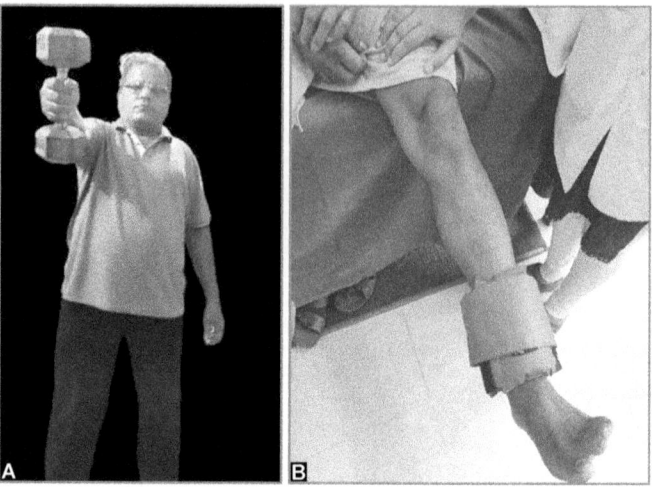

Figs. 30.49A and B: Strength training for muscles of upper and lower limbs.

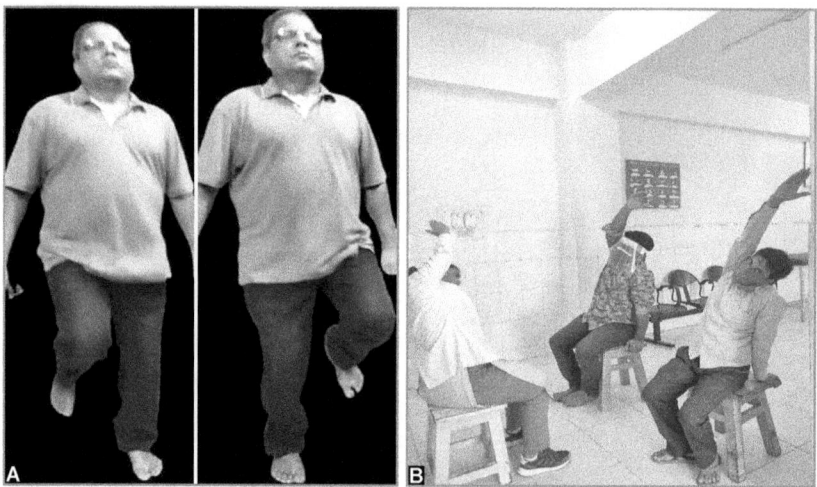

Figs. 30.50A and B: (A) Aerobic exercise involving lower limbs (jogging); (B) Exercise involving breathing combined with movement of upper limb and trunk.

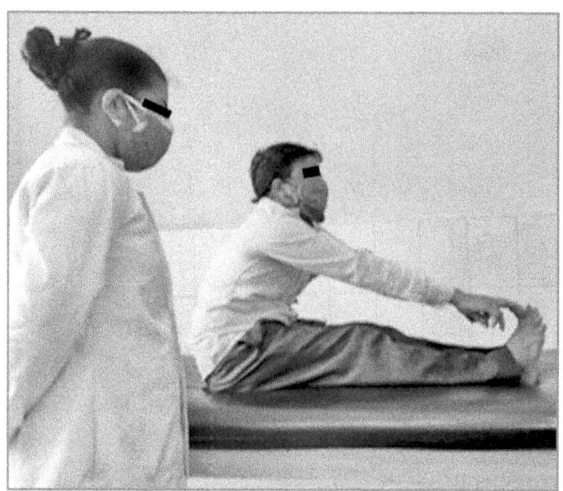

Fig. 30.51: Flexibility exercise for the body.

group sessions to educate the patient about the pulmonary disease, he/she is suffering from, and how to manage dyspnea, right way to take oxygen, if he is on home oxygen therapy, right way to take inhalers and the importance of quitting smoking.

Studies show that people who learn about their COPD/lung diseases and treatment plan are better able to spot symptoms of a flare-up and take the right action.

- ❖ **Nutritional counseling:** The patients with pulmonary diseases should be advised to take a healthy diet, as advised by the dietician.
- ❖ **Psychological/Emotional support:** People with severe COPD have a great chance of being depressed or anxious. Relaxation training and counseling included in the program helps to support the client to show interest in pleasurable activities.

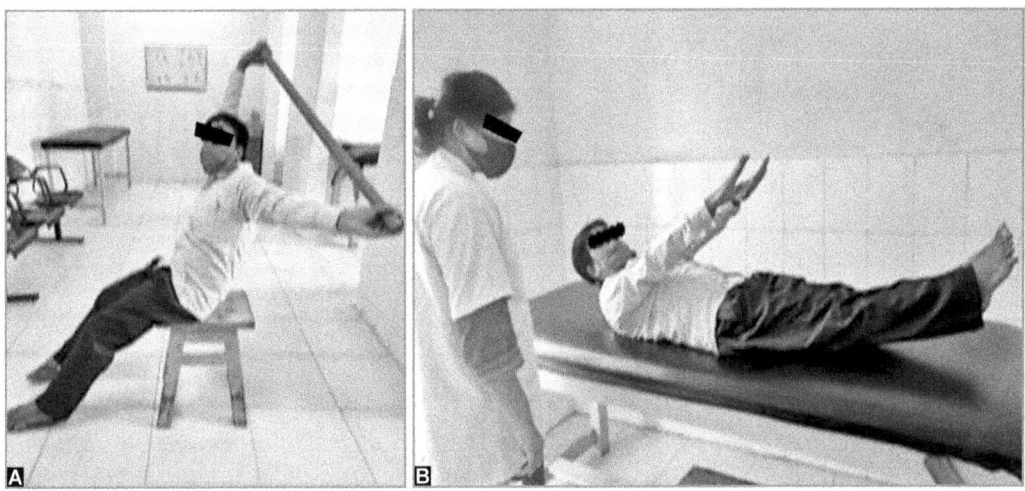

Figs. 30.52A and B: (A) Upper limb elevation with trunk extension during inspiration and trunk flexion and upper limb lowering during expiration; (B) Trunk flexion during expiration and trunk lowering (extension) during inspiration.

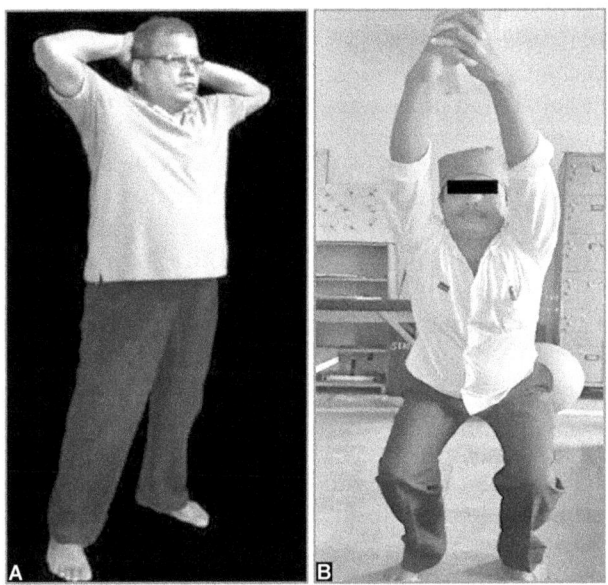

Figs. 30.53A and B: Cool down exercises.

- **Outcome measurement:** Periodically the client's blood oxygen saturation level, lung capacities (Spirometry), exercise tolerance and ability to participate in life roles should be evaluated and compared with pre-training status for making modifications in the program and to take a decision about advice on discharge and continuing home exercise program.

The clinical improvements in outcomes due to pulmonary rehabilitation are measurable through:
 – Exercise testing using exercise time.
 – Walk tests such as 6-minutes walk test.
 – Exertion and overall dyspnea using the Borg scale.

Cardiac Rehabilitation

INTRODUCTION

Cardiac rehabilitation is the use of exercise, education, as well as psychological and emotional support to facilitate a patient's recovery from heart disease or heart surgery.

It is a comprehensive medically supervised recovery program especially designed for patients with heart disease. Typically, the cardiac rehabilitation program begins with a careful analysis of patients' condition and needs with proper exercise stress testing, followed by a supervised progressive exercise regime, combined with education on a heart healthy lifestyle and medications. It may be beneficial for patients with any kind of heart condition, including coronary artery disease, angina, heart failure, heart attack, and cardiac surgeries. It is a structured program of exercise and education, designed to help the patient return to optimal fitness and function following an event such as heart attack/cardiac surgeries.

Cardiac rehabilitation is defined as the combined and coordinated use of medical, psychological, educational, vocational, and physical measures, required to ensure cardiac patients the best possible physical, mental and social conditions, so that, they may by their own efforts, resume and maintain as normal a place as possible in the community, maintaining an active and satisfying lifestyle.

It is an interdisciplinary team approach, and may include the cardiac physician/cardiac surgeon, nurse, physiotherapist, occupational therapist, exercise physiologist, nutritional specialist, and medicosocial worker. Cardiac rehabilitation begins in the hospital and extends indefinitely into the maintenance phase.

Until 1950s, patients who used to get heart attack, strict bed rest was thought to be the appropriate advice, and after discharge from hospital, moderately stressful activities such as climbing stairs, were discouraged for years, significantly affecting the person's life roles in family and society affecting the overall quality of life. After the cardiac rehabilitation emerged, the living of people having a heart attack, heart failure, heart valve surgery, coronary artery bypass grafting, etc., have become much comfortable.

The World Health Organization (WHO) defined cardiac rehabilitation in 1993 in a timeless way that is inclusive and sensitive to the psychosocial, biomedical, professional expertise and service delivery mode and location elements required of a contemporary cardiac rehabilitation service. It states cardiac rehabilitation as:

"The sum of activities required to influence favorably the underlying cause of the disease so that (people) may by their own efforts preserve, or resume when lost, as normal a place in the community...
...it must be integrated within secondary prevention services of which it forms one facet".

The coordinated, multifaceted interventions are designed by the rehabilitation team, to optimize a cardiac patient's physical, psychological, and social functioning, in addition to stabilizing, slowing or even reversing, the progression of the underlying atherosclerotic process, thereby reducing morbidity and mortality. Physiotherapists work as members of cardiac rehabilitation team, helping to evaluate cardiac function, assess impairments that may limit the client's mobility, performs exercise tolerance tests, and prescribe and implement progressive exercises and activities to help the patient return to normal lifestyle after a cardiac event.

Cardiac rehabilitation involves adopting heart healthy lifestyle changes to address risk factors for cardiovascular disease. It promotes lifestyle changes through improvement of cardiac function, focussing on exercise tolerance testing, exercise training, patient and care giver education on heart-healthy living, patient counseling to reduce stress and helping return to an active life.

Before starting the program, the rehabilitation team performs the following:

❖ Collect the patient's medical history
❖ Do a physical examination
❖ Perform tests such as ECG examination, cardiac imaging tests, simple tests like 6 minutes walk test/step test, symptom limited treadmill or static cycle exercise test (bicycle ergometry), measurement of cholesterol levels and blood sugar.

During cardiac rehabilitation, the patient is taught certain exercises with in safe limits to increase physical activities in a progressive manner. Though the length of time for cardiac rehabilitation depends on the patient's conditions, a standard cardiac rehabilitation program includes 36 supervised sessions over 12 weeks. If serious problems such as life-threatening heart rhythm problems, which are unlikely to occur during the supervised program, still occur, the physical activities should be stopped immediately, and appropriate treatment should be started by the physician/cardiologist.

INDICATIONS OF CARDIAC REHABILITATION

- Postmyocardial infarction.
- Postcoronary artery bypass grafting through open heart surgery.
- Angina pectoris.
- Percutaneous coronary intervention (PCI), also known as cardiac catheterization (a procedure to open blocked coronary arteries and restore blood flow to the heart muscles).
- Valve replacement or repair.
- Heart transplantation.
- Congestive heart failure. The requirement needs to be established through more research.

Absolute Contraindications to Exercises During Cardiac Rehabilitation

- Acute myocardial infarction.
- Unstable angina (feeling of chest pain even at rest).
- Unstable cardiac arrhythmia.
- Symptomatic severe aortic stenosis.
- Uncontrolled symptomatic heart failure.
- Acute pulmonary embolism/pulmonary infarction.
- Acute myocarditis/pericarditis.
- Active endocarditis.
- Acute aortic dissection.
- Acute noncardiac disorder that may affect exercise performance.
- Inability to obtain consent.

Relative Contraindications to Exercises in Cardiac Rehabilitation

- Left main coronary artery stenosis.
- Moderate stenotic valvular heart disease.
- Electrolyte disturbances.
- Severe hypertension (systolic 200 mm Hg, and/or diastolic 110 mm Hg).
- Tachyarrhythmia or bradyarrhythmia, including atrial fibrillation with uncontrolled ventricular rate.
- Hypertrophic cardiomyopathy.
- High degree atrioventricular block.
- Mental or physical impairments leading to inability to cooperate.

GOAL OF CARDIAC REHABILITATION

- To stabilize, slow down or even reverse the progression of cardiovascular disease.
- To address risk factors that lead to coronary heart disease, including high blood pressure, high cholesterol, obesity, diabetes, smoking, lack of physical activity, depression and other emotional health concerns.
- Enable the client adapt to healthy lifestyle changes such as increasing the physical activity level, taking healthy diet, reducing risk factors for future heart problems and increasing emotional health.
- To improve the overall quality of life of the individual.

BENEFITS OF CARDIAC REHABILITATION

- Eliminates the psychological and physiological complications of bed rest during hospitalization.
- Provide additional medical surveillance of patients.
- Enable the patient return to activities of daily living within the limits imposed by their disease.
- Prepare the patient and the support system at home to optimize recovery after hospital discharge.
- Reduces cardiovascular and total mortality.
- Improves myocardial perfusion.
- Reduces progression of atherosclerosis, when combined with appropriate diet.
- Improves exercise tolerance, without significant cardiovascular complications.
- Improves muscular strength and endurance.
- Decreases angina and congestive heart failure symptoms.
- Promotes favorable exercise habits.

ASSESSMENT OF PATIENT BEFORE EXERCISE TRAINING FOR CARDIAC REHABILITATION

- For low-to-moderate risk patients, and those who require low to moderate intensity exercise, clinical risk stratifications should be done.
- For high risk patients, and those requiring high intensity exercises ECG/echocardiography and exercise testing should be performed.
- Functional exercise capacity should be evaluated before and after completion of the exercise training. Functional capacity to exercise is the aerobic capacity which is measured in VO_2 max. This is a measure of the maximum amount of oxygen the body can use during a specified period or intense exercise.

Examination of Different Systems before Cardiac Rehabilitation

- Vital signs such as pulse rate, respiratory rate, blood pressure, oxygen saturation level (pulse oximetry), ECG findings
- Respiratory system examinations
- Circulatory system examinations
- Central nervous system examinations
- Musculoskeletal system examinations

Measurement of Different Parameters before Cardiac Rehabilitation

- **Exercise capacity:** Assessment of exercise capacity provides valuable information to guide exercise prescription. This includes subjective and objective assessment of an individual's exercise tolerance and objective test results, which can be used to calculate exercise intensity.
  Exercise capacity can be assessed by the following tests, as per availability of facilities.
  – *Exercise stress test (maximal test)/symptom limited exercise test):* This test shows how the heart works during physical activity. This may reveal problems

with the blood flow within the heart. The test involves monitoring the heart rate and rhythm, blood pressure, breathing while exercising on a treadmill or stationary bicycle. This test is performed under the supervision of a cardiologist, if the patient has signs and symptoms of coronary artery disease or irregular heart rhythm (arrhythmia).
- *Cardiopulmonary exercise test:* The cardiopulmonary exercise test (CPET), is a type of stress test, that examines, how well the lungs, heart and muscles work. This is a provocative test that combines standard methods of electrocardiogram (ECG), stress testing with indices of gas exchange. This is an exercise test, where an individuals' heart and lungs functions are carefully monitored during a steadily increasing work load. This test is recommended, when dyspnea or exercise limitation cannot be fully explained by simpler tests.
- *Submaximal test (6-minute walk test):* The 6-minute walk test is a submaximal exercise test that entails measurement of distance walked over a time span of 6 minutes. The 6-minute walk distance provides the measure for integrated global response of multiple cardiopulmonary and musculoskeletal systems involved in exercise. This test provides information regarding, functional capacity, response to therapy and prognosis across a broad range of chronic cardiopulmonary conditions. The 6 minutes walk test, is performed on a straight 30 meter track. The subject is asked to walk as far as possible for 6 minutes. The total distance covered at the end of the test is measured, along with recording of heart rate, blood pressure, rating of perceived exertion (RPE), recovery time, etc.
- *Submaximal treadmill test:* The Bruce submaximal treadmill test is the most common test used to assess cardiorespiratory fitness in clinical settings. The test is administered in 3-minute stages, until the client achieves 85% of his/her age predicted maximum heart rate.
- *Incremental shuttle walk test:* The test is a low risk test that measures, how often one can walk back and forth between 2 cones in a 10 meter track. The walking pace will be set and increased every minute. One length of 10 meters is called a shuttle, and every minute the individual completes at a fixed speed is called a level.

❖ **Intensity of exercise:** Three parameters such as oxygen consumption (VO_2 max), heart rate (target heart rate), and rate of perceived exertion are used for determining the intensity of exercise. Exercise intensity can be prescribed using a percentage of the maximum VO_2 achieved on an exercise tolerance test (ETT). While using a percentage of VO_2 may be the most accurate method of prescribing exercise from a graded exercise test, it does not give the clinician a means to monitor exercise intensity during actual performance of exercises. Exercise HR [target heart rate range (THRR)] is a practical choice for measuring and monitoring exercise intensity.

- *The target heart rate range (THRR):* It defines a wide, safe, and effective range of exercise intensity that can be performed during the treatment session. The target heart rate for a specific patient defines a more narrow HR (within the prescribed THRR) that will be most appropriate to ensure aerobic training and patient adherence.

A common method to determine a patient's THRR and the target heart rate (THR) is using the heart rate reserve (HRR) method or Karvonen's formula. The HRR is the difference between the resting HR (HR rest) in the seated position and the maximal HR (HRmax) achieved on an exercise tolerance test (ETT). To calculate the THRR, percentages (40% and 85%) of the HRR are added to the resting HR.

Karvonen's formula for determining the upper and lower limits of the THRR is:
» Lower limit of THRR = [(HRmax − HRrest) × 0.40] + HRrest.
» Upper limit of THRR = [(HRmax − HRrest) × 0.85] + HRrest.
- *Borg's rate of perceived exertion scale:* It is also considered as a measure of intensity of exercise, which is discussed in **Table 31.1**.

❖ **Quality of life survey:**
- *SF-12 health survey:* This survey asks the views of the patient about his/her health. This information will help keep track of how the patient feels and how well he/she is able to do the usual activities. Patient is asked to answer each question by choosing just one answer.
- *SF-36:* The 36-item Short Form Health Survey (SF-36) is a measure of health-related quality-of-life. The SF-36 has 36 items grouped in eight dimensions such as: Physical functioning, physical role, emotional role, bodily pain, vitality, social functioning, general health,

Table 31.1: Borg rating scale of perceived exertion.

Rate	Level of perceived exertion
6	No exertion
7	Extremely light
8	
9	Very light
10	
11	Light
12	
13	Somewhat hard
14	
15	Hard
16	
17	Very hard
18	
19	Extremely hard
20	Maximal exertion

mental health. It is a generic measure, as opposed to one that targets a specific age, disease, or treatment group.
- **Blood pressure**
- **Weight**
- **Waist circumference**
- **Lipid profile**
- **Blood glucose level/HbA1C**
- **Telemetry monitoring:** Telemetry monitoring is when healthcare providers monitor the electrical activity of the patient's heart for an extended time. This should be done during exercise sessions.
- **Nutritional survey**
- **Measurement of stress level**.

COMPONENTS OF CARDIAC REHABILITATION

Cardiac rehabilitation programs should focus on:
- Patient assessment
- Nutritional counseling
- Weight management
- Blood pressure management
- Lipid management
- Diabetes management
- Tobacco cessation
- Psychosocial management
- Physical activity counseling
- Exercise training

The **Figure 31.1** summarizes the components of cardiac rehabilitation.

Exercise Training in Cardiac Rehabilitation

The physiotherapist as an important member of cardiac rehabilitation team is mostly concerned with exercise testing, prescription and designing of exercises to meet the need of the clients.

Benefits of exercise in cardiac rehabilitation: Exercises and activities performed during cardiac rehabilitation are associated with the following benefits:

- Strengthens heart muscles
- Increases hemoglobin concentration in the blood
- Increases stroke volume, enabling the heart to pump blood more efficiently
- Enlarges and increases the number of arteries supplying blood to the heart, thereby increasing oxygen supply and reducing the tendency for blood clots.
- Increases body's metabolism, thereby assisting in weight loss
- Reduces and assists with the control of cardiac risk factors such as high blood pressure, high cholesterol and diabetes
- Increases muscle strength, flexibility and endurance
- Reduces psychological stress

Exercises Performed in Cardiac Rehabilitation
- Warm up exercises
- Flexibility exercises
- Breathing exercises
- Aerobic exercises using variety of equipment such as treadmills, static cycle, rowing machines, steppers, arm ergometers, etc. It also includes walking, running, ball throwing/kicking.
- Low intensity resistance training
- Cool down exercises

Intensity, Duration and Frequency of Exercise

Intensity of aerobic exercise may be prescribed by either HR or by subjective report, a rating of perceived exertion (RPE) discussed earlier. Subjective ratings of intensity of exertion have been used to quantify effort during exercise. The RPE scale consists of numbers ranging from 6 to 20, which patients use to rate their perceptions of how hard they are working. Descriptive words accompany the numbers, such as hard or very hard. Commonly, patients are asked to limit their exertion to between very light and somewhat hard.

A common aerobic exercise prescription based on HR is 70–85% of HRmax. However, the more deconditioned patient may be aerobically trained at as low as 40–60% of HRmax. HRmax of the patient should be determined by the symptom limited exercise tolerance test (ETT). ETT should always be done in the presence of the cardiologist.

The duration of aerobic exercise training sessions should vary from 30 to 40 minutes, with an additional 5–10 minutes of warm-up and an adequate cooldown as appropriate.

Exercises are commonly performed 3–5 times per week. The patient should not experience increased fatigue as a result of exercise. If fatigue does occur, the frequency and/or intensity of exercise should be decreased.

If a patient becomes symptomatic with angina during a physical therapy intervention, the immediate goal is to decrease maximum oxygen consumption (MVO_2); and the activity should be immediately stopped. The patient should sit or, if possible, lie down on a bed or plinth. The physiotherapist should take the patient's HR and BP and calculate the rate pressure product [RPP = HR × systolic blood pressure] as soon as possible to determine the MVO_2 at which the patient became ischemic, known as ischemic threshold.

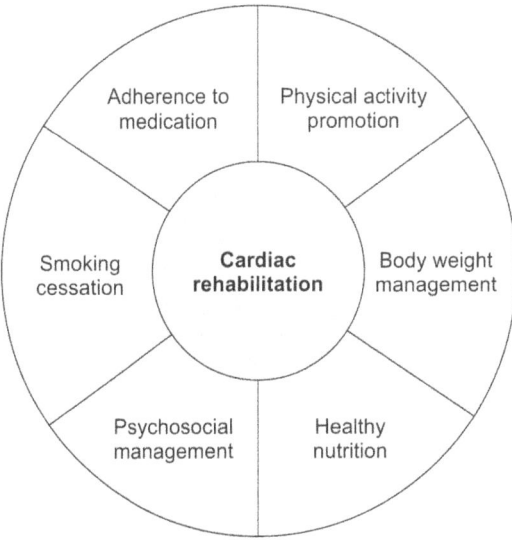

Fig. 31.1: The components of cardiac rehabilitation.

Exercises performed in cardiac rehabilitation include the following:
- Warm up exercises **(Figs. 31.2A and B)**
- Flexibility exercise **(Fig. 31.3)**
- Breathing exercises **(Fig. 31.4)**
- Aerobic exercises **(Figs. 31.5A to D)**
- Resistance training **(Figs. 31.6A and B)**
- Cool down exercises **(Figs. 31.7A and B)**

PHASES OF CARDIAC REHABILITATION

There are four phases of cardiac rehabilitation. The first phase called phase-I (in-patient phase) occurs in the hospital after the cardiac event, and the other three phases, i.e., phase-II—outpatient phase focuses on exercise training; phase-III—the maintenance phase occurs in a cardiac rehabilitation center or at home, once the patient has left the hospital; phase-IV—the long-term maintenance phase occurs in a cardiac rehabilitation center or a local leisure center. It should be kept in mind that the recovery after a cardiac event is variable; some people sail through each stage, while others may have a tough time getting back to normal.

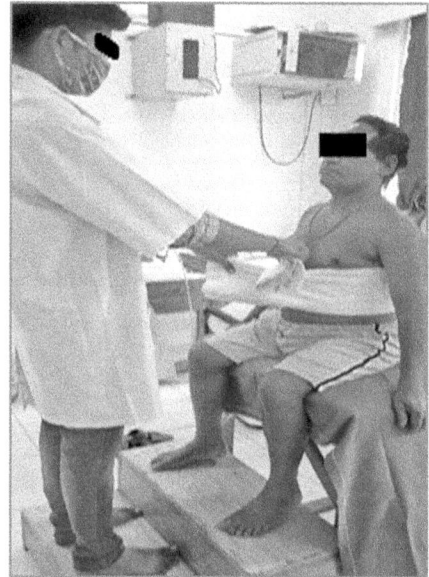

Fig. 31.4: Segmental breathing exercise using a towel.

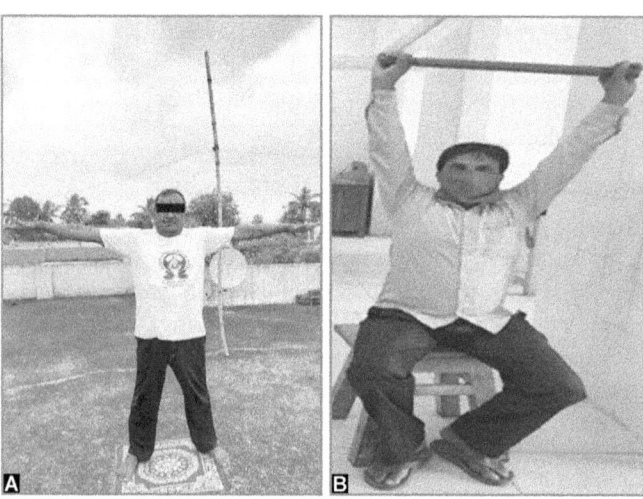

Figs. 31.2A and B: Warm up exercises.

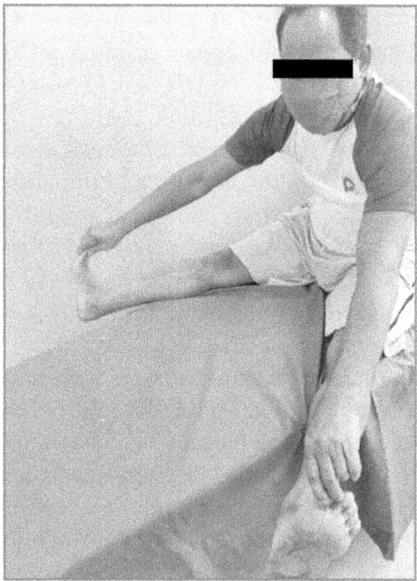

Fig. 31.3: Flexibility exercise.

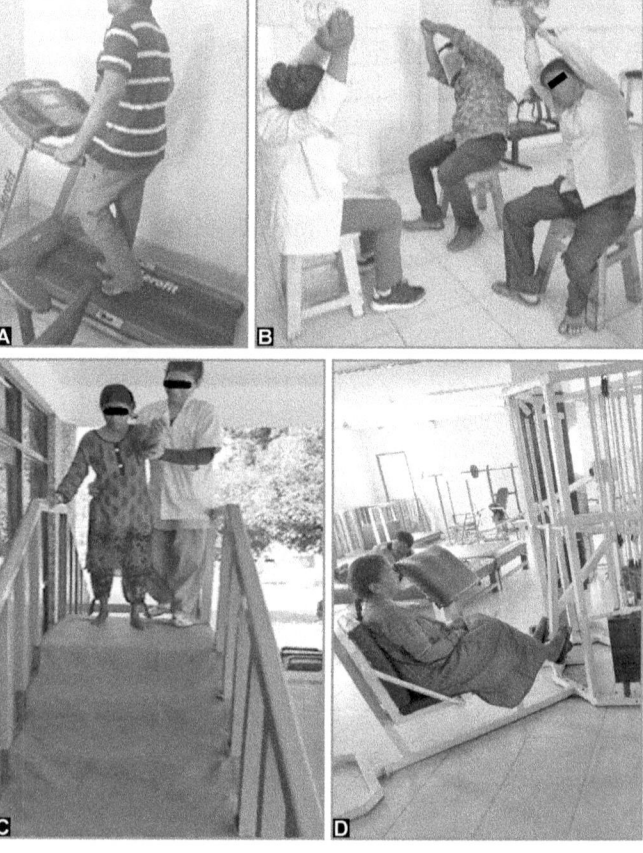

Figs. 31.5A to D: Aerobic exercises performed during cardiac rehabilitation.

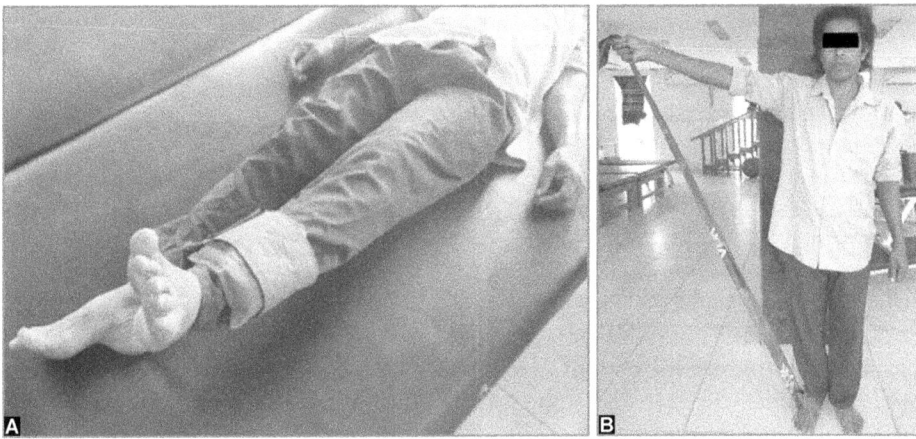

Figs. 31.6A and B: Low intensity resistance training in cardiac rehabilitation.

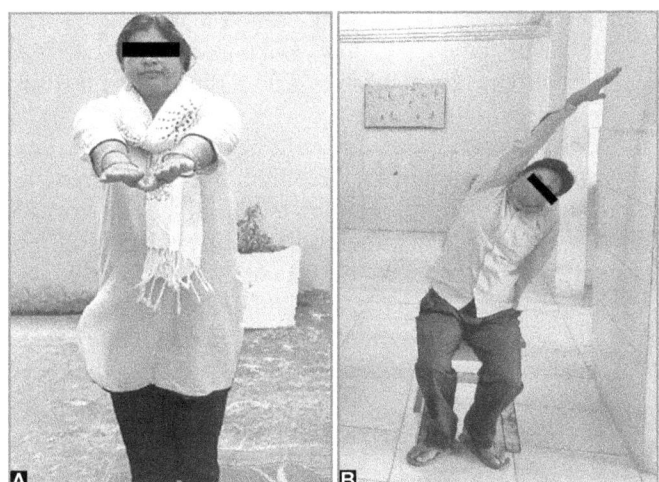

Figs. 31.7A and B: Cool down exercises in cardiac rehabilitation.

Phase-I

This phase lasts between 2 and 5 days, depending upon the patients' physical condition. Patients with acute heart conditions, such as those recovering from heart surgeries or heart attack, may be referred to the cardiac rehabilitation team, while still in the hospital.

The initial phase of cardiac rehabilitation occurs soon after the cardiac event. The physiotherapist working for stage-I, need to work closely with the physicians, nurses and other rehabilitation professionals, to help the patient regain mobility.

If the patient has a severe cardiac pathology/surgery, the physiotherapist starts working with the patient in the intensive care unit. Once the patient no longer requires intensive monitoring, he/she may be moved to a hospital ward.

Goals for Phase-I Cardiac Rehabilitation

The main goal of the first phase of the cardiac rehabilitation is to enable the patient leave the hospital and return home quickly and safely as possible. By the end of this phase, the patient should have:

- Learnt a safe, limited exercise plan to be followed at home
- An understanding of his/her problems and the need for cardiac rehabilitation
- Learnt to take precautions, if he/she has undergone open heart surgery
- Learnt the use of assistive devices such as a walking stick, if required
- Access to home oxygen therapy, if needed
- Knowledge of preventing secondary complications

Components of Phase-I Cardiac Rehabilitation

- **Assessment**: The physiotherapist along with other rehabilitation team members, focuses on the following components in the assessment of the patient:
  - Heart rate
  - Blood pressure
  - Oxygen saturation (pulse oximetry)
  - Upper extremity function, including range of motion (ROM) and muscle strength
  - Lower extremity ROM and muscle strength
  - Functional mobility for self-care and ambulation
- **Patient education**: Focuses on self-monitoring of heart function, management of cardiac pain, as well as psychological reactions (developing if any).
- **Physiotherapy**: The physiotherapist designs a carefully monitored progressive and very limited exercise program, such as gentle breathing exercises (protecting incision, if surgery in chest wall, i.e., thoracotomy/median sternotomy are done), getting up from bed and sitting, active ankle and foot exercises, standing and making the patient walk for a short distance in the hospital corridor.
- **Planning discharge**: Once the patient is found stable, and is able to walk, and the necessity for home oxygen therapy is not found, the therapist participates in discharge planning of the patient from hospital along with other team members. Educating the family members about the support to be given to the patient at home and carrying out simple exercises also are the components of discharge planning. Once significant healing has taken place, the patient may be discharged home to begin phase two cardiac rehabilitation.

Phase-II (Subacute Outpatient care: Post Discharge, Pre-exercise Period)

This phase is the subacute phase of cardiac rehabilitation, which starts after the patient has been discharged from the hospital. This phase requires intensive monitoring and supervision including ECG monitoring and intensive risk factor interventions. This is provided to the patient through an outpatient facility. Ideally, Phase II is initiated within 2 weeks of hospital discharge. This phase lasts from 3 to 6 weeks and involves continued monitoring of the cardiac responses to exercises and activities.

In this phase the patient/care givers are educated about proper exercise procedures, and how to monitor heart rate and exertion levels during exercise. The phase focuses upon safe return to functional activities while monitoring the heart rate. Toward the end of phase-II program, the patient should be ready to begin more independent exercises and activities.

Goals for Phase-II Cardiac Rehabilitation

- **Reinforce learning from phase-I**: The main goal for phase-II, is to support the patients learning from phase-I, and ensure that the patient has received all information about exercise/activity program.
- **Moving toward independence in self-care:** The patient in this phase should learn and perform activities for gaining more and more functional independence. He/she should be able to self-monitor the heart rate and exertion levels during exercises and activities.
- **Gaining independence:** The main goal is to increase the patients' level of independence, enabling him/her move into Phase-III.

Phase-III (Intensive Outpatient Rehabilitation)

This phase is the phase of intensive outpatient therapy. This phase involve more independent and group exercise therapy under supervision. This phase is sometimes referred to as "Exercise" phase, as it introduces more independent exercises and self-monitoring. It incorporates exercise training in combination with ongoing education and psychosocial and vocational interventions. It also emphasizes upon activities for return to work, hobbies and lifestyle, as well as management of depression and anxieties. The duration of this phase varies from 6 to 12 weeks, and the patient requires attending a cardiac rehabilitation unit 2–3 times weekly for structured exercise therapy and other lifestyle interventions. The patient should be able to monitor the own heart rate and symptomatic response to exercise as well as rate of perceived exertion (RPE). The physiotherapist guides the patient how to exercise more and more to increase the exercise tolerance, and monitors any negative changes that occur during exercise performance. In this phase, the patient is usually stable and and requires ECG monitoring only if signs and symptoms necessitate. Endurance training and risk factor modifications should continue.

Goals of Phase-III Cardiac Rehabilitation

The main goal of this phase of rehabilitation is to give the patient the tools to manage the heart condition, so that, he/she lives a healthier, happier life, through regular exercises, monitoring response of heart to exercises/activities, following heart healthy lifestyle and diet, etc.

The components of this phase of rehabilitation include:
1. **Assessment:** Before starting the program, the physiotherapist evaluates the patient, and the chief components of assessment include:
   - Joint ROM.
   - Scar tightness (if undergone any open surgery).
   - Muscle strength.
   - Resting heart rate.
   - Resting blood pressure.
   - Resting respiratory rate.
   - Endurance level/exercise tolerance.
2. **Exercises**: As the patient becomes more and more independent, the physiotherapist designs a series of exercises for the patient, such as exercises for flexibility, strength as well as aerobic exercises. The cardiac rehabilitation session starts with:
   - *Warm up exercises,* such as active free movements to lower limbs (shadow walking-alternate hip/knee flexion/extension), bilateral arm raisings, and breathing exercises as tolerated.
   - *Cardiovascular exercises,* such as static cycle exercises, upper limb ergometry, treadmill exercises, throwing/catching a ball, etc., as tolerated. Gradually progressive strength training program, using therabands/weight cuff to offer resistance can be started. While performing the exercises, the patient should be able to monitor his/her own response to exercise that include monitoring heart rate, blood pressure, level of exertion, etc.
   - *Cool down exercises,* which are the set of low intensity exercises like warm up exercises, performed before going to rest.
3. **Patient/care giver education:** Education of patient regarding maximizing the quality of life through intake of taking heart healthy diet, changing the lifestyle that include quitting smoking, exercising regularly, managing stress through breathing techniques and meditation, eliminating any underlying factor that promotes anxiety are imparted during this phase.

Phase-IV (Maintenance Phase)

This phase constitutes the components of long-term maintenance of lifestyle changes and professional monitoring of clinical status. This starts when the patients leave the structured phase-III exercise program. The patient is required to continue exercise and lifestyle modifications indefinitely. This may be facilitated in a cardiac rehabilitation unit or in a local leisure center. The patient may also prefer to exercise independently or he/she may decide to continue the exercises with the clinical team helping them to practice exercises safely.

Goals of Phase-IV Cardiac Rehabilitation

The goal of this phase of rehabilitation, is to continue to maintain the changes in lifestyle that was followed in phase-III, as well as continue the exercise program and manage stress and anxiety.

SECTION 6

Physiotherapy in Abdominal and Thoracic Surgeries

Section Outline

- Chapter 32: Physiotherapy in Abdominal Surgeries
- Chapter 33: Physiotherapy in Thoracic Surgeries

Physiotherapy in Abdominal Surgeries

INTRODUCTION

A physiotherapist is involved in the management of individuals undergoing various abdominal and thoracic surgeries for the following purposes:

* To prepare the patient mentally to undergo such surgery, by explaining him/her the procedures to be undertaken, need and purpose of pre- and postoperative physiotherapy, and how to achieve early mobility and return to home through advocation of timely postoperative physiotherapy.
* To provided adequate chest therapy, to enable the patient fit for general anesthesia.
* To teach the procedure/method to be followed for chest clearance, through huffing/coughing, protecting the site of incision.
* To explain the patient about the postoperative complications such as abdominal hernia, rupture of incisional wound, reduction of lung capacity, development of scoliosis/kyphosis in the spine, deep vein thrombosis (DVT), etc., and how such complications can be minimized/prevented through appropriate postoperative therapy.
* To provide and teach preoperative and postoperative physiotherapy.

COMMON ABDOMINAL SURGERIES

Common surgeries performed in abdomen and their therapeutic management are discussed here.

Cholecystectomy

A cholecystectomy is a surgery performed to remove the gallbladder (a specialized organ situated under the liver that stores the digestive enzyme—bile).

Indications for Cholecystectomy

The surgery may be indicated in the following conditions:
* Cholelithiasis (stones in the gallbladder).
* Choledocholithiasis (gallstones in the bile duct).
* Cholecystitis (inflammation of gallbladder).
* Large gallbladder polyps.
* Pancreatitis (inflammation of pancreas, due to gallstones).

Types of Surgeries Performed

There are two types of surgeries performed to remove gallbladder such as:

1. **Open (traditional) method:** In this method, 1 cut (incision), termed Kocher's incision, about 4–6 inches long is made in the upper right-hand side of the belly **(Fig. 32.1)**. The surgeon finds the gallbladder and takes it out through the incision. This method is followed, when laparoscopic removal of gallbladder is not possible.

   The surgeon incises the anterior rectus sheath along the length of the incision, and divides the rectus abdominis and lateral muscles (external oblique, internal oblique, and transversus abdominis) with the electrocautery. Then, the posterior rectus sheath and peritoneum are incised to enter the abdomen. After surgery, a drainage tube may be applied, which may be retained for 1–2 days.

2. **Laparoscopic method:** This method, which is less invasive, uses 3–4 very small incisions (one of the incision is slightly larger than others). It uses a long, thin tube called a laparoscope, which has a tiny video camera and surgical tools. The tube, camera and tools are put in through the incisions and surgeries are performed looking at a TV monitor. The gallbladder is removed through the large incision.

Appendicectomy

An appendicectomy, also termed as appendectomy, is a surgical operation in which the vermiform appendix (a

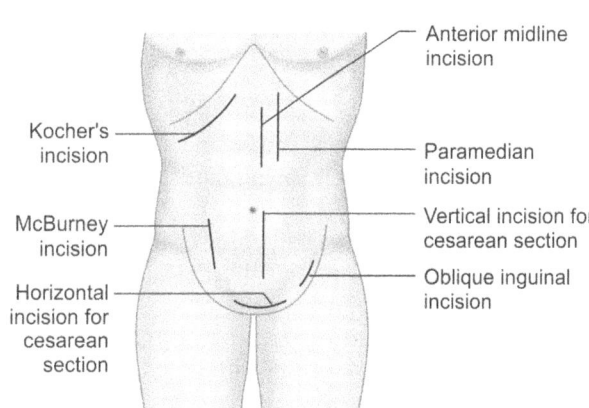

Fig. 32.1: The abdominal incisions.

portion of the intestine) is removed. Appendectomy is normally performed as an urgent or emergency procedure to treat complicated acute appendicitis.

There are two types of surgery to remove the appendix. The standard method is an open appendicectomy. A less invasive method is a laparoscopic appendicectomy.

1. **Open appendicectomy:** A cut or incision about 2-4 inches long, called McBurney's incision (**Fig. 32.1**) is made in the lower right-hand side of the abdomen. The appendix is taken out through the incision.
2. **Laparoscopic appendicectomy:** This method is less invasive. Instead of a large incision, 1-3 tiny cuts are made on the abdomen. A long, thin tube called a laparoscope is put into one of the incisions. It has a tiny video camera and surgical tools. The surgeon looks at a TV monitor to see inside the abdomen and guides the tools. The appendix is removed through one of the incisions.

The muscles cut in this incision are: External oblique, internal oblique and transverse abdominis muscles.

Laparotomy

This refers to the opening of the abdominal cavity for direct examination of its contents, e.g., to locate a source of bleeding or trauma. It may or may not be followed by repair or removal of the primary problem.

Cesarean Section Delivery

In this, incision is given in the abdomen and uterus to deliver the baby. The incision given is either a vertical incision (classical incision) between the umbilicus and pubic hair or more commonly a horizontal incision just above the pubic bone on the lower abdomen called bikini cut. No muscles are cut in cesarean section incision, only they are separated to get access to the uterus except in a few cases, where the rectus abdominis muscle is cut, when a horizontal incision is given. The vertical incision, though has more complications, gives the surgeon better access to the uterus, as compared to horizontal incision (most common incision performed).

PHYSIOTHERAPY IN ABDOMINAL SURGERIES

Preoperative Physiotherapy

It focuses on:
* Explanation regarding the nature of surgery, incisions, etc.
* Strengthening of abdominal muscles.
* Explanation about pain relieving modalities that may be required after surgery.
* Upper and lower limb strengthening exercises.
* Deep breathing exercises and chest clearance measures (if required).
* Advice on huffing and coughing after surgery, with protection to the incision site with a pad of towel/cloth (**Fig. 32.2**).
* Endurance training to improve cardiorespiratory fitness, such as exercises on treadmill, static bicycle, etc.

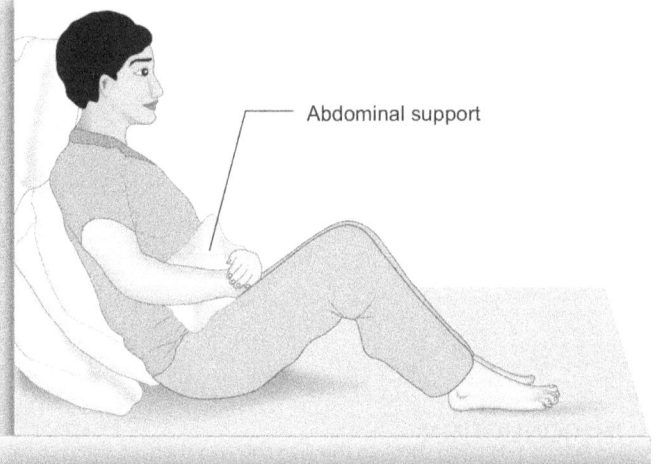

Fig. 32.2: Abdominal support while huffing/coughing.

* Guidance and preparation for rehabilitation after discharge from hospital.

Postoperative Physiotherapy

After surgery, the patient may be required to stay in the hospital for 1 week to 10 days (stitches are usually removed by 10 days). He/she may have the drainage tube, nasogastic tube, IV drip, and Foley's catheter placed in situ. During this time and after discharge from hospital, he/she is required to perform exercises to minimize complications and early return to function. The therapy schedule after surgery is as follows:

* **0–1 week:** The therapy focuses on:
  - Making the patient sit on bed with upper back supported, on the day of surgery/day following surgery. The time spent in sitting and inclination to achieve vertical sitting are gradually progressed as tolerated.
  - Walking with proper care of the drainage tube and catheter (if any), should be started on the day following surgery and is gradually progressed.
  - Cryotherapy surrounding incision to reduce swelling.
  - Pain controlling modalities, such as transcutaneous electrical nerve stimulation (TENS), if the intensity of pain is very high. High frequency low intensity TENS, should be applied, which should not cause any muscle contraction.
  - Gentle breathing exercises, huffing/coughing to loosen and remove secretions with proper abdominal support (if secretions accumulate in the airways)
  - Gentle anterior and posterior pelvic tilt exercises (**Fig. 32.3**)
  - Supine to sitting and sitting to standing transfers
  - Upper and lower limb strengthening exercises with more emphasis on ankle and foot exercises to prevent DVT.
  - Stair climbing may be started before the patient is discharged.

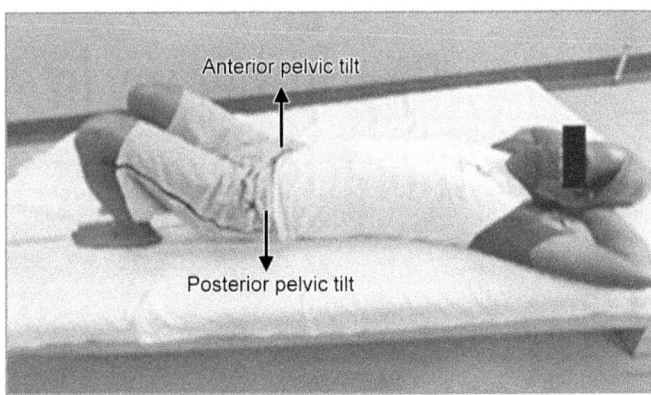

Fig. 32.3: Anterior and posterior pelvic tilt exercises.

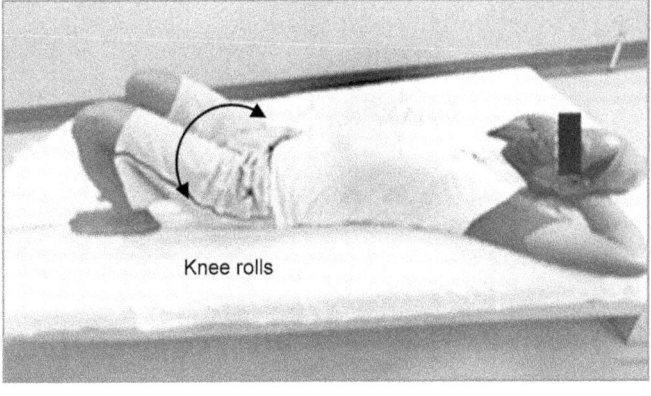

Fig. 32.5: The knee rolls.

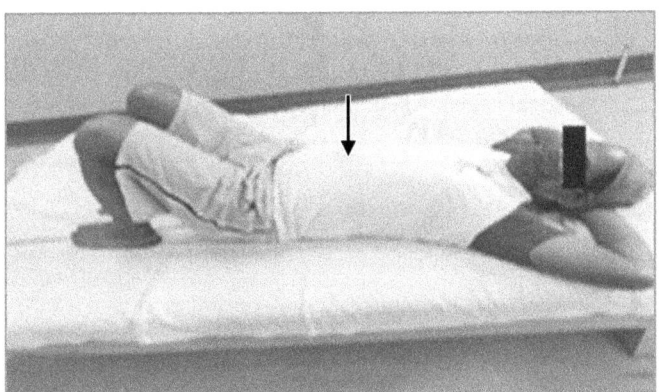

Fig. 32.4: Strengthening of transverse abdominis.

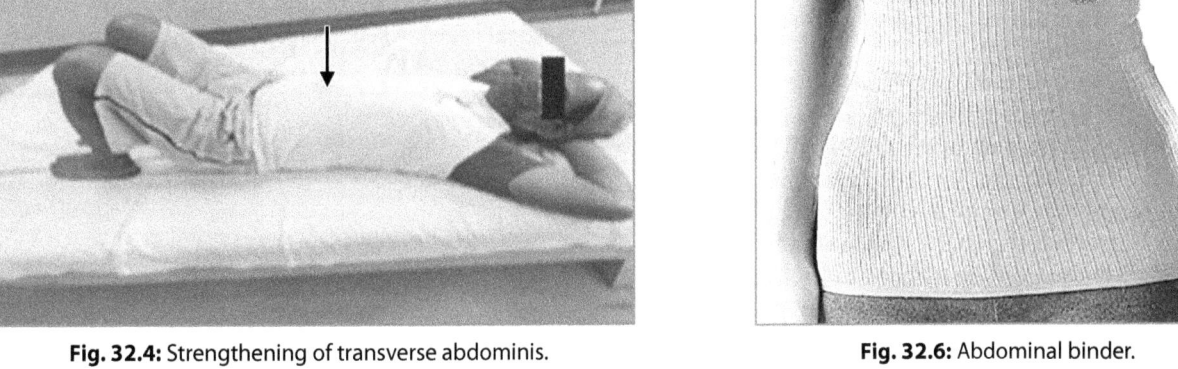

Fig. 32.6: Abdominal binder.

- **2–4 weeks:** By this time, the patient has been discharged from hospital and is at home. Physiotherapy during this time focuses on performance of exercises and activities performed during first week and the followings:
  - Abdominal strengthening exercises, with more emphasis on strengthening of transverse abdominis **(Fig. 32.4)** For this exercise, the patient is asked to place his hands under the buttock, and breath in through the nose and breath out gently through the mouth. As he/she breathes air out, pulls the tummy button down toward the spine and feel the contraction, which should be held for 3 seconds, and then relaxed. 15–20 contractions are performed twice daily.
  - Knee roll exercise **(Fig. 32.5)**
  - Treatment of back pain (if any using TENS)
  - Use of abdominal binder **(Fig. 32.6)** if there is tendency for incisional hernia
  - Deep breathing exercises
  - Upper and lower limb strengthening exercises
  - Exercises to improve pelvic stability
  - Endurance training
  - Emphasis on outdoor mobility with progressive walking with reference to certain markers, such as an electric pole/tree.
- **Week 5 onwards:**
  - Strengthening of abdominals to continue
  - Anterior and posterior pelvic tilt exercises to continue
  - Deep breathing exercises to continue and airways clearance techniques (if required)
  - Modalities to reduce low back pain (if any)
  - Posture correction
  - Endurance exercises
  - Gradual return to function. However, lifting heavy load is restricted till completion of 12 weeks.

33. Physiotherapy in Thoracic Surgeries

INTRODUCTION

Physiotherapists are closely associated in the management of patients, who undergo various surgeries in the chest wall for the treatment of pulmonary and cardiac diseases. Pre- and postoperative therapy is required to be given to patients who undergo such surgeries for minimizing pulmonary complications and return to function. The surgeries performed on the chest wall are:

- **Thoracotomy:** A thoracotomy is a surgical procedure in which an incision is made between the ribs to reach the lungs or heart for the purpose of diagnosis and treatment of cardiopulmonary diseases. Though many muscles are cut, depending upon the type of procedure, muscle sparing thoracotomy is the choice of many surgeons today.
- **Thoracoplasty:** Thoracoplasty is a surgical technique initially designed to permanently collapse tuberculous cavities by resection of ribs from the chest wall. In this procedure skeletal support of a portion of the chest is removed surgically, by subperiosteal removal of a varying number of ribs, resulting in sinking of the unsupported portion of the chest wall towards the mediastinum. At present, thoracoplasty is widely used for the treatment of empyema.

  Most thoracoplasties produce some degree of chest wall and shoulder deformities and other complications such as scoliosis, shoulder stiffness, progressive respiratory failure, which necessitate adequate pre- and postoperative physiotherapy.
- **Median sternotomy:** Median sternotomy is a type of surgical procedure, in which a vertical inline incision is made along the sternum, from supra sternal notch to tip of xiphoid process, to perform surgeries on heart and major blood vessels in the chest (**Fig. 33.1**). During open heart surgery, a median sternotomy (division of the sternum from top to bottom) is performed to allow surgeons to gain access to the heart. Appropriate pre- and postoperative physiotherapy in the form of cardiac rehabilitation should be followed. However, certain sternal precautions as compiled by Brocki et al., discussed below, should be followed during postoperative management.
  - Bilateral movements of the arms in the horizontal level, backward or over the shoulder level, should only be performed within pain-free limits during the initial 10 days following sternotomy or until the wound is healed.
  - Loaded movements of the arms should only be done at a pain-free level.
  - In general, patients should keep the upper arms close to the body for 6–8 weeks.
  - Patients with body mass index (BMI) ≥35 should wear a supportive vest to protect the sternum for 6–8 weeks.
  - Patients should be taught to hug a pillow over the surgical incision when coughing and sneezing for 6–8 weeks (**Fig. 33.2**).

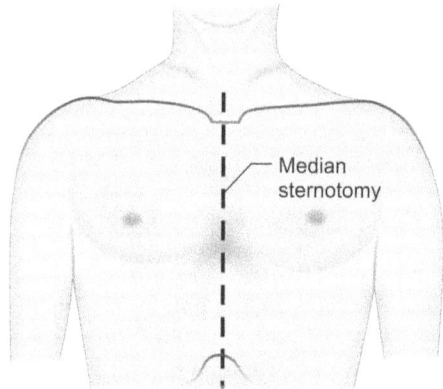

Fig. 33.1: Median sternotomy incision.

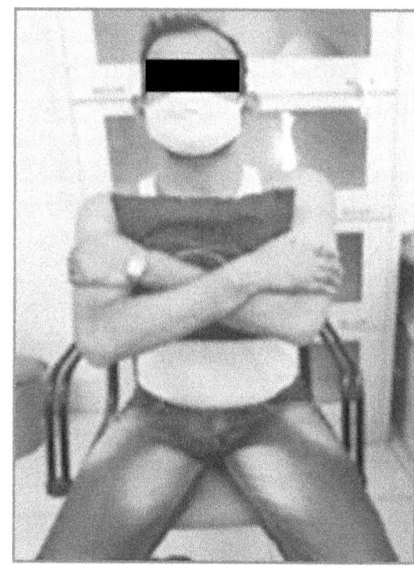

Fig. 33.2: Supporting the sternotomy incision by pillow.

- Patients who cough frequently should wear a sternal vest supporting the entire circumference of the thorax.
- Patients with large breasts should use a supportive brassiere that fastens in the front.

THORACOTOMIES AND ITS PHYSIOTHERAPY MANAGEMENT

Thoracotomies and its physiotherapy management are discussed here.

Over the past century, thoracic surgery (thoracotomy) has been the primary intervention used to treat pulmonary, pleural, chest wall, and mediastinal disorders. Thoracotomy could be of two types such as—(1) Posterolateral thoracotomy—most frequently used open procedure in thoracic surgery and is performed primarily for lung resections (lobectomy, pneumonectomy, wedge resections), repair of hiatus hernia; (2) Anterolateral thoracotomy—mostly performed for heart and lungs diseases, as well as for management mediastinal masses and pathologies of esophagus.

Indications for Posterolateral Thoracotomy

- **Posterolateral thoracotomy:** An approximate 6-inch incision is made below the inferior angle of scapula, typically between the fifth and sixth ribs. The incision is started along the inframammary crease and extend posterolaterally below the inferior angle of the scapula. It is then extended superiorly for a short distance between the spine and vertebral border of scapula. During the surgery, a drainage tube is inserted into the chest to drain excess fluid or air leaking into the chest.
  - A standard posterolateral thoracotomy incision (**Fig. 33.3B**) is given for:
    » Treatment of cardiac diseases
    » Treatment of diseases of esophagus
    » Treatment of diseases of mediastinum
    » Treatment of pulmonary conditions
  - The muscles cut in posterolateral thoracotomy are:
    » Latissimus dorsi
    » Serratus anterior
    » Trapezius muscle (mostly lower fibers)
    » Intercostal muscles

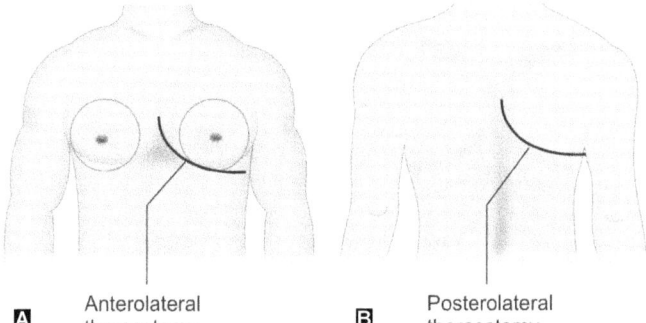

Figs. 33.3A and B: (A) Anterolateral thoracotomy incision; (B) Posterolateral thoracotomy incision.

- **Anterolateral thoracotomy:** The incision is made from the sternal edge under the mammary fold, in a curvilinear fashion towards the axilla, staying in close proximity to the 4th/5th intercostal space. Mostly performed on the left side (left anterolateral thoracotomy) to provide exposure to heart, aorta and left lung.
  - A standard anterolateral incision (**Fig. 33.3A**) is given for:
    » Treatment of pulmonary diseases.
    » Treatment of cardiac diseases (most commonly heart valve surgeries).
    » Treatment of diseases of esophagus.
    » Diseases of mediastinum.
  - The muscles cut in anterolateral thoracotomy are:
    » The serratus anterior muscle is sometimes not cut, it is only retracted.
    » Pectoral muscles.
    » Intercostal muscles.

Following thoracic surgery there is evidence of changes in lung function and associated clinical manifestations. The changes include characteristics reduction in lung volume which is primarily restrictive in nature, reduction in functional residual capacity, slowing of mucociliary clearance, and abnormalities in gaseous exchange, etc.

This leads to postoperative pulmonary complications such as atelectasis (partial or total collapse of lungs, when the alveoli are deflated or filled with alveolar fluid), consolidation of lungs, pleural effusion, persistent air leaks (pneumothorax), and pneumonia. Very often, post-thoracotomy pain syndrome and frozen shoulder on the affected side are also seen. Patients very often develop scoliosis/kyphoscoliosis (in antero-lateral thoracotomies) to prevent pain and injury to stitches.

Physiotherapy is widely considered to be important in limiting the development of postoperative pulmonary complications, which are associated with significant clinical and economic impact, and in the prevention and treatment of shoulder dysfunction, which has been reported extensively following thoracotomies. A physiotherapist is involved in preoperative assessment and therapy to the subjects selected for surgeries, as well as provides postoperative physiotherapy and pulmonary rehabilitation.

I. Preoperative physiotherapy for thoracotomy: Before surgery is undertaken, preoperative physiotherapy is provided for the following purposes:

- Explanation to the patient/caregiver about the nature of surgery, care of drainage tube, protection of incision while huffing/coughing to remove secretion and the importance of exercises to prevent DVT.
- Deep breathing exercises to increase lung capacities.
- Drainage of secretions through postural drainage/modified postural drainage.
- Upper and lower limb strengthening exercises.
- Endurance building exercises such as static cycle exercises, treadmill exercises, brisk walking, running, etc.

II. Postoperative physiotherapy:

Aims of postoperative physiotherapy:

- Proper positioning on bed/chair, to maintain as normal a posture, so that symmetrical chest expansion, and posture could be facilitated.
- Reduction of pain: The pain due to pleurisy, chest wall inflammation due to surgical trauma, periarthritis shoulder, that limit chest expansion and function using the affected upper limb, need to be reduced.
- Minimize/prevent pulmonary complications such as atelectasis, respiratory failure, pneumonia, aspiration after pneumonectomy (when the patient is placed in side-lying with the operated side up).
- Promote airway clearance: Secretions accumulating in the airways due to primary preoperative lung pathology, or due to general anesthesia and intervention in the lungs, need to be removed through postural/modified postural drainage techniques, active cycle of breathing techniques (ACBT).
- Prevent development of spinal deformities, such as scoliosis (bending toward the operated side to prevent stress on the incision) as seen in thoracotomies, as well as bending towards the collapsed side of rib cage as occurs in thoracoplasties).
- Prevent deep vein thrombosis (DVT).
- Prevent development of frozen shoulder.
- Improve endurance.
- Early return to function.

Postoperative assessment: Appropriate postoperative physiotherapy plans can only be designed based on an accurate initial assessment of postoperative patients. Following the initial assessment, a problem list for postoperative patients can be developed, which most commonly includes pain, a poor breathing pattern, reduced lung volume, ineffective coughing, retained secretions, and reduced shoulder range of motion, spinal deformities, reduced endurance and limitations of function.

Postoperative Physiotherapy Intervention

Postoperatively, once the patient is medically stable and recovered from anesthesia, physiotherapy can be started between 4 and 12 hours after recovery. 2-3 sessions of therapy comprising 30 minutes are conducted by the physiotherapists. The interventions include:
- **Transcutaneous electrical nerve stimulation (TENS) to reduce postoperative pain:** Pain associated with thoracotomy, may impair the patient's ability to take deep breath, causes retention of secretions and leads to complications like increase of respiratory and heart rate, increase of blood pressure (due to sympathetic stimulation). Pain can also induce anxiety, sleep disturbances and limits movement of shoulder leading to development of frozen shoulder. TENS has been found to be effective in reducing pain in patients of post-thoracotomy, when combined with analgesic medications.
- **Cryotherapy:** Application of cryopacks around the incision site during the first 24 hours, helps in reducing incisional pain and swelling, and facilitates deep breathing and movement of the affected upper limb.

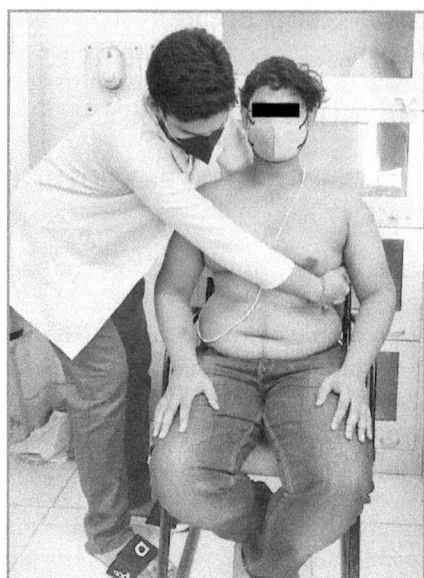

Fig. 33.4: Bear hug hold to protect the incision.

- **Protection to the incision site and drainage tubes:** It is very important to support the patient's incision and intercostal drain sites when breathing deeply and performing forced expiratory techniques (FET) such as huffing and coughing. To support the incision site, a bear hug hold **(Fig. 33.4)** is used, where the therapist stands on the contralateral side and places one hand on the anterior chest wall to stabilize the incision from the front, and places the other hand on the posterior side to protect the incision from the behind, with the forearms supporting the entire chest.

The patient is also taught, to hold a pillow firmly against the incision **(Fig. 33.5)** while huffing and coughing and taking a deep breath. An external thoracic support is sometimes required to be worn by the patient after the intercostal drainage tubes are removed.

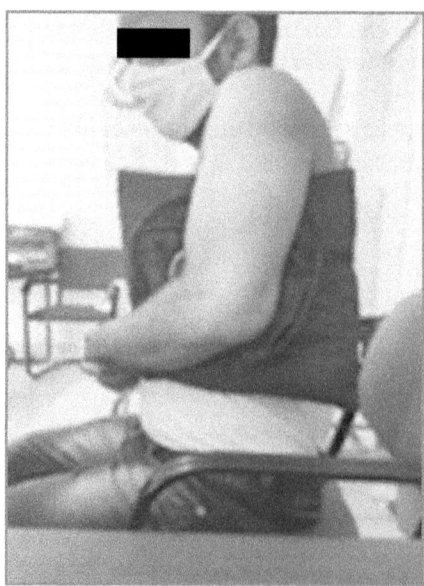

Fig. 33.5: Protecting the incision by pillow.

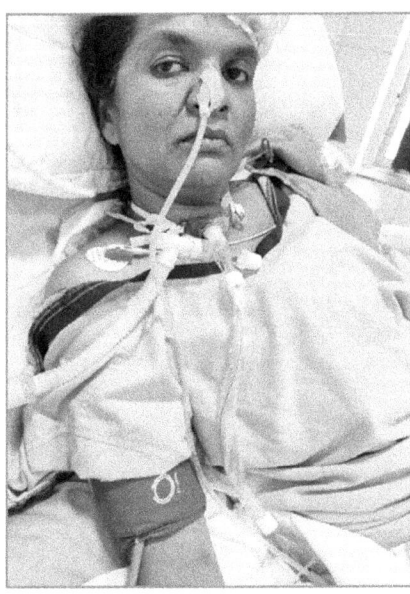

Fig. 33.6: Shows patient in half-lying with tracheostomy tube in situ.

- ❖ **Positioning:** Early upright sitting on bed with the endotracheal/tracheostomy and chest drainage tubes in situ, helps in proper excursion of diaphragm and chest wall, minimizes secretion accumulation by expanding all parts of the lungs. Sitting on bed is performed either on the day or on the next day after surgery. If the patient cannot sit on a chair, he/she should be made to sit on the bed with back support **(Fig. 33.6)**, or to adopt a high side-lying position with the operated side lung up (except when pneumonectomy is performed).

  However, after pneumonectomy, if the side-lying position is adopted for draining the remaining lung, the patient should be positioned on the operated side, because, if the patient lies on the sound side, the bronchial stump may be bathed with fluid, causing entry of the fluid into the bronchial stump.

- ❖ **Airways clearance:** The modified (horizontal) postural drainage position is used instead of the conventional head down position, as the later can lead to decreased arterial oxygenation and could induce more cardiovascular stress, carrying the risk of aspiration.

- ❖ **Mobility:** Early mobilization and exercise prescription for the patients should be done on the first postoperative day after consulting the treating surgeon. The aim of mobilization is to stress the cardiopulmonary system of the postoperative patient at a level sufficient to increase minute ventilation and cardiac output while still being within safe physiological limits. Mobilization and exercises started on the first postoperative day consists of:
  - Passive/active assisted/active free exercises to lower limbs in lying
  - Active free exercises to upper limbs
  - Deep breathing exercises (supporting the incision)
  - Making the patient sit on the edge of bed or in a chair.
  - Making the patient take short steps to walk around the bed. Upon standing, it is important to check for orthostatic hypotension, which can manifest by a drop in systolic blood pressure of >20 mm Hg and a drop in diastolic blood pressure of >10 mm Hg, and/or in the form of symptomatic dizziness or light-headedness. A graduated walking program should be adopted for mobilizing postoperative patients. When walking a patient with an underwater seal drainage tube still in place, the patient must receive appropriate analgesia prior to ambulation because chest drains can cause severe pain, limiting the patient's ability to ambulate and to cooperate with the physiotherapist. The use of breathing control during mobilization activities may improve exercise tolerance.

Mobilization should only be initiated for patients with clinically stable cardiopulmonary and cardiovascular conditions. Once a postoperative patient is able to sit unsupported on the edge of the bed for 5 minutes and can perform a full bilateral knee extension along with clinically acceptable vital signs, the patient can progress to standing and ambulation. A patient's clinical status is considered unstable if the vital signs exceed any of the following thresholds, i.e., heart rate <40/min or >140/min, respiratory rate <8/min or >36/min, oxygen saturation <85%, and blood pressure <80 or >200 mm Hg systolic or >110 mm diastolic. All patients' connections should be checked before mobilization and/or ambulation, and care should be taken not to pull any of the patient's lines, drains, or tubes during mobilization to avoid dislodgement. In case of accidental dislodgement of an intercostal drain, the patient is asked to immediately breathe out, and firm pressure with a sterile dressing is applied to the insertion site at the end of expiration and medical help should be sought. While maintaining pressure, the patient is asked to breathe normally till medical help arrives. Mobilization activities for patients who are connected to wall suction include bedside marching on the spot, besides upper and lower limb exercises and breathing exercises.

The physiotherapist must start low and go slow; that is, to start with sessions that are short (i.e., 3–5 minutes), more frequent (i.e., 2–3 times/day), and relatively non-intense [inducing a level of patient effort of <13 on the rating of perceived exertion (RPE) scale or at 60% of maximum heart rate (HR_{max})].

Stair climbing is initiated once the patient can walk for a considerable distance on a flat surface with optimum cardiovascular and cardiopulmonary stability. Stair climbing generally started on the fourth or fifth day after thoracic surgery.

The physiotherapist should make sure that the drainage system is working properly. Presence of symptoms of tachypnea, dyspnea, increased use of the accessory muscles, orthopnea, a restless or increased heart rate, or cyanosis may indicate malfunctioning of the drainage system.

When walking a patient who is receiving supplemental oxygen, the physiotherapist should monitor oxygen saturation during walking, and the amount of oxygen given to the patient must be enough to keep oxygen saturation ≥90% during ambulation.

Ambulation is contraindicated in postoperative patients with:
- Unstable vital signs.
- Patients who are not able to follow commands.
- Patients with untreated deep venous thrombosis or pulmonary embolism.
- Patients on high ventilatory support.
- Patients with hypotension, uncontrolled arrhythmia (e.g., atrial fibrillation), uncontrolled decompensated heart failure, or recent myocardial infarction, as these conditions can lead to severe compromise of cardiac output during ambulation activities.
- Patients with acute renal failure.

All patients unable to be mobilized and/or ambulated can start breathing exercises, circulatory exercises, and/or airway clearance techniques in bed.

- **Lung expansion programs:** After thoracic surgery, lung volume and functional residual capacity are reduced due to anesthesia, chest wall pain, and/or recumbency, which may lead to lung atelectasis, clinically manifesting as progressive hypoxemia, increased breathing frequency, dyspnea, increased heart rate, decreased breath sounds, fine late inspiratory crackles (crepitations), a dull note on percussion, and areas of opacification on a chest X-ray. Deep breathing exercises, incentive spirometry, and inspiratory muscle training (IMT), etc., are employed to reduce such complications.
    - *Deep breathing exercises:* Deep breathing exercises given in half-lying, side-lying or erect sitting helps to increase lung volume, improve ventilation and oxygenation, prevent basal atelectasis, reinflate collapsed lung regions, and reverse minimal postoperative atelectasis. Deep breathing exercises that can be prescribed to postoperative patients are 5-deep breaths with a 3-second end-inspiratory hold per every waking hour. Techniques for supporting the incision wound and drain sites during all deep breathing exercises can be taught to patients to allow them to take deep breaths comfortably. The breathing exercises comprise of:
        » Deep diaphragmatic breathing exercises: Deep diaphragmatic breathing should be practiced while the patient is sitting upright/half-lying **(Fig. 33.7)**, with his or her back supported and the pelvis in the posterior tilting position. The posterior pelvic tilt position optimizes the length-tension relationship of the diaphragm, which facilitates efficient diaphragmatic breathing. The patient is asked to relax the upper chest and shoulder and to breathe in from the nose as deeply as possible, then to exhale gently through the mouth.
        » Thoracic expansion exercises (lateral costal breathing exercises): Thoracic expansion exercises (TEEs) are deep breathing exercises that emphasize active inspiration with hold of breath for 3 seconds at the end of deep inspiration. The exercises include apical, middle, lower costal, and posterior basal expansion exercises, and can be unilateral or bilateral. Unilateral thoracic expansion exercises are preferable in

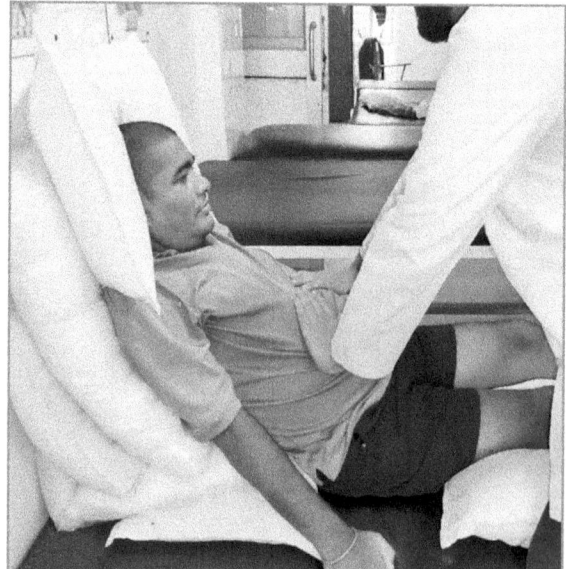

Fig. 33.7: Deep diaphragmatic breathing exercise in half-lying guided by therapist's hand.

postoperative patients after thoracotomy. These exercises are most efficiently performed in the high side-lying position, with the operated side on the top (except when pneumonectomy is done) and the arm on the involved side brought to abduction at the level of the head.
        » Sustained maximal inspiration (3-second hold at total lung capacity): This technique involves taking a deep breath, and holding the breath for 3 seconds after reaching deep inspiration. This is of great importance in facilitating more equal filling of the lung segments.
        » Deep breathing exercises coupled with arm or trunk movements: The patient may be taught to perform deep breathing with arm flexion, arm abduction, trunk extension, or trunk side flexion away from the operated side, while coordinating exhalation upon returning to the starting position. The incision site should be protected during this maneuver.
    - *Incentive spirometry:* It is a visual feedback system used to encourage and motivate postoperative patients to perform deep breathing and to engage in sustained maximal inspiration (i.e., a 3-second end inspiratory hold) to open up atelectatic alveoli. The patient is asked to breathe in slowly and deeply for as long as possible through the mouth piece of the device to maximally, distribute ventilation, and then holds the deep breath for a period of 5 seconds, which is then followed by a normal expiration.
    - *Inspiratory muscle training:* This technique which is a major component of pulmonary rehabilitation, is also helpful to postoperative thoracotomy patients. A study by Brocki et al., has shown that the addition of inspiratory muscle training to standard postoperative physiotherapy improved hypoxemic status in high-risk patients after lung cancer surgery, but had no additional benefit for preserving respiratory muscle strength.

- **Airway clearance techniques:** It refers to manual or mechanical procedures that are used to assist the mobilization of secretions from the airway after thoracic surgery. These include supported coughing, huffing, the forced expiration technique (FET), an ACBT, modified postural drainage positioning with or without vibration, and the positive expiratory pressure (PEP) therapy. The technique should be started as soon as the patient wakes on the day of surgery and/or on the first postoperative day. It should be repeated every 30 minutes, if persistent secretions are produced in the airways. Nebulized bronchodilators to open the airways, thinning the secretions by heated humidification, use of mucolytic agents and promoting systemic hydration by oral and intravenous fluid intake, help in cleaning the airways. The most suitable airway clearance technique should be selected for the patients. Protection of the incisional wound, use of ice packs around the incision help for effective airways clearance.
- **Forced expiratory techniques:** This is a combination of 1–2 forced expirations (huffs), followed by coughs and a period of breathing control. To carry out a huff or cough with high lung volume; the patient is asked to take a deep breath, and then to exhale forcibly, squeezing air out from the chest. It has been reported that the FET is the most effective component of chest clearance physiotherapy. The incision site should be protected during the FET.
- **Breathing control exercises:** It is tidal breathing at the patient's own rate and depth, while the patient adopts relaxed diaphragmatic (abdominal) breathing. For breathing control, the patient is instructed to rest one hand on the abdomen and to keep his or her shoulders and upper chest relaxed. Then, the patient is asked to let the air flow in through the nose (if possible), to feel the abdomen rise as he or she does so, and to feel it fall while he or she breathes out. In patients with bronchospasm or unstable/collapsed airways, a longer pause for breathing control is needed, while in other patients with no bronchospasm, the pause may be shorter.
- **Active cycle of breathing techniques:** It refers to a cycle of breathing control, thoracic expansion exercises and FET. It can be used in postoperative patients to clear excess bronchial secretions with or without assistance. The patient should start with breathing control for 20–30 seconds, followed by practice of thoracic expansion exercises, 3–4 times. The thoracic expansion exercises with a 3-second inspiratory hold allow the air to flow via collateral channels and to come in behind the sputum stuck in small airways and mobilize it towards the larger airways. The patient then restarts breathing control again (20–30 seconds or 6 breaths). Finally, the patient practices the FET.
- **The positive expiratory pressure technique:** Patients who use positive expiratory pressure (PEP) therapy only receive positive pressure at the end of the expiration. This therapy is most commonly applied with physiotherapy sessions once or twice daily to aid chest clearance. For the application of PEP application, the followings may be followed:
  - The patient sits upright or leans slightly forward with his or her elbows supported on a table and holds the mouthpiece or the mask firmly against his or her face.
  - The patient is asked to slowly take in a larger than normal breath with a short breath hold (3–5 seconds) and to exhale through the PEP device with active but not forced expiration against an expiratory resistor, giving a resistance that ranges from 6 to 25 cm H_2O.
  - The patient breathes for 10–20 breaths/cycle with a total of 4–8 cycles/session or for a maximum of 20 minutes.
  - After each cycle, the FET or supported coughing may be practiced by the patient to clear the already mobilized secretions.
  - *Modified postural drainage:* Modified positions are much more likely to be used postoperatively in patients where classical (head-down) positions are not well tolerated or may cause aspiration, vomiting, breathlessness, cardiovascular compromise, and/or pulmonary hypoxemia. The recommended modifications include approximating the position as closely as possible to the original classical position for postural drainage. Manual techniques such as percussion, vibration, shaking, etc., should be avoided over the operated side, in patients after thoracotomy.
- **Postural correction exercises:** As post-thoracotomy patients, tend to side flex their trunk toward the operated side, to avoid injury/pain at the incision site, they develop scoliosis in the spine. Initially, the patient should be given postural re-education exercises. Subsequently, as the incisional wound heals, gentle scar massage, myofascial release, positional stretching as tolerated, air shift maneuver should be performed. Patients developing kyphosis after median sternotomy, should be made to perform short arc upper trunk extension, with pillow under the abdomen, without causing pressure on the surgical site and without inducing marked pain.
- **Mobilization exercises to shoulder, spine and limbs:** After thoracotomy, majority of patients develop shoulder pain on the side of the incision, subsequently developing frozen shoulder. For this reason, autoassisted or active ROM exercises for the shoulder within pain limits can be started as early as possible, starting on the first postoperative day. The exercises are performed 3–4 times a day. However, shoulder abduction and external rotation are initially avoided to prevent increased stress on the incision.
  Relaxed passive exercises, active free lower limb exercises (i.e., quadriceps and ankle exercises) started on the first postoperative day to minimize circulatory stasis and to prevent circulatory problems such as deep vein thrombosis and pulmonary embolism should be continued.
  Gradually, thoracic mobilization exercises, in the form of thoracic extension in sitting, thoracic rotation and lateral flexion protecting the incision in sitting should be performed. Walking should be progressed gradually.
- **Discharge and home exercise program/pulmonary rehabilitation:** After removal of drainage tube and stitches, patients are usually discharged from inpatient hospital care. Those, who have no/minimal postoperative complications are advised home exercise program, however, those having marked cardio-pulmonary complications and functional impairment attend pulmonary/cardiac rehabilitation services.

SECTION 7

Ethics and Management and Special Techniques in Physiotherapy

Section Outline

- Chapter 34: Professional Ethics
- Chapter 35: Management for Physiotherapists
- Chapter 36: Motor Control, Motor Learning and Special Techniques of Therapy to Improve Function in Neurological Diseases/Disorders
- Chapter 37: Manual Therapy

Professional Ethics

INTRODUCTION

Physiotherapists, occupational therapists, and other healthcare professionals provide healthcare to individuals, who suffer from diseases and disabilities that require long-term intervention in the form of assessment and treatment. Most of the therapeutic interventions involve procedures where a therapist has to work with the patients for nearly 1 hour in a day, for months/years, where hands on techniques to apply exercises, mobilization, manipulation, along with application of electrodes on patient's body for electrotherapy are performed. Very often the patient and his family members become too much dependent on the therapists with trust and expectations. Sometimes during patient treatments, injury/burns, etc., may take place leading to medicolegal issues. To fulfill such expectations and to avoid medicolegal issues, it is essential that the therapists follow an ethical behavior and should show no sympathy to the patient/family members, and exhibit empathy, for proper delivery of therapeutic services.

MEDICOLEGAL ISSUES ARISING DURING PATIENT TREATMENTS

Malpractice

During treatment if any adverse effects/complications arise, which should not have occurred, had proper attention and care been given by the treating therapist/clinician, it is regarded as malpractice.

While treating patients, due to causation of any injury/burn, it may lead to healthcare malpractice liability on the treating therapist/clinician, if there is a legal basis to such malpractice. Malpractice liability occurs, when the clinician-patient relationship is breached due to patient injury, and the ethical principle of non-maleficence, i.e., do no harm to patients are severely breached.

Malpractice Liability

A healthcare provider is subjected to liability for patient care malpractice, if during performance of tests and measures and application of treatment interventions, the patient sustains injury, where no informed consent was taken from the patient/caregivers. The factors increasing healthcare professional's malpractice liability exposure include:

- New Government/Institution/Accreditation agency regulations.
- Constantly changing healthcare delivery techniques.
- Litigious nature of the public.
- The broadened scope of practice.
- Clinical specialty certification issues, where the care given by such specialists is considered superior, as compared to nonspecialists, who are sometimes blamed for such treatments.
- Using cross trained/multiskilled professionals.
- Using physiotherapy assistants/ward boys to provide therapy in place of the trained therapists.

The factors that lead to malpractice liability, causing patient injury are:
- Professional negligence.
- Breach of treatment related contractual promises.
- Intentional misconduct.
- Use of defective equipment.
- Use of faulty techniques.

Liability imposed on the healthcare provider, due to negligent conduct, causing injury to patients could be:
- **Primary liability:** It is the legal and financial responsibility on the individual healthcare provider for the negligent conduct by self.
- **Vicarious liability:** The term vicarious liability refers to indirect legal and financial responsibility on the clinician, for conduct of another person such as an employee or the ward boy or the students/trainees of physiotherapy.

Professional Negligence

Negligence can be considered as legally actionable carelessness by the clinician/therapist causing injury to patients. A professional is said to have committed negligence, if one or more of the following elements are proved.
- Violation of duties owed by the healthcare provider.
- The healthcare providers' negligent conduct has caused injury to the patients.
- Monetary compensation is required for the loss caused to the patient.

However, if the clinician/therapist works observing the principles and codes of ethics, and the injury caused is nonintentional/not caused by negligence, the injury so caused to the patient should not lead to malpractice liability. The clinician/therapist should have thorough understanding of codes of ethics applicable to therapists.

Ethics

A set of principles of right conduct to be exhibited by professionals. It is the moral philosophy that involves systematizing, defending and recommending concepts of right and wrong behavior.

According to Webster's dictionary ethics is a concept that deals with moral issues of good and bad, based on societal norms. Ethics, is the code written or unwritten that guides the behavior of human beings, in the context of different cultures and situations.

Types of Ethics

1. **Meta ethics:** It is the branch of ethics that seeks to understand nature of ethical properties, statements, attitudes and judgments.
2. **Normative ethics:** It describes a set of questions about, how one should act in his/her day to day activities.
3. **Applied ethics**: It is the philosophical examination from a moral stand point of particular issues in public and private lives that are matters of moral judgment. Applied ethics is divided into:
   – Professional ethics
   – Business ethics
   – Bio ethics
   – Machine ethics
   – Relational ethics
   – Military ethics
   – Public service ethics

It is understood from above given types, that everywhere starting from professional services such as clinicians, teachers to working in military and public services, one need to observe ethics for smooth discharge of duties and responsibilities.

Professional Ethics

It encompasses the personal and corporate standards of behavior expected from professionals, involved in vocations consisting of counseling and services to others after high educational training.

The components and qualities of professional ethics are:
- **Honesty:** It is a facet of moral character that denotes, positive, virtuous attributes such as truthfulness, straight-forwardness, integrity without lying, cheating or theft.
- **Integrity:** It is a concept of consistency of actions, values, methods, measures, principles, expectations and outcomes. The actions are to be performed as a whole, exhibiting the quality of honesty with strong moral principles.
- **Transparency:** It is a general quality, implemented by set of principles, practices and procedures, which allows citizens accessibility to various information about procedures adapted.
- **Accountability:** It is the acknowledgment and shouldering of responsibilities for actions, decisions and policies with answering for results.
- **Confidentiality:** It is the ethical principle of discretion associated with professions such as medicine, where the communications between the professional and the client (about the clients' medical condition), called privileged communications are not disclosed to anybody else.
- **Objectivity:** The clinician should exhibit strong faith in his/her techniques to achieve definite outcomes.
- **Respectfulness:** It is the specific feeling of regard to the profession and client to achieve the best outcome.
- **Obedience to law:** The professionals should work within the premises of laws, which are rules and guide lines to be observed while delivering professional services.

Three dimensions of professional ethics: A professional clinician need to follow 3 "R"s such as:
1. **Rules** and **regulations** for practice of the profession.
2. **Responsibility:** Should take responsibility to discharge the professional service efficiently.
3. **Respect:** Demonstrate respect to the profession, professional colleagues, seniors and clients.

Code of Ethics

The code of ethics is a guide of principles for specific group of professionals, to help them perform their roles, to know how to conduct themselves, and to know how to resolve various ethical issues. It helps the professionals to apply moral and ethical principles to the specific situations encountered by them during practice of professional services.

Every professional, whether in medicine, surgery, physiotherapy, occupational therapy, etc., need to follow the code of ethics laid down by the respective professional associations/professional bodies. These codes convey the rights, duties and obligations of the members of the profession. These codes provide the basic framework for ethical judgment of the professional and make him/her aware to realize what is right/wrong while discharging professional services.

Professional Association/Professional Body

A professional association (also called a professional body, professional organization, or professional society) is usually a nonprofit organization created to progressively develop a particular profession, the interests of individuals engaged in that profession and the interest of the public. This is constituted by a group of people (governing body) from the learned occupation, who are entrusted with maintaining control or oversight the legitimate practice of the occupation safeguarding public interest. It acts as the controlling body of the learned profession. The members of such bodies are the individual professionals. Some professional bodies have regulatory power on its members and it is mandatory for the members to register with such bodies. For example the National Medical Commission is a professional body, whose members, the medical practitioners are mandatorily required to register with the council to practice in the country. The Rehabilitation Council of India (RCI), is a professional body, where rehabilitation personnel like Prosthetists/Orthotists are required to register with this council for making practice in India.

For physiotherapists working in the country, the Indian Association of Physiotherapists (IAP) is the professional body for the Physiotherapists at present, where it is not mandatory to register with the association for practicing in the country. National Level Council for the profession is in the process of constitution, which has got approval from both the houses of parliament of the country. Once such Physiotherapy Council functions, it will have a strong controlling power on its members, who have to register with the council for practicing in the country. State level councils are getting formed in various states of India to regulate practice of Physiotherapists/Occupational therapists.

The functions of professional bodies include the following:
- Set and assess professional examinations.
- Provide support for Continuing Professional Development through learning opportunities and tools for recording and planning.
- Publish professional journals or magazines.
- Provide networks for professionals to meet and discuss their field of expertise.
- Issue Code of Conduct to guide professional behavior.
- Deal with complaints against professionals and implement disciplinary procedures.
- Be enabling fairer access to the professions, so that people from all backgrounds can become professionals.
- Provide careers support and opportunities for students, graduates and people already working.
- Promote research in the particular field.

In India, two types of professional bodies exist such as:
- **Constitutional bodies**: These are bodies that derive its authority from constitution. They are those bodies which find considerable mention in the constitution, in ways like having a part of the constitution or an article explaining their position. Example: Election Commission of India.
- **Non-constitutional bodies/Extra constitutional bodies**: Extra constitutional bodies derive their authority by a law created by the parliament, an ordinance promulgated by the president or an executive order. They are those bodies which do not find mention in the constitution. They are created by various methods which further explain their nomenclature. The extra constitutional bodies are of two types such as:
  1. **Statutory body**: They are those bodies which are created by a law passed by the parliament which explicitly mentions the objectives for creation, their composition, powers, etc. Example: Information Commission of India, Rehabilitation Council of India, National Medical Commission, etc.
  2. **Executive body:** They are those bodies which are created by an executive order, i.e., order of a ministry of union or state or registered with the Government. Such bodies have no constitutional or law backing them. Example: The Planning Commission of India (A government organization), Indian Association of Physiotherapists (A registred body).

International Professional Bodies

World Confederation of Physiotherapy

The World Confederation for Physiotherapy (WCPT) was founded in 1951. It is the sole international voice for physiotherapists. The confederation operates as a nonprofit organization and is registered as a charity in the United Kingdom.

World Confederation for Physiotherapy is committed to take the profession ahead, and improve global health through:
- Encouragement of high standard of physiotherapy education, practice and research across the globe.
- Supporting exchange of information among member organizations.
- Collaborating with national and international organizations. As WCPT was established on September 8, every year, on this date, World Physiotherapy Day is celebrated.

World Health Organization

The World Health Organization (WHO) is a specialized agency of the United Nations, responsible for international public health. It was founded on April 7, 1948, and has its headquarters in Geneva, Switzerland. It is an international professional body, which plays an essential role in the global governance of health and disease, due to its core global functions of establishing, monitoring and enforcing international norms and standards, and coordinating multiple actors toward common goals. Every year April 7 is celebrated as World Health Day.

The work of the WHO is defined by its Constitution, which divides WHO's core functions into three categories:
- **Normative functions,** including international conventions and agreements, regulations and nonbinding standards and recommendations.
- **Directing and coordinating functions,** including its health for all, poverty and health, and essential medicine activities and its specific disease programs.
- **Research and technical cooperation functions,** including disease eradication and emergency managements.

UNICEF

UNICEF, known as United Nations Children's Fund, is an agency of United Nations, responsible for providing humanitarian and developmental aid to children worldwide. It is recognized as one wide spread social welfare organization in the World. It was found on December 11th, 1946, in New York, United States, as its headquarter.

Functions of UNICEF

The main function of UNICEF includes the following:
* Providing immunization and disease prevention to children.
* Administering treatment for children and their mothers, affected by HIV.
* Strengthening child, childhood and maternal nutrition.
* Improving sanitization.
* Providing emergency relief in response to disasters.

Positive roles of code of ethics: The codes of ethics laid down by professionals associations/organizations work as a protective cover highlighting the boundaries within which a professional should work. It guides the professional to work, without damaging self, the profession and the clients. The codes of ethics have some positive roles such as:
* **Inspiration:** Ethical codes provide a positive inspiration to professionals for discharging their professional duties efficiently and honestly, exercising the obligations.
* **Guidance:** Ethical codes provide the guidelines for achieving success in professional matters.
* **Support for responsible conduct:** The ethical codes provide positive and potential support to the professional to practice a particular profession efficiently within ethical manner.
* **Education and promotion of mutual understanding**: The codes of ethics help in emphasizing the importance of moral issues in values among teachers and students, in educational institutions and promote mutual understanding to resolve professional issues.
* **Contributing to a positive public image of the profession:** The codes of ethics promote creation of a positive image of a particular profession, whose members are committed to provide service with dignity, taking accountability for their actions.
* **Promoting business interests:** The codes of ethics promote business interest by charging fees for professional services, which the client can afford to, considering the nature of services and period (days/months) for which the services are required, so that discontinuity in getting services by the clients can be eliminated.
* **Protects the status quo and suppress dissent within the profession:** The codes of ethics eliminate disputes within a profession and make the services run smoothly maintaining status quo.

Principles of Professional Ethics

* **Autonomy:** Autonomy of the client/patient to opt for or out of any treatment options should be available to him.
* **Beneficence:** Duty of the healthcare provider is to ensure that the client in his/her care is assured of all the benefits of his/her professional knowledge to help the person overcome the dysfunction.
* **Justice:** Duty of the health provider is to ensure that justice is done to the individuals in his/her care. This involves equal and unbiased care, respect for autonomy, and the duty to provide the correct information to the best of his/her knowledge if called upon by a court of law.
* **Non-maleficence:** It emphasizes upon doing no harm to the patient.
* **Confidentiality**: Maintain confidentiality about the patient's diagnosis. Do not discuss one patient's condition with another patient without the consent of the first party. Ensure that patient records are not kept in places of public access.
* **Dissipation of knowledge**: The patient has the right to get the information pertaining to his/her condition and treatment. He/she also has the right to change service providers and treatment procedures, if he/she so wishes.

ETHICS IN PHYSIOTHERAPY

Ethics in physiotherapy can be defined as the moral code of conduct that defines the relationship between the physiotherapist and his/her patient or client, and the therapist and other healthcare professionals based on mutual respect and trust.

It is the legal duty of a physiotherapist, to support the clinician or student to provide a "reasonable" standard of care to patients and to protect their safety.

Practitioners have a duty to make the care of patients or clients their first concern and to practice safely and effectively. Maintaining a high level of professional competence and conduct is essential for good patient care.

The Practitioners have ethical and legal obligations to protect the privacy of people requiring and receiving care. Patients or clients have a right to expect that practitioners and their staff will hold information about them in confidence, unless information is required to be released by law or public interest considerations.

Before applying any intervention, it is essential that, the therapist/clinician explains the patient/caregiver about the tests and measures to be performed and intervention to be applied including the costs of such procedures. After explaining these to the patients/caregivers, he/she should take informed consent from the patient/caregivers (if the patient is a small child, very old man or unconscious), expressing the willingness to perform the tests/measures on him/her and to take such treatments understanding the benefits and hazards.

Informed Consent

It is a process in which a healthcare provider, educates a patient or his/her relative, about the risks, benefits and alternatives of a given, test and measures and treatment intervention and take his/her (patient's/relatives) consent to undergo such tests/interventions in a prescribed format designed for the purpose. It is the duty of the healthcare provider, to make it clear that, the patient has understood the different elements of information regarding assessment and treatment, to take a decision about his/her assessment/treatment, and has signed the consent form without any pressure/force on him to agree to such interventions.

The elements of informed consent documentation are:
- Diagnosis of the disease/disorder and pertinent evaluation findings.
- The nature of the procedure/treatment interventions recommended.
- Material risks of serious harms/complications.
- The expected benefits of such treatment procedures.
- Reasonable alternatives available.
- Risk and benefits of alternatives.

It should be understood by all that failure to obtain patient informed consent constitutes healthcare malpractice. Professional negligence malpractice litigation, premised on a lack of informed consent is legally actionable only when the following take place:
- A patient injury takes place from an undisclosed risk.
- Patient/care givers complain that, had they known the details of such procedures before, they would not have consented for such procedures/treatments.

There are certain exceptions to obtain patient informed consent, such as:
- **Emergency doctrine:** Under this, when a patient presents for evaluation and treatments in life-threatening emergency situation, and is unable to communicate his/her desire to undergo such treatments/procedures, the clinician can start the intervention without waiting for consent, with presumptions that, the patient/caregiver would consent to such lifesaving interventions.
- **Therapeutic privilege:** Under this, a clinician may be justified in withholding from a patient information, about the patient's diagnosis/prognosis, when in the judgment of the clinician, the patient/care givers cannot deal psychologically with such information.

CODE OF CONDUCT FOR PHYSIOTHERAPISTS

Physiotherapists, as healthcare providers, are required to follow the code of conduct prescribed for their functioning to avoid medicolegal issues. A few codes of conduct are:
- Physiotherapists respect confidentiality, privacy, and security of patient information.
- Physiotherapists treat people fairly.
- Physiotherapists practice in a safe, competent and accountable manner.
- Physiotherapists act with integrity in all professional activities.
- Physiotherapists shall provide honest quality care, competent and accountable professional consultancy, and therapeutic services to any person who may seek or may be in need of the same.
- Physiotherapists should recognize the limits of their expertise and confine themselves to performing duties for which they are properly educated, trained, and qualified, making referrals when situations are outside their area of competence.
- Physiotherapists should not exploit, threaten, persuade the unwilling to accept forcefully, or sexually harass others.
- Physiotherapists should refrain from unjustified or unseemly criticism of fellow members, other programs and other organizations.
- Physiotherapists should take appropriate steps to enhance the safety and security of patients.
- Physiotherapists should provide accurate, complete, current, and unbiased information.
- Physiotherapists should respect the dignity and basic rights of patients and professional colleagues.
- Physiotherapists should make timely referral of the patient only, if required to appropriate specialists, for investigation and treatment if requirement arises.
- Physiotherapists should maintain secrecy of the patient's diagnosis and treatment, and can disclose the same before professional colleagues, during case discussions/seminars.
- Physiotherapists are required to explain the patient about the investigations and treatment to be undertaken, its potential benefits and dangers, reasonable alternatives available and take informed consent, before starting such intervention.
- Physiotherapists should apply an intervention to the patient, for which, he/she has expertise.
- Physiotherapists should not accept any gift from patients, intended to influence his/her treatments.
- Physiotherapists, while treating patients should have a feeling of internal kindness (empathy) to the patients rather than showing external kindness.
- Physiotherapists in private practice are required to charge reasonably for the services delivered.
- Physiotherapists are required to treat patients without any partiality, i.e., without considering, whether the patient is rich or poor, except, when especially detailed by the head of department (HOD) to treat a VVIP, and in such a case the therapist should arrange continuation of therapy for the regular patients also.
- Physiotherapists are required to attend seminars, conferences to get acquainted with the latest developments in the profession.
- Physiotherapists should participate in outreach services, to provide healthcare to people in the community.
- Physiotherapists involved in teaching, should use modern teaching technology and try to clear all doubts of the students.
- Male physiotherapists treating female patients should ensure that, a female attendant is available in the room during assessment and treatment.
- Physiotherapists should take appropriate measures for documentation and treatment of complications, if so arises.
- Physiotherapists should take advice of the HOD of the department, if any ethical dilemma arises.
- Physiotherapists should maintain proper documentation of the patients' records for follow-up and research.
- Physiotherapists should conduct researches and make publication in books and journals.

- Physiotherapists should make a thorough clinical reasoning, to select the appropriate modality/technique.
- Physiotherapists should make time management to complete the assessment and services in time.
- Physiotherapists should not make any discrimination among patients and students on the basis of cast, religion, etc.
- Physiotherapist should respond honestly to any enquiry conducted against allegations, and provide accurate information.
- Physiotherapists should provide high standards of clinical service and teaching to keep the profession at high levels.
- Physiotherapists involved in class room teaching should present themselves in a respectable manner.
- Physiotherapists should work ethically to keep the reputation of the profession, department, and institute at a very higher position.
- Physiotherapists should not make any public statements about the department/institution, except when he is assigned the responsibility to address media.

The Code contains important standards for practitioner behavior in relation to:
- Providing good care, including shared decision making among patients, care givers and different professionals.
- Working with patients or clients to resolve health/disability issues.
- Working with other practitioners to share his/her knowledge for achieving successful management of clients.
- Working within the healthcare system, to practice, what he/she has been trained for.
- Minimizing risk by using efficient, properly serviced equipment and selecting appropriate techniques through a thorough clinical reasoning.
- Maintaining professional performance at high standard.
- Observation of professional behavior and ethical conduct.
- Ensuring health and wellbeing of the practitioner (self).
- Teaching of professionals, supervising services of juniors and assessing the clients' progress.
  - Different professional associations/organizations [Indian Association of Physiotherapists, American Physiotherapists Association (APTA), etc.] have laid down code of ethics for its members. In India Physiotherapists are required to follow the code of ethics laid by IAP (IAP Code of Ethics). The physiotherapists, practicing in India and the students of physiotherapy are advised to read and follow code of ethics given by IAP.

Management for Physiotherapists

INTRODUCTION

As a family is managed by its head and associated members, the department of physiotherapy needs to be managed like a family for smooth functioning of its activities. However, the management of the physiotherapy department is more complex, than family management, as, the therapists are involved in providing services to patients through mobilization, manipulation, heat and electrotherapy, etc., which carries a risk of patient injury. Further the management of department becomes more complex, if the concerned department is involved in teaching and training. Such complexity of management can be minimized and smooth functioning is established, if the head of department and his/her subordinates have proper management skills. The students pursuing studies in technical/clinical courses should obtain complete knowledge of management, so that, he/she becomes competent in managing an establishment after completion of the course.

DEFINITION OF MANAGEMENT

Management is considered as a process of coordinating of all resources through the processes of planning, organizing, directing and controlling in order to achieve the organizational goals effectively and efficiently.

FUNCTIONS OF MANAGEMENT

It should be understood that management is an integrated concepts having so many aspects and functions. A good manager can only achieve these functions, making the organization progress. Joseph L Massie (1971) defines the following seven functions of management:

1. **Decision making:** The process by which a course of action is consciously chosen from available alternatives for the purpose of achieving a desired result.
2. **Organizing:** The process by which the structure and allocation of jobs is determined.
3. **Staffing:** The process by which managers select, train, promote and retire subordinates.
4. **Planning:** The process by which a manager anticipates the future and discovers alternative courses of action open to him/her.
5. **Controlling:** The process that measures current performance and guides it towards some predetermined goal.
6. **Communicating:** The process by which ideas are transmitted to others for the purpose of effecting a desired result.
7. **Directing:** The process by which actual performance of subordinates is guided toward common goals.

There are various aspects of management required to be followed for smooth functioning of a department, which are described here.

Resource Management

Resource management is considered as one important facets of management of any organization/department. It is the practice of planning, scheduling, and allocating people, money, and technology to a project or program to achieve the greatest organizational value. It is also the process of preplanning, scheduling, and allocating resources to maximize efficiency of performance to meet market needs.

Utilizing every resource intelligently is imperative for every organization, due to which it has become an integral part of organizations. Moreover, organizations spend a lot of time and cost in creating the right talent pool to manage its function and achieve maximum profit.

Different Types of Resources

The various types of resources to be managed in general are:
- Human resources
- Natural resources
- Water resources
- Environmental resources
- Energy resources
- Wild life resources
- Land resources
- Forest resources
- Agriculture resources

There are six steps for effective resource management, such as:

1. Determination of the required resources (i.e., understanding the demand).
2. Acquiring the resources.

3. Manage resources (assign people to that demand).
4. Control resource usage (track utilization and update the assignments).
5. Begin capacity planning.
6. Present the data to senior executives.

For the smooth functioning of the physiotherapy department, human resource management, water resource management (for hydrotherapy), energy resource management (for electrotherapy) and land resource management (utilization of premises for therapeutic services), inventory management (management of stores for procurement and supply of materials), etc., need to be made effectively, though human resource management is of utmost important.

Personnel Management/Human Resource Management

One of the key aspects of physiotherapy clinical leadership is the management of human resources/personnel, which facilitates effective clinical operations. Timely deployment of therapists for various functions of the hospital/department, such as OPD assessment clinics, OPD patients management, in-door patients management, out reach services, academic classes/seminars, etc., and arranging substitutes/alternatives, when certain faculty/staff is on leave are various challenges in personnel management, which an efficient manager/head of unit can discharge smoothly.

According to Brech, "Personnel Management is that part, which is primarily concerned with human resource of the organization."

Starting from training of students to recruitment through selection tests/interview and organization of professional development programs, the management of human resources is both time consuming and critically important to the success of the organization.

According to Flippo, "Personnel management is the planning, organizing, compensation, integration and maintenance of people for the purpose of contributing to organizational, individual and societal goals." It can be defined as obtaining, using and maintaining a satisfied workforce. It is a significant part of management concerned with employees at work and with their relationship within the organization.

Nature of Personnel Management done in any organization:
- Personnel management includes the function of employment, development of trained personnel and payments of incentives and compensation. These functions are performed primarily by the personnel manager in consultation with other departments.
- Personnel management is an extension to general management. It is concerned with promoting and stimulating competent work force to make their fullest contribution to the concerned establishment.
- Personnel management exists to advise and assist recruitment/placement of personnel in the sections of the establishment. The personnel department is considered as a staff department of an organization.
- Personnel management lays emphasis on action rather than making lengthy schedules, plans, and work methods. The problems and grievances of people at work can be solved more effectively through rationale personnel policies.
- It is based on human orientation. It tries to help the workers to develop their potential fully to meet the requirements.
- It also motivates the employees through its effective incentive plans, so that the employees provide fullest cooperation and participation for the growth and development of the organization.
- Personnel management deals with human resources for various units of concerned organization. In context to human resources, it manages both workers as well as the executives.

Role/Functions of Personnel Manager

Personnel manager is the head of personnel department. However, in the Department of Physiotherapy, the Head of Department acts as the Personnel Manager. He performs both managerial and operative functions of management. His role can be summarized as given below:
- **Personnel manager provides assistance to top management:** The top management are the people who decide and frame the primary policies of the concerned organization. All kinds of policies related to personnel or workforce can be framed out effectively by the personnel manager.
- He advices the Junior manager/Unit in-charges as a staff specialist, and assists the junior managers in dealing with various personnel matters.
- As a counselor, personnel manager attends problems and grievances of employees and guides them. He tries to solve the employees' issues to best of his capacity. Leaves to employees are sanctioned considering requirements/priorities, not as a matter of right to get leave.
- Personnel manager acts as a mediator between management and workers during crisis/strike call by employees.
- **Personnel manager acts as a spokesman:** Since he is in direct contact with the employees, he is required to act as representative of organization in committees appointed by government/concerned establishment. He represents the establishment/company in training programs.

Time Management

One important factor for good management, to increase productivity and service delivery in any work situation is time management. As physiotherapists are involved in assessment and treatment of different diseases and disorders and are also involved in teaching/training of personnel, effective time management is required for smooth functioning of the hospital/organization.

Definition: Time management is the process of planning, organizing, and exercising conscious control of time spent on specific activities, with an aim to increase effective outcomes, efficiency, and productivity.

It is the process of organizing and planning, how to divide and allocate time for specific activities. Good time management enables one to work smarter, without being exhausted. If one does not have the ability to manage time, he/she will work in high pressure, affecting his/her own health. For example, a physiotherapist working in a hospital set up, should have the time management skills, so that in between delivery of therapy to old patients attending therapy regularly, he/she should also find time in between therapy delivery to assess the new patients, attend to professional trainees, etc., and this will help him discharge duties efficiently without much tension.

There are five key elements of time management such as:
1. Conducive environment.
2. Setting priorities.
3. Eliminating nonpriorities.
4. Setting goal.
5. Developing the right habit.

Besides the above factors, the three "P"s of time management also help one to be more productive. The three **"P"**s are:
- **P**lanning properly before starting intervention.
- **P**rioritizing, the most difficult task to be performed first, followed by less difficult tasks.
- **P**erforming the tasks one after other, taking few minutes of rest between activities (energy conservation), helps one to complete the work in time, without much exhaustion.

Besides the three "P"s, the other strategies for effective time management are:
- Create a daily schedule of the functions to be discharged, preferably in the previous day.
- Develop intention to complete the work.
- Decide, which task is more important as per requirement.
- Group similar tasks together.
- Assign time limit for each task.
- Avoid distractions, while performing tasks.
- Organize all task elements in one place.
- Generate self-awareness.

Time management tools: The tools for effective time management include:
- Using specific software in machines for automatic on and off of devices
- Watch
- Alarm
- Calendar
- Diary

Quality Management

Quality management is a vital issue in any organization, dealing with healthcare delivery. Quality management ensures that an organization, product or service is maintained consistently at high standards. It is focused, not only on product and service quality, but also on means to achieve it. Quality management is very important in the physiotherapy department, as without qualitative services, quantitative achievements are not possible, which badly affects the reputation and functioning of the department/hospital.

Quality can be defined as fitness for intended use or, in other words, how well the product/service performs its intended function. Quality management is the act of overseeing all activities and tasks that must be accomplished to maintain a desired level of excellence. This includes the determination of a quality policy, creating and implementing quality planning and assurance, and quality control and quality improvement, which are briefly discussed below:
- **Quality planning:** A method for measuring the achievements of the quality objectives.
- **Quality assurance:** It is a part of quality management, focused on providing confidence that, quality requirements for the products/services will be fulfilled.
- **Quality control:** As part of quality management, it focuses on fulfilling quality requirements, in which quality of all factors involved in production/services are reviewed.
- **Quality improvement:** It refers to the combined and endless efforts of every worker in the organization, to make the products and services better and better.

Quality management ensures high quality products and services by eliminating defects and incorporating continuous changes and improvements in the system. High quality products/services in turn lead to loyal and satisfied customers who bring ten new customers along with them. A good quality service/education given in a specific physiotherapy clinic/institution attracts more patients/students to that organization.

Quality management is a central tenet of physiotherapy care. Quality indicators (QIs) as measurable elements of care are used to analyze and evaluate the quality of physiotherapy care. Quality indicators are tools that specify the minimum acceptable standard of practice. Quality indicators measure healthcare processes, organizational structures, and outcomes that relates to aspects of high quality care of patients.

Inventory Management

Inventory management refers to the process of procuring storing and supplying of materials to various units of an establishment for smooth functioning and service delivery.

Inventory management is the entire process of managing inventories/goods from raw materials to finished products.

It tries to efficiently streamline inventories to avoid both excessive supply and shortages of materials.

In physiotherapy department/hospital, the person dealing with the inventories/goods need to maintain three types of registers to document the procurements made, stock available, and supply made to various units. The materials should be categorized into: Consumables such as cotton rolls, ultrasound gels, etc., and Furnitures and equipments.

Two major methods for inventory management that should be followed are just-in-time (JIT) and materials requirement planning (MRP).

THEORIES OF MANAGEMENT

Management theories are a collection of ideas that recommend general rules for how to manage an organization/department or business. It addresses how supervisors (clinical supervisors/head of department in a physiotherapy department) implement strategies to accomplish organizational goals and how they motivate employees to perform at their highest ability.

Such theories are the set of general rules that guide the managers to manage an organization with effective management strategies. The theories focus on the role of supervision, organization, and group performance. These theories are an explanation to assist employees/clinicians/physiotherapists to effectively relate to the business goals/targets and implement effective means to achieve the same.

Benefits of Management Theories

Study of the management theories helps the leaders/head of organizations/departments to achieve the following benefits:
- **Increases productivity:** These theories help the heads of organizations to train their employees to improve performance for increasing productivity.
- **Simplify decision-making:** Management theories help leaders to develop strategies that speed up the decision-making process to enhance quality and quantity of production/delivery of services.
- **Enhances collaboration:** It helps leaders learn how to encourage employee participation and increase collaboration in the workplace to facilitate decision making and prompt delivery of services.
- **Increases objectivity:** Management theories encourage leaders to make scientifically proven developments in products and services to patients and public.

Kimani outlines four major management theories for the development of organizations, such as:
1. **Bureaucratic theory:** This theory of management proposes that the best way to run an organization/department is to structure it into a rigid hierarchy of officials/employees, governed by strict rules and procedures.
2. **Scientific management theory:** This theory of management analyzes and synthesizes work flow, with an objective of improving economic/clinical efficiency, especially enhancing productivity/service delivery abilities of its employees.
3. **Behavioral management theory:** This theory, also known as human relations movement, believes that a better understanding of human behavior at work, such as motivation, expectations and group dynamics enhances productivity/service deliveries.
4. **Human relations theory:** This theory is the school of organizational thoughts, which focuses on worker/professional's satisfaction, workplace organizations, and a means of influencing employee productivity/service and academic targets.

Qualities of a Good Manager/Head of Department/Head of Clinical Wing

A good manager/clinical supervisor/in-charge of the unit, should have the following criteria as per Robert Katz (1955):
- **Technical skills:** The manager should have proficiency in performing an activity in the correct manner with the appropriate techniques.
- **Human relationship skills:** The skill of cooperating with other members of the organization/department for efficient functioning.
- **Conceptual ability:** The ability to see individual matters as they relate to the overall picture.

All the three qualities need to be exhibited by the clinic head/head of physiotherapy department for effective discharge of function of the unit.

Organizational Chart

The organization chart also called an organogram is a diagram (**Flowchart 35.1**), showing graphically the relation of one official to another, of a company/Ministry and organizations/clinical establishment under it. It is also used to show the relation of one department to another, or of one function of an organization to another. This chart is valuable in that it enables one to visualize a complete organization, by means of the picture it presents.

MANAGEMENT OF PHYSIOTHERAPY DEPARTMENT

A physiotherapy department (**Flowchart 35.2**) is usually attached to a hospital, where the department needs to function adapting the policies of the hospital to which it is attached. In private and corporate hospitals, where collection of revenue is more emphasized through qualitative and quantitative therapeutic services, the head of the physiotherapy department needs to work with a good vision utilizing team spirit in the department to achieve success. The head of department of physiotherapy should understand policies of the hospital to which the department is attached, so that policies of the hospital are also followed in the department. In most hospitals/institutions, physiotherapy services and teaching (undergraduate/postgraduate) programs run concurrently, under the leadership of Dean/Director, where the Superintendent Physiotherapist, who is in-charge/HOD of clinical services, works with coordination with head of academic services for smooth functioning of service and teaching.

Organizing clinical services of physiotherapy department: The head of department should assign job responsibility to each therapist working under him/her understanding

Flowchart 35.1: Organizational chart of a rehabilitation center.

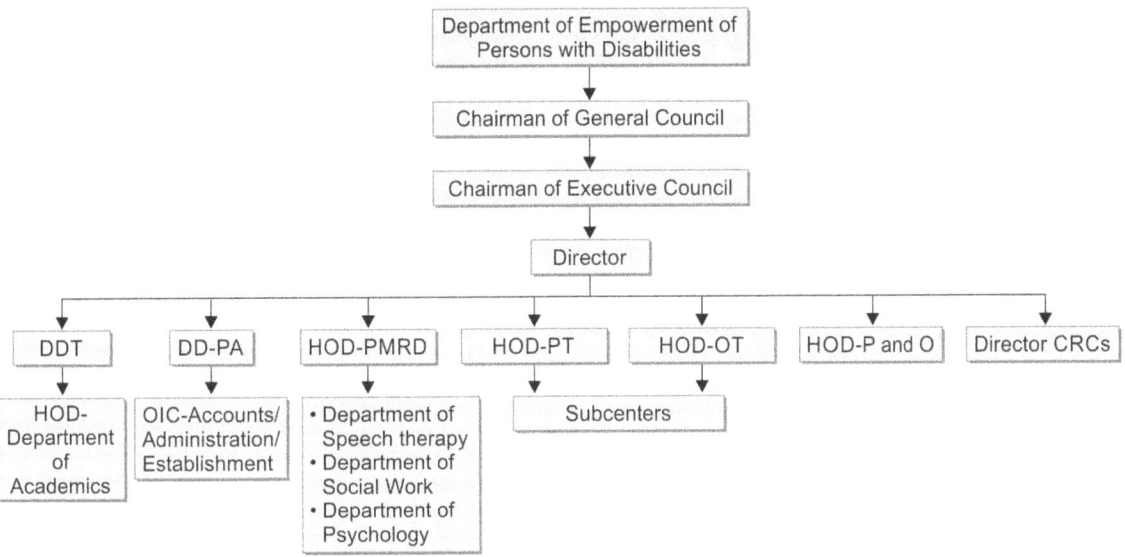

Flowchart 35.2: Working flowchart of a physiotherapy department.

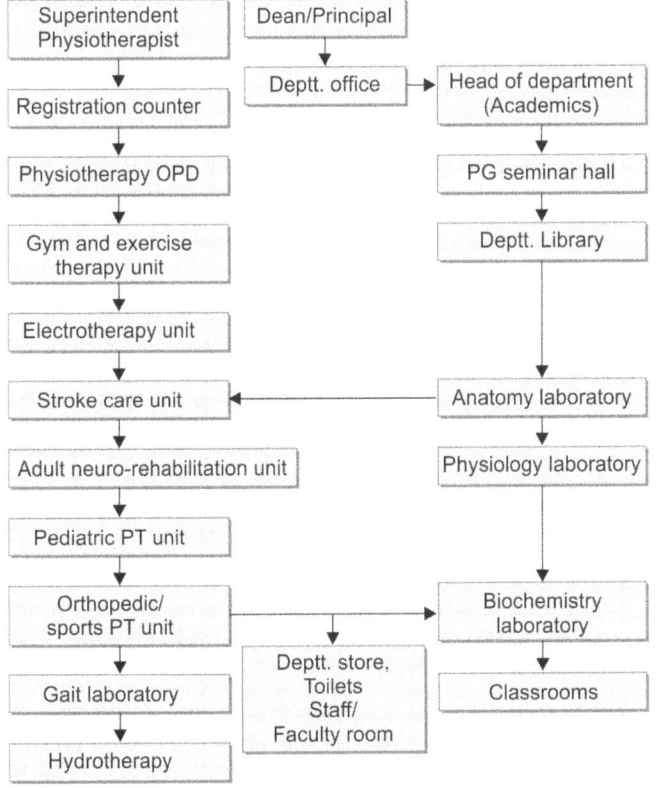

Decentralizing the works helps in the effective management of a department. Management of reception and accounts should be done by administrative/clerical staff. However, maintenance of equipment, allocation of duties for indoor and outdoor therapeutic services, etc., should be done by a senior level therapist under consultation with the head of department.

Documentation of the patients' records should be maintained properly by the administrative staff. The supervisor/head of department should avoid dictatorial approach (like, do it, or else action) and should follow the democratic approach where, the juniors are given opportunities to work independently, taking own decision, seeking the advice of seniors as and when required.

Management of accounts is very important, as the private hospitals depend on the revenue so collected from services, and for corporate and Government hospitals annual audit is done, where the revenue collected from patients are audited from records.

Management of physiotherapeutic services efficiently in physiotherapy department of any institution is a challenging issue. It is managed by a team comprising Physiotherapists, Senior Physiotherapists, Superintendent Physiotherapist, Nurses, Ward attendants, etc., for the clinical services. However, institutions involved in teaching undergraduate/postgraduate programs in physiotherapy also require a team of faculties and demonstrators. At the apex of the management hierarchy of the physiotherapy department, lies the head of the Department, whose dynamic leadership helps to manage a department smoothly. The management of different services of a physiotherapy department is achieved through the following:

❖ **Management of carpet area/land used for the services:** Depending upon the nature of services provided in a particular hall, the said hall need to be managed to meet the needs of the patients. For example, the electrotherapy

the competencies, of the particular therapist in specific categories of patient services. The duties and responsibilities of every member should be well defined by the head of department.

Besides the skills of organizing, the head of a physiotherapy department should also have the capabilities for planning, staffing, controlling and directing, for efficient management of different services. He/she should have good communication skills and supervising abilities.

hall should have insulated floorings to avoid earth shock, and the gait training laboratory, should have a gait mat, over which gait training can be given. There should be easy access to different floors through ramps, lift, etc. The halls should have enough lights and fans and the toilets attached should be free from barriers.

- **Management of infrastructure and equipment:** All the electrical/electronic equipment should be kept in air conditioned room and should be made dust free by daily cleaning. The mechanical equipment such as quadriceps table should also be cleaned daily for dusts. All the machines should be periodically serviced through Annual Maintenance Contract. The electrotherapy laboratory and gait laboratory should be provided with accessories and disposable substances. The water in hydrotherapy tank should have regular application with disinfectants and should have circulation of water at a particular temperature. Condemnation of old furniture and equipment should be done as per official norms.
- **Management of inventory:** It refers to the process of ordering, storing, and issuing the materials for use of patient services. The annual requirements of materials (both disposables and nondisposables) and equipment list should be prepared as annual action plan and after getting approval from the head of office, it should be provided to the central store of the organization at the beginning of the financial year for purchasing and supplying to the concerned department. After the materials are procured, it should be documented and supplied to various units as per written requisition. Sufficient stock of such materials such as cotton wool, ultrasound gel, etc., should be available in department's store for uninterrupted services.

  New equipment, furniture received from the central store should be numbered and documented in the stock register of the department. Damaged/defective equipment should be listed for condemnation.
- **Management of manpower/human resources efficiently:** With the current situation of cut in trained manpower, a good manpower management is essential to discharge various duties such as indoor therapy, outdoor therapy, etc. The supervisor should follow a democratic manpower management procedure using paternalistic approach, instead of dictatorial approach, so that activities of OPD services, outpatient therapy, Indoor patient's therapy can run smoothly. Leaves to the staff should be granted reasonably, realizing the importance.
- **Management of equipment services through Annual Maintenance Contract (AMC):** All the equipment must be serviced periodically through AMC for smooth functioning and for elimination of electrical hazards (electric shock). This procedure helps to eliminate medicolegal issues arising from use of defective and poorly serviced equipment.
- **Management of linen:** Management of linen involve sending the clothes for washing, maintenance of accounts, i.e., number of clothes taken for wash and number of clean clothes available for use along with number of clothes provided to various departments for services.
- **Management of documentation/record keeping:** The computerized system of documentation should be done as against the manual recording system done earlier. However, in hospitals, where manual filing of patients records are done, all the records of the patient should be preserved year and month wise in the medical record room for future follow up references.
- **Management of cleanliness/housekeeping:** All the therapy halls should be cleaned at least twice daily, i.e., in the morning and the afternoon sessions and the displaced machines, disposables should be kept in place by sweeper/housekeeping staff.
- **Management of security services:** If resources are available, security personnel should be engaged in OPD hall and the main entrance of the department for maintenance of discipline and preventing stealing.
- **Management of accounts:** Nowadays, all the services are chargeable, for which payment should be received from the patient as per exact slab and a receipt duly signed by the collecting clerk/accountant should be given to the patient.
- **Management of therapeutic services:** Allotment of duties to therapists for outdoor assessment clinic, outpatient department services, indoor services, allotment against leave/absence should be done by one senior therapist under consultation of HOD, for smooth management of services.
- **Management of academic activities:** Preparation of time table for classes, seminars, etc., should be done by one senior faculty under consultation with the Head of Department (Academics). In the absence of a faculty due to leave, arrangement classes should be organized from among the present faculties on that day.
- **Management of research cell:** As physiotherapy is a growing science, researches form the important methods for the progressive development. The research cell should have the appropriate instruments (measurement tools) for conducting research studies.

36. Motor Control, Motor Learning and Special Techniques of Therapy to Improve Function in Neurological Diseases/Disorders

MOTOR CONTROL

Motor control is the science that deals with the mechanisms of how movement is synthesized/organized by individuals who possess a nervous system. It explains, how complex interaction of multimodal sensory information from the environment interacts with the individual's physical systems to elicit necessary signals to recruit the muscles for production of goal directed movements. It talks how, posture and movements produced reflexively, can turn into voluntary, purposeful movements enabling individuals to hold a posture and produce purposeful functional movements. It also explains how, task and environment regulate one's posture and movements, so that, the body will either constrain or release the degrees of freedom to hold a posture to perform specific tasks.

All clinicians dealing with individuals with movement dysfunction, should have the knowledge of motor control for efficiently designing the treatment strategy for overcoming movement dysfunction.

Brooks (1986), referred Physiotherapists and Occupational therapists as: Motor control physiologists, as therapists spend a considerable amount of time retraining patients, who have motor control problems producing functional movement disorders. A therapist designs the strategies to improve the quality and quantity of movement essential for function. For the purpose of clinical practice, it is essential for the individual therapist to understands motor control.

It is found that, movement emerges from the interaction between individual, task and environment, which is described in the **Figure 36.1**.

The factors at the levels of individual, task and environment that influences production of movements are described in the **Figure 36.2**.

Constraints/Factors at the Level of Individual Regulating Movement Production

Three factors at the level of the individual influence production of movements, which include:

1. **Perception:** Perception is the integration of sensory impressions into psychologically meaningful information. Perception is essential to action, just as action is essential to perception. Sensory/perceptual systems provide information about the state of the body and features within the environment critical to the regulation of movement. The sensory/perceptual information is integral to the ability to act effectively within an environment.

2. **Cognition:** This process include, attention, motivation and emotional aspects of motor control that undertake the establishment of an intent or goal. Movement is not usually performed without such intent.

3. **Action:** Understanding the control of action, implies understanding the motor output from the nervous system to the body's effector system or muscles. This implies,

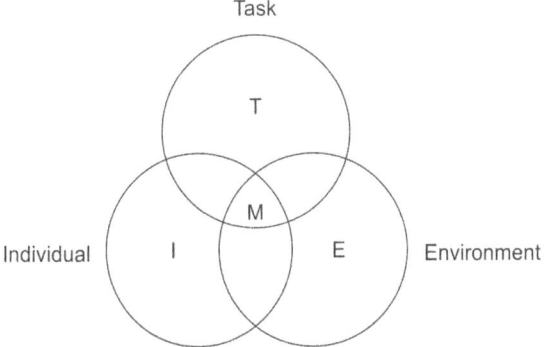

Fig. 36.1: Shows interaction of elements for movement production. (I: individual; E: environment; M: movement; T: task)

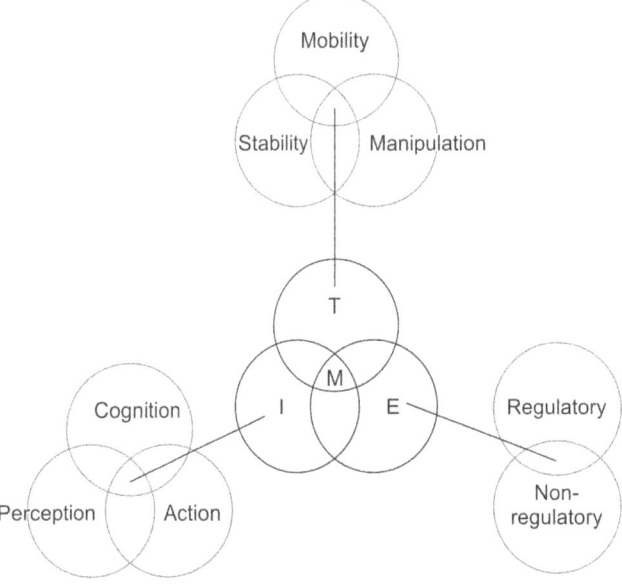

Fig. 36.2: Shows the factors essential for movement production. (I: individual; E: environment; M: movement; T: task)

how the nervous system organizes, the muscles and joints for co-ordinated movement called the various degrees of freedoms of body which are released to accomplish various functional tasks.

The interaction among perception (P), cognition and action in producing movement can be understood from **Figure 36.3**.

Task Constraints on Movement Production

Understanding the control of movement requires an awareness of how tasks regulate or constrain movement. Recovery of function following CNS damage requires that a patient develop movement patterns that meet the demands of functional tasks. Therapeutic strategies are to be designed that help the patient, learn or relearn to perform functional tasks essential to maximize recovery of functional independence. To establish a therapeutic environment for training of movement, the therapist should have an understanding of the nature of tasks to be taught. Functional tasks that are taught to patients include:

- Bed mobility task (rolling, supine to sitting etc).
- Transfer task (sit to stand, movement from chair to bed, movement onto and off a toilet etc).
- Activities of daily living (ADL), such as eating, grooming etc.
- Instrumental activities of daily living (IADL), such as writing, reading, cooking etc.
- Communication, which includes both verbal and non verbal methods of communicating with others.

Classification of Tasks based on Attributes

The task training given to patient are classified into the following types based on attributes/nature of the task such as:

- **Discrete and continuous tasks**. A discrete task has recognizable beginning and end (e.g. sit to stand), where as a continuous task has no recognizable beginning and end (e.g. running)
- **Stability and mobility tasks**: Stability task has fixed base of support (e.g. sitting), whereas mobility task has a mobile base of support (e.g. walking).
- **Manipulation continuum**: Movement tasks have also been classified, using a manipulation component. Manipulation tasks that require both speed and accuracy, increase the demand on the postural system to stabilize the body for task performance.
- **Attention continuum**: Attention of the performer plays an important role for the accomplishment of postural control tasks. Tasks such as sitting, standing, etc., requires lesser attentional demands as compared to mobility tasks such as walking, obstacle clearance, etc.
- **Open and closed tasks:**
  - *Closed tasks:* These are the fixed, habitual patterns of movement with minimum variation performed in a relatively fixed environment (taking food at the dinning table).
  - *Open tasks:* Open tasks are characterized by, tasks that are performed in a constantly changing unpredictable environment, making the ability to plan movement difficult (e.g. playing tennis).

Environmental Constraints on Movement Production

The environment that affects the performance of the task could be:

- **Regulatory:** Regulatory features specify aspects of the environment (shape, size, weight, positive reinforcement etc.) helping in shaping the movement.
- **Non-regulatory:** Non regulatory features of the environment (background noise, distraction, negative reinforcement etc.), may affect performance of task, where in it hinders the task performance.

Theories of Motor Control

Theories of motor control are groups of abstract ideas, that explain about the production and control of movement. Different theories of motor control have been developed over time and reflect current understanding and interpretation of nervous system function. The theories are described in brief as under:

Reflex Theory of Motor Control

This is the early theory of motor control, was given by Sir Charle's Sherrington. As per Sherrington, reflexes are the building blocks of complex behavior. As per him, movement results from a sequential stimulus—response event and the complex movements human beings produce result from the chaining together of a number of reflexes. He concluded that, with the whole nervous system intact, the reaction of the various parts of that system, the simple reflexes, are combined into greater actions that constitute the behaviour of the individual as a whole.

Clinical implications of reflex theory

Applying this theory into clinical practice, it necessitates for the therapist to apply various sensory stimuli as

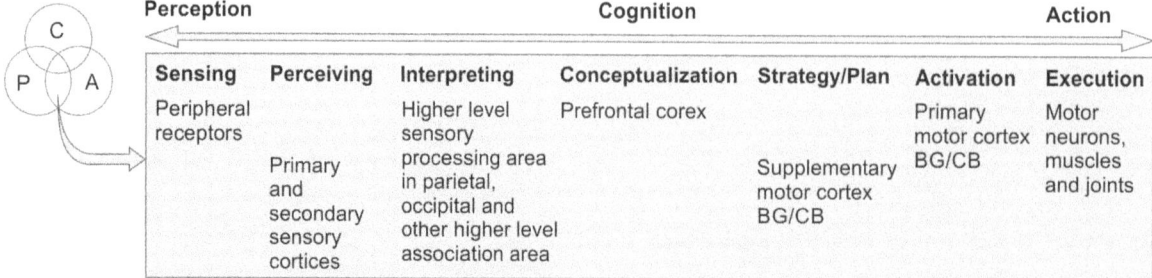

Model of interaction between perception action and cognition in motor control

Fig. 36.3: Shows interaction of essential components in the individual to produce movement.
(A: action; C: cognition; P: perception)

done in Vojta trigger point stimulation or Rood's sensory stimulation to get motor response. Once reflex response elicits movements, the same are gradually converted into voluntary motion through repeated practice integrating with task performance. Simple auditory/visual/tactile stimuli given in a planned manner help in producing movements in clients with CNS damage.

In pathological conditions, where the abnormal primitive reflexes affect movement production, the therapist designs strategies either to inhibit such reflexes and reactions (Bobath's NDT), or to facilitate such reflexes/reactions (Brunstrom's approach) to elicit movement.

Hierarchical Theory

The Hierarchical theory of motor control was given by Hughling Jackson, an English Physician, who stated that, the brain has higher, middle and lower levels of control. Hierarchical control implies an organizational control that is top down. Later Rudolf Magnus, who explored the function of the various reflexes, found that reflexes controlled by the lower levels of the neural hierarchy are present only when cortical centres are damaged, as the higher level hierarchy (CNS), that inhibits lower level reflexes is not functioning in such pathological states. The reflex theory in combination with the hierarchical theory is called the reflex hierarchical theory.

Clinical implications of reflex/hierarchical theory

Abnormalities of reflex organization are used to explain the disordered motor control found in subjects with cerebral palsy, brain stroke, etc. Signe Brunstorm, a physical therapist basing upon this theory stated that, when the influence of the higher centre is temporarily or permanently interfered with, normal reflexes become exaggerated, and the pathological reflexes appear. As per Berta Bobath, the abnormal postural reflexes found in children with cerebral palsy, brain stroke etc., result from the release of motor responses integrated at the lower level from restraining influences of the higher centers (cortex).

Motor Program Theory

This theory explains, how movement is possible in the absence of a stimulus, which is not explained by the Reflex theory of motor control. As per this theory, movement results from the motor programs.

A motor program/central motor pattern is defined as an abstract representation that store the rules of functional movements. When such representations are stimulated/initiated, results in the production of co-ordinated movement sequence. The motor program allows movement production in the absence of sensory input, by sending neural commands to different parts of the body for performing the desired task.

Clinical implications of motor program theory

This theory explains that abnormal movements found in brain injured, result from abnormalities of central pattern generators (motor programs). Movement will only emerge, when the motor programs are reconstructed through appropriate task practices.

Systems Theory of Motor Control

The system's theory proposed by Nicolai Bernstein, is based on the view that, motor control is the result of co-operative actions of many interactive systems, working to accommodate the demands of specific tasks. He suggested that, both internal factors (joint stiffness, inertia, movement dependent forces) and external factors (gravity) must be taken into consideration along with the functioning of body's multiple systems (nervous system, musculoskeletal system, cardiorespiratory system, cognitive-perceptual system, etc.) while planning movement. This theory is also called distributed model, as control of integrated movements is distributed throughout many interacting systems stated above, working co operatively to produce movements.

Considering the body as a mechanical system, Bernstein hypothesized that hierarchical control exists to simplify the control of the body's multiple degrees of freedom. The higher levels of the nervous system activate the lower levels, and the lower levels activate synergies (locomotors, postural and respiratory etc) to produce movements.

Clinical implications of the system's theory

It considers the fact that movement production is not determined solely by the out put of the nervous system, it also depends on the functioning of other body systems. The nervous system output channelized into the mechanical systems of the body help in movement production.

As it takes into account of the contribution of other systems, besides the nervous system, while working with a patient with CNS deficit, the therapist must be careful to examine the contribution of impairments in the other systems to overall loss of motor control.

Dynamic Action Theory

The dynamic action theory of motor control (Thelen et al 1987), began to see the moving person from a new perspective, which comes from the broader studies of dynamics or synergies within the physical world. It explains, how do a system of thousands of degrees of freedom are reduced to a few degrees of freedom, so that the system moves smoothly. As per this theory a system of individual parts come together making its elements work collectively in an ordered manner to produce movement. There is no need for a higher centre for issuing command to achieve co-ordinated action. This principle applied to motor control predicts that movement can emerge as a result of interacting elements without the need for specific commands or motor programs with in the nervous system.

This theory suggests that, new movements emerge because of a critical changes in one of the systems, called control parameter. A control parameter is a variable that regulates change in behaviour of the entire system. In the diagram that follows, the control parameter is **velocity**. The dynamic action perspective has deemphasized the notion of commands from the central nervous system in controlling movements. The changes in control parameters and corresponding changes of movement produced are shown in **Figure 36.4**.

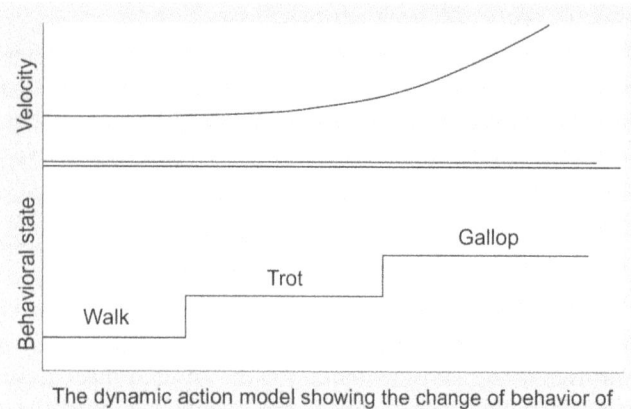

The dynamic action model showing the change of behavior of the moving animal as per the change of control parameter

Fig. 36.4: Shows how changes in control parameter (velocity) changes movement in a horse.

An important concept in describing movement from the perspective of dynamic action theory is the attractor state. An attractor state is an preferred pattern of movement used to accomplish common activity of daily life. An example of attractor state include, the desire of the individual to work at a preferred pace. The degree to which there is flexibility to change a preferred pattern of movement, is characterized as an attractor well. The deeper the well, the harder it is to change, the preferred pattern, suggesting a stable movement pattern. The shallow, the well, more is the flexibility to change **(Fig. 36.5).**

Clinical implications of Dynamic action theory

If the clinicians understand the physical or dynamic properties of the human body, these properties could be utilized to help patients regaining motor control. For example, velocity of movement is considered as an important contributor to the dynamics of the movement. A weak patient, not able to stand from chair sitting, when made to increase the velocity of trunk motion, is able to generate momentum/force production (as force is the rate of change of momentum), for being able to stand with weak glutei and quadriceps. A patient, walking very slowly, with freezing of degrees of freedom and consumption of more energy, can be made to walk efficiently, by increasing velocity of walking (establishing interaction between physical properties of body and velocity of movement). An unstable/ataxic patient walking very fast, and having frequent falls, can be made to walk slowly (reducing the velocity), so that, he/she can constrain the degrees of freedom and walk efficiently.

Ecological Theory

The Ecological theory of motor control was given by James Gibson (Psychologist) and expanded by his students. He explored the way in which our motor system allow us to interact most effectively with the environment to perform goal oriented behaviour. He found the importance of the environment in production of actions by controlling our movements.

It is stressed that, actions require perceptual information, that is specific to a desired goal directed action, performed with in a specific environment. The organization of action is specific to the task and the environment in which the task is being performed. As per Gibson, it is not the sensation but the perception of environmental factors, that is important for production of movement **(Fig. 36.6).**

Clinical implications of ecological theory

A patient with disordered motor control is helped to explore the possibilities, for achieving functional tasks in multiple ways. A patient with functional limitations, explores a range of possible ways to accomplish the task and develops the best solutions to them. A child, not able to walk, when perceives the presence of toys in the rack, tries to crawl to the rack, pulls self to standing holding the shelves and tries to remove the toys for playing. Cerebral palsy children, who are not able maintain neck in extension, can be placed on a wedge board with toys placed in front, so that, when the child could see the toys, tries to extend the neck more and more for playing with the toys.

Neuronal Group Selection Theory

As per the neuronal group selection theory for movement production, there is no central controller, there are no motor programs, there are no computations, in movement production as explained by the previous theories of motor

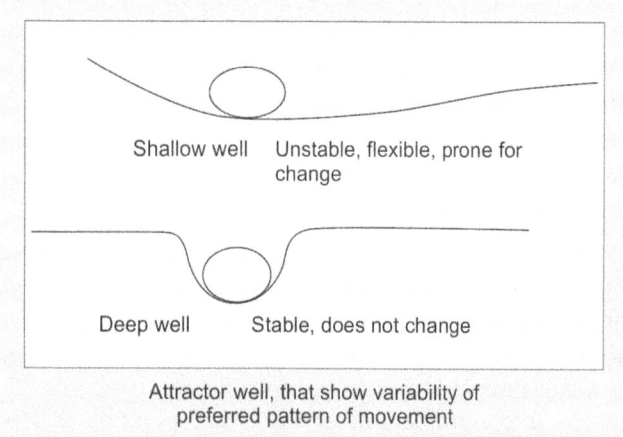

Attractor well, that show variability of preferred pattern of movement

Fig. 36.5: The attractor wells.

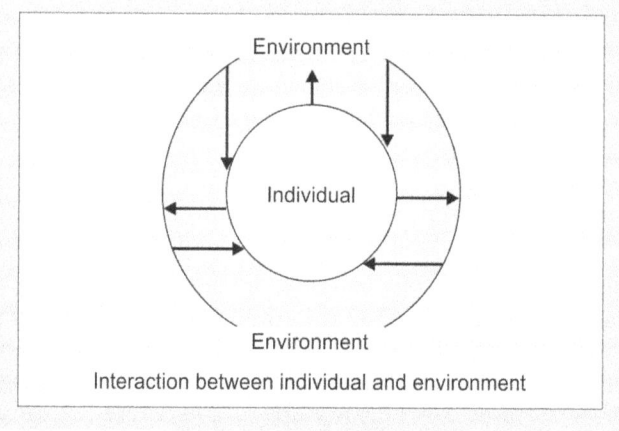

Interaction between individual and environment

Fig. 36.6: Shows interaction between individual and environment.

control. As per this theory brain development occurs through movement activating sensory receptors. The brain is not hard-wired and as a result has both individual uniqueness and life long plasticity. The degrees of freedom problem in movement control is solved through the selection of the most important neuronal groups, given the task and current status of the body systems, not through a computational process.

According to the NGST, the brain, i.e., the cortical and subcortical systems is dynamically organized into variable networks, the structure and function of which are selected by development and behavior. The units of selection are collections of hundreds to thousands of strongly interconnected neurons, called neuronal groups, which act as functional units.

Applying concepts of the NGST sheds new light on motor development. According to the NGST, variation is the keyword for normal development. The variation is not random, but determined by criteria set by genetic information. The variation has two forms: primary variability, which is not geared to external conditions, and secondary variability, in which motor performance can be adapted to specific situations. In both cases, selection on the basis of afferent information plays a significant role. Thus sensory information has an important function in motor development.

The NGST states that development starts with primary neuronal repertoires, with each repertoire consisting of multiple neuronal groups. The cells and the gross connectivity of the primary repertoires are determined by evolution (genetic factors). The secondary neuronal repertoires, responsible for movement production are acquired in nature. The changed connectivity within the secondary repertoire allows for a situation-specific selection of neuronal groups. Thus, the secondary neuronal repertoires and their associated selection mechanisms form the basis of mature variable behaviour which can be adapted to environmental constraints.

The theory explicitly states that development is neither exclusively governed by a genetically dictated neural substrate nor by environmental conditions. On the contrary, the theory highlights the notion that development is the result of a complex intertwining of information from genes and environment. Translating concepts of the NGST to the domain of human motor development results in a developmental progress with two different phases of variability.

Motor development starts during early fetal life with the phase of 'primary variability', which continues during infancy. All forms of goal-directed motor behavior start during infancy with the phase of primary variability. This is the time of life when (cortical) synaptogenesis is abundant. The resulting multifarious primary networks enable the most appropriate circuitries to be selected. The exploration and continuous processing of the concomitant afferent information gradually result in the selection of the most efficient movement patterns.

The creation of the secondary (sub)cortical repertoires is associated with extensive synapse rearrangement, the net result of synapse formation and synapse elimination. It is facilitated by increasingly shorter processing times which can be attributed in part to ongoing myelination. The long duration of the (sub)cortical developmental processes implies that it takes many years and experiences before the secondary neuronal networks are able to produce an efficient motor solution for each specific situation.

Clinical implications of neuronal group selection theory

A cerebral palsy child, not able to hold a posture and produce functional movements, can be thought to have the dysfunctions, due to inadequate primary neuronal repertoires. Such children should be given more and more environmental stimuli, so that, they develop secondary neuronal repertoires, enabling them hold a posture and produce movements.

MOTOR LEARNING

Motor learning is described as a set of processes associated with practice or experience leading to relatively permanent changes in the capability for producing skilled action. It involves learning new strategies for sensing as well as moving. Like motor control, it also emerges from a complex of perception-cognition-action process.

Types of Learning (Motor Learning)

Learning (motor learning) are of several types, such as:
- **Non-associative learning**: It takes place when subjects are given a single stimulus repeatedly, making the nervous system learn the characteristics of the stimulus. Example: Habituation, sensitization/desensitization exercises given to patients either to learn a single event/task (habituation) or to inhibit an abnormal response/reflex (desensitization) resulting in learning of normal posture/movement (sensitization).
- **Associative learning**: This enable the subject to associate ideas/establish relationship between stimuli, resulting in the performance of purposeful movement. This learning are of two types, such as:
  - *Classical conditioning:* In this the learner associates the applied stimuli and produces the desired response. A cerebral palsy child with impaired neck control can be made to develop neck control using the principles of classical conditioning, i.e., the therapist positioning the child on the wedge board when shows a toy in front of the child, the child tries to lift the head to look and enjoy the toy. In the next session, when the child sees the therapist try to lift the head associating the therapist's presence with presentation of toy (where a toy was not presented).
  - *Operant conditioning:* In this type of learning, the learner associates the reward presented at the end of performance to perform similar tasks in the next session anticipating to get a reward subsequently. A cerebral palsy child, who was presented with a toffee by the therapist for standing for few minutes with the help of a pair of elbow crutches, will try to stand more and more in the next session anticipating the reward from the therapist.

- ❖ **Declarative learning:** It involves learning through conscious recall, awareness, attention and reflection. Constant repetition leads declarative learning into procedural learning. With repetition of movement in motor training, the movement becomes an automatic motor activity, without the need of attention and monitoring. For example, while training gait to a patient, the therapist tells the patient to utter left and right while stepping the left and right legs respectively. After few days of training, without uttering/declaring, the patient becomes able to walk automatically like habit.
- ❖ **Procedural learning:** It involves learning tasks without conscious thoughts, like a habit. During motor skill acquisition, repeating a movement continuously, under varying circumstances typically lead to procedural learning. For example, a patient when made to practice an activity such as taking hand to mouth, after few days can take food to mouth with the hand while making conversation with a friend, as the activity has been learnt by him like a habit/procedure.

Theories of Motor Learning

The theories of motor learning are categorized into theories that describe the methods and stages of motor learning, which are described below briefly.

Theories Regarding Methods of Learning

Adam's closed loop theory

Adams (1971), a researcher in physical education was the first person to give a comprehensive theory of motor learning. The closed loop process, involve use of sensory feedback for on going production of skilled movement. The idea is that, in motor learning, sensory feedback from the ongoing movement is compared within the nervous system with the stored memory of the intended movement.

Two types memories are involved in the learning process, such as:
1. **Memory trace:** It is used for the selection and initiation of movement.
2. **Perceptual trace:** This builds up after a period of practice, which act as the internal reference of correctness.

It is stated that after the movement is initiated by the memory trace, the perceptual trace take over to carry out the movement and detect errors if any.

Clinical implications of Adam's close loop theory

A patient with CNS disorder, when learns a new movement, such as learning to pick up a glass, develops perceptual trace with practice, which serves as a guide for later movements through stimulation of memory trace. The more the practice of a particular movement, more stronger becomes the perceptual trace making the movement more accurate.

This theory suggests that when learning a motor skill, it is essential that, the patient practises the particular movement repeatedly with accuracy. The more the practice, the stronger the motor learning.

Schmidt's schema theory

This theory of motor learning was given by Richard Schmidt (Researcher in physical education). He proposed that, motor programs in the brain, do not contain the specifics of movement, but instead contain general rules for a specific class of movement. He predicted that, when learning a new motor program, the individual learns a general set of rules that can be applied to a variety of contexts.

Schema, an abstract representation stored in memory is the heart of his theory. The generalized motor program, that contain the rules for creating the temporal and spatial patterns of muscle activity, needed to carry out a given movement is the basis of this theory.

Schmidt proposed that, after an individual, makes a movement, four things are stored in the memory, such as:
1. Initial movement conditions.
2. The parameters used in the generalized motor program.
3. The outcome of the movement in terms of knowledge of results.
4. The sensory consequences of the movement.

The information about the movement is stored in the form of:
- ❖ **Recall schema (motor):** Used to select a specific response. When a person makes a given movement, the initial condition and the desired goal of the movement is the input to the recall schema.
- ❖ **Recognition schema (sensory):** This schema is used to evaluate the response of the movement performed. The sensory consequences and outcome of previous similar movement, coupled with the present performed movement is the input to this schema, enabling production of efficient movement.

When the movement is over, the error signal is fed back into the schema, and the schema is modified as a result of the sensory feed back and knowledge of results. Thus according to this theory, learning consists of the ongoing process of updating the recognition and recall schema, with each movement that is made. It is also theorised that, variability of practice improves motor learning, as it leads to stronger motor program rules.

Clinical implications of Schmidt's schema theory

As per this theory when a person is learning a new task, such as reaching for a glass of water with the affected upper limb, optimal learning occurs, if this task is practised under many conditions. This allows the patient, to develop a set of rules for reaching which can be applied for variety of reaching tasks. As the rules for reaching improves, the patient can perform the desired task more accurately and efficiently. If while drinking, the glass containing milk/water etc., is tilted, due to movement in co-ordination, resulting in seepage of the liquid, that information goes to the recognition schema, which subsequently is modified into an efficient recall schema resulting in holding the glass properly and avoiding seepage.

Ecological theory of motor learning

Karl Newell derived the ecological theory of motor learning from both the system's and ecological theory of motor control based on search strategies. Newell suggested that, motor learning is a process that increases the co-ordination between perception and action in a way consistent with task and environmental constraints. He proposed that, during practice there is a search for optimal strategies to solve the task.

Critical to the search for optimal strategies is the exploration of the perceptual motor workspace, which requires exploration of all possible perceptual cues to identify those that are most relevant to the performance of a specific task.

According to the ecological theory, perceptual information has a number of roles in motor learning. In a prescriptive role, perceptual information relates to understanding the goal of the task and the movement to be learned. The perceptual information provides feedback (knowledge of performance and knowledge of result).

Newell proposed the ways to augment skill learning as follows:
- The first is to help the learner to understand the nature of the perceptual motor workspace.
- The second is to understand the natural search strategies used by performers in exploring space.
- The third is to provide augmented information to facilitate the search.

In summary, the ecological theory of motor learning emphasises dynamic exploration of perceptual motor workspace to create optimal strategies for performing a task.

Clinical implications of ecological theory of motor learning
A patient with difficulty in reaching for a glass of milk, if given the scope to repeatedly practise the reaching task with a variety of glasses that contain variety of substances learns the appropriate movement dynamics for the task of reaching. The patient should not only be made to develop appropriate movement strategies, but also should be made to recognize the relevant perceptual cues (such as how slippery the glass is) and match them to optimal motor strategies. If, for example, the perceptual cue indicates the glass is heavy, the patient recruits motor strategies in such a way that the glass is held with more force. If the perceptual cue indicates the glass is full, the motor strategies are modified to avoid seepage. A cerebral palsy child, not able to reach for the toys, should be given opportunities, to find his own strategy to reach at the toys, with some perceptual cues if required.

Theories Regarding Stages of Motor Learning
These theories include:

Fitts and Posner three-stage model
Fitts and Posner, the two researchers in Psychology, described the stages involved in motor learning. The three stages so described include:
1. **Cognitive stage**: In this stage, the learner should understand the nature of the task, develop strategies that can be used to carry out the task, and has the skill to evaluate the task.
2. **Associative stage**: In this stage, the learner who has developed best strategy for the task, begins to refine the skill. In this stage there is less variability in performance and the task performance skill improves. The stage may last for days to weeks to months.
3. **Autonomous stage**: This stage, gives the learner automaticity in the task performance with low degree of attention towards the task.

Clinical implications of Fitts and Posner's three stage model
Initially, when the patient is given a task, he experiments with different strategies to accomplish the work. There might occur minimal damage, such as spilling of water/milk while reaching for the glass of the substance. Subsequently, the person goes to the second stage, where reaching for the glass is more refined and an optimal strategy has been developed. In the third stage the person can accomplish the task, even when he is carrying on conversation or doing some other task.

System's three stage model
This theory, like Bernstein's system's theory of motor control, emphasizes on controlling the degrees of freedom while learning a motor task. The three stages include:
1. **Novice stage**: In this stage, while learning a new skill such as standing by an infant, or balancing by a hemiplegic patient, the degrees of freedom of the body are constrained to make the task easier. As control develop the degrees of freedom are gradually released.
2. **Advanced stage:** The learner begins to release additional degrees of freedom, by allowing movement to occur at more joints involved in the task. The simultaneous contraction of agonists and antagonists in joints involved are reduced, and muscle synergies across number of joints are used to create well co-ordinated movements.
3. **Expert stage**: In this stage, the individual releases all the degrees of freedom necessary to perform the task, in the most efficient and best co-ordinated way.

Clinical implications of system's three stage model of motor learning
The systems three stage theory of motor learning explains why there is co-activation of muscles, during the early stage of acquiring motor skill. As the person practices the posture and movements, gradually, he/she releases additional degrees of freedom, pushing him/her to advanced and expert stages.

For example, the progression from all fours to upright kneeling to standing, is the result of gradual increase of number of degrees of freedom. As per this theory, initially while learning a new skill, external support, is given to patients with a co-ordination problem. As control develops, support can be systematically withdrawn, as the patient learns to control more and more degrees of freedom.

Gentile's two stage model of motor learning
Gentile proposed a two stage theory of motor skill acquisition, that describes the goal of the learner in each stage, which are discussed below briefly.
- **First stage:** In this stage, the goal of the learner is to develop an understanding of the task dynamics. At this stage, learners get the idea of requirement of the movement. This include, understanding the goal of the task, developing movement strategies appropriate for achieving the goal, understanding the environmental features crucial to the organization of movement, etc.
- **Second stage:** This is called the fixation/diversification stage, where the goal of the learner is to refine the movement. Refining movement includes both developing the capability of adapting the movement to the changing

task and the environmental demands and performing the task consistently and efficiently. The term fixation and diversification refer to the distinct requirements of open versus closed skills. Closed skills have minimal environmental variation requiring a consistent movement pattern (fixation). Open skills are characterized by changing environmental conditions requiring movement diversification.

Clinical implications of Gentile's two stage model of motor learning

A patient trying to pick up a glass of water, first need to understand the nature of the glass that contain water, how fragile it is, whether it is light or heavy, whether it is partially filled or with full of water.

Subsequently, the learner tries to initiate the movement to accomplish the task of taking water to mouth. If he/she is successful in taking water with the said glass containing the said amount of water, then he accepts the strategy for subsequent activities similar in nature. However, if the learner faces difficulty in performing the task, due either to the weight of the glass or the fear of spillage of water due to fullness of the glass, he/she tries to refine the skill either by filling the glass partially with water and taking it to mouth through several repetitions or selecting a glass that is lighter in weight and non fragile in nature. Gradually as skill develops, he/she becomes able to take a heavy glass filled with water to mouth.

MOTOR RELEARNING PROGRAM

The **motor relearning program (MRP)** was developed by the Australian physiotherapists Janet Carr and Roberta Shepherd, for management of individuals with brain stroke.

It is a task-oriented approach to improving motor control, focusing on the relearning of daily activities, through analysis of function and finding the missing elements, and establishing interaction between the performer and the environment to practice the missing components, followed by the whole task. It is strongly based on theories in kinesiology that emphasize a distributed (rather than a hierarchical) motor control model and is based upon the dynamic systems model of motor control. It acknowledges the critical role of cognition in motor learning. The movement patterns are taught in the context of task not simple exercises.

Gravity (movement is started first with the assistance of gravity/in the direction of gravitational pull, followed by movement with gravity eliminated and then movement against gravity), leverage (movement is started first with shorter weight arm, gradually progressing to longer weight arm as control of movement develops), type of muscle contraction (to start with eccentric/concentric gravity assisted) progressing to concentric gravity eliminated and concentric against gravity, are the guiding factors to elicit movement using the program. Once some movement is available, use of equipment, say stepping on and off over a short step to increase hip and knee flexion etc., should be made to improve functional skills.

Principles of Motor Relearning Program (MRP)

- The person is the active participant, whose goal is to relearn effective strategies for performing functional movements.
- Successful task learning occurs when the activities are performed by the patient efficiently and automatically.
- The learning of the skills does not follow a developmental sequence.
- Intervention is not focused on learning specific movements, but instead on learning general strategies for solving motor problems.
- Rehabilitation of stroke, using the program involve relearning of real life activities, which have meaning for the patient and not the practice of exercises.
- The treatment must take into account the needs of the individual patient, such as essential movement components of activities such as standing up and walking.
- Emphasis of MRP is on practice of specific activities, the training of cognitive control over muscles and movement components of the activities and conscious elimination of unnecessary muscle activity.
- The program assumes the brain's capacity for re-organization and adaptation and is aimed at either stimulating this or making the best possible use of it or both.
- The success of the program depends largely upon the therapists analysis of her patient's problems. Once each problem has been analyzed, and the therapist has made the necessary decisions, the program prescribes the methodology, that is the training regime.
- The program is based on three factors essential for learning of motor skill/essential for relearning of motor control following stroke, such as elimination of unnecessary muscle activity, feedback, practice.
- Relearning of the everyday activities contained in the program appears to involve the patient remembering the movement in which he was skilled before his stroke, helped by therapy, which triggers off previously learned motor programs and trains the muscular activity necessary for movements.
- For effective use of MRP, the therapist should have the problem solving skills, i.e., recognition, analyze, decision making, action taking and re-evaluation.
- The effectiveness of MRP depends to a large extent on the ability of the individual therapist to: Recognize and analyze the problem, select the most essential missing movement component, explain clearly to the patient by speech and demonstration, monitoring the patient's performance and give verbal feedback.
- Re-evaluation is done throughout each session, to find the effectiveness of therapist's own and the patient's performance.
- Progress the patient's level of performance as soon as he/she has grasped the idea of what he/she is practising.
- Ensure a positive environment with consistency of practice throughout the patient's day.

- Provide an enriched environment in which the patient will be motivated towards recovery of mental and physical abilities.

Sections of Motor Relearning Program

The program is made of seven sections comprising seven essential areas of daily living, such as:
- Orofacial function.
- Upper limb function.
- Supine to sitting.
- Sitting balance.
- Standing from sitting and vice versa.
- Standing balance.
- Walking.

The order in which the sections to be included for achieving function are unimportant. The therapist may start a treatment session with whatever section or part of a section is most appropriate for the patient. It is not necessary for a patient to perfect on one section, before going on to another section. Each treatment session should comprise material from all sections.

The program should commence as soon as the patient is medically stable. If he/she is confined to bed for a short period following stroke, he/she should start on part of the program which he/she can manage, such as orofacial function, upper limb function and extension of hip as preparation for standing. The various sections of the program will make up the patient's daily therapy session which should range from at least half an hour twice daily in the first few days to daily one hour session or preferably more. The activities the patient has been practising will need to be reinforced outside therapy sessions, and relatives and staff are encouraged to participate and trained to be consistent. A particular routine carried over from therapy sessions into rest of the patient's day is essential for consistency of performance and learning of motor control.

Steps of Motor Relearning Program

The following four steps are applied in practice of the program, starting from analysis of task, the patient is not able to perform and finding the missing elements in the task, to functional integration (transference of learning).
- **Step-1: Analysis of function and finding the missing components:**
  The procedures involved:
  - Observation.
  - Comparison.
  - Analysis.
- **Step-2: Practice of missing components:**
  The procedures involved:
  - Explanation + instruction.
  - Practice (with verbal feedback and manual guidance).
- **Step-3: Practice of activity** (whole task)
  The procedures involved:
  - Explanation + instruction.
  - Practice (with verbal feedback and manual guidance).
  - Progression: Increase complexity, add variety, decrease feedback +guidance.
- **Step-4: Transference of learning** (enabling the patient to perform activities in an open environment with a transition from closed to open environment).
  The procedures involved:
  - Opportunity for practice.
  - Consistency of practice.
  - Involvement of relatives and staff.
  - Positive reinforcement.
  - Stimulating environment.

There are three important points to be considered in the practice of MRP:
1. **Part practice followed by whole task practice**: Activities or motor tasks are either practised in their entirety or broken down into their components. Practice of each component being followed immediately by practice of the entire activity.
2. **Techniques:** Comprise of verbal and visual feed back and instruction and manual guidance.
3. **Methods of progression:** It is important that the activities of the patient are progressed to its limits. A patient should not be made to waste time, by practising what he can already do. As soon as the patient gains some control, the activities are progressed. Movements are made more complex by a decrease in manual guidance and feedback, by altering the speed of movement, and by adding variety

Equipment for the Practice of MRP

Very few equipment are necessary for practice of the program such as:
- A low bed of convenient height for the practice of standing up and sitting down.
- Several small steps starting from steps of 2 inch height to 6 inch height.
- Common objects for retraining hand function, such as spoon, fork, plastic balls of variable sizes, glasses of different shape and texture etc.
- Calico splint/gaiters.
- **Walking stick (if necessary):** To be selected very carefully for the patient as it promotes learned non-use. A patient who was using a walking stick before stroke, will need a walking stick for ambulation after stroke.
- Use of parallel bars, three-four point cane, splints for ankle and foot etc should be avoided as much as possible. If a hand splint/ankle foot orthosis is considered, it should be dynamic/functional.

Treatment Duration and Sessions

Daily therapy session should range from at least half an hour twice daily in the first few days to daily one hour session or preferably more.

Factors for improved quality of rehabilitation using MRP:
- **Early start**: Treatment should be started, as soon as the subject is medically stable (usually within 24-36 hours from onset of stroke).

- **Rehabilitation plan**: A general plan of rehabilitation, which includes, communication, socialization and motor skill acquisition, etc., should be made for each patient.
- **Consistency of goal:** The gain achieved through therapy sessions should be reinforced throughout rest of day by the caregivers/nurses/any other people dealing with the patient.
- **Motivational programs**: It Includes enrichment of the physical and emotional environment for motivation towards recovery.
- **Mental stimulation program**: As for the first few weeks following stroke, there is a feeling of slowness in thinking and concentration, the therapist should design mental stimulation programs, which demands the patients active participation enhancing the cognitive aspects involved in learning.
- **Educational program**: Educational programs consisting of lectures and group discussions should be organized for the patient and relatives. The success stories, while dealing with similar patients (if any), should be highlighted in the program.
- **Planning for discharge:** Before discharge of the patient is done from Hospital/Rehabilitation center, the patient's home environment need to be assessed for matching the physical needs of the patient. Any modification of home environment, if required should be done before the patient is discharged.

The impairment of various systems and their management using the program are briefly discussed below:

Section A: Orofacial Dysfunction and its Management

Orofacial function comprises of various events such as swallowing, chewing, jaw closure, facial expression, ventilation and the motor aspects of speech production. The orofacial problems are frustrating and embarrassing, as the patient in the early phase of stroke is fitted with a nasogastric tube, which grossly impairs feeding and speaking.

Step-I: Analysis of Orofacial function and finding the missing components

- Observation of sitting position, movement of lips, jaw and tongue, while eating or drinking.
- Intraoral digital stimulation of tongue and cheeks (to test threshold to touch and to establish whether the tongue offers the normal resistance to movement).

The followings may be observed leading to difficult swallowing:
  - Open jaw.
  - Poor lip seal **(Fig. 36.7A)**
  - Tongue too far forward and asymmetrically placed **(Fig. 36.7B)**.
  - Drooling.
  - Immobile and hypotonic tongue (tongue may be enlarged).
  - Food collecting between cheek and gums (could be due to lack of muscular activity in the buccinators and a hypo mobile tongue).

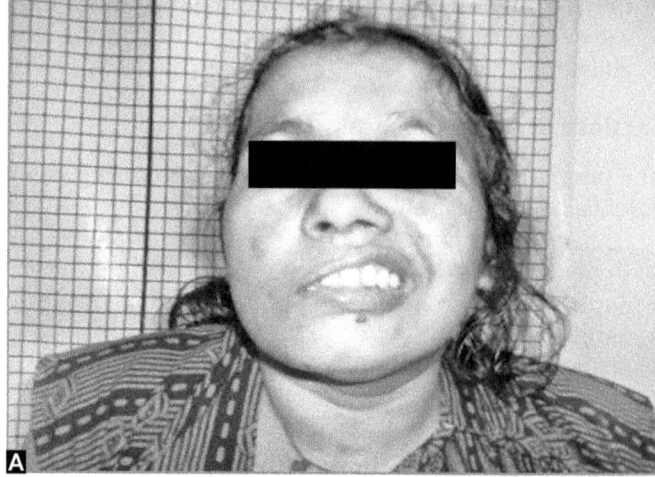
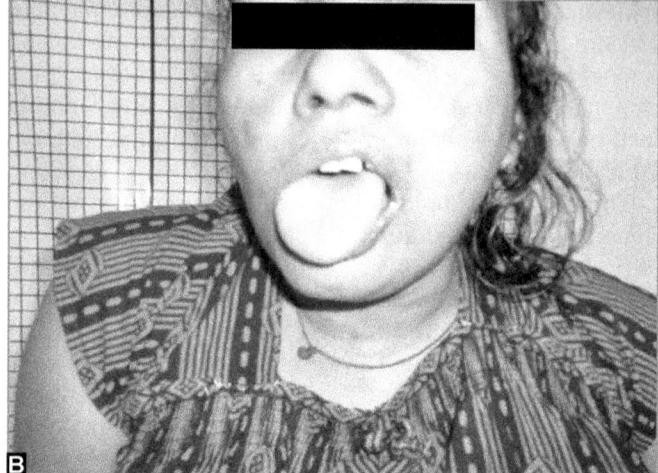

Figs. 36.7A and B: (A) Shows poor lip seal; (B) Shows tongue asymmetry.

  - *Asymmetry of facial expression:* This is the result of lack of motor control of the lower part of the face on the affected side, together with over activity and unopposed activity of the face in the intact side. The upper third of the face has bilateral innervations and is therefore not affected following stroke.
  - *Lack of emotional control:* Although not an Orofacial problem, lack of control over the physical manifestations of the emotions is frequently seen in the early phases following stroke. This lack of control is demonstrated by out bursts of uncontrolled crying, which are not necessarily related to sadness, or uncontrolled laughing, which is not related to happiness and which the patient has difficulty modifying or stopping.
  - *Poor breathing control:* This may result from a combination of factors including poor control over the soft palate, or motor impersistence, which is demonstrated by difficulty in taking a deep breath, holding the breath, and making a prolonged "ah" sound on expiration.

Step-II: Practice of missing components
- Ensure that that patient sits with his hips well back in the chair with his head and trunk erect.

- Do not persist too long with stimulation, as it may cause the patient desensitized and may result in failure to respond.
- Intraoral techniques should be interrupted frequently, with the fingers removed and the jaw held closed, in order to allow the patient to swallow.
- Facilitation of jaw and lip closure combined with improved muscular activity of the tongue, facilitates swallowing in the presence of saliva.
- Practice of lip closure, jaw closure, tongue movements, breath control are done as shown in the following figures:
  - *For lip closure (Fig. 36.8A):* The therapist holds the jaws closed with his/her fingers to indicate the patient that the affected side lips are open. Then he/she instructs the patient to try closing the lips while he/she assists in the process.
  - *For jaw closure:* The therapist closes the patient's jaws passively, with the head straight. Then he/she tells the patient to gentle open and close the jaw with assistance (if required). The tongue should be kept inside the mouth during the training.
  - *For tongue movements:* For training elevation of lateral border of tongue, the therapist uses the gloved index finger under the lateral aspect of the tongue on the affected side and assist the patient in elevating that border, telling the patient to make a tunnel with the tongue as if, he/she is swallowing food **(Fig. 36.8B)**
  - *For training of elevation of posterior part of the tongue:* The therapist puts the gloved index and middle fingers over the anterior aspect of the tongue and gives horizontal digital vibration to the anterior part of tongue with firm pressure to cause elevation of posterior part of the tongue **(Fig. 36.8C)**. The therapist's fingers should not remain in the patient's mouth for more than 5 seconds. After the fingers are removed, the patient should be told to try moving the tongue as if he/she is swallowing.
  - *Practice of facial symmetry:* The therapist, assists the patient pull the angle of mouth towards the affected side, at the same time assisting to elevate the lower lip and tells the patient try smiling **(Fig. 36.8D)**. This can best be done in front of a mirror.
  - *For training breathing control:* The patient sits inclined forward over pillows. He/she is told to take a deep breath through the nose and try expiring air through the mouth. During expiration, the therapist applies gentle pressure and vibration over the lower third of the posterior thorax to assist the expiration **(Fig. 36.8E)**. As the patient expires air, he/she is told to make sounds like "ah, ma, pa" etc, which will help him to produce speech sounds.

Step-III/IV: Practice of orofacial movements and transference of learning

The patient should be made to sit at a table for eating. The food should be palatable and should be semisolid in nature to avoid choking. The food should be chewable. If the patient has difficulty in chewing, the therapist/caregiver should hold his jaws lightly closed to assist in the act, and should remind the patient to keep the lips and jaw closed while swallowing the food. The therapist should assist the patient with his first few meals and should give the relevant part of the oro-facial section of the program, just before at least one meal a day, while such intervention is necessary.

The therapist should explain the nursing staff and the patient's relatives about the strategies to gain control over emotional outbursts (where the lips of the patient are to be tightly closed, and patient should be instructed to breath gently in and out through the nose)

The improvement of breathing control, a mobile tongue and the ability to breath with a prolonged expiration enables the speech therapist to improve further verbal communication.

Improved orofacial control and appearance helps the patient regain confidence in personal interaction with others. The orofacial problems are quickly overcome, if correct therapy is instituted with in the first few days of stroke, and opportunities for consistent practice are ensured by the therapist.

Section B: Upper Limb Dysfunction and its Management

Step-1: Analysis of upper limb function

Analysis of muscle activity around shoulder should be done with the patient in supine, until he can control his shoulder in sitting without compensation, analysis of muscle activity in hand is done with the patient sitting at the table **(Fig. 36.9)**.

Immediately following stroke many patients do not have easily observable motor activity in the upper limb and the muscles are either flaccid/hypotonic. The most common problems found in upper limb in stroke sufferers are:
- Poor scapular movement.
- Poor muscular control of glenohumeral joint, i.e lack of shoulder abduction and forward flexion. The patient may compensate by shoulder elevation and trunk lateral flexion.
- No elbow flexion/extension, or excessive and unnecessary elbow flexion, shoulder internal rotation, fore arm pronation (if the patient has developed spasticity).
- Difficulty grasping with wrist in extension and radial deviation.
- Difficulty in extending the MCP joint with IP joints in some degree of flexion.
- Difficulty with abduction and rotation of thumb for grasp and release.
- Inability to release an object without flexing the wrist (if the finger flexors are spastic).
- Excessive pronation of fore arm.
- Inability to hold different objects while moving the arm.
- Excessive ulnar deviation when using the hand.
- Difficulty in cupping the hand.

Besides the above, the following five common sequel of stroke need special attention.
1. Habitual posturing of the upper limb (in the spastic stage).
2. Neglect of the affected arm.
3. Compensation with the intact arm.
4. Use of the intact arm to move the affected arm.
5. Contracture of the soft tissues of the shoulder and wrist.

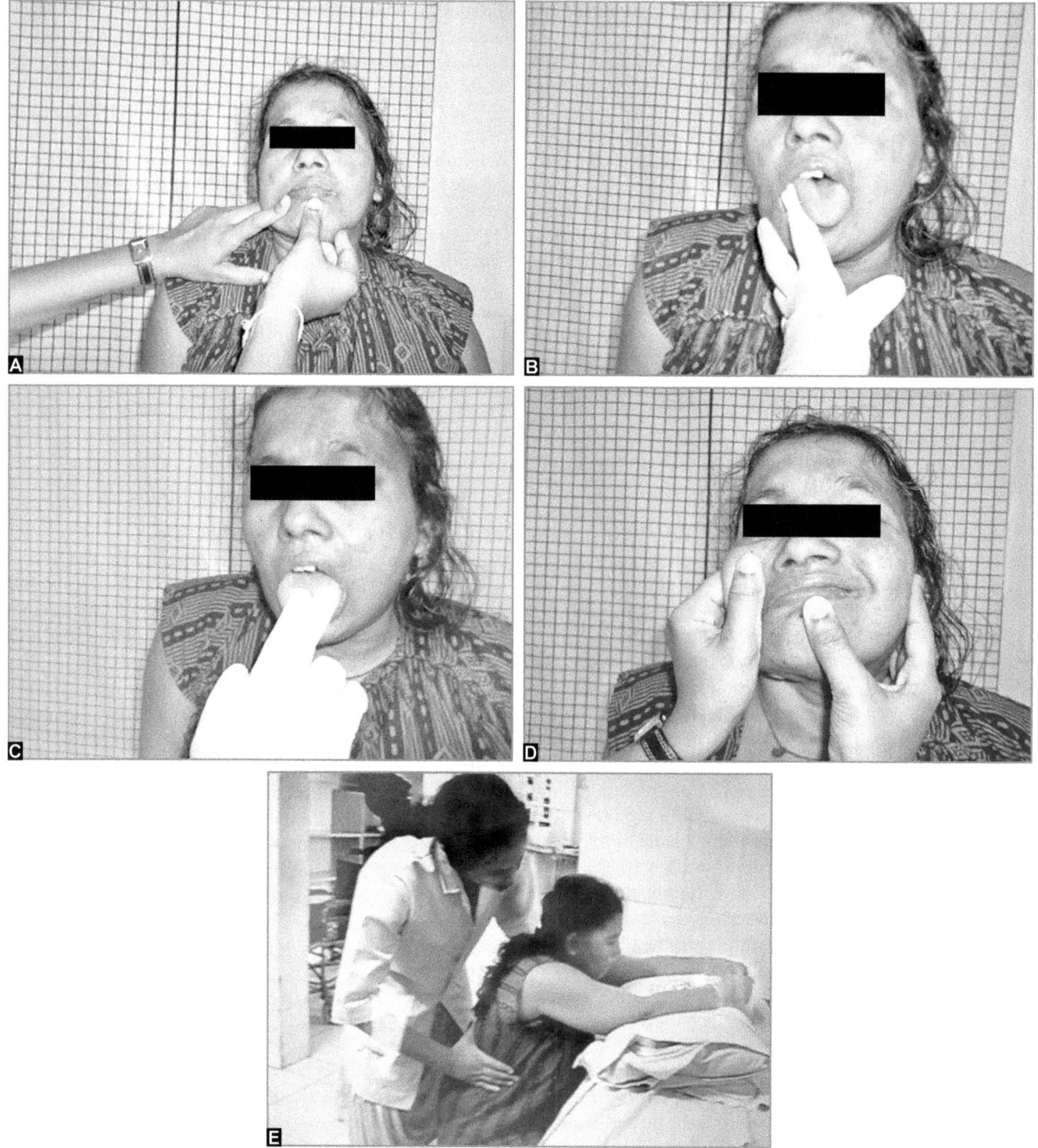

Figs. 36.8A to E: (A) Practice of lip/jaw closure; (B) Practice of elevation of lateral of tongue; (C) Practice of elevation of posterior part of tongue; (D) Practicing facial symmetry; (E) Practicing breath control exercise.

Step-II: Practice of missing components

To avoid failure of recovery of upper limb, the program suggests that, active therapy should be started without waiting for signs of recovery. Leverage pull of gravity and type of muscle contractions to be produced are the important factors to be considered in the stimulation of upper limb function.

Motor activity in the shoulder and elbow can be elicited early with the patient in supine lying and the upper limb elevated, i.e., arm vertical to body, where line of gravity is parallel to the upper limb, minimizing the influence of gravity **(Figs. 36.10A and B)**. The muscles are made to contract first eccentrically, rather than concentrically with in the inner half of the range. For scapula protraction, the therapist holds

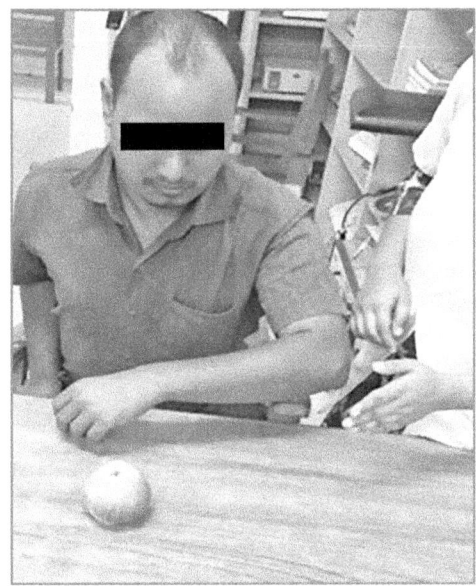

Fig. 36.9: Analysis of upper limb function in sitting.

the supine patient's elbow and hand with the upper limb vertical to bed, and asks the patient to move the arm upwards towards the ceiling (concentric contraction) **(Fig. 36.10A)** and slowly lower towards the bed (eccentric contraction). If no contraction of the scapular protractors are obtained, and the patient fails to move the arm towards ceiling, eccentric contraction, progressing to concentric with gravity eliminated, such as rolling a Swiss ball forward may be practiced, before making the patient push the arm towards the ceiling.

For shoulder, flexor/extensor, horizontal adductor/abductor, the position as shown in the **Figure 36.10B**, can be used to elicit activity in the muscles, where, gravity remains parallel to the arm and forearm, and the patient is made to contract the muscles, eccentrically in the inner range. Once muscle contraction could be elicited in this position, movements, should be started in side lying, followed by sitting, standing etc. For achieving shoulder abduction, side lying with the arm abducted to 90 degrees may be selected. For elbow, flexion and extension, the upper limb is held perpendicular to the bed, and the patient is assisted to lower the hand to the pillow in short arc (eccentric contraction of triceps) **(Fig. 36.10C)**, followed by assisted extension of elbow.

For achieving supination/pronation, the patient should be made to lie supine, with the elbow flexed to 90 degrees, and forearm vertically aligned to bed, so that gravity is parallel to the forearm and is eliminated **(Fig. 36.11A)**. The patient is assisted to rotate the forearm for supination and pronation. Subsequently, he/she should be made to sit on a chair, with the forearm placed on the table (in front) in the mid prone position. The patient is assisted to rotate the forearm towards supination with the help of gravity. Therapy putty/ball may be placed over the dorsal aspect of forearm to facilitate supination **(Fig. 36.11B)**.

Wrist extension and radial deviation: Radial deviation required for grasping objects, can be practiced, with the patient sitting on a chair, with the mid prone forearm placed

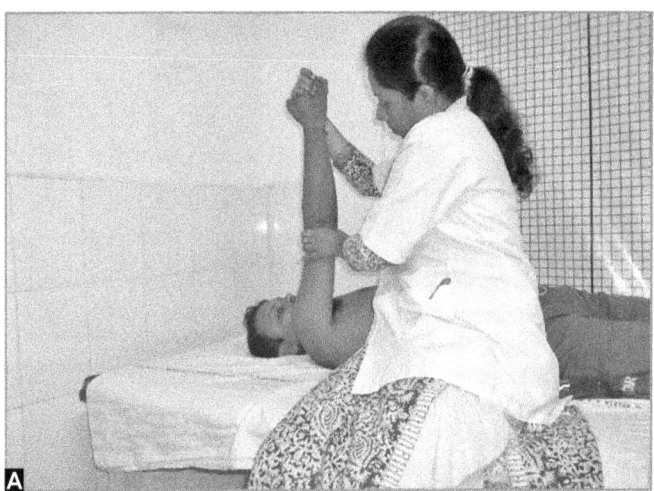

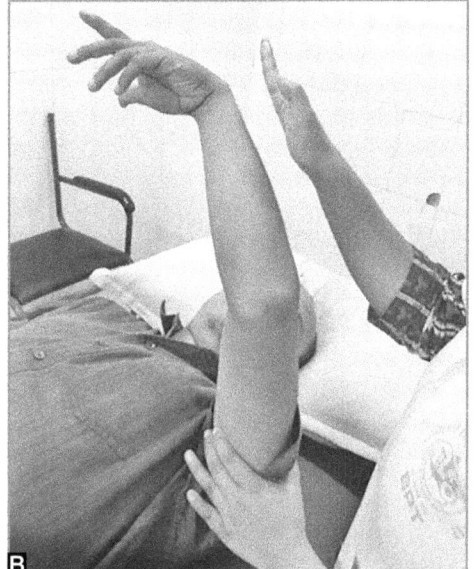

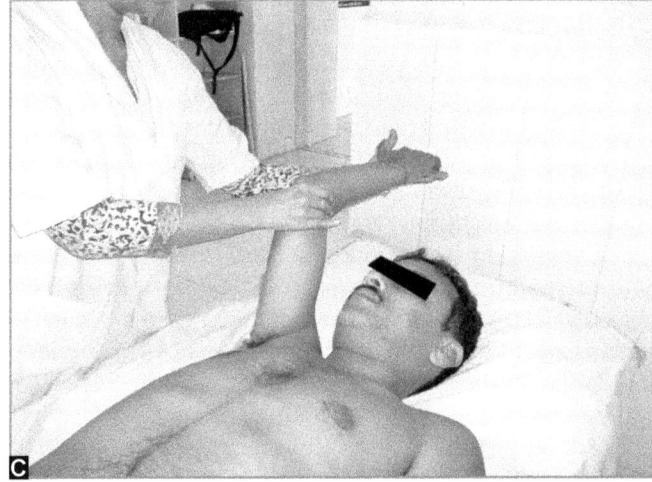

Figs. 36.10A to C: (A) Practice of scapular protraction (eccentric/concentric); (B) Shoulder flexion/extension horizontal adduction/abduction in supine lying with the arm vertical to body to minimize the influence of gravity (make gravity parallel to the upper limb); (C) Practice of elbow flexion/extension.

on the pillow. Initially eccentric, followed by, concentric assisted, concentric against gravity **(Fig. 36.12A)** is practiced. For wrist extension combined with radial deviation, the hand

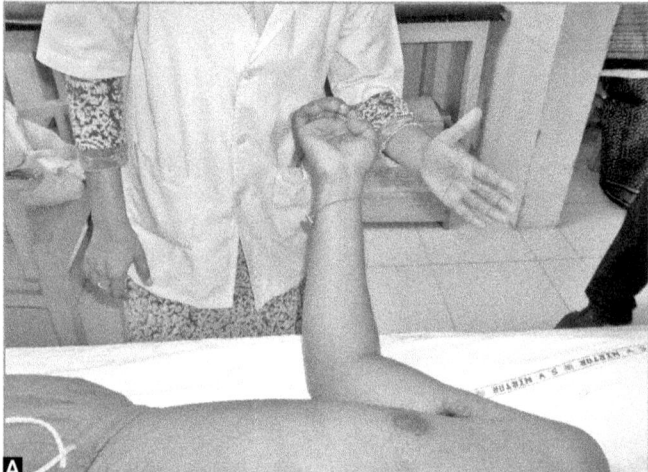

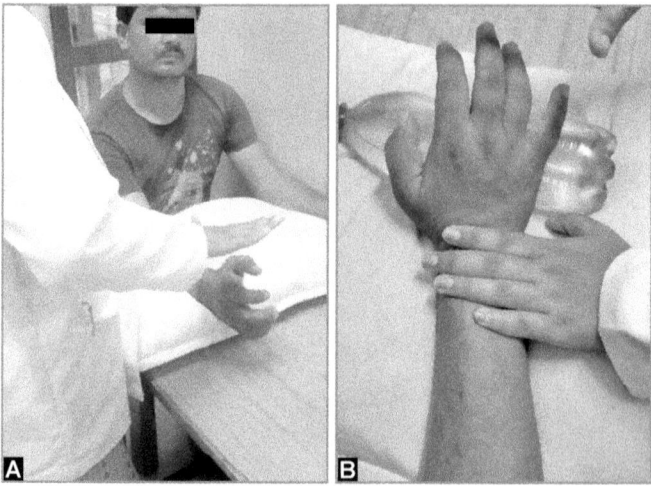

Figs. 36.12A and B: (A) Practice of radial deviation of wrist; (B) Practice of wrist extension and radial deviation.

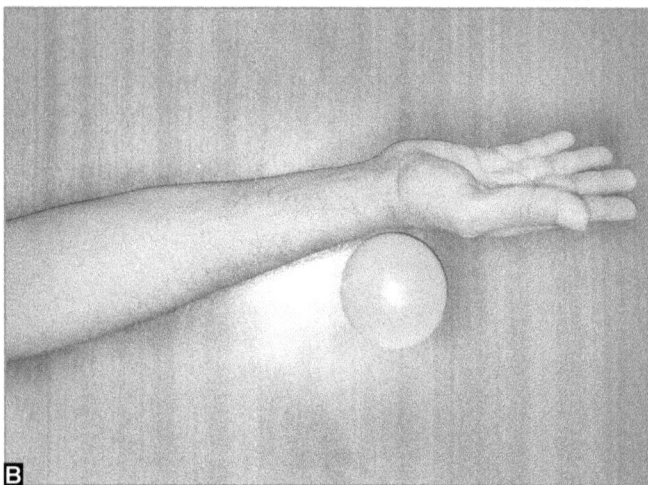

Figs. 36.11A and B: (A) Forearm supination/pronation in supine lying; (B) Forearm supination in sitting.

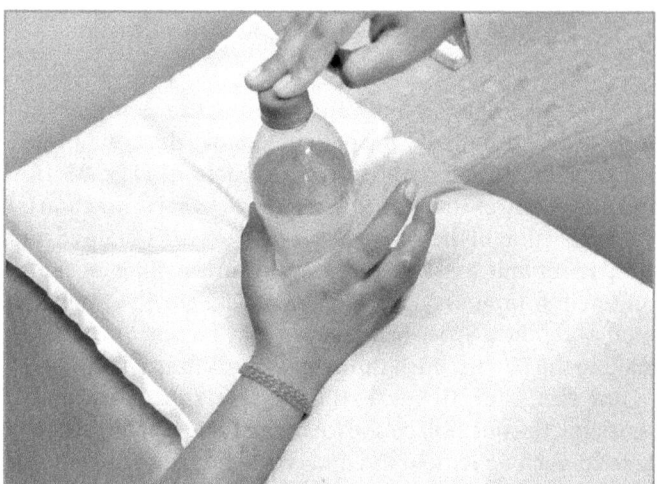

Fig. 36.13: Practice of wrist and finger flexion and extension.

is placed over a cylindrical object, say water bottle, placed on the table, The therapist guides the patient to extend and radial deviate the wrist against gravity **(Fig. 36.12B)**. If contraction of wrist extensors and radial deviators is not possible against gravity, eccentric contraction, progressing to concentric gravity eliminated should be performed, before making the muscles contract against gravity.

For fingers and thumb, the patient is made to sit on a chair, with the hand placed over a vertically placed cylindrical object, placed on the table. The patient is assisted/guided to extend and flex the fingers and thumb **(Fig. 36.13)**. Gradually, the diameter of the cylinder is reduced to achieve full flexion and extension of the fingers.

Spasticity/tightness (if any), affecting function, should be stretched using functional stretching, such as wall push **(Fig. 36.14)**.

Step-III: Practice of whole task using the upper limb
After practice of the missing components, the patient should be made to perform simple activities like picking up a glass (cupping action-cascade pinch) **(Fig. 36.15A)**, taking water to mouth using a paper/polystyrene glass **(Fig. 36.15B)**, eating with a spoon **(Fig. 36.15C)**, combing hair **(Fig. 36.15D)** etc.

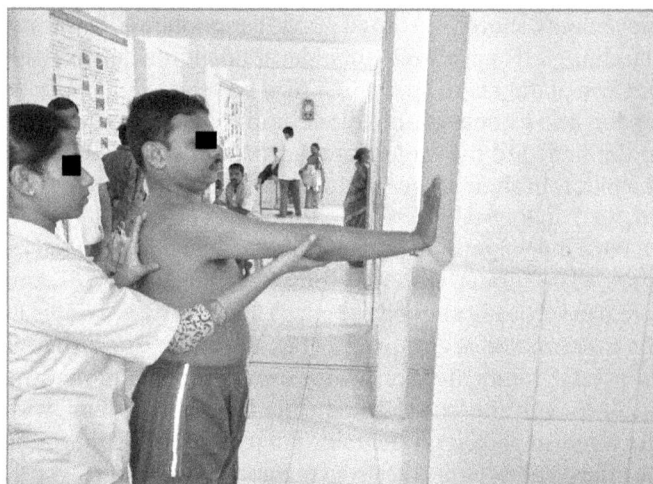

Fig. 36.14: Functional stretching of tight upper limb muscles.

Step-IV: Transference of learning
The patient should be encouraged to use the affected limb more and more for daily activities, with assistance (if

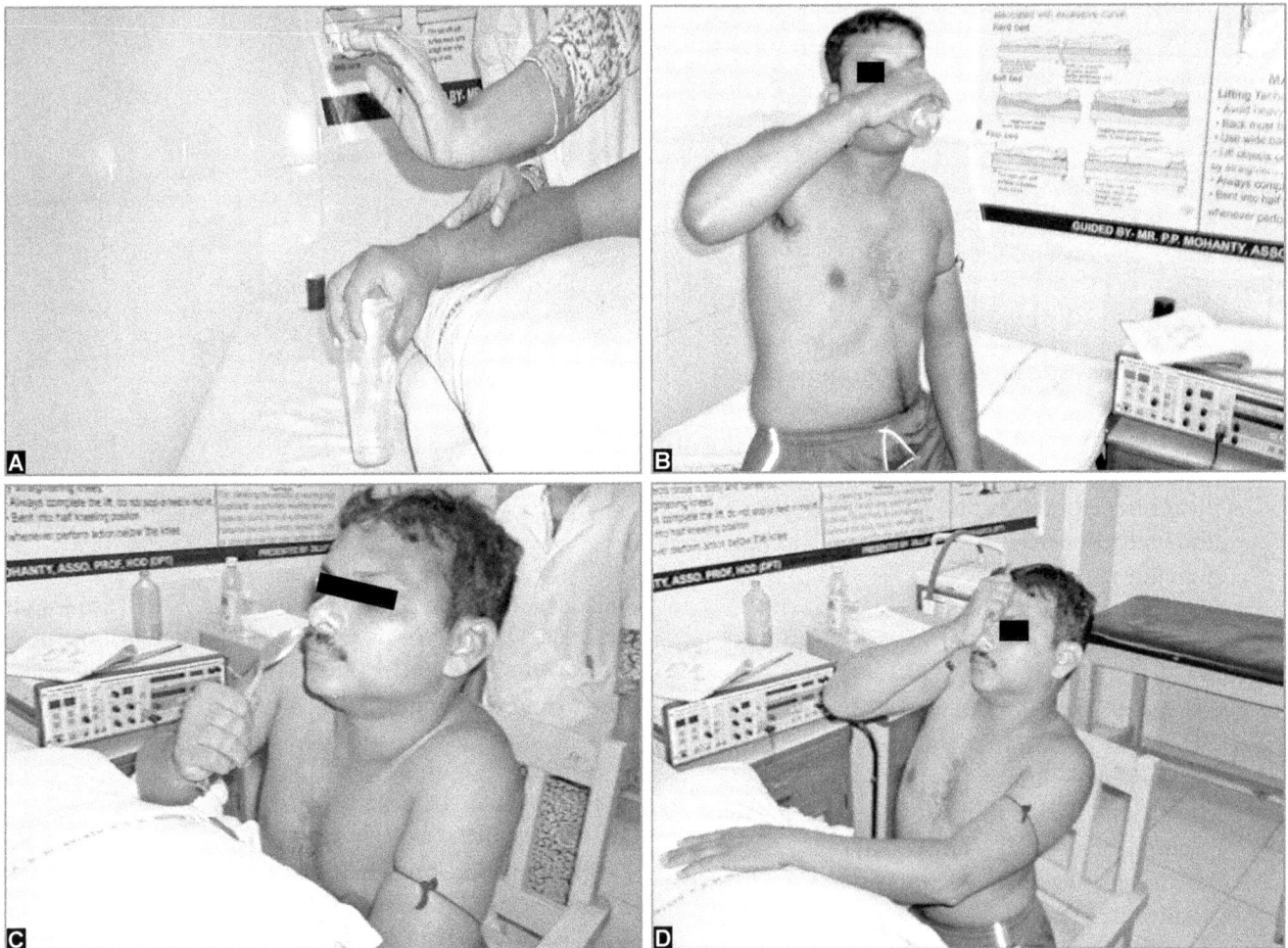

Figs. 36.15A to D: (A) Cupping action; (B) Using a polystyrene/paper glass for drinking; (C) Using a spoon for eating; (D) Combing hair.

required), and he/she should not be encouraged to use the sound limb for function, as it promotes learned non use of the affected limb. Mental practice of tasks should be encouraged before performance of the actual task, if the task performance is difficult. Habitual posturing of the upper limb should be corrected through repeated reminders to keep it as straight as possible.

Section C: Practice of Supine to Sitting

In the early stages following stroke, the patient should be helped to roll on to his intact side and to sit up from this position. It helps to avoid unrestrained use of the intact arm and is a quick and easy way for the patient to get up with minimal help from other persons. The therapist should apply leverage correctly at the patient's shoulder and pelvis enabling the patient side bend the trunk and lift the head laterally, and sit up without much effort.

Essential components of supine to sitting (Fig. 36.16)

- **Rolling to the side:**
  - Rotation and flexion of neck.
  - Hip and knee flexion.
  - Flexion of shoulder and protraction of shoulder girdle.
  - Rotation within the trunk.

- **Sitting up over side of bed:**
  - Lateral flexion of neck.
  - Lateral flexion of trunk.
  - Abduction of lower arm with gradual elbow extension, and pushing the body upward with the extended hand.
  - Lowering the legs over the side of the bed.

The procedure of supine to sitting involves

- **Step-1: Analysis of supine to sitting:**
  - Difficulty/Inability to flex and rotate the neck towards the normal side.
  - Difficulty/Inability to flex the affected hip and knees.
  - Difficulty/Inability to protract the affected side scapula and flex the shoulder.
  - Difficulty/Inability to rotate the trunk segmentally.
  - Difficulty/Inability to lateral flex, the neck and trunk on the affected side.
  - Difficulty/Inability to lower the legs at the edge of the bed.

- **Step-2: Practice of missing components:** It involves, practice of missing components for:
  - *Supine to side lying:* It includes practice of:
    » Neck flexion (initially eccentric, followed by concentric contraction)

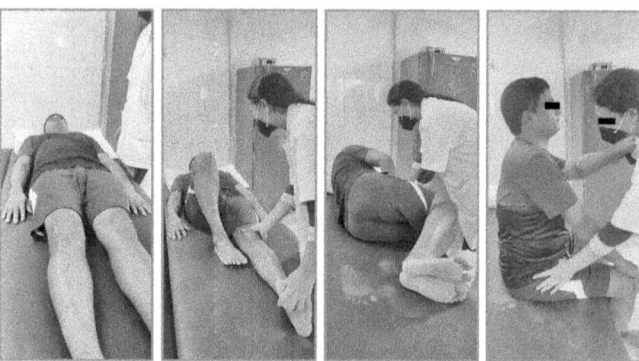

Fig. 36.16: Shows phases of supine to sitting.

- » Neck rotation (Starting with concentric gravity assisted, progressing to concentric free exercises)
- » Scapula protraction and shoulder flexion across the body (practiced as discussed under upper limb function).
- » Flexion of affected hip and knee.
- » Rotation within the trunk, i.e., lower trunk rotation, followed by rotation of the upper trunk.
- Side lying to sitting: It includes practice of :
  - » Neck side flexion (initially eccentric, followed by assisted concentric).
  - » Trunk side flexion (initially eccentric, followed by assisted concentric) **(Fig. 36.17A)**.
  - » Lowering of legs to the edge of bed and push with the sound hand to attain sitting **(Fig. 36.17B)**.
- ❖ **Step-3: Practice of Whole task, i.e., Supine to sitting:** After practice of missing components, the patient should be assisted to roll to the sound side and come to sitting, pushing with the sound hand **(Fig. 36.18)**.
- ❖ **Step-4: Transference of learning:** The patient should be encouraged and assisted to come to sitting from lying every time he/she desires to go to toilet, takes food etc with assistance as required.

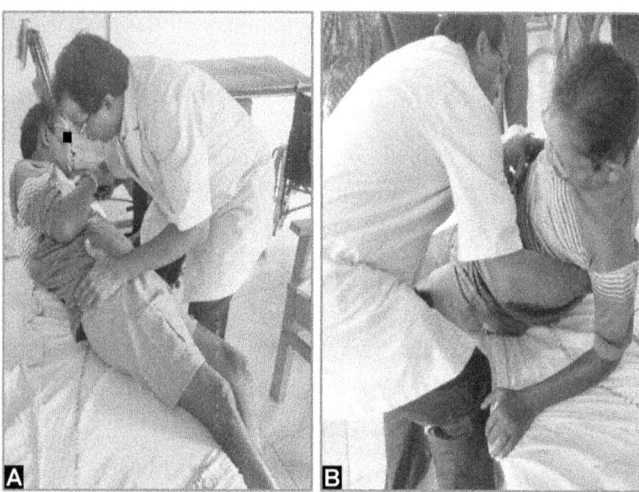

Figs. 36.17A and B: (A) Practice of trunk lateral flexion; (B) Practice of side-lying to sitting.

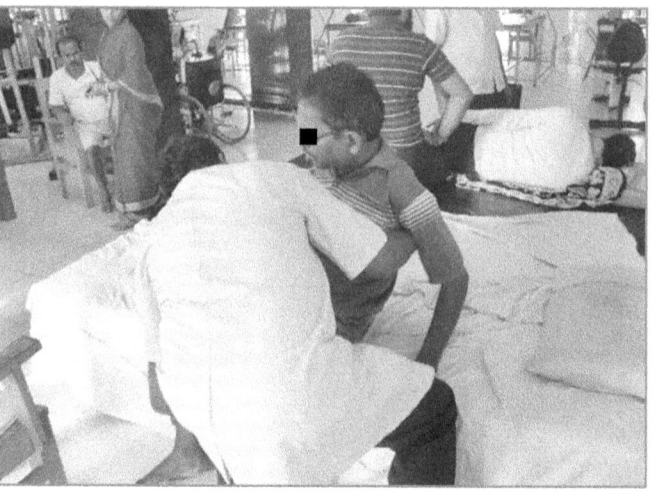

Fig. 36.18: Practice of supine to sitting.

Section D: Practice of Balanced Sitting

Balanced sitting involves, the ability to sit without using undue muscular activity, to move about in sitting and to move in and out of sitting position.

Essential components of balanced sitting (Static)
- ❖ Feet and knee close together.
- ❖ Symmetrical sitting.
- ❖ Flexion of hip with extension of trunk.
- ❖ Head balanced over shoulders.

Essential components of balanced reactions (dynamic balance)
- ❖ **Lateral shift in centre of gravity:**
  - Lateral flexion of neck, opposite to the direction of displacement of COG.
  - Lateral flexion of trunk, i.e., elevation of pelvis, depression of shoulder, opposite to the direction of displacement of COG.
- ❖ **Backward shift in centre of gravity:**
  - Forward flexion of neck.
  - Forward flexion of trunk.
- ❖ **Step-1: Analysis of balanced sitting**
  - *Static sitting posture:* The patient is usually found to sit with a head forward posture, with trunk bent to the affected side, affected shoulder depressed, affected hip laterally rotated, with inadequate flexion of hip and knee, and ankle aligned in plantar flexion **(Fig. 36.19)**
  - *Dynamic sitting balance:* It includes analysis of the ability, to control/prevent the displacement of the COG. As shown in the figure **(Fig. 36.20)**, when the COG is displaced from right to left, by giving perturbation from right side, the expected response, i.e neck and trunk lateral flexion opposite to direction of perturbation is missing **(Fig. 36.20)**.
- ❖ **Step-II/III: Practice of missing components and balanced sitting:**

   The postural muscles need to be facilitated through practice to help maintenance of sitting. A pad of towel need to be placed under the affected buttock to prevent pelvic retraction and maintain symmetry. Any shoulder

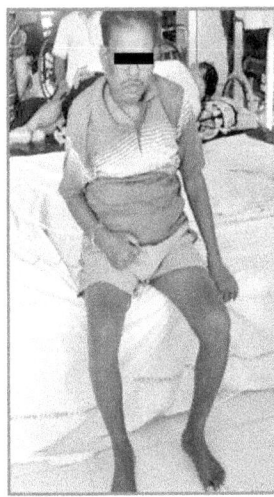

Fig. 36.19: Shows abnormal sitting posture.

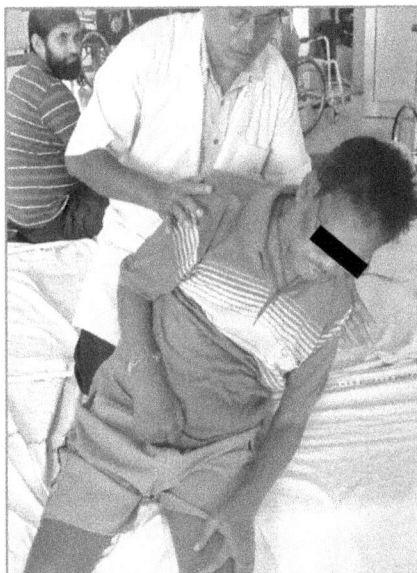

Fig. 36.20: Shows poor dynamic control in sitting, indicated by a failure to bend the neck and trunk to right side, to prevent displacement of COG to left side.

pain/subluxation existing need to be managed by proper shoulder splint/support. The height of the bed/ chair should be so adjusted, that the feet must touch the ground.

After some degree of static symmetrical sitting is achieved, perturbations in a progressive manner are to be given to develop dynamic sitting balance. For example, a patient with dynamic balance problems in sitting, may be asked to turn over left and right shoulder to look behind, to develop the skill of controlling/adjusting the displacement of centre of gravity. He/She may also be given perturbations in different directions to develop the skill of balancing as discussed below:

- Training the skill of prevention of displacement of COG, by bending the neck and trunk in the opposite direction to the displacement of COG **(Fig. 36.21A)**.
- Training the ability to control the displacement of COG, such as reaching for objects, without losing balance, turning over and look behind **(Fig. 36.21C)**.
- Training the advance aspects of balanced sitting, such as executing protective support on elbows and hands, when balance is disturbed **(Fig. 36.21B)**.

Complexities in sitting are increased through, activities such as picking up a ball from the floor, catching a volley ball from different directions, etc. As a preparatory measure for transitions to standing from sitting, the patient is made to practice trunk inclination forward and backwards at the hip joint in sitting as shown below **(Fig. 36.22)**.

❖ **Step-IV: Transference of learning:** Throughout the day, when the patient is sitting, he should sit on a chair from which it will be easier for him to get up with assistance (if required). He should be encouraged to do activities such as, eating, reading, writing etc as much as possible in sitting position.

Section E: Practice of Standing from Sitting and Vice Versa (Sitting from Standing)

The essential requirements include:
❖ Sitting symmetrically, with the feet placed posteriorly, so that, when the patient is asked to stand, resulting in

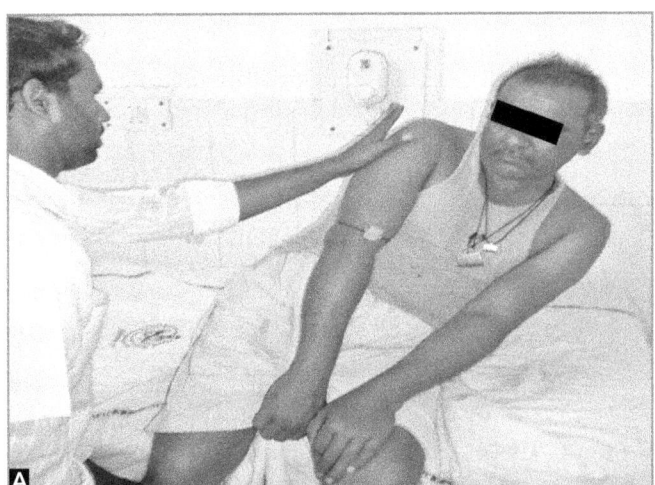

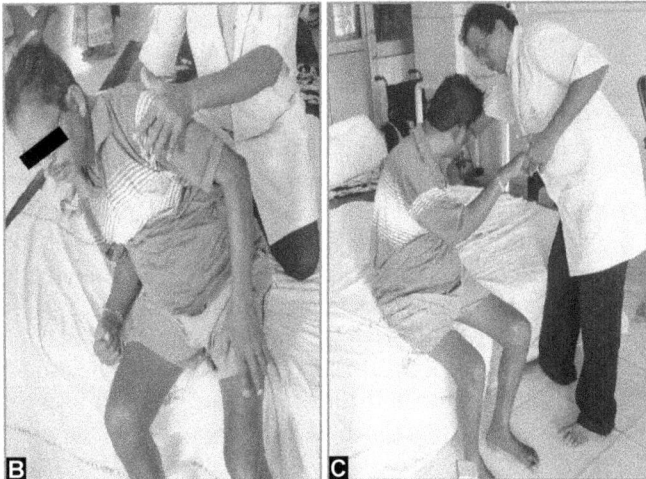

Figs. 36.21A to C: Practice of: (A) Prevention of COG displacement; (B) Protective extension, when balance is lost; (C) Training control of displacement of COG.

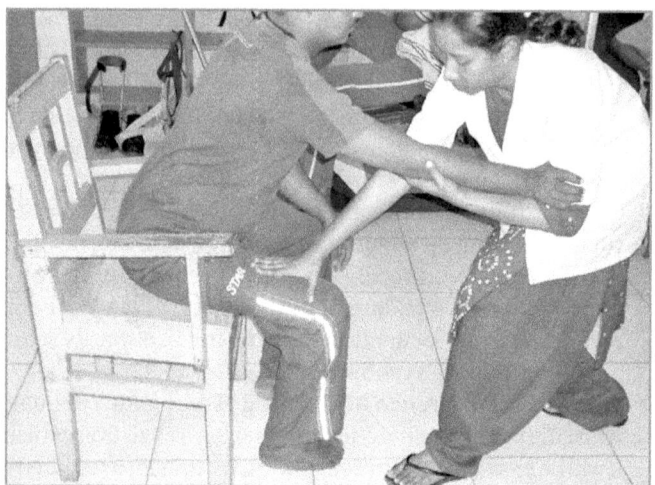

Fig. 36.22: Training displacement of COG forward and backward, with trunk inclination from hips.

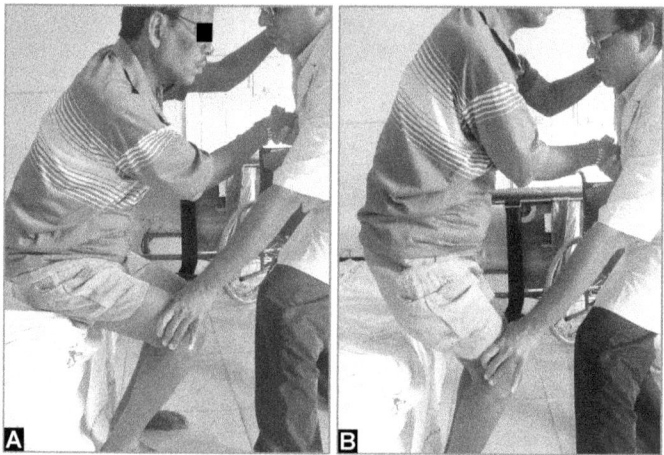

Figs. 36.23A and B: (A-B) Shows gradual progression in sitting to standing.

an anterior and upward displacement of COG, excessive anterior displacement of COG does not occur, resulting in alignment of line of gravity within the base of support.

The procedure of training involves:

- **Step-I: Analysis of standing from sitting and sitting from standing:** The problems found include:
  - *For standing from sitting:*
    » Inability/Difficulty to sit with adequate hip and knee flexion, ankle dorsiflexion and place the feet posteriorly.
    » Inability/Difficulty to bend the erect trunk forward and backwards from the hips.
    » Inability/Difficulty to extend the hips and knees and push the body anteriorly and upwards for standing.
  - *For sitting from standing:*
    » Inability/Difficulty to bend the trunk forwards from the hips.
    » Inability/Difficulty to flex the hip and knees and lower the buttocks to the bed/towards the floor.
- **Step-II/III: Practice of missing components and practice of standing from sitting and vice versa.**
  - *Practice of standing from sitting:* To start with, the patient should be made to sit on a high plinth/chair, so that feet touches the ground. The patient is made to move the trunk in an oscillatory manner in an increased order of velocity, to increase momentum and push the body to standing. The therapist applies pressure on the lower thigh in a downward and backward direction, assisting the patient stand up **(Figs. 36.23A and B)**. Gradually, the height of the plinth/chair, should be decreased, enabling the patient achieve standing from squat sitting.
  - *Practice of sitting from standing:* The patient should be made stand in front of a high plinth/chair. He/she should be asked to clasp both the hands, bend the trunk forward from the hips and slowly lower the buttocks to the couch. Once the patient is able to achieve independent sitting on the chair/bed of higher height, gradually, the height of the chair, should be decreased, till the patient is able to make squat sitting **(Figs. 36.24A and B)**.

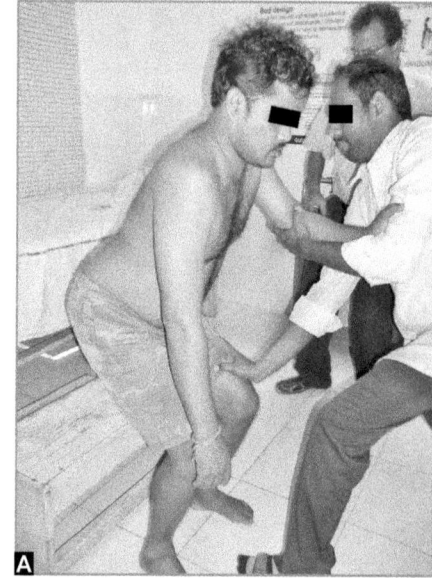

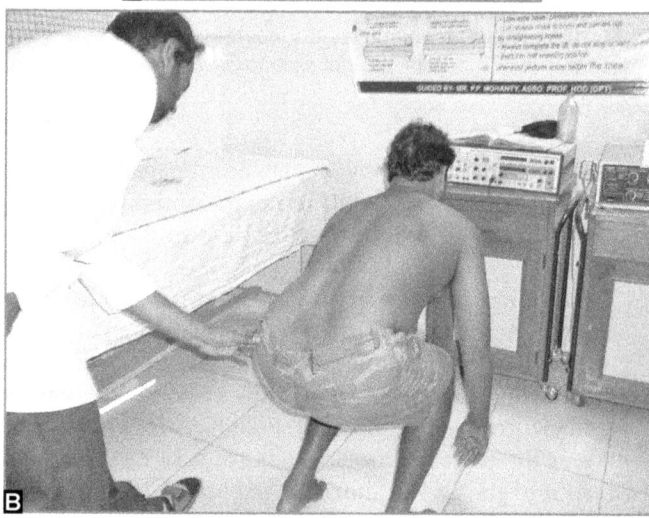

Figs. 36.24A and B: Shows gradual progression from standing to sitting.

- **Step-IV: Transference of learning:** Throughout the day, the patient should be assisted to sit and stand from bed/

chair/commode, so that the skill of standing from sitting and vice versa develops strongly, enabling him/her to sit and stand in an open and varying environment, such as home, office etc.

Section F: Practice of Standing Balance

Balanced standing involves the ability to stand without using undue muscular activity, to move about in standing, to move in and out of standing position and to walk, all without using the arms for support. In standing, the body continually sways, therefore there is a constant and accurately balanced movement of the centre of gravity, to keep the line of gravity to fall just in front of the ankles.

Essentials of balanced standing (Static)
- Feet few inches apart.
- Hips in front of ankles.
- Shoulders over hips.
- Head balanced on levelled shoulders.
- Erect trunk.

Essentials of balanced standing (Dynamic)
- **Lateral shift in centre of gravity:** Applied through perturbation from the sides. The strategies include:
  - Lateral flexion of neck to opposite side.
  - Lateral flexion of trunk on opposite side, i.e., elevation of pelvis and depression of shoulder.
- **Backward shift in centre of gravity:** Applied through perturbation from the front. The strategies include:
  - Flexion of neck.
  - Forward inclination of trunk at hips.
  - Extension of knees.
  - Dorsiflexion of ankles
- **Forward shift in centre of gravity:** Applied through perturbation from the back. The strategies include:
  - Extension of neck.
  - Backward inclination of trunk at the hips.
  - Flexion of the knees.
  - Plantar flexion of the ankles.

The procedure of training involves:

Step-1: Analysis of balanced standing (static). The following abnormalities may be found (**Fig. 36.25**):
- Affected foot too apart.
- Affected hip too posterior, i.e., behind the ankle joint.
- Affected shoulder depressed.
- Trunk bent to affected side.

Analysis of standing balance (dynamic)

When the centre of gravity is displaced anteriorly by a perturbation applied posteriorly on the trunk (**Fig. 36.26**), the required responses, i.e., neck and trunk extension, knee flexion and ankle plantar flexion are missing. In the same way, the response of the patient, when COG, is displaced laterally, posteriorly, should also be tested, and missing elements (if any) should be documented.

Step-II/III: Practice of missing components and practice of static and dynamic balance in standing: The essential requirements for static standing balance such as, adequate

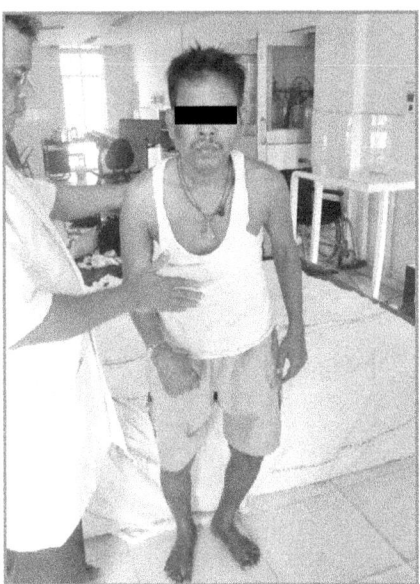

Fig. 36.25: Shows abnormal static standing posture in a right hemiplegic patient.

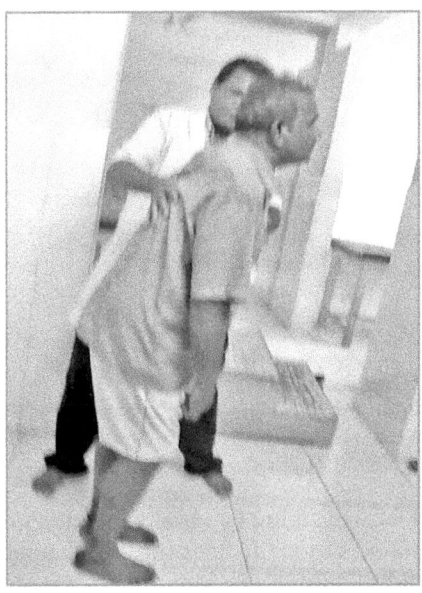

Fig. 36.26: Examination of dynamic balance in standing.

strength in the posterior chain muscles, such as neck and back extensors, glutei, quadriceps, ankle plantar flexors are facilitated/strengthened to make the patient stand symmetrically. The principle of facilitation of muscle contraction from a position of ease is followed, as evident from the **Figure 36.27A**, where, the hip extensor is made to contract concentrically with the assistance of gravity. After facilitation of different muscles for holding the standing posture, the patient should be made to stand as symmetrically as possible in front of a postural mirror. If the knee buckles during standing, a calico splint, such as knee immobiliser should be used to make the patient stand (**Fig. 36.27B**).

Practice of components of balanced standing (dynamic): Once the patient is able to maintain a static standing posture,

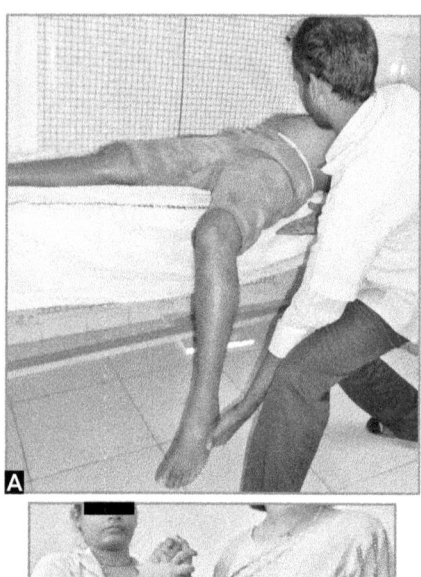

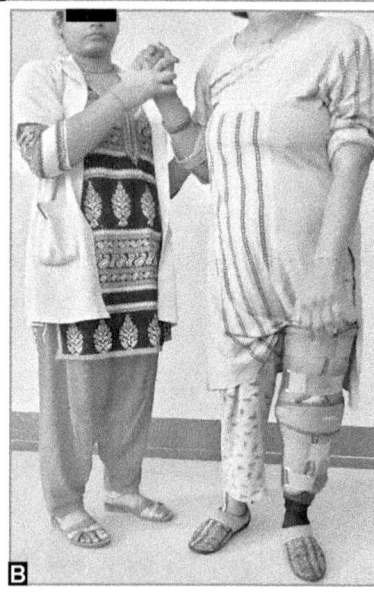

Figs. 36.27A and B: (A) Practice of missing components (hip extension in supine lying with gravity assistance); (B) Patient made to stand using knee immobiliser/calico splint.

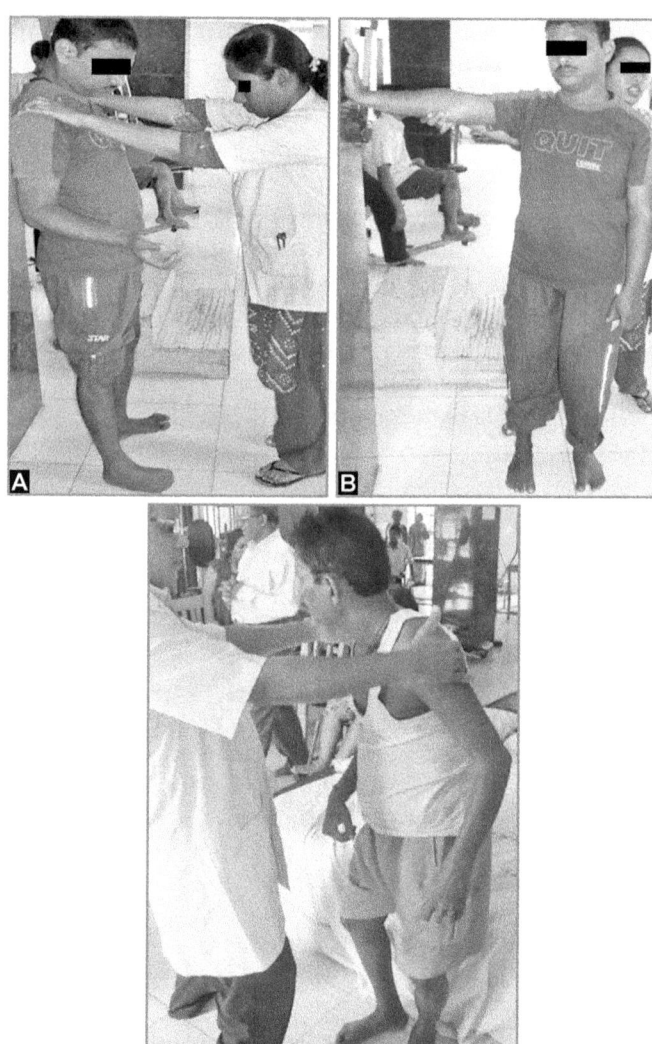

Figs. 36.28A to C: (A) Training ankle strategy; (B) Training protective reaction; (C) Training displacement of COG, through turning in standing.

activities such as reaching for objects in different directions, picking up objects from the floor, turning over left and right, catching and kicking balls, stepping on to steps etc are practised to improve dynamic balance in standing.

Stimulation of the ability to control the displacement of centre of gravity and stimulation of essential aspects of balanced standing such as strategy developments [Ankle strategy **(Fig. 36.28A)**/hip strategy/stepping strategy], training protective reactions in standing **(Fig. 36.28B)** are to be practised. The deficient ability to control the displacement of centre of gravity are also practised by giving challenges to the patient in standing, such as, standing turning backward over left and right **(Fig. 36.28C)**, reaching in standing, pushing and pulling in standing etc.

Increasing complexity: Once the patient regained some ability to stand statically, as well as dynamically, the activity needs to be progressed by making the standing more and more complex, such as bending in different directions and picking up different objects (light followed by heavy) from the ground, etc.

Step-IV: Transference of learning: The caregivers should be advised to make the patient perform various activities in standing throughout the day, such as picking up water bottle from dinning table, kicking a ball (swiss ball/volley ball) outside the home, etc, enabling the client stand and perform various activities in standing.

Section G: Training of Walking

Normal walking/Normal human locomotion is the series of rhythmic alternating movements of the trunk and extremities, resulting in a forward progression of centre of gravity. Normal walking should involve less and less muscular activities and should require less expenditure of energy. It should be rhythmical and symmetrical in nature. The kinetics and kinematics of normal gait have been described in chapter-1.

For the purposes of description, walking is divided into:

Stance phase

This phase begins with heel strike and ends with toe off. The hips and knees go through a series of flexion/extension moments in the various components of this phase. Extension

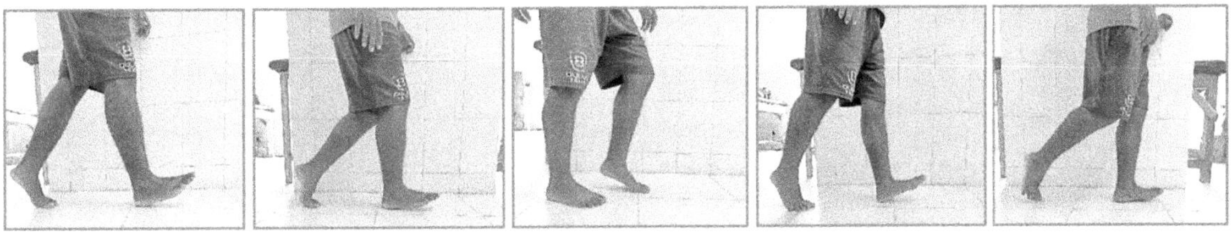

Chapter 36: Motor Control, Motor Learning and Special Techniques of Therapy to Improve Function...

Fig. 36.29: Different components of stance phase.

of the hip at the end of the stance phase, appears to be essential for the swing phase of that leg. The flexion- extension-flexion of the knee, gives walking its smoothness. As weight is shifted forward and laterally, the pelvis is prevented from dropping down on the swing side by contraction of hip abductors on the supporting side. The contraction of hip abductors of the standing leg, serves to control the amount of pelvic shift sideways, which is minimal and only as much as is necessary to shift the centre of gravity sufficiently laterally, to allow the opposite leg to swing through. The essential components of stance phase are:

Essential components of Stance phase:
- Extension of the hip and knee during loading (mid stance phase).
- Lateral horizontal shift of the pelvis and trunk (normal up to 4-5 cm in total)
- Flexion of knee (approximately 15 degrees) on loading response phase, followed by extension (5 degrees of flexion) in mid stance, then flexion prior to toe off.

The different components of stance phase are shown in **Figure 36.29**.

Swing phase
This phase begins with acceleration, proceeds through mid swing and ends with deceleration. Early flexion of knee, at the beginning of the swing phase, decreases the moment of inertia of the lower limb, which in turn decreases the amount of hip flexor activity required. The combined hip and knee flexion shortens the leg, and allows the swing foot to clear the ground following toe off. The early swing phase is characterized by hip flexion, knee flexion and dorsiflexion of ankle. The final period consists of knee extension prior to heel strike, ankle dorsiflexion, which terminates immediately following heel strike. The components of swing phase are shown in **Figure 36.30**.

Essential components of walking (swing phase):
- Flexion of hip, knee and dorsiflexion of ankle.

- Lateral pelvic tilt downwards (approximately 5 degrees) in the horizontal plane at toe off.
- Rotation of the pelvis forward on the side of the swinging leg (3-4 degrees on either side of the central axis).
- Extension of knee plus dorsiflexion of ankle, immediately prior to heel strike.

The procedure of training involves:
- **Step-1:** Analysis of walking and finding the missing components:
  - *Analysis of stance phase of affected leg:*
    » Lack of extension of hip.
    » Lack of controlled knee flexion from 0-15 degrees.
    » Excessive lateral horizontal shift of pelvis on the affected side.
    » Excessive downwards pelvic tilt on the intact side associated with excessive lateral pelvic shift to the affected side.
  - *Analysis of swing phase of affected leg:*
    » Lack of knee flexion at toe-off.
    » Lack of hip flexion, knee flexion and ankle dorsiflexion at mid swing.
    » Lack of knee extension plus ankle dorsiflexion on heel strike.
- **Step-II: Practice of missing components:**
  - *Practice of stance phase activities:*
    » Stimulation of hip extension **(Fig. 36.31)**: Patient supine, hip at the edge of the bed, therapist supports the foot and tells the patient to slowly lower the thigh producing hip extension. As the activity in

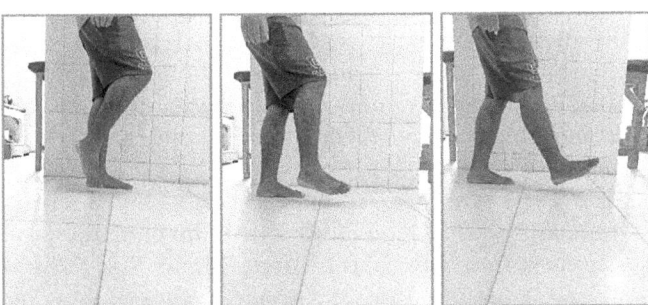

Fig. 36.30: The components of swing phase.

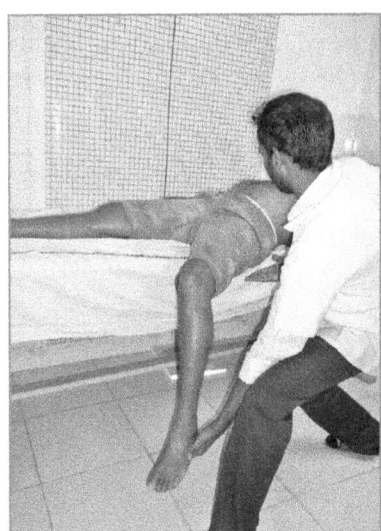

Fig. 36.31: Stimulation/facilitation of hip extension.

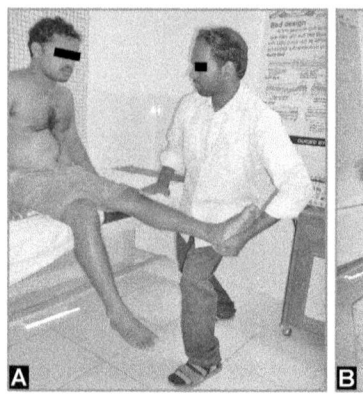
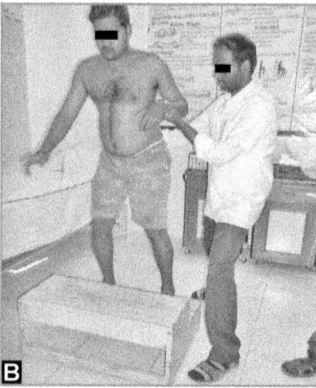

Figs. 36.32A and B: (A) Training controlled knee flexion in high sitting; (B) Training controlled knee flexion in standing.

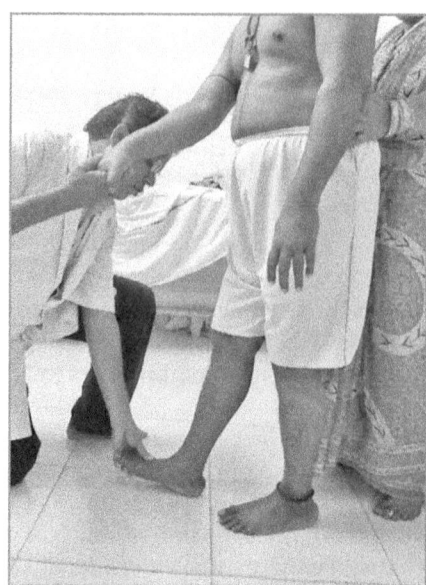

Fig. 36.34: Training knee extension and ankle dorsiflexion.

gluteus maximus is elicited, progression is made to concentric contraction in side-lying, concentric contraction in prone lying, concentric contraction in standing, such as, kicking a ball posteriorly.

» To train knee control: The patient is placed in high sitting. The affected knee is held in extension at the edge of the bed, by the therapist. The patient is asked to contract quadriceps, and try to prevent the drop of leg towards the ground **(Fig. 36.32A)**. The exercise can be progressed by, making the patient step on using the affected lower limb and hold the position for few seconds and then step off **(Fig. 36.32B)**.

» To train lateral horizontal pelvic shift **(Fig. 36.33)**: The patient is made to stand with normal stride width, in front of a postural mirror. The therapist places his/her hands on the pelvis and assists the patient shift the pelvis towards the sound side, to make the pelvis symmetrical.

» To train hip flexion and ankle dorsiflexion for heel strike, and knee flexion for pre swing: The muscles are made to contract eccentrically first, followed by concentric exercises in horizontal plane, and subsequently against gravity. However, for ankle dorsiflexion, emphasis should be laid on development of eccentric control of dorsiflexors required to hold the ankle in plantigrade during heel strike.

» To train knee extension and ankle dorsiflexion **(Fig. 36.34)**: The patient is made to stand, holding on to support/hand held by therapist. The therapist assists the patient to perform knee extension, with ankle dorsiflexion.

– *Practice of swing phase activities:*
  » To train flexion of knee at start of swing phase: Initially eccentric contraction of hamstrings is trained in prone **(Fig. 36.35A)**, and subsequently concentric contraction of hamstrings is practiced in side lying, followed by concentric contraction in prone lying and standing, i.e., stepping on and off to a step with affected lower limb/standing on the sound limb, flexing the affected knee etc. **(Figs. 36.35B and C)**. Knee flexion is subsequently trained by making the patient walk backwards **(Fig. 36.35D)**.
  » To train ankle dorsiflexion (eccentric contraction of dorsiflexors).
  » To stimulate knee extension and ankle dorsiflexion at late swing (for heel strike).

❖ **Step-III: Practice of walking:** After practice of stance phase and swing phase activities, the patient should be trained to walk in the same session. Arm swing is incorporated with limb movements to make walking efficient **(Fig. 36.36)**.

Increasing complexity: Once the patient is able to walk on plain surface, walking is made more complex by making the patient walk on uneven surface, walk up and down the incline surfaces, walk while making conversation, walk carrying a shopping bag, etc.

❖ **Step-IV: Transference of learning:** The therapist should give some time to walk with the patient on the way back from the therapy department. The patient should be enabled to set a goal for himself, how far he will walk on the first day and on subsequent days.

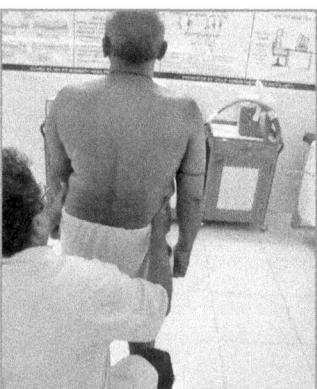
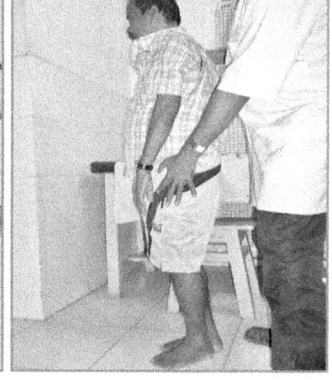

Fig. 36.33: Training lateral horizontal shift of pelvis.

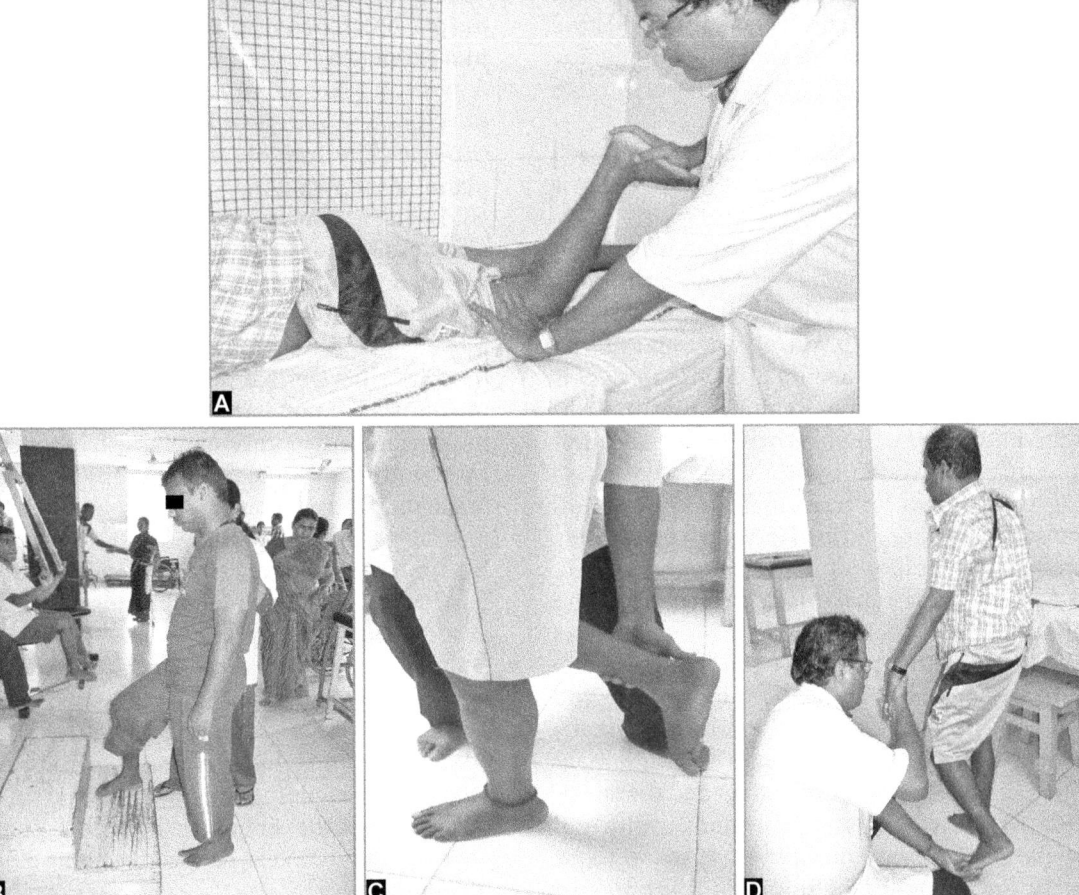

Figs. 36.35A to D: (A) Eccentric contraction of hamstrings in prone lying; (B) Stepping in standing; (C) Concentric knee flexion in standing; (D) Backward walking.

The patient should be given opportunity to either walk alone or walk with the assistance of other staff or care givers. Use of walking aids such as parallel bar, walking canes, tripod/tetrapod sticks, may be used if required (if the patient is too old, who was using walking aids before onset of stroke) aiming to have carryover into independent walking.

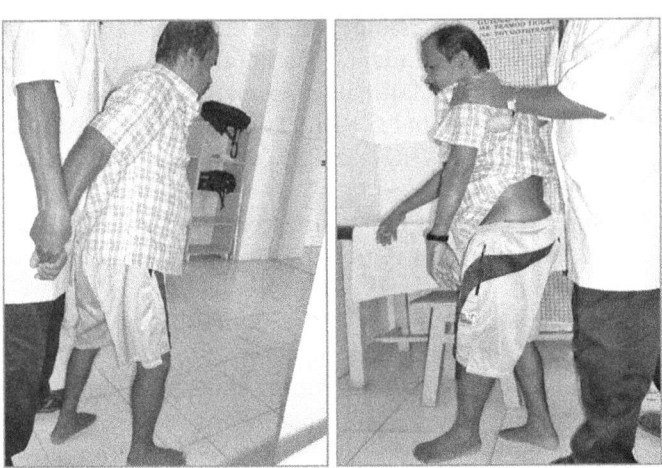

Fig. 36.36: Practice of walking with arm swings.

NEURODEVELOPMENTAL TREATMENT

Neurodevelopmental treatment (NDT), is an advanced hands-on approach to the examination and treatment of individuals with disturbances of function, movement and postural control due to a lesion of the central nervous system (CNS). It is a problem solving approach for the treatment of individuals with brain lesion, basing upon the dynamic systems's theory of motor control, using the selectionist model. This holistic interdisciplinary clinical practice model is informed by current and evolving research that emphasizes individualized therapeutic handling based upon movement analysis for habilitation and rehabilitation of individuals with CNS (brain) pathology.

The therapist uses the ICF model in a problem solving approach to assess activity and participation limitation due to impairment of various body systems and design strategies to overcome these limitations and set achievable outcomes in the clients with the help of relatives and caregivers.

It is an evolving approach which originated with the works of Dr Karel Bobath, a Neuropsychiatrist and his wife Mrs Berta Bobath a Physiotherapist in the late 1940s. The technique developed from observations, practical applications and desire to find better solutions for client's problems Bobaths introduced the revolutionary idea that a therapist could have an impact on client's functional movement by influencing the CNS through carefully guiding the motor output through handling

The approach has been modified through evolving research in the past years, and the current NDT, what we see today is the modified Bobath approach.

Though the original approach of Bobaths was based upon the Reflex Hierarchical model of motor control, the current NDT technique is based upon the dynamic systems model of motor control incorporating the Selectionist method. As per the current concepts of NDT, the CNS is not the controller of movement production, rather, it (CNS) determines the pattern of neural activity based on input from multiple intrinsic systems and extrinsic variables that establish the context for movement initiation and execution. Sensory feed back and feed forward mechanisms are considered equally important for movement control, as opposed to feed back mechanism described in the original Bobath approach. The negative signs such as muscle weakness, impaired postural control and paucity of movements are considered equally important as the positive signs (as per the original Bobath approach) such as spasticity, abnormal synergies for the functional limitations. Task goals, experience of patient and therapist, individual learning strategies, recruitment of normal movement synergies, energy and interest of patient and therapist determine the quality of final action, as opposed to the original view that (abnormal) muscle and postural tone determine the quality of posture and pattern of movement that determine the final action.

NDT techniques have been developed basing upon certain assumptions and principles, discussed below:

Assumptions of Neurodevelopmental Treatment (NDT)

The basic philosophy underlying all the NDT assumptions is that lesions in CNS produce problems in the coordination of posture and movement combined with atypical qualities of muscle tone that contribute directly to functional limitations. These functional limitations are changeable when the intervention strategies target specific system impairments in activities and contexts that are meaningful in the life of the person. The following ten assumptions were developed by the Bobaths, which were added with another ten assumptions through evolving research on motor science to complete the current therapeutic model of NDT.

- Impaired patterns of postural control and movement coordination are the primary problems in clients with CP, stroke.
- The system impairments in multiple systems are changeable and overall function improves when the problem of motor incoordination are treated by directly addressing neuromotor and postural control abnormalities in a task specific context.
- Sensorimotor impairments affect the whole individual – the person's function, place in the family and community, independence and overall quality of life.
- A working knowledge of typical adaptive motor development and how it changes across the life span provides the framework for assessing function and planning intervention.
- NDT clinicians focus on changing movement strategies as a means to achieve the best energy-efficient performance for the individual within the context of the age appropriate tasks and in anticipation of future functional tasks.
- Movement is linked to sensory processing. If a client could perceive what normal posture and movement feels like, he/she will be stimulated/motivated to hold a posture and move more and more to accomplish function.
- Intervention strategies involve the individual's active initiation and participation, often combined with therapist's manual guidance and direct handling.
- NDT intervention utilizes movement analysis to identify missing or atypical elements that link functional limitation to system impairments.
- Ongoing evaluation should be done throughout every treatment session.
- The aim of NDT is to optimize function.
- NDT accepts that, human motor function emerges from ongoing interaction among multiple internal systems of the individual, the characteristic of the task and the specific environmental context, each contributing different aspects of motor control.
- Movement is organized around behavioral goal, i.e., in motor planning, multiple systems are organized according to the inherent requirement of the task being performed and the current status (postural, motivational, emotional, cognitive etc.) of the individual.
- NDT assumes that, all individuals have competencies and strengths in various systems, that need to be explored and utilized.
- A hallmark of efficient human motor function is the ability of the individual to select and match various neuronal groups with a potentially infinite number of movement combinations that are attuned to the forces of gravity, forces generated by contracting muscles, and constraints posed by variety of environmental conditions.
- NDT uses a model of enablement/disablement based on the International Classification of Functions (ICF) developed by the WHO to categorize the individual's health and disability.
- Clinicians can best design interventions by establishing functional outcomes in partnership with the client and caregivers.
- Intervention programs are designed to serve clients throughout their lifespan.
- Learning and relearning motor skills and improving performance requires both practice and experience.
- Treatment is most effective during recovery and phase transitions.

- NDT clinicians assume the responsibility to provide the clients with the available evidence, related to all intervention methods, outcomes and service delivery systems.

Principles of NDT

There are principles of NDT examination/evaluation and intervention, which a clinician need to understand for best practice of the technique.

- **The principles of NDT examination/evaluation are:**
  - NDT examination process evaluates each client as a unique person with multiple competencies and limitations.
  - NDT examines each client in a life cycle framework.
  - NDT examination process incorporates an interdisciplinary therapeutic management team that includes and respects the client and the family as primary and active participants in decision making.
  - NDT examination begins the problem solving process that enables the clinician to make sound clinical decisions that combine evidence from clinical research with experience and judgement.
  - NDT examination and intervention incorporates principles from the study of motor control, motor learning and motor development.
  - NDT examination gives emphasis on components of posture and movements that are efficient or inefficient in persons with stroke or cerebral palsy.
- **The principles of NDT intervention are:**
  - Treatment plans should be established with anticipated outcomes that include specific, observable functions within a specific time frame under specific environmental conditions.
  - Therapy should utilize client's strengths, recognizing that each individual has competencies and disabilities.
  - Anticipated outcomes and impairment goals should be set in partnership with the family, the client, and the interdisciplinary team.
  - NDT intervention should construct a purposeful relationship between sensory input and motor output.
  - Therapeutic handling is a primary intervention strategy that therapist's use to assist the client in achieving independent function. The therapeutic handling used has three essential components, such as techniques of inhibition, techniques of facilitation and key point stimulation (hand placement).
  - Treatment strategies should include preparation and simulation of critical foundational elements (task components) as well as practice of the whole task.
  - NDT intervention should be designed to obtain active response from the client in goal directed activities.
  - Whenever possible, during treatment, movement should be initiated and actively performed by the client.
  - NDT intervention should allow the client to learn from errors that occur during movement.
  - NDT intervention should include planning and solving motor problems.
  - Repetition of task/activities should be one of the important component in motor learning.
  - An environment that is conducive to cooperative participation and support of the client's efforts should be created by the therapist.
  - Knowledge of the development of posture and movement components should be used in designing treatment strategies.
  - A single treatment session should progress from activities in which the client is most capable to activities that are more challenging.
  - NDT therapy sessions should provide motivation and purpose to engage the client fully in developing and reinforcing movement responses.
  - NDT intervention methods should include modifying the task, or the environment, and take into account the current level of the client's performance and capacity for function.
  - As the client is able to perform movement independently, the therapist should provide time during a treatment session for the client to move freely.
  - Individual treatment sessions should be designed to evaluate the effectiveness of treatment within the session.
  - The communicative intent of the client's motor behavior should be recognized and respected during treatment (e.g. An old patient, hesitant to adapt quadruped posture, indicates that he/she is doing so due to knee pain).
  - Families should be provided information regarding the client's problems and management of those problems, as they are able to understand and assimilate the information.
  - In an NDT approach, suggestions to the family should be as practical as possible.
  - NDT recommends an interdisciplinary model of service.
  - The therapist should coordinate with the goals and activities of all other medical, therapeutic, social, and educational disciplines to ensure a life-span approach to solving the client's problems.

Process/Methods of NDT Assessment

The focus of NDT assessment is to identify the client's abilities and limitations in order to tailor an individualized treatment plan for the client. The Assessment process consists of data collection from patient/caregiver, examination of various systems and evaluation.

The examination and evaluation should be done at the beginning and end of treatment session, as well as before and after completion of course of therapy.

The flowchart of the assessment process is shown below **(Fig. 36.37)**, which are briefly discussed below:

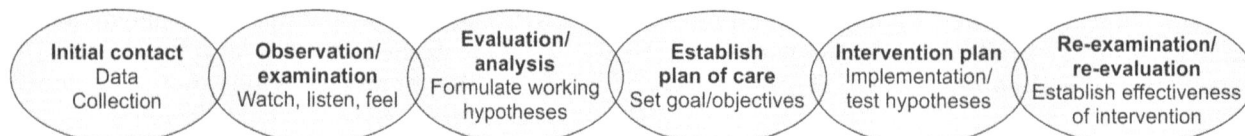

Fig. 36.37: The flowchart of assessment process.

- **Initial contact/Data collection:** It includes receiving the patient, noting the demographic details, diagnosis and reason for referral, taking medical history, collecting information on general level of function and noting family and environmental characteristics.
- **Examination:** The focus of examination is to identify constrains for function, including impairments in various systems that limit the client's ability to perform functional activities. It includes:
    - *Examination of gross motor function:* Posture and movement of body for functional activities such as: Transitions (e.g., supine to sitting), crawling, walking, etc.
    - *Examination of fine motor function:* Goal directed activities such as reaching, manipulation, exploration of objects, eating, drinking, playing, self care skills, work, school and leisure activities.
    - *Examination of oral motor function and communication:* Verbal and non-verbal communication, oral-motor abilities, facial expression, comprehension, etc.
    - *Examination of ability for control of behaviour and emotions:* Alertness, attention span, co-operation, tolerance for change, adaptability, perseveration, motivation, learning style, interpersonal interactions, ability to follow social rules etc.
    - *Examination of postural control and movement components:* Body alignment, relationship of base of support with center of mass, anticipatory postural control and weight shift, symmetry of body posture, movement strategies for manipulation, compensatory strategies (if any), oral motor function, gait etc.
    - *Examination of contextual factors:* Conditions and constraints on function, need for use of assistive devices (if any) to accomplish function, need for use of splints and orthosis (if any), are to be examined.
    - *Individual system review:* It includes brief examination of different systems of body such as neuromuscular, musculoskeletal, sensory, integumentary, cardiovascular, respiratory, gastrointestinal, cognitive-perceptual, limbic system, etc.
- **Evaluation:** It involves analysis of ineffective postures and movements that link functional impairments and their association with impairment of various systems and to make a working hypothesis for effective planning of intervention.
- **Plan of care (POC) and goal setting:** The plan of care consists of statements that specify the anticipated outcomes/goals, to be achieved when specific intervention strategies are designed and used specifying the duration and frequency of such interventions. The goals set after a thorough examination and evaluation should be observable and measurable. The goals set should be specific and achievable, and once achieved or if failed to achieve, it should be modified and another goal, matching the impairment status of the client should be set. The goals set are classified into:
    - *Short-term goal:* It includes functions such as neck control for a child with cerebral palsy, or supine to sitting for an adult with stroke. For children with cerebral palsy and similar disorders, the duration of achievement of short term goal is about 3 months. For adults with stroke or similar disorders the duration of achievement of short term goal is about 1 month.
    - *Long-term goal:* It includes functions such as achievement of creeping/crawling for a cerebral palsy child and achievement of walking for an adult with stroke. For children with cerebral palsy and similar disorders, the duration of achievement of long term goal is about 1 year, and for adult with stroke or similar disorders, the duration of achievement of long term goal is about 6 months.
- **Intervention plan:** After examination of impairment of various systems and linking the same to impairments of posture and movements and setting specific achievable goals, the therapist should design specific intervention strategies to inhibit abnormal postural tone, abnormal reflexes and reactions and facilitate movements as normally as possible, gradually incorporating the gained movements into functional tasks.
- **Re-examination/Re-evaluation:** After end of each session as well as at periodic intervals, the therapist should re-examine the various systems and subsequently evaluates the benefits achieved, evaluating himself/herself for applying the strategies effectively.

Techniques of NDT Intervention

Therapeutic handing is the primary intervention strategy in NDT intervention. Therapeutic handling in NDT takes the form of inhibition and facilitation of posture and movements to improve function. The therapist through contact with his/her hands tries to influence the posture and movements through:

- Directing, regulating and organizing tactile, proprioceptive and vestibular input.
- Directing the client's initiation of movements more efficiently and with more effective muscle synergies.
- Supporting or changing alignment of the body in relation to the base of support, and with respect to the force of gravity prior to and during movement sequences.

- Decreasing the amount of force the client uses to stabilize body segments.
- Guiding or re-directing the direction, force, speed and timing of muscle activation for successful task completion.
- Constraining or increasing the flexibility in the degrees of freedom needed to stabilize or move body segments in functional activities.
- Sensing the response of the client to the movement outcome and provide feedback as a reference of correction.
- Recognizing, when the client can become independent of the therapist's assistance and take over control of posture and movements.
- Directing the client's attention to meaningful aspects of motor task.

Therapeutic handling has three interactive components used by the therapist to develop as normal a posture as possible and produce goal directed functional movements, which are briefly discussed below:

Techniques of Inhibition

Techniques of inhibition are used to minimize the client's atypical postures and movements, that interfere with the development of motor patterns that support efficient performance. In the original Bobath approach, the term inhibition is referred to strategies for reduction of abnormally increased muscle tone and reflex activity that resulted from CNS dysfunction interfering with function. Currently, the inhibition strategies involve reduction of specific underlying impairments that interfere with function, which also includes the inhibition of abnormal tone and reflexes that resulted from impairment of neuromuscular system.

A clinician utilizes inhibition in treatment to:

- Prevent or re-direct those components of movements that are unnecessary and interfere with intentional, co-ordinated movements. For example, excessive forearm pronation, that unnecessarily interfere with the act of taking food to mouth need to be inhibited through designing of appropriate therapeutic strategies.
- To constrain the degrees of freedom to decrease the amount of force the client uses to stabilize posture. For example, the abnormal synergies/spastic patterns where movement in one component in the abnormal pattern, induces the whole movement pattern need to be controlled to maintain a specific joint position/postural alignment, reducing unnecessary expenditure of energy and making the posture and movements energy efficient.
- Balance antagonists muscle groups. For example, inhibiting the spastic elbow flexors to facilitate antagonistic elbow extensors, so that a stable elbow alignment that is required for reaching at an object away from the body could be achieved.
- Reduce spasticity or excessive muscle stiffness that interfere with functional movements. For example, the spasticity of the ankle plantar flexors that causes an equinus ankle, interfering with walking need to be reduced through appropriate techniques of inhibition.

As inhibition facilitates and facilitation inhibits, most often inhibition is applied in combination with facilitation and key point stimulation (therapeutic handling) to inhibit abnormal posture and movement and facilitate efficient posture and movement.

The techniques of inhibition include:

- **Passive elongation with proximal dissociation**: Slow and sustained stretching of spastic muscles to inhibit muscle tone/spasticity through autogenic inhibition (through stimulation of type-1b afferent from Golgi tendon organ, that inhibits the corresponding anterior horn cell) and elongating the actin-myosin cross bridge. It also reduces the bias of the muscle spindle to react, inhibiting hypertonicity. The elongation of spastic muscle groups promotes independent movements in distal segments over the proximal segments (proximal dissociation), as the abnormal pattern of movement are inhibited by weakening the abnormal muscle contraction through passive stretching/elongation. Orthotic and positional devices may be used to maintain sustained passive elongation if required.
- **Active movement**: Active movements at controlled velocities are performed in the antagonistic direction/pattern to reduce tone in spastic muscles and facilitate the antagonists.
- **Reflex inhibitory postures**: Based on the understanding of the law of shunting, Mrs Berta Bobath developed this special type of handling and manipulation to break through the abnormal motor pattern. The client is placed in postures that are roughly the opposite of those, the person with CNS lesion assume, when lying, sitting and standing. The positioning of the body parts (limbs and trunk) in postures opposite to the spastic/abnormal reflex postures help in inhibiting abnormal tone/reflex/movement patterns from developing strongly, as well as helping to inhibit such patterns if they have already developed. For example, Positioning a Cerebral palsy child with persistent Tonic labyrinthine reflex (TLR) inside a hammock, help in inhibiting the reflex gradually, promoting development of sitting. Various reflex inhibiting postures of the limbs that are commonly adopted after stroke/head injuries have been described in Chapter 19.

Positional devices, such as pillows, sand bags, orthotic devices (elbow/knee gaiters, polypropylene AFOs, etc) etc may be used to maintain the position. For example, a pillow placed under the head after onset of stroke or during the recovery stage when spasticity/abnormal reflexes are appearing may help in inhibiting extensor tone in the body through inhibition of TLR in supine.

Mrs Bobath, described Reflex inhibitory postures, simply not as static postures, rather these are components of functional movements. Passive positioning in reflex inhibiting postures produces decrease in muscle tone, but does not result in carry over into movement and function. As a patient tolerates reflex inhibiting postures, he/she should be encouraged to move from one posture to another posture, enabling performance of functional movement. For example, maintaining the elbow in extension and forearm in supination, the patient is assisted to reach forward and sideways to touch/manipulate objects.

- **Reflex inhibiting patterns**: The reflex inhibiting patterns are not simply the static postures, but are phases of movement away from the total patterns (abnormal synergistic/spastic patterns). Reflex inhibiting patterns evolved, as Mrs Berta Bobaths realized the importance of active movements to reduce muscle tone and improve function. The Bobaths called the patterns of inhibition, reflex inhibiting pattern to focus on movements rather than the static postures. These patterns are combined with key point stimulations, either to inhibit abnormal or facilitate normal patterns of movements. Guiding the client to produce movements in patterns opposite to abnormal synergistic patterns/spastic patterns/reflex patterns help in reducing abnormal muscle tone associated with the spastic muscle groups including inhibition of abnormal reflexes and reactions.

  Mrs Berta Bobath has presented five considerations for the therapist to keep in mind, when using reflex inhibiting patterns. They are:
  - The aim of this pattern is to reduce hypertonicity (spasticity/rigidity), as well as increase of postural tone.
  - The patterns of movement are introduced gradually, beginning proximally from head and progressing distally, it means all the abnormal components should not be broken at a time.
  - Handling must not start at the place on the body, where hypertonus is strongest.
  - The goal of this movement pattern is to enable the client gain their own control of abnormal postural reactions, so that they could attain independence from therapist's control.
  - It is important to give clients a great variety of postural patterns and to use similar combinations in different positions at certain stages of treatment.

- **Weight shifting (pressure tappings)**: Shifting of weights over joints covered with spastic muscles help in inhibiting spasticity, through alternate contraction of agonists and antagonists, using the Sherrington's principles of reciprocal inhibition. That, means while shifting weight over elbow joint in sitting, it result in loading (elbow extension) and unloading of elbow (elbow flexion). When elbow goes into extension from flexion, the spastic elbow flexor will be inhibited.

Techniques of Facilitation

Facilitation is the therapeutic handling that makes a posture and movement easier and efficient to perform function. During examination, the therapists examine the presence of atypical or abnormal movement components accountable for abnormal posture and movements and subsequently designs strategies to inhibit such abnormal components of posture and movements and facilitate normal posture and movements, enabling the patient adopt to developmental postures and perform efficient functional movements.

Facilitation modifies postural control by linking postural elements with movements. This is done by supporting body segments during movements, changing the demand on the postural system by altering the body position relative to the force of gravity, or changing the alignment of the body relative to the base of support (BOS). During treatment, the therapist sets up the environment, varies the task, and decides the components of posture and movements that can be made easier through facilitation to complement the motor learning process. A wide variety of sensory motor experiences (through functional task practice) are provided to the client gradually during the treatment, so that the client is able to build up movement repertoires and adapt posture and movements for similar functions in other context.

Facilitation techniques are applied from the very early stage, when the muscles are flaccid after onset of stroke/head injury and continues throughout the recovery phase. The techniques of facilitation are gradually progressed and are applied in the following manner:

- **Lower level facilitation**: This involves quick stretch, stroking, weight bearing (that produces co-contraction of muscles) to facilitate contraction of the flaccid muscles.
- **Middle level facilitation:** These techniques of facilitation were developed by the Bobaths to stabilize muscle tone and regulate reciprocal muscle function, through proprioceptive and tactile stimulation. The procedures involved are:
  - *Inhibitory tapping:* This is a facilitation technique that follows inhibition. Once spasticity or hypertonus has been reduced, the underlying muscle tone may be too low to support co-activation for stabilization or to allow normal balance between the agonists and antagonists for reciprocal interaction. Inhibitory tapping is applied directly to the muscles, keeping in view that spasticity does not increase.
  - *Sweep tapping:* This involves application of a strong tactile stimulus, sweeping over the muscles in the direction of movement to facilitate contraction of muscles and to produce movement.
  - *Alternate tapping:* This tapping technique is used to stimulate balanced contraction of agonists and antagonists, helping in stabilizing posture. In this technique the agonists and antagonist muscle groups are tapped alternately allowing little or no movements, making the muscles work in patterns of co-activation. While the tapping is applied, there is a moment, when the therapist's hands are completely off the client's body, allowing the individual to hold a posture.
  - *Pressure tapping:* This tapping involves weight bearing and compression/weight shifting through the joint to build up co-activation of agonists and antagonists, helping to hold a posture. Clinicians can assist the client's weight bearing in relationship with the support surface, prior to and during a movement sequence by using small weight shifts with pressure, requiring the client to adapt to the changes of centre of mass (COM), base of support (BOS) and the effects of gravitational

forces. The techniques can be practiced on a fixed supporting surface, as well as on a mobile surface, such as inflatable ball (Swiss ball), bolster etc.

Pressure is given through the joints to reinforce the client's sense of position, prior to movement initiation. For example, pressure is given through the knee joint of a child standing with support of a walker, to facilitate weight shift on the pressure applied leg, so that, the other leg could be moved to step forward.

Besides different tapping, resistance to active movements are used to give the client a stronger sense of direction or timing to make the client work harder to produce a successful action.

- **Higher level facilitation:** This includes placing, holding and eccentric lowering with distal dissociation. Placing is the ability to hold the body segment in precise alignment, relative to a place or object in the environment. Placing and holding which are essential requirements for performing functional movements are followed by eccentric lowering and movement of distal part (distal dissociation) of body enabling the body segments perform functional movements. For example, a stroke patient learning to put one leg through the sleeve of pant, need to hold the affected lower limb at a precise angle off the floor standing on the sound leg, and then lower the leg down and moves the ankle and knee (distal dissociation) through the sleeve of pant performing the function of dressing the lower body. Besides, placing and eccentric lowering, reflex inhibiting pattern of movements with key point stimulation are also used to facilitate movements out of spastic/synergistic pattern. While performing movements in reflex inhibiting pattern, the proximal key point stimulation is preferred first, as it keeps the distal part free to manipulate functional task. However, when spasticity in the distal part persists significantly, distal key point stimulation is also performed with reflex inhibiting patten. Distal key points are also stimulated to facilitate proximal movements. Stimulation of proximal and distal key points in a cerebral palsy child are shown in **Figures 36.38A and B).**

Techniques of Key Point Stimulation

Key points are parts of the body, where the therapists can most effectively, control and change patterns of posture and movements in other body parts. The key points **(Fig. 36.39)** include:
- **Proximal key points:** Head, Scapula, shoulder, pelvis, hip.
- **Distal key points:** Head, jaw, wrist and hand, ankle and foot.
- **Central key points:** Anteriorly: Xiphoid process, Posteriorly: T7-T8.

Besides these designated points, the Bobaths have said that, where, on the patients body, the therapist places his/her hands objectively and precisely to influence muscle tone and facilitate posture and movements, those are also considered as key points.

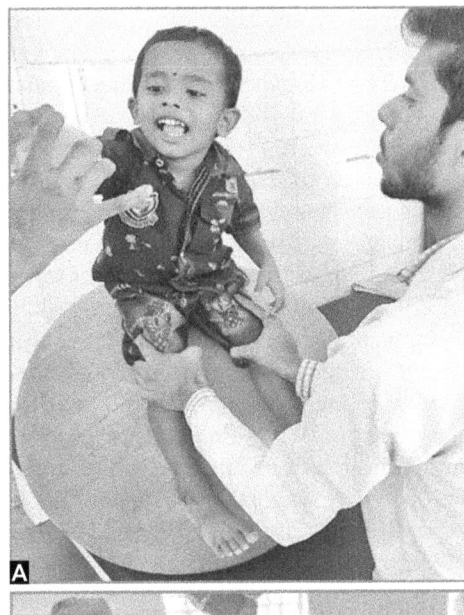
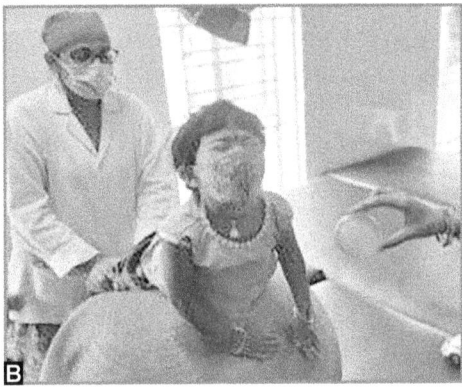

Figs. 36.38A and B: (A) Stimulation of proximal key point (lower thigh), to promote sitting and use of hand (distal key point) for playing; (B) Stimulation of distal key points (ankles/feet) to promote neck and trunk extension.

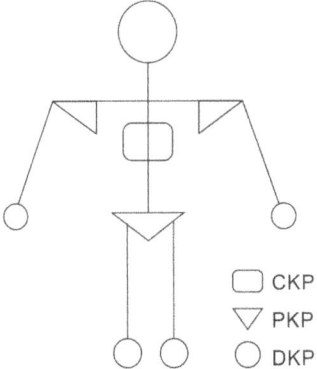

Fig. 36.39: Shows key points of control.

Phases of Inhibition and Facilitation

Though NDT is a task oriented approach, which aims at restoration of functional skills, inclusion of task components are not done at the start of therapy, and following three phases are adopted during therapy, gradually adding components of functional tasks till the client achieves maximum competency with assistance/

feedback from therapists/caregivers. Subsequently, the therapist/caregiver gradually withdraws support/assistance/feedback, so that the patient achieves independence in functional tasks. The three phases of training are:
1. **Phase of sensation:** This is the initial phase of training, where emphasis on practice of movements as normally as possible, inhibiting abnormal patterns of movements enabling the patient achieve sensation of normal posture and movements. No task is added at this phase of training.
2. **Phase of cognition:** As we know, every task demands cognitive input, and cognitive demand of the task stresses the body and mind, tasks demanding lesser cognitive input should be given to perform by the client, once the individual has achieved the ability to perform movements as normally as possible though he/she needs some assistance/feedback. Gradually tasks demanding increased cognitive input should be added.
3. **Phase of fading of control:** Once the individual achieves the skill of performing more and more complex tasks with assistance/feedback from therapist/caregiver, gradually, the support/assistance/feedback are withdrawn, enabling the client to achieve maximum functional independence.

ROOD'S APPROACH

This approach to treatment for neuro-muscular disorder was developed by Margaret Rood, a Physio-Occupational therapist. Margaret Rood drew heavily from the reflex and hierarchical models of motor control in designing her intervention approach.

Key components of the approach are the use of sensory stimulation to evoke motor responses and the use of developmental postures to promote changes in muscle tone. Sensory stimuli are applied to muscles and joints to elicit a specific motor response. Rood also described the use of specific developmental sequences believed to promote motor responses. These sequences were proximal to distal and cephalocaudal. Treatment strategies move the clients through these developmental sequences.

Assumption of Rood's Approach

- Motor patterns are developed from fundamental patterns/reflexes, which are refined and controlled as the individual matures.
- Sensory stimuli applied to muscles and joints lead to normalization of muscle tone producing the desired movement.
- Sensory motor control is developmentally based. Proper sensory stimuli applied to the appropriate sensory receptors, as it is utilized in normal sequential development leads to development of postures and purposeful movements.
- The movement produced by sensory stimulation should be purposeful.
- Repetition of sensorimotor response is necessary for motor learning.

Principles of Rood's Approach

- Tonic neck and labyrinthine reflexes can assist or retard the effect of sensory motor stimulation.
- Stimulation of specific receptors produce specific response. Rules of sensory input are:
  - A fast brief stimulus produce a large synchronous movement.
  - A fast repetitive stimulus produce a maintained response.
  - Slow, rhythmical repetitive sensory input deactivates the body.
  - Maintained sensory stimulus produces maintained response.
- Muscles have different duties. Heavy work muscles act as stabilizer helping for maintenance of posture. Light work muscles work as mobilizers and help in production of skilled movements repetitive and rhythmical in nature involving the distal part of body.
- Heavy work muscles should be integrated before the light work muscles.
- Development is cephalo-caudal, therefore treatment is head to toe.
- Ontogenic developmental sequences such as: Supine flexion (supine withdrawal), roll over to side-lying, pivot prone (prone extension), neck co-contraction, prone on elbows, quadruped, standing, walking, are used in the treatment.
- Movement is directed towards function.
- Repetition is necessary for motor learning.
- Treatment should begin at the developmental level of functioning.

Rood's Technique

Facilitatory and inhibitory techniques are used in the therapy to improve posture and movements. The techniques are briefly discussed below:
- **Rood's facilitatory techniques:** These techniques are used to increase tone of the flaccid muscles. The techniques include:
  - *Light moving touch:* Mediated by Aδ sensory fibers. Applied with fingertips/camel hairbrush/cotton swab. 3-5 strokes are applied with 30 seconds of rest between strokes to prevent over stimulation. Activates low threshold hair end organ and free nerve endings.
  - *Fast brushing:* Mediated by C-fibers. Fast brushing (high intensity stimulus) is the brushing of skin over the muscle/or over the dermatome of the same segment, that supplies the muscle, by soft paint brush or battery operated brush. The stimuli are applied for 3-5 seconds, and repeated after 30 seconds.
  - *Icing:*
    » A-icing/quick icing: Mediated by A fibers. Application of quick swipes of ice cubes (3 swipes) is made to evoke reflex withdrawal similar to light touch. The water should be blotted with a towel between swipes.

» C-icing: Mediated by C-fibers. Applied by ice cube pressed for 15–20 minutes either on muscle belly or dermatome area. Facilitates a maintained postural response.
- *Proprioceptive facilitatory techniques:*
  » Heavy joint compression/joint approximation: Facilitates co-contraction of the muscles around the joints combined with developmental patterns. It can be given manually or through the use of weights and sandbags, or using weight bearing positions, e.g-prone on hand.
  » Vibration: It can be used as tactile stimulation to desensitize the hypersensitive skin and to produce tonal changes in muscles. Vibratory stimuli applied over a muscle belly to activate the type- Ia afferent of muscle spindle, causing contraction of that muscles and suppression of the stretch reflex. This response is called the tonic vibration reflex and is best elicited by a high frequency vibrator that delivers stimuli at 100-300Hz. The duration of the vibration should not exceed 1-2 min per application because heat and friction will result. The prone position may be best while vibrating flexor muscle groups and the supine position may enhance the extensor muscles.
  » Stretch: Activates the proprioceptors in selected muscles and imply the principle of reciprocal innervations. It is applied in the following forms:
    ♦ Quick stretch: Low threshold stimulus which activates phasic response of the same muscle stretched. It produces immediate effect.
    ♦ Intrinsic stretch: It promotes stability of the scapulohumeral region, while bearing more weight on the ulnar side of the hands and promoting resistive grasp.
    ♦ Stretch pressure: Effects both exteroceptors and type- Ia afferents of the muscle spindle. Pressure on muscle belly places stretch on muscle spindles and hence activates stretch response.
    ♦ Secondary ending stretch: Combination of resistance and stretch to facilitate ontogenic patterns. Once a muscle is put on a full stretch, secondary nerve endings which are facilitatory to the flexors and inhibitory to the extensors are stimulated.
  » Resistance to muscle contraction: Heavy resistance is used in the technique to stimulate both primary and secondary endings of the muscle spindle. It is used in developmental fashion to influence the stabilizers. When a muscle contracts against resistance, it assumes a shortened length that causes the muscle spindle to contract so they readjust to the shortened length. This is called "biasing" the muscle spindle so it is more sensitive to stretch
  » Tapping: Tapping over tendon or muscle belly is useful in facilitating the muscle. With the fingertips percussion is done 3-5 times before or during the time the patient is voluntarily contracting the muscles. This stimulus acts on the afferents of the muscle spindles and increases the tone of the underlying muscles.
  » Vestibular stimulation: The vestibular system is found to activate the antigravity muscles. The system affects tone, balance, directionality, protective response, cranial nerve function, bilateral integration, auditory language development and eye pursuits. It is stimulated through linear acceleration and deceleration in horizontal and vertical planes and angular acceleration and deceleration such as spinning, rolling or swinging. Exercises on vestibular ball/wobble board, helps to facilitate the postural muscles. Fast stimulation tends to stimulate while slow rhythmical rocking tends to relax.

❖ **Rood's inhibitory techniques:** The following techniques have been used by Rood's to inhibit muscle hypertonus and induce relaxation.
  - *Slow rolling:* Patient is rolled slowly from a supine lying position to prone and back in a rhythmical pattern. Used on both sides of the body.
  - *Neutral warmth:* Affects the temperature receptors in the hypothalamus and peripheral sensory nerve receptors. It is used for patients with hypertonia. Patient in recumbent position and wrapped with a blanket for 5-20 minutes. Patient feels relaxed with decrease in tone.
  - *Slow stroking:* Patient in prone, while the therapist provides a rhythmical, moving deep pressure over the dorsal distribution of the posterior rami of the spine. It is done from occiput to coccyx and alternated and should not exceed 3 minutes because it causes a rebound phenomenon.
  - *Tendinous pressure:* Manual pressure when applied to the tendinous insertion of a muscle, helps in inhibiting that muscle (due to autogenic inhibition). It can be used for spastic muscles.
  - *Light joint compression/approximation:* Joint compression less than or equal to body weight is applied to inhibit spastic muscles around the joint.
  - *Maintained stretch:* Maintenance of an elongated position of the muscle for a period of time ranging from several minutes to several weeks causes lengthening of the muscle, including the lengthening of the muscle spindle, thereby reducing its bias to undergo stretch-contraction. The afferents of the muscle spindle are set to a longer position, so that they become less sensitive to stretch
  - *Rocking:* Shifting the weight forward and backward, progressing to side to side and then in diagonal patterns.

VOJTA APPROACH

Dr Vaclov Vojta, a Neurologist, came upon certain trigger points by chance, when he was examining babies in the course of his routine work, which is the basis of the therapy described by him. He found that, when the healthy baby's body is touched at certain points, the two basic forms of locomotion, i.e., reflex creeping in prone and reflex rolling in supine were triggered. Dr Vojta's thought was, a child not able to move at all, if could be stimulated to move reflexly, and the reflex locomotion is combined with purposeful activities like reaching for a toy to play etc., after a course of therapy, the child, without any physical stimulus applied on him, may start to move towards the toy, leading to conversion of reflex locomotion into voluntary motion.

Dr Vojta emphasized on early identification of babies, who carry the risk of turning into cerebral palsy, through testing of various postural reactions briefly mentioned below. Dr Vojta used postural reactions to identify babies having a disturbance of central co-ordination. He categorized babies into: Mildest cerebral palsy, Mild cerebral palsy, moderate cerebral palsy, severe cerebral palsy, depending on the presence of nos of abnormal postural reactions (discussed below).

As per the technique, a thorough assessment of the child's physical levels is carried out and the problems of the child need to be diagnosed before therapy is started. As per Dr Vojta, the process of evaluation and therapy can be started in the first few days after birth, by diagnosing a child with disturbance in central co-ordination, who is expected to be diagnosed as cerebral palsy in future

Dr Vojta analysed the following seven main postural reactions in every child for normal or abnormal responses and found that a child with central movement disorder demonstrated stereotyped uniform postural reflexes/reactions with poverty of movements. The pathological reactions seen in an infant, with a central disturbance are analogous to the fixed pathological movement patterns of a fully developed cerebral palsy child.

The seven main postural reactions tested on babies by Dr Vojta are:
1. Traction response.
2. Landau's reaction.
3. Axillary suspension reaction.
4. Vojta's side-tilt reaction.
5. Colli's horizontal reaction.
6. Peiper and Isbert's vertical suspension reaction.
7. Colli's vertical suspension reaction.

As per Dr Vojta, cerebral palsy may develop from the disturbances of central co-ordination, and the condition may be categorized from mildest to severe, depending upon the presence of number of abnormal postural reactions. The following grading scale was used by Dr Vojta for grading the disorder.
- **Mildest:** Presence of 1,2, or 3 abnormal postural reactions.
- **Mild:** Presence of 4 or 5 abnormal postural reactions.
- **Moderate:** Presence of 6 or 7 abnormal postural reactions.
- **Severe:** All seven postural reactions are abnormal, along with existence of severe disturbance of muscle tone.

Dr Vojta's observation was that, children categorised under mildest to mild types normalize spontaneously, hence do not require any therapy, but they should be followed up regularly to monitor their development. For infants categorized under moderate or severe disturbances therapy should be started at once.

Instead of using a month by month account of motor development, Dr Vojta divided the first year of life of the infant into trimesters and noted the principal physical achievements in each trimester as described under **(Table 36.1)**:

Table 36.1: Physical achievements in various trimesters of a growing child.

Trimester	Duration	Achievements
I	1-3 months	Holding of prone position
II	3-6 months	Elbow and knee posture Start of active rolling
III	6-9 months	Includes hands and knee position and rotation into sitting
IV	9-12 months	Standing and walking

Dr Vojta has described 18 trigger points **(Fig. 36.40)** 9 points on left half of the body and 9 points on right half of the body. Besides these 18 trigger points, he also described an auxiliary trigger point, located under the chin, used to encourage and improve jaw, tongue and swallowing movements, and to control drooling.

The 9 trigger points described on each side:
- **Trigger points on the upper limb:**
  - Root of spine of scapula.
  - Tip of acromion process.
  - Medial epicondyle of humerus.
  - Just above the styloid process of radius.
- **Trigger point on the trunk:**
  Between 7th and 8th rib in line with the nipple.
- **Trigger points on the lower limb:**
  - Anterior superior iliac spine (ASIS).
  - Gluteus medius.
  - Medial condyle of femur.
  - Lateral border of calcaneum.

The trigger points are stimulated in supine to promote reflex turning, and in prone to stimulate reflex creeping. There are no specific trigger points for specific movements. Whichever trigger points produce the desired movements are stimulated, which depends on experience of the therapist and response of the client.

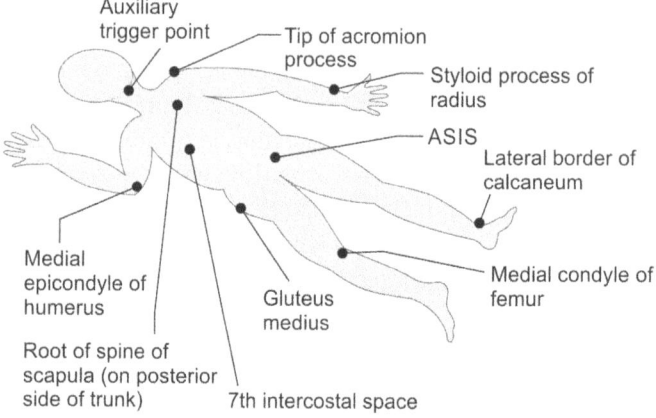

Fig. 36.40: Trigger points on body, as per Dr Vojta.

To help identify the starting positions for the exercises, Dr Vojta used the expression 'facial side' and occipital side. In both reflex creeping and reflex turning, the head is always turned by approximately 30 degrees, to one side, i.e., on the facial; side. Dr Vojta has distributed the trigger points to either facial or occipital sides, and described the direction of pressure at these points in order to elicit increased stability of the trunk and proximal joints **(Fig. 36.41)**.

For Vojta Therapy to be successful, it must as a rule be performed several times a day (up to four times where necessary). A therapy session lasts between five and twenty minutes. Since parents or caregivers perform the therapy daily, they play a significant role in the application of Vojta Therapy.

SENSORY INTEGRATION THERAPY

Sensory integration is the ability to take in information through the senses of touch, movement, smell, taste, vision, and hearing, and to combine the resulting perceptions with prior information, memories, and knowledge already stored in the brain, in order to derive coherent meaning from processing the stimuli. It is a process that senses and organizes sensation from ones own body and surroundings. Sensory integration focuses primarily on three basic senses, i.e: Tactile, Vestibular and Proprioceptive.

Clients with brain lesion such as stroke, traumatic brain injury, cerebral palsy, etc. have significant impairment of sensory integration, resulting in lack of ability in maintaining efficient posture and balance as well failing to produce purposeful co-ordinated movements. Sensory integration problems are also common manifestations in children with autistic spectrum disorders (ASD). To overcome the problems of sensory integration, sensory integration therapy was developed by A Jean Ayres, an occupational therapist in 1970s to help children with sensory processing problems to cope with the difficulties faced by them in processing sensory input.

Ayres recognized that some children with cerebral palsy have difficulties with attention, behavior and visual perception. These difficulties are related to sensory integration problems. The basic goal of this therapy is to teach clients

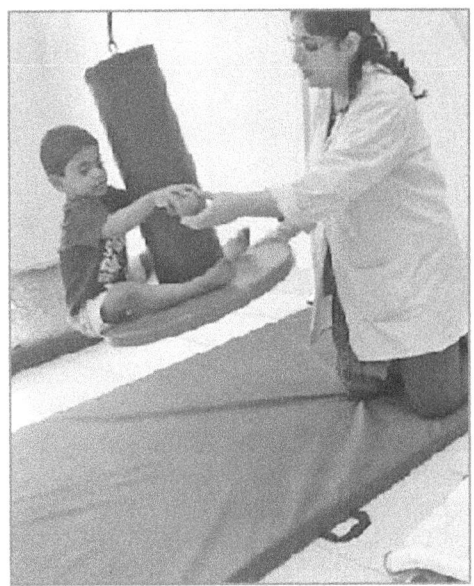

Fig. 36.42: Sensory integration therapy in progress to a child with ASD.

(CP/Stroke/TBI etc.) how to integrate their sensory feedback and then produce useful and purposeful motor responses to accomplish function.

Activities such as catching a ball in different positions may be used as a way of stimulating and requiring integration of visual, vestibular, and joint proprioception feedback systems at the same time **(Fig. 36.42)**. Typical stimuli include vestibular stimulation and tactile stimulation by brushing, rubbing, as well as joint compression and traction. Educating the parents/caregivers is recognized as an important aspect of the treatment. The theory underlying this system is that sensory input followed by appropriate motor function will contribute to the improved development of higher cortical motor and sensory function.

CONDUCTIVE EDUCATION THERAPY

Conductive education is a comprehensive method of learning in which individuals with mobility impairment learn to specifically and consciously perform actions, that children without such impairment learn through normal life experiences. It is an educational system, that incorporates learning into activities helping children and adults with movement impairment perform goal directed functional movements. This system of therapy was developed by Hungarian Professor Andras Peto to help children with movement disorder such as Cerebral palsy, to overcome their limitations for motor functions with direct teaching and learning. The technique can also be applied to adults with movement disorders such as Stroke. The application of the technique has been discussed separately for cerebral palsy in Chapter 18 and stroke in Chapter 19.

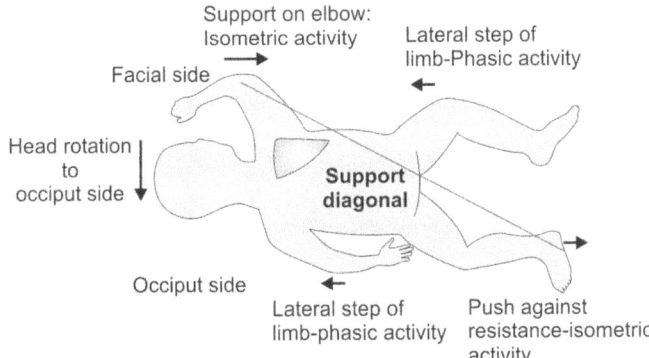

Fig. 36.41: Shows the trigger point stimulation on facial and occipital sides with direction of pressure to elicit muscular activity for reflex creeping.

Manual Therapy

Healing touch is always considered beneficial for disorders affecting musculoskeletal/neuromuscular systems. From the early laying on hands for therapy such as massage therapy, developed in Ancient China, many advanced manual therapy techniques have evolved and used by Physiotherapists today. However, the therapist should have adequate knowledge in anatomy, biomechanics and clinical pathophysiology affecting musculoskeletal and neuro muscular systems as well as adequate hands on training/practice for application of the techniques.

The various manual therapy techniques have been discussed briefly as under. However, the reader is advised to refer manual therapy books, and journals and should undergo specific hands on training before application of the techniques to patients.

MCKENZIE METHOD

The McKenzie method of treatment for the spinal disorders was developed by, New Zeland based physiotherapist, Robin McKenzie. The acronym for this method of treatment is mechanical diagnosis and therapy (MDT).

This therapeutic approach, requires the patient to move through a series of test movements to interpret the patient's pain response. The information gained from the test movements are used to develop an exercise program designed to centralize/alleviate pain (i.e., to move the pain from the legs to the back), and to reduce stiffness (dysfunction) and postural abnormalities (if any).

According to McKenzie, the pain of spinal origin can be classified into three syndromes, such as:

1. **Postural syndrome**: This is caused by mechanical deformation of soft tissues as a result of postural stresses. As per this syndrome, mechanical deformation due to prolonged stress produces pain, and the pain eases only with a change of position or after postural correction.

    Treatment for postural syndrome: The treatment includes:
    - Patient education.
    - Correction of posture, by restoring normal biomechanics of spine, say lumbar/cervical lordosis and/or normal thoracic kyphosids.
    - Avoiding provocative postures, that produce prolonged tensile stress on normal structures.

2. **Dysfunction syndrome**:
    This is caused by mechanical deformation of soft tissues affected by adaptive shortening. The cause of dysfunction may be a previous trauma, inflammation (spondylitis)/ degenerative disorder of spine (spondylosis). Due to the dysfunction, there might be a tissue contraction, scarring, adherence or adaptive shortening. The pain is brought on as soon as shortened structures are stressed by end positioning/ end range movements and stops almost immediately, when the stress on the joint/soft tissues is released. Dysfunction may occur in articular/contractile tissues.

    Treatment of dysfunction syndrome: The treatment includes:
    - Mobilizing exercises in the direction of dysfunction, or in the direction that reproduces the pain. For example, in spondylitis of lumbar spine, if flexion is limited and painful, patient is taught lumbar flexion exercises (**Fig. 37.1**).
    - The aim of the treatment is to remodel/lengthen the tight/dysfunctional tissue, which limits movements, through exercises, so that it becomes pain free over time.

3. **Derangement syndrome:** This is caused by mechanical deformation of soft tissues, as a result of internal derangement. Alteration of the position of nucleus pulposus and the surrounding annulus fibrosus within the disc, causes a disturbance of normal resting position of the two vertebrae that enclose the disc. The mechanical deformation produced by altered position of the inter vertebral disc, increases mechanical deformation producing pain. For example, prolapsed intervertebral disc (PIVD) of lumbar and cervical spine.

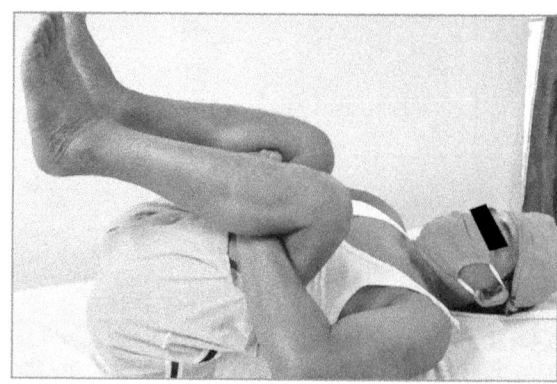

Fig. 37.1: Exercise for flexion dysfunction.

Treatment of derangement syndrome: The treatment includes:
- Examination of the patient's symptomatic and mechanical response to repeated movements or sustained positions, because the chosen treatment depends on the clinically induced directional preference. It describes the situation, when movements in one direction, reduces the pain and limitation of ROM, whereas movements in the opposite direction cause signs and symptoms to worsen.

The phenomena produced during testing of movements are typed into:
  » **Centralization:** This describes the phenomenon, in which, the limb pain emanating from the spine is progressively reduced in a distal to proximal direction, in response to therapeutic loading strategies, i.e., performing repeated movements. For posterior derangements like a central disc bulge/postero lateral disc bulge, repeated movement in the direction of extension should reduce limb pain by correcting the derangement **(Fig. 37.2)**. Flexion exercises should be avoided in posterior/postero lateral derangements of spine. However, for anterior derangement (which is rare) repeated flexion should reduce the symptoms, and extension of the spine should be avoided. The spine pain that persists during this process, gradually reduces by performing the exercises repeatedly.
  » **Peripheralization:** This describes the phenomenon by which, the pain emanating from the spine, spreads distally into the limb, when the test movement is performed. If the pain is produced in the limb, spreads distally/increases distally and remains worse, the loading strategy/exercise/movements that worsens the pain should be avoided.

Different McKenzie exercises are discussed below:
❖ **McKenzie exercises for lumbar spine:**
  – McKenzie exercises for posterior/postero lateral derangement of lumbar spine:
    » Lying on stomach: Patient is asked to lie in prone with arms at sides and hold the position for 2-3 minutes and repeat the position several times in a day as per need **(Fig. 37.3)**.
    » Lying on a pillow: Patient is asked to lie in prone over a pillow under abdomen and thorax, with arms

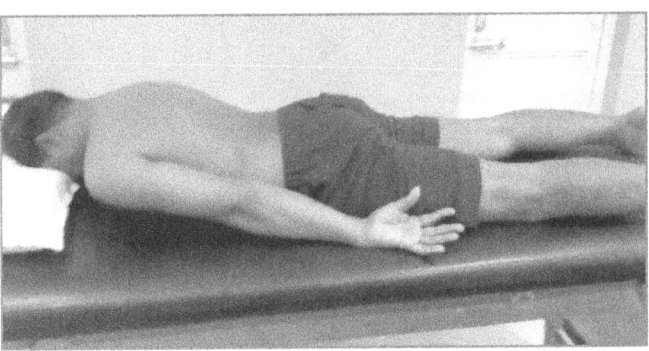

Fig. 37.3: Lying on stomach.

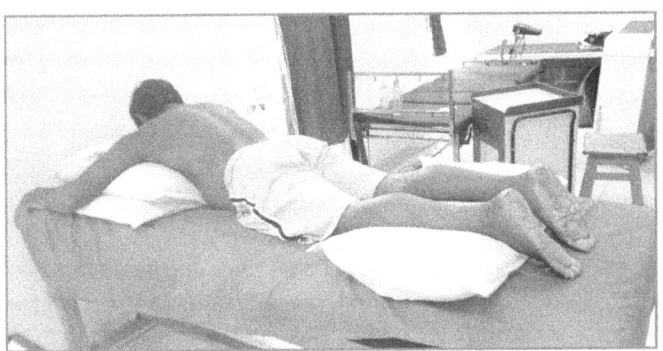

Fig. 37.4: Lying on pillow.

at sides and hold the position. The duration of lying on pillow and repetitions depends on the relief of symptoms **(Fig. 37.4)**.
  » Prone on elbows: This exercise helps to restore the natural curve of the low back. The patient in prone is asked to prop himself/herself on the forearms, with the shoulders above the elbows, hold for 2-3 minutes and then lower to bed. The exercises are repeated for several times in a day as per need **(Fig. 37.5)**.
  » Prone press up: This exercise also helps to restore the natural curve of the low back. The patient in prone is asked to prop himself/herself on the hands, with the hands under the shoulders. The position is held for 2 second and then lowered to bed. The exercises are repeated 10 times for several times in a day as per need **(Fig. 37.2)**.
  » Extension in standing: The standing patient is asked to place the hands on the buttocks and bend backwards as far as possible with the knees straight.

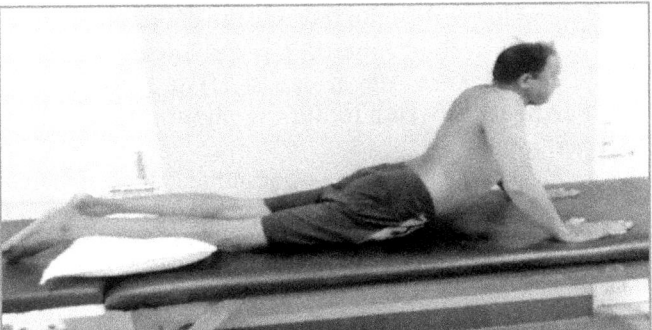

Fig. 37.2: McKenzie extension exercises in prone.

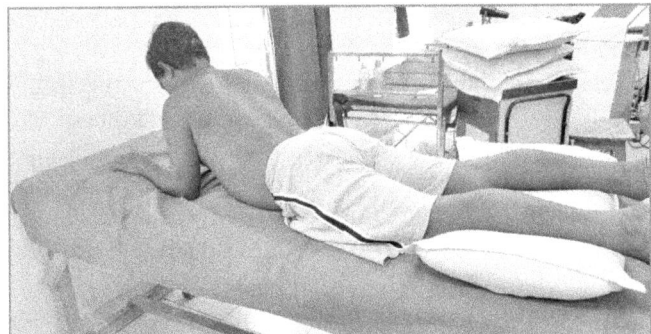

Fig. 37.5: Prone on elbows.

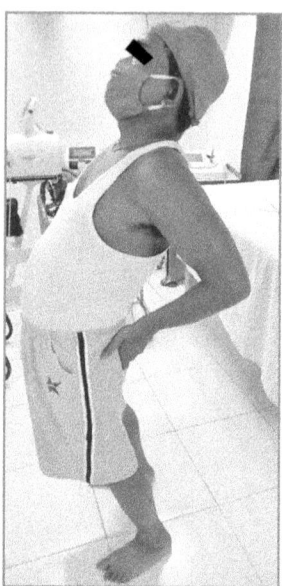

Fig. 37.6: Extension in standing.

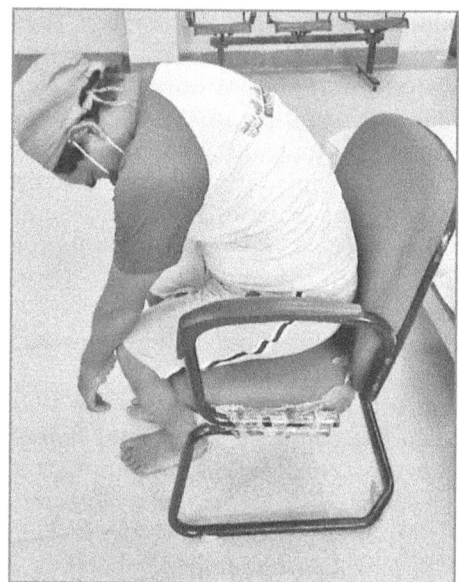

Fig. 37.7: Flexion in sitting.

The position is held for 2 seconds and again brought to vertical position. 10 repetitions of exercise for several times in a day as per need are performed **(Fig. 37.6)**.

- **McKenzie exercises for anterior derangement/flexion dysfunction of lumbar spine:**
  » Flexion in lying: Lying flexion is the first step in restoring the bending forward motion of the lower back. Once the back pain has improved, begin with this exercise in order to regain range of motion. Patient is made to lie down on the back, with the feet flat on the floor, hip-width apart. He/she is asked to pull both the knees towards the chest, keeping the tail bone on the bed/ground and hold the position for 2 seconds, followed by returning to starting position. 6 repetitions of exercise, several times a day as per need is performed, if there is a relief from the symptoms **(Fig. 37.1)**.

❖ **Flexion in sitting:** This exercise helps to restore the forward bending motion of the lumbar spine. The patient is made to sit on the edge of the chair, with the back straight and feet flat on the floor. He/she is asked to bend forwards and stretch the hands towards the floor, hold the bent posture for 2 seconds and then return to vertical position. 6 repetitions of exercise, several times a day as per need are performed **(Fig. 37.7)**.

❖ **Flexion in standing:** This exercise increases the spines ability to bend forwards. The patient is asked to stand with the feet shoulder width apart and bend forward at the hips, towards the floor keeping the knees straight. The position is held for 1–2 seconds and reversed to starting position. 6 repetitions of exercise several times a day as per need are performed **(Fig. 37.8)**.

❖ **McKenzie exercises for neck pain:** The exercises selected depends on the cause of neck pain, i.e., postural, dysfunction or derangement.

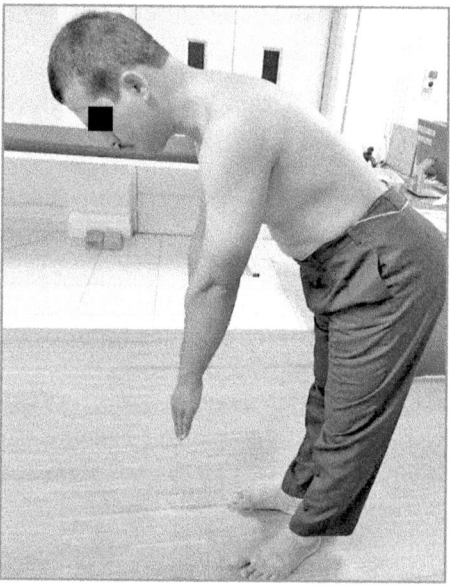

Fig. 37.8: Flexion in standing.

- **For postural neck pain:**
  » Neck retraction/Chin tucks: Patient is asked to sit with back straight, head vertically over the shoulders, and lower the chin towards the chest and hold for 15–30 seconds and then relax. A few repetitions, several times a day are advised **(Fig. 37.9)**.
- **For neck pain due to derangement:** The exercises performed are:
  » Neck retraction exercises described above, if there is no peripheralization of symptoms.
  » Neck extension in supine: The supine patient is made to lie with the neck and head at the edge of bed towards the head end. The head is supported by the clinician/care giver, and the patient is asked to tuck the chin back and extend the neck. The position

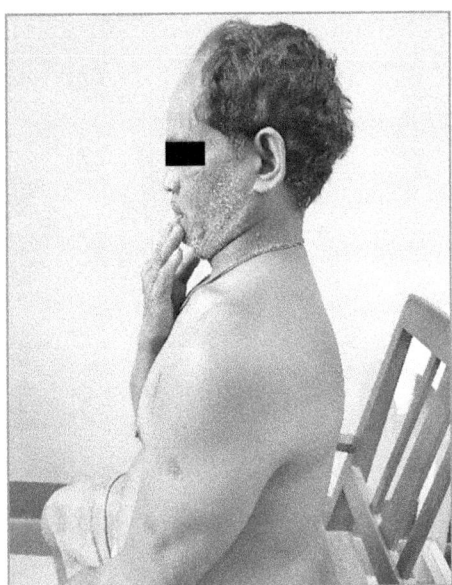

Fig. 37.9: Neck retraction/chin tuck exercise.

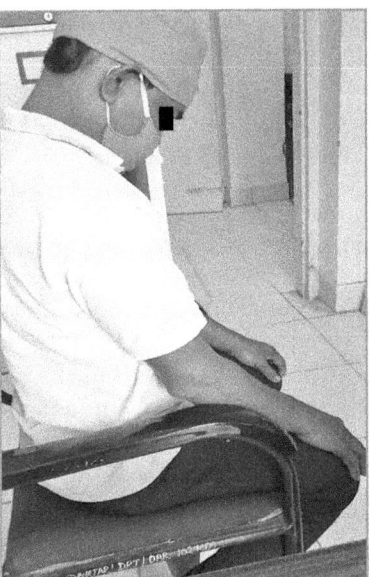

Fig. 37.11: Neck flexion exercise in sitting.

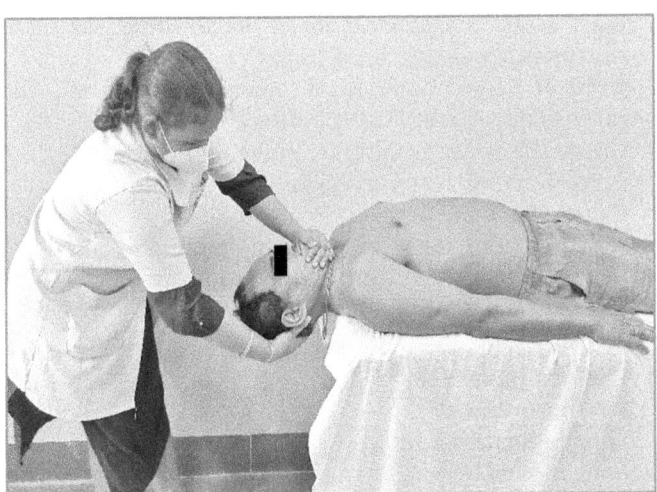

Fig. 37.10: Neck extension in supine.

is held for few seconds and brought to the initial position by the clinician. The same are performed several times in a day **(Fig. 37.10)**.
» Neck extension in sitting: The sitting patient with the back straight and head vertical over the shoulders is asked to tuck the chin and bring the base of the skull towards the back, hold for few seconds and repeat the same for several times.
– **For pain due to cervical dysfunction**:
  » Neck extension exercises: The exercises selected depends on the type of dysfunction. If extension dysfunction exists, exercises described above for the cervical derangement can be performed, provided, there is no radicular pain in the upper limbs (As commonly occurs in advanced cervical spondylosis).
  » Neck flexion exercises: The sitting patient with head vertical over the shoulders is asked to bend the neck forward, apply over pressure at the end and sustain the pressure for 3-4 seconds. The exercises are repeated several times in a day **(Fig. 37.11)**.
  » Neck side flexion exercises: Patient sitting with neck retracted. He she is asked to guide the head with own hand towards the direction of movement limitation, till a gentle stretch is felt on the opposite side muscles followed by returning to neutral position. Five repetitions on each side several times a day are performed.
  » Neck rotation exercises: Patient sitting with neck retracted. He/she is asked to rotate the neck to one side, brings the nose over the shoulder and then return to neutral position. Five repetitions on each side several times a day are performed.

Contraindications for McKenzie's Method

❖ If in the examination, no position or movement can be found which reduces the presenting pain, the patient is unsuitable for this mechanical therapy.
❖ Patients having saddle anaesthesia and bladder incontinence are contraindicated.
❖ Patients who exhibits signs of extreme pain.
❖ Developmental or acquired anomalies of bone structures, which may lead to instability of mechanical articulations.
❖ Architectural faults, such as spondylolisthesis, should be excluded from the mechanical therapy.

MAITLAND APPROACH

The concept of treatment is named after its pioneer GD Maitland in 1950s, who was seen as a pioneer in musculoskeletal physiotherapy. The Maitland concept of manual therapy, emphasizes a specific way of thinking, continuous evaluation and a total commitment to the patient, while delivering therapy. It mainly deals with the concept of examination, treatment and assessment by passive movement. The passive movements applied to reduce pain and increase ROM are of two types, such as:

1. **Physiological movements**: Movements produced in the joints in the cardinal planes of body, which can be measured and produced actively are the physiological movements. Flexion/extension, abduction/adduction, external rotation/internal rotation are the physiological movements.

    The body levers that become dysfunctional are moved passively in a graded manner to restore movement, which are subsequently maintained by active exercises.
2. **Accessory movements**: The movements, which are associated with physiological movements, without which active/passive physiological movements are not possible are the accessory movements. These include joint play movements such as rolling, gliding, spinning, traction, distraction, etc.

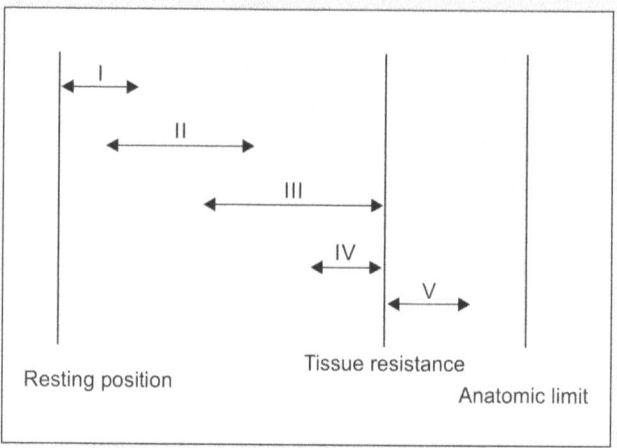

Fig. 37.12: Grades of Maitland mobilization.

The treatment is based upon, a detailed subjective and objective examinations. The aims of subjective examination are:
- To identify, how the patient is affected by the disorder.
- To establish the extent of physical examination and desired effect of treatment based on SIN (Severity, Irritability, Nature).
- To generate hypothesis.

SIN factor, which is an important determinant of therapy has the components such as:
- **Severity**: Refers to the intensity of symptoms, and the extent that they limit normal activity. It can be rated using different pain rating scales, such as: 0–10 Numerical pain rating scale/visual analogue scale.
- **Irritability**: Refers to the ease in which the symptoms are produced and the time it takes to settle. For example, onset of symptom immediately on movement or after sustained activities, such as the symptoms persisting for 10–15 minutes after the patient stands up straight.
- **Nature**: It refers to type and extent of injury producing symptoms. For example:
    - *Type:* Aching, throbbing, burning, stabbing, sharp, dull, deep, superficial, etc.
    - *Symptom behavior:* Radiating, referred, local, etc.
    - *Tissue and injury:* Sprain, degenerative joint disorder, fracture, osteoporosis, multi tissue trauma, neural tension.
    - *Degree of injury:* Mild to severe, etc.

Principles of the Techniques

Techniques of treatment are based on the passive movements that provokes or relieves patient's symptoms based on SIN. The direction and grades of mobilization depends on the desired effect, i.e., to reduce pain or stiffness.

Grades of Mobilization

Five grades of mobilization are used (**Fig. 37.12**). Lower grades (I and II) are used to reduce pain and irritability. Higher grades (III and/or IV) are used to stretch the joint capsule and passive tissues which support and stabilise the joint so increase range of movement. Grade-V is the manipulation. The grades of mobilization are briefly discussed below:
- **Grade I:** Small amplitude movement at the beginning of the available range of movement (small amplitude out of resistance).
- **Grade II:** Large amplitude movement within the available range of movement(large amplitude out of resistance).
- **Grade III:** Large amplitude movement that moves into stiffness or muscle spasm (Large amplitude into resistance)
- **Grade IV:** Small amplitude movement stretching into stiffness or muscle spasm(Small amplitude into resistance).
- **Grade V:** High velocity thrusts, between physiological and anatomical limits.

The passive accessory movements given include:
- A-P (anteroposterior)
- P-A (posteroanterior)
- Longitudinal caudad
- Longitudinal cephalad
- Joint distraction
- Medial glide
- Lateral glide

Passive accessory inter vertebral movements of the spine can be symbolically represented as under (**Figs. 37.13A and B**):

Rates and rhythm of mobilization: The rate and rhythm of mobilization could be:
- **Sustained**: Where pressure is applied without any oscillations. It is applied for painful conditions, where the patient can not tolerate oscillatory movements, as well as for stiff joints, where a sustained force is applied to elongate soft tissues through creep.
- **Smooth rhythmical oscillations:** The rhythmical movements given are categorized into three types such as:
    1. **Slow:** 1 oscillation for 2 seconds, i.e., 30 oscillations per minute are given. This is selected for more acute conditions.
    2. **Medium:** 1 oscillation per second, i.e., 60 oscillations per minute.
    3. **Fast:** In this 2 oscillations are given in a second, which are used for more chronic conditions.

the structures responsible for patient's pain. Lesions of contractile tissue (muscles, musculotendinous junction, body of tendons, teno-osseus junction, bone at insertion of tendon) are established by resisted isometric contractions (RIC), whereas lesion of inert structures are established by passive movements. If passive elongation is painful, but resisted isometric contraction is painless, the inert tissues are at fault, whereas, pain in passive elongation, combined with pain on resisted isometric contraction, mostly indicates pathologies in contractile structures (muscles/tendons).

- **Resisted isometric contraction (RIC):** For resisted isometric contractions, the joint should be held in mid-range, so that, no inert structures are stretched. The patient should be asked to produce a maximal contraction of the muscles, against the resistance offered by the clinician. The results of RIC, should be interpreted as follows:
  – Strong and painless—normal.
  – Strong and painful—minor lesion in muscles or tendon.
  – Weak and painful—significant lesion in muscle/tendon, possible fracture.
  – Weak and painless—complete rupture or nerve lesion.
- **Passive movements:** Assessment of lesions of inert tissues (structures that lack the capacity to contract and relax such as capsule, ligaments, bursa, fascia, neural tissues and cartilage) are tested by passive stretching/squeezing. The findings of passive movements are:
  – **Capsular/non-capsular pattern of limitations:** If the limitation of movement is in a capsular or non-capsular pattern, the inert structures are at fault. The capsular pattern of limitation of various joints have been described in Chapter 1.
  – **End feels:** It is the perception of tissue resistance at the end of passive movements. Different types of pathological end feels imply different disorders. The normal and pathological end feels have been described in Chapter 1.
  – **Pain behavior of different tissues:**
    » Bone → Minimum reference with local area of tenderness.
    » Capsules, ligaments, bursa → Refer pain strongly.
    » Muscles, tendons → Minimal reference.
- **Tests performed by Dr Cyriax for spine:** It focuses on examinations to establish the presence of:
  – *Bone signs:* Any deviations of vertebrae (scoliosis), erosion of vertebrae, tenderness, etc.
  – *Joint signs:* Limitation of movements if any, and cause of the limitation. For example, if flexion limitation in lumbar spine exists in an individual below the age of 60 years, it could be due to a lesion of the lumbar disc. However, in individuals above 60 years, if lumbar flexion reduces symptoms, it may be a severely eroded hard disc lesion, with significant reduction of intervertebral space and laxity of posterior longitudinal ligament (when bent forward, the PLL, becomes tight, reducing the disc protrusion).
  – *Dural signs:* Straight leg raise test, straight leg raise test combined with neck flexion, if increases pain, involvement of dura mater is confirmed.

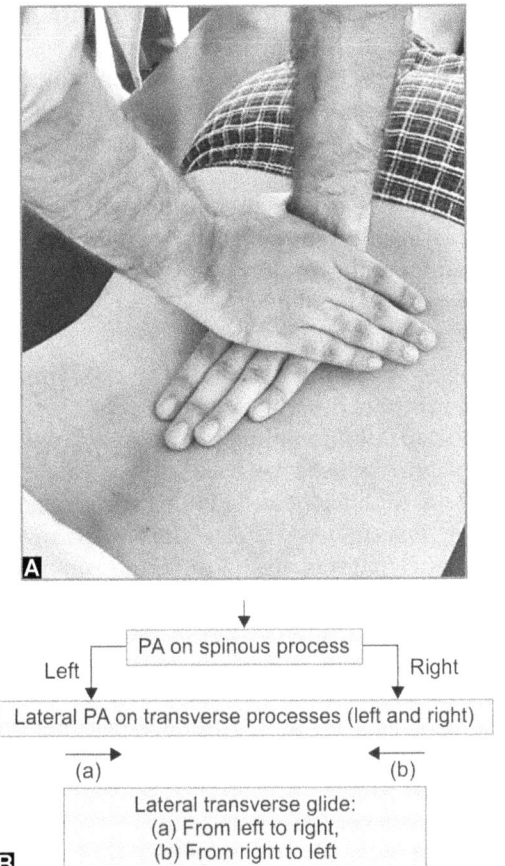

Figs. 37.13A and B: Shows symbolic representation of accessory mobilization of spinal column: (A) Central PA mobilization, (B) Lateral PA and Lateral transverse mobilization.

Contraindications of Maitland mobilization: It includes red flags such as cancer, recent fracture, open wound or active bleeding, infective arthritis, joint fusion, etc.

CYRIAX APPROACH

James Cyriax an orthopaedic Surgeon in England has developed a system of Orthopedic medicine over an extended period starting in the early 1920s. The scope of his treatment includes lesions of ligaments, tendons, bursa, and muscles along with lesions of cervical, thoracic and lumbar spines.

The basic principles/philosophy of Cyriax orthopaedic medicine are:
- Every pain has an anatomical source.
- Treatment must reach that anatomical source.
- Treatment must benefit the source in order to relieve the pain.
- A specific diagnosis leads to successful treatment.

Cyriax's methods of management focusses on assessment and management of dysfunctions in peripheral and spinal joints.

- **Tests performed in the technique for peripheral joints:**

Selective tissue tension tests: The test consists of active-range of motion, passive range of motion, and resistive tests, followed by palpation of anatomical structures, to identify

- *Nerve root mobility:* Straight leg raise test for sciatic nerve, prone knee bend test for femoral nerve, etc., should be performed to establish, whether the nerve roots are moving freely (in normal situations) or there is restriction with mobility of the nerve root due to a displaced disc/projecting osteophytes.
- *Nerve root conduction:* Motor, sensory and deep tendon reflex examinations should be made to establish the nerve root conduction. For example, a weak quadriceps, combined with reduced knee jerk and sensory impairment in the front of thigh (L3 dermatome), suggests reduced conduction in L3 root.
- *Cord sign (if any):* Presence of spasticity/extensor plantar response (if any) should be noted, as these contradict manipulation.

❖ **Assessment of patient using Cyriax principle:**
  - Complain and demographic data:
  - Subjective examination:
  - Nature of symptoms/pain (site and spread, onset and duration and behavior)
  - Objective examination
  - Observation of posture and movements:
  - Inspection: Skin color, wasting, deformity, swelling.
  - Palpation: Warmth, swelling, synovial thickening.
  - Active movements: Tests for inert and contractile tissue. Active range of motion, pain, willingness to produce movement.
  - Passive movements: Tests for inert tissues.
  - Resisted movements: Tests for contractile tissues.
  - Establishment of soft disc and hard disc lesion: As per Dr. Cyriax, after the age of 60, the nucleus pulposus, becomes hard and disappears and the disc becomes uniform (i.e., annulus fibrosus and nucleus pulposus structurally become same)
  - Neurological tests: To find abnormal root signs/cord signs, saddle anesthesia, etc.
  - Investigations: X-ray, ultrasound scan/CT scan/MRI, EMG, blood tests.
  - Interpretation/Evaluation: Identification of anatomic structures associated with lesion. It includes and specifies whether the spinal disc lesion is soft or hard type, whether the limitation of movement is due to pain, muscle/ligament/capsular tightness/loose body in the joint, etc. It also establishes the source of pain (if any).

In lumbar disc lesion, if pain comes first in the legs, suggests primary posterolateral disc bulge (where manipulation is contraindicated). If back pain and leg pain occur simultaneously, metastatic lesions should be excluded.

Presence of cord signs (spasticity and extensor plantar response), if any should be tested in pathologies involving cervical/thoracic/lumbar (L1 and above) spines (as this contradicts manipulation).

❖ **Treatment:** The components of treatment include:
  - Injection.
  - Transverse friction massage: Deep transverse friction massage, is a very useful technique for the treatment of traumatic and overuse soft tissue lesions. It imposes cyclic loading, without bringing too much tension on the healing longitudinal structures of tendons and ligaments, and is found to be beneficial.
  - Manipulation: It consists of rapid, small amplitude, thrusting passive movements (grade-C mobilization), used to reduce small cartilaginous displaced fragments, both in the spine and peripheral joints (loose bodies).
  - Mobilization: Grade-A, B mobilizations are used to stretch capsular adhesions, and to improve the function of ligaments and tendons.
  - Exercises and modalities.
  - Patient education.

The methods of treatment used by Cyriax, important to Physiotherapists are described below.

❖ **Mobilization/Manipulation:** Three grades of mobilization/manipulation are used, such as:
  - *Grade-A:* Mobilizations within pain free range.
  - *Grade-B:* Sustained stretch at the end of range,
  - *Grade-C:* High velocity low amplitude manipulation at the end of the range.

Grade "A" and "B" mobilizations are movements of low velocity with varying amplitude, remaining within the physiological limit and within the patients tolerance and control, where as a grade "C" mobilization/manipulation usually consists of a single thrust of high velocity and low amplitude, performed at the end of the passive movement, after the slack has been taken up.

Traction during Manipulation

Most of the manipulations described by Cyriax, are performed under traction. For the cervical and thoracic spines, traction is applied by the therapist/manipulator with the help of a fixing belt, or by an assistant, where as for the lumbar spine traction is already built into the maneuver.

General summary of manipulation: Though the procedures vary from joint to joint, the purpose and common techniques are briefly summarized below.
❖ The purpose of manipulation is to reduce a displacement in the peripheral and spinal joints.
❖ The techniques involve:
  - Application of manual traction.
  - Moving the joint into extreme range (to take the slack).
  - Application of overpressure.

Manipulation of Peripheral Joints

Manipulative reductions of displacements/loose bodies in elbow, wrist, hip, knee and ankle have been described by Cyriax. The principles involved are:
❖ The clinician applies long axis traction to distract the joint surfaces, allowing room for the loose fragment to move.
❖ Then, the joint is twisted in an endeavour to shift the loose fragment.
❖ The patient is then re-examined, to see, if the displacement, now lies in a more favourable position.

Indications of spinal manipulation described by Cyriax:
❖ The sole indication for spinal manipulation is reduction of a cartilaginous disc displacement, found in 2/3rd of sufferers

with lumbar disc displacement under the age of 60 years and for all patients over the age of 60 (hard disc lesion).
- Primary posterolateral protrusion (sciatica without immediately preceding backache) under the age of 60 is the nuclear protrusion (soft disc lesion), which should not be manipulated.

Manipulative Techniques for Spine

- **Lumbar spine:**
  - **Rotation strains:** Though engagement of the facet joints greatly limit rotation of the lumbar spine, a rotation strain is a highly effective way of achieving reduction at lower lumbar disc lesions. Rotation strains applied are:
    » Rotation strain-I.
    » Rotation strain-II.
    » Rotation strain-III.
    » Rotation strain-IV.
    » Rotation strain-V
  - **Extension strain:** The extension strains are mostly applied to elderly people, and those having minor protrusions. Extension strains applied are:
    » Forced extension-1.
    » Forced extension-2.
    » Forces extension-3.
    » Forced extension-4.
    » Forced extension-5.
  - **Correction of lateral deviation;**
    » **Correction of lateral deviation-1:** The patient is placed in supine and made to flex both hips. If the deviation is to left, the left thigh is supported over the right, and the clinician pushes the lower knee (right knee in the example), and pulls the upper knee (left knee in the example) **Figure 37.14**. This is done several times (approximately 10 minutes, until the spine stays vertical after the patient has stood for a while).

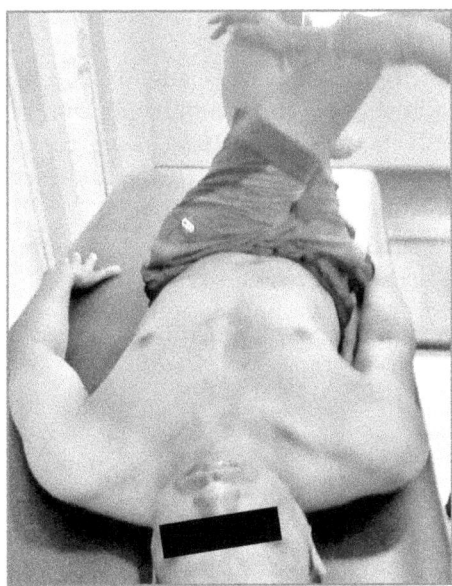

Fig. 37.14: Correction of lateral deviation.

» **Correction of lateral deviation-2:** In the standing posture, the manipulator put his/her hands round the patient's pelvis on the convex side and places his/her chest against the patient's arm on the concave side. Then he/she pulls the pelvis towards himself, and repeats the movement several times and holds the corrected posture for few minutes.

- **Thoracic spine:**
Rotation strains applied to relieve blocked thoracic joints are of the following types:
  - Rotation during traction-1.
  - Rotation during traction-2.
  - Rotation during traction-3.
  - Rotation during traction-4.

- **Cervical spine:** The treatment of cervical disc lesion (except postero-central disc protrusion) is immediate manipulative reduction. The principles of manipulation are:
  - Manual traction is applied throughout.
  - Overpressure is administered, during continued traction.
  - The neck should never be manipulated in flexion. It should be held either in neutral position or slight extension.
  - The patient should be re-examined after the manoeuvre. The cervical manipulations performed are:
    » Rotation during traction-1.
    » Rotation during traction-2.
    » Side flexion during traction.
    » Antero-posterior glide during traction.
    » Lateral gliding without traction.
    » Traction with leverage.

- **Transverse friction massage (TFM):** It is a technique devised by Cyriax, whereby repeated cross-grain massage is applied to muscle, tendon, tendon sheath or ligament to increase the mobility and extensibility of individual musculoskeletal tissues and to help prevent and treat inflammatory scar tissue. This type of massage is indicated for acute or sub acute ligament, tendon, or muscle injuries, chronically inflamed bursae and to break adhesions in ligaments, muscles and inter tissue structures.
  - **Duration of massage:**
    » **In acute conditions**: The duration of transverse friction massage is: Gentle massage up to 10 minutes.
    » **In chronic conditions** : Deep transverse friction massage up to numbness plus 10 minutes of massage there after.

  Transverse friction massage can also be applied before performing a manipulation or strong stretch to desensitize and soften the tissues.
  Transverse friction massage has the following therapeutic effects:
    » **Traumatic hyperaemia:** According to Cyriax, longitudinal friction to an area increases the flow of blood and lymph, which, in turn, removes the chemical irritant by-products of inflammation. In addition, the increased blood flow reduces

venous congestion, thereby decreasing edema and hydrostatic pressure on pain-sensitive structures.
- » **Pain relief**: The application of transverse friction massage stimulates type I and II mechanoreceptors, producing presynaptic anaesthesia. This presynaptic anesthesia is based on the gate theory of pain control.
- » **Mobilizing scar tissue**: The transverse nature of the friction assists with the orientation of the collagen in the appropriate lines of stress and also helps produce hypertrophy of the new collagen. Given the stages of healing for soft tissues, light transverse friction massage should only be applied in the early stages of a sub acute lesion, so as not to damage the granulation tissue. These gentle movements theoretically serve to minimize cross-linking and so enhance the extensibility of the new tissue. Following a ligament sprain, Cyriax recommends immediate use of gentle transverse friction massage to prevent adhesion formation between the tissue and its neighbours, by moving the ligamentous tissue over the underlying bone.
- ❖ Modalities such as Cryotherapy/Heat therapy to reduce inflammation and pain. Range of motion exercises, strengthening exercises to maintain mobility and function are emphasized.
- ❖ Patient should be educated about his/her pathology and the need for maintenance program after receiving therapy.

Contraindications of Cyriax Mobilization

- ❖ Contraindications to Transverse friction massage:
  - Ossification/calcification of soft tissues.
  - Bacterial and rheumatoid type tendinitis, tenosynovitis, tenovaginitis.
  - Skin ulcers/blisters/psorias.
  - Bursitis.
  - Hematoma (large).
- ❖ Contraindications to mobilization/manipulation:
  - Hypermobile joints.
  - Bleeding disorders and anticoagulant therapy.
  - Spinal tumors (including hemangiomas).
  - Severe osteoporosis.
  - Unstable fractures.
  - Bone infections (osteomyelitis).
  - Rheumatoid arthritis/psoriatic arthritis/ankylosing spondylitis.
  - Cord signs/neurological deficits.

KALTENBORN'S ORTHOPEDIC MANUAL THERAPY

Kaltenborn technique uses a combination of traction and mobilization to reduce pain and to mobilize hypomobile joints. According to Kaltenborn, all joint mobilizations when performed correctly, should be made parallel or at right angles to the plane of joint motion. The mobilizing force applied by Kaltenborn is sustained in nature, as compared to oscillatory forces applied by Maitlands. The treatment primarily focuses on joint capsule. A common goal in orthopedic manual therapy (OMT) is to restore the gliding component of roll-gliding to normalize movement mechanics, as rolling movements in the absence of gliding can be damaging to the joint.

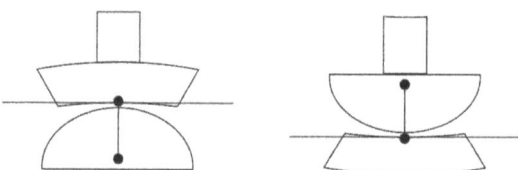

Fig. 37.15: Shows Kaltenborn's treatment plane.

Kaltenborn's methods supplemented traditional physical medicine approaches with treatment techniques for pain relief, reduction of muscle spasm, and stretching tight structures in joints.

Kaltenborn's treatment plane: The treatment plane passes through the joint and lies at right angle to a line running from the axis of rotation in the convex bony partner, to the deepest aspect of the articulating concave surface (**Fig. 37.15**). The treatment plane remains with the concave joint surface, whether the moving joint partner is convex or concave. Testing of joint play, or joint mobilization is done by moving the bone parallel to or at a right angle to the Kaltenborn treatment plane.

Translatoric (linear) joint play movements: Translatoric joint play movements used in the technique are:
- ❖ Traction.
- ❖ Compression.
- ❖ Gliding.

There are two methods of determining the direction of restricted joint gliding, such as:
- ❖ **The glide test**: Passive translatoric gliding movements are applied in all possible directions to determine in which directions joint gliding is restricted, and what is the end feel. Gliding tests should be performed in the joint's resting and non-resting positions.
- ❖ **Kaltenborn concave-convex rule**: When convex surface moves over concave surface, roll and glides occur in the opposite direction (**Fig. 37.16A**). When, concave surface moves over convex surface, roll and glide occurs in the same direction (**Fig. 37.16B**).

Grades of translatoric movement of Kaltenborn: There are three grades of movements (**Fig. 37.17**). The grades are determined by the amount of joint slack (looseness and resistance) in the joint. The slack is taken up when testing

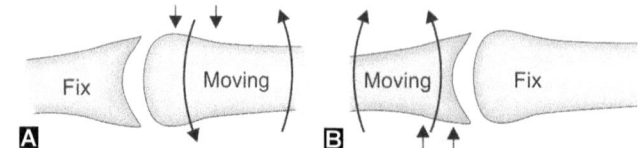

Figs. 37.16A and B: Demonstrates concave-convex rule: (A) Convex surface moving over concave; (B) Concave surface moving over convex.

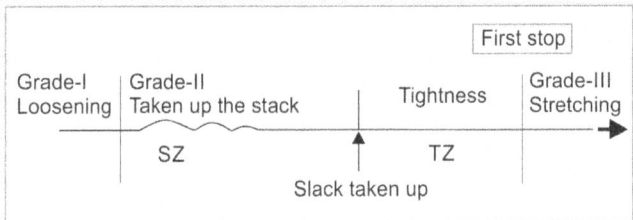

Fig. 37.17: Shows grades of translatory movements.
(SZ, slack zone; TZ, transition zone)

and treating joints with gliding or traction. When gliding is performed, the slack is taken up in the direction of joint gliding. When traction is performed, slack is taken up in the direction of traction. The criteria of different grades are briefly discussed below:
- In the grades I and II, slack zone (SZ) range, the therapist senses little or no resistance.
- In the grade II, transition zone (TZ), the therapist senses gradually increasing resistance.
- At the first stop, the therapist, senses marked resistance, as the slack is taken up, and all tissues become taut.
- In grade III, Stretching occurs beyond first stop.

Clinical Uses of Translatoric Grades

- **Grade-I (Loosen):** Relieves pain.
- **Grade-II (Tighten):** Initial treatment, maintains joint play.
- **Grade-III (Stretch):** Stretches joint and increases joint play.

Indications of Kaltenborn's Translatory Mobilization

- Restricted joint play (hypomobility).
- Abnormal end feels.

Contraindications (Absolute)

- Malignancy in treatment area.
- Infectious arthritis.
- Metabolic bone disease.
- Ankylosis.
- Osteomyelitis.
- Fracture/ligament rupture.
- Hypermobility.

Contraindications (Relative)

- Excessive pain or swelling.
- Arthroplasty.
- Pregnancy.
- Spondylolisthesis.
- Rheumatoid arthritis.
- Vertebro basilar insufficiency.

MENNEL'S APPROCH

Dr. John Mennell introduced the theory of joint play as a therapeutic manual medicine technique. As per him, loss of normal joint movement or joint play, can lead to dysfunction, and joint manipulation can restore normal joint play movements.

Dr. Mennell defined joint play, as small movements, within a synovial joint, that are independent of voluntary muscle contraction, but essential for maximal pain free movements of joints. As per Dr. Mennell, the prime fault of joint dysfunction in synovial joints is the impaired joint play. When the prime faults, can be corrected, this leads to correction of secondary abnormalities.

The movements such as rolls, glides, spins, distraction, etc., can not be produced by voluntary muscle contraction. All anatomical movements individuals produce, are the summation of joint play, and physiological movements produced by voluntary muscle contractions. These small movements, which are involuntary in nature, measure not more than 1/8th inch in any plane, and follow the contour of the opposing joint surfaces. Although small, the integrity of joint play movements, greatly affects the production of gross voluntary movements in synovial joints. After joint play evaluation, Joint mobilization is used to treat joint dysfunction.

Examination of joint-play movements: The joint play, that are examined passively, could be hypomobility, normal or hypermobility, which are graded as follows:
- **Hypomobility:**
  - Grade-0: No movements (ankylosis).
  - Grade-1: Considerable decreased movements.
  - Grade-2: Slightly decreased movements.
- **Normal:** Grade-3.
- **Hypermobility:**
  - Grade-4: Slightly increased movements.
  - Grade-5: Considerable increased movement.
  - Grade-6: Complete instability.

Dr. Mennell clearly defined 10 rules for joint play examination and treatment. These include:
- The patient must be relaxed.
- The therapist must remain relaxed. Therapeutic grasp must be firm, painless and protective.
- One joint must be examined and mobilized at a time. Complex joints should be broken into component joints, for example, examination and treatment of wrist joint must involve, radiocarpal, ulnocarpal and intercarpal articulations.
- One movement in a joint should be restored at a time.
- One aspect of the joint should be stabilized, while moving the other aspect.
- Extent of movement is same as assessed in the same joint on the opposite side.
- No forceful or abnormal movement should ever be used.
- The manipulative movement is a sharp thrust with velocity, to result in 1/8th inch gapping or sliding in the joint being treated.
- Therapeutic movements occur, when all of the slack, has been taken up in the joint.
- No therapeutic maneuver is done in the presence of joint inflammation/disease.

Joint dysfunction once identified, treated by the techniques/strategies described under. Dr. Mennell highlighted four basic principles/facts in practice such as:
1. When a joint is not free to move, the muscles that move the joint can not be free to move.
2. Muscles can not be restored to normal, if the joints that they move are not free to move.
3. Normal muscle function is dependent on normal joint movements/joint play.
4. Impaired muscle function may cause deterioration in abnormal joints.

Treatment strategies:
- Manipulation
- Mobilization
- Exercise and modalities
- Patient education.

MUSCLE ENERGY TECHNIQUE

The origin of the technique is credited to Fred Mitchell. The techniques require the active participation of the patient and are thus viewed as mobilization techniques, which utilize muscular facilitation and inhibition.

It is a form of manual therapy, that uses muscle's own energy, in the form of gentle isometric contractions, to relax the muscles through autogenic/reciprocal inhibition mechanisms, causing lengthening of muscles. If a submaximal contraction of the muscle is followed by stretching of the same muscle, it is called autogenic inhibition, whereas, if a submaximal contraction of a muscle, results in lengthening of the opposite muscles, it is termed as reciprocal inhibition.

When a muscle contracts, after 7-10 seconds, the increased muscle tension, activates the Golgi tendon organ (GTO), causing inhibition of contraction (lengthening) of the agonist, and facilitation of the antagonists. When the agonist groups are lengthened, the muscle spindles are also lengthened, making the muscle lengthen further, as the reactivity of the spindle to undergo shortening is reduced.

The techniques, involve positioning a restricted muscle-joint complex at its restricted barrier, and making the muscle contract isometrically/concentrically/eccentrically, against the resistance offered by the clinician. After the muscle contracted, enough time should be given for the muscle to relax. It can be used to mobilize joints, strengthen weakened muscles, and stretch adaptively shortened muscles and fascia.

The amounts of force and counterforce are governed by the length and strength of the muscle group involved, as well as by the patient's symptoms. The clinician's force should match the effort of the patient, thus producing an isometric contraction and allowing no movement to occur, or it may overcome the patient's effort, thus moving the area or joint in the direction opposite to that in which the patient is attempting to move it, thereby incorporating an eccentric or isolytic contraction. An isolytic contraction occurs, where the clinician's force, overcomes the contraction of the muscle, thereby forcing it to lengthen.

The technique helps to manage somatic dysfunction, where harmony and rhythm of the body is disturbed due

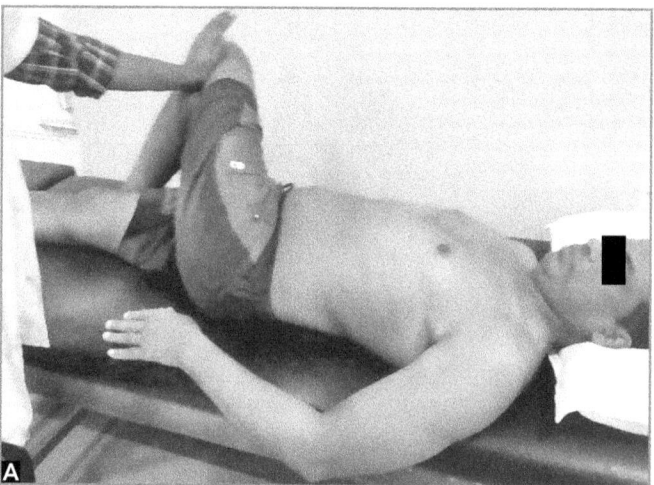

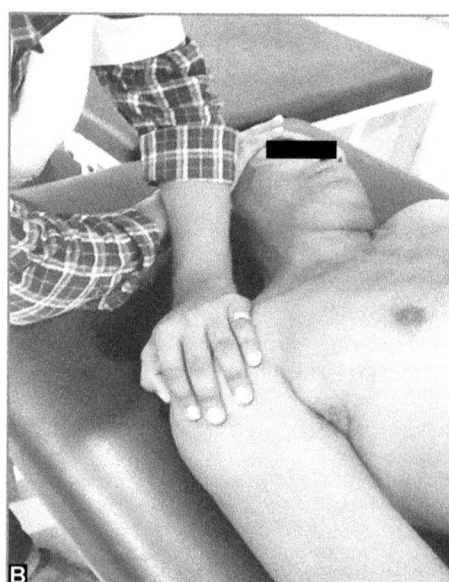

Figs. 37.18A and B: MET for: (A) Piriformis; (B) Upper trapezius.

to involvement of the musculoskeletal system causing asymmetric pattern of motion, pain and impairments. Somatic dysfunctions (where the motion barrier is encountered before the physiological barrier is reached) are treated by restoring the muscles around a joint to their normal neurophysiologic state, through either stretching or strengthening the agonist and antagonist muscle groups. **Figures 37.18A and B** show application of muscle energy technique (MET) to piriformis and upper trapezius muscles.

STRAIN/COUNTER STRAIN (POSITIONAL RELEASE TECHNIQUE)

Strain-Counterstrain is a passive positional technique used in the treatment of musculoskeletal pain and related somatic dysfunction. It was developed in 1955 by an osteopathic physician, named Lawrence Jones. It is an effective and extremely gentle technique, because, its action for treatment moves the patient's body, away from the painful, restricted direction of motion **(Fig. 37.19)**. The technique uses a position of comfort of the body, its appendages and tissues to resolve

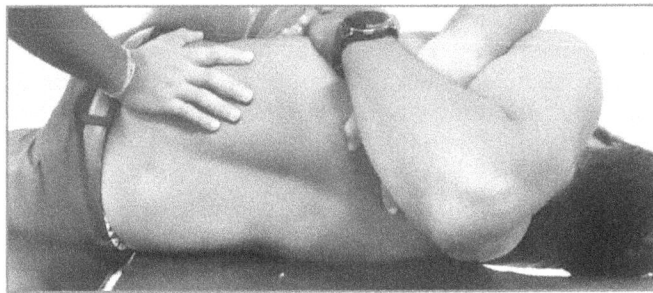

Fig. 37.19: Positional release technique for myofascial bands in left buttock and sacroiliac joint.

somatic dysfunction. The painless and delicate approach, makes the technique suitable for treating people with acute painful states.

Jones (1973), proposed that, as a result of somatic dysfunction, tissues often become kinked, or knotted, resulting in pain, spasm and loss of range of motion. The technique, unkinks tissues much, by gently twisting and pushing the tissues together, to take tension off the knot.

The therapist first identifies the myofascial trigger points/tender points on ligaments/muscles/joints on the client's body, and then applies a firm constant pressure, to this point, until the client experiences a subjective level of discomfort (4-5 in the 0-10 scale). The therapist then moves the tender body part away from the restricted motion barrier, towards the most comfortable position, where the point should no longer feel tender. The precise position should be held for 90 seconds (musculoskeletal conditions) to 3 minutes (for neurological disorders).

A possible neurophysiologic explanation of how and why these techniques work was first suggested by Korr, who postulated that an injured joint and its related tissues behaved differently from those of an uninjured joint in that the γ motor neuron activity in the former became increased. Bailey, later refined the theory by suggesting that an inappropriate high "gainset" of the muscle spindle resulted in changes characteristic of somatic dysfunction. Thus, the techniques of strain-counterstrain appear to serve to effect the muscle spindle-γ loop, by allowing the extrafusal muscle fibers to lengthen to their normal relaxed state, thereby decreasing spindle output and interrupting the pain-spasm cycle. Strain-counterstrain is also thought to improve blood flow to the area through a circulatory flushing of previously ischemic tissues.

The skill and success of strain-counterstrain techniques relies on the ability of the clinician to find the tender point and then to position, or move, the patient in such a way as to release muscular tension as well as relieve pain. This gentle and painless technique is a very effective treatment for a wide variety of orthopaedic conditions such as myofascial trigger points, fibromyalgia, sciatica, tendinitis, chronic neck pain, and post-surgical condition.

MYOFASCIAL RELEASE

Myofascial release (MFR) is a holistic, therapeutic approach to manual therapy, popularized by John Barnes. The technique offers a comprehensive approach for the evaluation and treatment of the myofascial system, the system of tissues and muscles in the body. This technique is designed to release restrictions such as trigger points, muscle tightness, and dysfunctions in soft tissue that may cause pain and limit motion in all parts of the body. It increases range of motion, reduces pain and enhances fascial mobility.

The technique involves application of gentle sustained pressure to the deep fascia, in order to release fascial restrictions, thereby restoring normal pain-free function. Clinicians use the elbow, knuckle, or fingertips creating localized hyperemia through deep friction. The technique relies entirely on the feedback received from the patient's tissues, with the clinician interpreting and responding to the feedback. This feedback is based on the Upledger concept of the natural body rhythm, called the craniosacral rhythm. It is this rhythm that is theorized to guide the clinician as to the direction, force, and the duration of the technique. It is not unusual for a patient to experience muscle soreness following the techniques. This soreness is thought to result from postural and alignment changes or from the techniques.

The soft tissue techniques used in myofascial release, help to break up the cross restrictions of the collagen of the fascia. The maneuvers used in the technique are:

- **J-stroke**: This technique is used to increase skin mobility. Counter pressure is applied with the heel of one hand, while a stroke in the shape of the letter "J" is applied in the direction of soft tissue restrictions, with 2 or 3 fingers, which creates some torque at the end of the stroke.
- **Vertical stroke:** The purpose of vertical stroking is to open up the length of vertically oriented fascia. As in the J stroke, counter pressure is applied with one hand, while the stroking is performed with the other.
- **Transverse stroke**: The stroking force is applied in a transverse direction to the body. The force is applied downwards into the muscle with the finger tips of both hands, and the force is applied slowly and perpendicular to the muscle fibers.
- **Cross-hands technique**: This technique is used for the release of deep fascial tissues. As shown in **Figure 37.20**

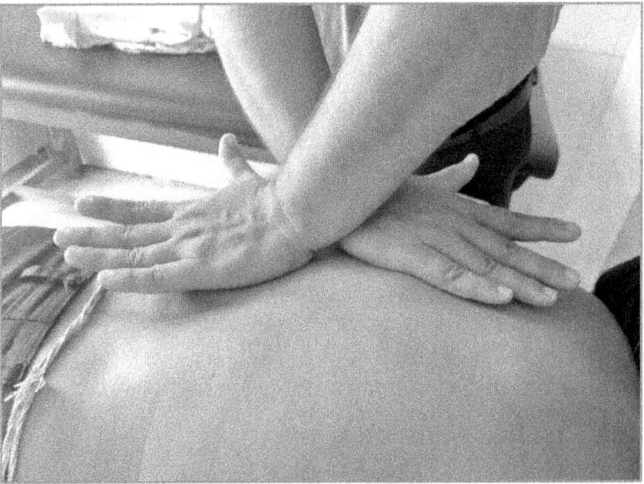

Fig. 37.20: Myofascial release (cross hand technique).

the clinician places the crossed hands over the site of tissue restrictions and stretches the elastic components of the fascia until the barrier is met. At the point of the barrier, the clinician maintains a consistent gentle pressure for approximately 90-120 seconds. Once the release of fascial restrictions are felt, the clinician reduces pressure.

- **Sustained pressure:** The technique is applied to the center of the restricted tissues, at exact depth, direction and angle of tissue restrictions. The technique can also be modified by applying force in either a clock wise or anti clock wise direction, while maintaining sustained pressure. The spiral motion so developed, increases tissue tension in one direction, while easing it in the other. The sustained pressure can also be applied perpendicular or parallel to the restricted tissue.
- **Ischemic compression:** Ischemic compression (where a sustained pressure is applied) can be applied on both the active and inactive trigger points. It is believed that, the ischemic compression deprives the trigger points of oxygen, rendering them inactive and breaking the cycle of pain-spasm-pain. The pressure is usually applied for 30–90 seconds. The treatment is repeated, if reduction of pain (both local and/or referred pain) is reported by the patient. If the pain does not subside, the pressure need to be adjusted and still if no benefit is obtained, this treatment should be stopped and alternative treatment should be applied.

Indications of the Technique

MFR can be used to treat pain and increase mobility in patients with a wide range of conditions, including back pain, neck pain, and fibromyalgia.

Contraindications

It is not applied in malignancy, aneurysm, acute rheumatoid arthritis, advanced diabetes, severe osteoporosis, and healing fractures.

Mulligan's Approach

Brian R Mulligan has developed the manual therapy technique such as natural apophyseal glides (NAGs), sustained natural apophyseal glides (SNAGs), mobilization with movements (MWMs) for extremities and spine, for practice by therapists, as well as a self treatment for spine and extremities for public. Mobilization with movement (MWM) is a manual therapy technique based on the analysis and correction of any minor positional fault in a joint. According to Mulligan, positional faults are due to various soft tissue and/or bone lesions in/around the joint.

Mulligan's Concept

- Injury to joints leads to positional faults and is responsible for limitation of physiological movements.
- The mobilization technique, when applied, overcomes joint tracking problems/positional faults.

Principles of Mulligan's Mobilization

- Pain free passive accessory gliding movements are applied as per Kaltenborn's principles.
- A thorough assessment to identify the comparable signs as described as Maitland, such as loss of joint movements/pain associated with movements/specific functional movements, should be done by the therapist.
- During mobilization, a continuous monitoring should be made for patients reaction, to ensure that no pain is reproduced.
- While sustaining the accessory glides, the patient should be requested to perform the comparable sign, which should improve with therapy.
- Failure to achieve improvement, indicates that, the therapist has not found the correct treatment plane, or the technique is not indicated.
- During treatment, the painful movement/activity is repeated by the patient, while the therapist applies the appropriate accessory glides.
- Mobilization with movement (MWM) is the concurrent application of sustained accessory mobilization applied by the therapist, while an active physiological movement to the end range is produced by the patient. Passive end of range over pressure/stretching is then applied by the therapist without pain as a barrier.
- Mobilization with movement (MWM), while applied as an assessment before treatment, PILL (Pain free, Instant, Long Lasting result), should be observed.
- The selected technique should not be applied in the absence of PILL response, and the principles of CROCKS, i.e., Contraindications (No PILL response), Repetitions (3 repetitions on day-1), Overpressure, Communication, knowledge of treatment planes and pathologies, Sustaining the mobilization throughout the movement should be followed.

Techniques of Mulligan's Mobilization

- **Sustained natural apophyseal glides (SNAGs):** It can be applied to spinal joints **(Fig. 37.21)**, rib cage and sacroiliac joints. The procedure involves:
- Application of appropriate accessory zygapophyseal glides by the therapist, while the patient performs the desired

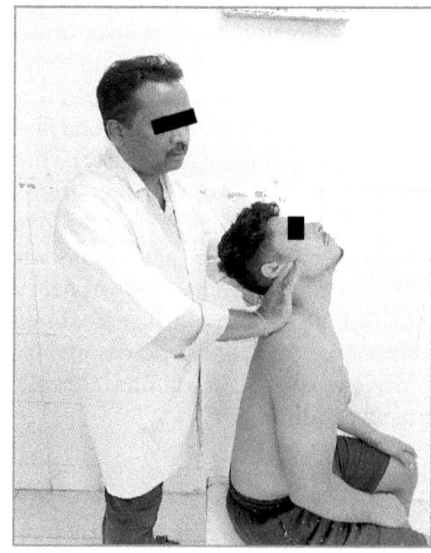

Fig. 37.21: SNAG to improve neck extension.

symptomatic movements. The resultant movement should be pain free.
- The techniques are usually performed in weight bearing positions. They can be adapted for use in the non-weight bearing positions also.

SNAG for Headache

Headache mostly affecting the occipital and parietal area (supplied by greater auricular-C2, C3, Greater/lesser occipital-C2, third occipital-C3 roots) is a presentation in pathologies, such as cervical spondylosis, affecting the upper cervical segments. SNAG applied to upper cervical spine in sitting is helpful in reducing such symptoms.

The procedure involves, the therapist standing on the side of the seated patient, cradles his/her (patient's) head between own body and forearm. The manoeuvre is started by placing the index, middle and ring fingers of the stabilizing hand (left hand in the figure), at the base of the occiput. The middle phalanx of the little finger of same hand is placed over the spinous process of C2. The lateral border of thenar eminence of the other hand is then placed on the top of the little finger of the hand placed over C2, and a gentle pressure is applied in a ventral direction on the spinous process of C2, keeping the patient's head steady as shown in **Figure 37.22**.

Natural Apophyseal Glides (NAGs)

This is applied for pathologies involving the cervical and upper thoracic spines, where movements are grossly restricted. It is the application of oscillatory mobilizations, instead of sustained glides. Mid to end range oscillatory antero-posterior facet joint mobilizations are applied along the treatment plane of C2 to T3 vertebrae as shown in **Figure 37.23**.

Mobilization with Movements (MWM) for Peripheral Joints

This could be mobilizations (glides and physiological movements) in weight bearing/non-weight bearing positions **(Figs. 37.24A and B)**, which largely depends on SIN factor.

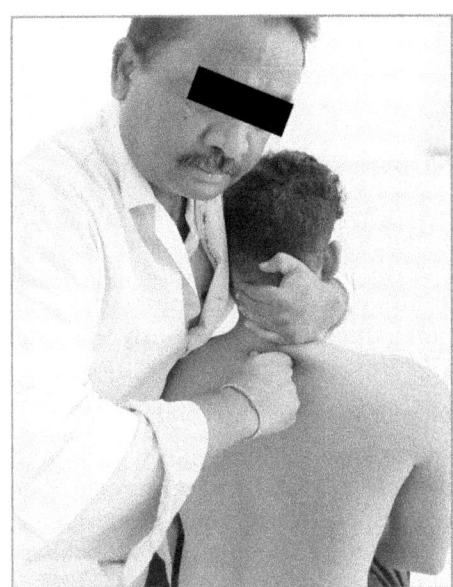

Fig. 37.23: NAG to cervicothoracic spine.

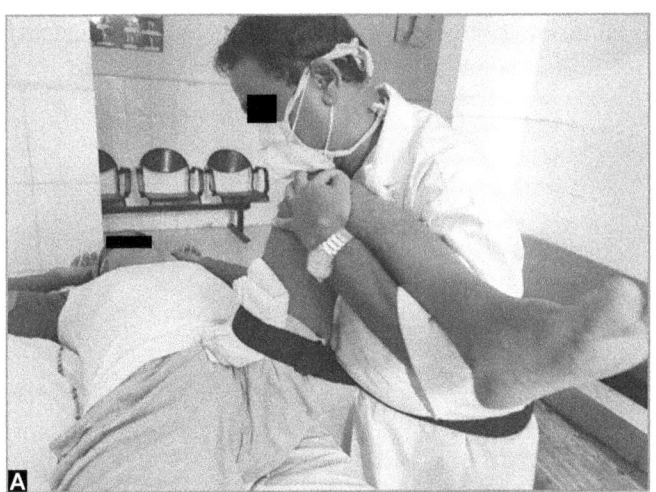

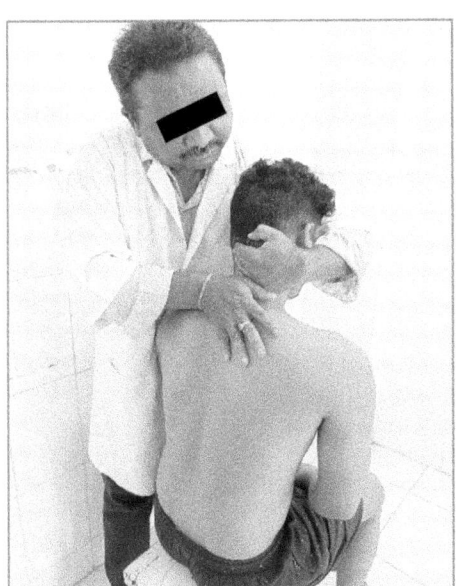

Fig. 37.22: SNAGs for headache.

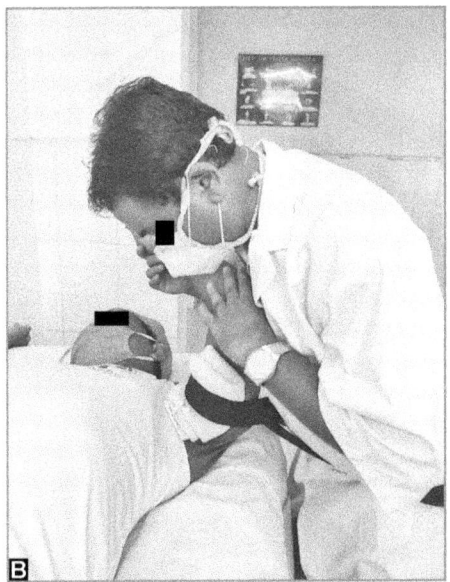

Figs. 37.24A and B: Mulligan's mobilization in non-weight bearing position for: (A) Hip rotation; (B) Shoulder rotation.

Once the glide has been chosen, it must be sustained, throughout the physiological movements, until the joint returns to its original starting position. The mobilizations are always into tissue resistance and should be pain free.

Spinal Mobilization with Limb Movement

If restriction of movement of the spine is also associated with restriction of movement of the joints of the limbs (in close proximity), the therapist while applying transverse pressure to the spine, asks the patient to concurrently move the limb, through the previously restricted range of movement.

Mobilization with Movement for Lumbar Spine

- **Extension in sitting:** The therapist stabilizes the pelvis with the belt **(Fig. 37.25)**, places one of his/her hands on the anterior aspects of the shoulder, and applies superior-anterior force on the spinous process of lumbar spine with the other hand, assisting in extension.
- **Flexion in sitting:** The therapist puts one of his/her hand on the back of the thorax, and pushes the spinous process of the lumbar spine superiorly, with the hook of the pisiform bone of the other hand. The pelvis is stabilized by a belt, connecting the pelvis of patient and therapist **(Fig. 37.26)**.

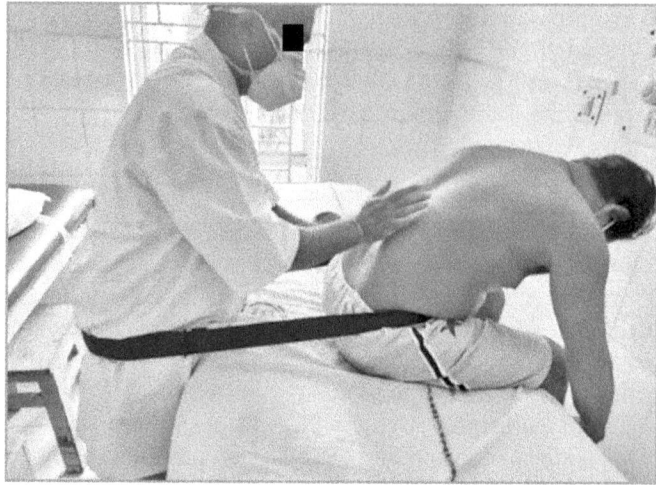

Fig. 37.26: Mulligan's mobilization to improve spinal flexion.

- **Extension in supine:** The therapist places both the hands around the lumbar spine, and compresses the hands. The patient extends the back, taking assistance from pushing with own hands.

Parameters for Practice of Mobilization with Movements

- **Repetitions/sets:** 10 repetitions, 3 sets in a session. A rest period of 30 seconds to 2 hours between sets should be followed.
- **No of sessions:** 3 to 6 sessions in a week.

Indications for Mulligan's Mobilization

- Painful conditions (non-inflammatory type), such as ankle sprain, tennis elbow, frozen shoulder, etc.
- Stiffness due to arthritis.
- Post surgical stiffness.
- Headache and dizziness due to cervical pathologies

Contraindications of Mulligan's Mobilization

- Joint hypermobility.
- Pregnancy.
- Osteopenia/osteoporosis.
- Vascular pathologies.
- Neurological deficits (multilevel PIVD, cervical myelopathy).

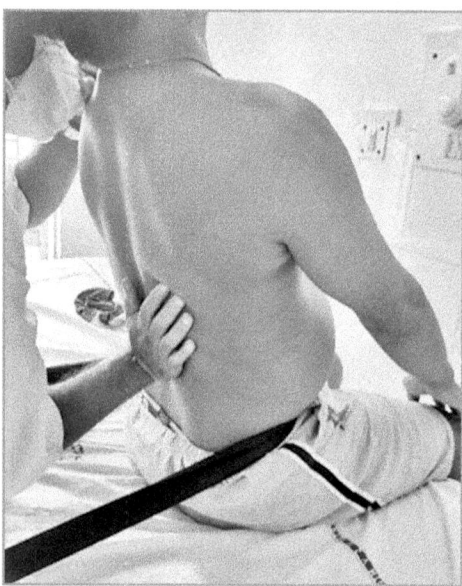

Fig. 37.25: Mulligan's mobilization to improve spinal extension.

Index

Page numbers followed by "*f*" refer to figure; and "*t*" refer to table.

A

Abdominal
 binder 480*f*, 491*f*, 541*f*
 incisions 539*f*
 reflex 33*f*, 396
 strengthening 127*f*, 480*f*
 support 540*f*
 surgeries 539
 thrust 515
Abduction 22, 24, 53, 54
 type fracture 299
Accessory movements 43, 600
 effects of 43
 joint movements, grading of 34, 34*t*
 use of 43
Active assisted exercise 39, 404*f*
Active exercises 34, 494
Active free exercise 37, 148
 effects of 38
 for shoulder flexors 38*f*
 use of 38
Active
 postures 12
 resisted exercise 39
 stretch of knee flexors 184*f*
 stretching 44
 test for medial epicondylitis 240*f*
Activity, assessment of 398
Acupressure 487
Acute inflammatory demyelinating polyneuropathy 467, 469
Acute motor axonal neuropathy 467
Acute motor sensory axonal neuropathy 467
Acute postoperative physiotherapy 266
Acute soft tissue injuries 52
Acute tennis elbow 235*f*
Adam's forward bending test 256
Adaptive postural control 6
Adduction 22, 24, 53, 54
 deformity of hip 30*f*
 type fracture 299
Adductor muscles 67*f*
Adductor strain 150
Adhesive capsulitis 226
 clinical features of 227
 diagnosis of 227
 management of 227
 pathophysiology of 227
 pathophysiology of 227
Adjunct devices 353
Adjustable ROM elbow orthosis 295*f*
Advanced lateral spine movements 259*f*
Aerobic exercises 534, 534*f*
Agnosia 364
Agonist contraction 45
Air mattress 400*f*
Air shift maneuver 515
Airplane splint 445*f*
Airway clearance 517
 techniques 547
Airway suctioning 519
Airways clearance 545
Alexander technique 134, 135*f*
Ambulation training 161
American Spinal Injury Association Motor score 389
American Thoracic Society grading 506
Amputation
 causes of 264
 incidence of 264
 indications for 264
 types of 264, 265
Amputee rehabilitation 266
Amputee rehabilitation, phases of 266
Amyotrophic lateral sclerosis 438
Aneurysm 359
Angular osteotomy 355
Ankle 23
 disorders of 196
 dorsiflexion 23*f*, 584*f*
 equinus, secondary 329*f*
 foot orthoses 351, 409
 jerk 32*f*
 joint 55, 192, 192*f*, 338
 ligaments, sprain of 196
 plantar flexion 23*f*
 special tests for 193
 sprain
  mechanism of 196*t*
  types of 196*t*
 strategy 13, 14*f*, 582*f*
  assessment of 368*f*
  development of 16*f*
 traction strap 274*f*
Ankylosing spondylitis 283
 management of 285
 types of 283
Anosognosia 364
Antalgic gait 78
Anterior apprehension test 214, 214*f*
Anterior basal segments 520*f*
Anterior cord syndrome 390, 391*f*
Anterior cruciate ligament injury
 grading of 175
 physiotherapy for 176
 rehabilitation 175
 surgical management for 177
 treatment 176
Anterior dislocation 149*f*
Anterior fibers of deltoid ligament 194*f*
Anterior opening type walker rollator 78*f*
Anterior pelvic tilt exercises 541*f*
Anterior shoulder pain 230*f*
Anterior trunk bending gait 78
Anterolateral thoracotomy 543
 incision 543*f*
Anteromedialization 173
Anthropometric measurements 339
Antispastic pattern of upper limb 379*f*
A-O screw 300*f*
Aphasia 365
Apical expansion exercise 513*f*
Apley's grinding test 163, 164*f*, 212, 213*f*
Apneustic breathing 505
Apoplexy 358
Apparent limb length measurement 29, 30*f*
Appendicectomy 539
Appendicectomy, open 540
Apprehension test for patella 163, 163*f*
Aquatic therapy 350
Aquired syphilis 282
 latent syphilis 282
 primary stage 282
 secondary stage 282
 tertiary syphilis 282
Arterial blood gas analysis 509
Arteriovenous malformation 359
Arthritis 271
 chronic 278, 279
 mutilans 280
Arthrodesis 355, 448
 of shoulder 448*f*
Arthrokinematics of 88, 137, 192
 ankle joint 192
 elbow joint 232
 knee joint 162
 radioulnar joints 233
 shoulder joint 209
 wrist joint 242
Arthroscopic repair 217
ASH brace 418*f*
Ashworth scale, modified 334*t*
Assisted hip abduction 156
 exercise 157*f*
Assistive devices 386
Asthenia 472
Asymmetric tonic neck reflex 363
Ataxia
 assessment of 473
 causes of 471
 clinical features of 471
 diagnosis of 473
 management of 473
 telangiectasia 472
 types of 471
Ataxic breathing 505
Ataxic cerebral palsy 320, 321*f*
Ataxic disorders 471
Ataxic gait 332
Athetoid dance gait 333
Atlantoaxial joint 88
Atlanto-occipital joint 16*f*, 88
Attention continuum 564
Attractor wells 566*f*
Auchincloss modified radical mastectomy 493
Auscultation 507
Autoassisted lumbar extension 113
Automated motion analysis 73*f*
Automatic bladder, management of 405
Automatic movement reactions 336
Autonomic dysreflexia 393
Autonomic nervous system 83
Autonomous bladder, management of 405
Avascular necrosis of head of femur 147, 148
Avulsion 444
 fracture 288
Axillary crutches 74, 74*f*, 267*f*
 measurement of 74
Axillary pad 387*f*
Axillary web syndrome 493
Axonotmesis 442

B

Babinski's sign 396
Back extensors 343*f*
 strengthening exercises 117
Baker's cyst 273, 273*f*
Balanced
 and agility exercises 184
 assessment of 14, 396
 efficacy scale 14
 evaluation systems test 14
 sitting, practice of 578
 standing
  essentials of 581
  practice of components of 581
 training 16*f*, 344*f*, 425*f*
 virtual therapy for 376*f*
 with crutches, development of 74
Ballistic stretching 44, 45*f*
Bankart's
 lesion 220*f*
 procedure 226
Barlow maneuver 138
Barlow test 152
Barrel chest 504*f*
Barton's fracture 296, 296*f*
Basal expansion exercise, lateral 512
Basal ganglia circuit 413*f*
 direct pathway 412*f*
Beating 82
 massage 82*f*
Beatty's maneuver 140
Bechterew's disease 284
Becker muscular dystrophy 431*f*, 433
Bed mobility exercises 376*f*
Beevor's sign 434
Bell's palsy 450
 causes of 450
 diagnosis of 451
Bell's sign, positive 451*f*
Bend standing 7*f*
Bennett's fracture 297, 298*f*, 298
Berg balance scale 14, 368
Bertolotti syndrome 133
Bicep
 jerk 32*f*
 brachii 36*f*
  eccentric contraction of 36*f*
  tendinitis with transverse humeral ligament test 214
Birth trauma 443
Bladder 365
 dysfunction 393
 function 422
 problems 105
 symptoms 428
 training 405
Blood test 432
Body 21
 and brings clarity 515
 axes 4*f*

chart 312f
position and mechanics 60
scheme disorders such
 asomatognosia 364
systems 4f
weight-supported walking 344f
 device with treadmill 408f
Bones of leg 307f
Bony procedures 354
Borg dyspnea scale, modified 506
Borg rating scale of perceived exertion 532t, 532
Boston brace 262f
 for scoliosis 353f
Botulinum toxin injections 404
Boutonniere deformity 279f
Bow string test 111
Bowel
 dysfunction 394
 involvement 365
 management 406
Boyd's amputation 265
Brachial neuralgia 93
Brachial plexus injury 443, 443f
 causes of 443
 classification of 443
 management of 445
 pathophysiology of 444
 surgical management of 446
Brachialgia and cord syndrome 90
Bradykinesia 415f
Bragards sign 110, 110f
Braiding pattern 68f, 69
Brain attack 358
Brain death 422
Breast cancer
 clinical presentation of 492
 management of 492
 surgeries for 492
Breast stroke swimming 116f
Breathing
 boosts energy levels and improves
  stamina 516
 control
  exercise 512, 547, 574f
  poor 572
  tranining 573
 detoxifies and releases toxins 515
 elevates moods 516
 exercise 526, 534, 469f
  benefits of 515
  conscious 46
  types of 511
 game 528f
 improves
  endurance 516
  lung function 516
  nervous system 515
  posture 515
  quality of blood 515
  tissue healing 516
 increases digestion and
  assimilation of food 515
 massages vital organs 515
 mechanics of 499
 pattern 504
 releases tension, relaxes mind 515
 relieves emotional problems 515
  pain 515
 sounds, normal 507t
 strengthens immune system 515
 technique, active cycle of 487, 513f, 547
 training 526
Breathlessness, grading of 505

Breech position 152
Bridging exercise 117
 unilateral 379f
Bridging of pelvis 149
Brisk walking 144
Bristow procedure 226
Bronchitis, chronic 521, 522f
Bronchodilators 522
Bronchopulmonary segments 517f
Brown-Sequard syndrome 90, 288, 390, 391f
Brunnstrom approach 383
Brunnstrom's stages of recovery 367
 of hand function in stroke 367
Bryant's triangle 30, 31f
Bucket handle tear 183f
Buckled fracture 288
Bulbar palsy, progressive 439
Bulge test 162
Bullectomy 522
Bunion splint 281f
Buoyancy 56
Burn
 causes of 311
 chemical 313
 clinical features of 312
 cold 313
 deeper fourth degree 312
 degrees of 311t
 electric 312, 312f
 full thickness 312
 heat (thermal) 312
 injuries, types of 311
 management of 313
 partial thickness 311
 percentage of 312, 312f
 physiotherapy techniques 315
 superficial 311
Bursitis, types of 146
 acute 146
 chronic 146

C

Cadence 72
Calcaneal spur 200f
Calcaneo fibular ligament 195f
Calcaneus fracture 308f, 309
Calcium supplements 92
Calf muscles, pseudohypertrophy of 432f
Camel back sign 170f, 170
Capsular pattern 87, 89, 137, 162, 209, 242
Capsular pattern of limitation of 192
 elbow joint 232
 radioulnar joint 233
 thoracic spine 88
Capsular shift 226
Card test 454f
Cardiac rehabilitation 530, 531, 533, 534f, 535, 535f
 benefits of 531
 components of 533, 533f
 indications of 531
 phases of 534
Cardiomegaly 510f
Cardiopulmonary exercise test 532
Cardiorespiratory system 3
Cardiovascular fitness, assessment of 397
Carpal compression test 246
Carpal tunnel syndrome 243, 245, 245f, 458
 management of 246

Cat and camel exercise 116f, 134
Cauda equina involvement 123f
Cauda equina syndrome 391
Cavus foot 204f, 205f
Cemented
 tibial and patellar component 189
 total knee arthroplasty 189
Center of
 mass 5, 5f
 pressure 5f
Central cord syndrome 90, 390, 390f
Central disc bulge 128
Central nervous system 412, 427
 pathology of 320
Central processing 5
Centralization 597
Centre of gravity 72
 backward shift in 581
 changes of 590
 forward shift in 581
 horizontal displacement of 72
 lateral shift 581
Cerebellar ataxia 471
Cerebral haemorrhage, primary 359
Cerebral palsy 89, 169, 319, 320, 329f, 333, 335t, 350f, 352f
 assessment process 333fc, 334fc
 assistive devices for 351
 chairs 354f
 classification of 320
 clinical features of 322, 323t
 diagnosis of 340
 epidemiology 319
 gait 332
 management of 340
 mild 322
 moderate 322
 risk factors 319
 severe 322
 surgery in 354
 topographical types of 321
Cerebral vascular accident 358
Cerebrovascular accident 358
Cervical cord injuries 392
Cervical disc bulge, management of 98
Cervical disc prolapse, clinical features of 96
Cervical extension, measurement of 27f
Cervical flexion, measurement of 27f
Cervical manipulation 99
Cervical pillow 92f
Cervical prolapsed intervertebral disc 95
Cervical roll 98f, 315f
Cervical roots 90
Cervical rotation 27
Cervical spine 27, 88, 93f, 94f, 603
 distraction test for 97f
 fracture 288, 290
Cervical spondylosis 89, 92f, 94f
 course of 89
Cervical stabilization exercises 103f
Cervical traction 18f, 93f
Cervical vertebral segments 96f
Cervicothoracic muscles 99f
Cervicothoracic spine 609f
Cesarean section delivery 486, 489, 540
Chair test 234, 234f
Charcot's joints 282
Chemical burn 313f
Chest
 care 315
 circumference 339t
  measurement of 339

expansion 270, 506
 measurement of 506f
 inspection of 503
 muscle exercise 484, 485f
 pain 506
 percussion, cupped hands for 517f
 secretion clearance techniques 525
 symmetry and deformity 503
 tightness 493
 vibration, application of 517f
 wall pain 506
 wall percussion 507f
Cheyne-Stokes respiration 505
Child walking 332f, 333f
Chin tuck 99f
 exercise 599f
Cholecystectomy 539
 indications for 539
Cholecystitis 539
Choledocholithiasis 539
Cholelithiasis 539
Chondromalacia patella 166, 167f
Chromosomal theory 206
Chronic inflammatory demyelinating polyneuropathy 467, 470
 etiology 470
 pathophysiology 470
Chronic obstructive pulmonary disease 521
Circuit interval training 430f
Circular friction 81
Circumduction gait 78
Circumductory gait 332, 333f
Clam shell exercise 158
Clapping 81
Clapping massage 82f
Clarke's sign 167
Claw hand deformity 450f
Closed fracture 288
Closed kinematic chain exercise 37
Closed kinetic chain 177
 exercise 218f
Closed pack position 192
Clubbing of finger 504f
Clubfoot 206f
 serial casting for 207f
Clutton's joint 282
Cobb's angle 257, 258, 263
 measurement 256, 257f
Coccydynia 135, 135f, 481
 cushion 136f
 pillow 481f
Coccygodynia 135
Codman's exercises 218f
Coffee cup test 235f
Cognitive
 behavioral therapy 315, 429
 dysfunctions 364
Cold burn 313f
Cold immersion 375f, 376
Coleman block test 196f
Collateral injury management, lateral 186
Collateral ligament 186
Colles fracture 296, 296f
Coma 362, 421
Comminuted fracture 288
Complete basilar artery syndrome 360
Complex degenerative tear 183f
Complexity, increasing 582, 584
Compound fracture 288
Compound muscle action potential 468
Compression test 97f
Concave-convex rule 604f

Concentric
    exercise 35, 36f, 241f
    knee flexion 585f
    muscle work 19
    resisted adductor strengthening 173f
    work of elbow flexors 20f
Conductive education 349, 383
    program 384f
    therapy 595
Condylar fractures 303, 304
    lateral 294f
Condyles of femur 302
Congenital talipes equinovarus
    epidemiology 206
    etiologies 206
Congestive heart failure 510f
Consciousness, level of 422
Contact sports 443
Continuous ultrasound therapy 236
Contraction 20
Contract–relax
    direct treatment) 67
    indirect treatment) 67
Contracture 366
Contralateral stage 345
Contrast method 47
Controlled sensory input for facilitation 385
Controlled walking 113
Contusion of brain 520f
Conventional exercises 375
Conventional exercises in acute stage 372
Cool down 4
    exercises 529f, 534, 535f
Cooper's test 397
Cord sign 602
Core muscle strengthening exercise 116, 132f, 260f
Core strengthening exercises 132
Corner stretch exercise 286f
Corticospinal 90
Costal expansion, lateral 512
Cozen's test 234, 234f
Crab walking 159f
Cranial nerve integrity 334
Crawling 347f
Crede's maneuver 405
Creeping 347f
Crepe bandage, application of 197f
Crook
    lying 10, 11f, 483f
    sitting 10, 10f
Cross hand technique 607, 607f
Crouch
    gait 78, 332, 332f
        two-point 75f
    length of 74
    palsy 462
    sitting 10, 11f
    walking
        preparation for 74
Crutches 74, 155
Cryotherapy 544
Cunningham method of reduction 219
Cyclic stretching 44
Cylindrical pop cast 172f
Cyriax
    approach 601
    deep transverse friction 236
    listing correction 115f
    method 114
    mobilization, contraindications of 604
Cystic fibrosis 522

D

Daily adjusted progressive resisted exercise technique 42
De Quervain's disease 247, 248f
Dead bug 124
    exercise 125f
Dead Butt syndrome 151
Decerebrate posture 422f
Decorticate posture 422f
Deep brain stimulation 419
Deep breathing exercises 103, 155, 287f, 433, 483, 546
Deep diaphragmatic breathing exercise 546f
Deep massage 83
Deep tendon reflexes 32f, 335, 396
    grading of 31, 335t
Deep transverse friction massage 81
Deformity 47, 366
    auto correction of 258
    positions of 279
Degenerative spondylolisthesis 122
Delorme and Watkins technique 41
Deltoid ligament stress test 193
Demonstration 75
Denis brown splint 207f
Derangement syndrome 596
    treatment of 597
Derived postures 6
Diabetes mellitus 360
Dial test 166
Diaphragmatic
    breathing exercise 511f
    muscle training using weight 513f
Diastasis recti abdominis 479f
Digital Allen's test 243, 244f
Digital stimulation 406
Diplegia 321
Disability 444
    degree of 50
Disc bulge
    posterolateral 96f
    types of 95, 95f
Discharge planning 270
Discrete and continuous tasks 564
Dislocated patella 171f
Dislocation
    of hip joint 340f
        congenital 152
    of patella 171
    posterior 149f
    reduction of 219
Displaced fracture 288
Displacement, posterior 288f
Distal interphalangeal predominant psoriatic arthritis 280
Distal key points, stimulation of 591f
Distal muscular dystrophy 435
Distal realignment 173
Distal upper extremities 439f
Dog clip 52, 52f
Dorsal blocking splint 253f
Dorsal rhizotomy 357f
Dorsiflexion 23
    eversion of ankle 61f
Drawer test 165f, 165, 175, 193f, 193, 215f
    anterior 164f, 164, 193f, 193, 215f
    posterior 215
Drop arm test 211, 211f
Drug therapy 414
Duchenne muscular dystrophy 431, 431f
Duga's test 213, 213f
Duputryen's

amputation 265
    contracture 250, 250f
        stage of 251t
Dymphysis pubis, diastasis of 480
Dynamic
    action theory 565
    balance exercise 13, 15, 396, 429f, 578
        examination of 581f
    muscle work 19
    postural control 13, 15
Dysarthria 365
Dyskinetic cerebral palsy 320, 320f
Dysphagia 365
Dysplasia of hip, development of 152, 153
Dysplastic spondylolisthesis 122
Dyspnea
    grading of 505
    observation of 505
Dyssynergia 472

E

Ears 6
Eccentric
    contraction 35
    muscle work 20
ECG graph, parts of 511f
Ecological theory 566
Edema control 83, 445
Effector component 6
Egawa test 455f
Eirene collis 345
Elastic support stockings 480f
Elbow 25
    crutch 75, 76f, 408f
        measurement of 76
    disorders of 232
    extension 25, 62f, 297f, 383f
    flexion 25, 62f, 270, 297f, 385f
    flexion deformity of 295f
    flexion of 17f
    flexors, eccentric work of 20f
    gaiter 387f
    joint 53, 232, 232f
    kneading 80f, 104f
    motion of 233t
    pain 233
    stump length
        above 265
        below 265
Electrical stimulation 376
Electrocution 311
Electromagnetic motion analysis systems 73
Electromyography 140, 468
Electrophysiological studies 454
Electrotherapy 225
Eley's test for rectus femoris 337f
Eliciting joint line tenderness 163f
Ely's test 139, 139f
Embryonic theory 206
Emery-Dreifuss muscular dystrophy 436, 437f
Emotional
    control, lack of 572
    disturbances 365
Emphasis, timing for 60, 61f
Emphysema 510f, 521, 522f
Empty can test 210, 211f
End feel, normal 33t
Endoskeletal design 269f
Endurance test 414
Endurance training 57

Energy conservation techniques 279
Energy consumption, measurement of 73
Energy cost analysis 73
Energy expenditure, physiological cost of 73
Environmental assessment 398
Epidural analgesia 356
Episodic ataxia 472
Equilibrium reaction 331f
Equinus 206
Erb's palsy 448, 448f, 449f
    diagnosis of 448
Erector spinae stretch 124, 125f
Ergonomic measures 258, 279
Escharotomy 314
Ethics
    in physiotherapy 554
    positive roles of code of 554
    professional 551, 552
    types of 552
Evoke potential studies 428
Executive body 553
Exercises 113, 131, 173, 455, 536
    and mobilization 236
    assisted 148
    capacity 531
    classification of 34
    during pregnancy 482
    for flexion dysfunction 596f
    frequency of 483
    help for uncomplicated labor 482
    help to prevent diastasis recti abdominis 482
    improves
        cardiorespiratory fitness 482
        psychological well-being 482
    intensity of 532
    on ankle exerciser 309f
    on leg press device 303f
    on multigym 381f
    prevents
        and improves low back pain 482
        urinary incontinence 482
    progression of 48
    repetition of 48
    speed of 41
    testing 525
        and training 525, 533
    therapy 3, 15, 18f, 21, 429
Expiration 500
Expiratory reserve volume 500
Extension 22, 27, 53, 52, 54
    adduction 66f
    and rotation test 90
    loading test 130f
    measurement of 28
    pattern 289
    resistance test 168
    strain 603
Extensor
    stretching 249f
    zones of hand 251f
Extra constitutional bodies 553
Extracapsular
    femoral neck fractures 299f
    fracture 299f, 299
Extracorporeal shock wave therapy 235, 315
Extremities, inspection of 506
Eye hand coordination exercises 429f
Eyes 6

F

Fabrication 268
Face mask 517f
   ventilator 516
Facetectomy 121
Facial exercises 452f
Facial expression 503
Facial motion, promote 68
Facial symmetry 574f
Facilitation of
   abdominals 374f
   back extensors 374f
   hip extension 583f, 378f
   knee extensors 373f
   knee flexion 379f
   phases 591
   upper limb muscles 374f
Facilitatory technique 384
Facioscapulohumeral muscular dystrophy 434, 434f, 435f
Fajersztajn test 110
Fall hanging 12
Fallout
   sitting 10, 11f
   standing 8f, 8
Faradic
   stimulation 172f, 226f, 260f, 344f, 374f, 375f
   type currents 375
Faradism under tension 236
Fatigue, prolonged 13
Feagin test 215, 215f
Femoral head 152
Femoral nerve tension test 111, 111f
Fibrocartilage complex, triangular 242f, 242
Fibromyalgia 105
Fibrous arthroplasty 154
Fibula 306f
Field tests 397
Figure-8 strap 291f
Finger gutter splint 281f
Finger pulleys 252, 252f
Finger spring 249f
Finkelstein test 243, 244f
Fire
   breakout of 311
   hydrant exercises 483, 483f
Fitness training 379, 410, 418
Fitts and Posner three-stage model 569
Fixation point 53, 54
Fixators 21
Fixed pulley 18
Flat foot 201f
   causes of 201
   clinical features of 201
   deformity 201
   management of 202
   physiotherapy 202
   types of 201
Flexbar 238f
   exercise 237, 238f
Flexibility
   and joint mobilization exercises 184
   exercise 202, 415, 534, 534f
Flexible ankle brace 197f
Flexible shoulder support 216f
Flexion 22, 23, 27, 52, 53, 54, 598f
   abduction, diagonal of 66f
   adduction-internal rotation test 140f
   dysfunction of lumbar spine 598
   in sitting 598
   in standing 598
   lateral 27
   measurement of 28
   pattern 289
Flexor synergy pattern, abnormal 362f
Flexor synergy, use of 384f
Foot 23, 192
   deformities 205
   disorders of 196
   inversion eversion 23
   joint 338
   lateral radiograph of 202f
   orthosis 352
   special tests for 193
Foramina stenosis 109
Foraminotomy 121
Forced adduction test 212, 213f
   on hanging arm 213
Forced expiratory technique 513, 547
Forearm 25
   motion of 233t
   pronation 25, 25f, 270, 576f
   supination 25, 25f, 576f
Forward head posture 100
   diagnosis of 101
Fracture 52, 288, 302
   and around condyles of femur 302
   around ankle 308
   around femoral condyles, management of 303
   around foot 308
   bones of
      forearm 296
      hand 297
   both bones of leg 307
   clavicle 291
   complications of 296
   dislocation 289
   forearm bones 295
   greater tuberosity of humerus 293f
   hand 298
   head of radius 296f
   humerus 292
   medial condyle of tibia 30
   metatarsals 309
   metatarsals 310
   mid shaft of clavicle 291f
   neck
      of femur 299
      management of 300f
   open 288
   patella 304, 304f, 305f
   pathological 288
   pelvis 298, 298f
   phalanges 309
   proximal humerus 292
   scapula 291, 292f
   shaft and condyles of femur 302
   shaft and lower end of humerus 294
   shaft of femur 302, 302f
   shaft of humerus 294f
   simple 288
   spine 288
   surgical neck of humerus 294f
   talus 309
   tarsal bones 309, 310
   tarsals 309
   tibial condyles 306
   transverse process 289
   trochanters 301
   tuberosities 292
   upper limb 291
Freiberg sign 140
Frenkel's exercise 47, 48f, 48, 50f
   benefits of 50
   indications of 48
Friction 81
Friction massage 455
   transverse 603
Friedreich's ataxia 473
Froment's sign 243, 244f
   positive 454f
Frontal ataxia 472
Frontal axis 4
Frontal plane 4
Frost bite 311
Frozen shoulder 226, 227
   causes of 227
   classification of 227
   primary/idiopathic 227
   secondary 227
   stage of 227, 227t
Fulcrum 21
Function, retraining of 491
Functional
   arm brace 446f
   balance grading scale 14
   electrical stimulation 409
   reach test 14
   residual capacity 500
   stretching of upper back 104f
   training 416
   use of upper limb 270, 379f
Fundamental postures 6
Funnel chest 504f

G

Gait 413
   abnormal 366
   analysis 72, 340f
   assessment of 340
   cycle 70f
   determinants of 72
   ladder 378f
   pathological 78
   training 70, 344f, 377f, 378f, 416, 418f, 425f, 470f
   with walking stick 77
Galeazzi fracture 295, 296f
Galeazzi sign, positive 152f
Galeazzi test 152
Gallow's traction 302
Gastrointestinal complications, management of 491
Gear shift exercise for shoulder 229f
Gentile passive exercises 149
Gentile's two stage model of motor learning 569
Genu varum 273f, 276f
Girdle stone arthroplasty 154
Glasgow Coma Scale 421
Glossopharyngeal breathing 514f, 514
Gluteus maximus strengthening 178f
Gluteus medius 151, 177
   strengthening 177f
Golfer's elbow 239, 239f, 240f
   splint 240f
   test 239,
      active test 239
      passive test 239
Goniometry for 21
   Cervical
      lateral flexion 28f
      rotation 28f
   elbow
      extension 25f
      flexion 25f
   eversion 24f
   hip
      abduction 22f
      extension 22f
      flexion 22f
      lateral rotation 22f
      medial rotation 22f
   inversion 24f
   knee
      extension 23f
      flexion 23f
   shoulder
      abduction 25f
      adduction 25f
      extension 24f
      flexion 24f
      lateral rotation 25f
      medial rotation 25
Gouty arthritis 282, 283f
Gouty tophi 283f
Gower's maneuver 432f
Gower's sign, positive 432f
Gracilis 337f
Grasshopper sign 170
Great toe, abduction ROM of 24f
Greater trochanter 301
Greenstick fracture 288
Gritti-Stoke's amputation 265
Groin
   strain 150
   stretch 485f
   in tailor sitting 484
Ground reaction force 5f
Group therapy 350f
Guillain-Barré syndrome 467
   classification 467
   clinical features 468
   diagnosis 468
   pathophysiology 467
   treatment 468
Gutter crutch 76, 76f, 279f
   measurement of 76

H

Hacking 81
   massage 82f
Half circle bodied goniometer 21f
Half kneeling 8, 9f, 144f, 348f
Half standing 8f, 8
Half-crook lying 11f, 11
Half-lying 11, 11f, 45
Halo device 401, 401f
Halo vest immobilization 289f
Hamstring stretching 169f
   curls 186
   eccentric contraction of 585f
   exercise 133f, 134
Hand 26
   cuff neuropathy 462
   disorders of 242, 245
   flexor
      muscles of 240f
      zones of 251f
   function
      adaptive devices to improve 410
      development of 348f
      training 344f
   injury 251
   placement of 513
   special tests for 242
   splint 353, 450f
      for Klumpke's palsy 450f
   to knee gait 78
Hard cervical collar 92f

Index

Hawkin's Kennedy impingement test 210, 211f
Head and spinal injury 56
Head circumference 339t
    measurement 339
Head of femur 148
Headache 609, 609f
Hearing, development of 328t
Heart
    disease 360
    problems 278
    sounds 508t
    therapy 113
    thump test 194, 194f
Height loss, measurement of 257
Heimlich maneuver 515
Hematoma 420f
Hemiarthroplasty 154, 300f
    of hip 154f
Hemivertebrae 256f
Hemophilic arthritis 44
Hemorrhagic stroke 359, 369
Hennepin technique 220
Heterotopic ossification in hip joints 398f
Hey's amputation 265
Hierarchical theory 565
High heeled shoes 205
High power laser therapy 104f, 236
High-velocity low amplitude 236
Hill-Sachs lesion 220f
Hinged knee
    brace 178f
    cap 276f
Hip
    abduction 157f
        exercise 485f
        in side lying 484
        orthosis 352, 352f
            trilateral 160, 161f
        test 140
    abductor 39f, 173, 300f, 469f
        strengthening 149f, 151f
    arthroplasty 153
    assumes flexion abduction 159
    dislocation, management of 149
    dislocations 148
        types of 148
    extension 582f
    extension-abduction 66f
    flexion deformity of 354f
    flexion-adduction 66f
    flexors 145f, 342f
        right 126f
    joint 22, 54, 137, 336
        special tests for 137
    MRI of 146f
    replacement arthroplasty 154
    rotation 609f
    specific disorders of 139
    strategy 14, 14f
    surgery 355
Hippo therapy 153, 349, 429
Hirayama disease 439f
Hoffmann's reflex 396
Homan's sign test 194f, 194
Homolateral limb synkinesis 364
Homolateral stage 345
Homolateral synkinesis, right sided 364f
Honeymoon palsy 462
Hoover's sign 504, 505f
Hornblower sign 212f, 212
Horner's syndrome 444
    presence of 444

Hughes test 140
Hughston's plica test 166f
Human locomotion, normal 70
Human resource management 558
Humeral
    cuff 387f
    flexion 270
Hybrid prosthesis 189f
Hydromechanics 56
Hydrostatic pressure 56
Hydrotherapy 56, 115, 116f, 161, 287f, 315, 350, 374f
    advantages of 57
    clinical applications of 56
    contraindications for 57
    objectives of 56
    pool 57f, 350f, 411f
        features of 57
    precautions for 57
    principles of 56
    use of 57
Hypermobile joints 52
Hyper-lordosis 105
Hypermobility 44, 605
Hypertrophied scar 314f
Hypomobility 605
Hypothermia, therapeutic 400
Hypotonic cerebral palsy 321
Hysterectomy 494, 495f
    indications for 494

I

Ideational 364
Ideomotor 364
Idiopathic
    clubfoot 206
    pulmonary fibrosis 524
Iliac apophysis 256, 257f
Iliopsoas crosses 145
Iliotibial band syndrome 141f, 141
Inactive posture 12
Incentive spirometry 262f, 514f, 546
Incision
    transverse 490f, 495f
    types of 489, 490f, 495f
Inclined prone kneeling 9f, 9
Incomplete injury 390
Incontinence, presence of 506
Indwelling catheter 362f
Infections 278
Inferior apprehension test 215
Inferior radioulnar joints 232
Inflammation, acute 44
Inflammatory spinal diseases 105
Infraspinatus lesion 212
Infraspinatus test 211
Infra-trochanteric length 30
Inhaled steroids 522
Inhibition, phases of 591
Inhibitory tapping 590
Inhibitory technique 386
Injection palsy, prevention of 464f
Injury, complete 390
Inserting suppository 406
Inspiratory
    capacity 500
    muscle training 546
    reserve volume 500
    resistance training 514f
Integumentary system 3
Intensity 35, 45
Intensive outpatient rehabilitation 536
Interindividual variability 41
Intercarpal joints, mobilization of 246f

Intercondylar fracture 294f, 304f
    of tibia 306f, 306, 307
Interferential therapy 227, 235
Intermittent lumbar traction 120f
Intermittent stretching 44
Internal carotid artery syndrome 359
Internal rotation 54
International Professional Bodies 553
International Standards for Neurological Classification of Spinal Cord Injury 389
Interpelviabdominal amputation 265
Interphalangeal joints 193
Interscapulothoracic amputation 265
Intertrochanteric fracture 299f, 301f
Intervertebral
    disc 95f
    foramina 90
    joint 88
Intraarticular hip derangement 145
Intracapsular femoral neck fractures 299f
Intracapsular fracture 299
    of neck of femur 299f
Intracerebral hemorrhage 359
Intrathecal baclofen therapy 404
Intrauterine malposition 152
Invasive ventilator 516
Inventory management 559
Iontophoresis 113, 236
Irradiation 60
    and reinforcement 60
Irritability 600
Ischemic
    compression 608
    stroke 358, 369
Ischial bursitis 146
Isokinetic dynamometer 36f
Isometric exercise 34, 36t, 36, 93f, 124f, 124, 183, 300
    limitations of 35
    precaution of 35
Isometric
    flexion 93f
    gluteal contractions 114
    gluteal exercise 148, 156f, 190f
    hamstring exercise 181f, 305f
    hamstrings sets 183
    lateral flexion 93f
    muscle work 19, 20f
    quadriceps exercise 35f, 148, 156f, 169f, 181, 190f, 275f
    quadriceps sets 183, 190
    rotation 93f
    shoulder
        abductor strengthening 221f
        extensor strengthening 221f
        flexor strengthening 221f
    spinal extension exercise 124f
    strengthening of
        flexor muscles 240f
        lower abdominals 118
        shoulder adductors 221f
        shoulder lateral rotators 222f
        shoulder medial rotators 222f
Isotonic exercises 35
Isthmic spondylolisthesis 122

J

Jaw closure 573
Jobe's test 210
Johnstone approach 386
Joint
    angle 35

compression, application of 386f
laxity 480
lesions in congenital syphilis 282
line tenderness 163
mobility 38
mobilization 43, 184
    passive 44
movement, velocities of 335t
play movements, examination of 605
positioning 402
protection 279
range of motion assessment 396
space, reduction of 108f
stiffness 444
structures 6
symmetrical involvement of 278f
unloading knee brace 276f
Jugular vein, distension of 504f
Jump knee gait 78, 332, 332f

K

Kaltenborn concave-convex rule 604
Kaltenborn's
    orthopedic manual therapy 604
    translatory mobilization, indications of 605
    treatment plane 604f, 604
Karvonen's formula 532
Kegel's exercise 480, 483f, 483, 488, 489
    benefits of 483
Keloid 314f
Key muscle strength grading 389
Key sensory point grading 389
Kinematic analysis, methods for 73
Kinematics 70
Kinetics 70
    analysis of gait 73
    approach 74
Kitchen sink exercises 416, 417f
Klapp exercise 260
    for scoliosis 261f
Kleiger's test 195
Klisic's test 152, 152f
Klumpke's palsy 448f, 450, 450f
    diagnosis of 450
    management of 450
Knee
    ankle and foot interactions 72
    CPM machine for 42f
    flexion deformity of 354f
    MRI of 180f
Knee effusion 162f
Knee exercises 191
Knee extension 23, 63f, 66f, 484f
    in sitting 484
    training 584f
Knee flexion 23, 63f, 66f, 301f, 303f, 385t
    during stance phase 72
Knee gaiter 352f, 352
Knee immobilizer 172f, 176f, 352f
Knee jerk 32f
Knee joint 23, 55, 162, 168f, 275f
    and leg 336
    medial compartment of 272f
Knee ligaments 175f
Knee mobilization 190, 190f, 305f
Knee orthoses 351
    types of 352
Knee orthosis 351
Knee rehabilitation 183

Index

Knee rolls 119f, 489f, 541f
  above 265
  below 265
Knee to chest 131
  exercise 134f
Kneel sitting 9, 9f
Kneel standing 343f, 348f
Knight spinal brace 402f
Knuckle bender splint 446f
Kocher's method 219
Krukenberg's amputation 265f, 265
Kussmaul's respiration 505
K-wire fixation 309f
Kyphoscoliosis deformity 329f
Kyphosis 105

L

Labor, stages of 486
Lachman test 164, 164f
Lacunar stroke 360
Laminectomy 121
Laminotomy 121, 133
Landau reaction 324f, 331f
Landau reaction, absence of 324f
Landouzy-Dejerine disease 434
Laparoscopic appendicectomy 540
Laparoscopic hysterectomy 494
Laparotomy 540
Large gallbladder polyps 539
Larrey's amputation 265
Lasegue test 110, 111f
Latarjet procedure 226
Lateral deviation, correction of 603f
Lateral epicondylitis
  management of 235
  surgical management of 239
Lateral flexion, measurement of 29
Lateral horizontal shift of pelvis, training 584f
Lateral medullary syndrome 360
Lateral sclerosis, primary 439
Lateral trunk bending 78
Latex bands 19f
Latex tubes 19f
Lax stoop standing 8f, 8
Learning, transference of 576, 580, 582, 584
Learning, types of 567
Leg press exercise 178f
Leg press-double leg 186
Legg-Calve-Perthes disease 158
Leg-prone lying 11f, 11
Lesion
  determination of level of 388
  per site of 443
  severity of 443
Lesser trochanter 301
Levator scapulae 102f
Lever 15, 16f
  first order 16f, 16
  second order 16, 17f
  third-order 17, 17f
Lhermitte sign 97f
Liability
  primary liability 551
  vicarious liability 551
Lift-off test 211, 211f
Ligament instability 34t
  four grading of 34
Ligamentum patellae, length of 169f
Light
  moving touch 592
  weight resistance training 490f
Limb amputation

levels of 264f
  site of 264
  types of 264f
Limb girdle muscular dystrophy 436, 436f
Limb length
  discrepancy 155
  measurement 29, 31f
Limb movement 610
Limb synergies, abnormal 362
Limp 159
Lingular (left) expansion exercise 512
Lithotomy position 487f
Locomotor training 416
Lofstrand and Canadian crutch 75
Long adductors of hips 342f
Long cock up splint 387f
Long patellar tendon 169
Long sitting 10, 10f
Long weight arm 18f
Loose body in joint 44
Low back pain 105
  assessment of 107
  classification of 106
  clinical features of 107
  diagnosis of 107
  epidemiology of 105
  etiology of 105
  pathophysiology of 106
Low intensity resistance training 429f
Lower abdominals 124f
Lower body exercise 526f, 526
Lower crossed syndrome 106f
Lower limb 29, 265, 363t, 372f
  ergometry exercise 374f, 411f
  fractures 298
  preparation for 74
Lower trapezius
  exercise 222f, 223f
  strengthening in prone 222f
Lower trunk 52
  pattern 64f
  rotation 65f, 134
Low-intensity laser therapy 227
Lumbar and sacral nerve injuries 393
Lumbar canal stenosis 128
  diagnosis of 130
  etiology of 128
  management of 130
Lumbar extension exercise 117f
Lumbar flexion in kneel sitting 132, 132f
Lumbar flexion in supine 117f
Lumbar lordosis 432f
Lumbar puncture 428, 468
Lumbar spine 87, 118f, 603
  fractures 290
  posterolateral derangement of 597
Lumbar spondylolisthesis 121, 123f, 127f
  clinical features of 122
Lumbar spondylosis 108f, 131t
  management of 118
Lumbar traction 123f
Lumbarization 133
Lumbarization
  complete 134
  types of 133
Lumbopelvic rhythm 87
Lumbosacral
  angle 87f
  belt 112f
  extension 120f
  flexion 120f
  spine, range of motion of 109

Lumbrical grip 61f
Lung
  capacities, normal 500f
  compliance 500
  disease 278
    restrictive 501f, 501t
  expansion programs 546
  function 257
    tests 521
  nodule 510f
  transplantation 522
  volumes 501f
Lunge exercise 144f
Lunge sideways standing 8, 8f
Lurching gait 78, 332
  posterior 78
Lycra weight jacket 425f
Lying
  on stomach 597f
  supine 45
Lymphedema 493
Lymphedema of left upper limb 493f
Lymphoma 278

M

Mac Queen technique 42
Maitland
  approach 599
  finger deformity 279f
  mobilization, grades of 600f
Management
  for physiotherapists 557
  functions of 557
  human resource 558
  inventory 559
  of academic activities 562
  of accounts 562
  of carpet area 561
  of cleanliness/housekeeping 562
  of documentation/record keeping 562
  of equipment services through annual maintenance contract 562
  of infrastructure and equipment 562
  of inventory 562
  of linen 562
  of manpower/human resources efficiently 562
  of physiotherapeutic services 561
  of physiotherapy department 560
  of research cell 562
  of security services 562
  of therapeutic services 562
  personnel 558
  quality 559
  role/functions of personnel manager 558
  theories of 560
  types of resources 557
Manipulative techniques for spine 603
Manual
  contact 60
  muscle testing 31, 396
  therapy 596
  traction 99f
Marie-Strumpell disease 283
Massage 47, 79, 455
  classification of 79
  contraindications for 84
  lower abdomen 406
  lubricants 84
  picking up 80f

tapping 82, 82f
  therapeutic uses of 83
  therapy 487
Mastectomy, incision site for 492f
Mat exercises 342, 343f
Maudsley's test 234f, 234
Maximal resistance 60
McConnell's test 168
McKenzie approach 98
McKenzie exercises
  for lumbar spine 597
  for neck pain 598
McKenzie extension exercise 597f
  for thoracolumbar spine 286f
McKenzie flexion exercise 120f
McKenzie program 113
McKenzie's method 110f, 114, 596
  contraindications for 599
  of assessment 98
  of treatment 99
McMurray test 163
  for medial meniscus 163f
Mechanical back pain 106
Mechanical block theory 207
Mechanical ventilation 516, 516f
Medial collateral ligament 185
  injury 184
Medial column injury 185
Medial condyle fracture 294f, 304f
Medial elbow pain, site of 239f
Medial epicondylitis 239
Medial hamstrings 337f
Medial ligament sprain, combination therapy for 198f
Medially extended heel 203f
Median medullary syndrome 360
Median nerve injury 457
  assessment of 458
  diagnosis of 458
  high 458
  laboratory tests for 459
  low 458
  management of 459
Median sternotomy 542
  incision 542f
Medical management 217, 341, 369, 370, 468
Medical Research Council Dyspnea scale 505
Medical Research Council grading scale 31t
  modified 506
Medicine ball exercise 527f
Medicolegal issues 551
Meniscal lesions 182
  clinical features 183
  diagnostic procedure 183
  epidemiology/etiology 182
  types of 182
Meniscal tears, types of 183f
Meniscectomy 184
Meniscus injury
  management of 183
  types of 182
Mennel's
  apparatus 173f
  approch 605
Mental attitude 13
Mental stimulation program 572
Meralgia paresthetica 143
Metabolic bone disorders 129
Metabolic equivalents 482
Metacarpal fractures 297, 298f, 298
Metallic implant 401f
Metatarsal bar 206f

Metatarsal fracture 308f
Metatarsalgia 205
Metatarsalgia 205
Metatarsophalangeal joint 193
  of great toe 283f
Miami brace 262f
Microwave diathermy 225, 227
Middle cerebral artery stroke 359
Midtarsal joints 192
Milch maneuver 219
Mill's
  manipulation 236, 236f
  test 234, 234f
Miller fisher syndromes 467
Milwaukee brace 262f, 263
Minerva jacket 289f, 402f
Mini open repair 218
Mini squat position 483f
Mini wall squats 178f
Minimally invasive surgery 133
Mini-open muscle resection
        procedure 241
Mirror therapy 374f
Missing components, practice of 582f
Mixed ataxia 472
Mixed cerebral palsy 320
Mobility 545
Mobility exercises 222
Mobilization
    exercises 105, 547
    grades of 600
    rates and rhythm of 600
Mobilize secretions in lungs 84
Mobilize shoulder 292
Moist hot pack 142
Monomelic amyotrophy 439
Monoplanar method 236
Monoplegia 321
Monteggia fracture 296f
    dislocation 295
Moore's pin 300f
Moro reflex 331f
Morton's disease 205
Morton's neuroma 205f
Motor
    assessment scale 396
    control 563
    dysfunction 90
    examination 367
    imagery 429
    integrity 334
    learning 563, 567
        ecological theory of 568
    neuron disease 431, 437
    program theory 565
    programming deficits 364
    relearning program 382, 570
        equipment for 571
        principles of 570
        principles of 570
        sections of 571
        sections of 571
        stages of 571
        steps of 571
    syndrome 90
    system 83
        theory of 565
Mouth, angle of 451f
Movement
    for lumbar spine 610
    for peripheral joints 609
    in frontal plane 4f, 5f
    in transverse plane 5f
    limitation of 284f
    planes of 4f

production 563, 563f, 564
speed of 48
Moving arm 21
Muller's test 165f, 165
Mulligan's
    approach 608
    concept 94, 608
    mobilization 94, 120f, 237f, 286f,
        609f, 610f
        contraindications for 610
    exercise 229f, 237
    indications for 610
    principles of 608
    spinal mobilization with arm
        movement 94
Multiangle isometrics 34, 35f
Multiple sclerosis 427f
    clinical features 428
    diagnostic tests in 428
    epidemiology 427
    etiology 427
    management 428
    pathophysiology 427
    physiotherapy assessment 429
Murmurs 508
Murphy's sign 243, 244f
Muscle 6
    biopsy 432
    cramps 481
    endurance 40
    energy technique 240, 606
    group action of 20
    normal 433f
    of upper back 104f
    of upper limb 373f
    of ventilation 500t
    power 38, 40, 368
    setting exercises 34
    spasm and pain 84
    strength 39, 186
    strength, assessment of 396
    tone, reduce 68
    wasting 438f, 439f
    weakness 13, 365
    work, range of 19, 20, 20f
    work, types of 19
Muscular atrophy
    progressive 439, 439f
Muscular dystrophy 431
    clinical features 431
    congenital 435
    etiopathology 431
Muscular weakness 335
Musculoskeletal
    impairments 428
    pain 106
    system 3
Musculotendinous groin injuries 150
Myofascial bands 607f
Myofascial release 81, 99f, 115f, 119f,
        143f, 262f, 607, 607f
    techniques 82f
Myogenic theory 206
Myopathic muscles 433f
Myotomes 31
    of body 31t
Myotonic muscular dystrophy 435

N

Nasogastric tube 362f
Natural apophyseal glides 609
    movements 94
Navicular fracture 308f

Nebulization and steam inhalation
    517
Neck
    extension 60f, 99f, 599f
    extensors 20f
    flexion exercise 599f
    inspection of 503
    pain 100
        due to derangement 598
    pattern 63f
    retraction 599f
        exercise 99f
    righting reaction 330f
    rotation
        exercise 484f
        in sitting 484
Neer's impingement test 210f, 210
Negative pressure ventilator 516
Neonatal reflexes 324t
Nerve
    conduction velocity 468
    cross section of 442f
    fiber 442f
    gliding exercises 456f
    injuries, classification of 442
    injury 443f
    normal 427f
    root conduction 602
    root mobility 602
    roots 444t
    structure of 442
Neural transplantation 419
Neurodevelopmental therapy 381
Neurodevelopmental treatment 346,
    585
    assumptions of 586
    phases of inhibition and
        facilitation 591
    principles of 587
    process/methods of 587
    techniques of 588
Neurogenic
    claudication 129
    theory 206
Neurological diseases 471, 563
Neuroma 268, 444
Neuromotor development 345
Neuromuscular
    coordination 38
    inhibition techniques 44
    system 3
Neuron, structure of 442f
Neuronal group selection theory 566
Neuroplasticity 367
Neuropraxia 442, 444
Neuroprosthesis 409
Neurosurgery 356, 446
Neurotmesis 442
Neutral warmth 593
New York Heart Association Grading
    505
Night splint for
    ankle 315f
    foot drop deformity 465f
    hand 315f
Noble compression test 142
Nondisplaced fracture 288
Noninvasive ventilator 516
Nonmechanical back pain 106
Nonradiographic axial
    spondyloarthritis 284
Nonspecific back pain 106
Nonsteroidal anti-inflammatory drugs
    92, 227

Nonweight-bearing isotonic exercises
    183
Normal gait, parameters of 71
Nuclear bulging 108
Nutritional counseling 528
Nystagmus 471

O

Ober's test 138, 138f, 142, 146
Obesity 118
Oblique fracture 288
Oblique tear 183f
Obstetrics brachial plexus injuries 448
Obstructive lung diseases 501f
Occipital headache 100
Occupational stress 13
Oculopharyngeal muscular dystrophy
    437, 437f
Oligoarthritis, asymmetrical 280
Open kinematic chain exercise 37f
Open reduction and internal fixation
    for
    calcaneal fracture 309f
    Pott's fracture 309f
Opposition stretch exercise 249f
Optical motion analysis systems 73
Optical righting reaction 331f
Organizational chart 560
    of rehabilitation center 561fc
Orofacial dysfunction 572
    analysis of 572
    management 572
    practice of 573
        missing components 572, 574
Orthopedic surgery 354, 354f, 433, 447
    types of 355
Orthotic
    consideration 401
        for ambulation 409
    devices 386
    use of 375f
    management 351, 470
Ortolani maneuver 138f
Ortolani's test 138, 152
Osgood-Schlatter disease 173
    types of 174
Osteitis pubis 480
Osteoarthritis 271, 272f
    knee 271, 273f
Osteogenic theory 207
Osteokinematics 88, 137, 192
    of ankle joint 192
    of elbow joint 232
    of knee joint 162
    of lumbar spine 87
    of midtarsal joints 192
    of radioulnar joint 232
    of shoulder joint 209
    of wrist joint 242
Osteophytes, formation of 272f
Osteoporosis 278, 481
    severe 44
Oxford technique 42
Oxygen
    saturation, monitoring of 400
    therapy 522

P

Pace sign 140
Paget's disease 129
Pain 13, 159, 366, 428
    assessment of 397
    control 445

due to cervical dysfunction 599
in plantar fascia 199
management 407
reduction of 291
Painful arc sign 212, 213f
Pallidotomy 419
Palmar abduction 27f
Palmar kneading 80f
Palpation 506
Pancake splint 446f
Pancreas, inflammation of 539
Paper glass 577f
Parachute reaction 331f
Paradoxical breathing 505
Paraffin wax bath 172
Paraparesis 388
Paraplegia 388
in extension 392
in flexion 392
Parascapular muscles 104f, 119f
Parkinson's disease 412, 414f
clinical features 413
diagnosis of 414
epidemiology and etiology 412
features of 413f
pathophysiology 412
stages of 413, 414t
treatment 414
Parrot's syphilitic osteochondritis 282
Pars interarticularis 122f
Partial curl 124, 125f
Partial hip replacement arthroplasty 154
Partial knee replacement 188f
Partial lumbarization 133
Partial squatting 159f
Partial weight-bearing
ambulation 161
crutch gait 75f
Participation, assessment of 398
Passive knee extension 191f
Passive lumbar extension test 130f
Passive manual mobilization techniques 43
Passive movements, classification of 42
Passive stretching 44, 47
contraindications for 44
Passive test 240f
Patella alta 169, 170f
Patellar alignment brace 168f, 171f
Patellar grinding test 167
Patellar movement 170
Patellar stabilization brace 172f
Patellar tap 162
Patellar tap test 162f
Patellar tendon 355f
Patellectomy 170
Patey's operation 493
Pathological end feels 34t
Pathological flexor synergy pattern 362t, 363t
Patrick's test 139, 139f
Pavlik harness 153f
Peak oxygen consumption test 397
Pedicular screw, application of 129f
Peg board activities 50
Pelvic bridging 343f, 483f
Pelvic bridging exercise 117f, 149f, 372f, 418f, 494f
Pelvic dip 72
Pelvic floor
dysfunction 480
exercise 488, 489
muscle rehabilitation 496

muscle strengthening exercise 489f
squeeze 494f
strengthening exercise 494f
Pelvic inflammatory disease
causes of 496
management of 496
Pelvic swing 488f
Pelvic tilt exercise 124, 134f, 489f, 489
posterior 125f, 480f, 541f
Pelvic tilt, lateral 72
Pelvis 496f
distraction test for 72
in transverse plane, rotation of 72
lateral displacement of 72
rotation of 72
squaring of 30, 30f
Pencil-in-cup deformity 281f
Pendular suspension 52
Pentaplegia 321
Pentaplegic cerebral palsy 322f
Perceptual dysfunction 364
Perceptual system 3
Percussion 81, 516
Perfecting technique 483
Perinatal
history 334
period 486
physiotherapy 485
Periodization protocol 41
Peripheral joints, manipulation of 602
Peripheral nerve injuries, causes of 442
Peripheral nerves 442
Peripheral vascular disease 131f, 360
Peripheralization 597
Peroneal nerve 464f
Personnel management 558
Personnel manager, role of 558
Perthe's disease 159
Pes cavus 204
clinical features and types of 204
deformity 204
management of 205
pathomechanics of 204
Pes planus 201
Petrissage 80
Phalanx fracture 297, 298, 298f
Phalen's test 243, 244f, 246
reverse 243, 244f, 246
Phantom limb
pain 265
sensation 265
Philadelphia cervical collar 402f
Philadelphia collar 92f, 289f
Phonation and cough, observation of 505
Phonophoresis 236
Phosphodiesterase-4 inhibitors 522
Physiotherapists, code of conduct for 555
Physiotherapy 160, 174, 187, 278, 285, 291, 292, 298, 300, 301, 308, 309, 315, 341, 414, 445, 468, 485, 524
after hysterectomy 494
after radical mastectomy 492
assessment 429
department, working flowchart of 561
during time of child birth 486
following a hysterectomy 495
for amputees 264
for ankle 192
for avascular necrosis 148

for burn 311, 314
for congenital dislocation 153
for foot 192
for hip 137
for muscular dystrophies 431
for pelvic inflammatory disease 496
for peripheral nerve injuries 442
for shoulder 209
for SMA 440
for spinal cord injury 388
for spinal disorders 87
for spinal fractures 290
for stroke survivors 373
for thoracolumbar spine fractures 290
for total hip replacement arthroplasty 154
in abdominal surgeries 539, 540
in arthritis 271
in ataxia 471, 473
in fractures 288
in Guillain-Barré syndrome 467
in gynecological diseases 492
in inflammatory phase 197
in multiple sclerosis 427
in obstetrics 479
in pelvic inflammatory disease 496
in proliferative phase 197
in remodeling phase 197
in rotator cuff tear 217
in scoliosis 256, 258
in thoracic surgeries 542
intervention 415, 501
management 101
methods 450
postoperative 118, 179, 190, 226, 489, 495, 540
after selective dorsal rhizotomy 357
intervention 544
prenatal 481
preoperative 178, 190, 266, 494, 540
role of 266
techniques 433
treatment 370
strategies 429
Pigeon chest 504f
Pilate 490f
Pilate exercise 260f
Piriformis 115f, 606f
muscle 139f
Piriformis stretching exercise 133f
Piriformis syndrome 139
management of 140
primary 139
secondary 139
Pirogoff amputation 265
Pivot shift test 164, 164f
Plank exercise 117f
Planovalgus feet 338f, 338
Plantar fascia 199, 199f
normal 199f
Plantar fasciitis 198
Plantar flexion 23
Plaster of Paris 152
bandage 266f
Plate and screw fixation 291f, 302f
Pleural effusion 510f
Plica stutter test 166f
Plica syndrome 187
clinical features 187
diagnostic procedures 187

epidemiology/etiology 187
management 187
Plyometric exercises 37, 37f
Pneumonia 510f
Police man's tip hand 449f
Poly hill sign 434, 435f
Polypropylene shoulder orthosis 387f
Polystyrene 577f
Ponseti method 207t
Poor lip seal 572f
Poor working environment 105
Pop boot and bar 299f
Popliteal angle, assessment of 338f
Positional release technique 606
Positional stretching
for rhomboids 102f
of piriformis 141f
Positioning in
sitting 372
supine lying 370f
Positioning on bed 371
in side lying over affected side 371
in side lying over sound side 371
supine lying 371
Positive expiratory pressure technique 547
Positive-pressure ventilation 516
Posterior apprehension test 214, 214f
Posterior basal expansion exercise 512f
Posterior cerebral artery stroke 359
Posterior cord syndrome 391, 392f
Posterior cruciate ligament injury
acute 180
chronic 180
diagnosis 180
grades of 180
postoperative physiotherapy 182
rehabilitation 179
surgical management of 181
Posterolateral thoracotomy
indications for 543
indications for 543
Postganglionic brachial plexus lesions 444f
Postganglionic lesion, pathophysiology of 444
Postnatal
history 334
physiotherapy 488
Postural control 5
mechanism 6f
Postural correction exercises 547
Postural drainage 516, 519f, 520f
aim of 516
contraindications for 516
indications of 516
modified 547
procedure for 518
Postural neck pain 100, 598
clinical features of 100
Postural reflex 6, 6f
Postural sway 13
Postural syndrome 596
Posture 5
classification of 6
correction exercises 258
Pott's fracture 308, 308f
Pounding massage 83f
Power wheel chair 407f
Preganglionic
brachial plexus lesions 444f
lesion, pathophysiology of 444
Pregnancy 479
Prenatal tests 432

Preprosthetic rehabilitation 266
Pressure manipulation 79
Pressure sore
   management 405
   prevention 401
   treatment 405f
Pressure tappings 590
Pressure ulcer 397f, 402f
   assessment/grading of 397
   prevent development of 402
Primitive reflexes 335
   release of 363
Professional association 552
Professional body 552
Pronator teres syndrome 458
Prone
   falling 12
   knee bend test 110f, 111
   kneeling 9, 9f
   lying 11f, 11, 45, 286f, 345
   on elbows 114f, 597f
Proper breathing assists in weight control 516
Proprioceptive neuromuscular facilitation 59, 60f, 345, 383, 426
   basic principles of 59, 60
   clinical application of 67
   philosophy of 60
Prosthesis, above
   elbow 269f
   knee 269f
Prosthesis, use of 268
Prosthetic
   prescription 268
   training, use of 268
Protection to incision site and drainage tubes 544
Protective
   extension 331f
   knee pad 175f
Proximal dissociation, passive elongation 589
proximal key point, stimulation of 591f
Pseudohypertrophic muscular dystrophy 431
Psoriasis 280f
Psoriatic arthritis 280
   symmetric 280
   types of 280
Psoriatic spondylitis 280
Psychological stress 13
Psychological therapy 406
Pulley rope system 51f
Pulmonary complications, management of 491
Pulmonary diseases 521
Pulmonary function tests 509
Pulmonary rehabilitation 499, 521, 524, 526f, 547
   benefits of 525
   components of 525, 525f
   contraindications for 525
   focus of 525
   indications for 524
   objectives of 525
   program 522
   settings for 525
Pulmonary system, examination of 503
Pulmonary tuberculosis 510f
Pulsed
   lip breathing 505, 515f
   lip breathing exercise 514
   microwave diathermy 227
   oximetry 509, 509f
   shortwave diathermy 227
   ultrasound therapy 315
Pusher's syndrome 365
Putti-Platt procedure 226

Q

Q-angle, measurement of 163
Quadriceps 173, 183
   active test 165, 165f
Quadriceps lag 305
Quadriparesis 388
Quadriplegia 321, 388
Quadripod 77f
Quadruped
   arm and leg raises 125, 126f
   position 480f
Quadruped weight shifting 343f
Quality management 559
Quick stretch 60

R

Radial deviation 576f
   of wrist 576f
Radial nerve injury 461
   management of 462
   surgery for 463
Radial nerve
   palsy, diagnosis of 462
   sensory functions of 461
Radial tear 183f
Radiation, exposure to 311
Radical mastectomy 492, 492f, 493f, 493
   modified 492
Radicular pain 90, 106
Radioulnar joint
   inferior 232
   superior 232
Raimiste's phenomenon 364
Ramirez's test 194
Range of motion 137, 162t, 368
   ankle joint 192t
   cervical spine 88t
   hip joint 137t
   thoracolumbar spine 87, 87t
Readymade lumbosacral brace 129f
Reciprocal gait orthosis 409f
Reciprocal inhibition 60
Reciprocal innervations 60
Recovery, late 367
Reflex
   inhibiting patterns 381f, 590
   inhibitory postures 589
   integrity 335
   locomotion 348
   theory of motor control 564
Regular passive movements 315, 402
Rehabilitation 176
   after total knee replacement 188, 189
   of burn injury 314
   phase 403
   postoperative 456
   protocol, postoperative 190
Relaxation 38, 45
   additional methods of 46
   degrees of 45
   exercises 415
   progressive 46, 47f
   techniques 487
Relaxed half lying 46f
Relaxed passive exercise
   effects of 43
   principles of 42
   use of 43
Relaxed prone lying 46f
Relaxed supine lying 46f
Relaxing shoulders 47
Remplissage procedure 226
Replacement arthroplasty 154, 300
Research and technical cooperation functions 553
Residual volume 500
Resistance exercise, progressive 41
Resistance training 534
Resisted ankle plantar flexion exercise 158f
Resisted concentric exercise 181f
Resisted
   exercise
      effects of 42
      use of 42
   hip abduction 159f
      exercise 158f
   hip flexion 150f
   isometric tests 34t
      results of 34
   knee extension 301f
      exercise 158f, 174f
   knee flexor strengthening 177f
Respiratory care 314, 401
Respiratory dysfunction 428
Respiratory function
   assessment 397
   impairments 393
Respiratory physiology 500
Respiratory system 499, 499f
   assessment 502
   effect on 83
Rest and activity modification 98
Restful atmosphere 46
Resting hand splint 254f
Retrolisthesis 108f
Rheumatoid arthritis 276
   diagnostic criteria for 277
   progression of 277, 277t
Rheumatoid nodules 278
Rhomboids 101f, 104f
Rhythmic stabilization of shoulder 66f
Rib angle 504f
Rib fracture 510f
Ride sitting 9, 9f
Rigid ankle brace 197f
Rigidity 414
Risser sign 257f
Road traffic accident 288
Robotic device 387f
Robotic rehabilitation 386
   of brachial plexus injury 446
Robotic therapy 350, 350f
Romberg test 14
Rood's approach 384, 592
   assumption of 592
   principles of 592
Rood's facilitatory techniques 592, 593
Rooting reflex 329f
Rotation
   external 54
   measurement of 29
   pattern 289
   strains 603
Rotational osteotomy 355
Rotator cuff injury 215
   management of 216
Rupture 444
Russian stimulation 186

S

Sacral sparing 390
Sacralization 133
   types of 133
   unilateral 134f
Sacroiliac joint 607f
Sacroiliitis, grades of 285f
Sag sign 164f, 164
Salter's osteotomy 153
Sarcoidosis 523
Sarcoidosis 523
   management 524
Sarmiento's amputation 265
Saturday night palsy 462
Sausage finger 281f
Scaphoid fracture 297, 298f
Scaphoid pads 203
Scapular abduction 270
Scapular protraction, practice of 575f
Scapular setting exercises 222, 225
Scapulohumeral rhythm 209
Scar
   massage 315
   mobilization 83
   tissue 444
Schmidt's schema theory 568
Schober method, modified 29
Schober test, modified 29f
Schroth therapy 260
Sciatic 256
Sciatic nerve 139f, 464f
Sciatic nerve injury 463
   causes of 464
   diagnosis of 465
   features of 464
   surgery for 466
Sciatic scoliosis 109
Scissoring gait 332, 332f
Scissoring gait 78
Scoliosis 105, 107f, 257f
   assessment of 256
   auto correction of 259f
   clinical features 256
   congenital 256f
   epidemiology/etiology 256
   management of 257, 258t
   surgery for 263
Scott-Craig orthosis 409f
Seddon's classification 442, 443f
Sedentary lifestyle 118
Segmental breathing 511
   exercise 534f
Selective dorsal rhizotomy 356
Selective obturator neurectomy 357
Self-stretching 44
   exercises 258
   of gluteus maximus 147f
   of hamstrings 120f, 128f, 147f, 173f, 274f
   of left gluteus maximus 126f
   of left scalene muscles 102f
   of levator scapulae 94f
   of neck extensors 103f
   of pectorals-corner stretch 103f
   of piriformis 120f, 141f
   of right levator scapulae 102f
   of thumb flexor and adductor 246f
   of upper trapezius 94f
Semi-Fowler position 120f, 123f, 483f
Sensorimotor impairments 586
Sensory
   assessment 334
   ataxia 472
   dysfunction 90
   examination 414

impairment 365, 428
innervation of hand 453*f*
integration therapy 348, 349*f*, 384, 385*f*, 595, 595*f*
nerve action potential 468
processes 5
system 83
Serratus anterior
　exercise 225*f*
　anterior strengthening 223*f*
Serum creatinine phosphokinase 432
Sexual
　dysfunction 365, 394
　　treatment for 406
　function, assessment of 397
　symptoms 428
Sexuality and infertility, management of 406
Shaking 517
Shockwave therapy for tennis elbow 236*f*
Shoe inserts 200
S-hook 52, 52*f*
S-hook splint 451*f*
Short adductors 337*f*
　of hip 342*f*
Short arc
　knee flexion 305*f*
　quadriceps exercise 184*f*
Short weight arm 18*f*
Shortwave diathermy 225, 227
Shoulder
　abduction 220
　abduction of 18*f*
　abductor 217*f*
　after reduction of dislocation 220
　circumduction exercise 291*f*
　depression 270
　dislocation 218
　　clinical features 219
　　diagnosis 219
　　etiology of 219
　　management of 219
　extension 575*f*
　external rotators 217*f*
　flexion 220, 575*f*
　　practice of 383*f*
　flexor 35*f*, 217*f*
　　facilitation 374*f*
　　strengthening 224*f*
　hand syndrome 375*f*, 377
　immobilizer applied after reduction of dislocation 220*f*
　injuries, common 215
　internal rotation 223, 229*f*
　internal rotation of 213*f*
　joint 23, 53, 209, 209*f*, 230*f*, 293*f*
　　replacement 226
　　special tests for 210
　ladder 229*f*
　lateral rotating of 220, 213*f*
　　strengthening 221, 222
　medial rotators 217*f*
　mobilization 18*f*
　muscles strengthening exercise using theraband 223
　pulley exercise 218*f*
　rotation 53, 609*f*
　sling 292*f*
　stiffness of 100, 493
　strengthening 221, 224*f*
　subluxation 366, 366*f*
　support 372
　wheel exercise 218*f*, 229*f*, 286*f*

Side
　falling 12
　flexion 52
　lying 46
　plank 117
　plank exercise 117*f*, 126*f*
　sitting 9
　stepping exercise 485*f*
Signe brunnstrom 345
Silfverskiold test 338*f*
Silicon arch support 203, 204*f*
Silicon heel cup 200*f*
Silicon insole 200*f*, 206*f*
Sill sign 122*f*
Silver ring splint over pip joint 279*f*
Simmond's test 194
Single rope system 51*f*
Sinuses 52
Sit lying 12, 12*f*
Sitting 91
　ability, assessment of 340
　balance score 396
　flexion exercise 121*f*, 131, 131*f*
　from standing, practice of 580
　posture
　　abnormal 579*f*
　　prolonged 118
Sitz bath 136*f*
Sjogren's syndrome 278
Skeletal traction 290
Skin diseases 52
Skin grafting for burns 314
Skin rolling massage 81*f*
Slack zone 605
Sleep apnea 360
Slight knee flexion 170
Slings 51
　triangular 216*f*, 371*f*, 445*f*
　used for suspension therapy 51*f*
Slocum's test 165
Slump test 111, 111*f*
Smith's fracture 296, 296*f*
Smooth rhythmical oscillations 600
Snapping hip syndrome 144
Sodium biurate crystals, deposit of 283*f*
Soft cervical collar 92*f*
　use of 354*f*
Soft tissue
　effect on 83
　problems 278, 354
Somatosensory system 13
Somi brace 402*f*
Sotator cuff tear, assessment of 216
Souques' phenomenon 364
Space occupying lesions 128
Spastic cerebral palsy 320*f*
Spastic diplegic cerebral palsy 321*f*
Spastic hemiplegic cerebral palsy 321*f*
Spastic patterns 363
　in lower limb 363*f*, 363*t*
　in upper limb 363*f*, 363*t*
Spastic quadriplegic cerebral palsy 322*f*
Spasticity
　grading of 31
　management 404
　of gastrocnemius 338*f*
　of hand, reduce 375*f*
Spatial
　parameters of gait 72*f*
　relations disorder 364
　summation 60
Speech, development of 328*t*
Speed test 214, 214*f*

Spinal brace 126
Spinal canal 129*f*
　stenosis 126, 131*f*
Spinal column 601*f*
Spinal cord 129*f*, 389*f*
　anatomy of 388
　independence measure 398
　injury 388, 390
　　ASIA system of assessment of 395*f*
　　assessment of 394
　　classification of 389
　　clinical features of 391
　　management of 398
　　pain 394
　　unit 400
Spinal decompression surgeries 121
Spinal deformity 105, 493
Spinal extension exercise 260*f*
Spinal extensor strengthening exercise 118*f*
Spinal flexion 286*f*
　exercise 260*f*
Spinal fusion surgery 263*f*
Spinal mobilization 610
Spinal movements, abnormal 118
Spinal muscles 259
Spinal muscular atrophy 431, 439
　clinical features 439
　diagnosis 440
　epidemiology/etiology 439
　physiotherapy 440
　treatment of 440
　types of 440
Spinal orthosis 353
Spinal segment 389*t*
Spinal shock, stage of 391
Spinal stabilization 401*f*
　for spondylolisthesis 129
　surgery 121
Spinal stenosis 105
Spinal tap 468
Spinal tracts 389*t*
　ascending 389*t*
Spine
　board 400*f*
　disorders of 89
　surface landmarks of 89*t*
　surgery 355
Spinocerebellar ataxia 473
Spiral fracture 288
Spirometry 509*f*
Splint for
　carpal tunnel syndrome 246*f*
　Dupuytren's contracture 251*f*
　trigger finger 250*f*
Split transfer 355
Spondylitis 105
Spondylolisthesis 108*f*, 123*f*, 109
　epidemiology of 122
　etiology of 122
　grading of 122*t*
　management of 123
　surgical management of 126
　types of 122
Spondylolysis 105, 108*f*, 109
Spondylotic changes 89
Spontaneous amputation 265
Sports specific exercises, training of 237
Spring back test 212, 212*f*
Spurling sign 90*f*, 90
Sputum, color of 505*f*
Square sign test 246
Stability and mobility tasks 564

Stabilization exercise 34
Stabilizing reversals 65
Stable fractures managed conservatively 290
Staheli's prone extension test 337*f*
Stance phase
　different components of 583*f*
　essential components of 583
Standing balance
　analysis of 581
　development of 417*f*
　practice of 581
　training 470*f*
Standing extension exercise 132*f*
Standing from sitting, practice of 580
Standing hip abduction 150
　exercise 151*f*
Standing hip flexion and extension 149
Standing knee raise 149
Standing lumbar extension 132
Standing lumbar flexion exercise 131, 132*f*
Standing wall press 484, 485*f*
Star excursion test 14
Static balance 13, 396
Static cervical traction 98*f*
Static cycle exercise 287*f*, 469*f*, 526*f*
Static muscle work 19
Static postural control 13, 15
Static posture 12
Static progressive stretching 44
Static strengthening exercises 221
Static stretching 44
Stationary arm 21
Stationary bicycle exercise 177, 178*f*
Statutory body 553
Stem cell therapy 357, 387
Step sign 122*f*
Stepping exercises 484
Stepping reflex 329*f*
Stepping strategy 14, 14*f*
Stereotaxic surgery 357
Steroids, use of 400
Stethoscope 507*f*
Sticks, use of 77
Stiff knee gait 332
Stiffness, reduction of 291
Still pose 47*f*
Stoop
　sitting 10, 11*f*
　standing 8
Straight leg raise test 140, 190
Strain injuries 150
Strength training 42
Strengthening ankle
　dorsiflexor 198*f*
　plantar flexor 198*f*
Strengthening exercises 173, 202, 343*f*, 415, 488*f*
Strengthening hip abductors 143*f*
Strengthening of
　deep abdominal muscles 126*f*
　hamstrings 171*f*, 267*f*
　lower trapezius 103*f*
　muscles 291
　quadriceps 267*f*, 344*f*
　rotator cuff muscles 231*f*, 293*f*
　serratus anterior 103*f*
　shoulder
　　abductors 224
　　extensors 224, 224*f*
　　external rotators 225*f*
　　flexors 224, 231*f*
　　medial rotators 225*f*

tibialis posterior 203f
transverse abdominis 541f
wrist extensors 238f
Stress fracture 288
Stretch standing 7f
Stretching exercises 342, 342f
　determinants of 45
　types of 44
Stretching of
　hamstring muscle 188f
　hip flexors 128f
　left hip flexors 144f
　left piriformis 140f
　left upper trapezius muscle 102f
　piriformis 132
　plantar fascia 200f
　quadriceps 171f
　right hip flexors 144f
　spine 259f, 261f
　trunk lateral flexors 261f
Stride length 72
Stride sitting 9
Stride width 72
Stroke 358
　assessment of 367
　classification of 358, 359
　clinical features of 361
　direction of 33f
　early recognition of 361
　epidemiology and etiology 358
　massage 79, 79f
　pathophysiology of 360
　recovery of 366, 367
　rehabilitation 372
　silent 360
　transverse 607
　unit 369
Stump bandaging
　above elbow 268f
　above knee 268f
　below elbow 268f
Stumps, ideal length of 265f
Stupor 362
Subarachnoid hemorrhage 359
Subgluteus maximus bursa 146
Submaximal arm tests 397
Subscapularis test 211
Substantia nigra pars compacta 412, 413
Subtalar joint 192
Subtotal hysterectomy 494
Sucking reflex 336f
Sudeck's osteodystrophy 297
Sulcus sign 366f
Sulcus test 215, 215f
Sunderland's classification 442
Superficial reflexes 32t, 335
　examination of 32
Superior radioulnar joints 232
Supine heel drag 179f
　exercise 157f
Supine hip abduction 149
Supine hip flexor stretching exercise 159f
Supine, phases of 578f
Supporting ropes 50
Supporting sternotomy incision 542f
Supra pelvic tilt 30f
Supracondylar fracture 294f, 302, 303, 304
　of femur 303f
Supracondylar knee-ankle-foot orthosis 352
Supramalleolar orthosis 204, 204f, 353f

Surface tension 56
Suspension frame 50, 51f
Suspension therapy 50, 148
　advantages of 50
　contraindications for 52
　disadvantages of 50
　for elbow 54f
　for hip abduction 54f
　for hip adduction 54f
　for hip extension 54f
　for hip flexion 54f, 157f
　for hip rotation 55f
　for knee extension 55f
　for knee flexion 55f
　for lower limbs 54
　for shoulder abduction 53f
　for shoulder adduction 53f
　for shoulder extension 217f
　for shoulder extension 53f
　for shoulder flexion 53f, 217f
　for shoulder rotation 54f
　for trunk side flexion 52, 53f
　for upper limb 53
　for upper trunk side flexion 53f
　indications for 52
　principles of 50
Sustained pressure 608
Swain test 165, 165f
Swan neck deformity 279f
Swedish massage 83
Swing phase 71, 270, 583
　activities, practice of 584
　components of 583f
Swing to gait 75, 408
Swiss ball 15f, 261f, 344f, 380f, 382f, 483f
　balancing on 376f
Syme's amputation 265
　modified 265
Syndesmophytes 285f
Syndesmosis of ankle 196f
Synergistic movement pattern 345
Synergists 20
Syphilis, congenital 282
Syphilitic arthritis 282

T

Talar tilt test 194, 195f
Talipes equinovarus, congenital 206
Talus fracture 308f, 309
Tape measure for neck
　extension 28f
　flexion 28f
　rotation 28f
　side flexion 28f
Tape measure for trunk
　extension 28f
　flexion 28f
　side flexion 29f
Tapotement 81
Tardieu scale 334, 335t
　modified 335, 335f
Tarsal bones 309
Tarsal joints, transverse 192
Tarsometatarsal joints 193
Task, independent performance of 382f
Taylor's brace 402f
Tear
　acute 182
　bucket handle 182
　chronic 182
　longitudinal 182

　oblique 182
　radial 182
Technique of
　facilitation 590
　Frenkel's exercise 48
　goniometry 21
　inhibition 589
　key point stimulation 591
　mulligan's mobilization 608
　physiotherapy 217
　progressive resisted exercise 41
　proprioceptive neuromuscular facilitation 63
　relaxation 45
　resisted exercise 41
Telescopic test 137, 138f
Temporal summation 60
Temporomandibular joint pain 100
Tendinitis of rotator cuff muscles 293
Tendo-Achilles 274f, 342f
　lengthening 433
Tendon
　gliding exercises 247f
　healing, phases of 253t
　injuries of 252
　　assessment of 252
　lengthening 355
　repair 253
　　early 44
　transfer 355
Tennis elbow 233, 236f
　splint 235f
　taping for 238f
Tenodesis action 410f
Tenodesis grasp 469f
Tenodesis splint 410f
　use of 409
Tenotomy, simple 355
Tens electrodes, placement of 129f, 487f
Teres minor test 212, 212f
Tertiary genu recurvatum 329f
Test for
　anterior cruciate ligament 164
　anterior rotator instability of knee 165
　Babinski sign 33f
　deltoid ligament 196f
　effusion in knee 162
　extension 109f
　femoral anteversion 337f
　flexion 109f
　forward head posture 101f
　meniscus injury 163
　patellar instability 162
　plica syndrome 166
　posterior cruciate ligament injury 164
　posterolateral knee instability 166
　shoulder joint 210t
　vertebra basilar insufficiency 90
Tetraplegia 388
Tetraplegic hand 410f
　management of 409
Thalamotomy 419
Theophylline 522
Theories of motor
　control 564
　learning 568, 569
Theraband exercise 127f, 485, 486f, 527f
　for shoulder 19f
Therabands, progressive use of 19f
Thermal burn 313f
Thermoplastic splint for

thumb 254f
wrist 254f
Thomas heel 203f
Thomas test 138, 138f, 336f
Thompson's test 194, 195f
Thoracic cord injury 393
Thoracic expansion exercise 513, 546
Thoracic spine 88, 603
　fractures 290
Thoracolumbar spine 28, 258, 289
Thoracoplasty 542
Thoracotomies 543
Thoracotomy 542
　incision, posterolateral 543f
　posterolateral 543
　preoperative physiotherapy for 543
Thromboprophylaxis 401
Thumb 26
　kneading 80f
　muscle strengthening 254f
　spica splint 248f, 281f
Tibia 306f
Tibial condyle fractures 306
Tibial inlay procedure 182
Tibial torsion test 195
　measurement of 195f, 338f
Tibial tuberosity
　apophysis of 174f
　osteotomy 170
Tibial tunnel method 182
Tightness 47, 366
　of ankle plantar flexors 375f
　of hip flexors 336f
Tilt table standing 404f
Timed up and go test 14
Tinel's sign test 243, 245f, 246, 444
Toe out, degree of 72
Toe standing 17f
Tone grading scale 334t
Tongue
　asymmetry 572f
　cyanosis of 504f
　movements 573
　posterior part of 574f
Tonic
　labyrinthine reflex 363
　lumbar reflex 363
　neck reflex, symmetric 363
　thumb reflex 364
Total abdominal hysterectomy 494
Total hip arthroplasty, indications of 154
Total hip replacement 154f
Total knee arthroplasty 189f, 189
Total knee replacement arthroplasty
　contraindications for 188
　indications of 188
　types of 188
　weight bearing schedule 189
Total knee replacement
　contraindications for 188
　indications of 188
　rehabilitation 189
Total lung capacity 500
Trachea position 506
Tracheostomy tube in situ 545f
Traction 113
　and approximation 60
Training, transfer of 41
Transcutaneous electrical nerve stimulation 227
　to reduce postoperative pain 544
Transfemoral amputees 269
　stubbies for bilateral 267t

Transient synovitis of hip 143
Transition zone 605
Translatory
   grades, clinical uses of 605
   joint play movements 604
   movement of Kaltenborn, grades of 604
Translatory movements, grades of 605
Transtibial amputees 270
Transverse abdominis strengthening exercises 495f
Transverse lesion syndrome 90
Trauma 443
Traumatic brain injury 420
   assessment of 422
   clinical features 421
   diagnostic tests in 421
   etiology 420
   management of 423
   mechanism of 420
   mild 420
   moderate to severe 420
   types of 420
   types of 420
Traumatic hyperaemia 603
Traumatic spondylolisthesis 122
Treadmill test 142
Tremor 415f
Trendelenburg gait 152
Trendelenburg test 137, 140
   positive 137f
Treponema pallidum 282
   hemagglutination 282
Triceps jerk 32f
Trigger finger 249, 249f
Trigger points 594f
   on stimulation 348
   on trunk 594
   on upper limb 594
   stimulation 595f
Trigger thumb 249, 249f
Trimalleolar fracture 308, 308f
Triplegia 321
Trochanteric bursitis 145, 146f, 146
   management of 146
True limb length discrepancy, measurement of 30f
Trunk asymmetry, measurement of 257
Trunk bending, posterior 78
Trunk lateral flexion, practice of 578f
Trunk lateral flexor stretching 258f
Trunk prone lying 12f, 12
Tumors and cancer treatments 443
Turn buckle splint 295f

U

U-cast 293f
Ulnar nerve 456t
Ulnar nerve injury 452, 455f
   causes of 453
   management of 455
Ultrasound therapy 101f
Underberg test 91, 92f
Universal goniometer 21f
Upper abdominal muscle 118
Upper abdominals 124f
Upper back pain 101
Upper back strengthening exercises 105f
Upper back stretching 488f
Upper body exercises 526
Upper cross syndrome 100f
Upper limb 264, 362f, 362t, 372f, 374f
   deformed attitude of 449f
   dysfunction 573
   elevation 262f
   examination of 339
   exercises 380f
   function 417f
      analysis of 573, 575f
   movements 415f
   muscles 576f
   normal alignment of 375f
   pattern 424f
   preparation of 74
Upper lobes
   apical segments of 518f
   posterior segments of 518f
Upper trapezius 606f
Upper trunk 52

V

Vaginal delivery 485
Vaginal hysterectomy 494
Valgus stress test 165, 165f, 243, 244f
Varicose veins 480, 480f
Varus stress test 165, 243, 244f
   for knee 166f
Vas scale 108f
Vascular complications, management of 491
Vascular theory 206
Vasopressor suppor 400
Vaulting gait 78, 332
Vegetative state 421
Veneral Disease Research Laboratory Test 282
Ventilation, mechanics of 499
Ventilatory muscle training 513
Vertebral artery compression test 90
Vertebrobasilar artery syndrome 359
Vertebrobasilar insufficiency 90
Vertical incision 490f
Vertical stroke 607
Vertical suspension 52
Vestibular ataxia 472
Vestibular stimulation 593
Vestibular system 13
Vibration 516
Vibratory massage 82
Videography 73
Viscosity 56
Visual analogue scale 108
Visual biofeedback 268
Visual disturbances 428
Visual system 13
Vital capacity 500
   measurement 400
Vital functions, stimulation of 67
Vocal fremitus 506
Vocational assessment 398
Vocational rehabilitation programs 410
Vojta approach 593
Vojta's trigger point stimulation 349f
Volkman's ischemic contracture 294, 295f
Voluntary motor control grading 368
von Rosen splint 153f

W

Waddling gait 78, 332, 432f
Walk standing 7f
Walk-aid system 378f
Walker 354f
   measurement of 77
Walking
   aids 70, 74
   essential components of 583
   frame, simple 77f
   index for spinal cord injury 398
   lunge 484
      exercise 484f
   on gait ladder 418f
   pattern 345
   practice of 584
   stick 76, 77f, 571,
   training 344f, 582
Wall ladder exercise 229f
Wall slide squatting exercise 484f
Wall slides 191f
Wall squats 117
Wallenberg test 91, 92f
Wallenberg's syndrome 360
Wand exercises 218f, 228f, 534
Warmth of water 56
Warm-up 3
   exercises 526, 526f, 534f
Wedge compression fracture 290f
Wedge fracture 288
Weight bearing 299, 372f
   exercises 225, 226f
   resistive exercises 184
   schedule 189
Weight chart 339t
Weight cuff 150f, 301f
Weight shifting 590
Well leg-raise sign 111
Wertheim's hysterectomy 494
William's lumbar flexion exercises 127f
Williams flexion exercises 126
Wiltse classification 122
Windlass mechanism 199
Windlass test 199
Wing standing 7f
Wobble board 15f, 376f
Wooden cleat 51, 52f
World Confederation of Physiotherapy 553
Wound, open 52
Wringing massage 81f
Wrist 26
   disorders of 242, 245
   drop deformity 462f
   extension 26, 26f
      and radial deviation 575
      practice of 576f
   extensors, eccentric exercise for 238f
   flexion 26, 26f
   flexor 241f, 249f
   joint 54, 242f
   radial deviation 26f
   special tests for 242

X

Xiphoid process 542
X-ray 272f, 281f, 283f, 309f
   of cervical spine 97f
   of dislocated hips 153f
   of hip 148f, 149f
   of knee 171f
   of neck 92f
   of normal hips 153f
   of pelvis 340f
   of shoulder dislocations 219f

Y

Yard standing 7f
Yergason test 214
Yergason test 214f

Z

Zinovieff 42
Zone of
   extensor tendon injuries 253t
   partial preservation 390
Zygapophyseal joints 88

EU GSPR Authorised Reprsentative
Logos Europe, 9 rue Nicolas Poussin
1700, La Rochelle, France
Phone: +33 (0) 6 67 93 73 78
E-mail: contact@logoseurope.eu

www.ingramcontent.com/pod-product-compliance
Ingram Content Group UK Ltd.
Pitfield, Milton Keynes, MK11 3LW, UK
UKHW050458150426
5217IPUK00025B/1743